Thieme

Clinical Epidemiology of Orthopaedic Trauma

Second Edition

Yingze Zhang, MD
President
The Third Hospital of Hebei Medical University
Shijiazhuang, Hebei
PRC

With contributions by
Yanling Su, Wei Chen, Juan Wang, Jiandong Hao

1926 illustrations

Thieme
Stuttgart • New York • Delhi • Rio de Janeiro

Library of Congress Cataloging-in-Publication Data
Names: Zhang, Yingze, author. | Su, Yanling, contributor. | Chen, Wei, 1981 January 23- contributor. | Wang, Juan, 1982- contributor. | Hao, Jiandong, contributor.
Title: Clinical epidemiology of orthopaedic trauma / Yingze Zhang; with contributions by Yanling Su, Wei Chen, Juan Wang, Jiandong Hao.
Other titles: Clinical epidemiology of orthopedic trauma.
Description: Second edition. | Stuttgart; New York: Thieme, [2016] | Includes index. | Preceded by Clinical epidemiology of orthopedic trauma / Yingze Zhang; with contributions by Yanling Su, Jiandong Hao, Michael Punsoni. c2012.
Identifiers: LCCN 2015044656| ISBN 9783131658821 (hardcover: large print) | ISBN 9783131660428 (eISBN)
Subjects: | MESH: Fractures, Bone.
Classification: LCC RD101 | NLM WE 180 | DDC 617.4/71044-dc23 LC record available at http://lccn.loc.gov/2015044656

This book is an authorized and updated translation from the Simplified Chinese language edition published by People's Medical Publishing House (PMPH), Beijing, PRC. Title of the original Chinese edition:
临床创伤骨科流行病学, © 2009. All Rights Reserved.

Thieme Publishers Stuttgart
Rüdigerstrasse 14, 70469 Stuttgart, Germany
+49 [0]711 8931 421, customerservice@thieme.de

Thieme Publishers New York
333 Seventh Avenue, New York, NY 10001 USA
+1 800 782 3488, customerservice@thieme.com

Thieme Publishers Delhi
A-12, Second Floor, Sector-2, Noida-201301
Uttar Pradesh, India
+91 120 45 566 00, customerservice@thieme.in

Thieme Publishers Rio, Thieme Publicações Ltda.
Edifício Rodolpho de Paoli, 25º andar
Av. Nilo Peçanha, 50 - Sala 2508
Rio de Janeiro 20020-906 Brasil
+55 21 3172 2297 / +55 21 3172 1896

Cover design: Thieme Publishing Group
Typesetting by DiTech Process Solutions, India
Printed in Germany by Aprinta Druck GmbH 5 4 3 2 1

ISBN 978-3-13-165882-1

Also available as an e-book:
eISBN 978-3-13-166042-8

Contents

Foreword by Liming Li

Epidemiology's research field and application scope are expanding constantly as methods of medical research to study the distribution of disease and health status and their determinants, and to study the strategies and measures for preventing and treating diseases as well as promoting health. The epidemiology of orthopaedic trauma is an interdiscipline of epidemiology and orthopaedic trauma, using the principles and methods of epidemiology to study the incidence, prevalence, and constituents of traumatic fractures, and explore the possible causes of fractures, thus providing scientific basis for the prevention and treatment of traumatic fractures. The epidemiologic research of orthopaedic trauma can clearly describe the distribution of gender, age, location, time, and severity of fractures, as well as investigate the etiology of fracture by finding clues to possible cause and verifying the hypothesis, in order to provide scientific evidence for the prevention and treatment of traumatic fractures in the population.

We are very pleased to see that Professor Zhang Yingze and his team have carried out an in-depth and detailed research work of the epidemiology of fractures in our country over 11 years. In 2009, they published the *Clinical Epidemiology of Orthopaedic Trauma*, the first book of our country in this field, analyzing the distribution of age, sex, site, and severity of fracture of over 60,000 patients (65,267 fractures), and systematically expounding the constituent ratio of various sites and types of fracture. This book has been well received by the readers. Its English version was published by Thieme Medical Publishers in 2012.

On this basis, Professor Zhang Yingze led the research group to carry out the national fracture epidemiology investigation. The difficulty of epidemiological study of a large sample population is selecting the representative sample and controlling the mixed factors effectively.

Under the premise of considering the socioeconomic situation, urban–rural differentials, the level of hospital, and the ethnic distribution, the research group selected 83 hospitals with excellent representativeness from 31 provinces and autonomous regions (except Hong Kong, Macao, and Taiwan) using multistage random sampling methods. The data of all traumatic fractures treated in those hospitals from January 2010 to December 2011 was collected, and epidemiological analysis of 431,822 fractures of 414,935 patients was performed, comprehensively reflecting the epidemiological characteristics of traumatic fracture in China. They have established an epidemiological database of the largest domestic and foreign sample volume of orthopaedic trauma. Their data collection and analysis of traumatic fracture in the whole country have revealed the common laws and the specific characteristics and laid the scientific foundation for the prevention, diagnosis, and treatment of fractures.

The data in this book are visually presented to the readers by means of pie charts, curve graphs, and bar graphs in order to minimize the description text. The text of fracture classification is supplemented by color schematic diagrams and radiographs, making it easy to understand and grasp for clinical orthopaedic surgeons. The epidemiological characteristics of fractures are reflected intuitively and concisely by pictures with addition of actual data. Furthermore, the new theory and new technology in the field of orthopaedic trauma in recent years are briefly introduced in this book, which can expand the readers' perspective and help young orthopaedic surgeons master the essentials of the diagnosis and treatment of fractures.

Clinical Epidemiology of Orthopaedic Trauma is the most important achievement of large scale epidemiological investigation of orthopaedic trauma in recent decades. It has filled the domestic gap in the epidemiological study of fracture, and improved the system of epidemiology of orthopaedic trauma in China.

I felt delighted after reading the first edition of *Clinical Epidemiology of Orthopaedic Trauma* 5 years ago, with great admiration for the author's hard work of processing more than 60,000 cases. Now, Professor Yingze and his team have completed the second edition, enriched by their insurmountably meticulous survey work with wide region and large sample size. It is a great honor and pleasure for me to be invited to write this foreword.

Liming Li, MD
Chairman of the China Association of Epidemics
College of Public Health of Peking University
Chinese Academy of Medical Sciences,
Beijing Union Medical College Secretary
and Deputy Chief Institutions

Foreword by Guixing Qiu

At present, epidemiological data of fractures in Chinese literature mainly refer to foreign research, partially with unknown or unverifiable sources. As China is a multinational country with such a large population, development levels vary greatly in different regions of the country, and the cause of injury is always complicated and changeful. For this reason, foreign data is not able to reflect the characteristics and distribution of fractures in our country, especially when the incidence and types of the fractures in our country have changed greatly in recent years. Therefore, a large-scale domestic epidemiological investigation of fractures with large sample size is much needed.

Dr. Zhang and his collaborators have done a lot of research work on the epidemiological characteristics of the fractures in our country by stages since 2003. In the first stage, this team systemically analyzed the data of 65,267 fracture cases treated in the third hospital of Hebei Medical University from 2003 to 2007, according to the AO/OTA classification system and other commonly used or accepted classifications. Their work was published by the People's Health Publishing House in 2009 as the first monograph of clinical epidemiology of traumatic fractures. This book was translated into an English edition and published by Thieme Medical Publishers in 2012, which introduced the great achievement of our country's fracture epidemiology to the whole world.

On this basis, Professor Yingze Zhang led his team to extend the research to 31 provinces and autonomous regions in China. They investigated and analyzed 431,882 fractures of 414,935 patients from 83 hospitals, and built an epidemiological database of orthopaedic trauma with the world's largest sample size to date. The results have been included in the second edition of *Clinical Epidemiology of Orthopaedic Trauma*. Epidemiological characteristics of, as well as diagnosis and treatment techniques for, fractures of the trunk and limbs in our country are comprehensively illustrated in this edition. Each chapter contains an overview of the diagnosis and treatment for the fracture of various parts, accompanied with the latest technology progress, which is helpful to young orthopaedists' study of injury characteristics and essentials in diagnosis and treatment of various fractures. The second edition is still dominated by pictures and figures, consistent with the first edition in style and form. Age, gender, and type distribution of the fractures are displayed by the charts, and the injury characteristics of various types of fractures are presented to the readers via the combination of color sketches and X-rays.

Clinical Epidemiology of Orthopaedic Trauma is an indispensable tool for orthopaedic surgeons, with abundant content, precise diction, detailed materials, excellent pictures and text, and comprehensive instruction. The new edition of this book makes our country's academic field more glorious and resplendent. I sincerely congratulate the authors for the publication of this book, and hope it can play a proper role and be published in more foreign languages, so as to disseminate the new development of clinical epidemiology research of orthopaedic trauma in China to the orthopaedists and epidemiologists of other countries in the world.

Guixing Qiu, MD
China Academy of Engineering
Professor of Peking Union Medical College
Peking Union Medical College Hospital Surgery Department
Department of Orthopaedics Director

Foreword by Robert D. D'Ambrosia

I am honored to write a foreword to Professor Zhang's book, *Clinical Epidemiology of Orthopaedic Trauma*. He is well known to me personally and in orthopaedic academia in the United States. I was privileged to hear his presentations in Denver, Colorado; also at the "Current Concepts Course" in Orthopaedics in Kwai, Hawaii, 2015; and at the Chinese Orthopaedic Association meeting in Beijing, China, this past year.

He is president-elect of the Chinese Orthopaedic Association and the current president of the Third Hospital of Hebei Medical University. He is an accomplished orthopaedic surgeon with a wide and varied experience in orthopaedic trauma in his position as chair of Orthopedic Trauma at Hebei University.

His book is practical, well-illustrated, and will be an essential reference book for the experienced orthopaedic surgeon, residents, and medical students. He has drawn upon his wide experience as an orthopaedic researcher who has been remarkably productive—authoring 22 books and over 400 publications. This book, in its second edition, includes 414,936 cases from 83 hospitals and 31 provinces across China. It is a comprehensive epidemiology study of orthopaedic trauma on a national scale with a huge sample size, which has worldwide implications. His orthopaedic team, under his guidance, has done an outstanding job in the tedious work on AO/OTA classification of each fracture. The diagrams are easy to understand and the illustrations demonstrate the superb results that could be obtained.

Through the study, the world now has a better understanding of fracture care in different areas of China, which will be very beneficial in allocating valuable resources accordingly. Professor Zhang and coworkers are to be congratulated on a valuable treatise in orthopaedic trauma that will serve as a reference and database for the present and well into the future. It is a monumental contribution to the world of orthopaedic trauma.

Robert D. D'Ambrosia, MD
Professor and Chair
Department of Orthopaedics
University of Colorado

Foreword by Roy Sanders

Clinical Epidemiology of Orthopaedic Trauma by Professor Zhang is an outstanding resource. This is one of the few, if not the only, books collating this information in one volume. Comprehensive in nature and amply illustrated with diagrams, charts, and drawings, it evaluates every fracture seen and treated at a major international trauma center—complete with AO/OTA classification, demographic information, among other important data. Clearly and rationally organized, and in great detail, the authors lay out the individual fractures, their patterns, diagnosis, mechanism of injury, and treatment options. Beyond the orthopaedic surgeon's interest in such information, this book should be of inestimable value to researchers, residents, and students of all disciplines. In short, a must-have reference book for the serious orthopaedic researcher. Dr. Zhang is to be congratulated on an outstanding achievement.

Roy Sanders, MD
Editor-in-Chief
Journal of Orthopaedic Trauma
Tampa, Florida

Preface

The *Clinical Epidemiology of Orthopaedic Trauma* is the first monograph on fracture epidemiology. It was first published by People's Medical Publishing House 5 years ago, and translated into English by Thieme Medical Publishers and distributed worldwide in 2012. The book has received extensive positive reviews for its unique writing style, which combined knowledge in both theory and practice. Prof. David E. Parker from North Carolina wrote a book review and considered it an excellent textbook with reasonable structure, abundant illustrations and pictures, and concise description.

The first edition was based on a retrospective review of 60,266 patients (65,267 fractures) treated in our trauma center over a 5-year period from 2003 to 2007. Given very large differences in natural and social environments in China, we performed a large-scale, multicenter study to get a comprehensive understanding of the features of orthopaedic trauma epidemiology. Based on the first edition, advanced research throughout the nation was carried out.

Eighty-three hospitals from 31 provinces nationwide were selected with a stratified multistage random sampling method and 414,835 patients (431,822 fractures) were identified from all levels of trauma center and included into the study. Our research teams were composed of orthopaedic surgeons, radiologists, and epidemiologists. Survey forms, data collection, and analysis scheme were designed in detail. All researchers were trained to classify the fractures accurately and consistently. The AO classification is adapted in this edition, because it has been recognized worldwide with its practicality, uniformity, and comparability. Meanwhile, other special fracture classifications are adapted as well to reflect the features of fracture comprehensively. Two senior orthopaedic surgeons and one radiologist are responsible for the high quality of the work. The second edition of *Clinical Epidemiology of Orthopaedic Trauma* is completed after tallying the results.

This book introduces the epidemiological features of individual types of fracture concisely and yet comprehensively. The new trends and changes were documented as well. Although the structural organization is consistent with the last edition, the sample size is increased largely to reflect more authentic and accurate trends and changes in the epidemiological features of fractures in China as a nation. The easy-to-understand but exceptional graphics, with corresponding X-ray films and fracture line graphs, are retained. Magnetic resonance imaging or computed tomography images are added to complicated fractures to fully illustrate the characteristics of the injuries. For the purpose of the clinical and scientific research, the sections DIAGNOSIS and TREATMENT were updated with the latest developments and progress. The omissions and mistakes are unavoidable due to the heavy workload and tight schedule. We are looking forward to your valuable comments and suggestions, which will be a generous help to our endeavors to create a consummate monograph.

All participants have clinical and scientific research backgrounds. They spent great efforts on this book, which made this publication possible. My deepest gratitude and respect to all of them!

Yingze Zhang

Acknowledgments

A special note of thanks to the following people for their efforts at various stages in shaping this book.

Yanling Su, MD, PhD, MPH
Department of Orthopedic Surgery
The Third Hospital of Hebei Medical University
Shijiazhuang, Hebei
PRC

Wei Chen, MD, PhD
Emergency Center of Trauma
The Third Hospital of Hebei Medical University
Shijiazhuang, Hebei
PRC

Juan Wang, MD, PhD
Department of Joint Surgery
The Third Hospital of Hebei Medical University
Shijiazhuang, Hebei
PRC

Jiandong Hao, MD, PhD
Emergency Center of Trauma
The Third Hospital of Hebei Medical University
Shijiazhuang, Hebei
PRC

The authors wish to thank the following colleagues for their assistance in the collection and analysis of the radiographic images and data.

Contributor	Hospital
Haitao Zhao	The Third Hospital of Hebei Medical University
Ran Sun	The Third Hospital of Hebei Medical University
Tao Sun	The Third Hospital of Hebei Medical University
Haili Wang	The Third Hospital of Hebei Medical University
Bing Yin	The Third Hospital of Hebei Medical University
Song Liu	The Third Hospital of Hebei Medical University
Yanbin Zhu	The Third Hospital of Hebei Medical University
Jiaxiang Cheng	The Third Hospital of Hebei Medical University
Ruyun Zhang	The Third Hospital of Hebei Medical University
Yansen Li	The Third Hospital of Hebei Medical University
Guohui Xu	The Third Hospital of Hebei Medical University
Tao Zhang	The Third Hospital of Hebei Medical University
Lei Liu	The Third Hospital of Hebei Medical University
Jiayuan Sun	The Third Hospital of Hebei Medical University
Zongyou Yang	The Third Hospital of Hebei Medical University
Xiao Chen	The Third Hospital of Hebei Medical University
Bo Liu	The Third Hospital of Hebei Medical University
Guang Yang	The Third Hospital of Hebei Medical University
Ye Tian	The Third Hospital of Hebei Medical University
Fei Zhang	The Third Hospital of Hebei Medical University
Chi Zhang	The Third Hospital of Hebei Medical University

Yanjiang Yang	The Third Hospital of Hebei Medical University
Ming Li	The Third Hospital of Hebei Medical University
Wenjuan Wu	The Third Hospital of Hebei Medical University
Haotian Wu	The Third Hospital of Hebei Medical University
Changchun Zhang	The First Affiliated Hospital of Bengbu Medical College
Chunwan Ye	Hefei Orthopaedics Hospital
Zhonghua Xie	Funan People's Hospital
Tuo Ba	The Yanzhaomeng Hospital of Bayinguole
Yongneng Xu	Bazhou People's Hospital
Feng su	The First Affiliated Hospital of Hebei North University
Junlin Zhou	Beijing Chao-Yang Hospital
Hongbin Han	Peking University Third Hospital
Jichen Du	The Beijing Aerospace Center Hospital
Ruchen Peng	Beijing Luhe Hospital
Rengui Wang	Beijng Shijitan Hospital
Qing Cui	Cangzhou Hospital of Integrated Traditional And Western Medicine
Yongqing Xu	Kumming General Hospital of Chengdu Military Command
Yijian Liang	The Third People's Hospital of Chengdu
Leiting Chi, Wenbo Li	Chengdu First People's Hospital
Dianming Jiang	The First Affiliated Hospital of Chongqing Medical University
Xiaofei Chi	The Second People's Hospital of Dalian
Dewei Zhao	Affiliated Zhongshan Hospital of Dalian University
Haihua Li,Fuge Sui	Daqing Longnan Hospital
Jianzhong Xu	The Southwest Hospital of The Third Military Medical University
Jinhua Wang	The People's Hospital of Dingxi
Zhiwen Li	The First Hospital of Nanping
Huanghui Wu	The Hospital of Ningde, Fujian
Qi Zhu, Bin You	The Second Hospital of Fuzhou
Cheng Zhou	Gansu Provincial Hospital of TCM
Junqiang Chen	The First Affiliated Hospital of Guangxi Medical University
Xianhua Cai	Wuhan General Hospital of Guangzhou Military
Bin Zhao	The Forth People's Hospital of Guiyang
Xiaobin Tian	Guizhou Province Osteological Hospital
Qiping Deng	Guizhou Provincial People's Hospital
Zhenggang Bi	The First Affiliated Hospital of Harbin Medical University
Shou Zhang	Haikou Municipal People's Hospital
Jiangning Shen	Hainan General Hospital
Min Zhang	Luoyang Orthopedic-Traumatological Hospital
Shengwu Kan	The Orthopedic Hospital of Wuhan, Hubei
Kaihu Xu	Xianning Central Hospital
Ji'an Li	Xiangxiang City Second People's Hospital
Zhongli Gao	The Third Hospital of Jilin University
Xuecheng Cao	Jinan Military General Hospital
Fuqing Li	The 273 Hospital of The Chinese Liberation Army
Wenzhong Xie	Kaifeng Central Hospital
Jianlu Zhang	Korla People's Hospital

Langsuo Bianba	The People's Hospital of Lhasa
Weigao Chen, Chunhua Lu	The Second Affiliated Hospital of Nanchang University
Xiangzuo Xiao	The First Affiliated Hospital of Nanchang University
Dadi jin, Shaolin Li	The Third Hospital of Southern Medical University
Fan Li	Affiliated Hospital of Nantong University
Hongjun Huo	The Second Affiliated Hospital of Inner Mongolia Medical University
Zhongkui Ma	The First Affiliated Hospital of Inner Mongolia Medical University
Long Lv	Inner Mongolia People's Hospital
Hongyi Hao	Ningxia People's Hospital
Zili Wang	General Hospital of Ningxia Medical University
Haibin Lin	The Affiliated Hospital (Group) of Putian University
Peng Zhang	The Orthopedic Hospital of Qingdao
Fuan Li	The Affiliated Hospital of Qinghai University
Dongsheng Zhou	Shandong Provincial Hospital
Lu Sun	Teaching Hospital of Shandong University of Traditional Chinese Medicine
Xiaochun Wei	The Second Hospital of Shanxi Medical University
Weiwu Yao	Shanghai Sixth People's Hospital
Maoquan Li	Shanghai Tenth People's Hospital
Yi Xiao	Shanghai Changzheng Hospital
Yue Wang	Sichuan Provincial People's Hospital
Jingcheng Wang	Subei People's Hospital of Jiangsu Province
Gang Zhao	The Second Hospital of Tangshan
Wen Shen	Tianjin First Centre Hospital
Xinlong Ma, Baotong Ma	Tianjin Hospital
Kezao Fang	The People's Hospital of Pingyang
Licheng Zhang	Ruian People's Hospital
Xiaoshan Guo	The Second Affiliated Hospital & Yuying Children's Hospital of Wenzhou Medical University
Kunzheng Wang	The Second Affiliated Hospital of Xi'An Jiangtong University
Junding Hao	Xi'an Honghui Hospital
Zuoming Yin	The General Hospital of Tibet Military Command
Guoxuan Wang	Hospital of Xinjiang Production & Construction Corps
Zhanyong Wu	Jizhong Energy Xingtai Mig General Hospital
Baoshan Duan	Yangquan Coalmine Group General Hospital
Yunhui Li	The People's Hospital of the Country of Meng
Zhong Chen	The Red Cross Hospital of Yunnan
Zengkuan Li	The People's Hospital of Zhengzhou
Chuanhui Liu	Zhengzhou Orthopedic Hospital
Jinzhao Geng	Wangjing Hospital of CATCM
Wenzheng Li	Xiangya Hospital Central South University
Jianwang Wang	The Sixth Affiliated Hospital of Sun-Yaisen University

How to Use This Book

The authors of this book retrospectively reviewed radiographic images of 431,882 fractures in 414,935 patients obtained from 83 hospitals in 31 provinces of China, and performed fracture classification and statistical studies based on the AO/OTA system and other commonly used classification systems. The book comprises 10 chapters organized according to the coding system proposed by AO/OTA fracture classification. The first chapter presents an outline of the book and provides an introduction to the coding of bones used by OA/OTA and to fracture classification principles. The remaining nine chapters deal with features occurring at different anatomical locations arranged in ascending order according to the OA/OTA coding system: humerus, radius/ulna, femur, tibia/fibula, spine, pelvic ring/acetabulum, hand, foot, and others (including patella, clavicle, and scapula). Each chapter is divided into sections that deal with segments within the bone. The final section of each chapter describes other commonly used fracture classification systems and their epidemiological characteristics.

The epidemiological features of each type of fracture contain such information as the number of fractures and patients and gender and age distribution, which is displayed in tables, pie charts, bar charts, and so on.

Please note that percentages are often displayed with two digits of precision after rounding up, therefore the numbers in the tables may not always add up to 100% as a result of possible rounding differences.

1 General Information

Fractures Overview

Bone fractures occur when there is a break in the continuity and integrity of the bone as a result of excessive force. Fractures usually begin with intensive pain and swelling at the site of injury, along with some degree of loss of function. Furthermore, fractures can also present with shock and fever as seen in severe cases. Characteristics of fractures include deformities, abnormal movement, bony crepitus, and a perception of friction between fracture fragments. Fractures that result in a deformed limb and severe pain often require immediate surgical intervention. In severe fractures, the circulation may become disrupted and lead to a loss of pulse distal to the fracture site. Fractures involving articulation sites may result in subsequent dysfunction of the joint.

Fractures can be classified into different categories based on the impact of the fracture. For example, they can be classified as open or closed, depending on the integrity of the skin tissue and mucosa; as complete or incomplete, depending on the severity of the fracture; or as stable or unstable in terms of displacement, angulation, and shortening. Fractures can also be described as traumatic or nontraumatic—the latter more commonly seen as a pathologic fracture. Traumatic fractures are seen more frequently in clinical practice than nontraumatic fractures.

Radiographic examination should include anteroposterior (AP) and lateral views of the fractured bone, along with the nearest joint. Some fractures require additional radiographic views, such as AP and oblique views for metacarpus and metatarsus, lateral and axial views for calcaneus, and AP and ulnar deviations for scaphoid. Sometimes, if the injury is difficult to determine, comparison views of the contralateral uninvolved side will be helpful in reaching an accurate diagnosis. In cases with a clinically suspected fracture and negative or inconclusive findings on initial radiography, a radiographic examination should be repeated 2 weeks later, when the fracture line will emerge as healed fragments, as seen in carpal scaphoid fractures. For fractures adjacent to a joint or a complex anatomical structure, X-ray examination provides limited information, therefore computed tomography (CT) or magnetic resonance imaging (MRI) are highly recommended to provide a clear depiction of the fracture.

The overall principles of fracture management are: restoration of anatomy, stable fracture fixation, and early mobilization of the limb and patient. Fracture reduction is a procedure to restore anatomy by positioning displaced bone fragments in the correct alignment, and to encourage healing and normal use of the bone and limb. Fixation is an attempt to maintain proper alignment of the fracture site until the bone becomes strong enough to support the union. Functional exercise must be started as soon as possible to restore the functional ability of muscle, tendon, and joint ligaments without compromising the fixation hardware.

Fracture Classification

To understand the injury mechanism, select proper treatment option, and compare the outcomes of different treatment regimes, it is important to have a system of fracture classification. Numerous fracture classification systems have been proposed in orthopaedics. A standardized and widely accepted fracture classification system would facilitate communication between physicians and assist documentation and research. For clinical relevance, it should reflect the complexity of treatment planning and have prognostic value for patient outcome. Maurice E. Müller indicated that a classification is useful only if it considers the severity of the bone lesion and serves as a basis for treatment and for evaluation of results. The AO classification is currently in use along with conventional classification. The latest version of the Müller AO classification was published in 1996 in the form of a supplement to volume 10 of ***The Journal of Orthopaedics Trauma***, where the classifications for the long bones, spine, and pelvis were comprehensive; however, smaller bones such as those of the hand and foot were listed only with numbers indicating location. The Müller AO classification has become widely accepted and applicable in practice not only because of the great impact the AO Foundation has had over the years in the field of orthopaedics, but also because of scientific validation of the classification system itself. The strength of Müller's system is that it provides a framework within which a surgeon can recognize, identify, and describe long bone injuries. The Orthopaedic Trauma Association (OTA) has established its own classification system, with the AO system as a reference. Essentially, the OTA system added to the AO system by classifying those bones that were never classified in the AO system, ultimately leading to the formation of the AO/OTA system. The OTA published the latest version of fracture classification in December 2007 in a supplement to volume 21 of ***Journal of Orthopaedics Trauma***. The OTA adopted the AO system of classifying long bones, spine, and pelvis, and significantly revised the classification for the clavicle and scapula, foot and hand, and patella.

The AO Foundation should be mentioned whenever the AO fracture classification system is discussed. In 1958, a group of Swiss general and orthopaedic surgeons led by Maurice E. Müller, Martin Allgower, and Hands Willenegger established the AO Foundation. The AO "pioneers" proposed a method of absolute stability through compression between fracture fragments to achieve a goal of rigid internal fixation of fractures. This concept may be less than perfect by modern standards, but caused a revolution in the treatment of fractures. The most important contribution of the AO Foundation is to promote these original principles, which not only are of great practical and scientific value but also can be continually refined and improved with use. Over the past 10 years, the AO principles of fracture management have evolved in various ways, and have begun to advance internal fixation methods. Today, almost 60 years after its establishment, the AO principle for operative fracture fixation and the bone-healing concept are accepted worldwide. As research in the biomechanics of fractures has advanced, the AO principles and the hardware for internal fixation have seen dramatic improvement, with emphasis shifting from strong internal fixation based on pure mechanics to fixation based on biomechanics. The latest AO principles stress the pathophysiology and biology of the bone-healing process rather than its mechanics.

The AO classification system adopted a five-element alphanumeric code to describe each fracture as the following: ■■-□□.□. The first two elements of the alphanumeric code describe the location (bone segment), followed by an alphabetic character for the fracture type (A, B, C), and lastly two numbers for morphological characteristics of the fracture (group and subgroup) (**Fig. 1.1**).

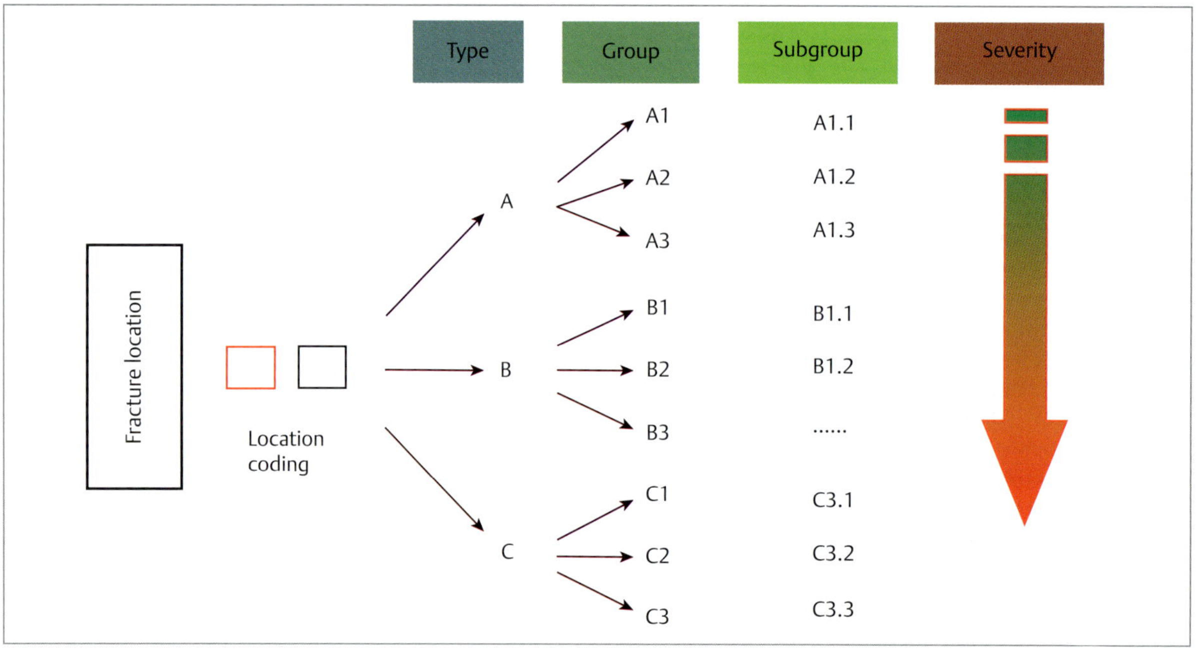

Fig. 1.1 AO classification of fractures.

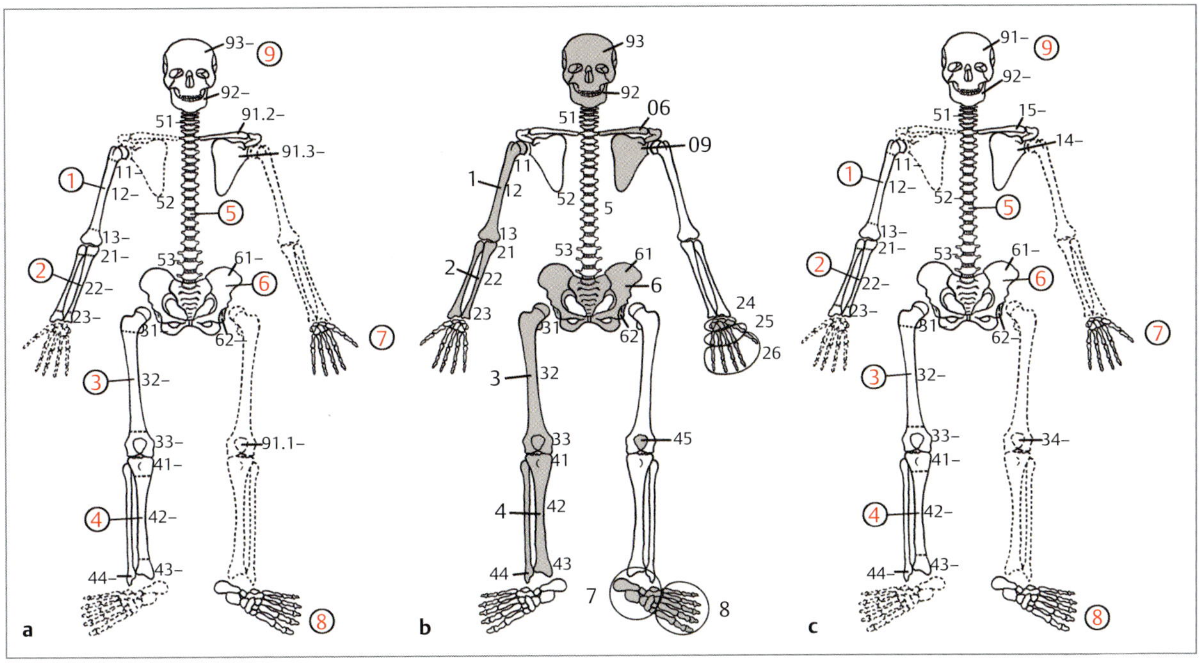

Fig. 1.2 Principles of the AO/OTA classification of fractures. All bones are coded by numbers that indicate the anatomical location. **(a)** The Müller AO classification system. **(b)** The OTA classification system. **(c)** The new unified classification system.

Bones

The numeric coding for every bone is seen in **Fig. 1.2**. It should be noted that the ulna/radius, tibia/fibula are each considered one long bone pair.

Segments

Each long bone is divided into three segments: proximal, diaphysis and distal, and numbered 1 to 3. Due to the complexity of a distal fracture of the tibia/fibula, the ankle joint is listed separately as segment 4. The anatomical delineation of the segments, proximal and distal, is performed according to Heim's square (**Fig. 1.3**): a square whose lateral sides equal the maximum width of the epiphysis, and delineate the proximal and distal segments of each bone (except for 31 and 44).

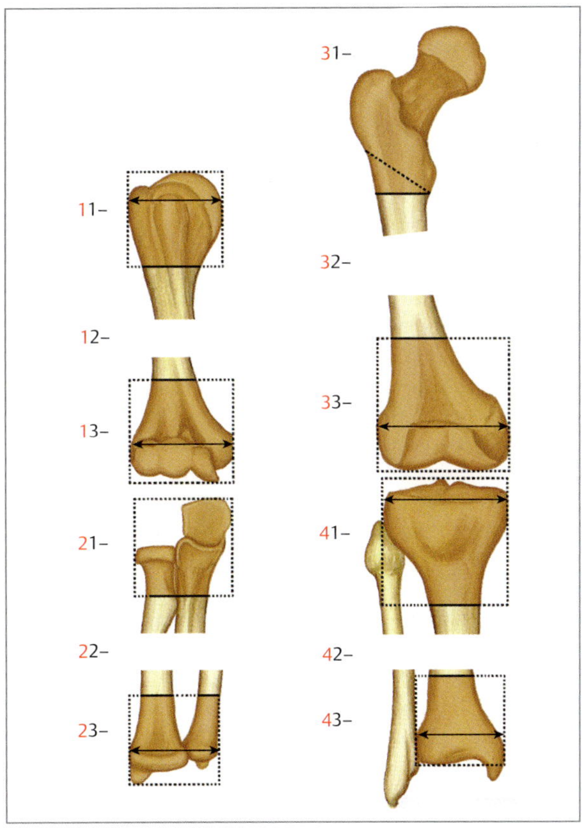

Fig.1.3 Delineation of the proximal and distal segments of a long bone (Heim's square).

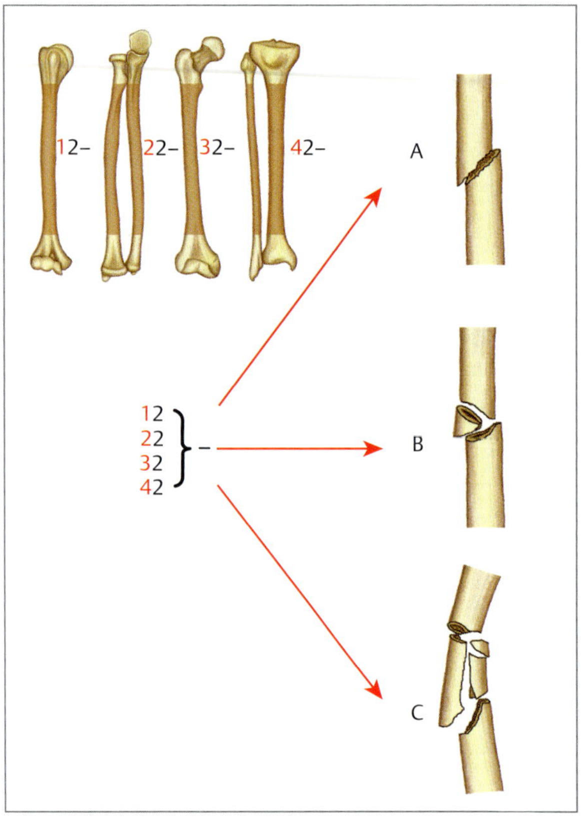

Fig. 1.4 Types of diaphyseal fractures of the long bones.

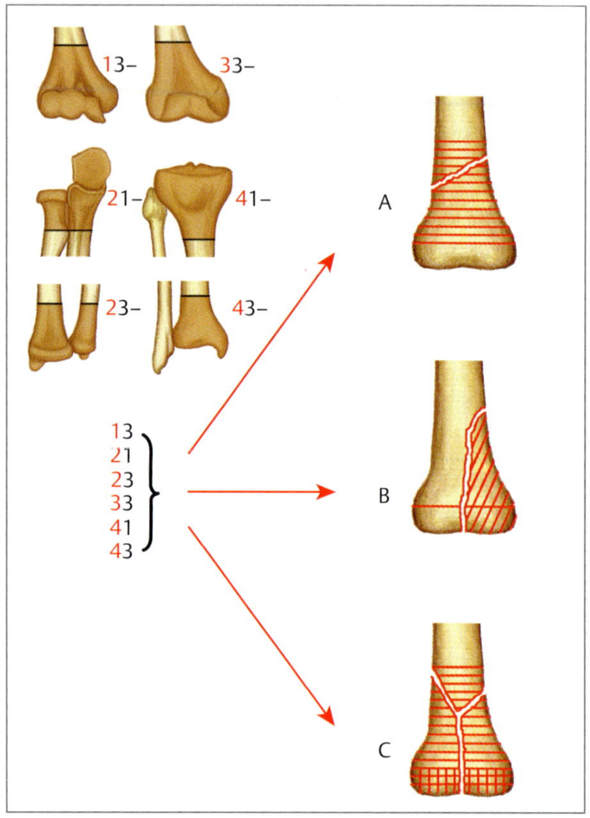

Fig. 1.5 Fracture type of the proximal and distal segments, and intra-articular fracture.

Types

Fractures are divided into three types and coded with the letters A, B, and C, which indicate increasing severity.

- ***Diaphyseal fractures of the long bones:*** based on surface contact between the main fragments after the fracture is reduced (**Fig. 1.4**).
  - *Type A:* simple fracture; there is 90% surface contact between the main fragments
  - *Type B:* wedge fracture; there is minimal surface contact between the main fragments
  - *Type C:* complex fracture; there is no surface contact between the main fragments
- ***Fractures of the proximal and distal segments:*** based on the involvement of the articular surface (**Fig. 1.5**).
  - *Type A:* extra-articular (or nonarticular) fracture; the fracture line does not pass through the articular surface
  - *Type B:* partial articular fracture; the fracture line passes through the articular surface, with a portion of it still connected to the diaphysis
  - *Type C:* complete articular fracture; the fracture line passes through the articular surface and separates it completely from the diaphysis

Group and Subgroup

When fractures occur, they can be divided into groups based on morphologic features once their location and fracture type are determined. Each group can then be further divided into subgroups, indicating increasing severity. The division of groups and subgroups varies at different segments of each bone, and is introduced in detail in the corresponding chapters of this book. For clinical practice, division by group is sufficient for appropriate diagnosis and treatment, while division by subgroup would be needed for research investigation.

Epidemiological Study of Fractures

A number of large-scale epidemiologic studies of fractures have been conducted in several countries over recent years. With the help of the AO Foundation, a group of talented orthopaedic surgeons based in Spain conducted a retrospective review of 54,280 fractures obtained from the AO database over a 5-year period. All 54,280 fractures were updated using the AO classification system, a statistical study of fracture incidence according to each type and subdivision was also conducted. However, this study was limited by using the AO system exclusively throughout, while other classification systems commonly used in clinical practice were barely referenced. In current Chinese literature, there are few systemic studies or reports on the incidence of fractures based on a large sample size. The statistical data referred to in China are mostly from publications from other countries. A handful of similar studies conducted in China have been limited either by a small sample size or by over-generalization due to specific targeting of particular populations or a specific fracture location. The Chinese research study of fracture incidence with the largest sample size to date was conducted by Dr. Liu Li-ke at Huaxi Medical University in Sichuan province. The author randomly selected 10,930 residents of Chengdu city aged over 50 years and conducted a retrospective review of their past fracture history. Risk factor analysis of fractures performed on 1,639 of the 10,930 residents concluded that the highest incidence of fracture was found in the forearm, followed by the spine, and finally the femoral neck; and the incidence of fracture is higher among women than men and in urban more than rural areas. Factors such as the level of physical work, amount of sleep a person has, and heredity may have an impact on the occurrence of fractures. Dr. Chen Wenchang at the Fujian Provincial Hospital examined 3,688 patients with fractures or joint injury, the largest study, to date, of patients with fractures. Statistical analysis of the injury mechanism, fracture location, age, and treatment led to the conclusion that fractures are most likely to occur at the wrist, ulna/radius, tibia/fibula, and distal radius. At the end of 20th century, a project named "An investigation on the current status and characteristics of common health conditions resulting from aging" was performed in China. However, the results of this project cannot be applied to the general population as it solely targeted osteoporosis in the elderly population. The studies and investigations mentioned above fail to accurately reflect the incidence and features of fracture among the general population, due to limited sample size, age-restricted target population, and lack of analysis on the variation of fracture incidence.

The third hospital of Hebei Medical University is a grade III class A hospital according to the grading system in China. As a full service hospital, it specializes in orthopaedic medicine and draws patients mainly from the local, surrounding area. The authors have reviewed radiographic images of 65,267 fractures treated at this hospital over a 5-year period from 2003 to 2007. Fracture classification and statistical studies were performed based on the AO/OTA system, with application of the picture archiving and communication systems (PACS). This extensive review also permitted statistical studies on fracture incidence based on commonly used classifications other than the AO/OTA system, which involve fractures occurring in bones of the extremities, spine, and pelvis. In 2009, we published a book to describe the epidemiological characteristics of 65,267 fractures. Based upon the above-mentioned work, we conducted a nationwide survey to investigate the epidemiological characteristics of fractures of the trunk and four extremities of China. The current study consisted of 414,935 patients (431,822 fractures) obtained from 83 hospitals across China. To the best of our knowledge, this is a comprehensive epidemiological study on fracture incidence on a national scale, with the largest sample size to date. It reflects the epidemiological status of fractures of China.

Statistical studies were conducted after fractures of long bones in the extremities, spine, and pelvis, which had also been coded according to the AO classification system, while the remaining fractures were also classified based on the OTA classification system. In an effort to secure accurate diagnoses and appropriate treatment, statistical analyses were also performed on the incidence of fracture in a specific location based on other commonly used classifications, such as the Robinson classification for clavicle fractures and the Denis classification for thoracolumbar spine fractures.

Currently, the AO/OTA classification system is widely accepted and used for fracture classification in adults, while its pediatric system is still in development. Consequently, all statistical data were collected from patients aged over 16 years when the AO/OTA system was indicated, whereas the incidence of pediatric fractures was analyzed by other classification systems.

A patient can sustain one or more fractures when an injury occurs; therefore, the total number of fractures is greater than the total number of injured patients. To achieve scientific statistical analysis, the numbers of patients and of fractures (fracture location) are discussed separately. All fractures are classified and analyzed based on the number (location) of fractures. For example, if a patient received an injury that resulted in a unilateral humeral fracture and bilateral tibia/fibula fractures, the number of fractures is counted as three, while the number of patients is one.

The present statistical study is based on a total of 414,935 patients (431,822 fractures): 257,764 male and 157,171 female including 360,300 adults (374,396 fractures) and 54,635 children (57,426 fractures), obtained between January 2010 and December 2011 from 83 hospitals selected from 31 provinces of China. A summary of key points found in this book follows.

Incidence of Sex-specific Fractures

- In general, the incidence of fracture is higher in males than in females (**Fig. 1.6**)
- Line charts of age and sex distribution of fractures of the trunk and four extremities (**Figs. 1.7–1.17**).

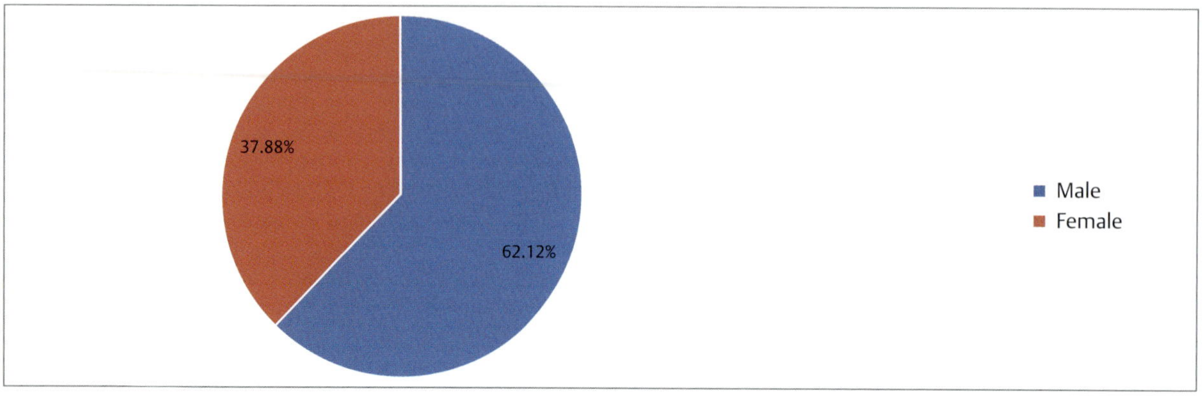

Fig. 1.6 Sex distribution of 414,935 patients with fractures treated from 2010 to 2011 at 83 hospitals in China.

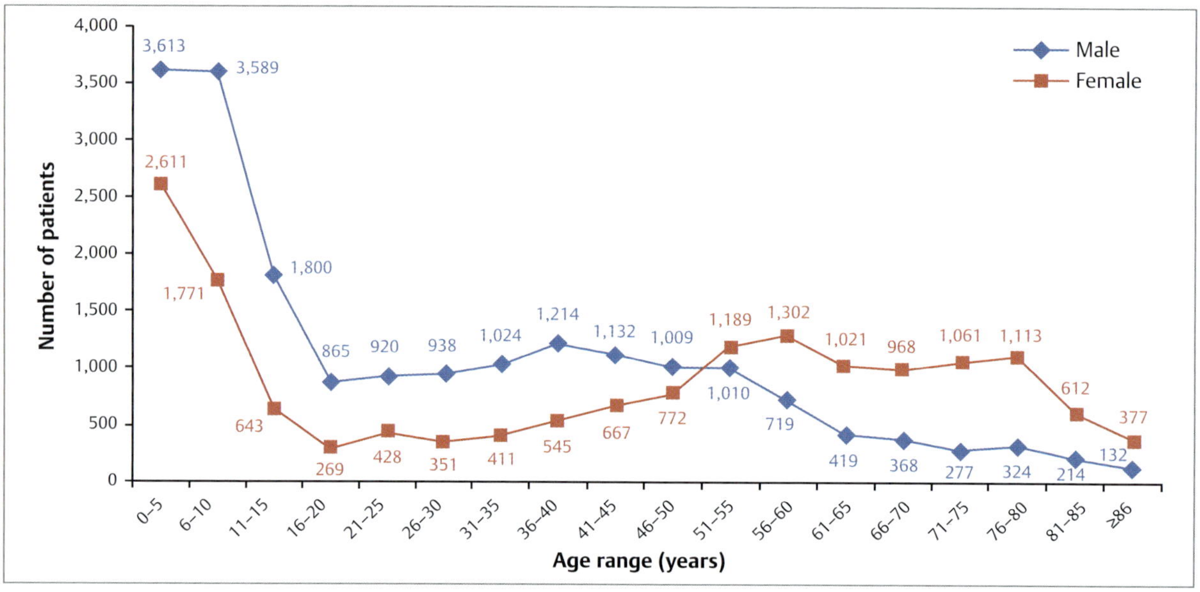

Fig. 1.7 Age and sex distribution of 35,678 patients with humeral fractures.

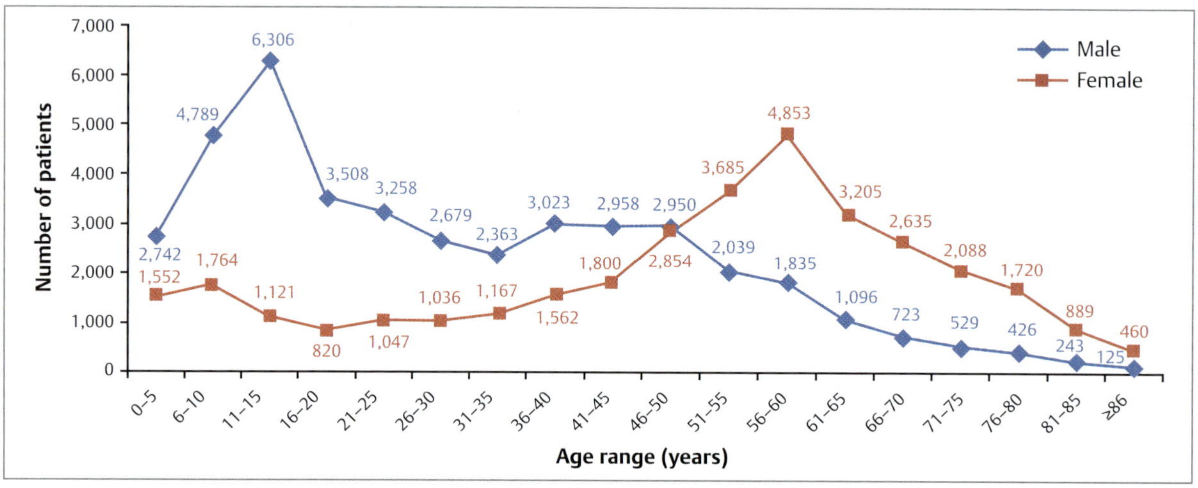

Fig. 1.8 Age and sex distribution of 75,850 patients with radius/ulna fractures.

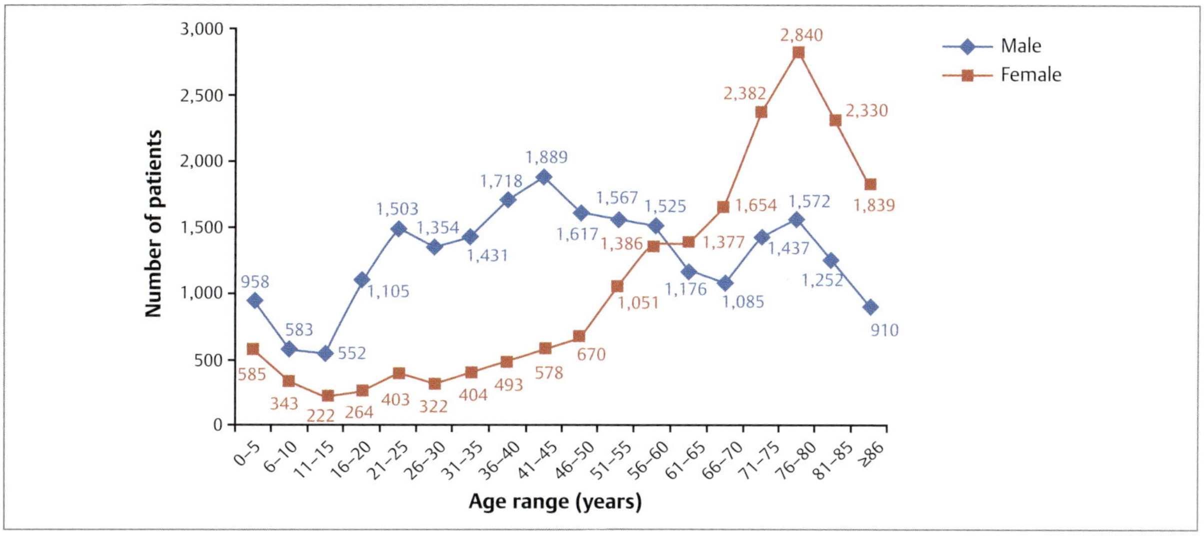

Fig. 1.9 Age and sex distribution of 42,377 patients with femur fractures.

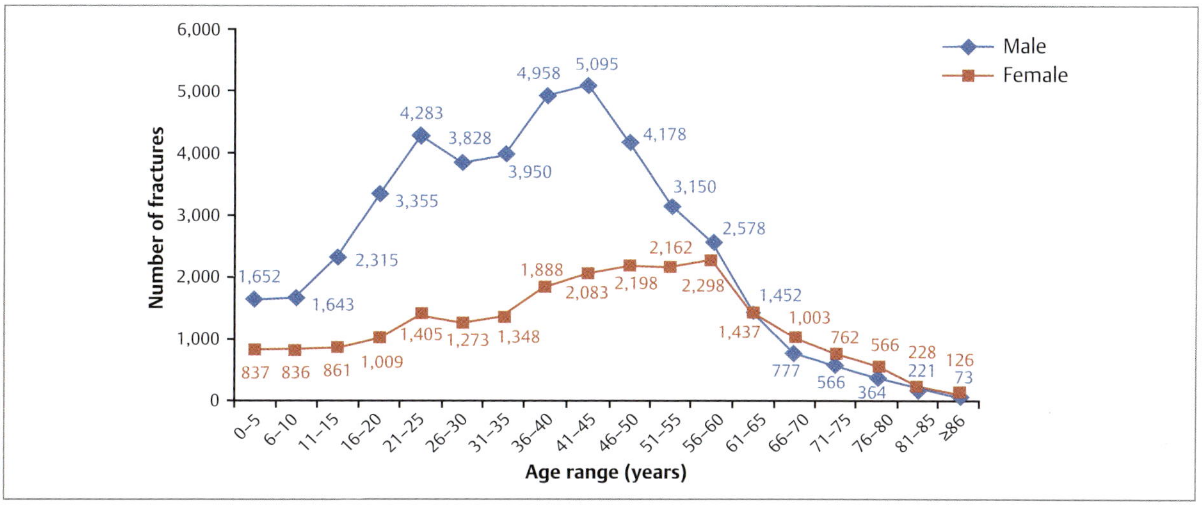

Fig. 1.10 Age and sex distribution of 66,758 patients with tibia/fibula fractures.

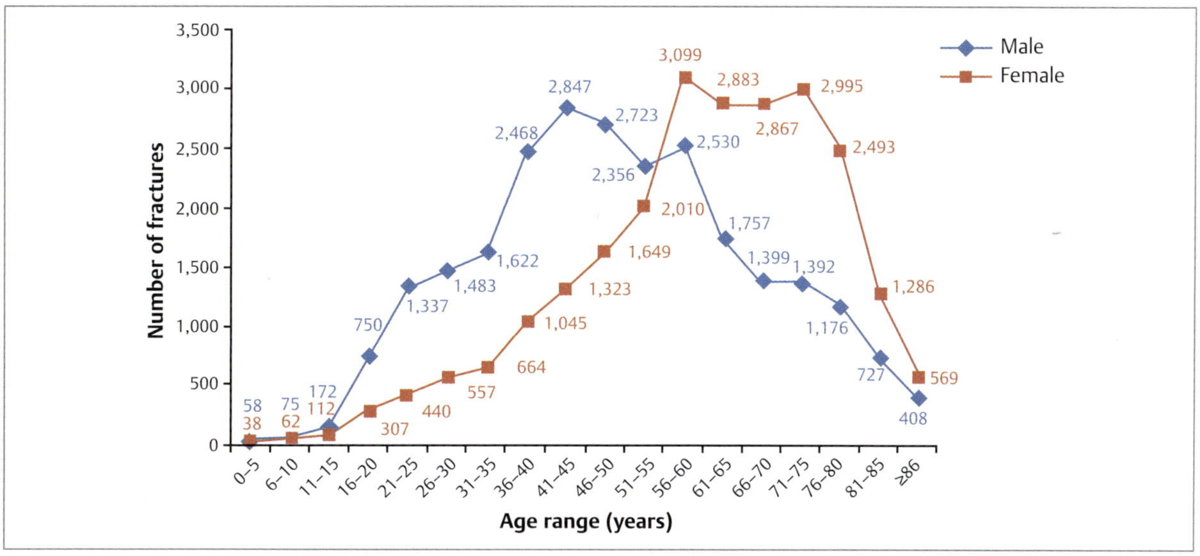

Fig. 1.11 Age and sex distribution of 49,679 patients with spinal column fractures.

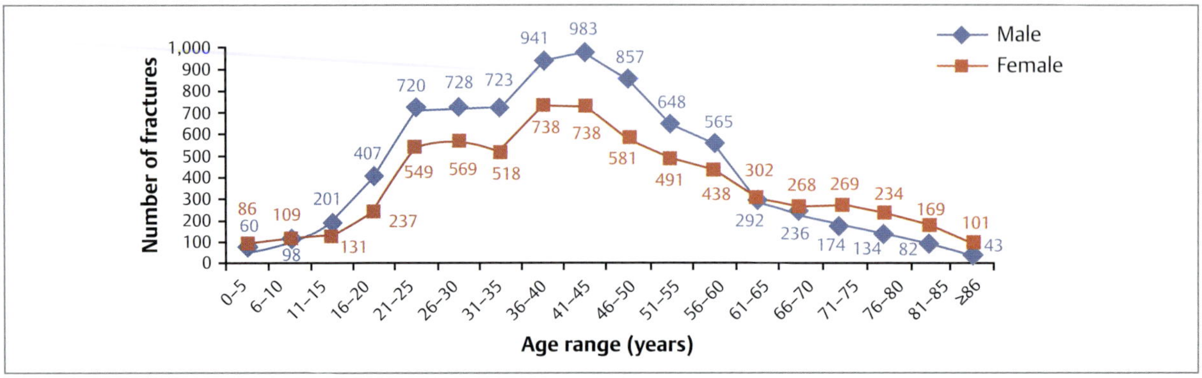

Fig. 1.12 Age and sex distribution of 14,420 patients with fractures of the pelvic ring and acetabulum.

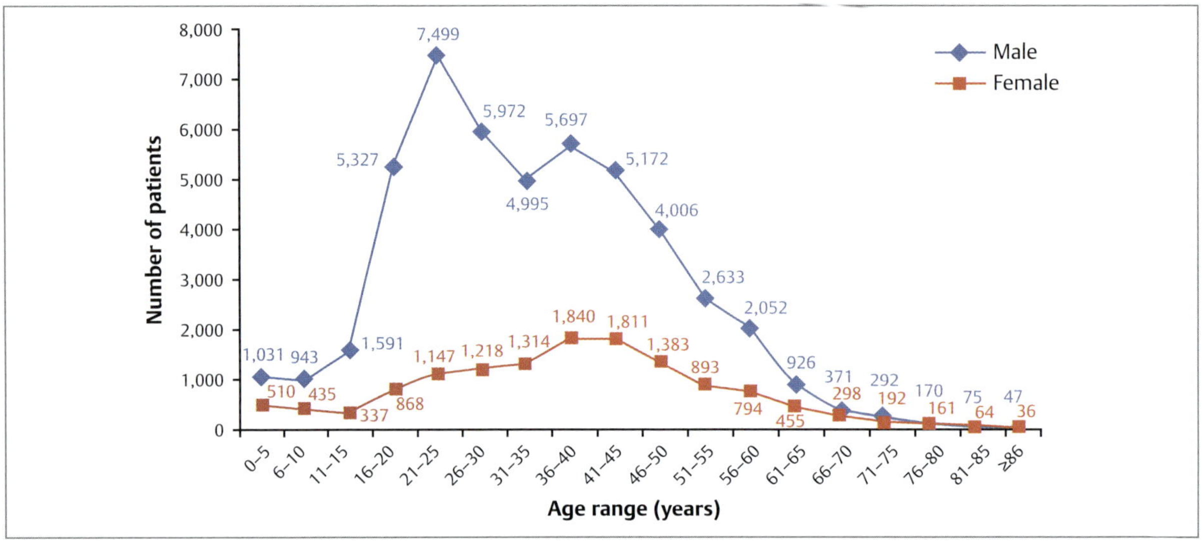

Fig. 1.13 Age and sex distribution of 62,555 patients with hand fractures.

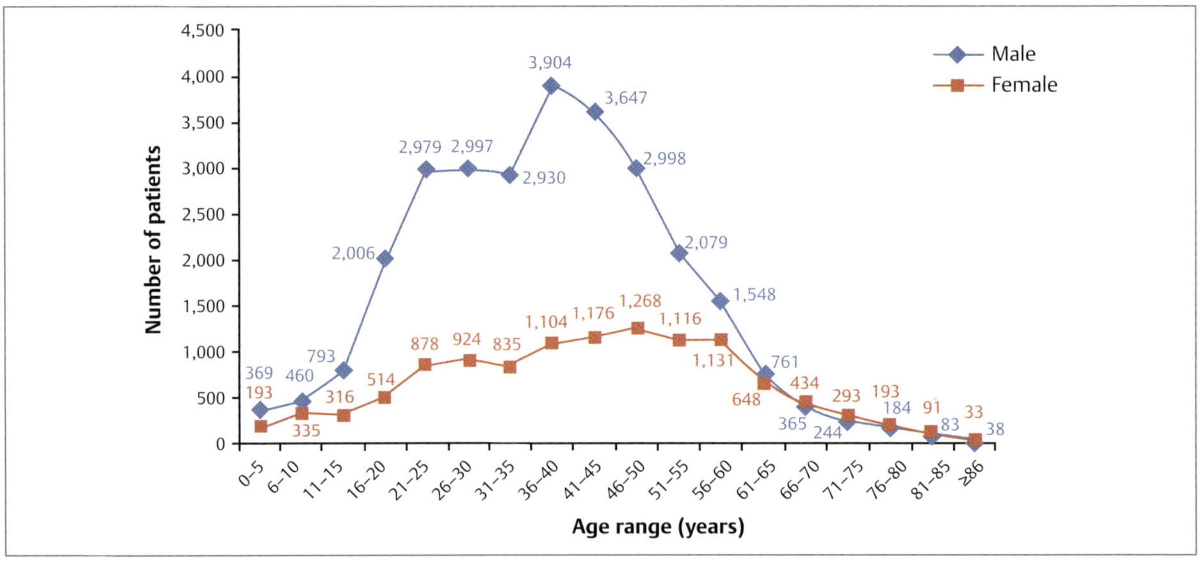

Fig. 1.14 Age and sex distribution of 39,867 patients with foot fractures.

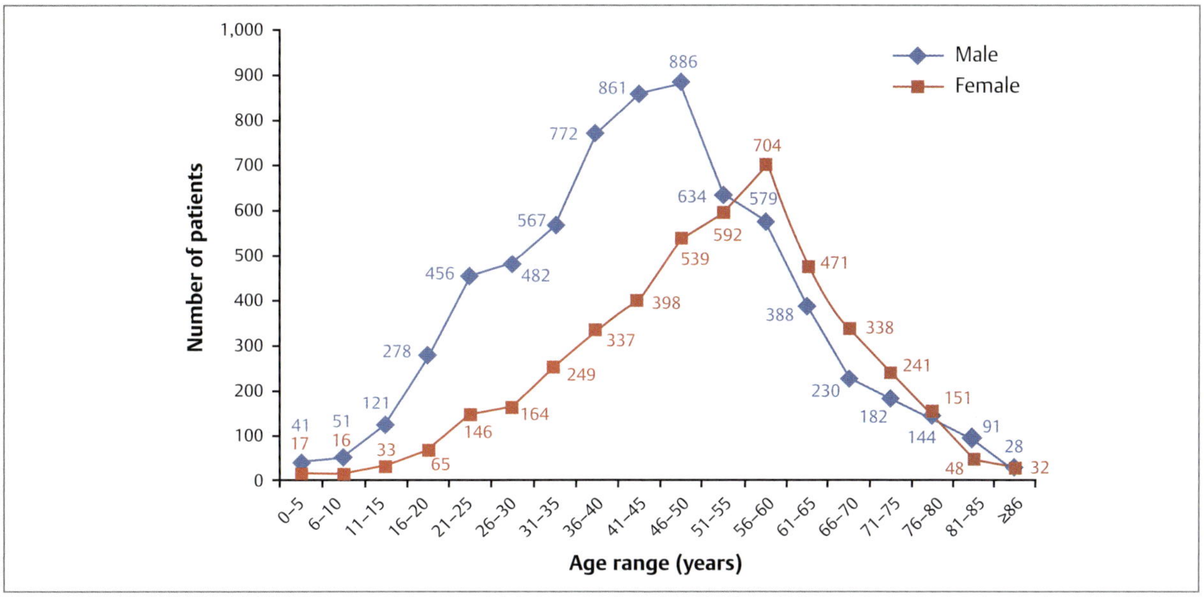

Fig. 1.15 Age and sex distribution of 11,332 patients with patellar fractures.

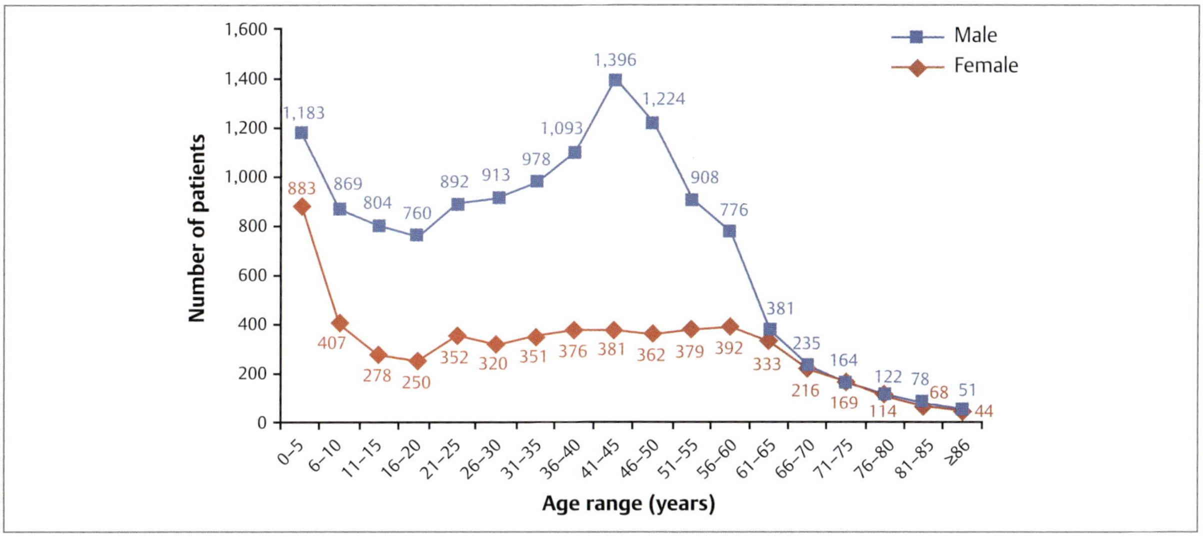

Fig. 1.16 Age and sex distribution of 18,502 patients with clavicle fractures.

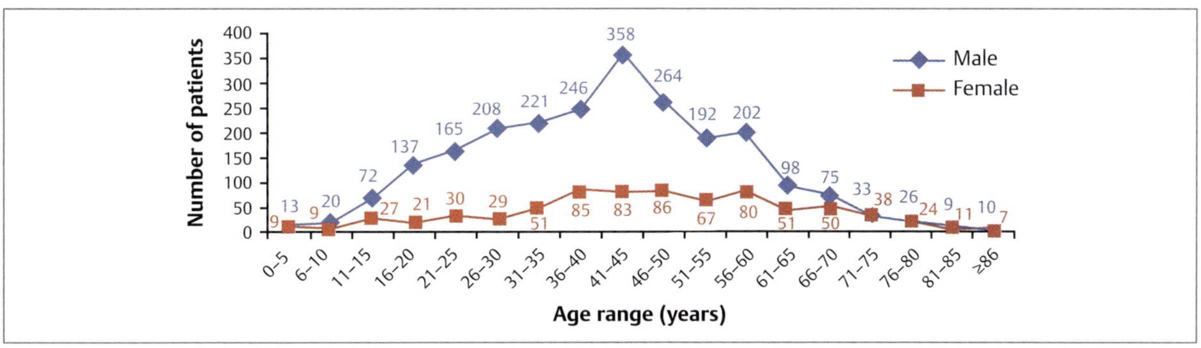

Fig. 1.17 Age and sex distribution of 3,107 patients with scapular fractures.

Fracture Location

Fractures more frequently occur in tibia/fibula, ulna/radius, and hand (**Table 1.1** and **Fig. 1.18**).

Table 1.1 Distribution of 420,125 patients by fracture locations and by gender

	Humer-us	Ulna/Radius	Femur	Tibia/Fibula	Spine	Foot/Ankle	Hand	Pelvis/acetabulum	Clavicle	Scapula	Patella	Total
Male	19,567	41,592	23,234	44,438	25,280	28,385	48,799	7,892	12,827	2,349	6,791	261,154
Female	16,111	34,258	19,143	22,320	24,399	11,482	13,756	6,528	5,675	758	4,541	158,971
Total	35,678	75,850	42,377	66,758	49,679	39,867	62,555	14,420	18,502	3,107	11,332	420,125
%	8.49%	18.05%	10.09%	15.89%	11.82%	9.49%	14.89%	3.43%	4.40%	0.74%	2.70%	100.00%

Note: Since a patient may sustain one or more fractures of different locations, the total number of patients summarized according to locations is 420,125, greater than the total number of 414,935 patients.

Unit: patient

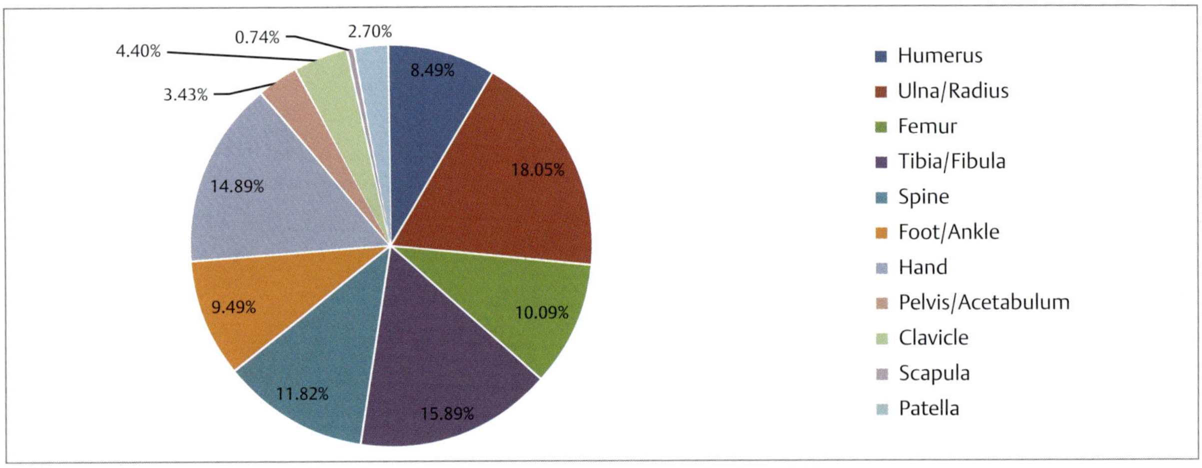

Fig. 1.18 Fracture distribution of the 420,125 patients summarized according to locations.

Fractures in Children

Fracture characteristics in children are different than in adults, with ulna/radius, humerus, and tibia/fibula being bones with the highest fracture incidence. The locations with the highest risk of fractures are distal humerus, distal ulna/radius, clavicle, and diaphysis of tibia (**Table 1.2**).

Table 1.2 Distribution of fracture locations in children and adults

	Humer-us	Ulna/Radius	Femur	Tibia/Fibula	Spine	Foot/Ankle	Hand	Pelvis/Acetabulum	Clavicle	Scapula	Patella	Total
Children	14,041	18,334	3,282	8,264	564	2,502	4,881	687	4,430	151	290	57,426
Adults	21,769	58,216	39,696	60,614	54,533	38,634	58,849	13,868	14,157	2,972	11,088	374,396
Total	35,810	76,550	42,978	68,878	55,097	41,136	63,730	14,555	18,587	3,123	11,378	431,822

Unit: fracture

2 Fractures of the Humerus

Overview

Anatomical Features

The humerus (**Plate 2.1**) is the longest and largest bone of the arm, and is divided into a body and two extremities. The proximal humerus is part of the radiographic anatomy of the shoulder. The humeral head is nearly hemispheric in shape, and articulates with the glenoid cavity of the scapula. The greater tubercle, situated lateral to the head, has three areas of muscle insertion: the supraspinatus superiorly, the infraspinatus in the middle, and the teres minor inferiorly. Situated in front of the head is the lesser tubercle, into which the tendon of the subscapularis inserts. The tubercles are separated from each other by a deep groove named the intertubercular groove, which contains the long tendon of the biceps brachii. The articular surface of the head is called the anatomical neck, and provides attachment for the articular capsule of the shoulder joint. The surgical neck is the narrowing below the tubercles and is frequently the site of fracture of the proximal humerus. The body runs from the tubercles, is almost cylindric in its upper half, and gradually flattens and gains a prismatic shape. The radial nerve winds around the posterior aspect of the humerus, running laterally in the radial sulcus toward the forearm. The lower extremities are flattened, broad, and thin proximally, while they are thicker at the two tuberculated eminences (lateral and medial epicondyles). The trochlea and the capitulum of the humerus articulate with the semilunar notch of the ulna and the margin of the radial head, respectively, to form the humeroulnar articulation and the humeroradial articulation.

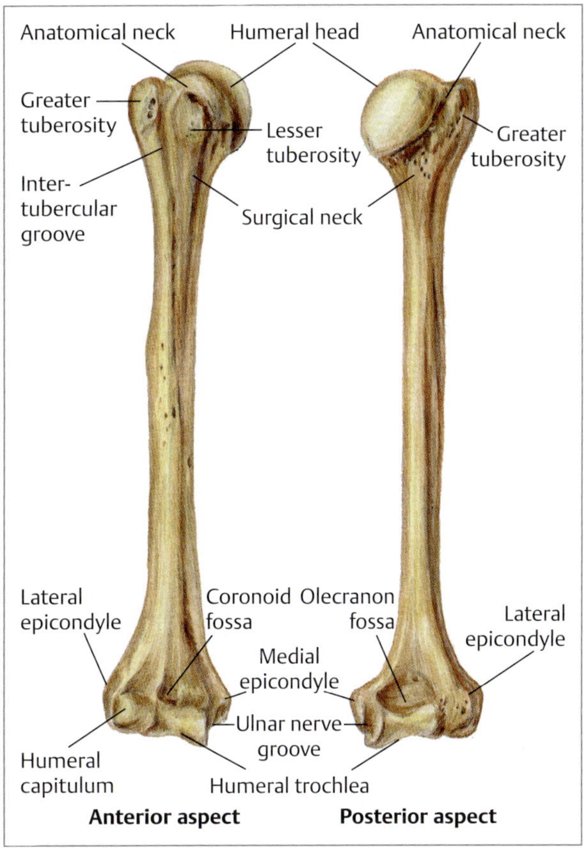

Plate 2.1

AO Classification and Coding System for Humeral Fractures

The humerus is assigned the number 1 based on the AO system and is further divided into three zones: 11, proximal fracture; 12, shaft fracture; and 13, distal fracture (**Plates 2.2** and **2.3**).

Clinical Epidemiologic Features of Humeral Fractures

A total of 35,678 patients with 35,810 humeral fractures were treated in 83 hospitals in China over a 2-year period from 2010 to 2011. All cases were reviewed and statistically studied; the fractures accounted for 8.6% of all patients with fractures and 8.29% of all types of fractures. Among 35,678 patients, 14,027 were children with 14,041 fractures, and 21,651 were adults with 21,769 fractures.

The epidemiologic features of humeral fractures are as follows:

- More males than females
- More left sides involved than right sides
- The highest-risk age groups are 0–5 years and 6–10 years
- In adults, fractures occur most frequently in the proximal humerus; in children they occur most frequently in distal humerus.

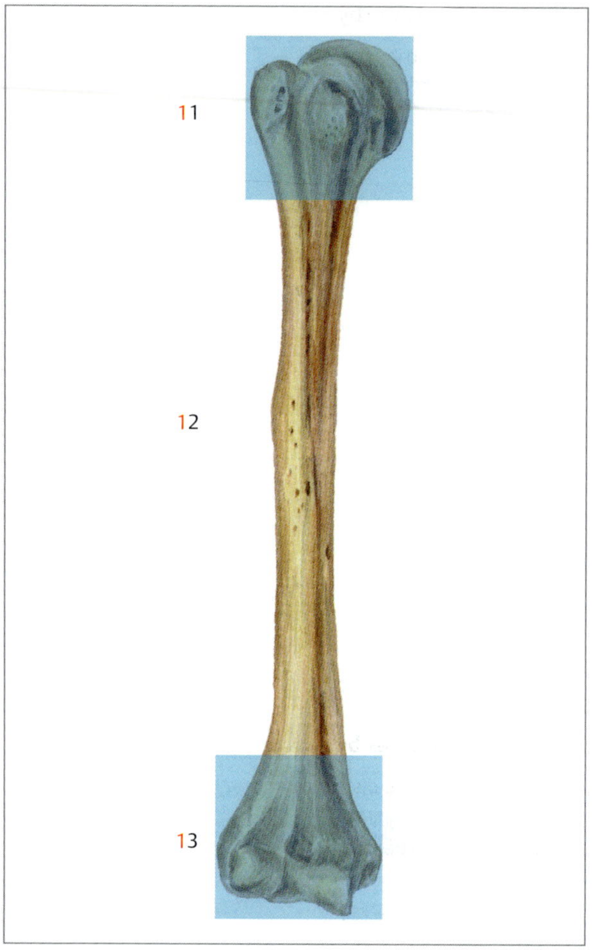

Plate 2.2

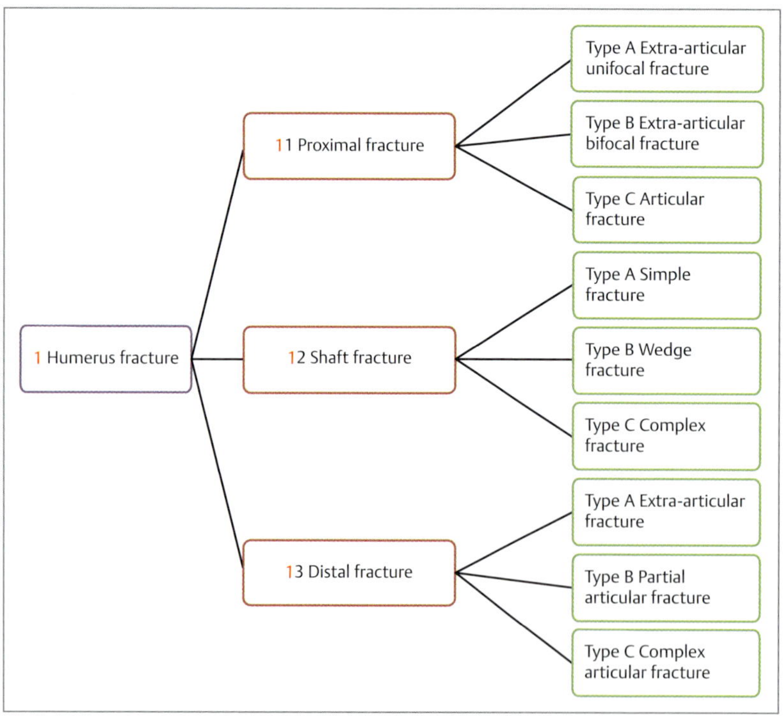

Plate 2.3

Humeral Fractures by Sex

Table 2.1 Sex distribution of 35,678 patients with humeral fractures

Sex	Number of patients	Percentage (%)
Male	19,567	54.84
Female	16,111	45.16
Total	35,678	100.00

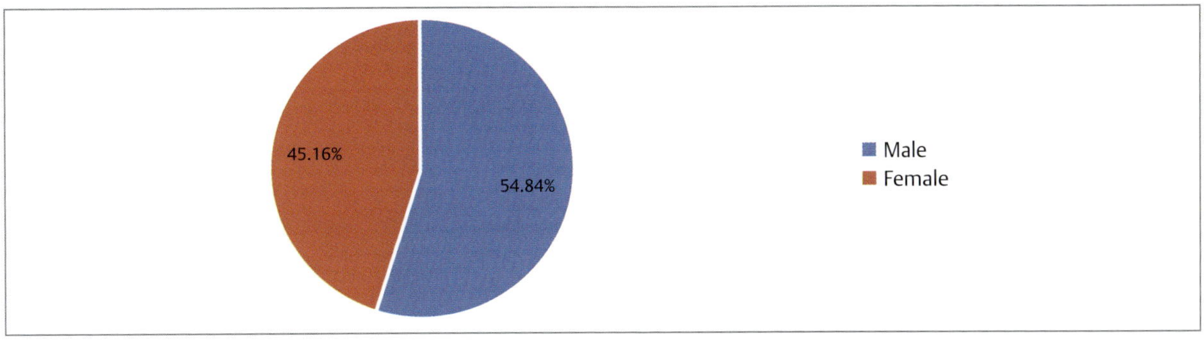

Fig. 2.1 Sex distribution of 35,678 patients with humeral fractures.

2

Humeral Fractures by Injured Side

Table 2.2 Injury side distribution of 35,678 patients with humeral fractures

Injured side	Number of patients	Percentage (%)
Left	18,809	52.72
Right	16,827	47.16
Bilateral	42	0.12
Total	35,678	100.00

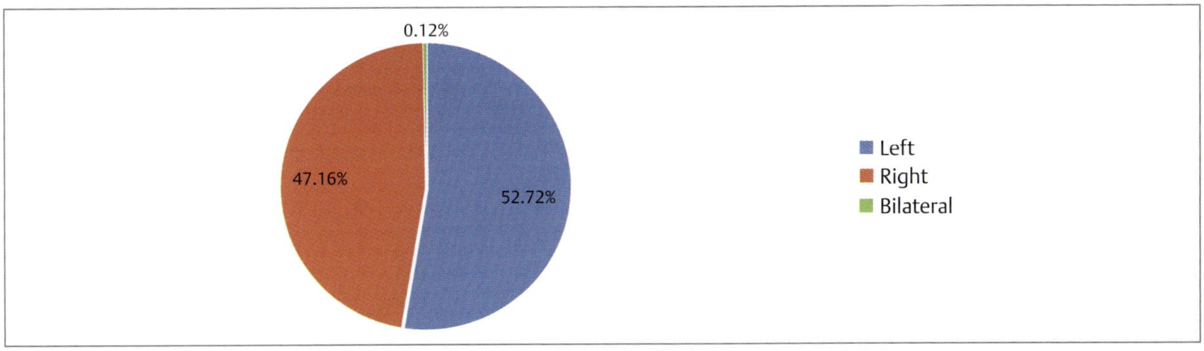

Fig. 2.2 Injury side distribution of 35,678 patients with humeral fractures.

Humeral Fractures by Age Group and Sex

Table 2.3 Age and sex distribution of 35,678 patients with humeral fractures

Age group (years)	Male	Female	Total	Percentage (%)
0–5	3,613	2,611	6,224	17.44
6–10	3,589	1,771	5,360	15.02
11–15	1,800	643	2,443	6.85
16–20	865	269	1,134	3.18
21–25	920	428	1,348	3.78
26–30	938	351	1,289	3.61
31–35	1,024	411	1,435	4.02
36–40	1,214	545	1,759	4.93
41–45	1,132	667	1,799	5.04
46–50	1,009	772	1,781	4.99
51–55	1,010	1,189	2,199	6.16
56–60	719	1,302	2,021	5.66
61–65	419	1,021	1,440	4.04
66–70	368	968	1,336	3.74
71–75	277	1,061	1,338	3.75
76–80	324	1,113	1,437	4.03
81–85	214	612	826	2.32
≥86	132	377	509	1.43
Total	19,567	16,111	35,678	100.00

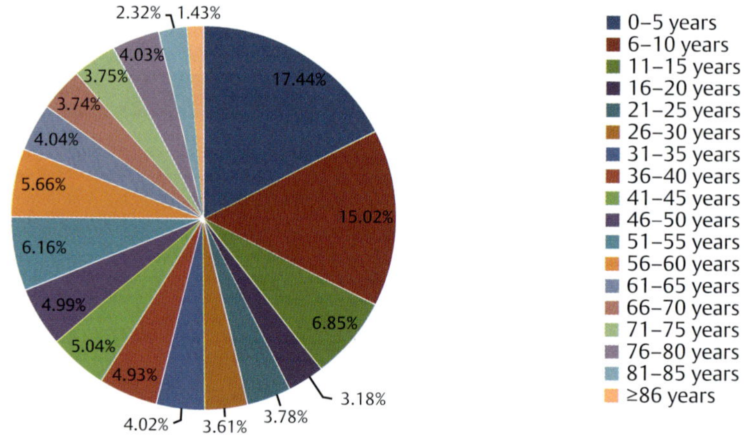

a

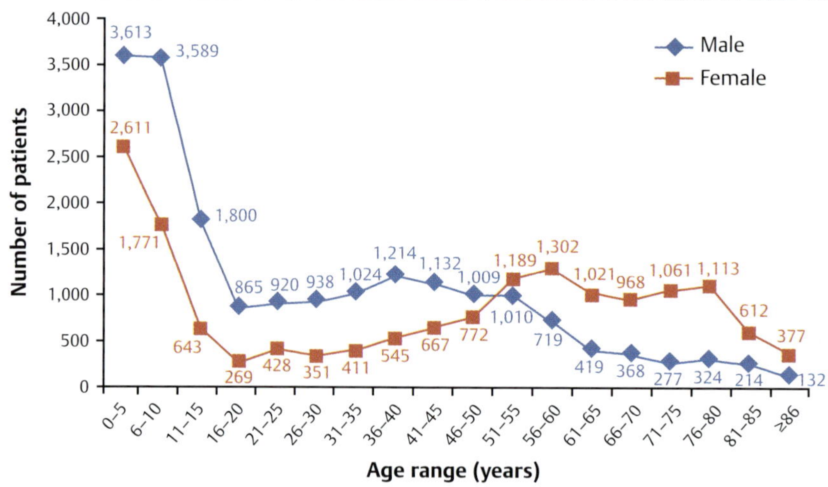

b

Fig. 2.3 **(a)** Age distribution of 35,678 patients with humeral fractures.
(b) Age and sex distribution of 35,678 patients with humeral fractures.

Humeral Fractures by Location

Distribution of Humeral Fractures by Segments in Adults Based on AO Classification

Table 2.4 Segment distribution of 21,769 humeral fractures in adults based on AO classification

Segment	Number of fractures	Percentage (%)
11	12,959	59.53
12	5,049	23.19
13	3,761	17.28
Total	21,769	100.00

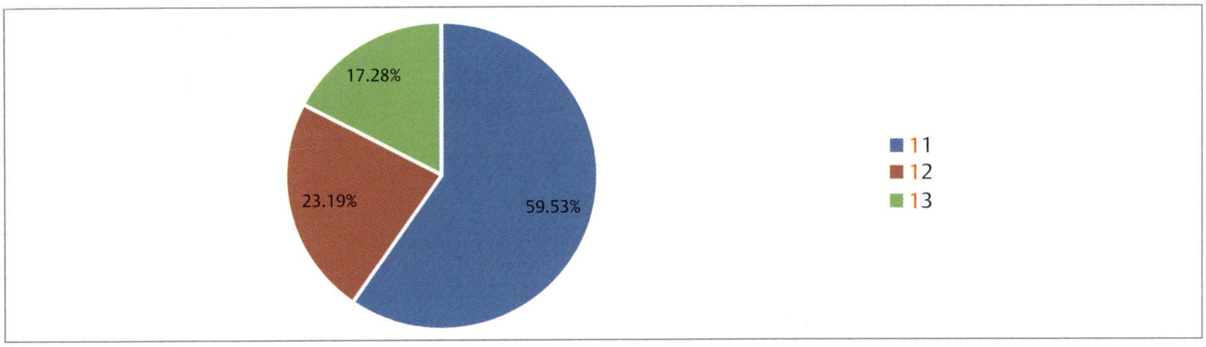

Fig. 2.4 Segment distribution of 21,769 humeral fractures in adults based on AO classification.

Distribution of Humeral Fractures by Segments in Children

Table 2.5 Segment distribution of 14,041 humeral fractures in children

Segment	Number of fractures	Percentage (%)
Proximal	1,618	11.52
Diaphysis	923	6.57
Distal	11,500	81.90
Total	14,041	100.00

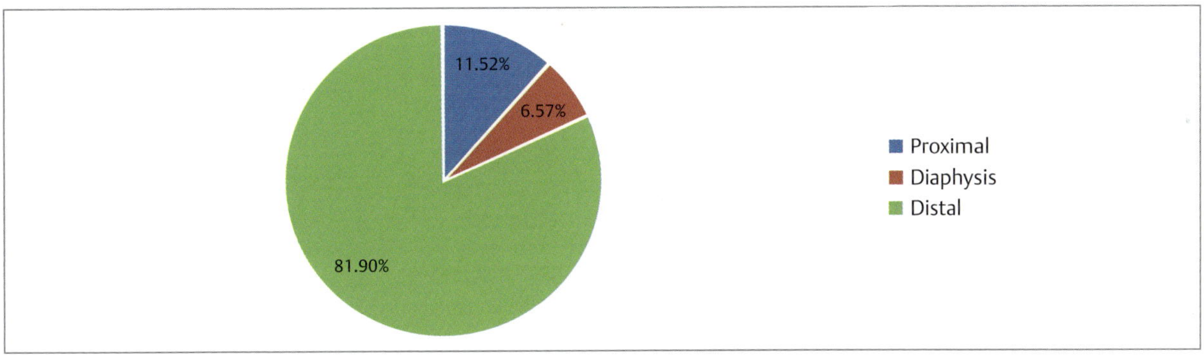

Fig. 2.5 Segment distribution of 14,041 humeral fractures in children.

Proximal Humeral Fractures (Segment 11)

Anatomical Features

The proximal part of the humerus consists of the head, two eminences, the greater and lesser tubercles, and the surgical neck (**Plate 2.4**). The humeral head has a hemispherical shape, which has a superior, medial, and posterior aspect. The narrow groove separating the head from the tubercles is the anatomical neck, where fractures rarely occur but there is a high incidence of avascular necrosis due to the disruption of blood supply to the main head fragment. The narrowing below the tubercles, called the surgical neck, is the junction of the two tubercles with the cylindric shaft. It is frequently fractured because the cortex at this part of the bone abruptly becomes quite thin. The greater tubercle is situated laterally and posteriorly to the proximal humerus, and provides insertion points for the supraspinatus, infraspinatus, and teres minor. The ridge descending down the shaft from the root of the greater tubercle is called the crest of the greater tubercle, into which the pectoralis major muscle inserts. The lesser tubercle, situated anteriorly, represents the center of the humeral head and provides an insertion point for the subscapularis. The crest descending from the lesser tubercle has attachments to the latissimus dorsi and the teretiscapularis. The intertubercular groove lodges the long tendon of the biceps brachii (**Plates 2.5** and **2.6**).

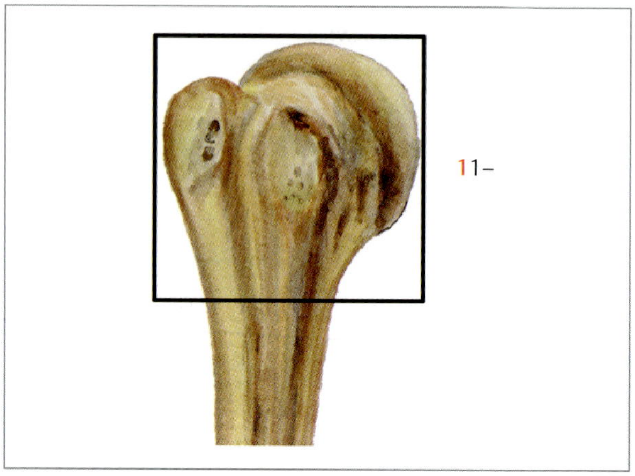

Plate 2.4

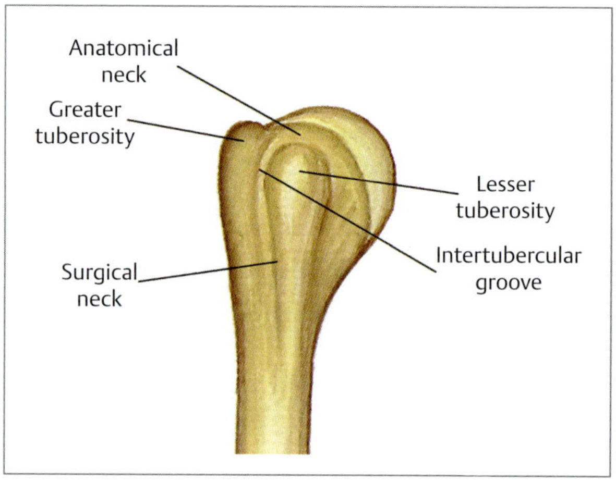

Plate 2.5

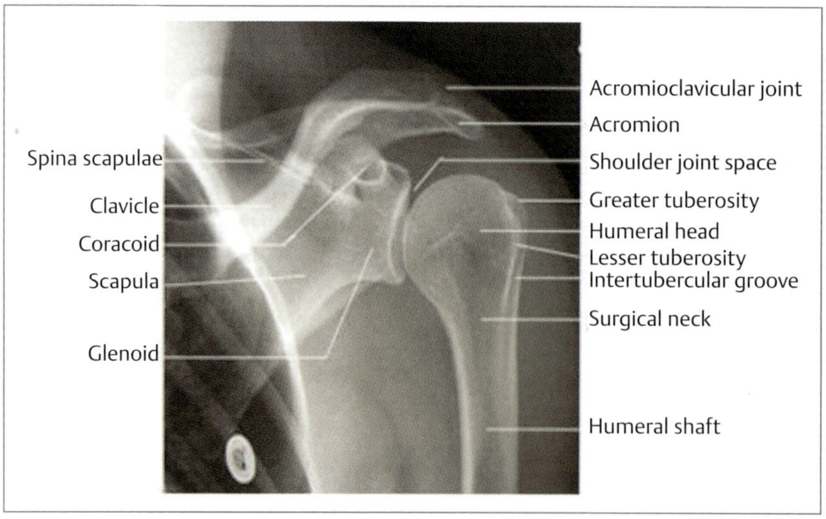

Plate 2.6

AO Classification of Proximal Humeral Fractures

Based on AO classification, the proximal end of the humerus is delineated by a square with its lateral side equal to the maximum width of the epiphysis. The AO coding of a proximal humeral fracture is 11, and is further divided into three categories based on the severity of injury: types A, B, and C (**Plate 2.7**).

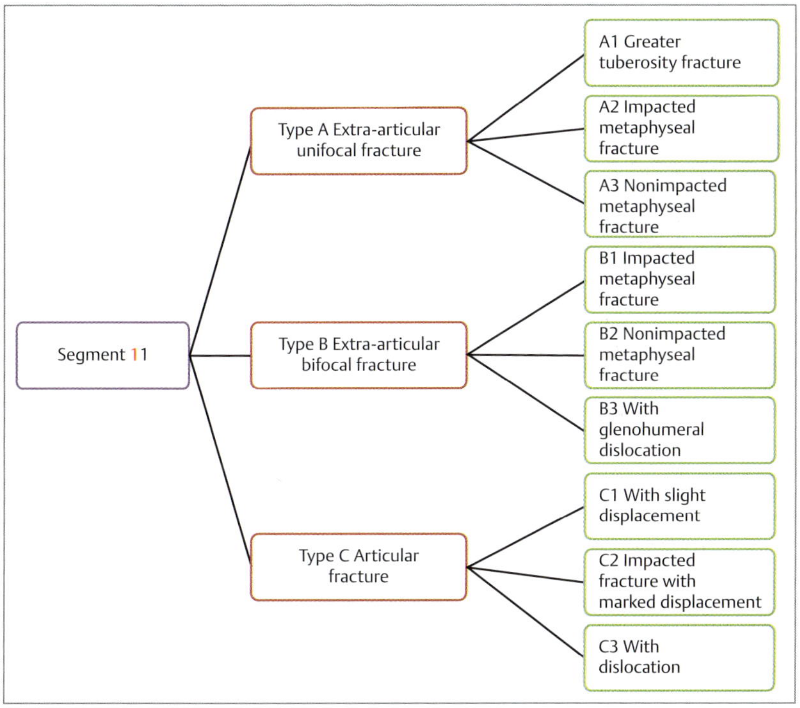

Plate 2.7

Clinical Epidemiologic Features of Proximal Humeral Fractures (Segment 11)

A total of 12,959 adult proximal humeral fractures (segment 11) were treated in 83 hospitals in China over a 2-year period from 2010 to 2011. Each case was reviewed and statistically studied; the fractures accounted for 59.53% of adult humeral fractures. The epidemiologic features are as follows:

- More females than males
- The high-risk age group includes ages 51–55 years, specifically ages 51–55 years for males and ages 56–60 years for females
- The high-incidence type is 11-A, and is the same for both males and females
- The high-incidence group is 11-A1, and is the same for both males and females.

Fractures of Segment 11 by Sex

Table 2.6 Sex distribution of 12,959 fractures of segment 11

Sex	Number of fractures	Percentage (%)
Male	5,247	40.49
Female	7,712	59.51
Total	12,959	100.00

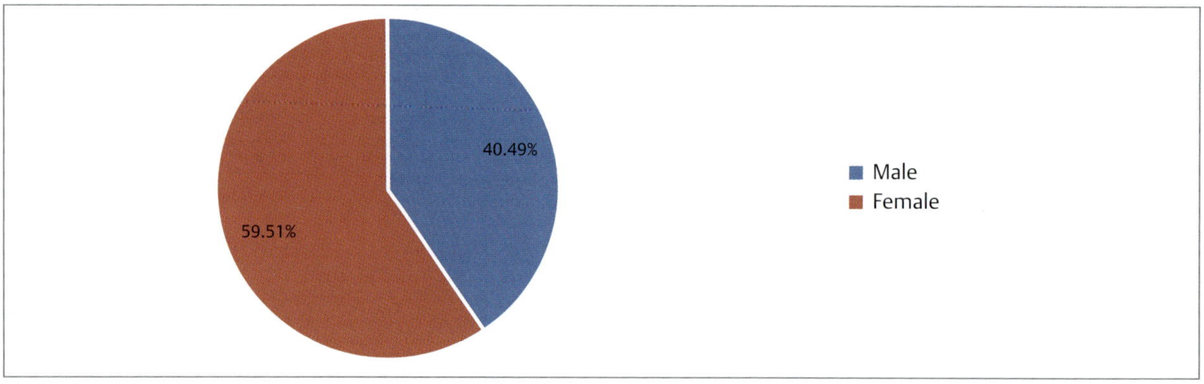

Fig. 2.6 Sex distribution of 12,959 fractures of segment 11.

Fractures of Segment 11 by Age Group

Table 2.7 Age and sex distribution of 12,959 fractures of segment 11

Age group (years)	Male	Female	Total	Percentage (%)
16–20	236	86	322	2.48
21–25	218	153	371	2.86
26–30	334	164	498	3.84
31–35	448	197	645	4.98
36–40	568	295	863	6.66
41–45	582	401	983	7.59
46–50	574	526	1,100	8.49
51–55	634	920	1,554	11.99
56–60	411	977	1,388	10.71
61–65	273	779	1,052	8.12
66–70	255	752	1,007	7.77
71–75	204	837	1,041	8.03
76–80	235	863	1,098	8.47
81–85	174	482	656	5.06
≥86	101	280	381	2.94
Total	5,247	7,712	12,959	100.00

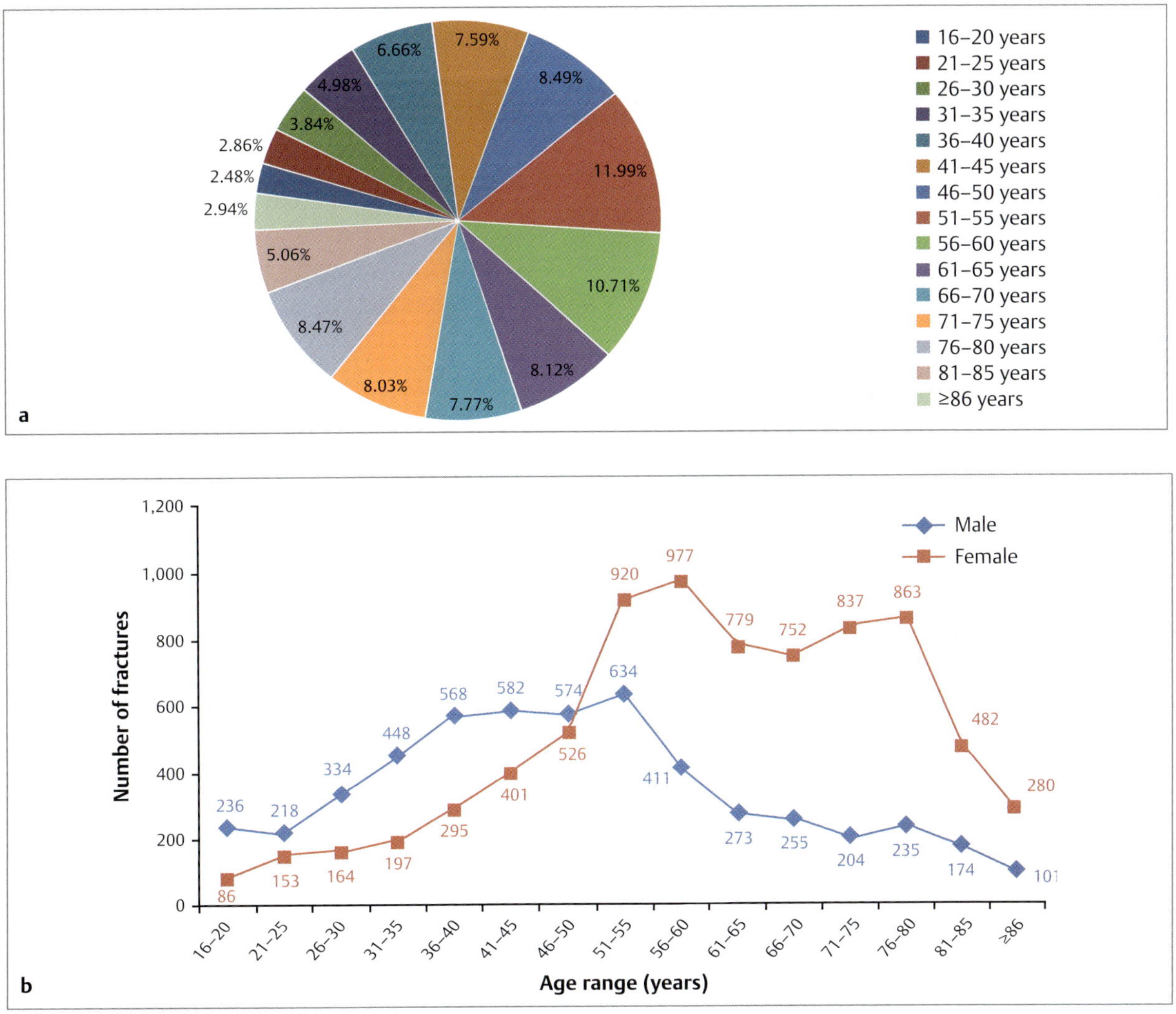

Fig. 2.7 **(a)** Age distribution of 12,959 fractures of segment 11.
(b) Age and sex distribution of 12,959 fractures of segment 11.

Fractures of Segment 11 by Fracture Type

Table 2.8 Sex and fracture type distribution of 12,959 fractures of segment 11

Fracture type	Male	Female	Total	Percentage of segment 11 (%)	Percentage of adult humeral fractures (%)
11-A	3,718	5,085	8,803	67.93	40.44
11-B	1,038	1,801	2,839	21.91	13.04
11-C	491	826	1,317	10.16	6.05
Total	5,247	7,712	12,959	100.00	59.53

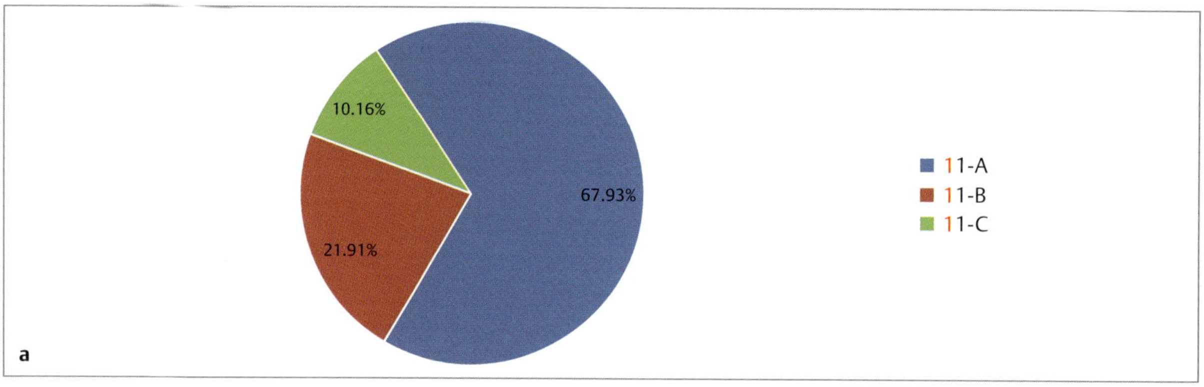

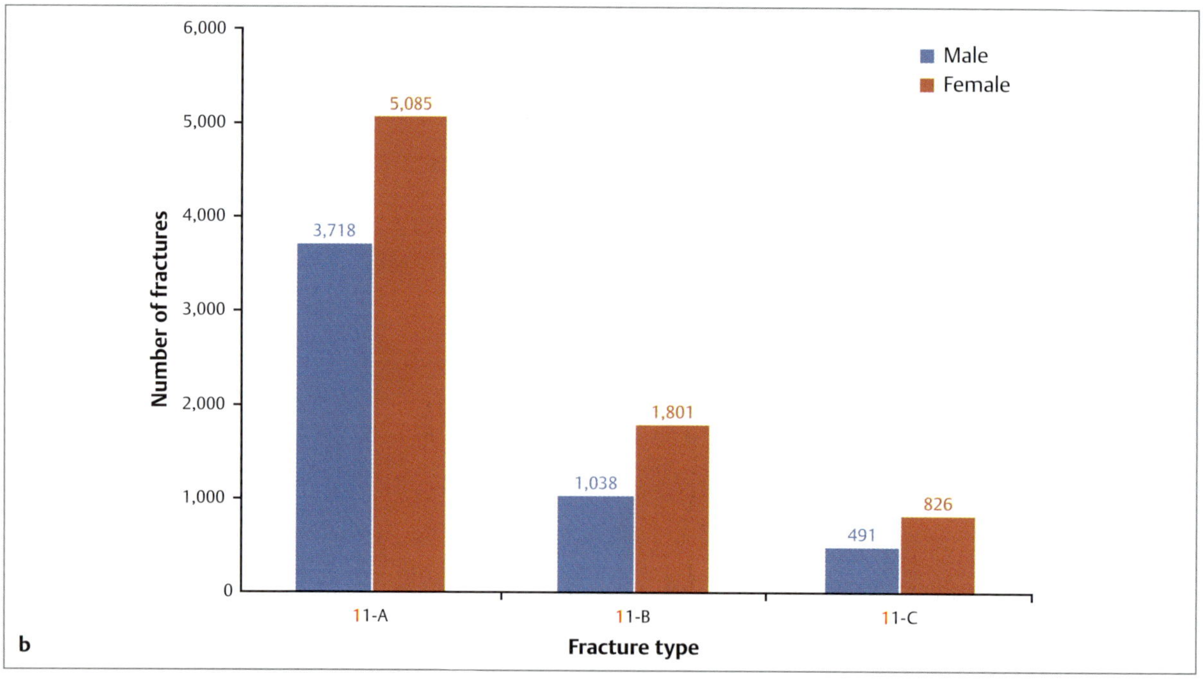

Fig. 2.8 **(a)** Fracture type distribution of 12,959 fractures of segment 11.
(b) Sex and fracture type distribution of 12,959 fractures of segment 11.

Table 2.9 Sex and fracture group distribution of 12,959 fractures of segment 11

Fracture group	Male	Female	Total	Percentage of segment 11 (%)	Percentage of adult humeral fractures (%)
11-A1	2,302	2,841	5,143	39.69	23.63
11-A2	865	1,468	2,333	18.00	10.72
11-A3	551	776	1,327	10.24	6.10
11-B1	524	960	1,484	11.45	6.82
11-B2	385	616	1,001	7.72	4.60
11-B3	129	225	354	2.73	1.63
11-C1	169	295	464	3.58	2.13
11-C2	166	291	457	3.53	2.10
11-C3	156	240	396	3.06	1.82
Total	5,247	7,712	12,959	100.00	59.53

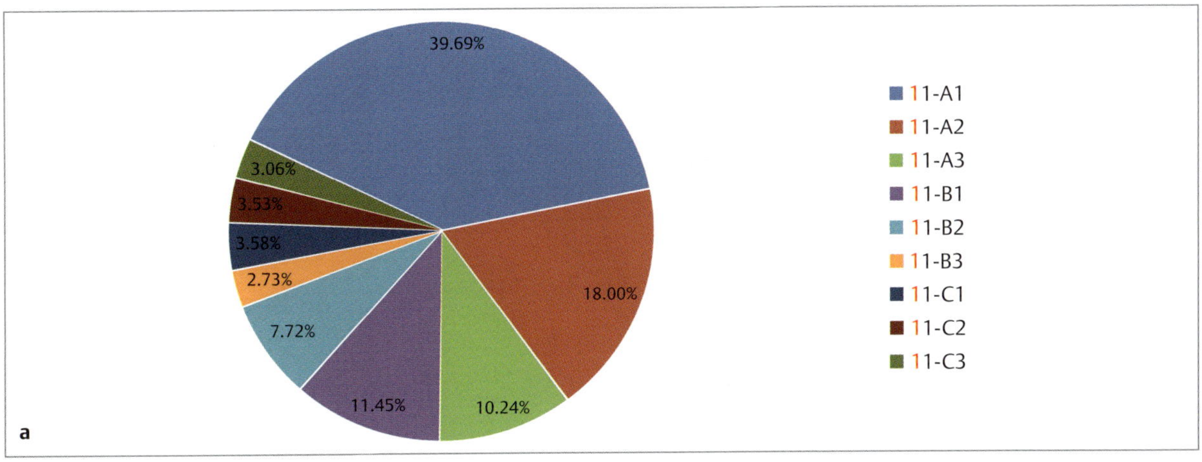

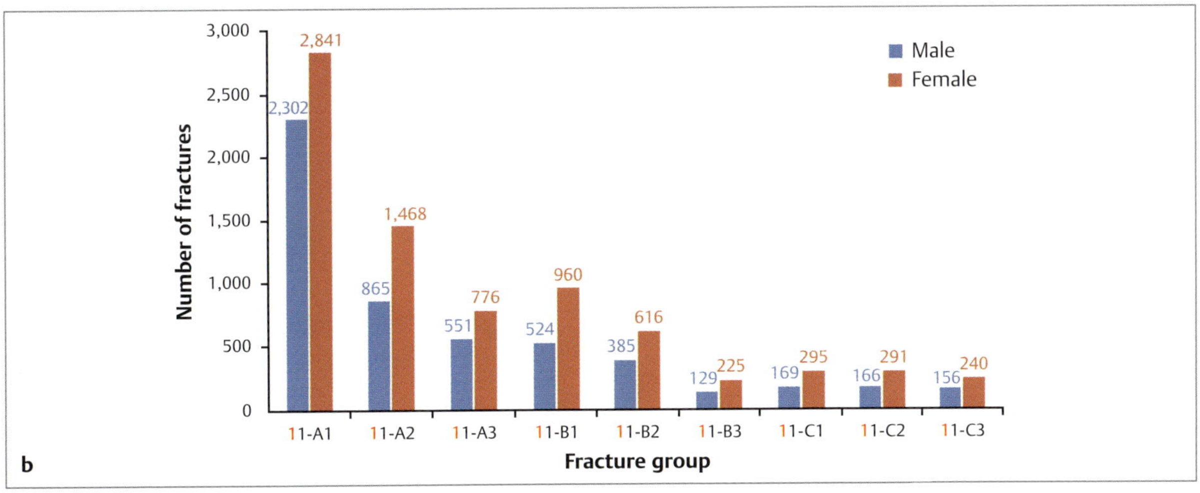

Fig. 2.9 **(a)** Fracture group distribution of 12,959 fractures of segment 11.
(b) Sex and fracture group distribution of 12,959 fractures of segment 11.

2

11-A Humerus proximal extra-articular fractures, unifocal

11-A1
Humerus proximal extra-articular, greater tuberosity fracture
5,143 fractures
M: 2,302 (44.76%)
F: 2,841 (55.24%)
1.37% of total adult fractures
23.63% of adult humeral fractures
39.69% of segment 11
58.42% of type 11-A

11-A1.1

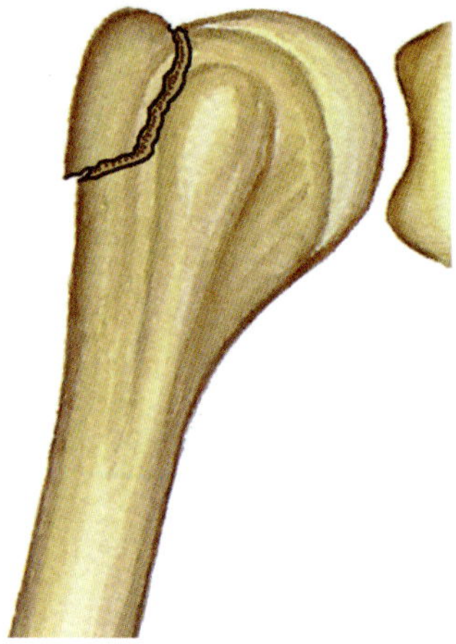

Greater tuberosity fracture without displacement

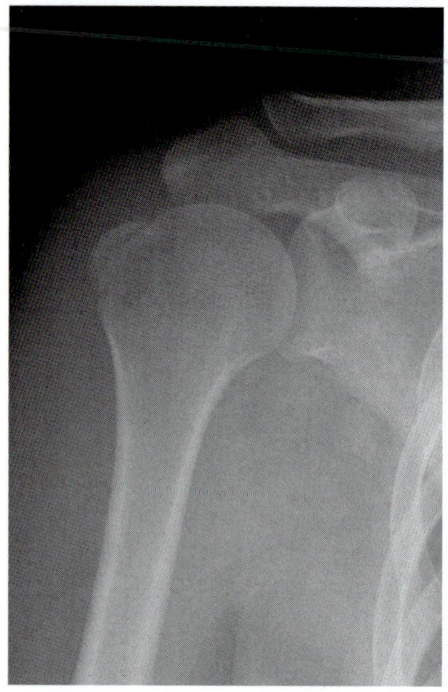

11-A1.2

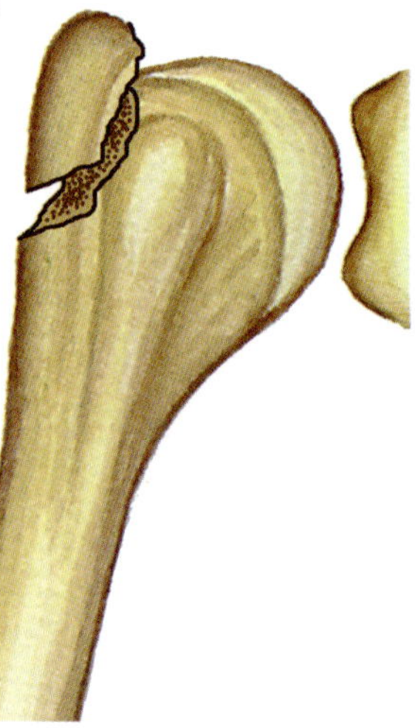

Greater tuberosity fracture with displacement

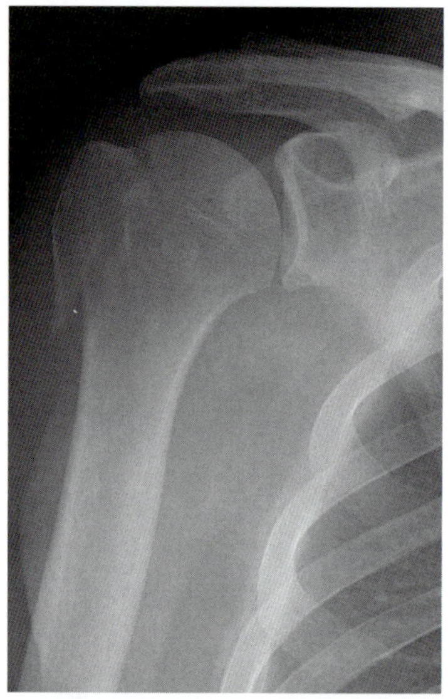

11-A1.3

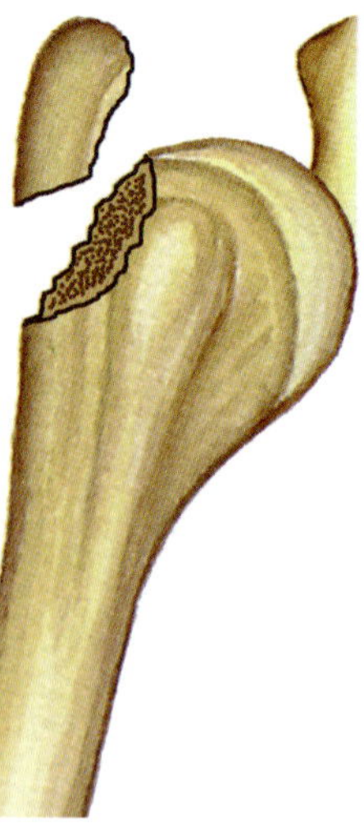

Greater tuberosity fracture with glenohumeral dislocation

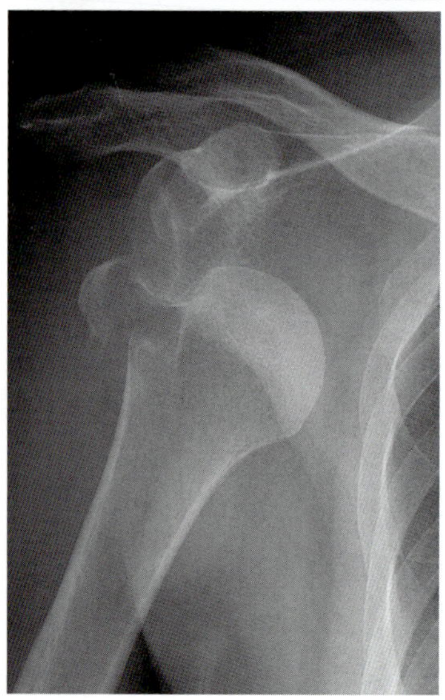

11-A Humerus proximal extra-articular fractures, unifocal

11-A2
Humerus proximal extra-articular fracture with impacted metaphysis
2,333 fractures
M: 865 (37.08%)
F: 1,468 (62.92%)
0.62% of total adult fractures
10.72% of adult humeral fractures
18.00% of segment 11
26.50% of type 11-A

11-A2.1

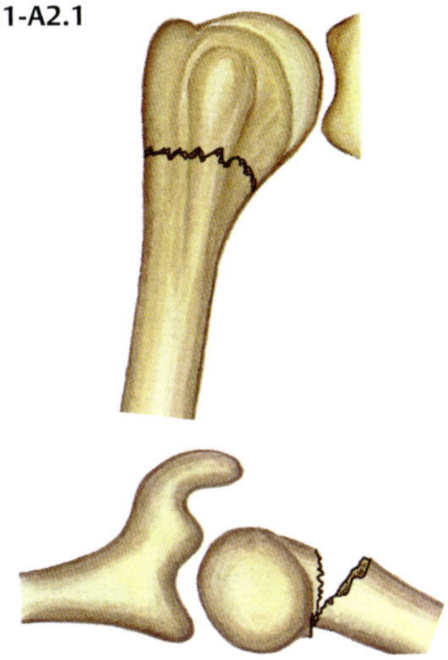

With frontal malalignment

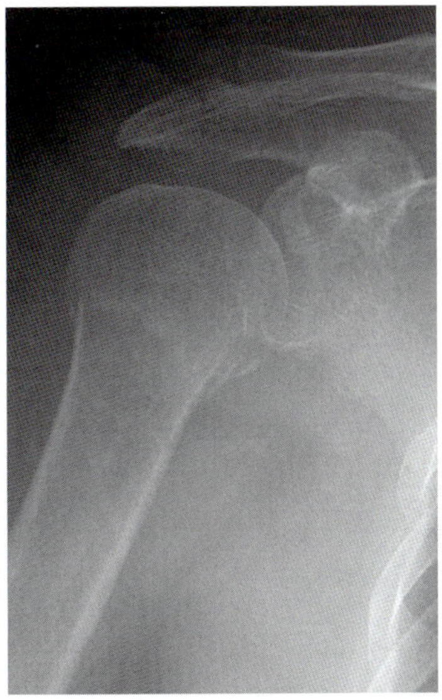

11-A2.2

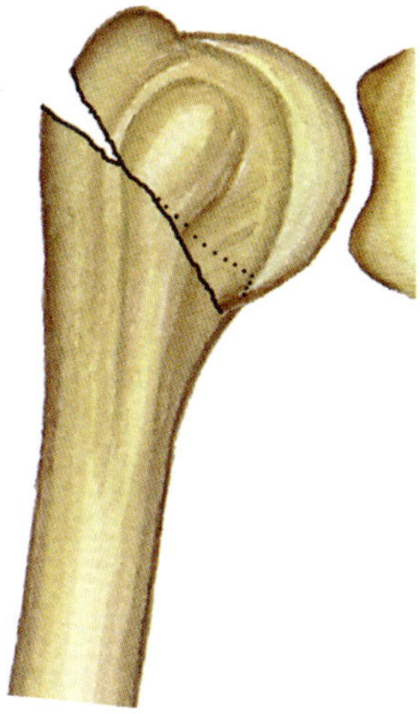

With varus malalignment

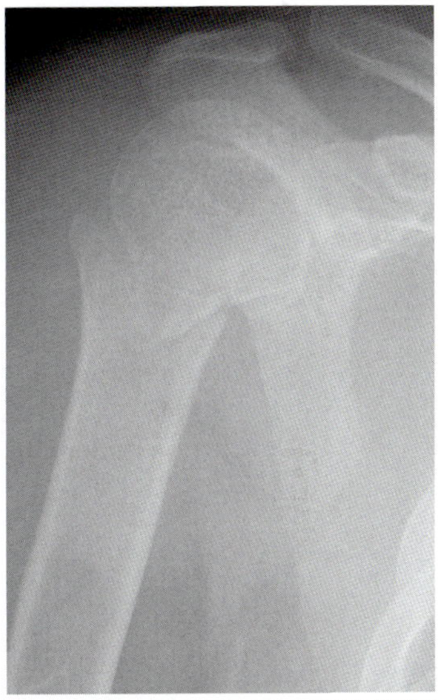

11-A2.3

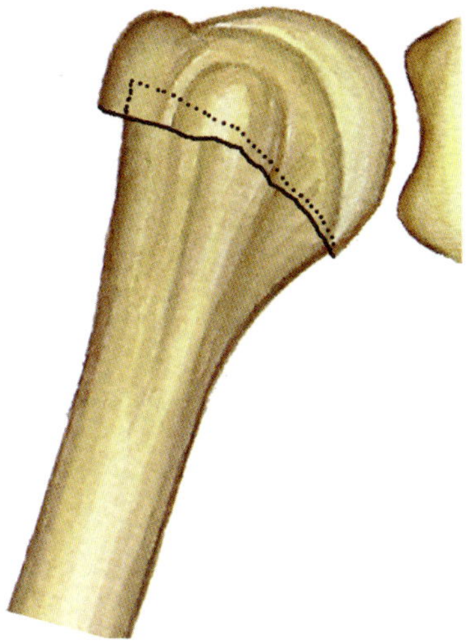

With valgus malalignment

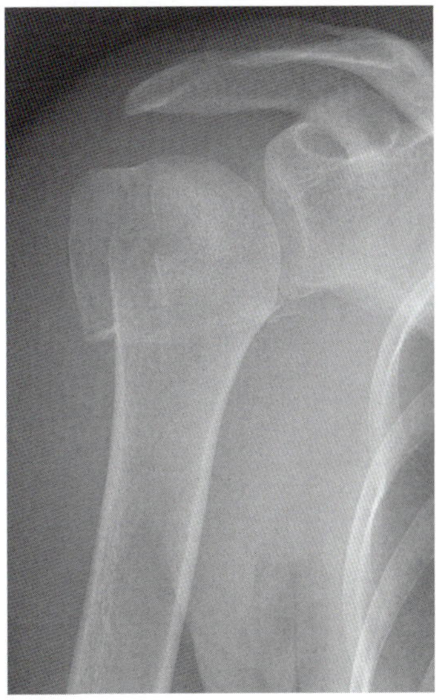

11-A Humerus proximal extra-articular fractures, unifocal

11-A3
Humerus proximal extra-articular fracture without impacted metaphysis
1,327 fractures
M: 551 (41.52%)
F: 776 (58.48%)
0.35% of total adult fractures
6.10% of adult humeral fractures
10.24% of segment 11
15.07% of type 11-A

11-A3.1

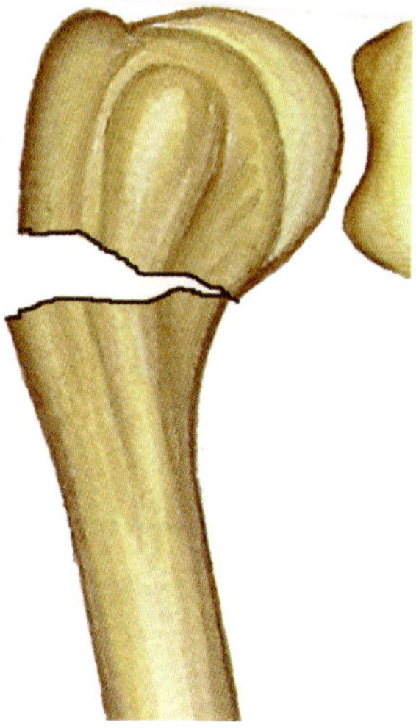

With angulation

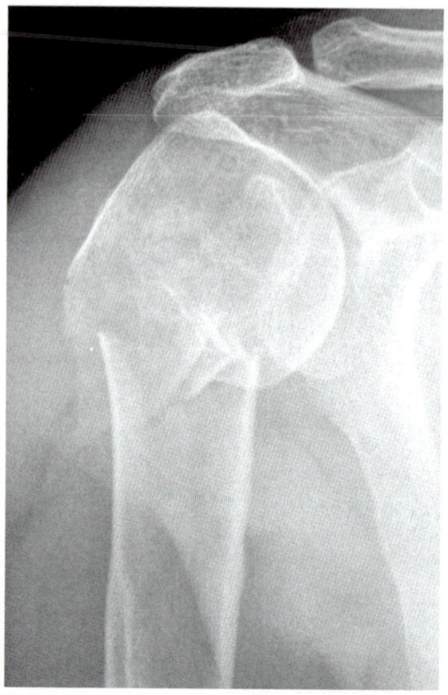

11-A3.2

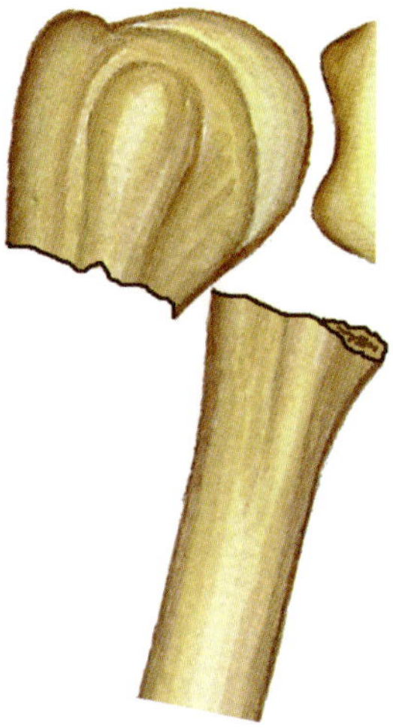

With translation

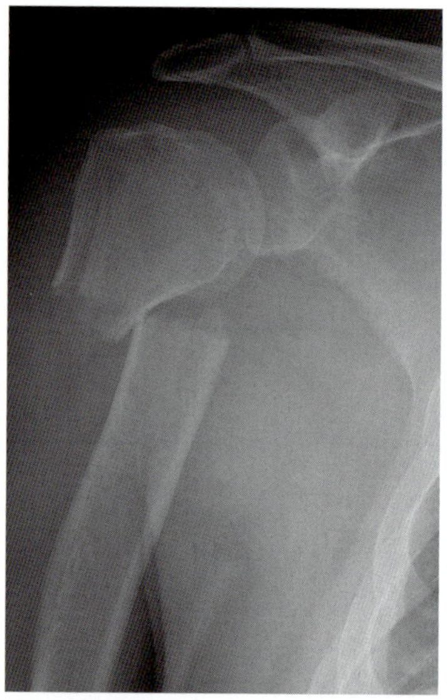

11-A3.3

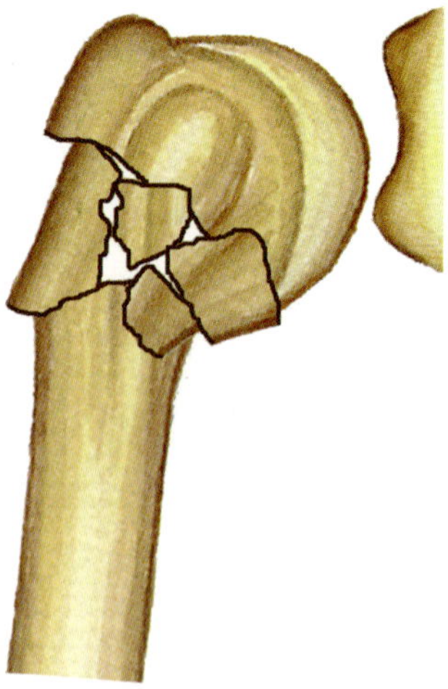

Multiple fragments

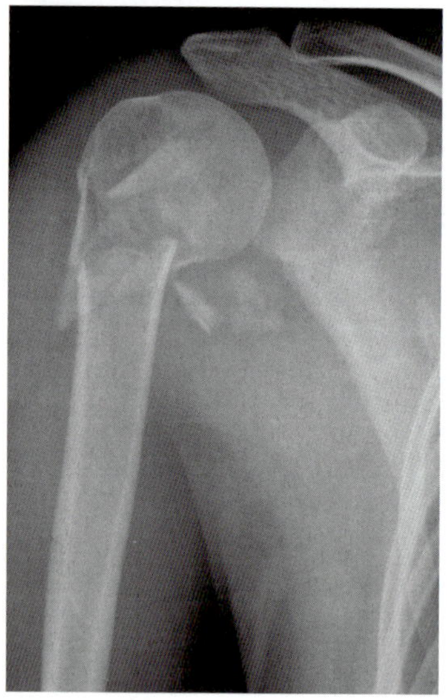

11-B Humerus proximal extra-articular fractures, bifocal

11-B1

Humerus proximal extra-articular bifocal fracture with impacted metaphysis

1,484 fractures
M: 524 (35.31%)
F: 960 (64.69%)
0.40% of total adult fractures
6.82% of adult humeral fractures
11.45% of segment 11
52.27% of type 11-B

11-B1.1

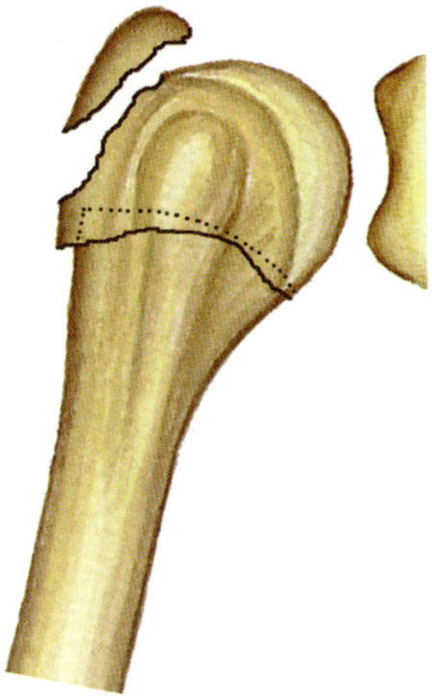

Lateral and greater tuberosity fractures

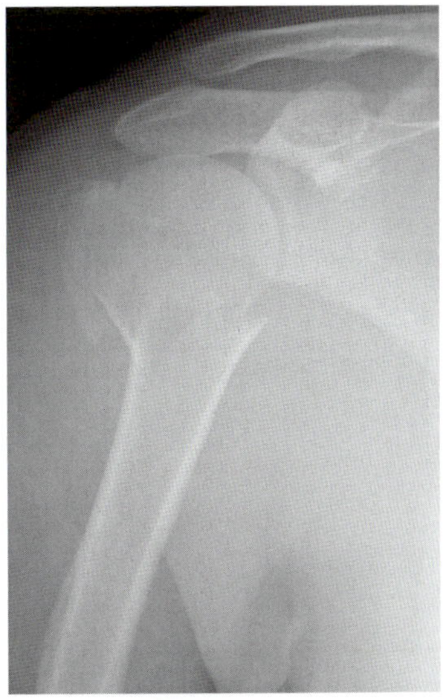

11-B1.2

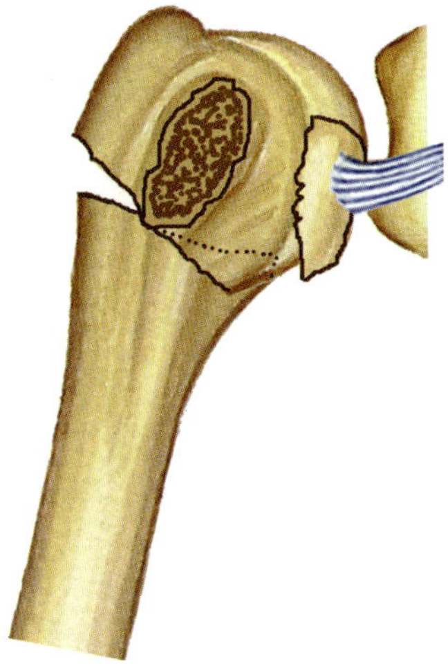

Medial and lesser tuberosity fractures

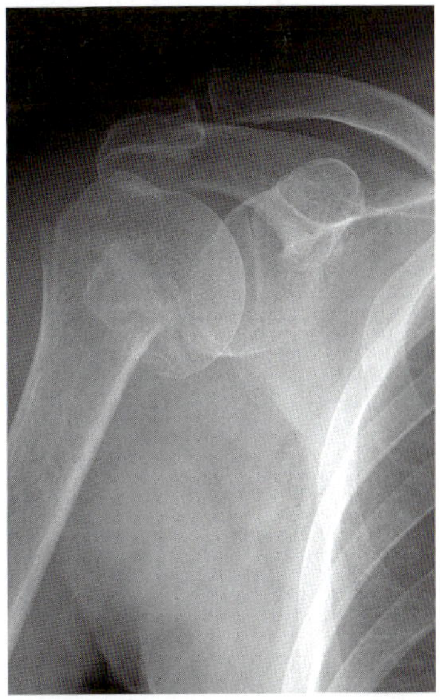

11-B1.3

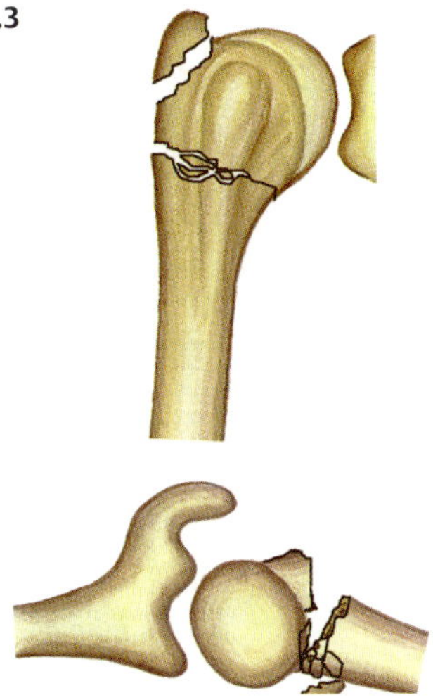

Posterior and greater tuberosity fractures

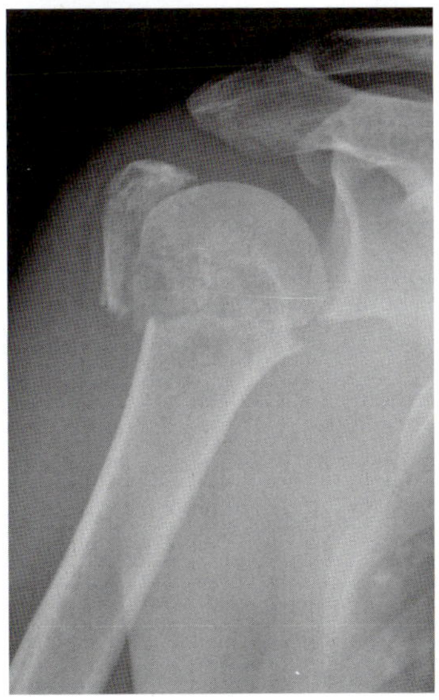

11-B Humerus proximal extra-articular fractures, bifocal

11-B2
Humerus proximal extra-articular bifocal fracture without impacted metaphysis
1,001 fractures
M: 385 (38.46%)
F: 616 (61.54%)
0.27% of total adult fractures
4.60% of adult humeral fractures
7.72% of segment 11
35.26% of type 11-B

11-B2.1

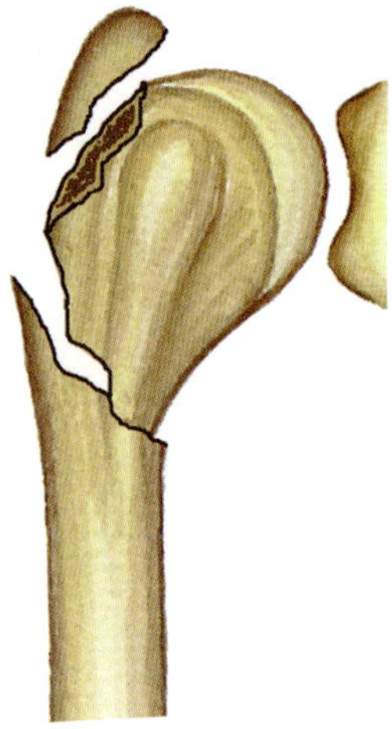

Without rotatory displacement of the epiphyseal fragment

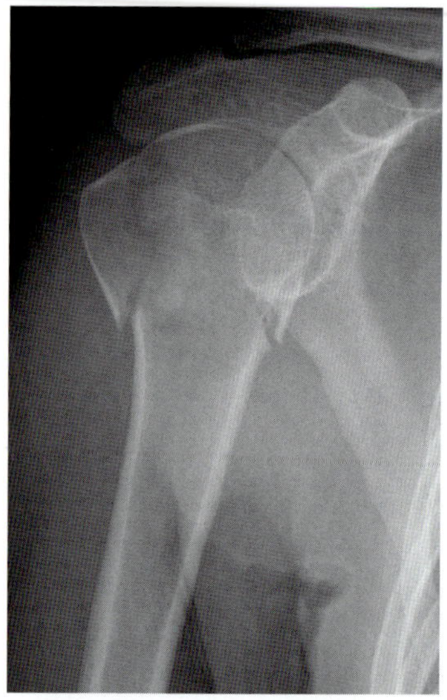

11-B2.2

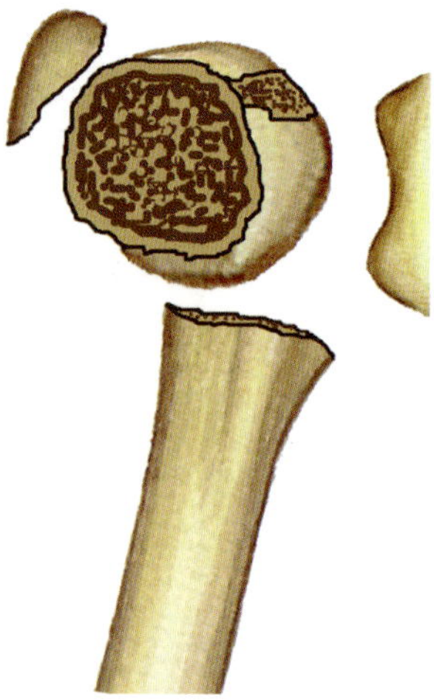

With rotatory displacement of the epiphyseal fragment

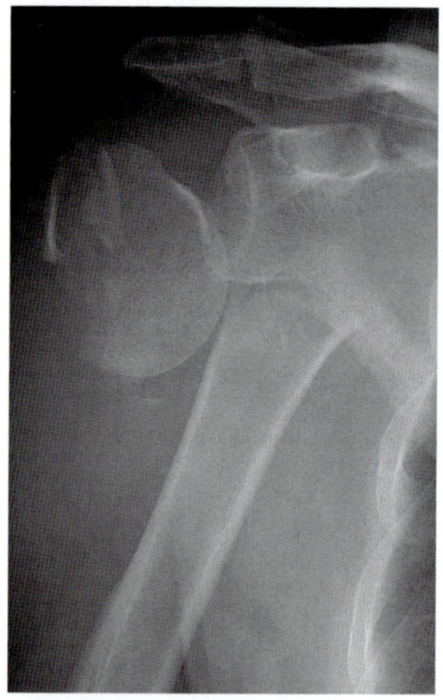

11-B2.3

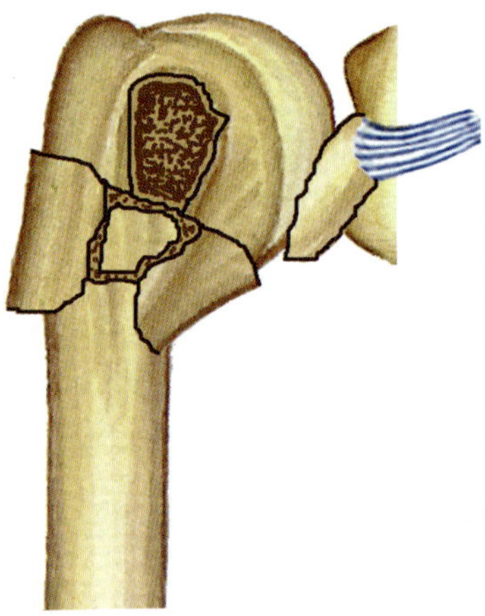

Multiple fragments with fracture of one tuberosity

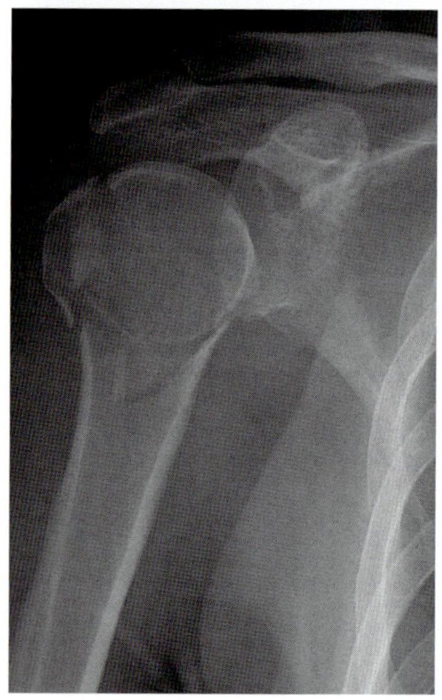

11-B Humerus proximal extra-articular fractures, bifocal

11-B3

Humerus proximal extra-articular bifocal fracture with glenohumeral dislocation

354 fractures
M: 129 (36.44%)
F: 225 (63.56%)
0.09% of total adult fractures
1.63% of adult humeral fractures
2.73% of segment 11
12.47% of type 11-B

11-B3.1

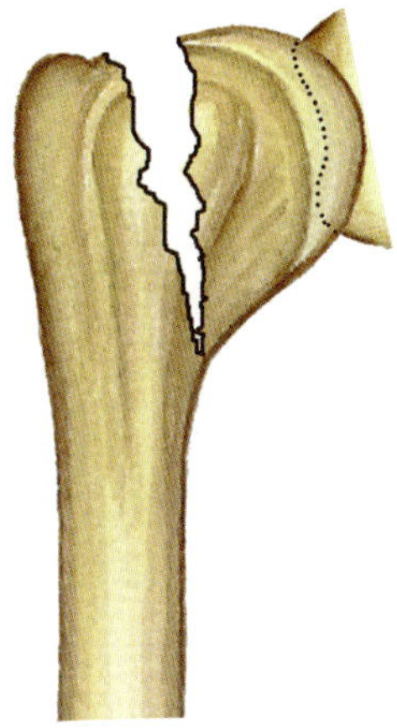

Vertical cervical line;
greater tuberosity intact;
anterior medial dislocation

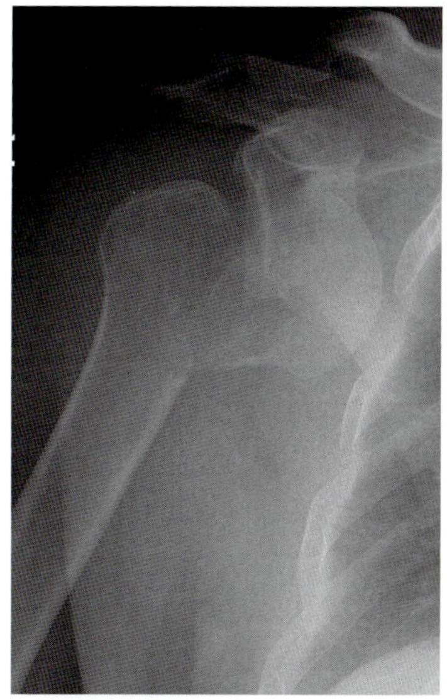

11-B3.2

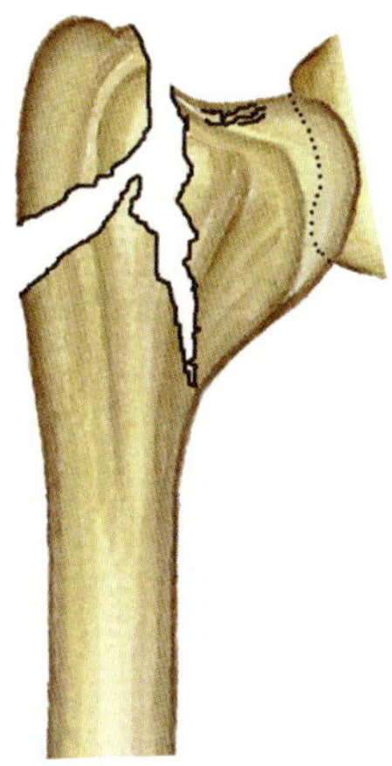

Vertical cervical line;
anterior medial dislocation;
greater tuberosity fractured

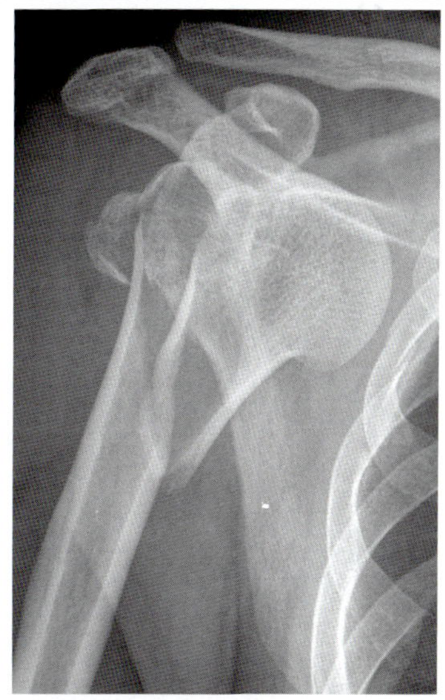

11-B3.3

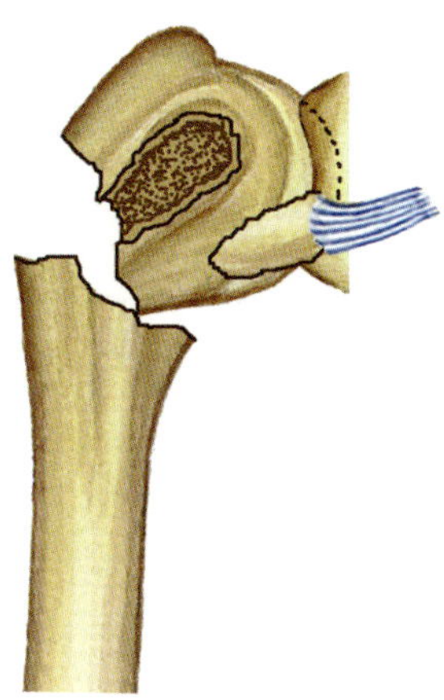

Posterior dislocation;
lesser tuberosity fractured

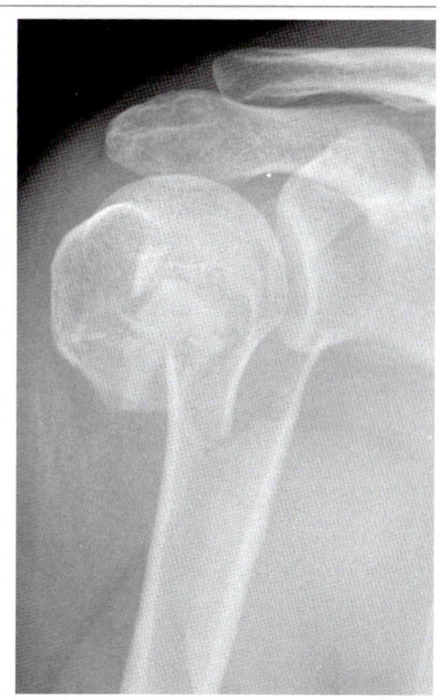

11-C Humerus proximal articular fractures

11-C1
Humerus proximal articular fracture with slight dislocation

464 fractures
M: 169 (36.42%)
F: 295 (63.58%)
0.12% of total adult fractures
2.13% of adult humeral fractures
3.58% of segment 11
35.23% of type 11-C

11-C1.1

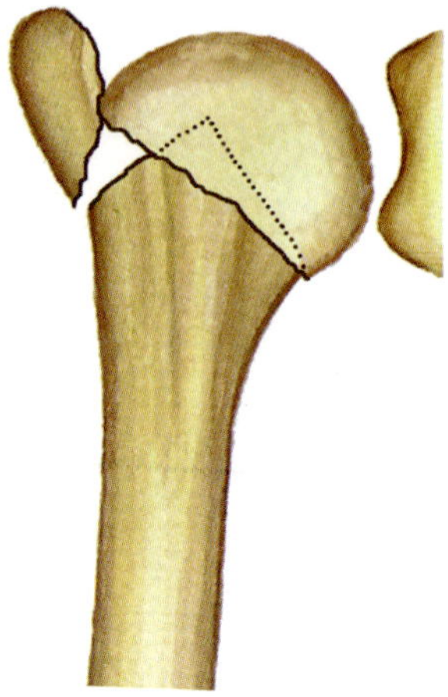

Cephalotubercular, with valgus malalignment

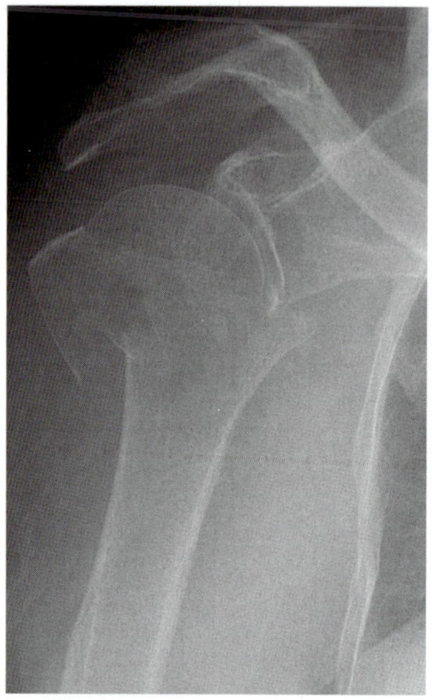

11-C1.2

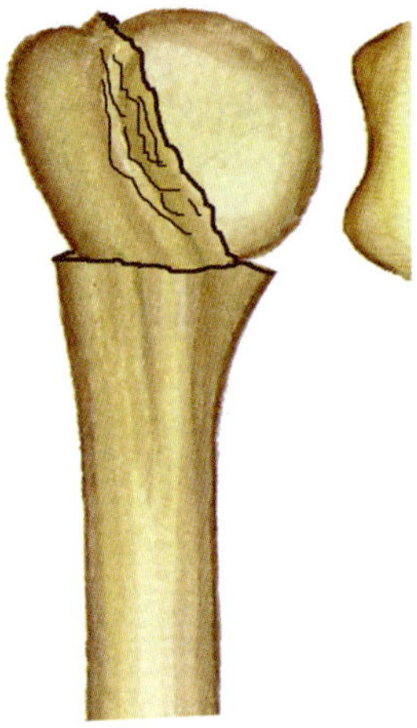

Cephalotubercular, with varus malalignment

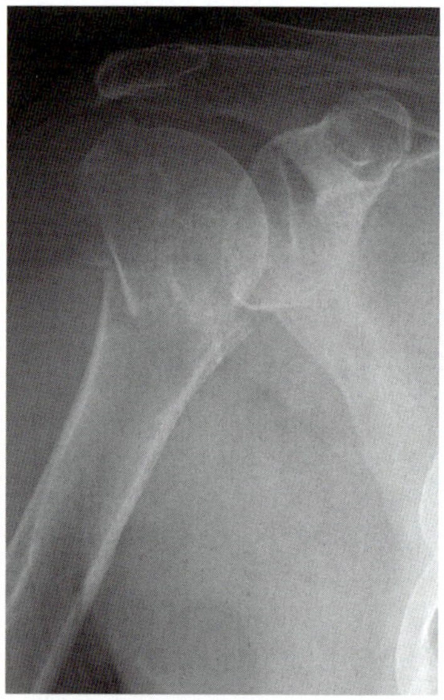

11-C1.3

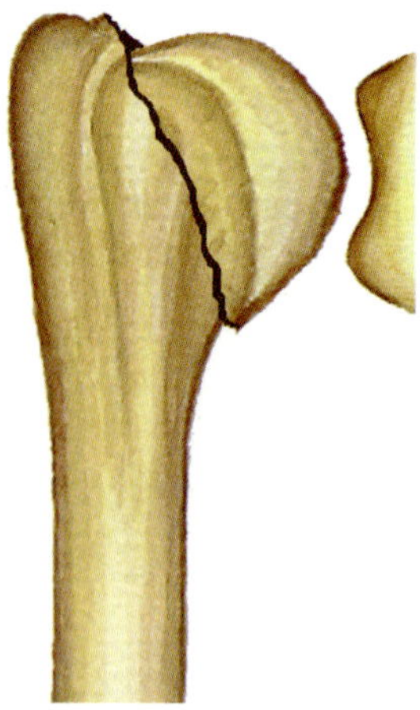

Anatomical neck

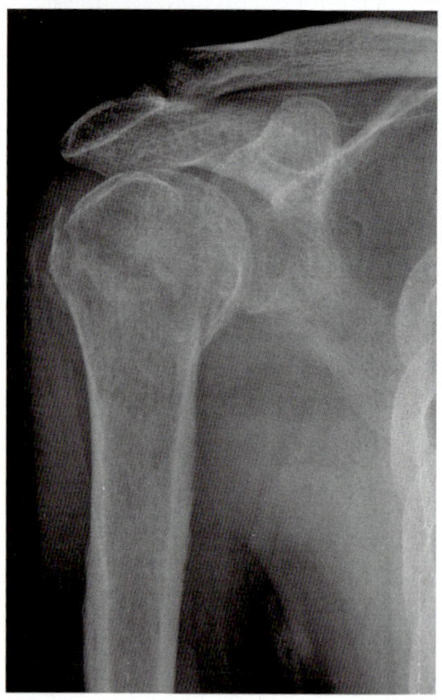

11-C Humerus proximal articular fractures

11-C2

Humerus proximal articular fracture, impacted with marked displacement

457 fractures
M: 166 (36.32%)
F: 291 (63.68%)
0.12% of total adult fractures
2.10% of adult humeral fractures
3.53% of segment 11
34.70% of type 11-C

11-C2.1

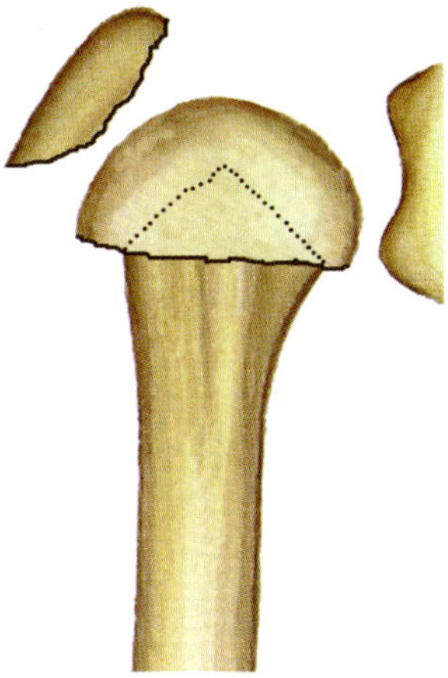

Cephalotubercular, with valgus malalignment

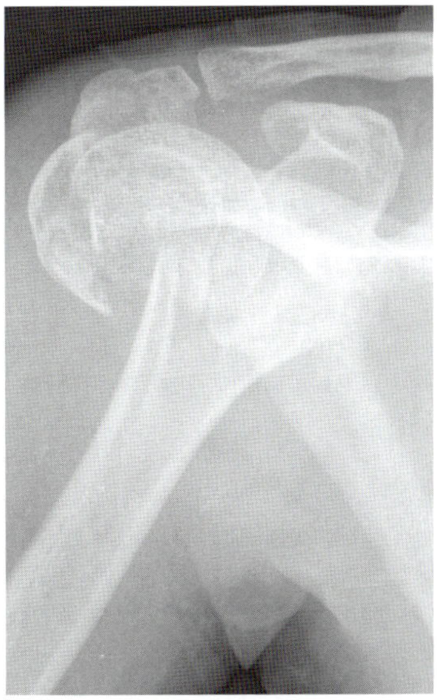

11-C2.2

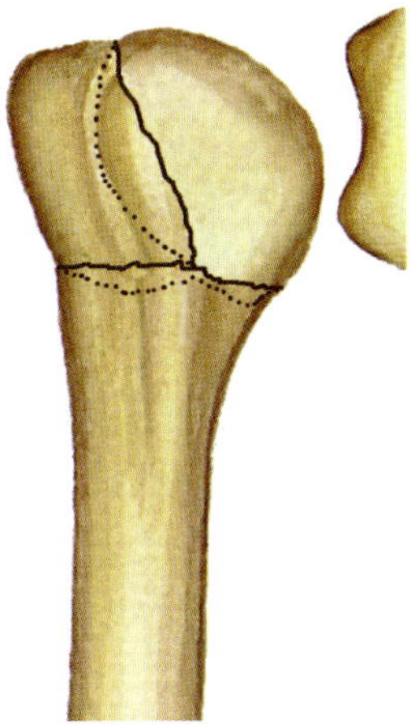

Cephalotubercular, with varus malalignment

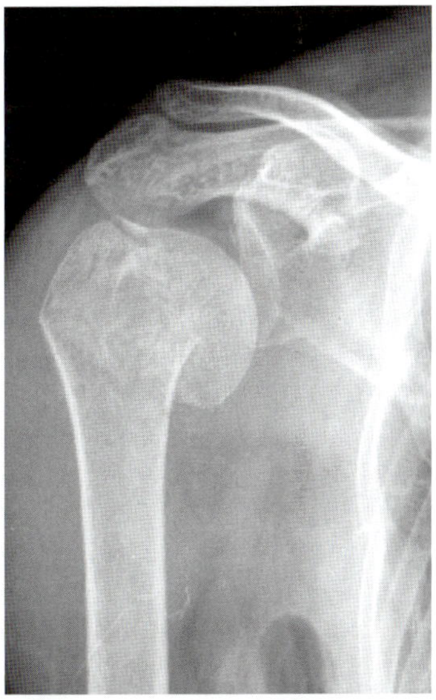

11-C2.3

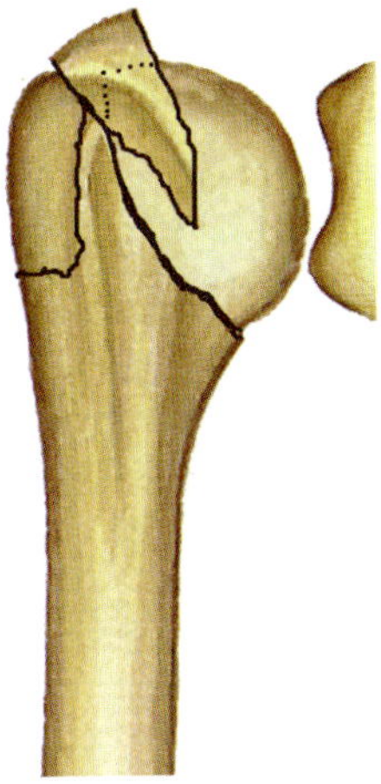

Transcephalic and tubercular, with varus malalignment

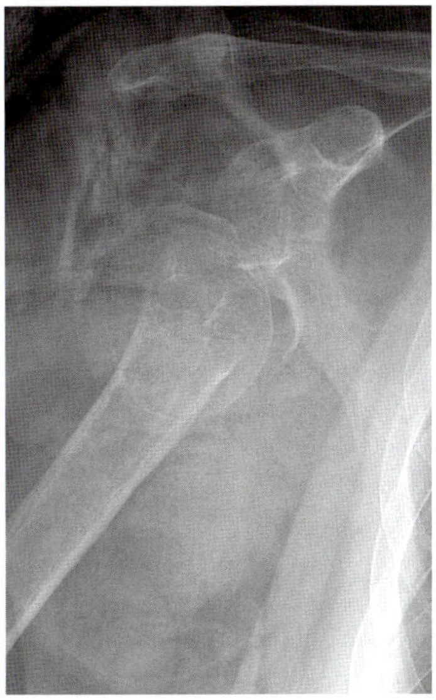

11-C Humerus proximal articular fractures

11-C3
Humerus proximal articular fracture with dislocation
396 fractures
M: 156 (39.39%)
F: 240 (60.61%)
0.11% of total adult fractures
1.82% of adult humeral fractures
3.06% of segment 11
30.07% of type 11-C

11-C3.1

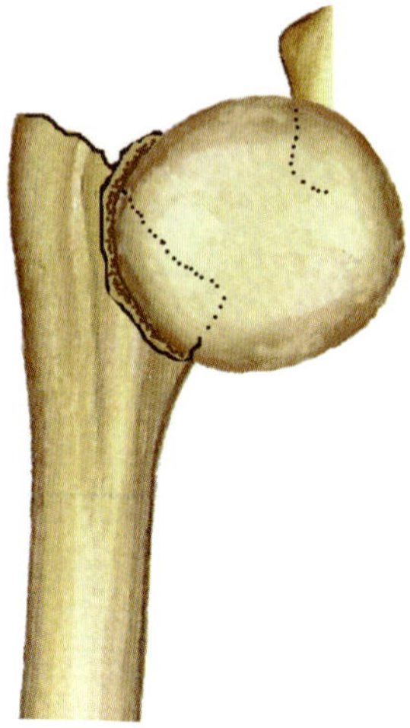

Anatomical neck

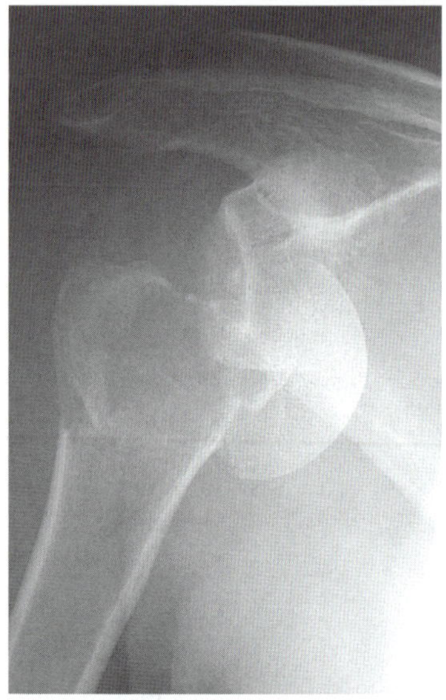

11-C3.2

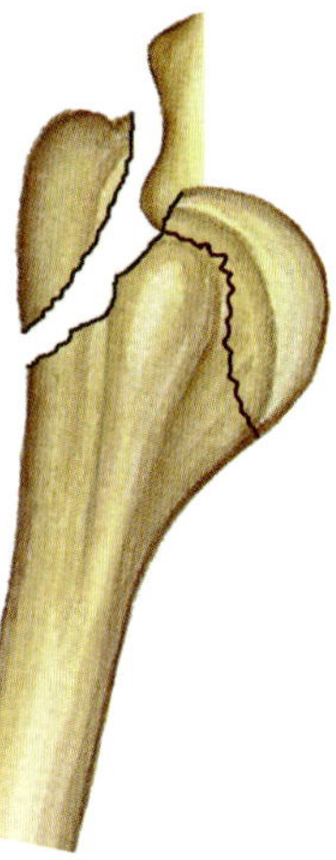

Anatomical neck and tuberosities

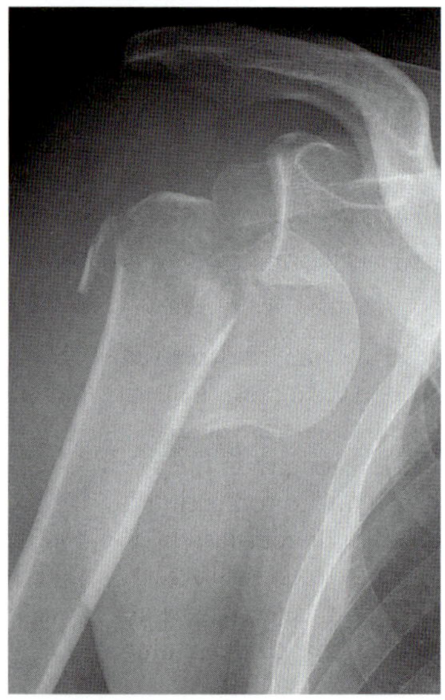

11-C3.3

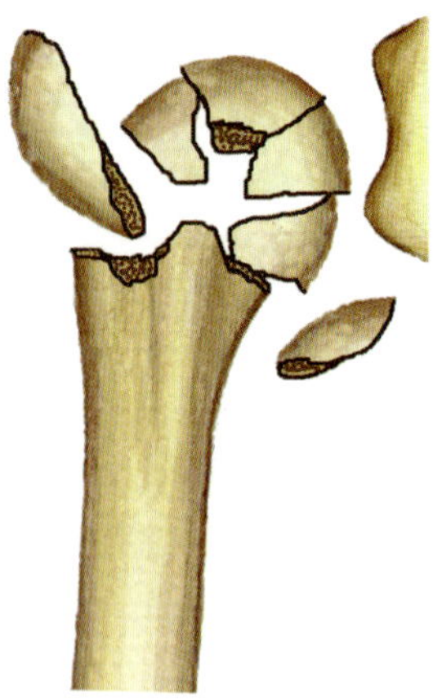

Cephalotubercular fragmentation

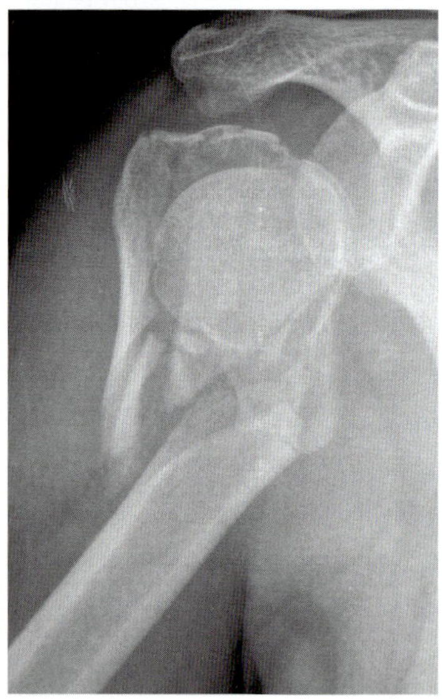

Injury Mechanism

Proximal humeral fractures are often caused by indirect force. In elderly patients, fractures are usually associated with osteoporosis, and can be caused by low or moderate force, such as that seen in falls from a standing position. For example, during a fall with an upper extremity in the outstretched position, when one's hand touches the ground the lateral shoulder is subjected to an upward directed force, and this may result in a proximal humeral fracture. Young patients often receive fractures from high-energy and direct-force impact to the proximal humerus.

When fractures occur, the greater tuberosity fragment is usually pulled superoposteriorly by the supraspinatus, infraspinatus, and teres minor. In contradistinction, the lesser tuberosity fragment usually moves medially due to traction from the subscapularis. When surgical neck fractures occur, the proximal fragment is usually shortened and displaced due to traction from the deltoid, and the distal fragment is pulled medially by the pectoralis major.

The *black arrows* on **Plate 2.8** indicate the directions of displacement of three anatomical structures (1, greater tuberosity; 2, lesser tuberosity; 3, humeral shaft) after fracture, under traction of the rotator cuff muscles, deltoid, and pectoralis major.

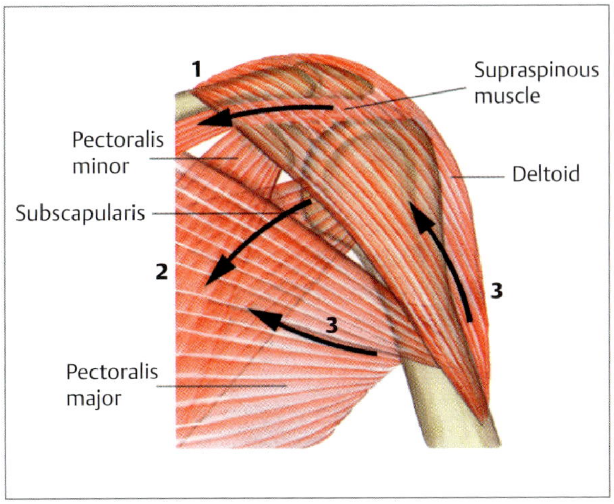

Plate 2.8

Diagnosis

Pain, swelling, and restricted motion are usually present when fracture of the proximal humerus occurs. If the fracture involves the articulation site, with minimal or no displacement, then the swelling and deformity may not be visible, due to protection from thick soft tissue around the shoulder. Tenderness of the shoulder and bone crepitus indicate a fracture. If a fracture fragment becomes displaced, a palpable cavity in the glenohumeral joint will be noted. It is essential to determine the presence of any associated neurovascular injury. The axillary artery and axillary nerve are most commonly injured in proximal humeral fractures.

The trauma series of radiographic evaluation for suspected proximal humeral fractures consists of anteroposterior (AP) and lateral views in the scapular plane and an axillary view.

- When obtaining an *AP view* (**Plate 2.9**), the patient stands in a position with the shoulder to be examined in contact with the examining table. The scapula should lie parallel to the cassette and the X-ray beam must be tilted 40 degrees to the plane of the thorax. Good visualization of the subacromial space should be obtained with no overlap of the humeral head and glenoid cavity, resulting in the anterior and posterior rim of the glenoid fossa being superimposed.
- To obtain an outlet view (**Plate 2.10**), the patient stands in an anterior oblique position, with the anterior aspect of the examined shoulder in contact with the cassette, and the X-ray beam parallel to the scapular spine with the body tilted 40 degrees.

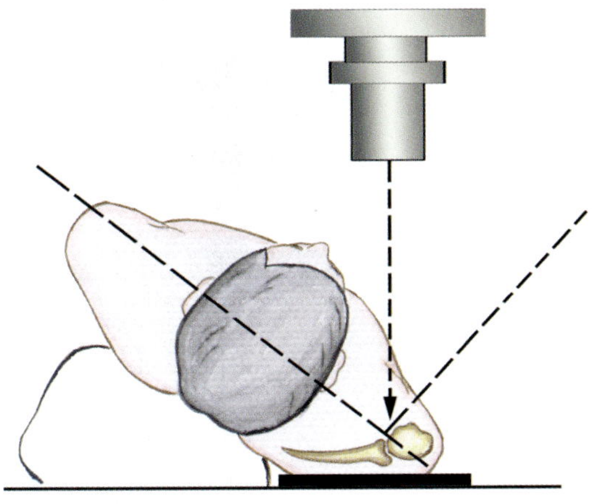

Anteroposterior view of scapula.

Plate 2.9

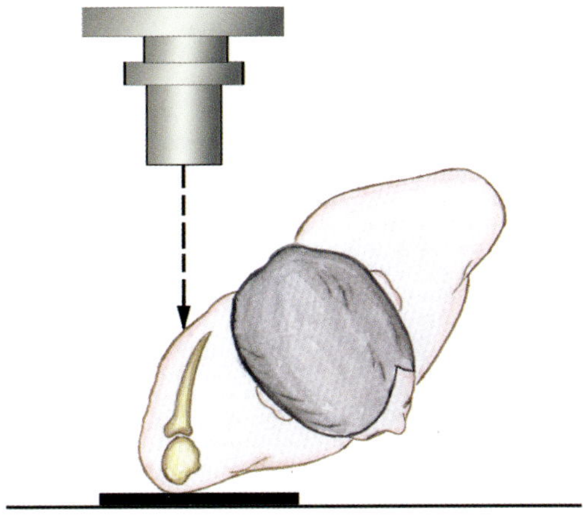

Outlet view of scapula.

Plate 2.10

Since the plane of the scapula is 30–40 degrees anterior to the coronal plane of the body, the glenohumeral joint inclines anteriorly, and the glenoid fossa directly faces the humeral head posteriorly. The common AP view and transthoracic lateral projection of the shoulder both provide a lateral view of the shoulder joint, neither of which are true reflections of the displacement, angulation, or dislocation of the proximal humeral fracture (**Plate 2.11**).

- To obtain an *axillary view* (**Plate 2.12**), the patient is placed in a supine position with his or her arm abducted 70–90 degrees. The cassette is placed on the superior aspect of the shoulder and the beam can be centered on the axilla. In recently occurring fractures, since abduction of the shoulder is markedly restricted due to the pain, a modified axillary view, known as a Velpeau view (**Plate 2.13**), is used. In this view, the patient is in a standing position and is tilted backward ~30 degrees over the cassette on the table. The X-ray beam is then projected vertically from above the shoulder onto the cassette. This view is limited by unavoidable overlapping of structures; thus, a supine projection is the recommended choice of imaging in practice.

If the radiographic evaluation is equivocal or if there is soft tissue damage, computed tomography (CT) or magnetic resonance imaging (MRI) can be a good imaging choice to provide more accurate information for early diagnosis and proper treatment. Doppler ultrasound or angiography can be of great assistance if the proximal humeral fracture is associated with dislocation or with vascular injury.

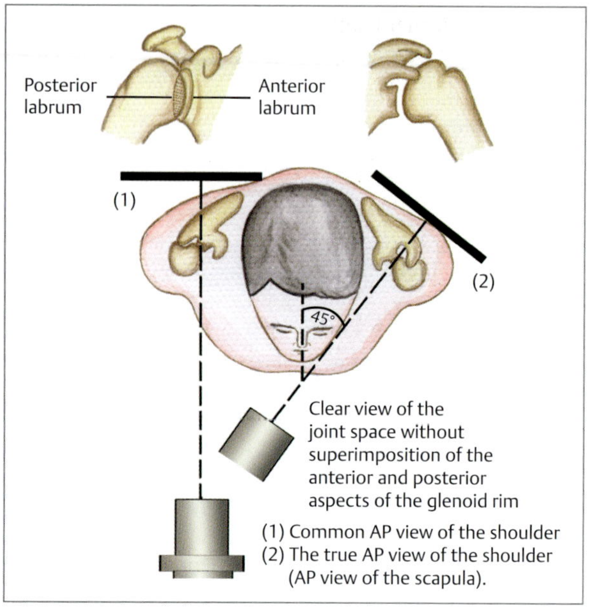

Plate 2.11

Treatment

Proximal humeral fracture with minimal or no displacement may be treated nonoperatively with satisfactory results. However, for patients older than 50 years, minimally invasive

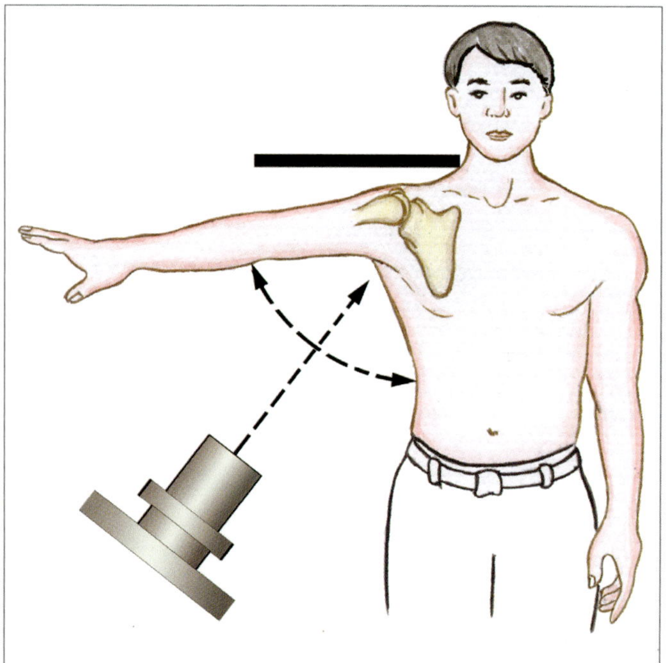

Axillary view of scapula

Plate 2.12

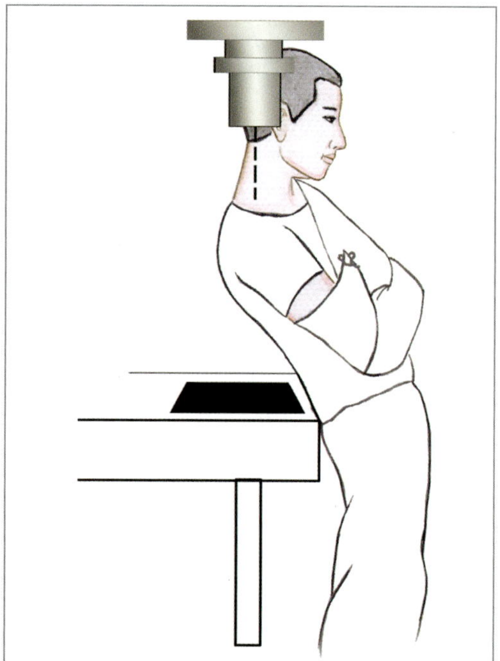

Velpeau view

Plate 2.13

surgery for internal fixation is recommended to avoid the occurrence of traumatic periarthritis of the shoulder joint. An unstable fracture, or one with marked displacement, requires surgical stabilization. Surgical management in patients with osteoporosis or severely comminuted fractures cannot achieve satisfactory results by reduction and stabilization; therefore, prosthetic replacement for the joint should be applied for such patients.

Humeral Shaft Fractures (Segment 12)

Anatomical Features

The shaft of the humerus (**Plate 2.14**) extends from the upper border of the pectoralis major insertion site to the supracondylar ridge distally. The proximal aspect of the humeral shaft is cylindric on cross-section; distally, its anteroposterior diameter narrows. The medial and lateral intermuscular septa divide the arm into anterior and posterior compartments. The anterior compartment contains the biceps brachii, coracobrachialis, and brachialis muscles. The brachial artery and vein and median, musculocutaneous, and ulnar nerves course along the medial border of the biceps. The triceps brachii muscle and radial nerve are contained in the posterior compartment. The radial nerve winds around the radial sulcus in between the medial and lateral heads of the triceps brachii, perforating the lateral intermuscular septum at the junction of the middle and distal thirds of the humeral shaft and entering the anterior aspect of the arm, which makes it an easy target when fractures and dislocations occur at this location.

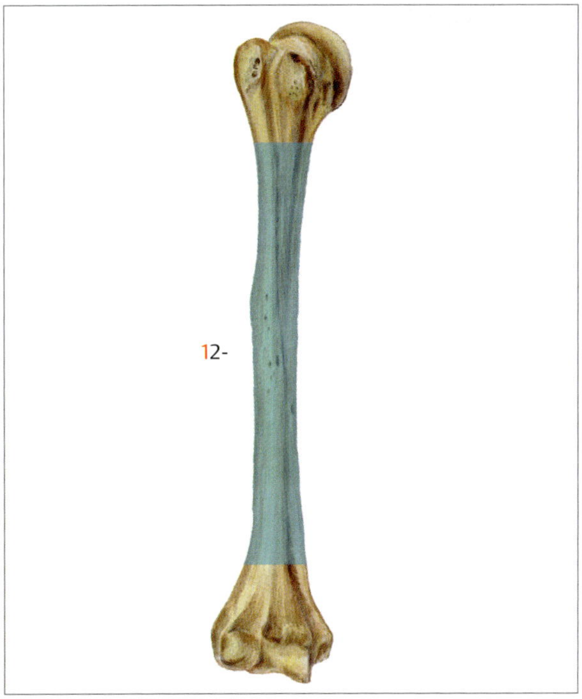

Plate 2.14

AO Classification for Humeral Shaft Fractures

The humeral shaft segment is coded as number 12 based on the AO classification, and is further divided into three main types depending on fracture morphology: types A, B, and C (**Plate 2.15**).

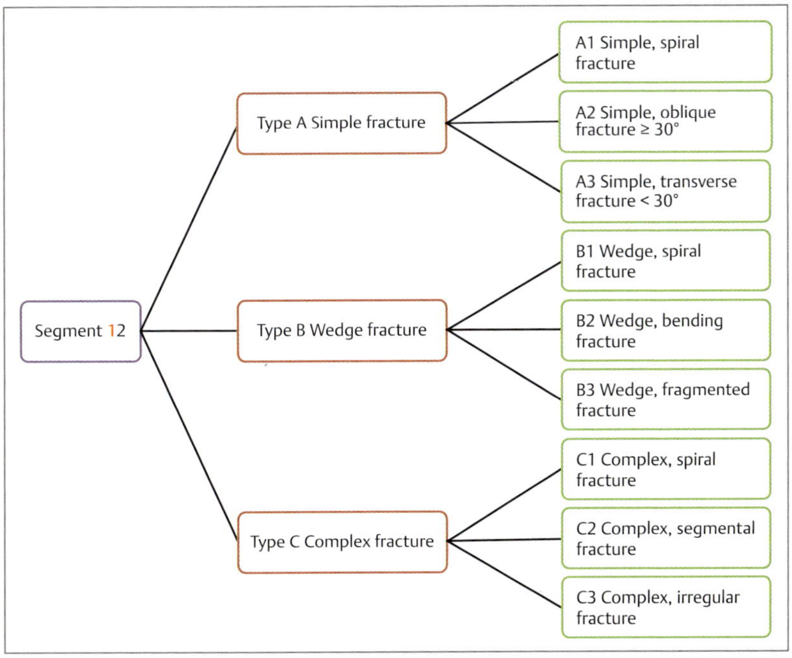

Plate 2.15

Clinical Epidemiologic Features of Humeral Shaft Fractures (Segment 12)

A total of 5,049 adult fractures of the humeral shaft (segment 12) were treated in 83 hospitals in China over a 2-year period from 2010 to 2011. All cases were reviewed and statistically studied; the fractures accounted for 23.19% of adult humeral fractures. The epidemiologic features are as follows:

- More males than females
- The high-risk age group is 21–25 years; 21–25 years for males, 41–45 years for females
- The high-incidence fracture type is 12-A, and is the same for both males and females
- The high-incidence fracture group is 12-A3; 12-A3 for males, 12-A1 for females.

Table 2.10 Sex distribution of 5,049 fractures of segment 12

Sex	Number of fractures	Percentage (%)
Male	3,267	64.71
Female	1,782	35.29
Total	5,049	100.00

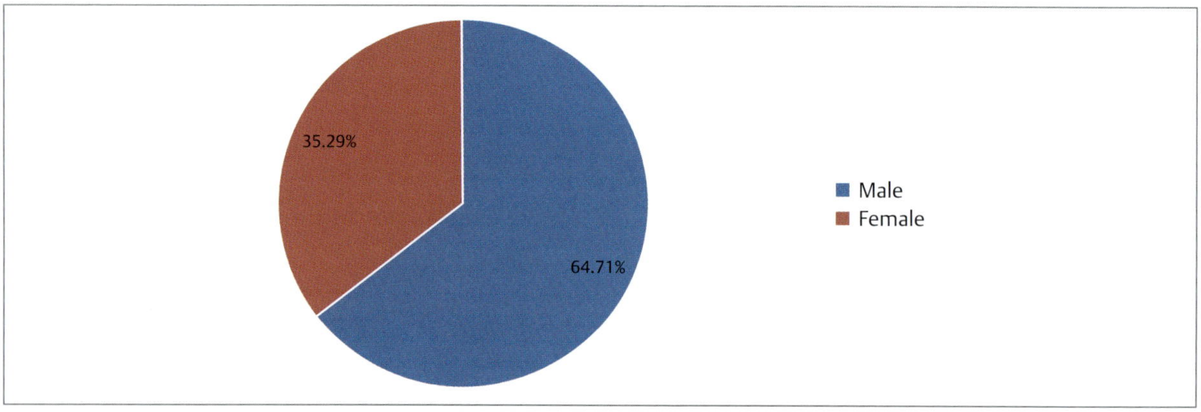

Fig. 2.10 Sex distribution of 5,049 fractures of segment 12.

Fractures of Segment 12 by Sex

Table 2.11 Age and sex distribution of 5,049 fractures of segment 12

Age group (years)	Male	Female	Total	Percentage (%)
16–20	252	75	327	6.48
21–25	434	155	589	11.67
26–30	388	121	509	10.08
31–35	364	117	481	9.53
36–40	414	152	566	11.21
41–45	382	160	542	10.73
46–50	294	148	442	8.75
51–55	231	139	370	7.33
56–60	208	152	360	7.13
61–65	95	120	215	4.26
66–70	69	99	168	3.33
71–75	47	106	153	3.03
76–80	52	147	199	3.94
81–85	21	52	73	1.45
≥86	16	39	55	1.09
Total	3,267	1,782	5,049	100.00

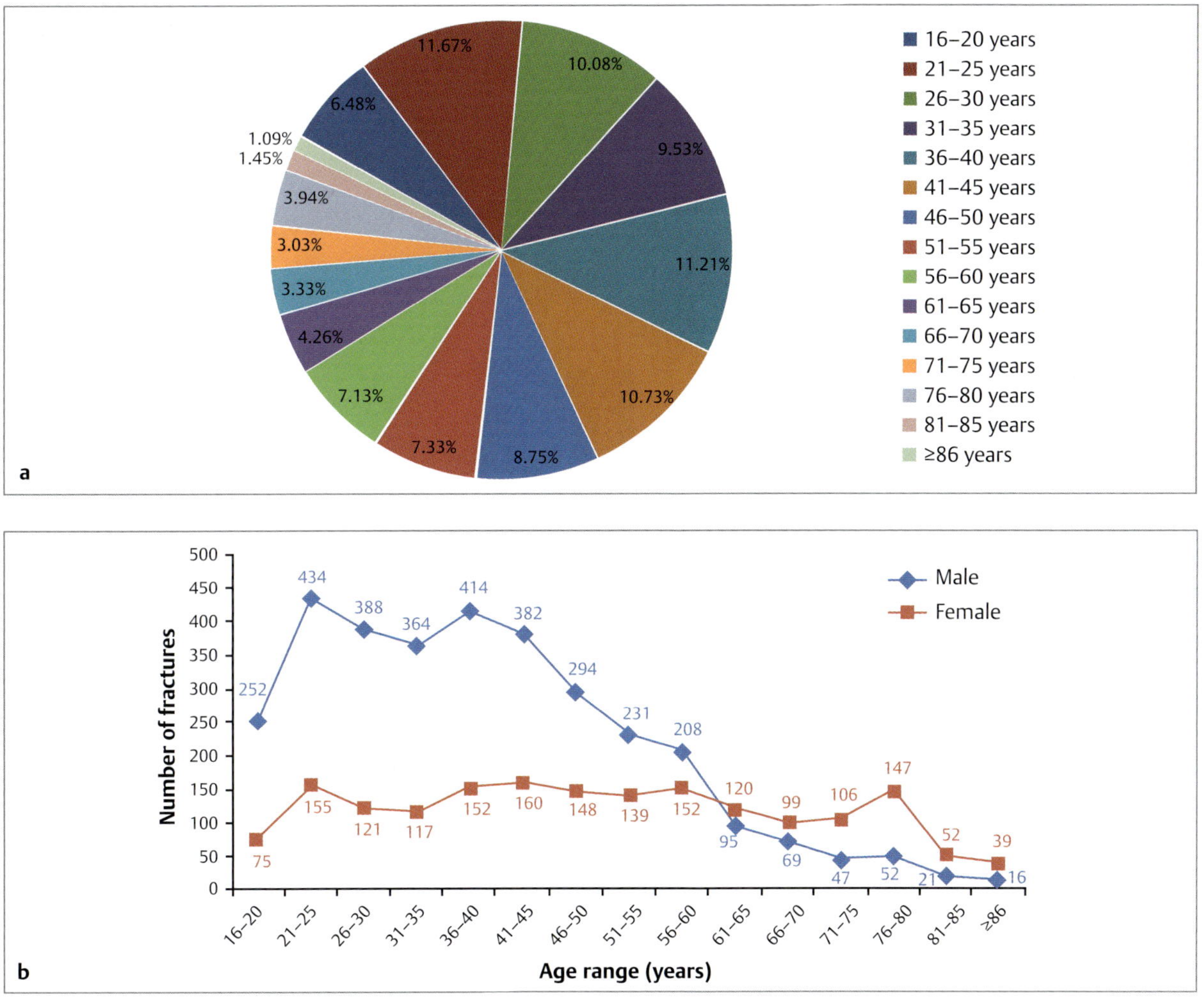

Fig. 2.11 **(a)** Age distribution of 5,049 fractures of segment 12.
(b) Age and sex distribution of 5,049 fractures of segment 12.

Fractures of Segment 12 by Fracture Type

Table 2.12 Sex and fracture type distribution of 5,049 Fractures of segment 12

Fracture type	Male	Female	Number of fractures	Percentage of segment 12 fractures (%)	Percentage of adult humeral fractures (%)
12-A	1721	945	2,666	52.80	12.25
12-B	1249	657	1,906	37.75	8.76
12-C	297	180	477	9.45	2.19
Total	3,267	1,782	5,049	100.00	23.19

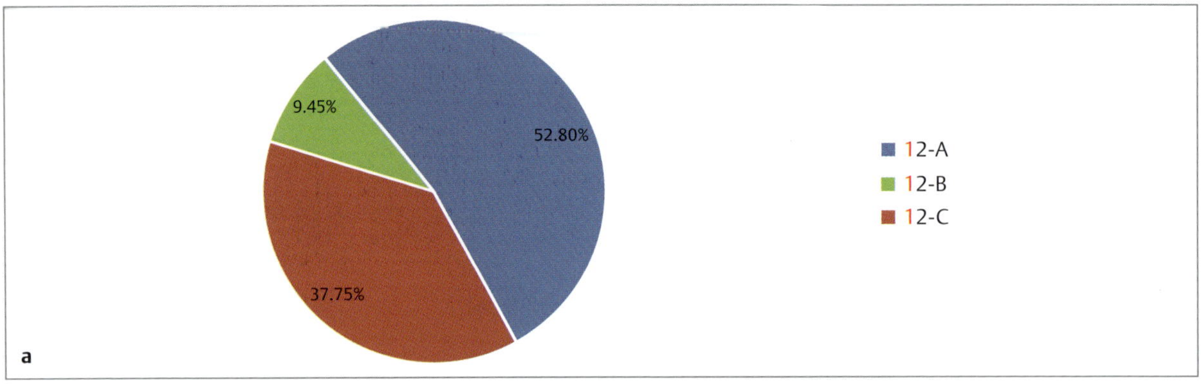

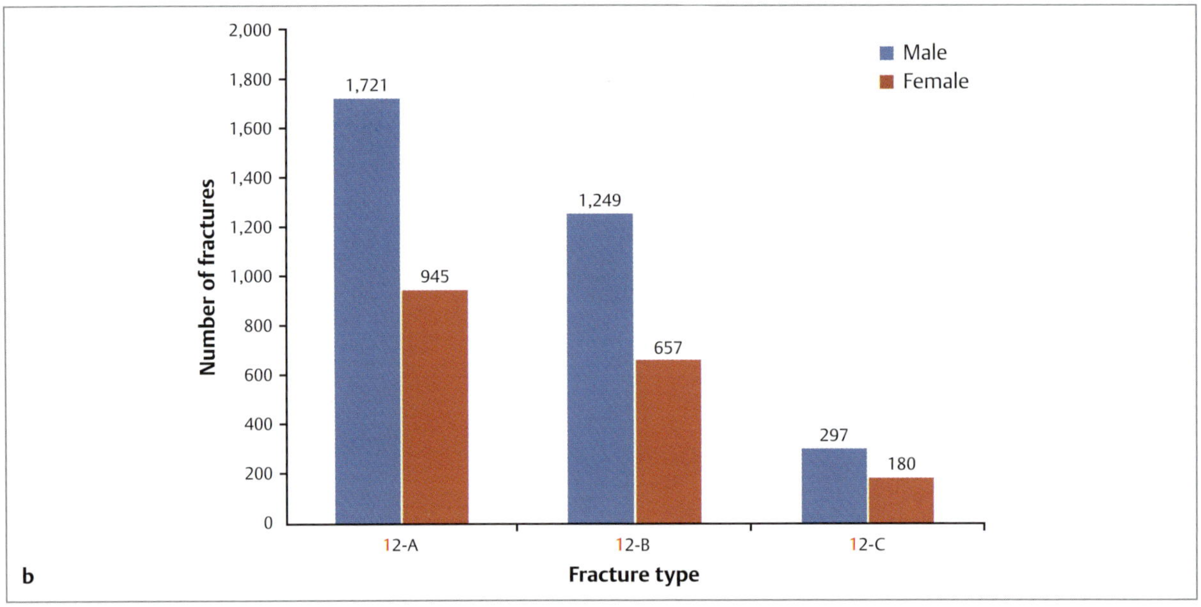

Fig. 2.12 **(a)** Fracture type distribution of 5,049 fractures of segment 12.
(b) Sex and fracture type distribution of 5,049 fractures of segment 12.

Fractures of Segment 12 by Fracture Type

Table 2.13 Sex and fracture group distribution of 5,049 fractures of segment 12

Fracture group	Male	Female	Total	Percentage of segment 12 fractures (%)	Percentage of adult humeral fracture (%)
12-A1	408	378	786	15.57	3.61
12-A2	609	275	884	17.51	4.06
12-A3	704	292	996	19.73	4.58
12-B1	418	285	703	13.92	3.23
12-B2	609	282	891	17.65	4.09
12-B3	222	90	312	6.18	1.43
12-C1	126	107	233	4.61	1.07
12-C2	62	26	88	1.74	0.40
12-C3	109	47	156	3.09	0.72
Total	3,267	1,782	5,049	100.00	23.19

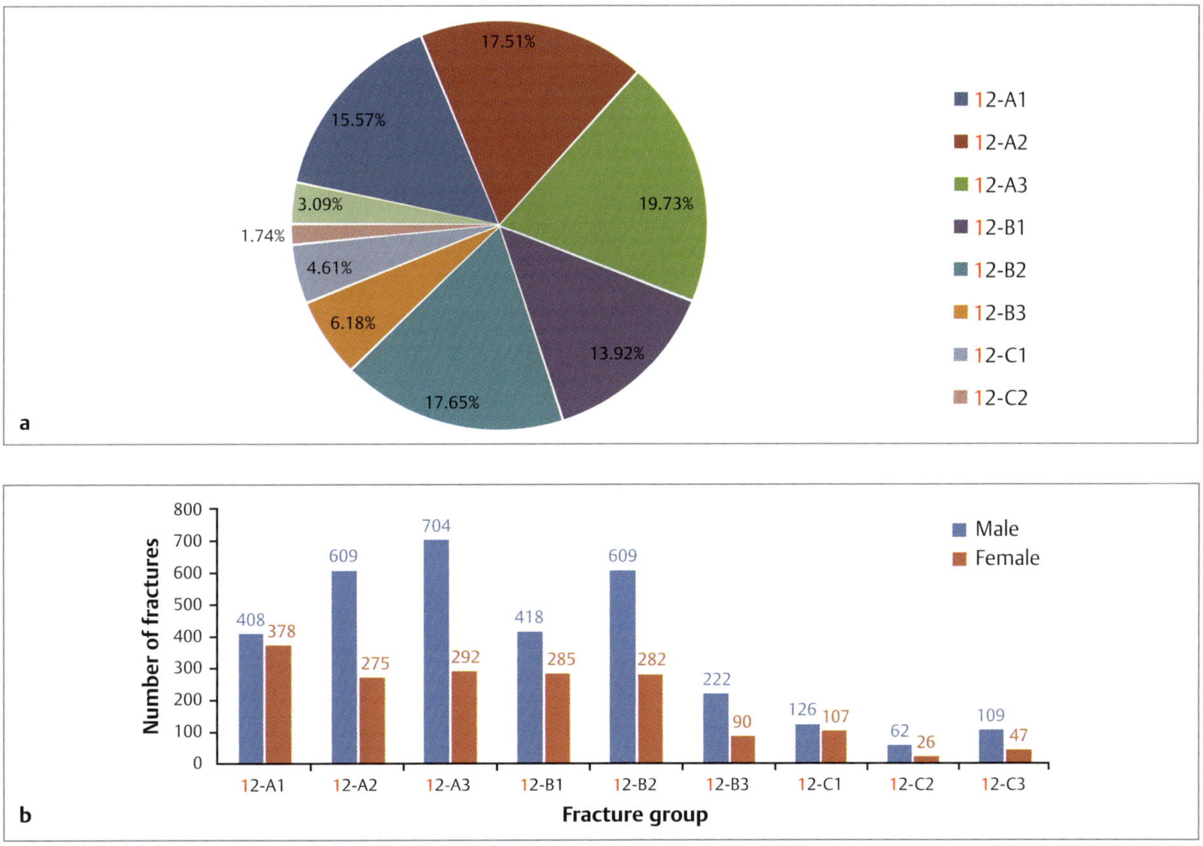

Fig. 2.13 **(a)** Fracture group distributions of 5,049 fractures of segment 12.
(b) Sex and fracture group distribution of 5,049 fractures of segment 12.

12-A Humerus diaphysis simple fracture

12-A1
Humerus diaphysis simple fracture, spiral fracture
786 fractures
M: 408 (51.91%)
F: 378 (48.09%)
0.21% of total adult fractures
3.61% of adult humeral fractures
15.57% of segment 12
29.48% of 12-A

12-A1.1

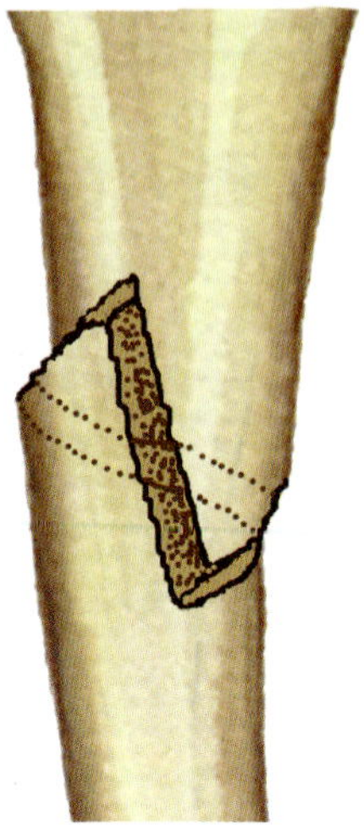

Proximal third

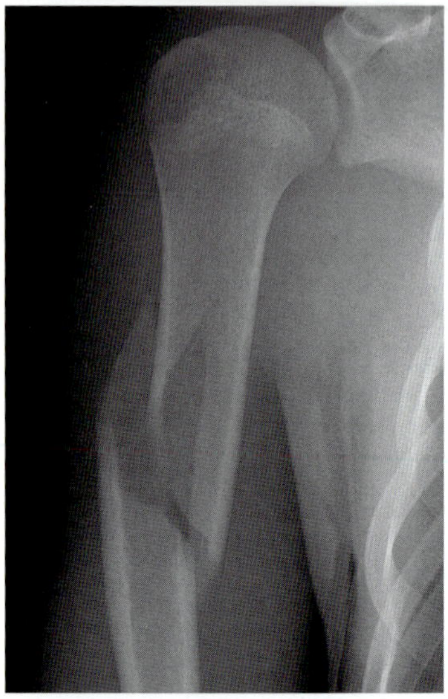

12-A1.2

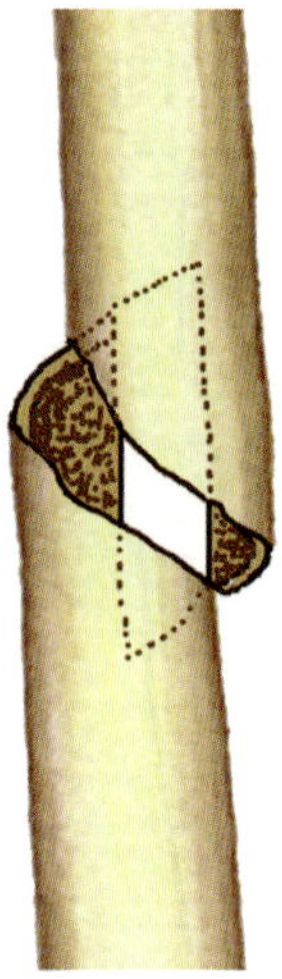

Middle third

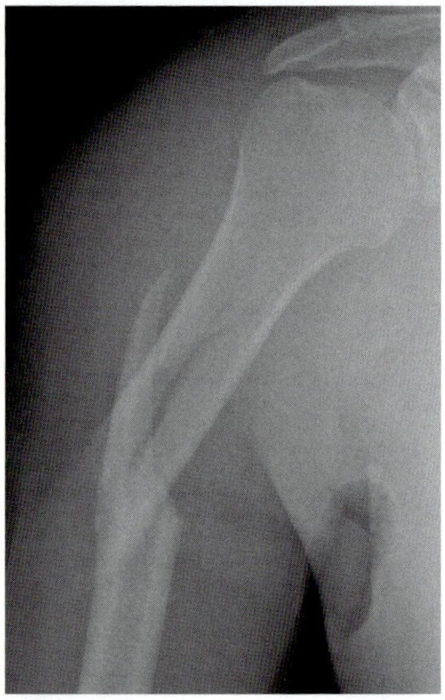

12-A1.3

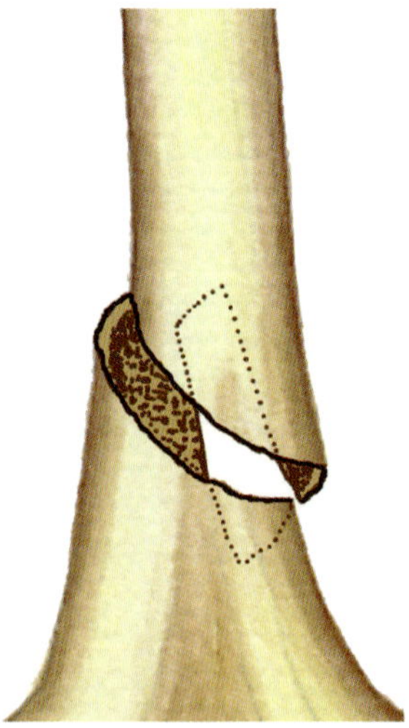

Distal third

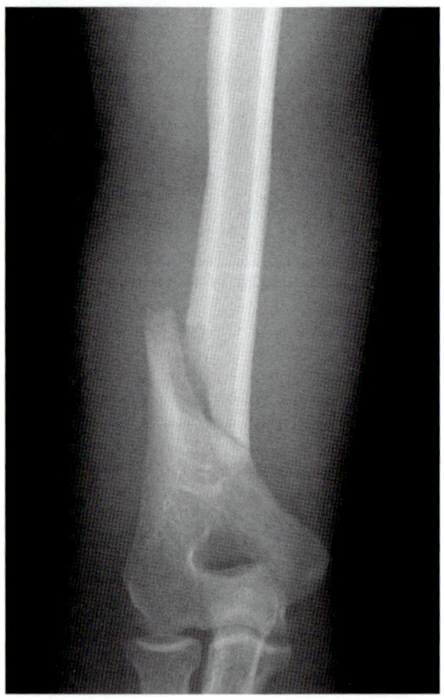

12-A Humerus diaphysis simple fractures

12-A2
Humerus diaphysis simple fracture, oblique fracture (≥ 30 degrees)
884 fractures
M: 609 (68.89%)
F: 275 (31.11%)
0.24% of total adult fractures
4.06% of adult humeral fractures
17.51% of segment 12
33.16% of 12-A

12-A2.1

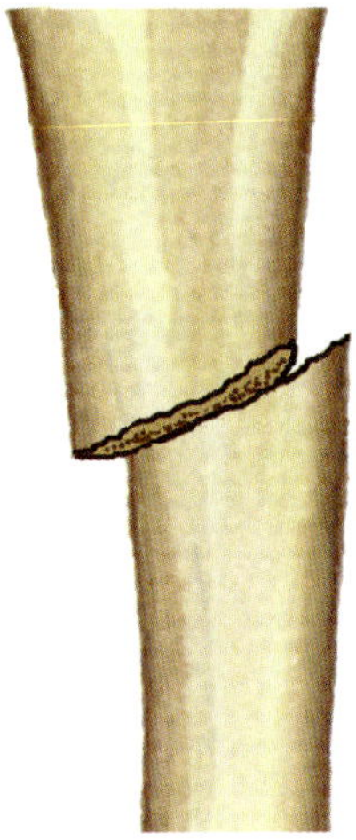

Proximal third

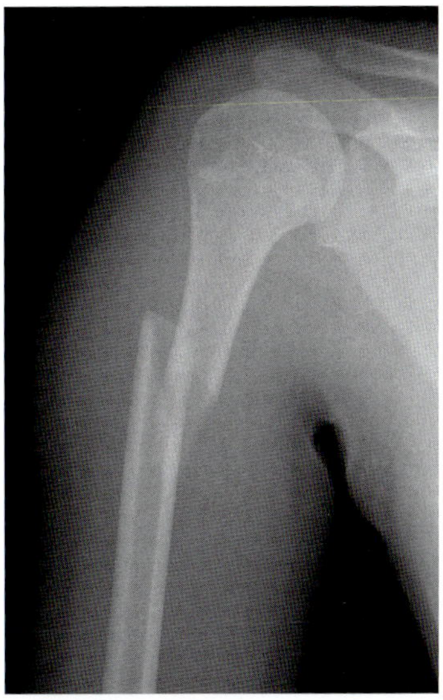

12-A2.2

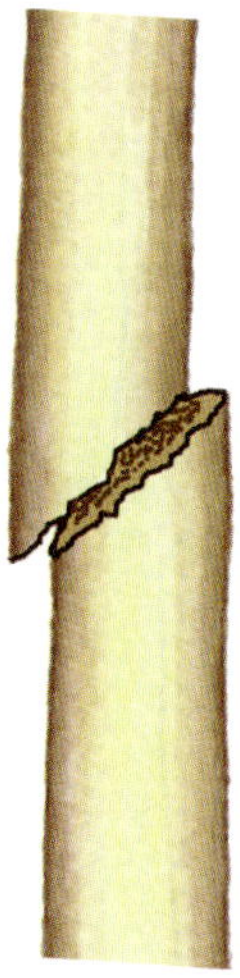

Middle third

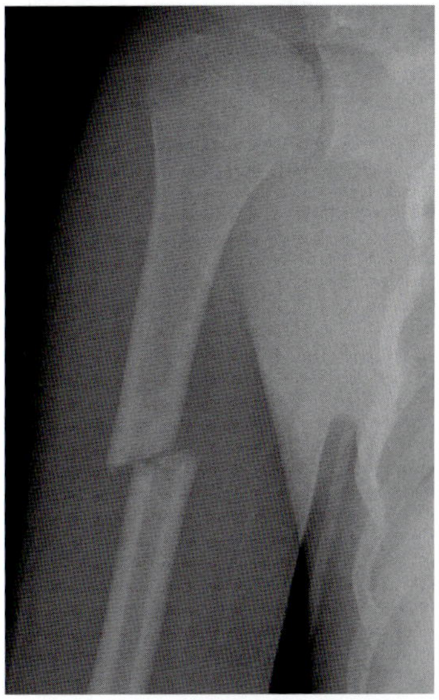

12-A2.3

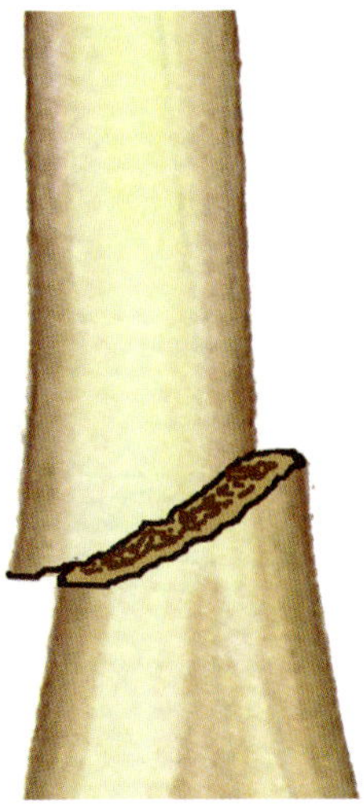

Distal third

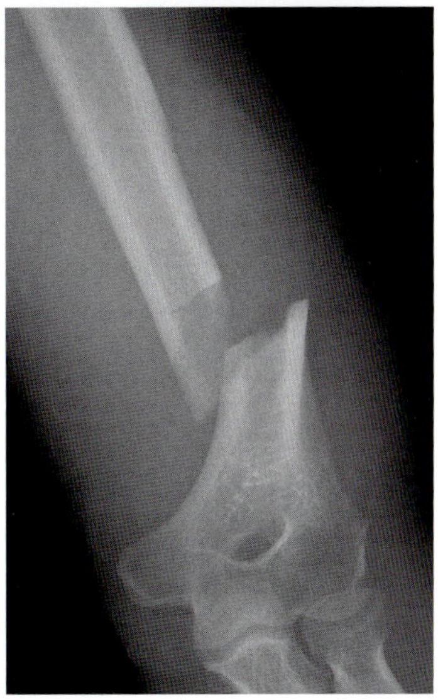

12-A Humerus diaphysis simple fractures

12-A3
Humerus diaphysis simple fracture, oblique fracture (≥ 30 degrees)
996 fractures
M: 704 (70.68%)
F: 292 (29.32%)
0.27% of total adult fractures
4.58% of adult humeral fractures
19.73% of segment 12
37.36% of 12-A

12-A3.1

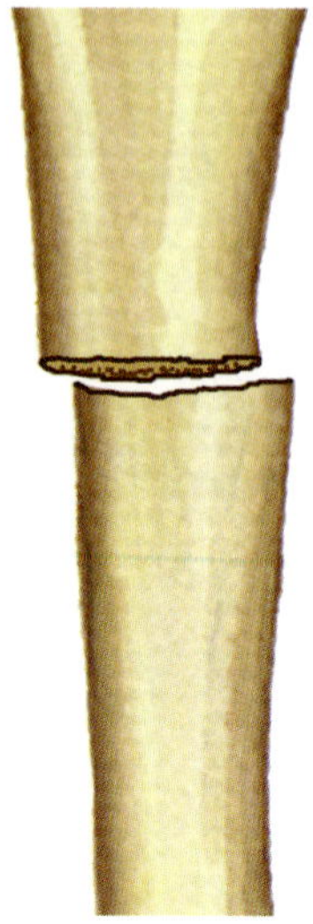

Proximal third

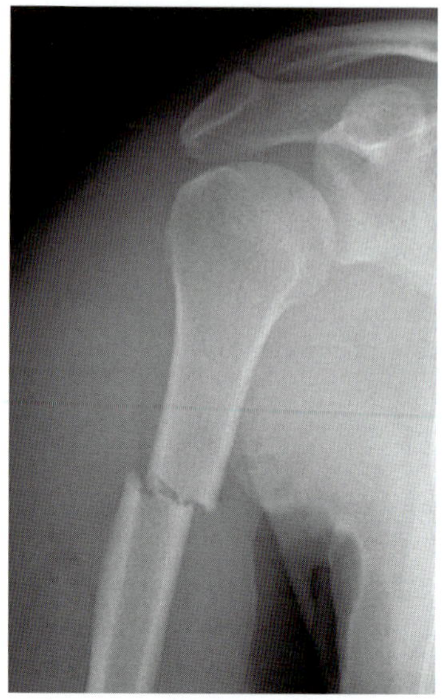

12-A3.2

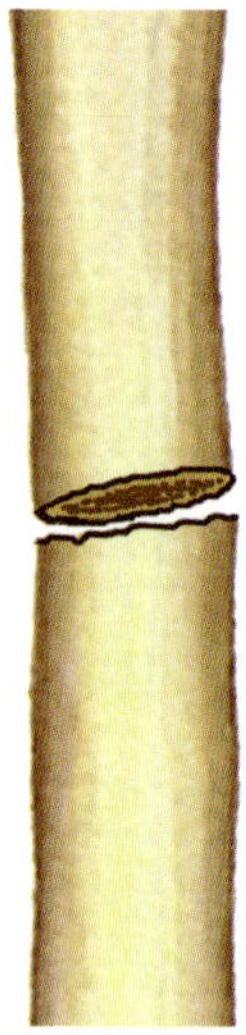

Middle third

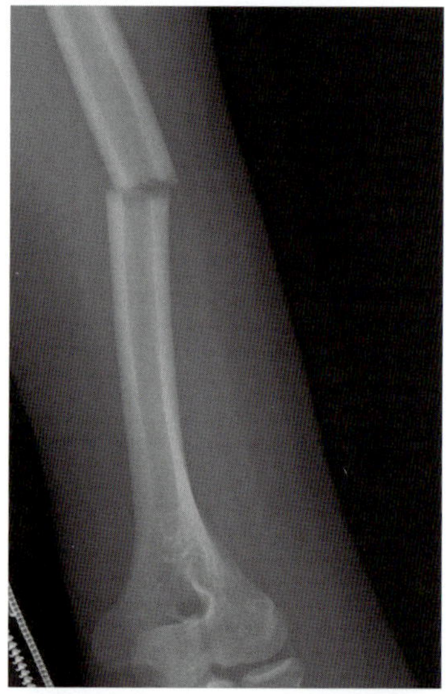

12-A3.3

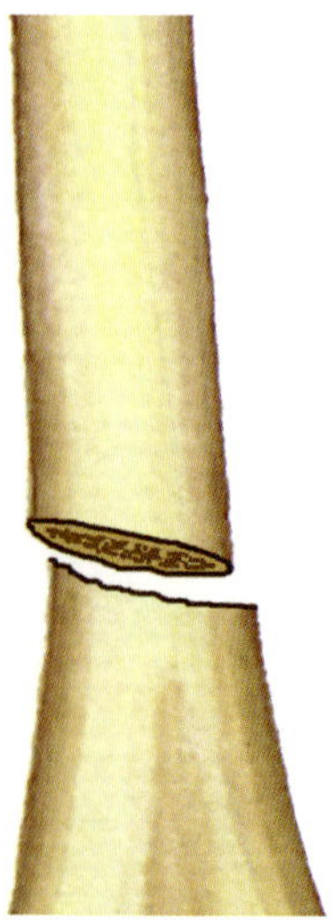

Distal third

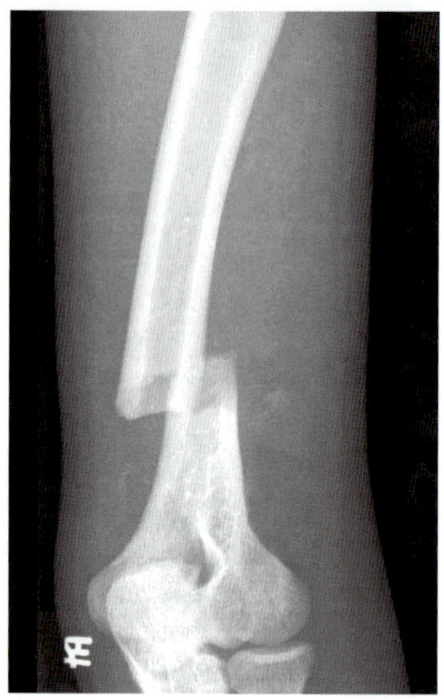

12-B Humerus diaphysis wedge fractures

12-B1
Humerus diaphysis wedge fracture, spiral fracture
703 fractures
M: 418 (59.46%)
F: 285 (40.54%)
0.19% of total adult fractures
3.23% of adult humeral fractures
13.92% of segment 12
36.88% of 12-B

12-B1.1

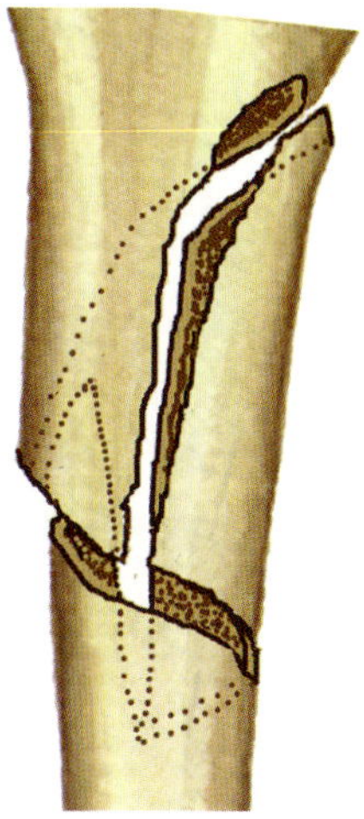

Proximal third

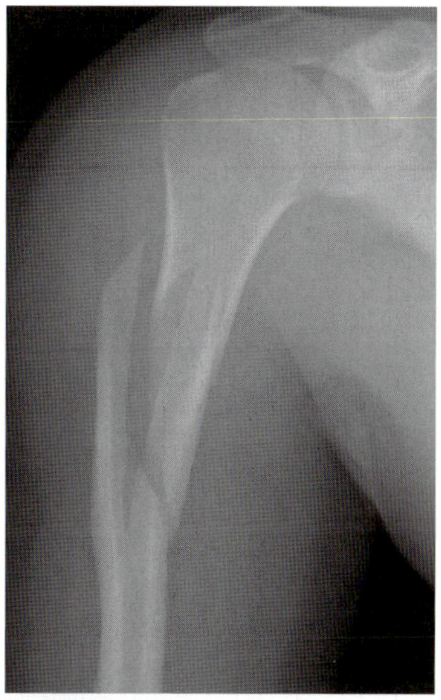

12-B1.2

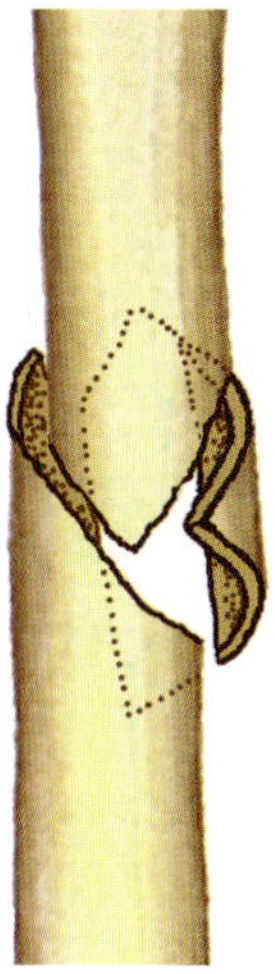

Middle third

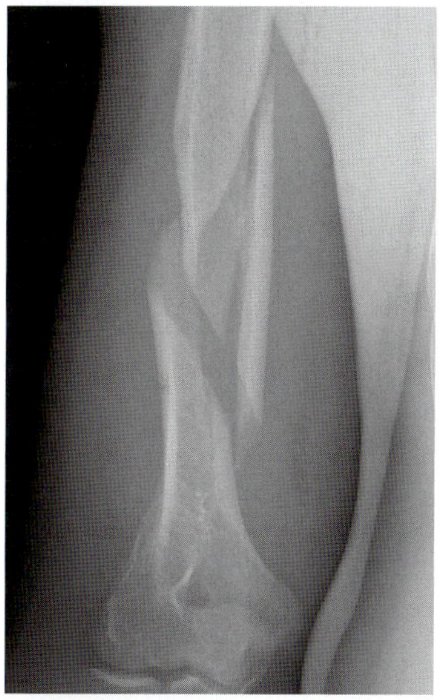

12-B1.3

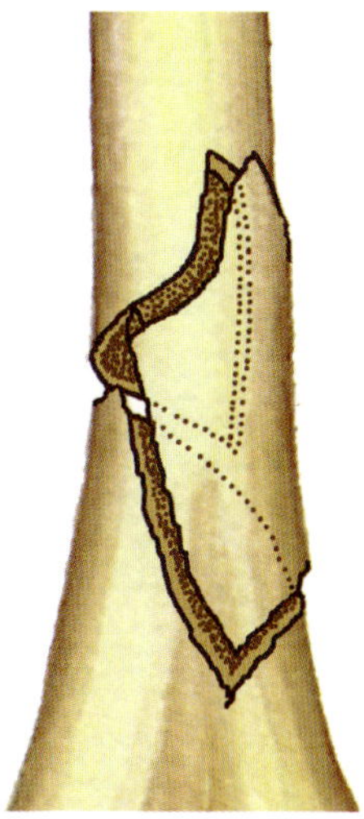

Distal third

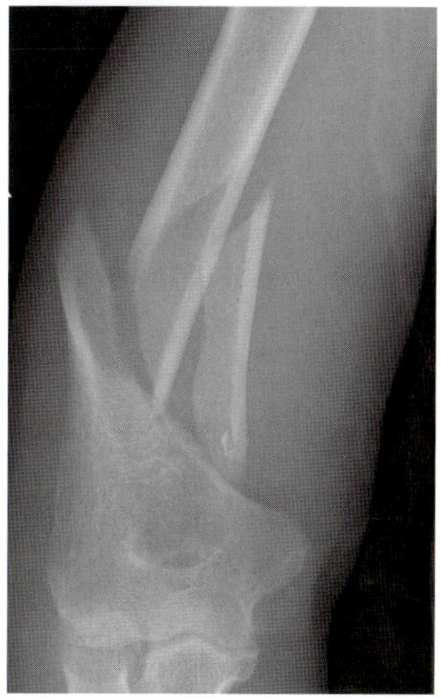

12-B Humerus diaphysis wedge fractures

12-B2
Humerus diaphysis wedge fracture, bending fracture
891 fractures
M: 609 (68.35%)
F: 282 (31.65%)
0.24% of total adult fractures
4.09% of adult humeral fractures
17.65% of segment 12
46.75% of type 12-B

12-B2.1

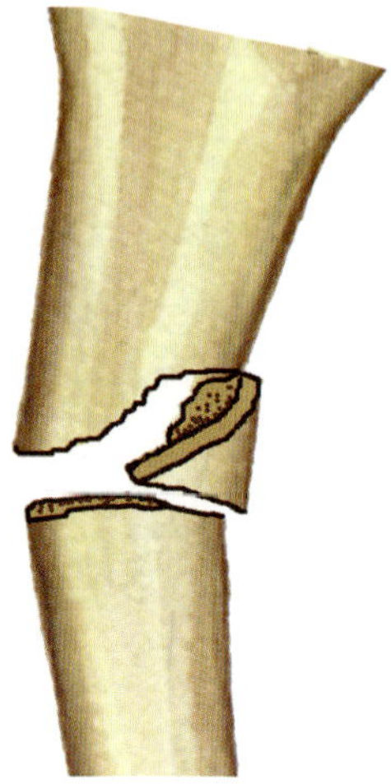

Proximal third

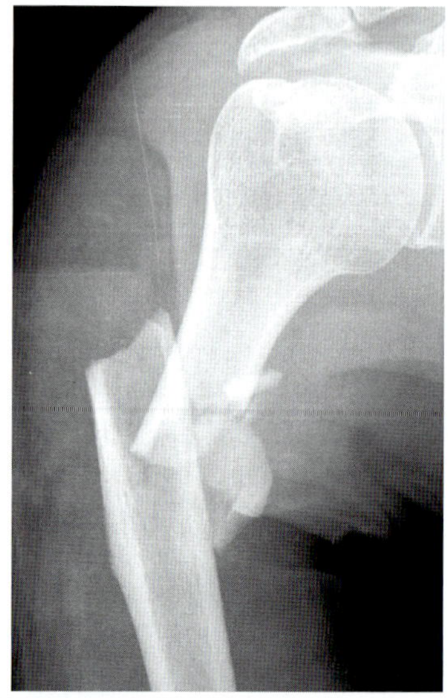

12-B2.2

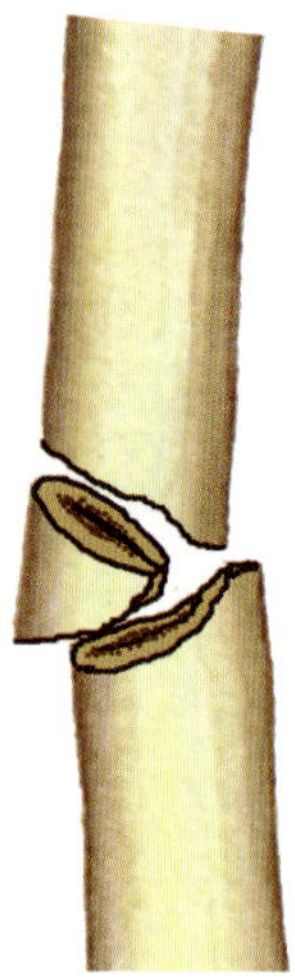

Middle third

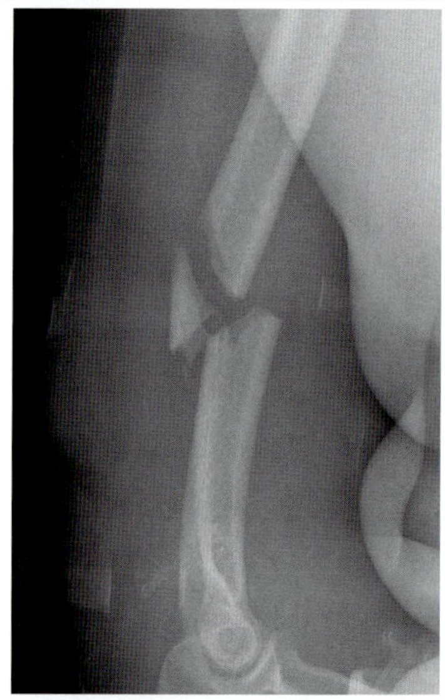

12-B2.3

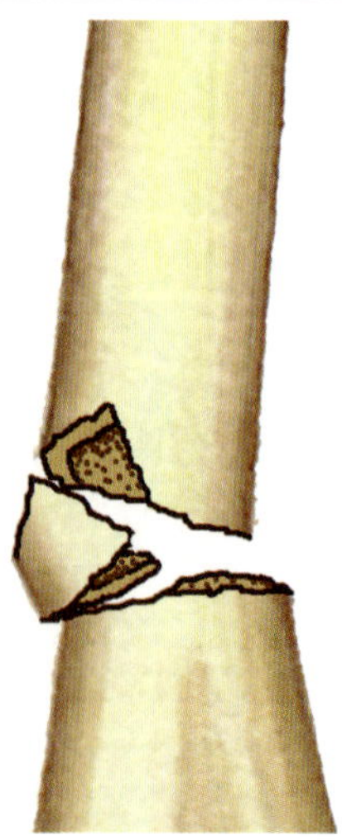

Distal third

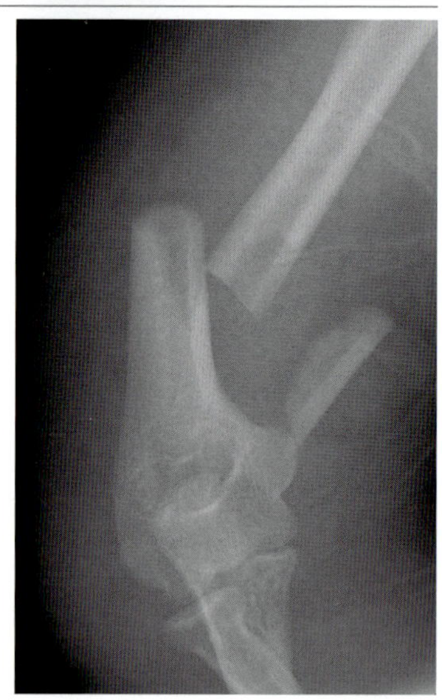

12-B Humerus diaphysis wedge fractures

12-B3
Humerus diaphysis wedge fracture, fragmented fracture
312 fractures
M: 222 (71.15%)
F: 90 (28.85%)
0.08% of total adult fractures
1.43% of adult humeral fractures
6.18% of segment 12
16.37% of 12-B

12-B3.1

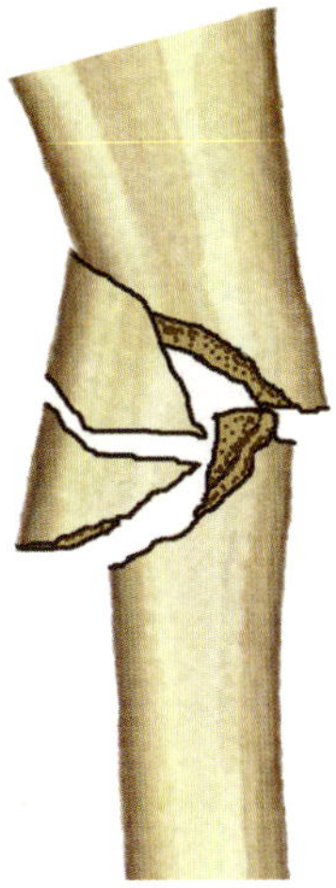

Proximal third

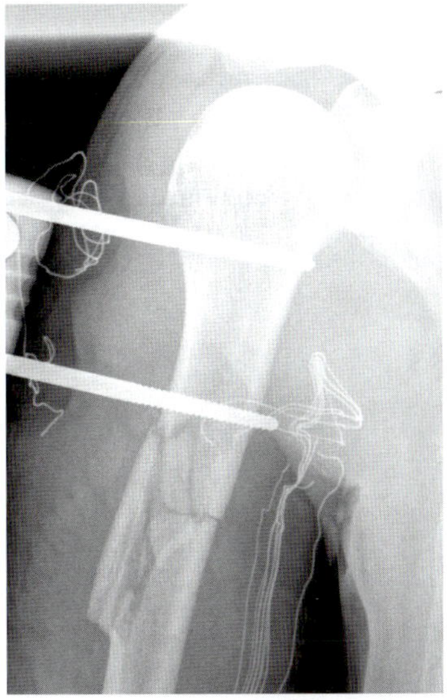

12-B3.2

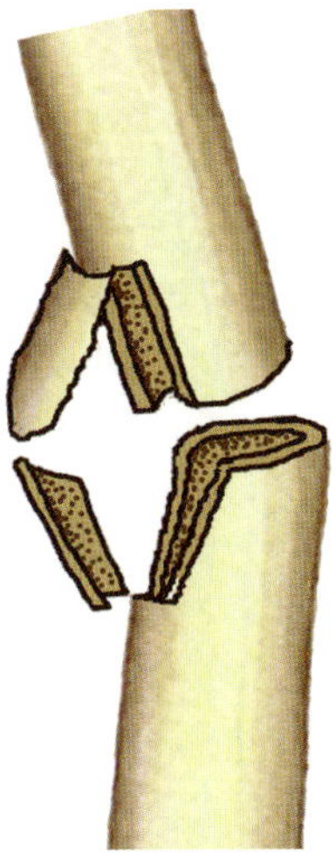

Middle third

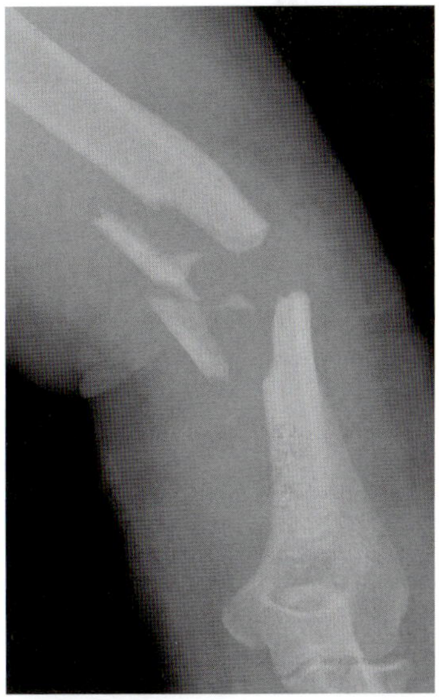

12-B3.3

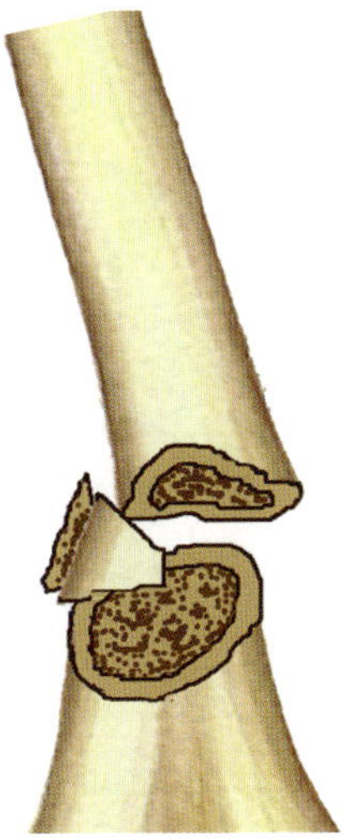

Distal third

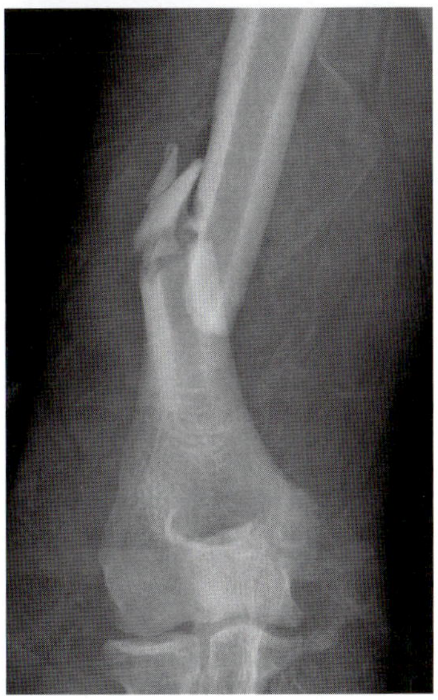

12-C Humerus diaphysis complex fractures

12-C1
Humerus diaphysis complex fracture, spiral fracture
233 fractures
M: 126 (54.08%)
F: 107 (45.92%)
0.06% of total adult fractures
1.07% of adult humeral fractures
4.61% of segment 12
48.85% of 12-C

12-C1.1

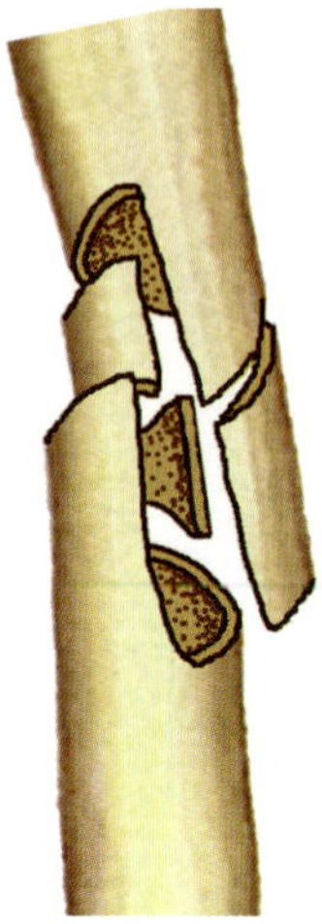

With two intermediate fragments

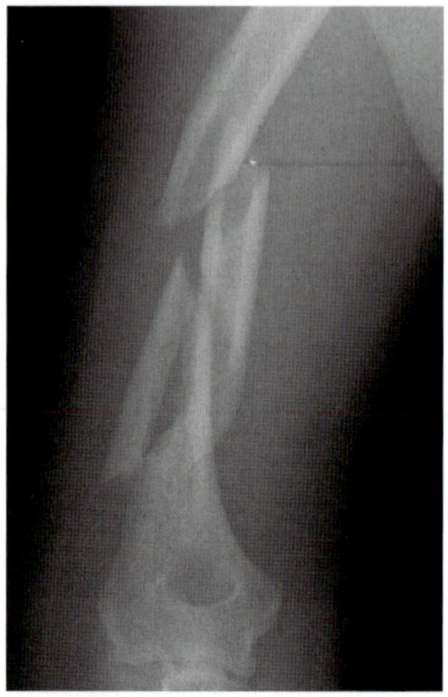

12-C1.2

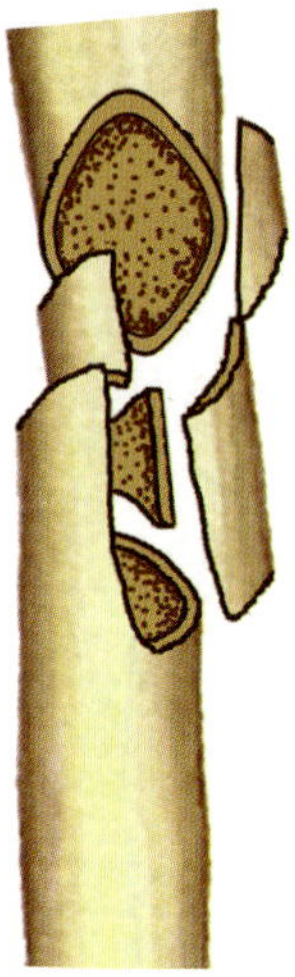

With three intermediate fragments

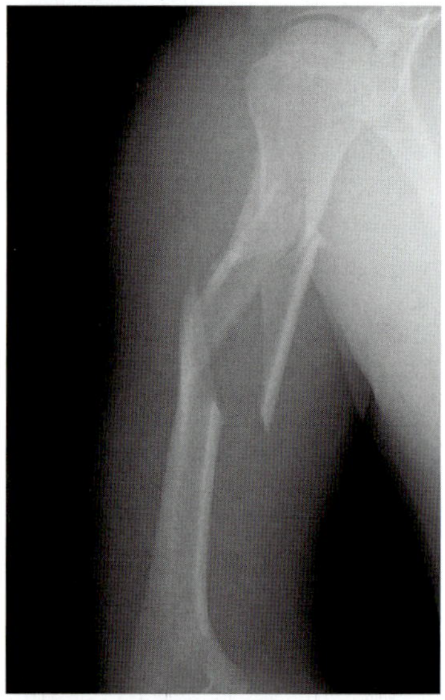

12-C1.3

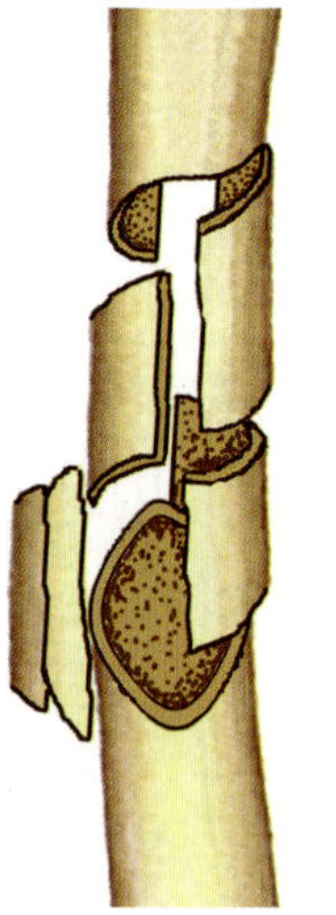

With more than
three intermediate fragments

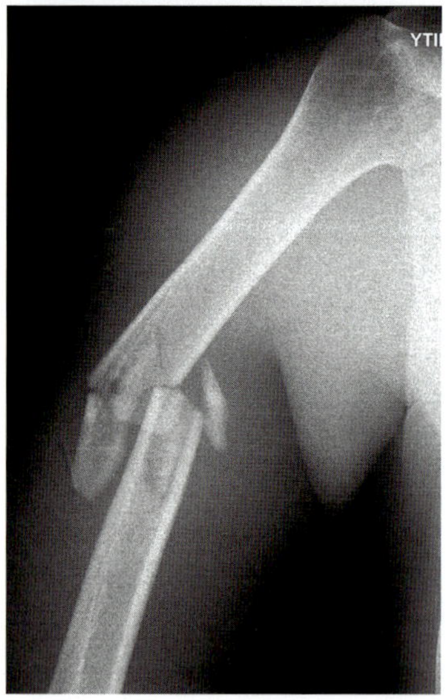

12-C Humerus diaphysis complex fractures

12-C2
Humerus diaphysis complex fracture, segmental fracture
88 fractures
M: 62 (70.45%)
F: 26 (29.55%)
0.02% of total adult fractures
0.40% of adult humeral fractures
1.74% of segment 12
18.45% of 12-C

12-C2.1

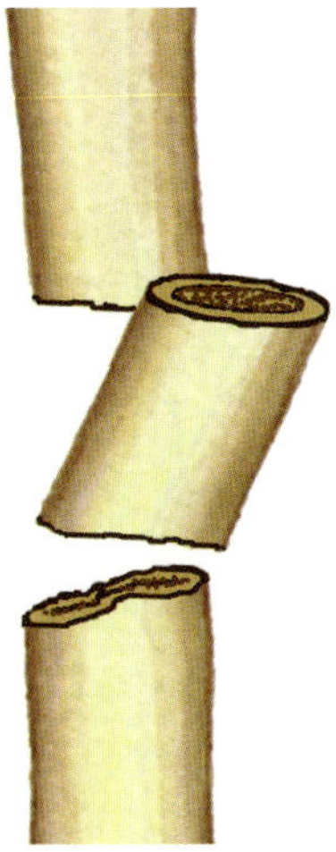

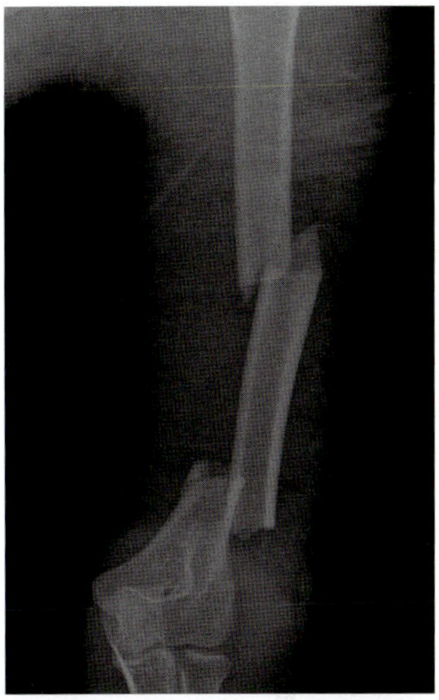

With one intermediate segment

12-C2.2

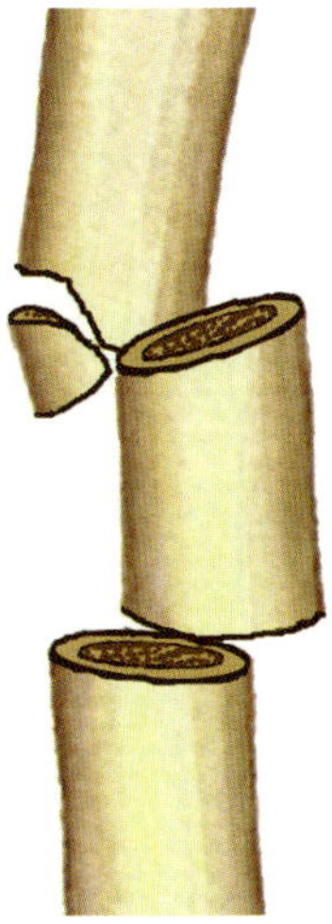

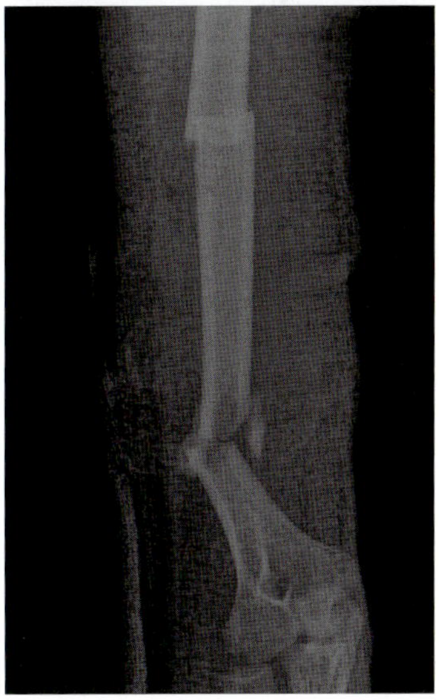

With one intermediate segment and additional wedge fragment

12-C2.3

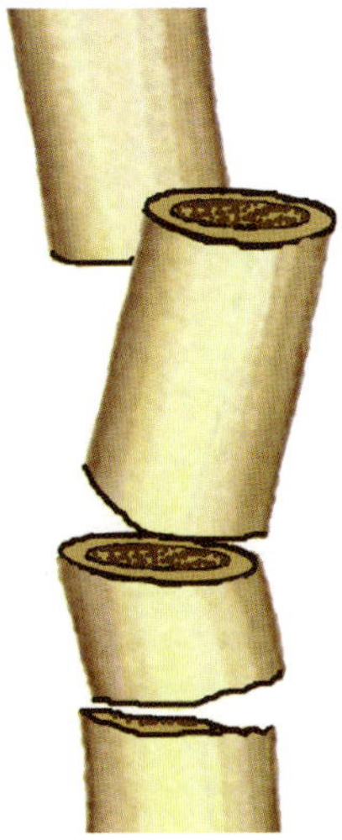

With two intermediate segments

12-C Humerus diaphysis complex fractures

12-C3
Humerus diaphysis complex fracture, irregular fracture
156 fractures
M: 109 (69.87%)
F: 47 (30.13%)
0.04% of total adult fractures
0.72% of adult humeral fractures
3.09% of segment 12
32.70% of 12-C

12-C3.1

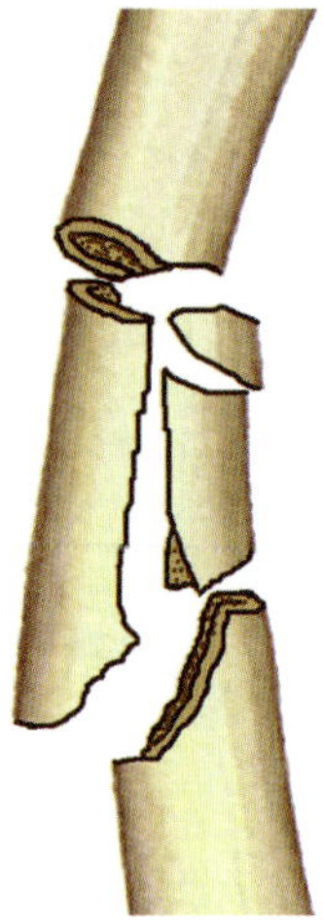

With two or three intermediate fragments

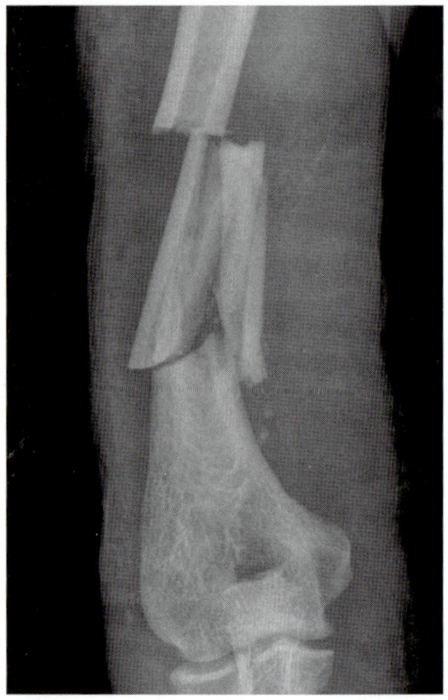

12-C3.2

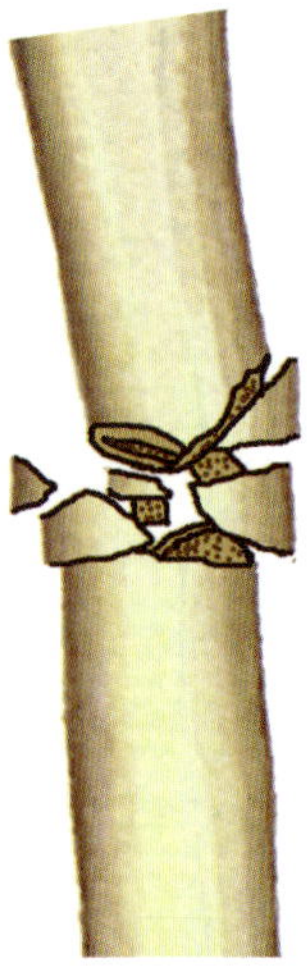

With limited shattering (< 4 cm)

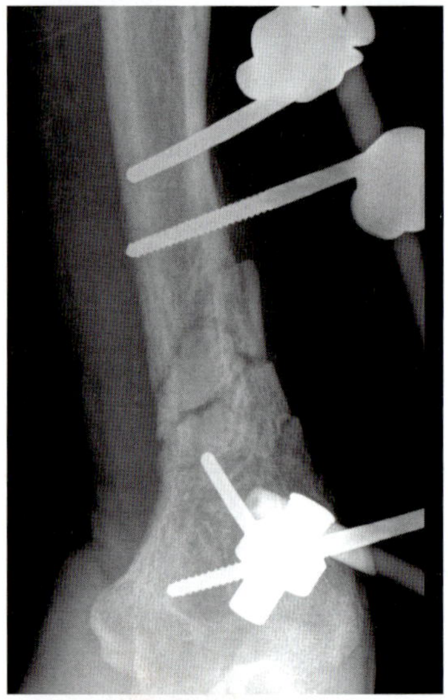

12-C3.3

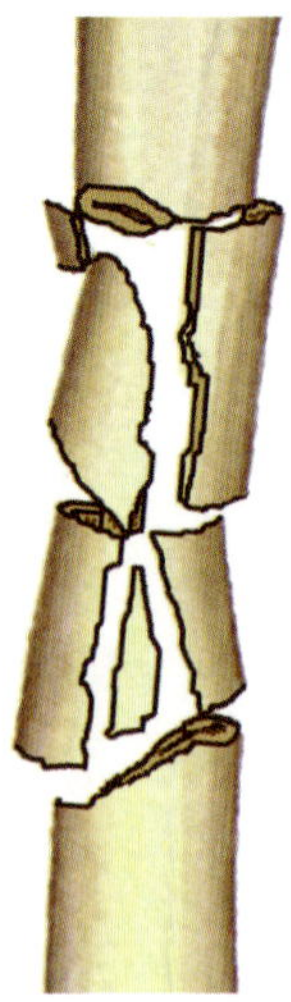

With extensive shattering (> 4 cm)

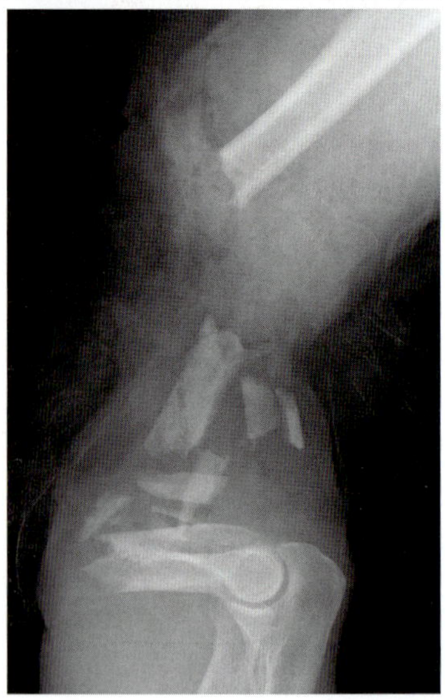

Injury Mechanism

There are several mechanisms that result in humeral shaft fractures:

- Direct force is the most common mechanism of injury, such as in a direct blow, a compression force, or a gunshot wound—all of which usually produce transverse, comminuted, or open fractures.
- Indirect mechanisms involve a fall where the hand or elbow touches the ground. The fall usually involves a twisting motion to the remainder of the body, or the attached muscles may contract asymmetrically, leading to a greater incidence of spiral or oblique fractures.
- Spiral injuries typically occur in the junction of the middle, distal third of the humeral shaft, caused by military training or athletic activities such as throwing or arm wrestling. When engaged in such activities, the attached muscle contracts abruptly and the axial load increases, leading to a spiral fracture.

The fractured arm usually presents with typical deformity under the influence of the attached muscle. For example, when the fracture line is proximal to the insertion of the pectoralis major, the traction of the rotator cuff muscles results in abduction and internal rotation of the proximal fragment, while the distal fragment is displaced medially by the pectoralis major. When fractures occur between insertions of the pectoralis major and deltoid, the distal fragment is displaced laterally by the deltoid, while the proximal fragment is pulled medially by the pectoralis major, latissimus dorsi, and teres major. Fractures below the deltoid insertion will result in abduction and flexion of the proximal fragment, and the proximal displacement of the distal fragment (**Plate 2.16**).

Diagnosis

Patients with humeral shaft fractures present with arm pain, swelling, and deformity. Abnormal movement and crepitus can be observed. A careful neurovascular evaluation of the affected limb should be performed, especially checking for compartmental pressure and the presence of the distal pulse if the limb is swollen. A test for sensory and motor function should be performed as well.

The radiographic evaluation for humeral shaft fractures should include an AP and a lateral view of the entire humerus to clarify fracture locations and types.

Treatment

The treatment of choice for humeral shaft fractures depends on several factors, including the patient's physical status, age, comorbidities, soft tissue damage, and fracture type.

Most humeral shaft fractures can be treated successfully with nonoperative management. Multiple closed techniques are available, including use of the hanging arm cast, U plaster, sling/swathe, abduction humeral/shoulder spica cast, and functional brace, as well as the use of skeletal traction.

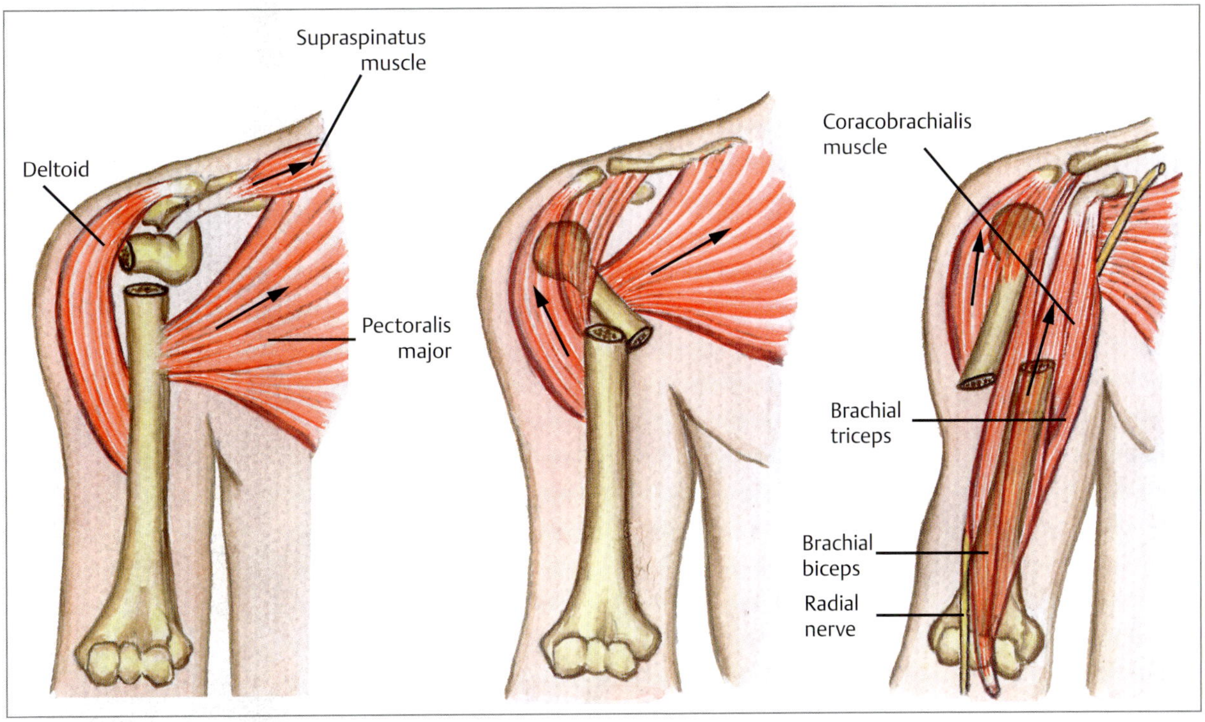

Plate 2.16

Operative intervention is indicated in special circumstances, including failure of closed treatment, open fracture, vascular injury, floating elbow, segmental fractures, bilateral fractures of the humerus, and polytrauma such as multiple fractures. Radial nerve injury can be seen in 18% of humeral fractures, often caused by traction injury, 90% of which resolve to normal function in 3–4 months. Nerve exploration is required for unresolved radial nerve injury. An indication for early nerve exploration also includes compromised radial nerve function associated with the treatment of closed manipulation itself. It is generally accepted that up to 3 cm of shortening and 20–30 degrees of varus, anterior, or rotational deformity will result in an acceptable upper extremity function. The fracture fixation devices include intramedullary nails, plates, and external fixators—the choice of which to use is most often based on clinical experience and the fracture type.

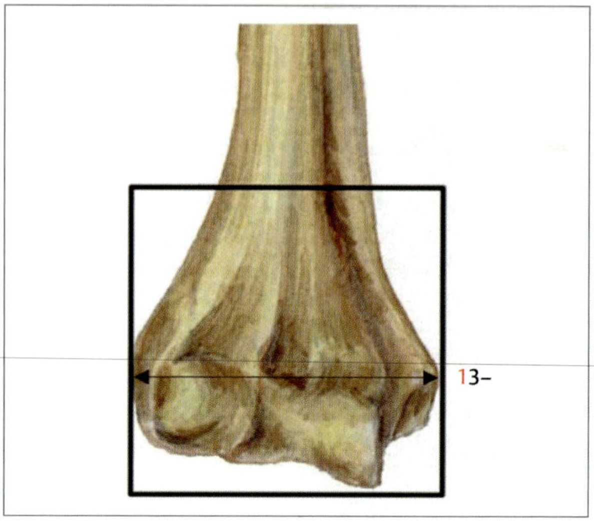

Plate 2.17

Distal Humeral Fractures (Segment 13)

Anatomical Features

The distal end of the humerus is flattened and bears two articulations: the trochlea for the ulna and the capitellum for the radius (**Plate 2.17**). There are three depressions: the radial fossa and coronoid fossa above the anterior part of the trochlea receive the radial head and coronoid process of the ulna during the flexion of the forearm, while posteriorly the back part of the trochlea is the olecranon fossa, which receives the olecranon during extension of the forearm (**Plate 2.18**).

The lateral epicondyle is a tuberculated eminence and provides an attachment site for the extensor muscle of the forearm. The medial epicondyle, larger and more prominent than the lateral one, provides an attachment site for the flexor muscles of the forearm, while the ulnar nerve runs in a groove on the back of this epicondyle. The capitulum of the humerus, a portion of the articular surface that extends lower than the lateral epicondyle, articulates with the cup-shaped depression on the head of the radius (**Plate 2.19**). The grooved portion on the trochlea's articular surface fits precisely within the ulna's semilunar notch, a large depression formed by the coronoid process anteriorly and

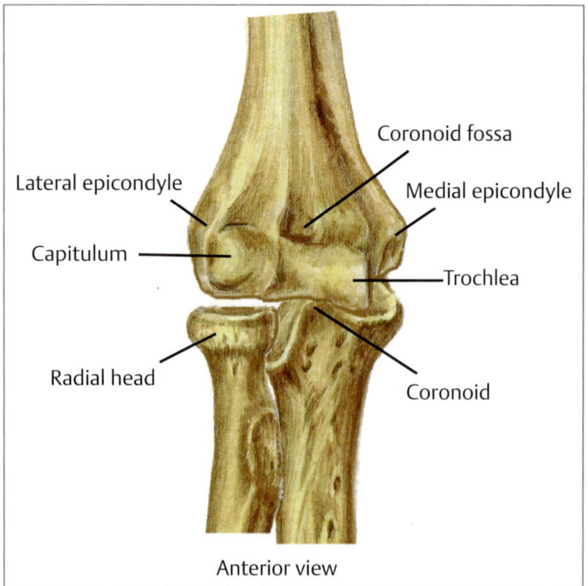

Plate 2.18

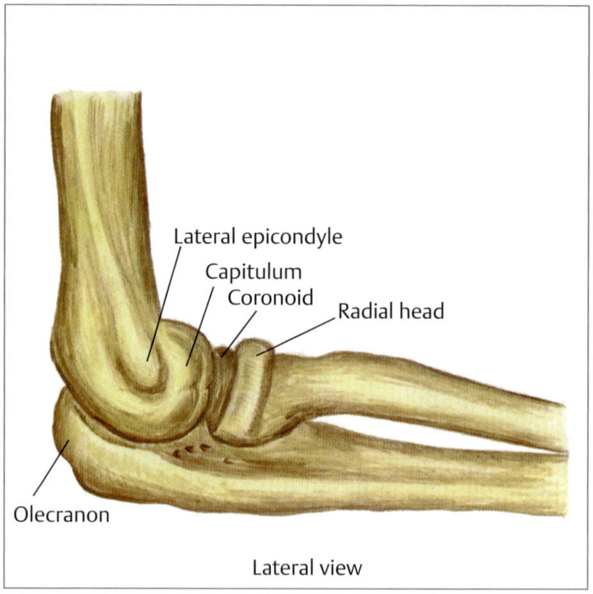

Plate 2.19

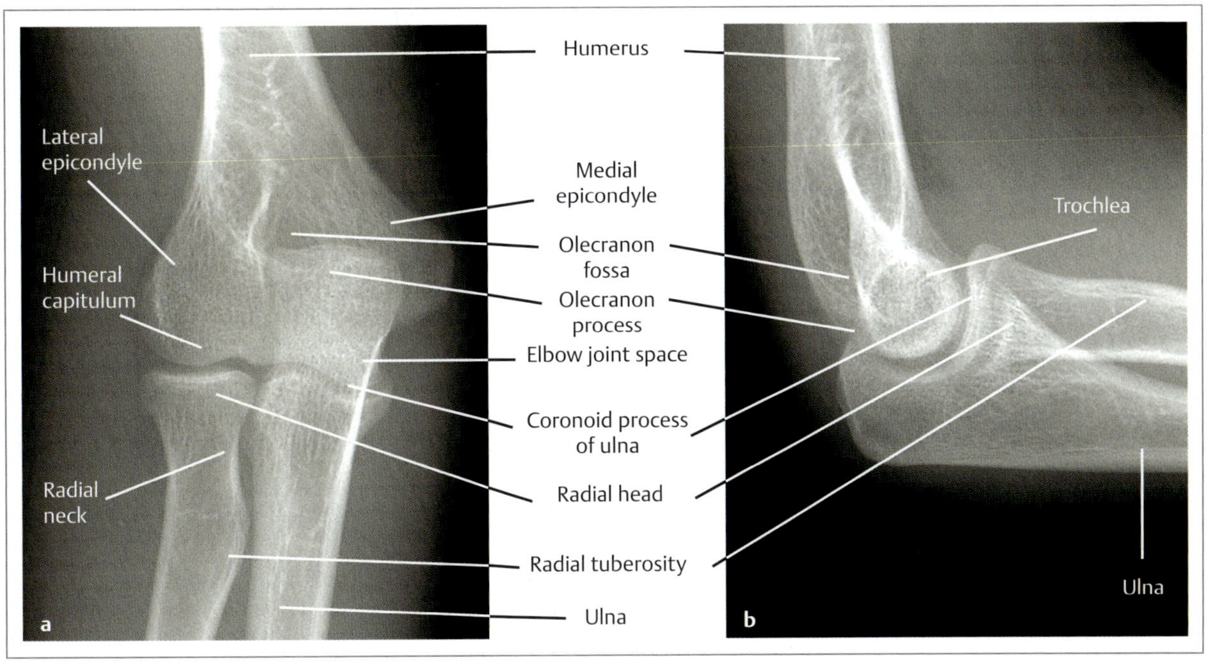

Plate 2.20

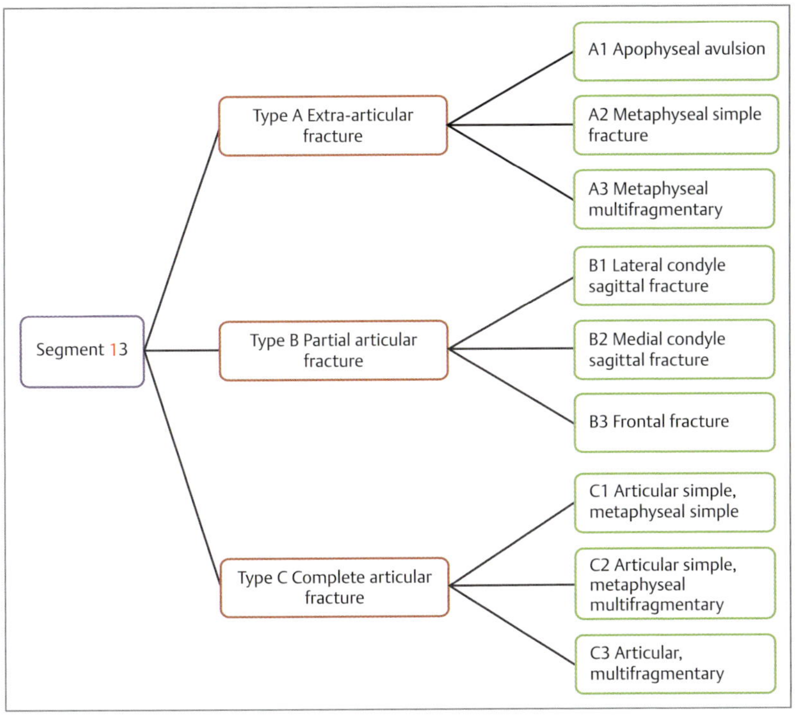

Plate 2.21

the olecranon process posteriorly (**Plate 2.20**). When the arm is extended with the palm facing up, the supplementary angle to that between the longitudinal axis of the arm and of the forearm is called the carrying angle or the valgus angle. Malreduction of fractures in the distal humerus can lead to changes in the carrying angle, and consequently a valgus or varus deformity of the elbow.

AO Classification of Distal Humeral Fractures

The distal end of the humerus is delineated by a square whose side is equal to the maximum width of the distal humerus based on the AO classification, and the location coded as number 13. Classification is by three types, depending on the involvement of the articulation: 13-A, extra-articular fracture; 13-B, partial articular fracture; and 13-C, complete articular fracture (**Plate 2.21**).

Clinical Epidemiologic Features of Distal Humeral Fractures (Segment 13)

A total of 3,761 adult fractures were treated in 83 hospitals in China over a 2-year period from 2010 to 2011. All cases were reviewed and statistically studied; the fractures accounted for 17.28% of all humeral fractures in adults. The epidemiologic features are as follows:

- More males than females
- The high-risk age group is 16–20 years; 16–20 years for males, 56–60 years for females
- The high-risk fracture type is 13-A, and is the same for both males and females
- The high-risk fracture group is 13-A1, and is the same for both males and females.

Fractures of Segment 13 by Sex

Table 2.14 Sex distribution of 3,761 fractures of segment 13

Sex	Number of fractures	Percentage (%)
Male	2,114	56.21
Female	1,647	43.79
Total	3,761	100.00

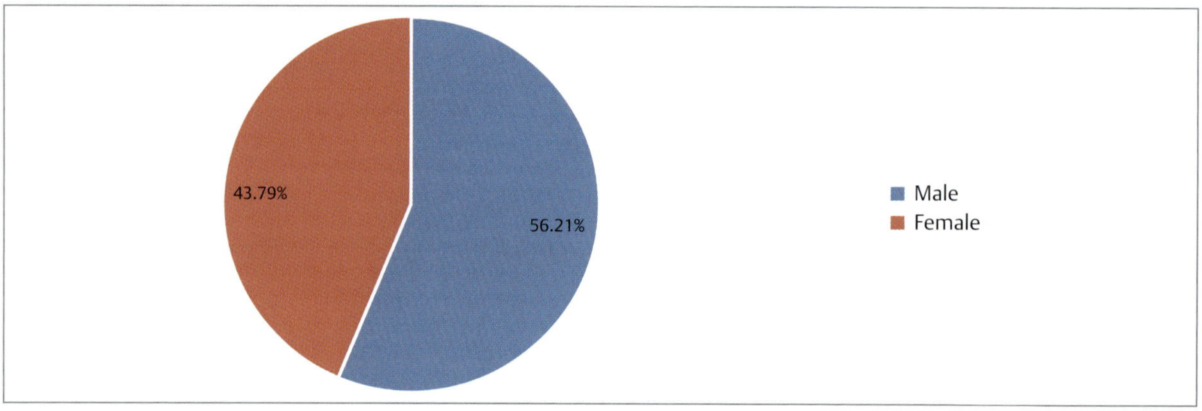

Fig. 2.14 Sex distribution of 3,761 fractures of segment 13.

Fractures of Segment 13 by Age Group

Table 2.15 Age and sex distribution of 3,761 fractures of segment 13

Age group (years)	Male	Female	Total	Percentage (%)
16–20	381	111	492	13.08
21–25	275	123	398	10.58
26–30	229	68	297	7.90
31–35	218	97	315	8.38
36–40	236	98	334	8.88
41–45	177	110	287	7.63
46–50	145	102	247	6.57
51–55	149	142	291	7.74
56–60	107	178	285	7.58
61–65	51	128	179	4.76
66–70	45	121	166	4.41
71–75	27	120	147	3.91
76–80	37	111	148	3.94
81–85	20	79	99	2.63
≥86	17	59	76	2.02
Total	2,114	1,647	3,761	100.00

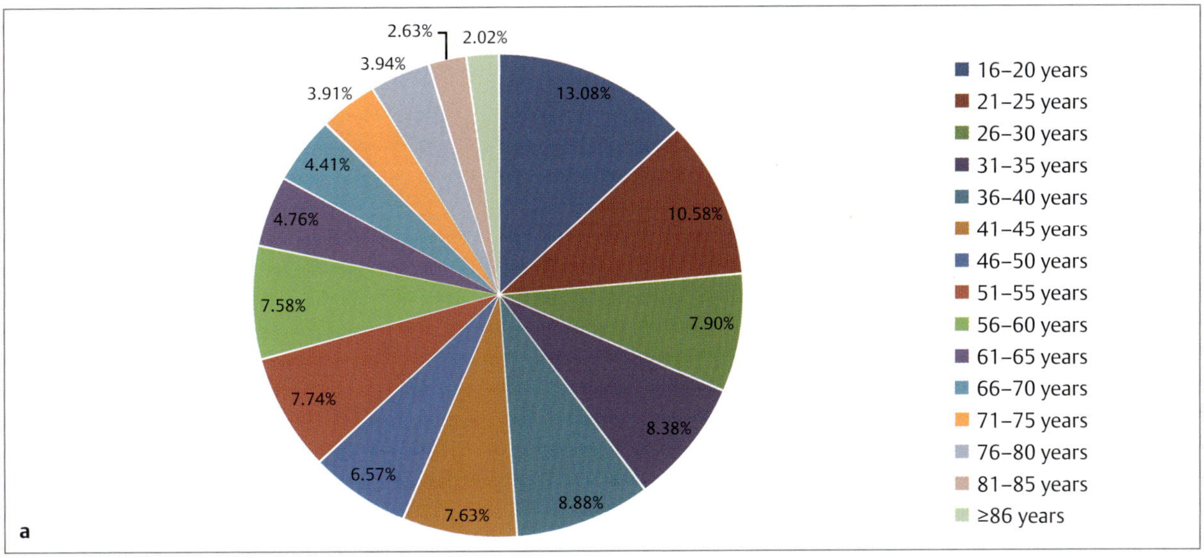

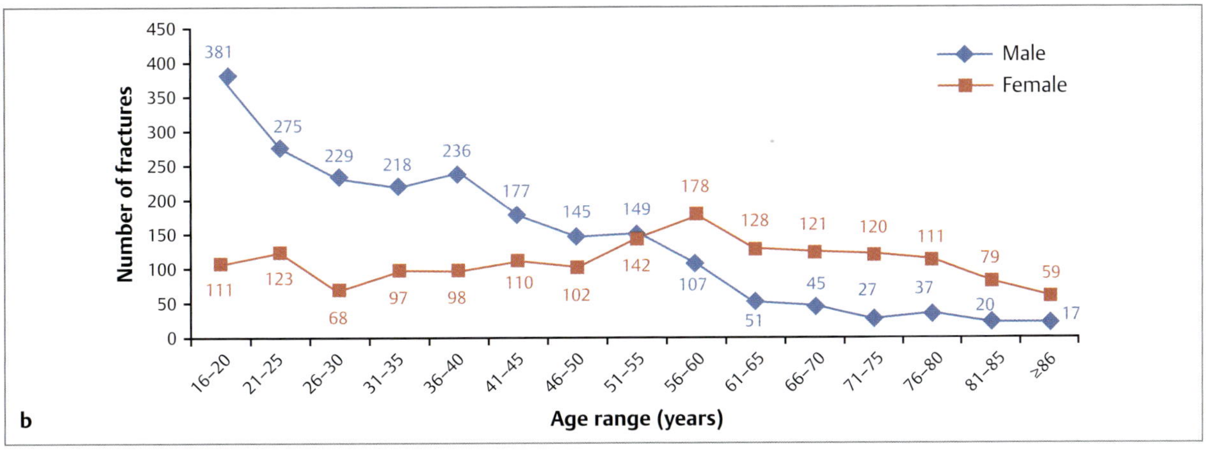

Fig. 2.15 **(a)** Age distribution of 3,761 fractures of segment 13.
(b) Age and sex distribution of 3,761 fractures of segment 13.

Fractures of Segment 13 by Fracture Type

Table 2.16 Sex and fracture distribution of 3,761 fractures of segment 13

Fracture type	Male	Female	Number of fractures	Percentage of segment 13 fractures (%)	Percentage of adult humeral fracture (%)
13-A	1,157	834	1,991	52.94	9.15
13-B	534	412	946	25.15	4.35
13-C	423	401	824	21.91	3.79
Total	2,114	1,647	3,761	100.00	17.28

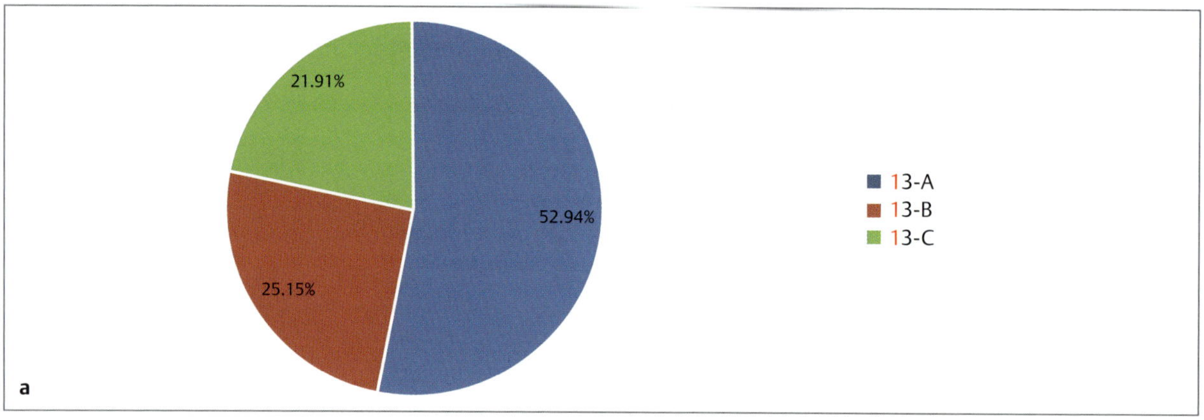

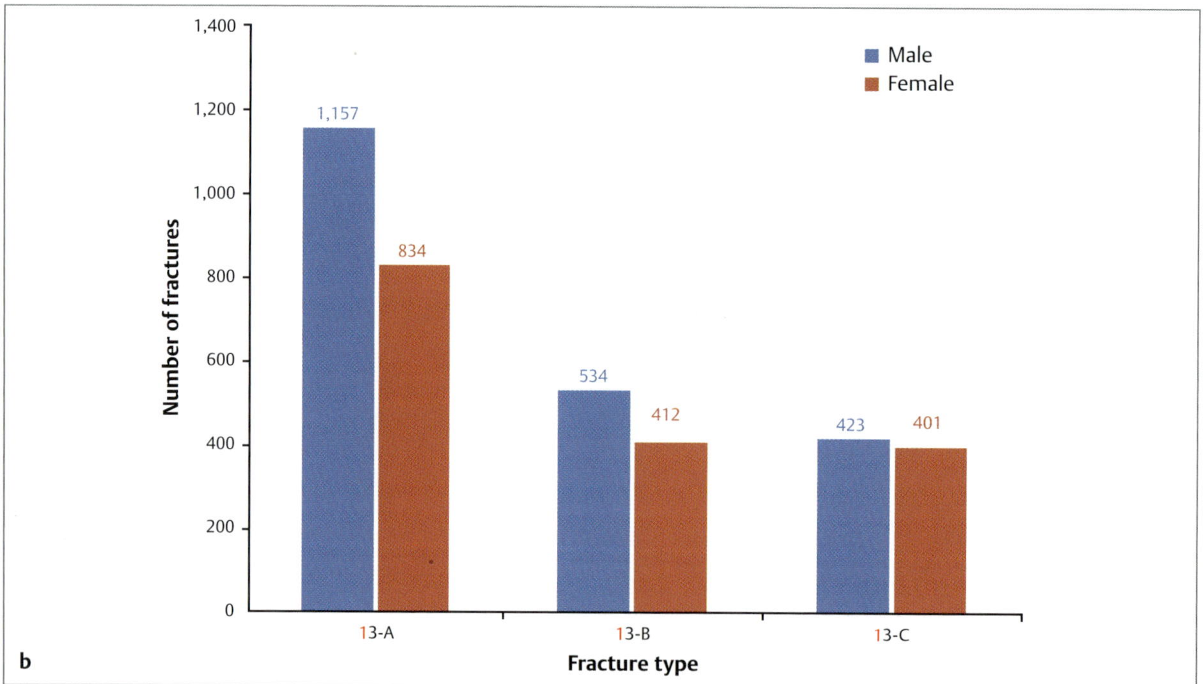

Fig. 2.16 **(a)** Fracture type distribution of 3,761 fractures of segment 13.
(b) Sex and fracture type distribution of 3,761 fractures of segment 13.

Table 2.17 Sex and fracture group distribution of 3,761 fractures of segment 13

Fracture group	Male	Female	Total	Percentage of segment 13 fractures (%)	Percentage of adult humeral fracture (%)
13-A1	687	373	1,060	28.18	4.87
13-A2	349	346	695	18.48	3.19
13-A3	121	115	236	6.27	1.08
13-B1	291	208	499	13.27	2.29
13-B2	174	141	315	8.38	1.45
13-B3	69	63	132	3.51	0.61
13-C1	117	128	245	6.51	1.13
13-C2	149	144	293	7.79	1.35
13-C3	157	129	286	7.60	1.31
Total	2,114	1,647	3,761	100.00	17.28

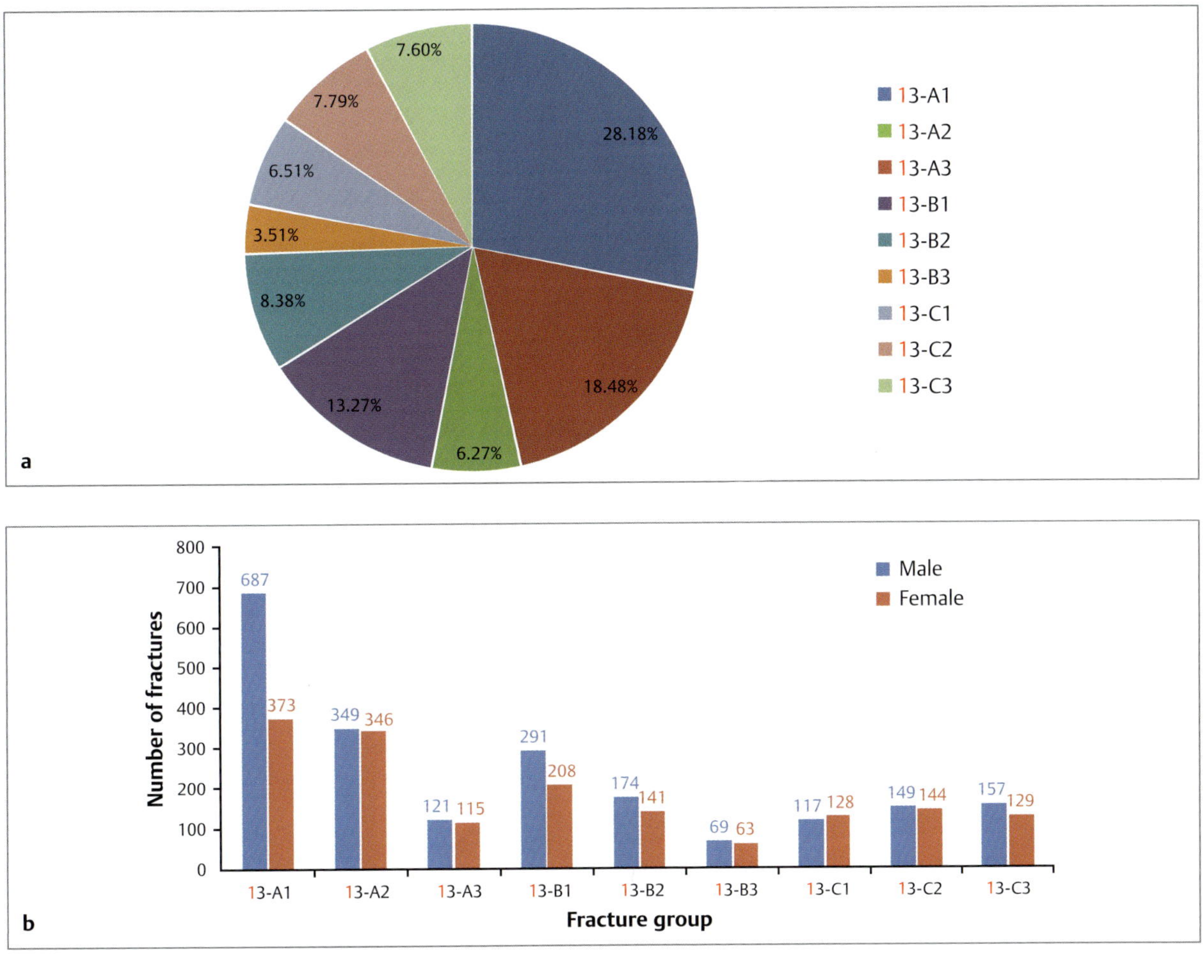

Fig. 2.17 **(a)** Fracture group distribution of 3,761 fractures of segment 13.
(b) Sex and fracture group distribution of 3,761 fractures of segment 13.

13-A Humerus distal extra-articular fractures

13-A1
Humerus distal extra-articular fracture, apophyseal avulsion
1,060 fractures
M: 687 (64.81%)
F: 373 (35.19%)
0.28% of total adult fractures
4.87% of adult humeral fractures
28.18% of segment 13
53.24% of type 13-A

13-A1.1

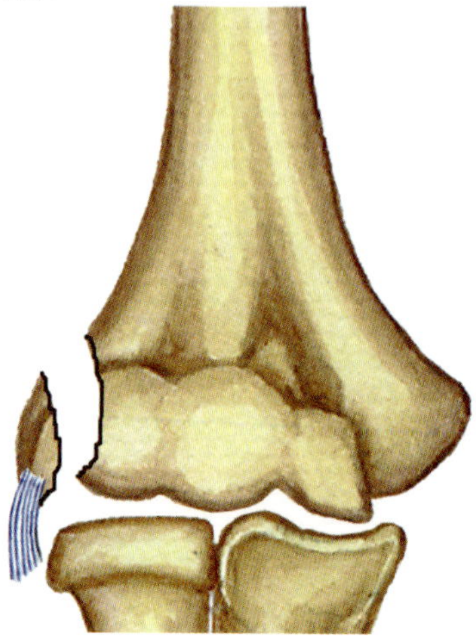

Lateral epicondyle

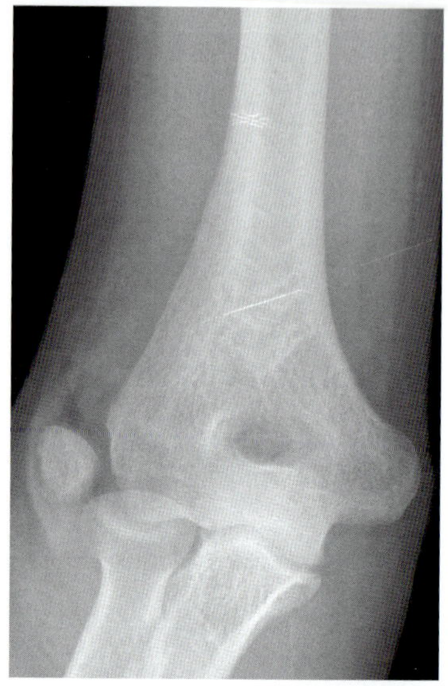

13-A1.2

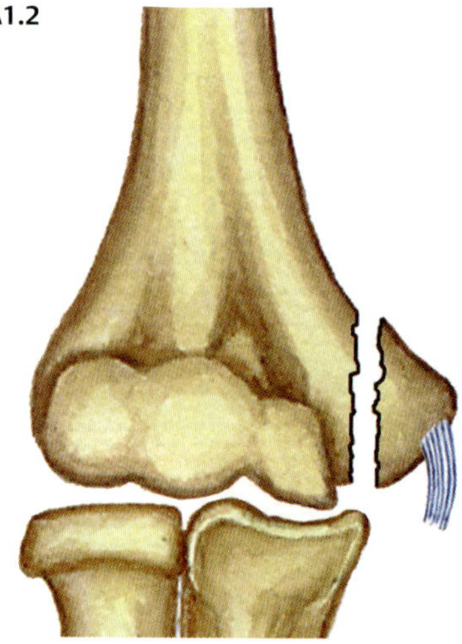

Medial epicondyle with no incarcerated fragment

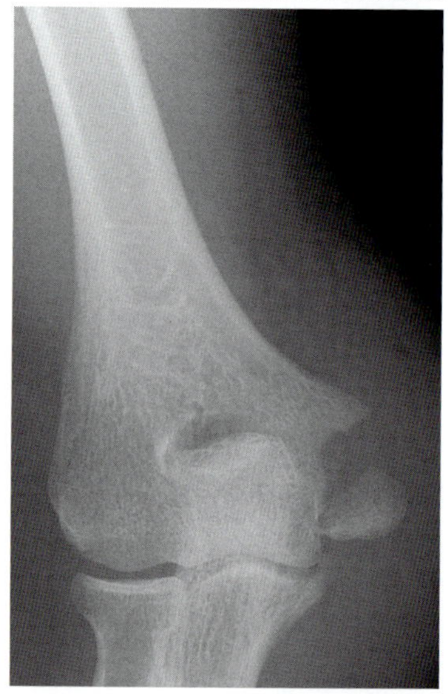

13-A1.3

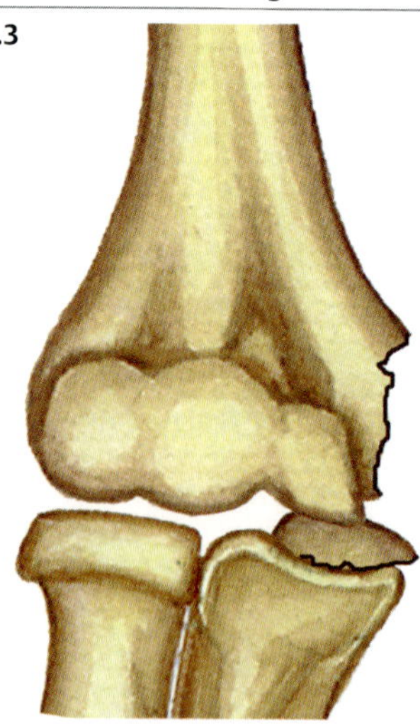

Medial epicondyle with incarcerated fragment

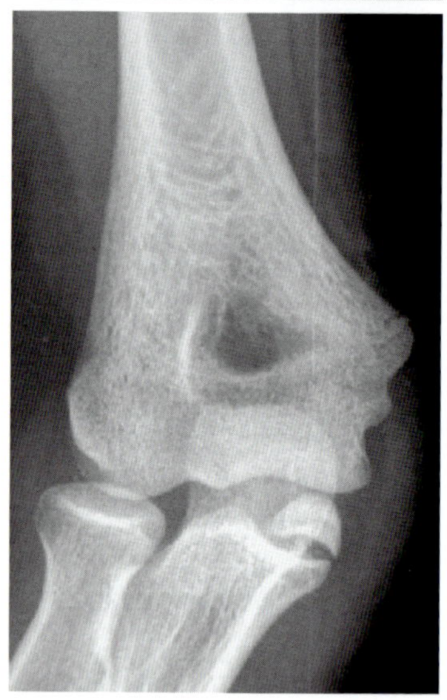

13-A Humerus distal extra-articular fractures

13-A2

Humerus distal extra-articular fracture, metaphyseal simple fracture

695 fractures
M: 349 (50.22%)
F: 346 (49.78%)
0.19% of total adult fractures
3.19% of adult humeral fractures
18.48% of segment 13
34.91% of type 13-A

13-A2.1

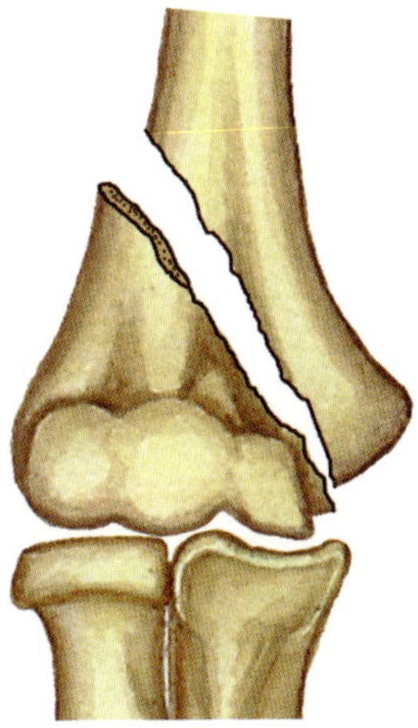

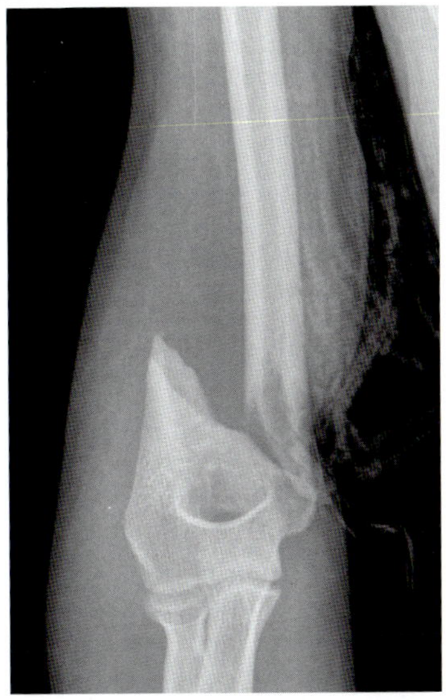

Oblique downward and inward

13-A2.2

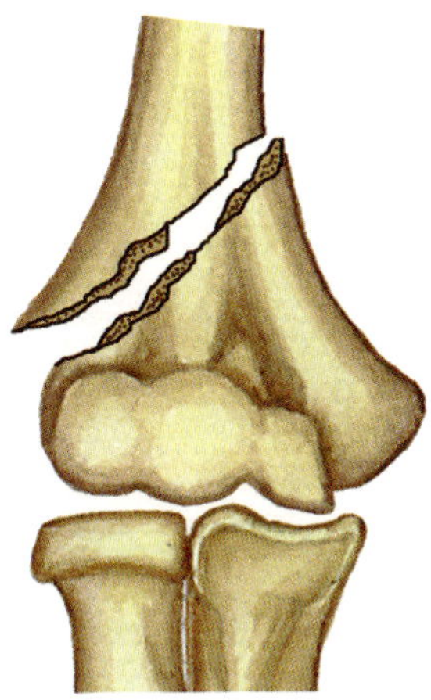

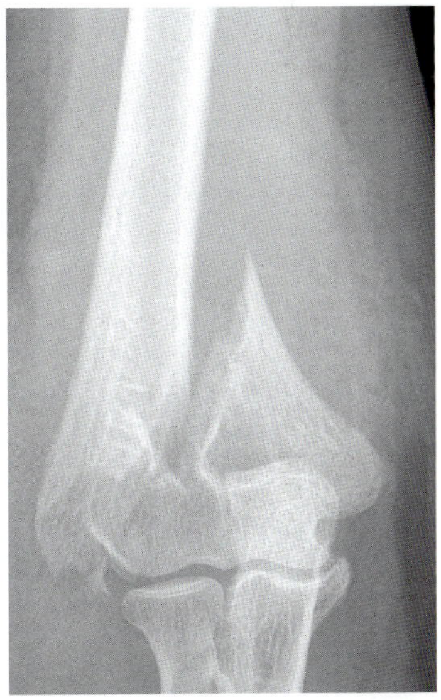

Oblique downward and outward

13-A2.3

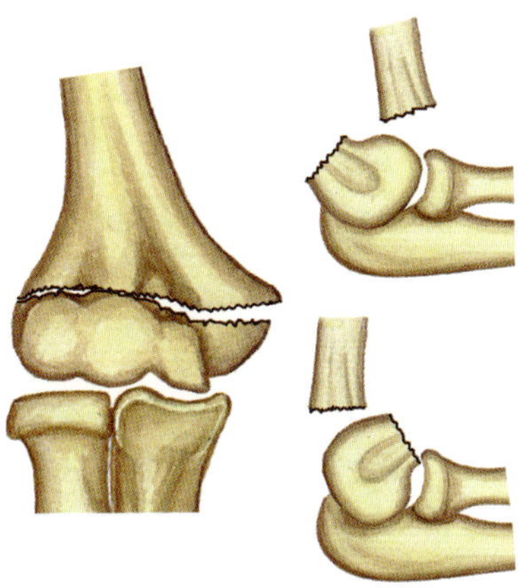

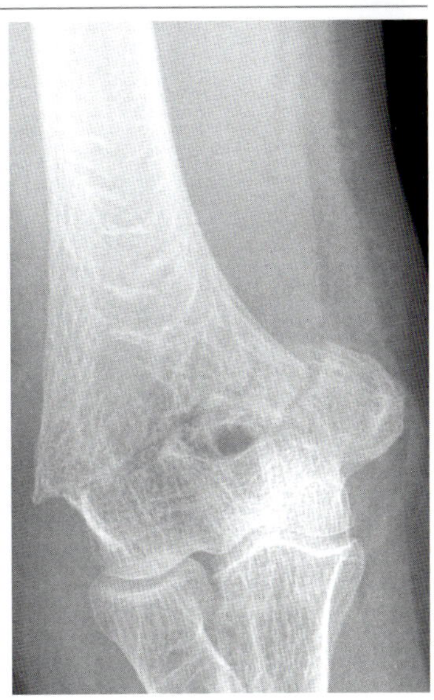

Transverse

13-A Humerus distal extra-articular fractures

13-A3
Humerus distal extra-articular fracture, metaphyseal multifragmentary fracture
236 fractures
M: 121 (51.27%)
F: 115 (48.73%)
0.06% of total adult fractures
1.08% of adult humeral fractures
6.27% of segment 13
11.85% of type 13-A

13-A3.1

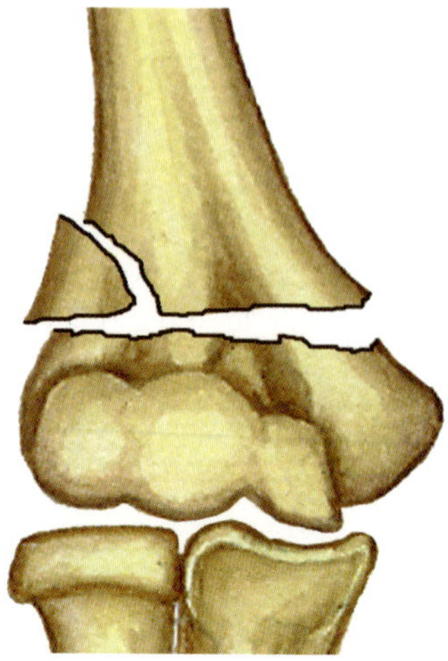

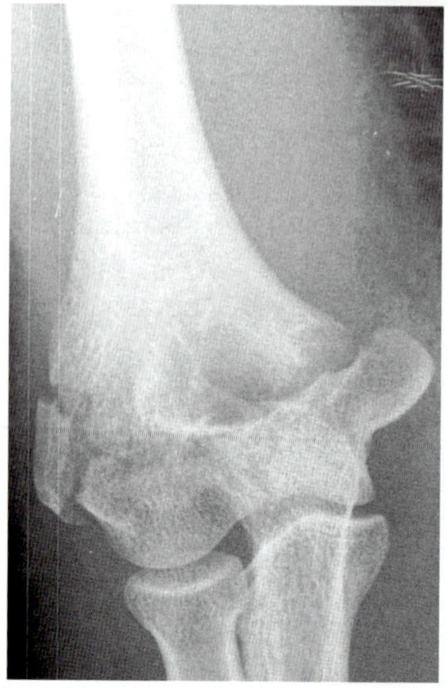

With intact wedge

13-A3.2

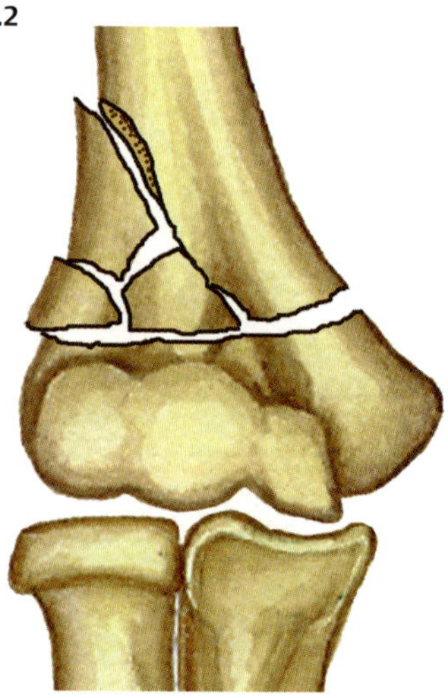

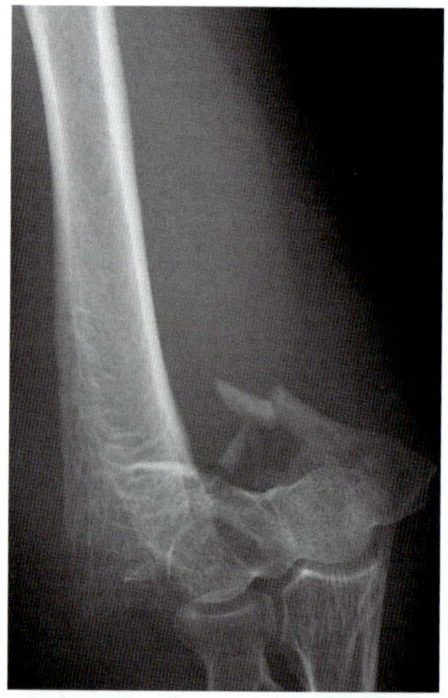

With a fragmented wedge

13-A3.3

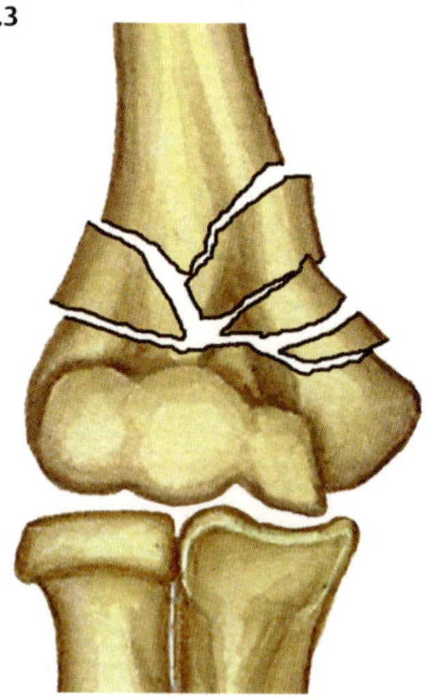

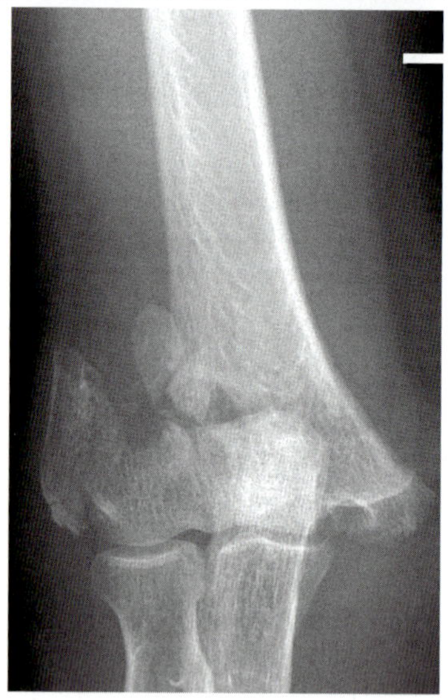

Complex

13-B Humerus distal partial articular fractures, single condyle

13-B1
Humerus distal partial articular fracture, lateral condyle sagittal fracture
499 fractures
M: 291 (58.32%)
F: 208 (41.68%)
0.13% of total adult fractures
2.29% of adult humeral fractures
13.27% of segment 13
52.75% of type 13-B

13-B1.1

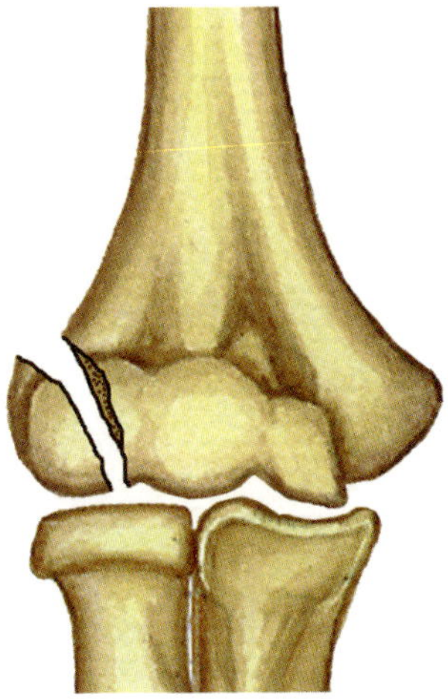

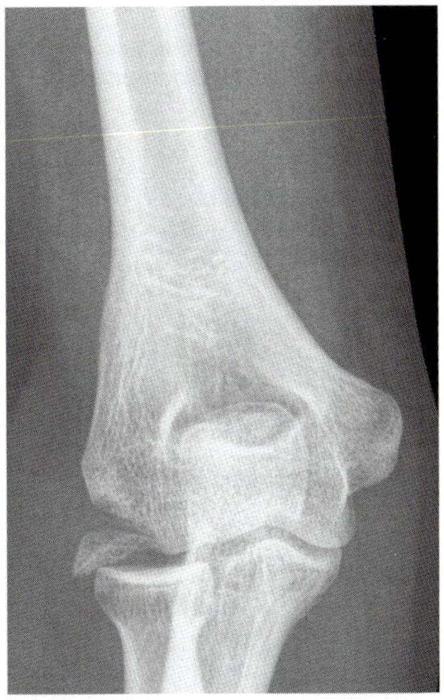

Capitellum

13-B1.2

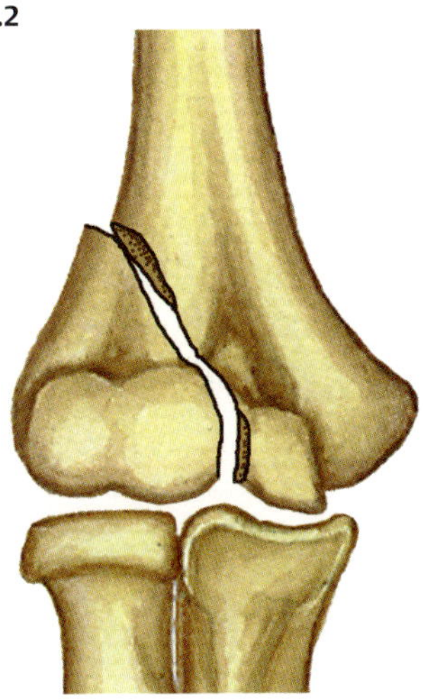

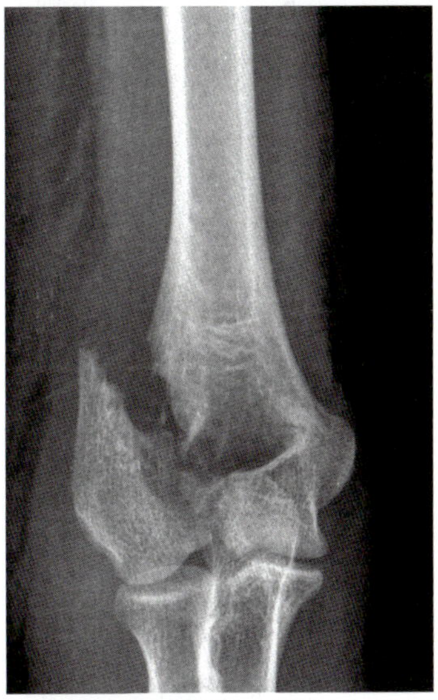

Transtrochlear simple

13-B1.3

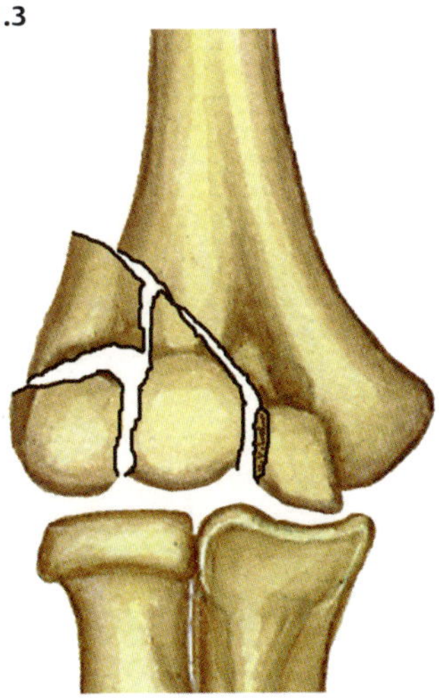

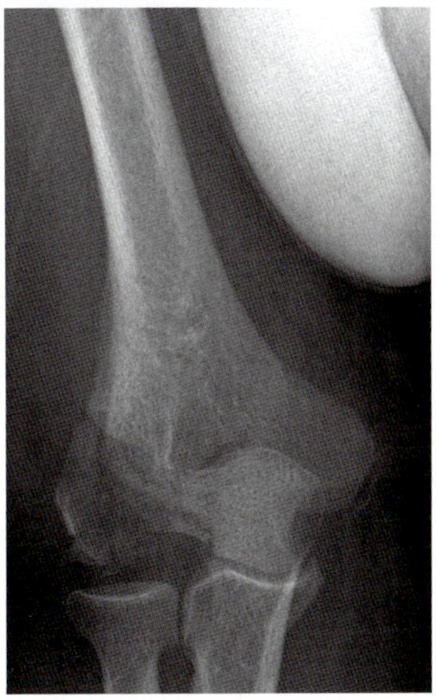

Transtrochlear multifragmentary

13-B Humerus distal partial articular fractures, single condyle

13-B2
Humerus distal partial articular fracture, medial condyle sagittal fracture
315 fractures
M: 174 (55.24%)
F: 141 (44.76%)
0.08% of total adult fractures
1.45% of adult humeral fractures
8.38% of segment 13
33.30% of type 13-B

13-B2.1

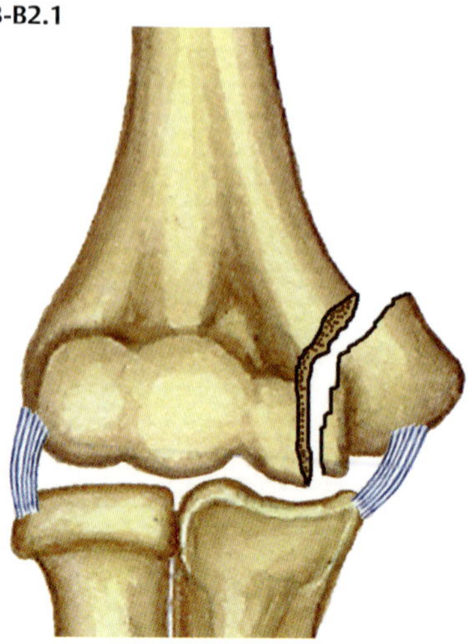

Transtrochlear simple, through the medial condyle

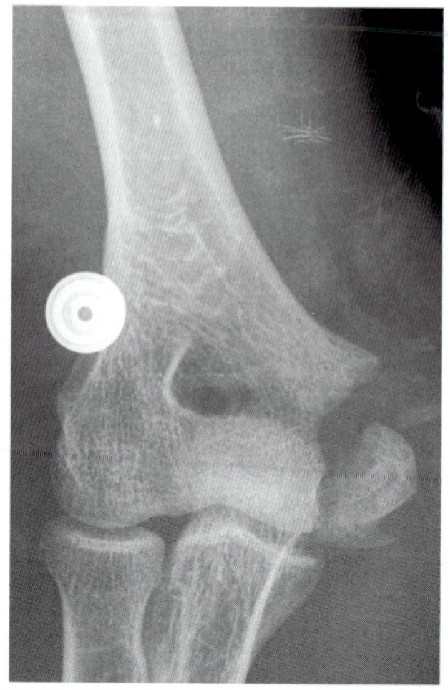

13-B2.2

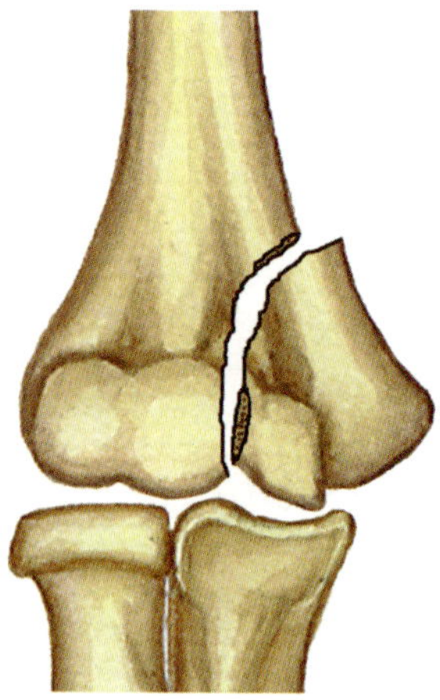

Transtrochlear simple, through the groove

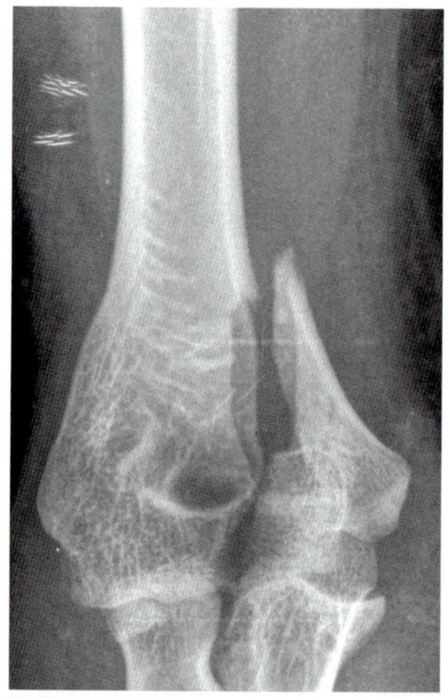

13-B2.3

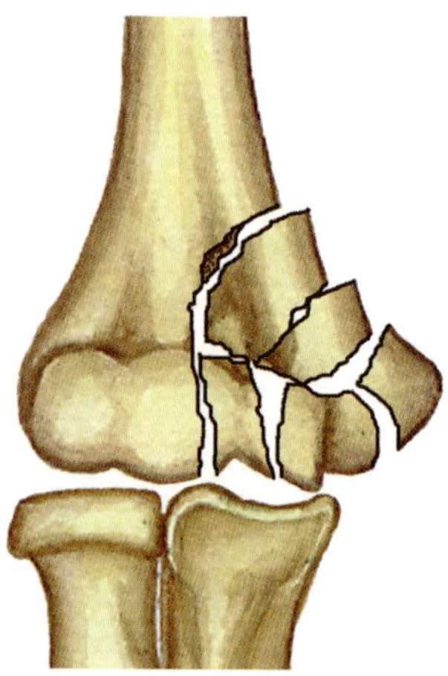

Transtrochlear complex

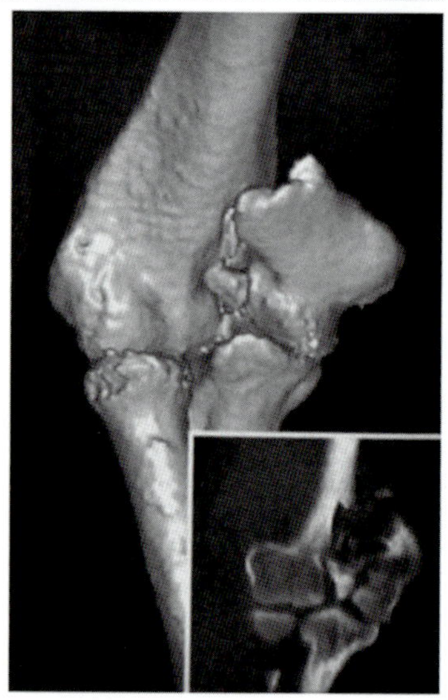

13-B Humerus distal partial articular fractures, single condyle

13-B3
Humerus distal partial articular fracture, single condyle, frontal fracture
132 fractures
M: 69 (52.27%)
F: 63 (47.73%)
0.04% of total adult fractures
0.61% of adult humeral fractures
3.51% of segment 13
13.95% of type 13-B

13-B3.1

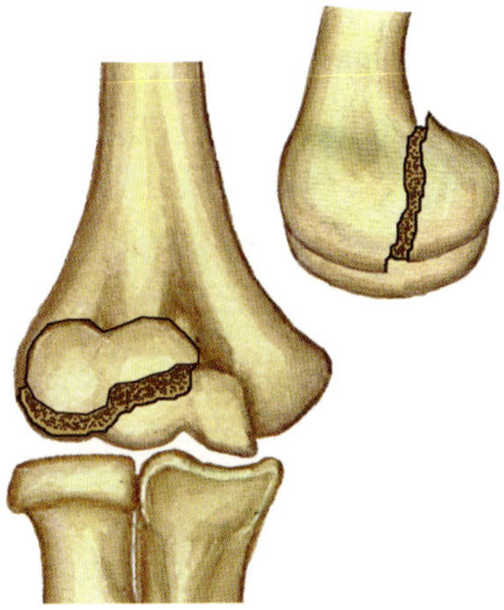

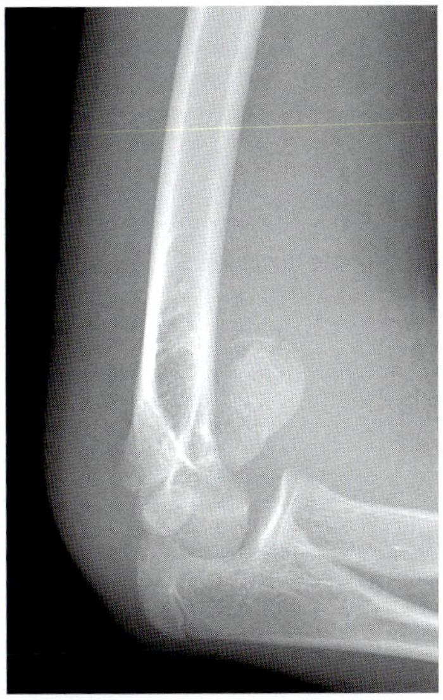

Capitellum

13-B3.2

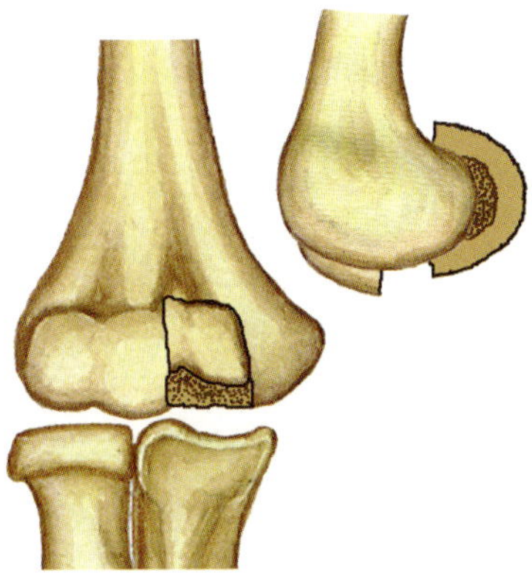

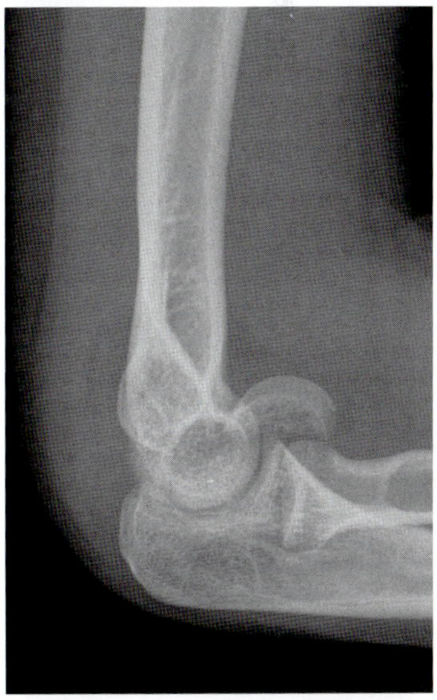

Trochlea

13-B3.3

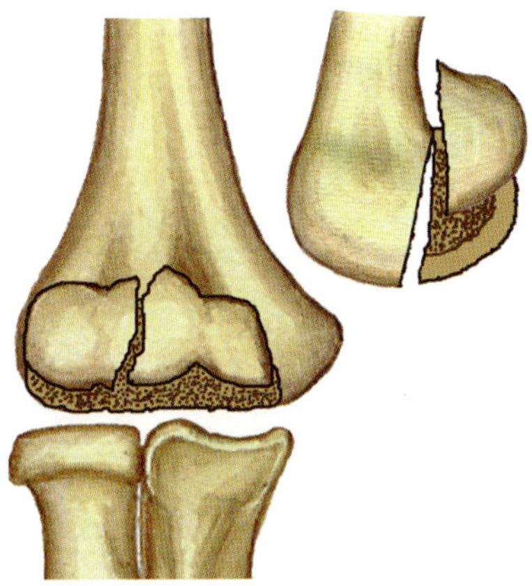

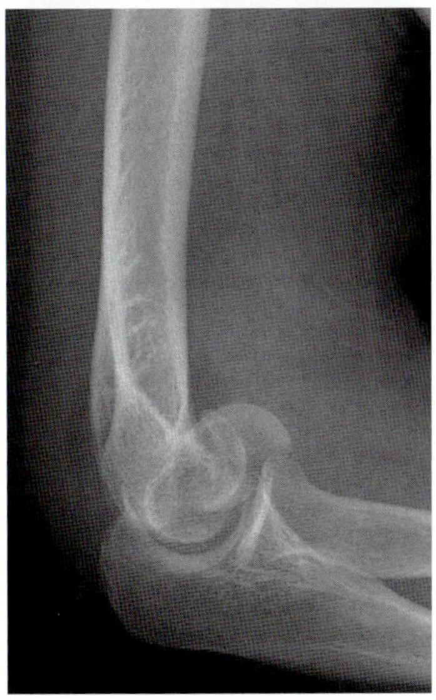

Capitellum and trochlea

13-C Humerus distal complete articular fractures

13-C1
Humerus distal complete articular fracture, simple, metaphyseal simple
245 fractures
M: 117 (47.76%)
F: 128 (52.24%)
0.07% of total adult fractures
1.13% of adult humeral fractures
6.51% of segment 13
29.73% of type 13-C

13-C1.1

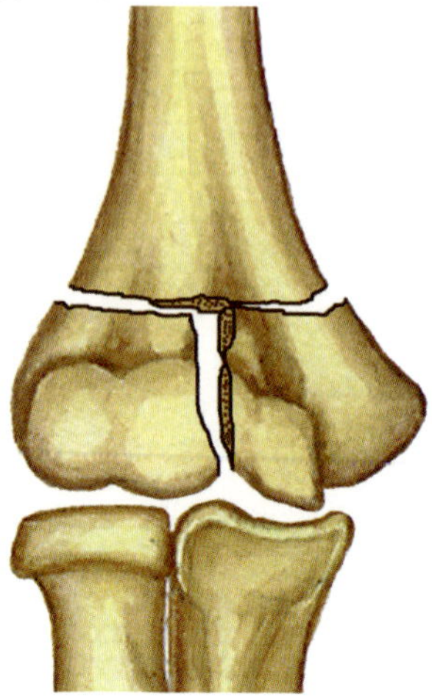

With slight displacement

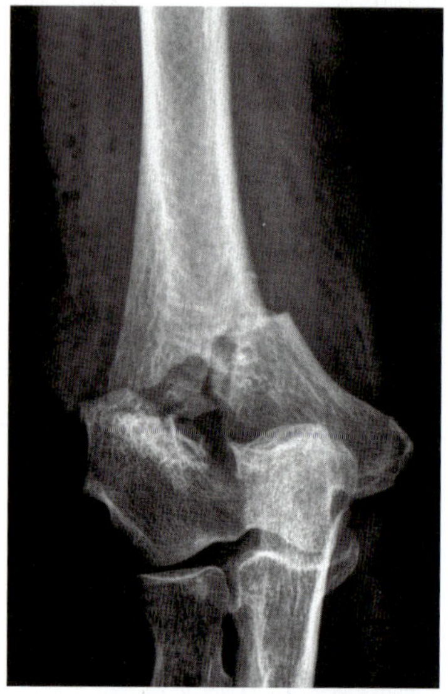

13-C1.2

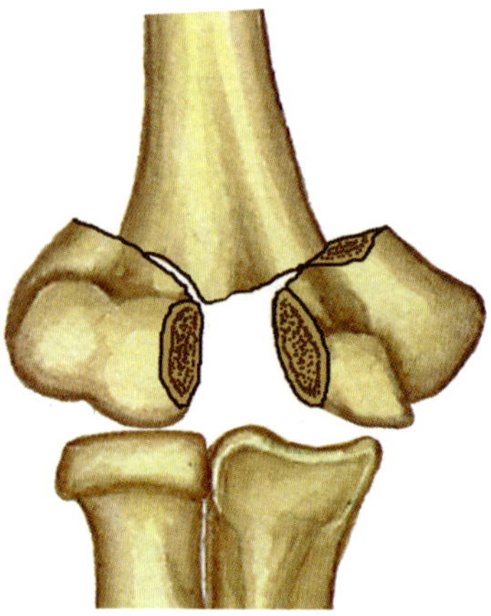

With marked displacement

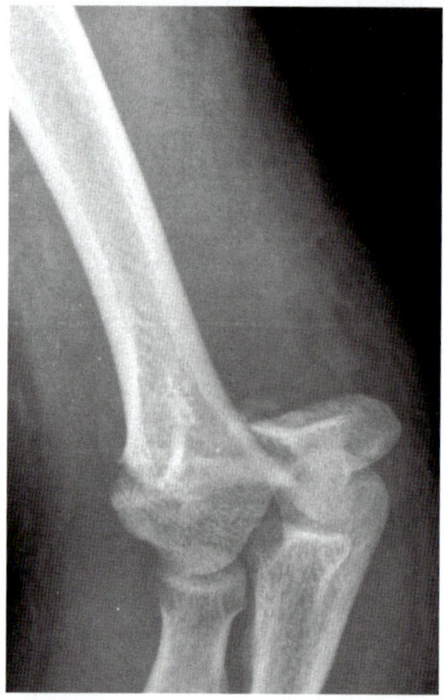

13-C1.3

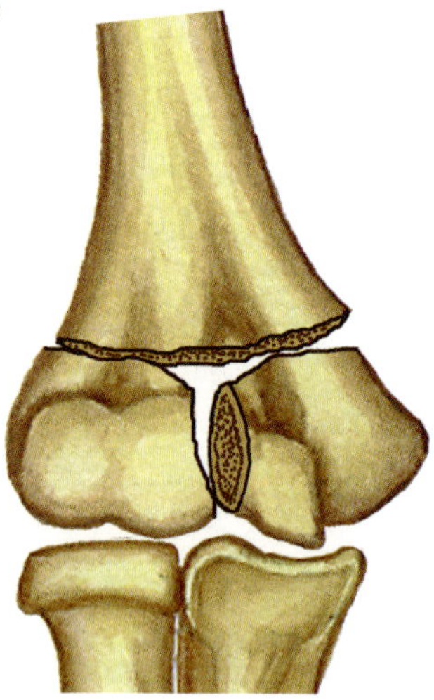

T-shaped epiphyseal

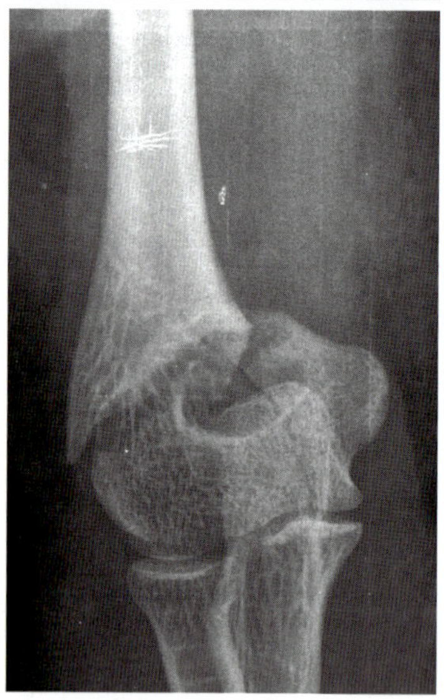

13-C Humerus distal complete articular fractures

13-C2
Humerus distal complete articular fracture, simple, metaphyseal multifragmentary
293 fractures
M: 149 (50.85%)
F: 144 (49.15%)
0.08% of total adult fractures
1.35% of adult humeral fractures
7.79% of segment 13
35.56% of type 13-C

13-C2.1

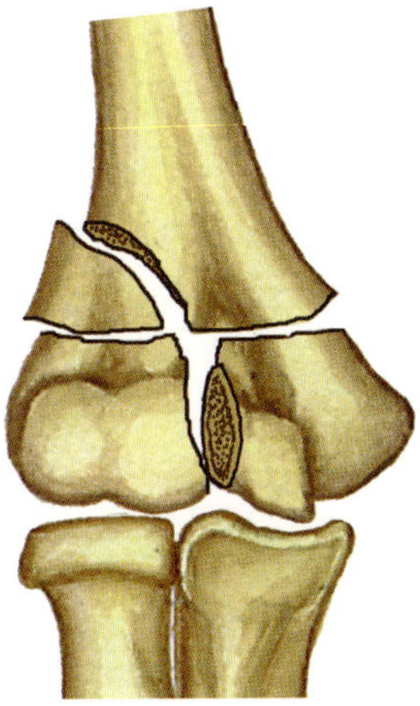

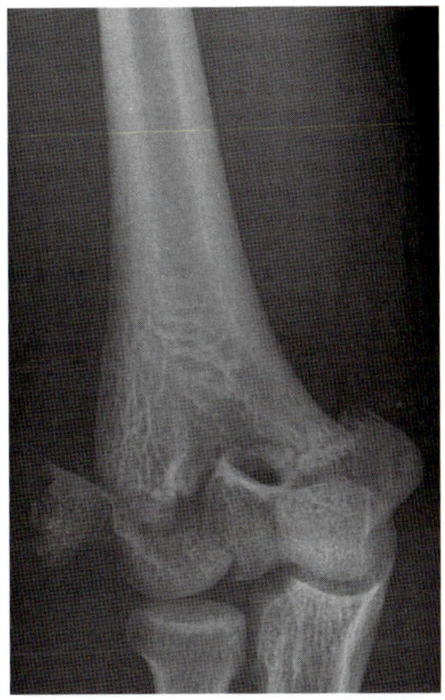

With an intact wedge

13-C2.2

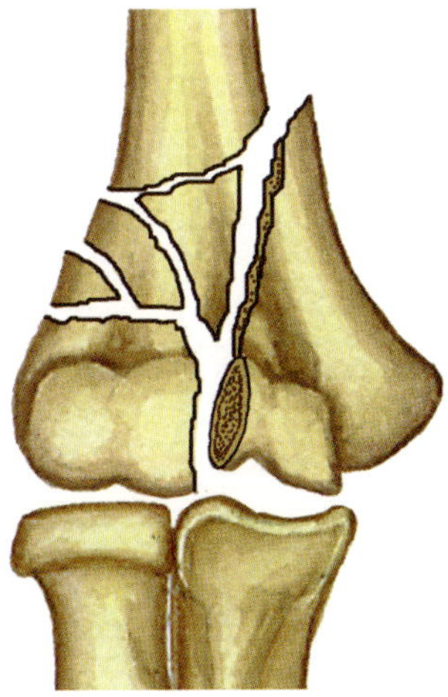

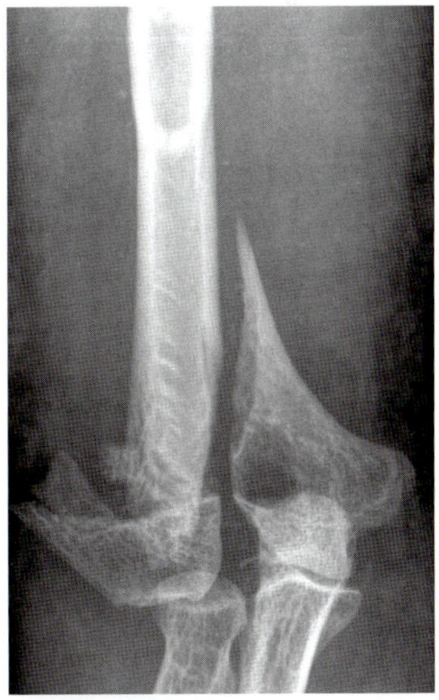

With a fragmented wedge

13-C2.3

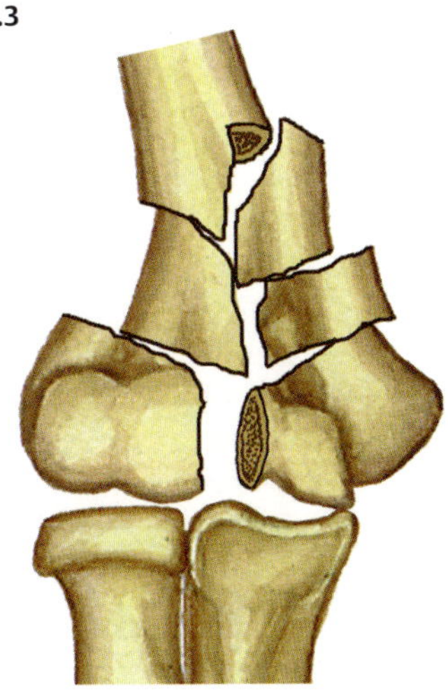

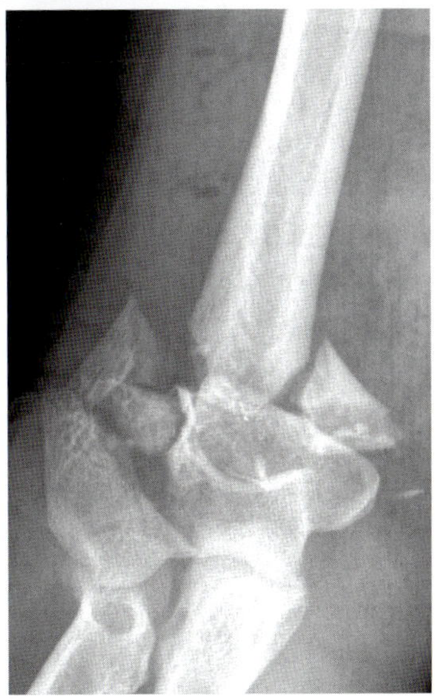

Complex

13-C Humerus distal complete articular fractures

13-C3
Humerus distal complete articular fracture, multifragmentary
286 fractures
M: 157 (54.90%)
F: 129 (45.10%)
0.08% of total adult fractures
1.31% of adult humeral fractures
7.60% of segment 13
34.71% of type 13-C

13-C3.1

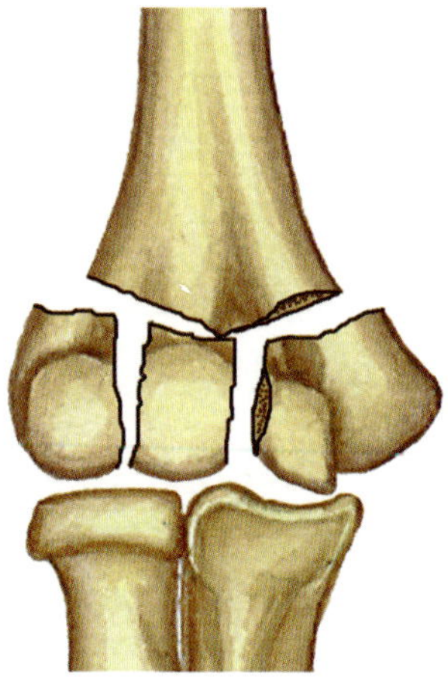

Metaphyseal simple

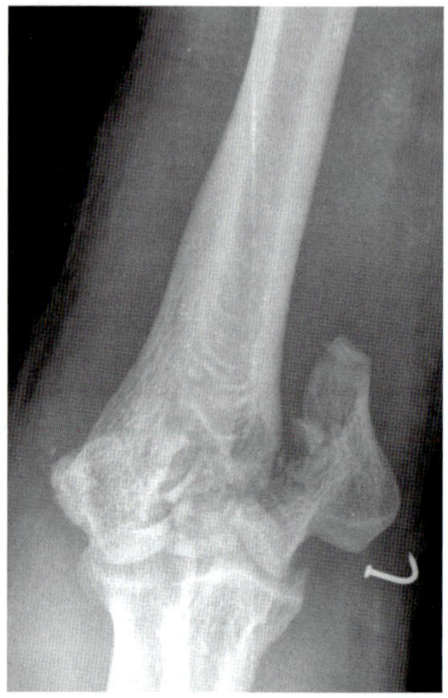

13-C3.2

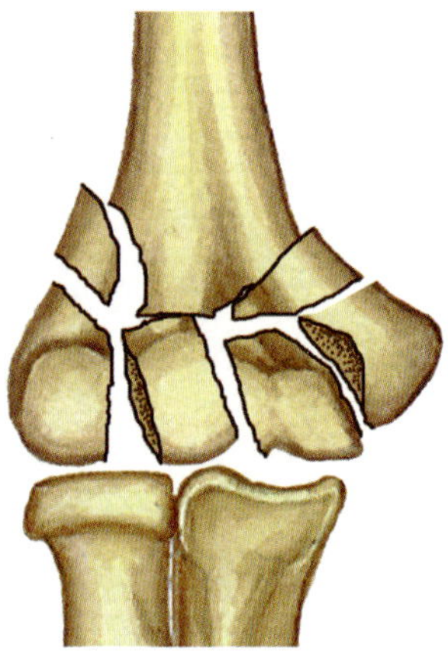

Metaphyseal wedge

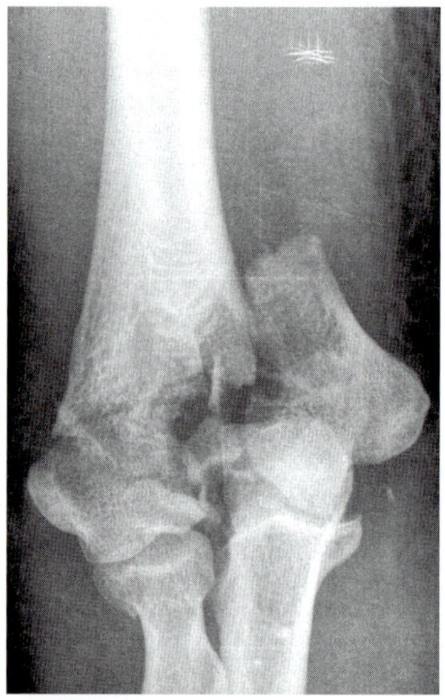

13-C3.3

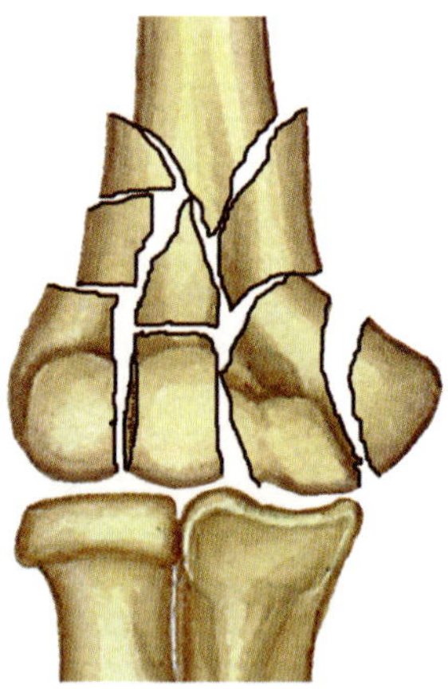

Metaphyseal multifragmentary

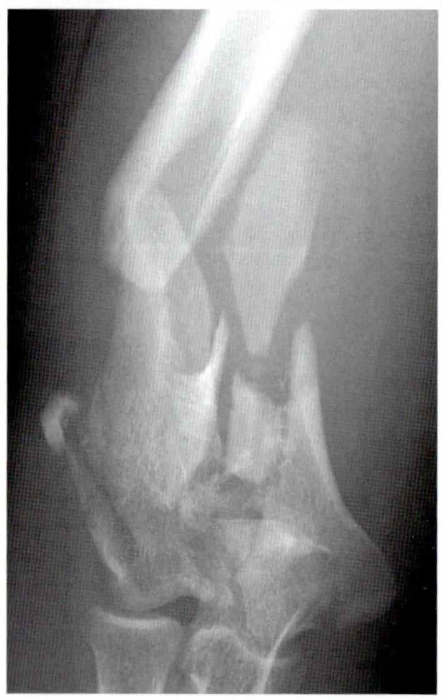

Injury Mechanism

- *Supracondylar fractures*: there are two types of supracondylar fractures: extension and flexion. The extension type accounts for most cases, and is often caused by a fall on the outstretched hand with hyperextension of the elbow, in which case the distal fragment is displaced posteriorly. The flexion type occurs less frequently, usually from a fall with the elbow flexed as it hits the ground, resulting in a fracture with anterior displacement of the distal fragment.
- *Single condylar fracture*: commonly occurs from a fall on the outstretched arm, with the elbow forced into valgus or varus position. A direct blow can also lead to single condylar fracture.
- *Capitellar fracture*: fractures of the capitellum are rare, usually caused by an axial load on the capitellum through the radius, and may be associated with radial head fractures and posterior dislocation of the elbow.
- *Bicondylar fractures*: this type of fracture is caused by a direct force applied to the elbow, especially on the olecranon when the joint is flexed about ~ 90 degrees.

Diagnosis

The patient with a fracture of the distal humerus presents with pain, swelling, and restricted motion. Deformity of the elbow may be present if there has been marked displacement. Thorough examination of the limb should be performed, including a neurovascular examination and X-rays, since such fractures may be associated with an injury of the median nerve, ulna, or brachial artery.

Radiographic evaluation for distal humeral fracture includes AP and lateral views of the elbow. CT or MRI will be required to clarify the diagnosis if there are complex fractures or severe soft tissue injuries surrounding the affected area. Angiogram or Doppler ultrasonography for evaluation of arterial injury may be indicated if Doppler pulses are absent or greatly diminished compared with the normal side and swelling is present around the fractured area.

Treatment

Most fractures with minimal or no displacement can be treated with a nonoperative approach. Closed reduction can be attempted as a first step to treat displaced fractures, and should be performed with slow, gentle, sustained maneuvers. Multiple attempts at closed reduction may be associated with a high risk of neurovascular impairment, and therefore should be avoided. Emergent operation must be performed if there is impaired circulation. For unstable fractures or after multiple failed attempts at closed treatment, surgical management should be considered, such as percutaneous pin fixation, external fixation, or open reduction with internal fixation. Since the region of the elbow is the most common site to develop myositis ossificans and malfunction postoperatively, minimal invasive surgery and internal fixation is highly recommended. In elderly patients with osteoporosis, total elbow replacement as a primary or secondary procedure has been suggested if fractures are severe.

Other Classifications of Humeral Fractures

The Neer Classification of Proximal Humeral Fractures

Overview

In 1970, Neer described his classification system for fractures of the proximal humerus into four segments of classification depending on the segment involved in fractures and the degree of displacement, and his classification system is the most commonly used for proximal humeral fracture.

Based on the presence or absence of significant displacement of one or more of the four major bone segments—humeral head, shaft, greater tuberosity, and lesser tuberosity—the Neer system classifies fractures of the proximal humerus into four types. According to Neer, a fracture is displaced when there is more than 1 cm of displacement and 45 degrees of angulation between any of the four segments in relation to one another. The Neer classification addresses the number of displaced fragments, instead of fracture lines. For example, a fracture with less than 1 cm displacement and 45 degrees of angulation is considered as a one-part fracture. The Neer system is based on several factors such as the anatomical structure where fractures occur, degree of displacement, and different combinations of displacement; therefore, the system is able to identify all possible types of proximal humeral fractures. In addition, the Neer system can help show the impact of the attached muscle on the fracture displacement and assess the blood supply to the humeral head to provide better guidance in treatment and estimate the prognosis of patients with proximal humeral fractures.

- *Type I*: one or more fractures occur in one or more of the four segments, but with minimal or no displacement, in which a segment is displaced < 1 cm or angulated/rotated < 45 degrees. Though the soft tissue and blood supply to the fragment remain intact, this group accounts for the majority of all proximal humeral fractures.
- *Type II*: fractures occur in one or more of the four segments, with one fracture fragment displaced > 1 cm and angulated/rotated > 45 degrees. In this group, displaced surgical neck fractures are most commonly seen.

2

- *Type III*: fractures occur in one or more of the four segments, with two fracture fragments displaced > 1 cm, and angulated/rotated > 45 degrees. Glenohumeral dislocation (fracture-dislocation) is included in this group.
- *Type IV*: all the humeral segments are displaced, including dislocation of the humeral head. In this group, the humeral head is isolated and its main blood supply is disrupted.

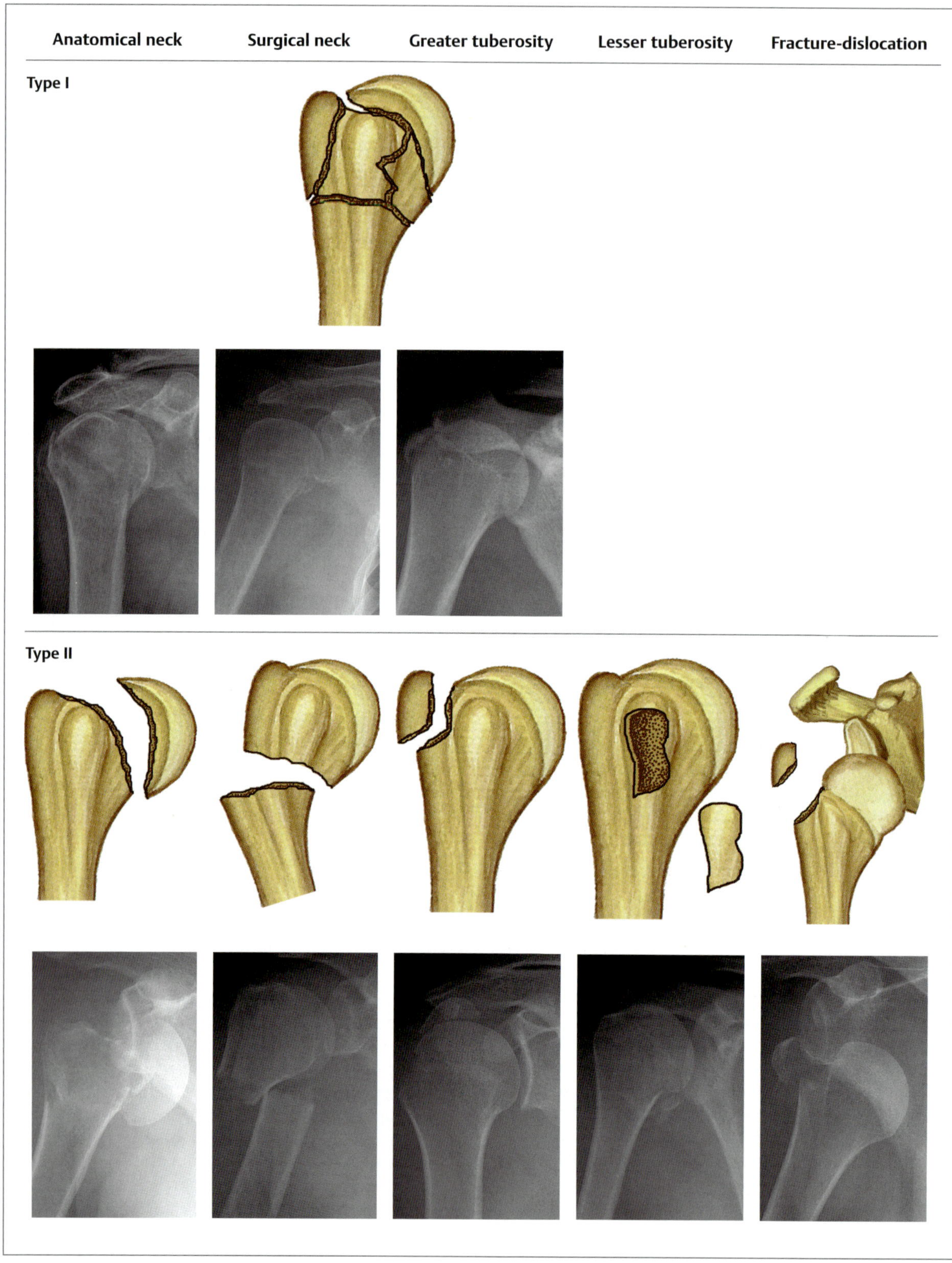

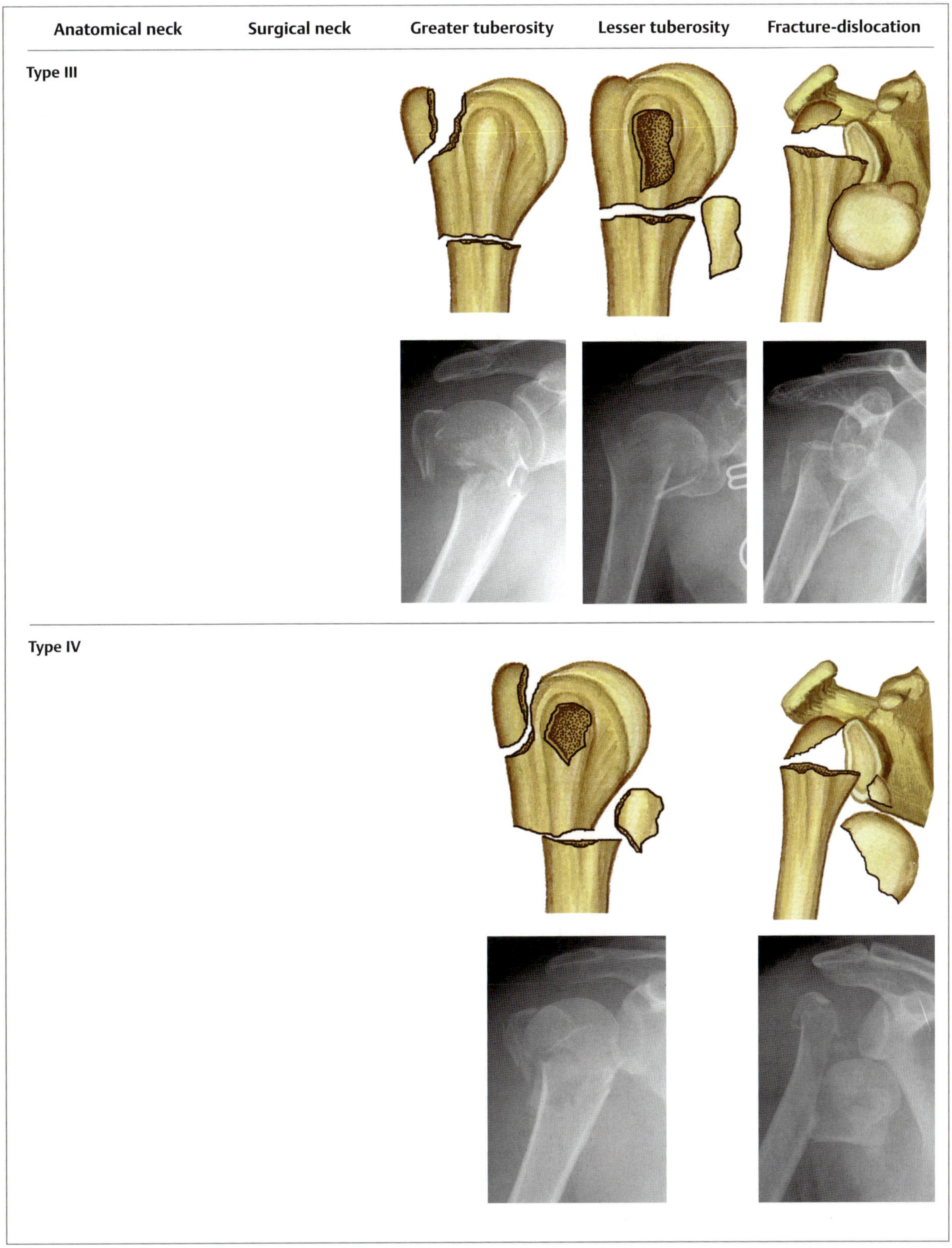
Anatomical neck
Surgical neck
Greater tuberosity
Lesser tuberosity
Fracture-dislocation
Type III
Type IV

Clinical Epidemiologic Features for Neer Classification

A total of 13,361 proximal humeral fractures based on the Neer classification were treated in 83 hospitals in China over a 2-year period from 2010 to 2011. All cases were reviewed and statistically studies were performed; the fractures accounted for 91.66% of all the proximal humeral fractures. The epidemiologic features are as follows:

- More females than males
- Type I fractures account for most cases.

Table 2.18 Sex and fracture type distribution of 13,361 proximal humeral fractures by Neer classification

Fracture type	Male	Female	Number of fractures	Percentage (%)
Type I	2,958	3,969	6,927	51.84
Type II	1,781	2,469	4,250	31.81
Type III	620	1,065	1,685	12.61
Type IV	212	287	499	3.73
Total	5,571	7,790	13,361	100.00

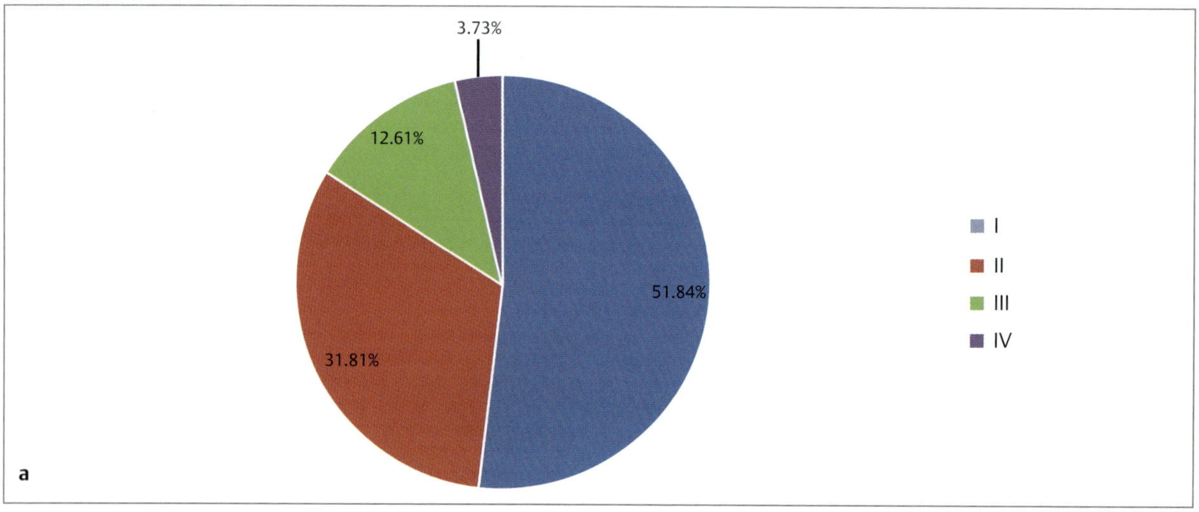

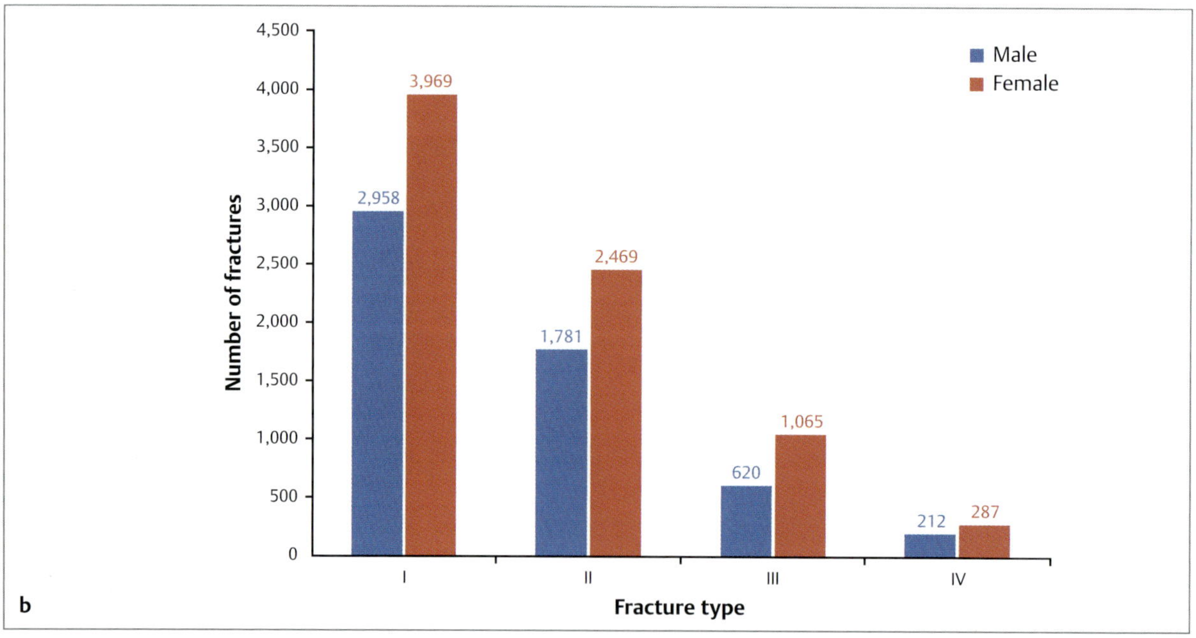

Fig. 2.18 **(a)** Fracture type distribution of 13,361 proximal humeral fractures by Neer classification. **(b)** Sex and fracture type distribution of 13,361 proximal humeral fractures by Neer classification.

Classification of Humeral Fractures by Fracture Location

Supracondylar Humeral Fractures

Overview

Supracondylar humeral fracture is mostly caused by indirect force on the elbow, with various injury mechanisms and fracture patterns. There are two types of supracondylar fractures, extension and flexion type, both based on the mechanism of the injury.

Extension Type

The extension type fracture is caused by a fall on an outstretched hand when the elbow is hyperextended. When a fall occurs, the impact force from the ground transmits to the elbow through the forearm and results in a fracture. The distal fragment of the humerus will displace posteriorly, with anterior displacement of the proximal fragment. The fracture line runs obliquely downward from posterior to anterior. When the displacement is severe, the proximal fracture fragment often injures the brachial muscle, median nerve, and brachial artery (**Plates 2.22, 2.23, 2.24,** and **2.25**).

Flexion Type

The flexion type of fracture is rare, and is caused by a fall on the olecranon when the elbow is flexed. The impact force on the olecranon transmitted vertically to the condyle can result in supracondylar fractures. The distal fragment will displace anteriorly, and the proximal fragment posteriorly. The fracture line runs obliquely downward from anterior to posterior (**Plates 2.26, 2.27, 2.28,** and **2.29**).

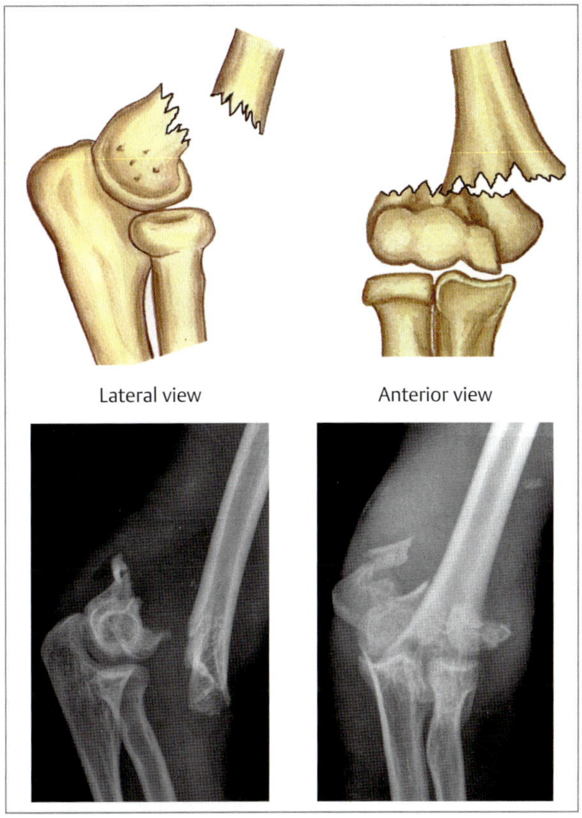

Plates 2.22–2.25

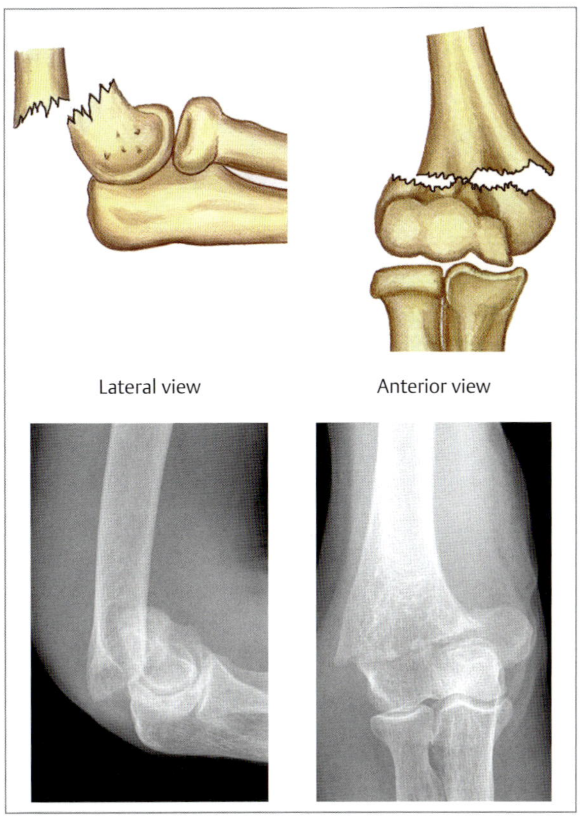

Plates 2.26–2.29

Clinical Epidemiologic Features of Supracondylar Humeral Fractures

A total of 6,323 supracondylar fractures of the humerus were treated in 83 hospitals in China over a 2-year period from 2010 to 2011. All cases were reviewed and statistically studied; the fractures accounted for 17.66% of all humeral fractures. The epidemiologic features are as follows:

- More males than females
- The high-risk age group is 0–5 years
- Extension types of fractures account for the majority of cases.

2

Supracondylar Humeral Fractures by Sex

Table 2.19 Sex distribution of 6,323 supracondylar fractures of the humerus

Sex	Number of fractures	Percentage (%)
Male	3,865	61.13
Female	2,458	38.87
Total	6,323	100.00

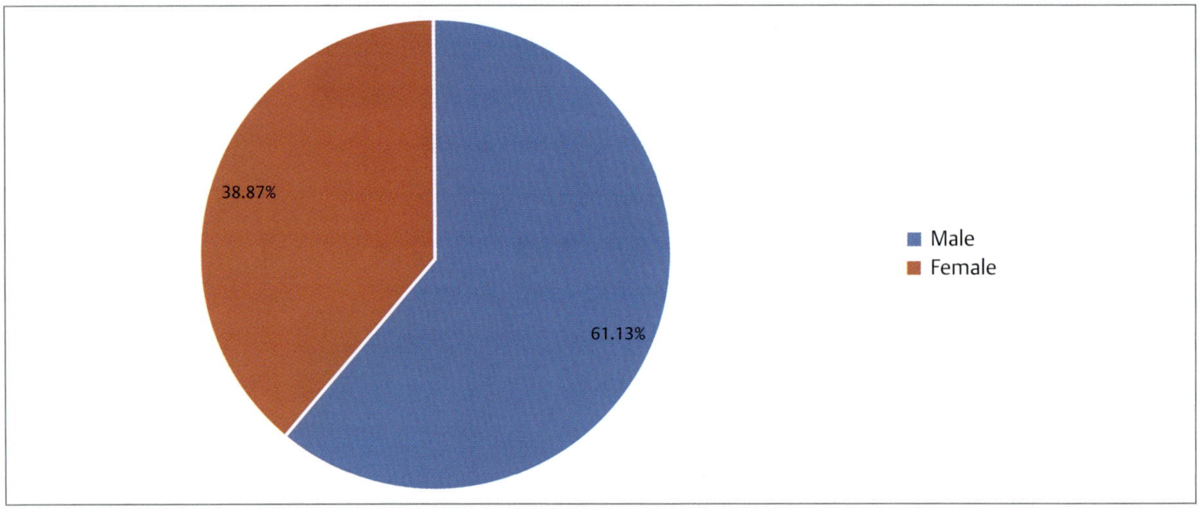

Fig. 2.19 Sex distribution of 6,323 supracondylar fractures of the humerus.

Supracondylar Humeral Fractures by Age Group

Table 2.20 Age and sex distribution of 6,323 supracondylar fractures of the humerus

Age group (years)	Male	Female	Number of fractures	Percentage (%)
0–5	1,500	1,174	2,674	42.29
6–10	1,561	761	2,322	36.72
11–15	441	146	587	9.28
16–20	53	19	72	1.14
21–25	29	26	55	0.87
26–30	37	15	52	0.82
31–35	36	21	57	0.90
36–40	38	20	58	0.92
41–45	21	14	35	0.55
46–50	29	10	39	0.62
51–55	48	30	78	1.23
56–60	23	38	61	0.96
61–65	12	25	37	0.59
66–70	9	27	36	0.57
71–75	5	30	35	0.55
76–80	13	39	52	0.82
81–85	6	38	44	0.70
≥86	4	25	29	0.46
Total	3,865	2,458	6,323	100.00

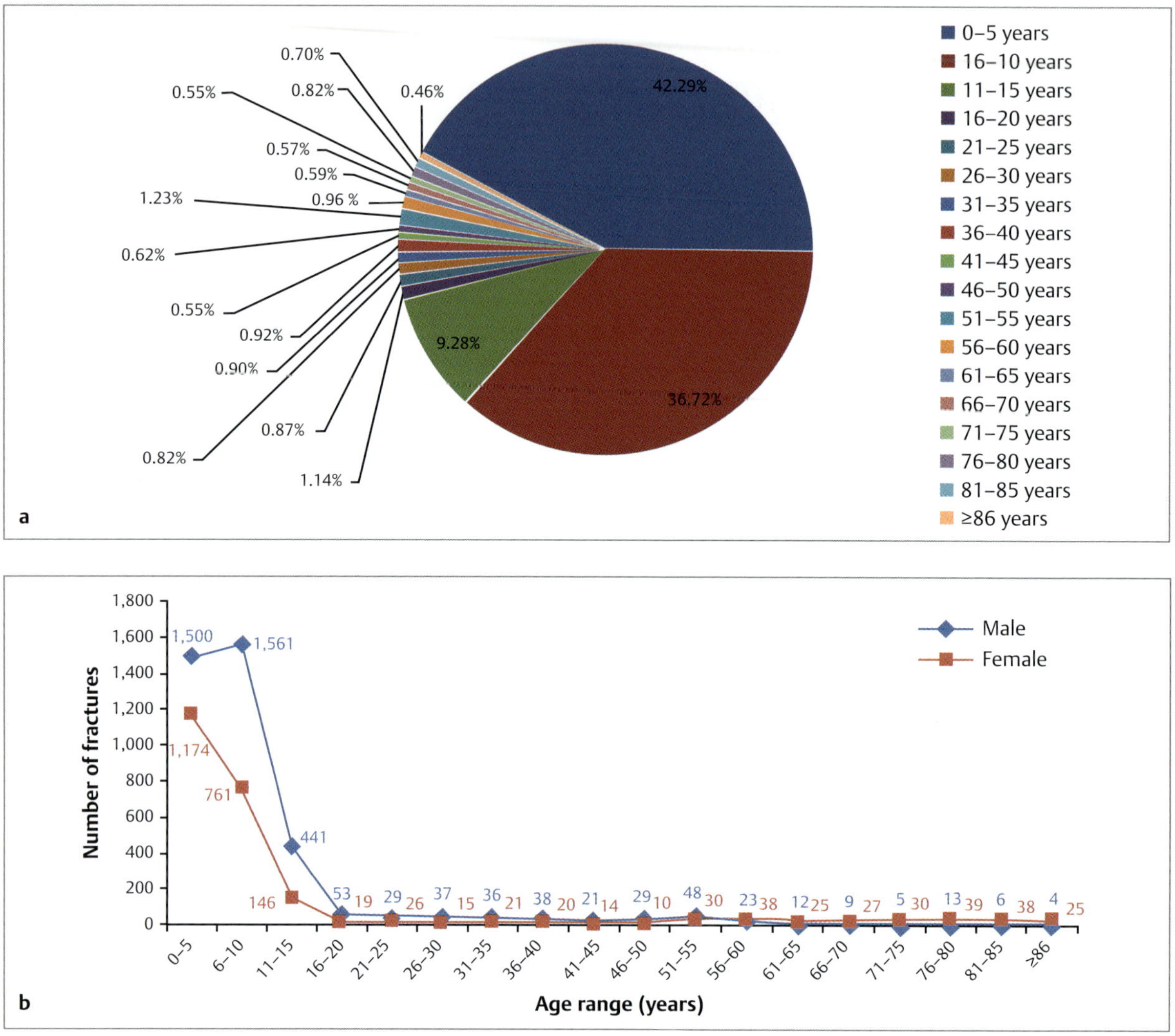

Fig. 2.20 **(a)** Age distribution of 6,323 supracondylar fractures of the humerus.
(b) Age and sex distribution of 6,323 supracondylar fractures of the humerus.

Supracondylar Humeral Fractures by Fracture Pattern

Table 2.21 Sex and fracture pattern distribution of 6,087 supracondylar fractures of the humerus

Fracture pattern	Male	Female	Number of fractures	Percentage (%)
Extension	2,914	1,859	4,773	78.41
Flexion	792	522	1,314	21.59
Total	3,706	2,381	6,087	100.00

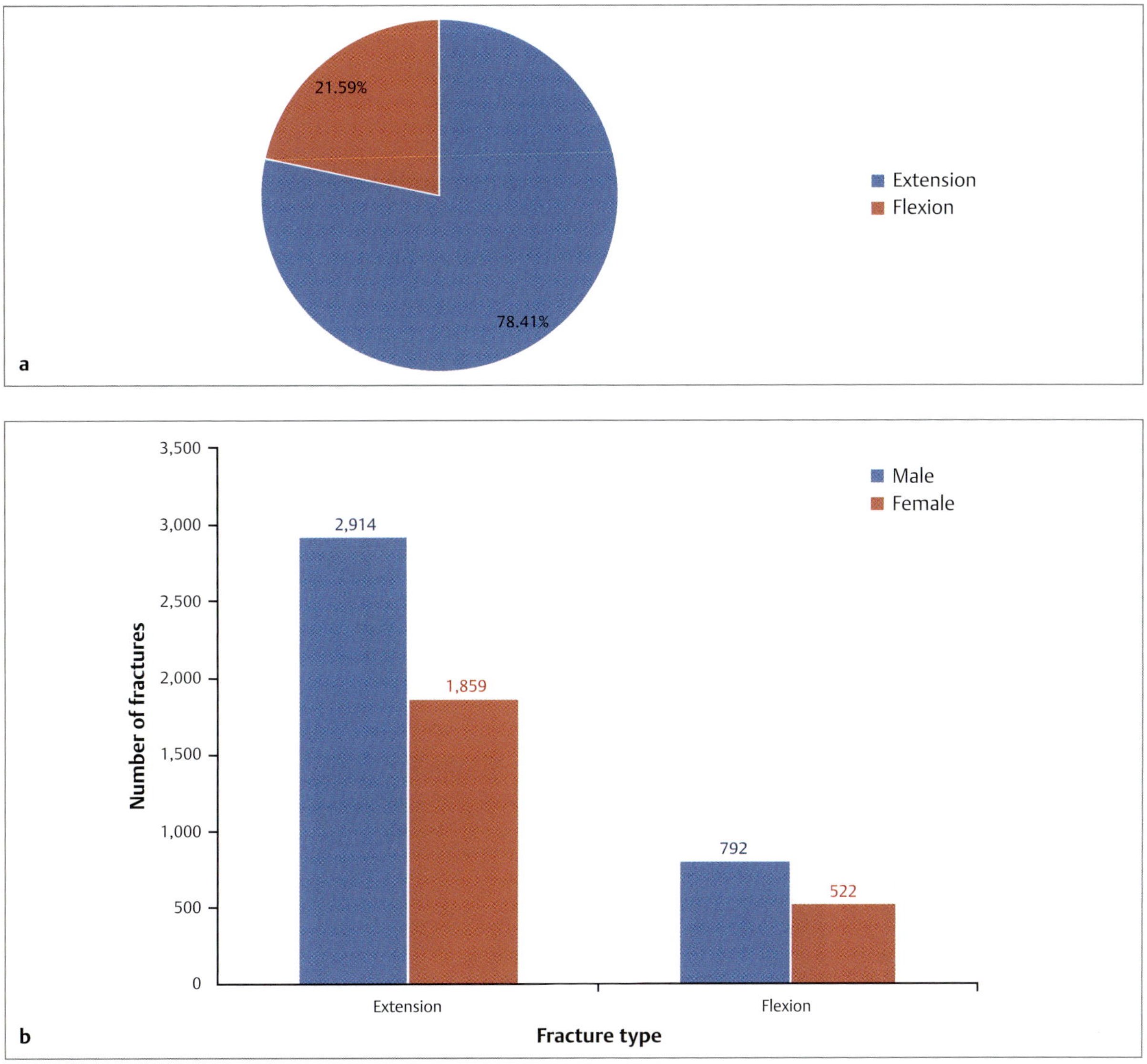

Fig. 2.21 **(a)** Fracture pattern distribution of 6,087 supracondylar fractures of the humerus. **(b)** Sex and fracture pattern distribution of 6,087 supracondylar fractures of the humerus.

Intercondylar Humeral Fractures

Overview

Rise classified intercondylar fractures of the humerus into four types, based on the degree of fracture displacement (**Plates 2.30, 2.31, 2.32, 2.33, 2.34, 2.35, 2.36,** and **2.37**).

- *Type I*: with minimal or no displacement, congruity of the articular surface remains.
- *Type II*: displacement between the trochlea and capitellum; the articular surface is nearly intact with no rotation of either fracture fragment.
- *Type III*: displacement and separation of fragments with rotation; congruity of the articular surface is compromised.
- *Type IV*: multifragmentary fractures with significant displacement and severely damaged articular surface. The fracture fragment may penetrate through the skin to form open fractures.

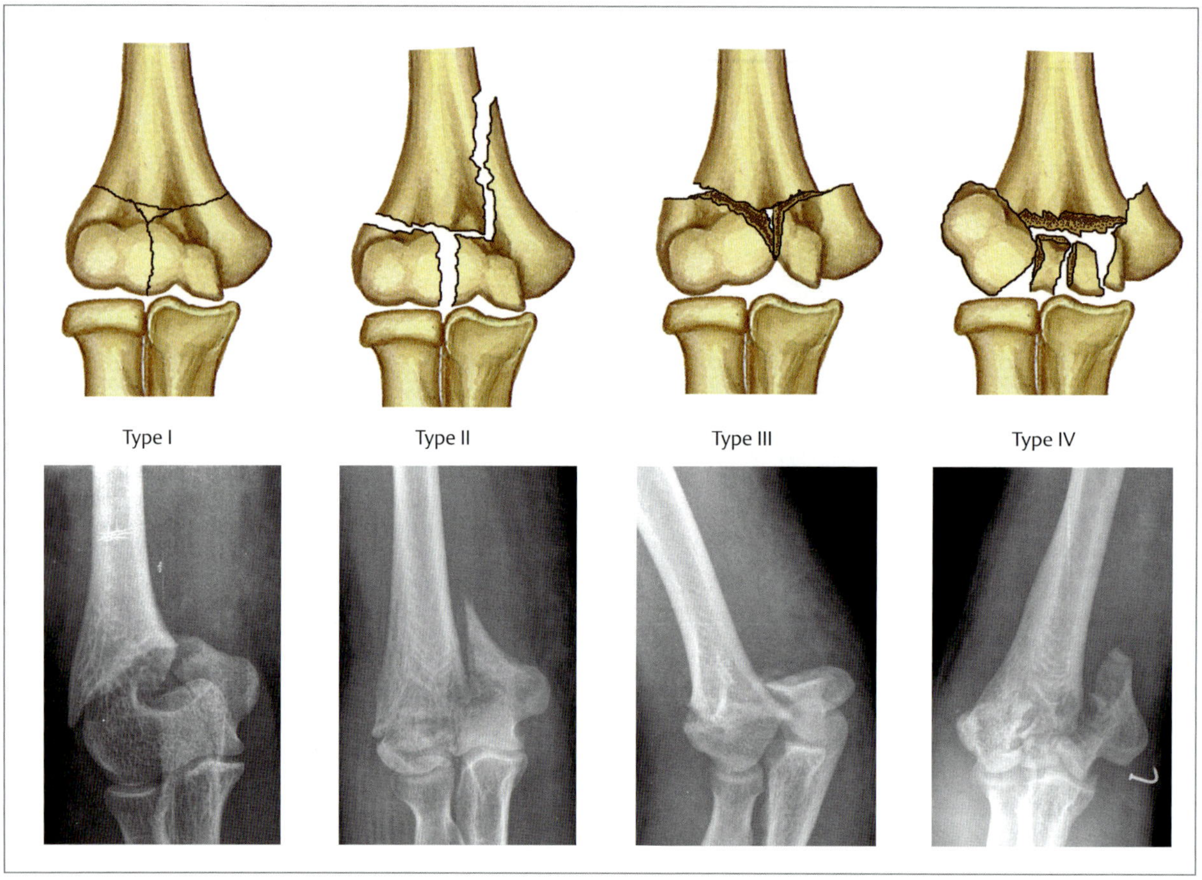

Plates 2.30–2.37

Clinical Epidemiologic Features of Intercondylar Humeral Fractures

A total of 1,318 intercondylar fractures of the humerus were treated in 83 hospitals in China over a 2-year period from 2010 to 2011. All cases were reviewed and statistically studied; the fractures accounted for 3.68% of all humeral fractures. The epidemiologic features are as follows:

- More males than females
- The high-risk age group is 0–5 years and 6–10 years; 0–5 years and 6–10 years for males, 0–5 years for females.

Intercondylar Humeral Fractures by Sex

Table 2.22 Sex distribution of 1,318 intercondylar fractures of the humerus

Sex	Number of fractures	Percentage (%)
Male	752	57.06
Female	566	42.94
Total	1,318	100.00

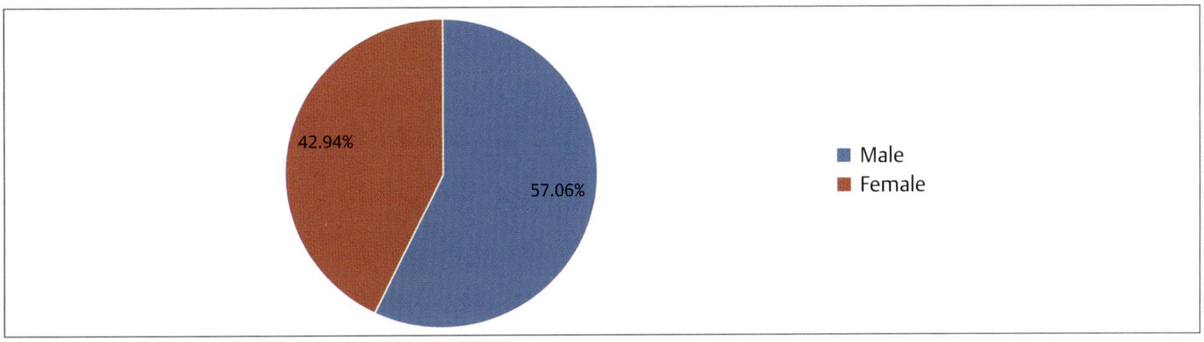

Fig. 2.22 Sex distribution of 1,318 intercondylar fractures of the humerus.

2

Intercondylar Humeral Fractures by Age Group

Table 2.23 Age and sex distribution of 1,318 intercondylar fractures of the humerus

Age group (years)	Male	Female	Number of fractures	Percentage (%)
0–5	132	105	237	17.98
6–10	134	55	189	14.34
11–15	68	33	101	7.66
16–20	46	24	70	5.31
21–25	39	35	74	5.61
26–30	38	10	48	3.64
31–35	61	19	80	6.07
36–40	58	17	75	5.69
41–45	44	23	67	5.08
46–50	38	18	56	4.25
51–55	29	28	57	4.32
56–60	30	38	68	5.16
61–65	14	43	57	4.32
66–70	7	31	38	2.88
71–75	4	31	35	2.66
76–80	4	29	33	2.50
81–85	2	17	19	1.44
≥86	4	10	14	1.06
Total	752	566	1,318	100.00

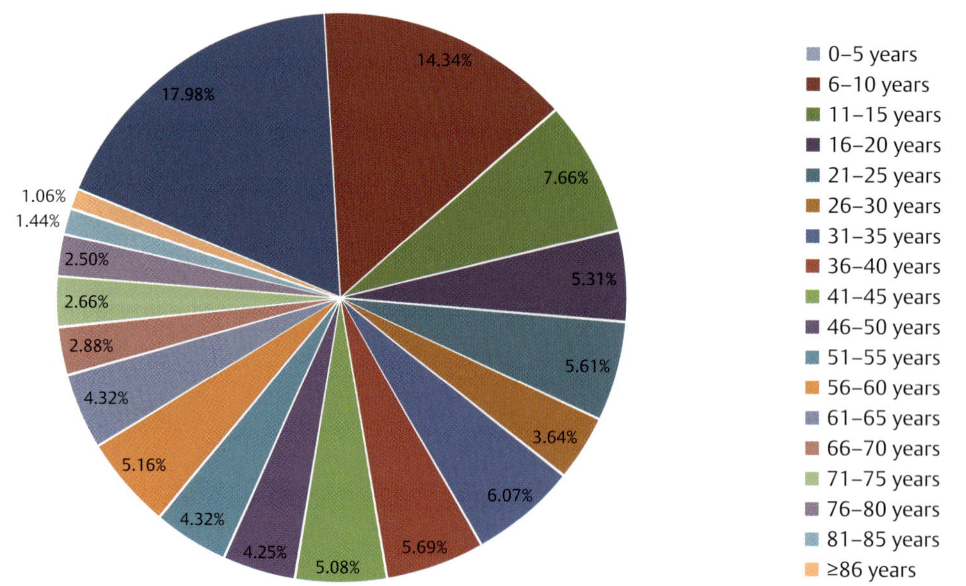

a

Fig. 2.23 **(a)** Age distribution of 1,318 intercondylar fractures of the humerus.

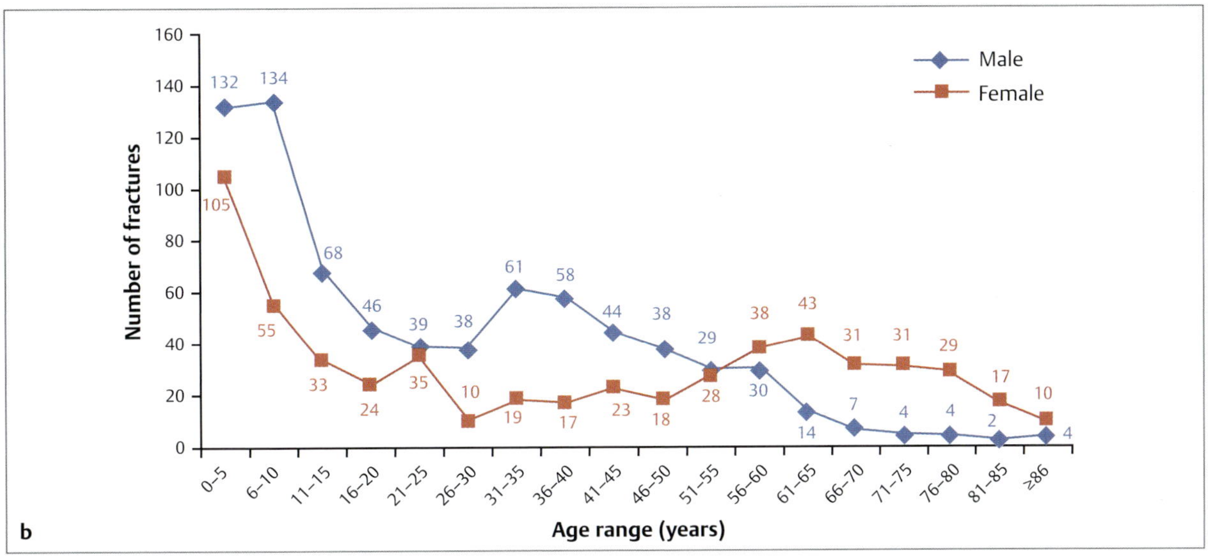

Fig. 2.23 (*continued*) **(b)** Age and sex distribution of 1,318 intercondylar fractures of the humerus.

Lateral Humeral Condylar Fractures

Overview

Lateral condylar fracture of the humerus is often caused by a fall on the outstretched arm with the forearm in abduction, which transmits a force through the forearm extensor musculature to its attachment on the lateral condyle. This type of fracture may also result from a fall onto the extended hand, leading to impaction of the radial head into the lateral condyle. The same force may also lead to impaction of the coronoid process of the ulna into the trochlea, and consequently result in fractures in the lateral aspect of the trochlea. Because the elbow position varies as the injury occurs, the direction of fracture displacement and size of the fragment are markedly different from each other.

Lateral humeral condylar fracture is classified into four types, based on the degree of fracture displacement (**Plates 2.38–2.45**).

- *Type I* (nondisplaced): with minimal or no displacement
- *Type II* (lateral displacement): the fracture fragment is displaced laterally and posteriorly without rotation
- *Type III* (rotatory displacement): complete displacement with rotation. The rotation of the fragment can be 90 degrees, or 180 degrees in severe fractures.
- *Type IV* (fracture dislocation): the lateral condylar fragment is displaced laterally, often associated with dislocation of the elbow, which may be medial, lateral, or posterior.

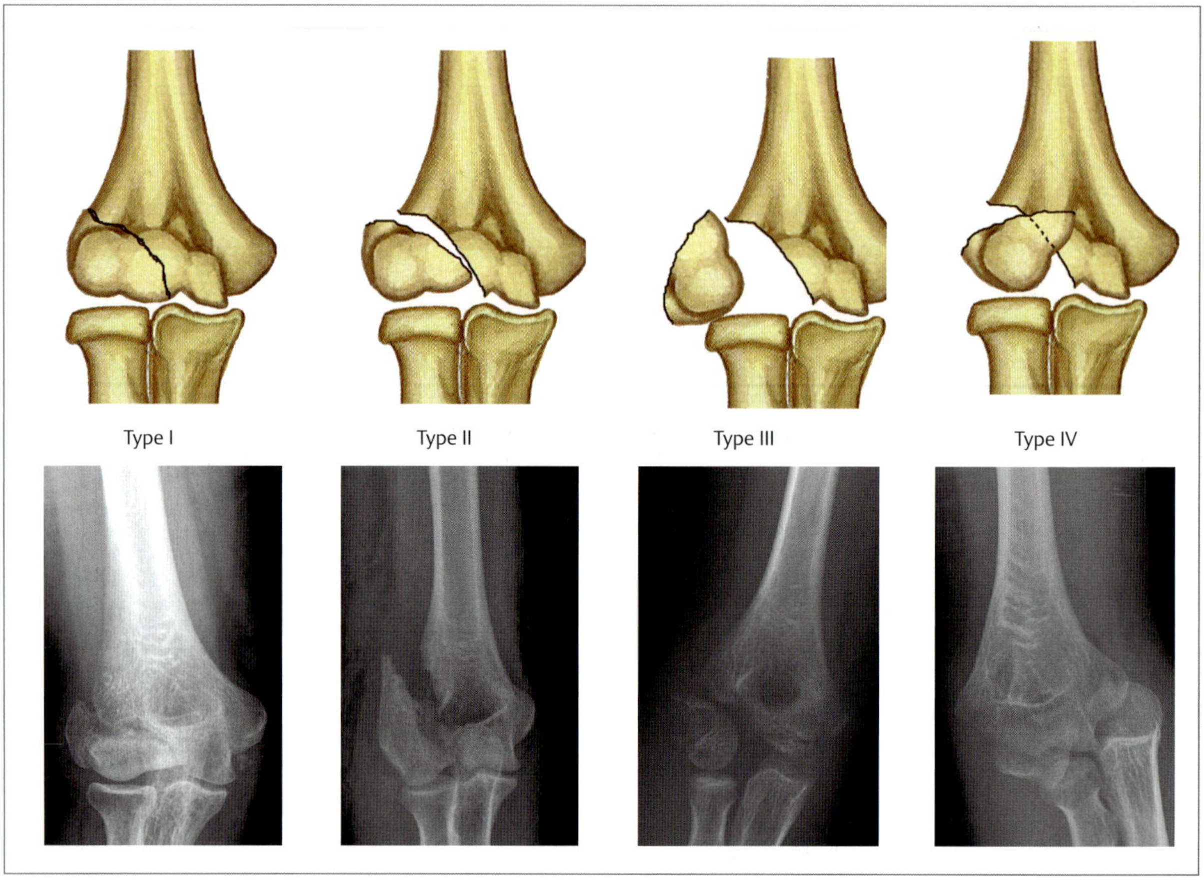

Plates 2.38–2.45

Clinical Epidemiologic Features of Lateral Humeral Condylar Fractures

A total of 1,971 lateral humeral condylar fractures were treated in 83 hospitals in China over a 2-year period from 2010 to 2011. All cases were reviewed and statistically studied; the fractures accounted for 5.50% of all humeral factures. The epidemiologic features are as follows:

- More males than females
- The high-risk age group is 0–5 years and 6–10 years.

Lateral Humeral Condylar Fractures by Sex

Table 2.24 Sex distribution of 1,971 lateral condylar fractures of the humerus

Sex	Number of fractures	Percentage (%)
Male	1,326	67.28
Female	645	32.72
Total	1,971	100.00

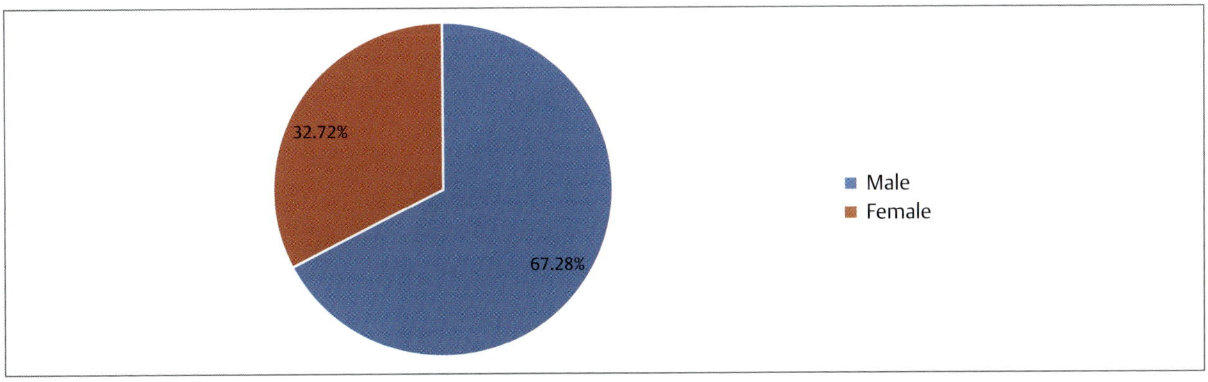

Fig. 2.24 Sex distribution of 1,971 lateral condylar fractures of the humerus.

Lateral Humeral Condylar Fractures by Age Group

Table 2.25 Age and sex distribution of 1,971 lateral condylar fractures of the humerus

Age group (years)	Male	Female	Number of fractures	Percentage (%)
0–5	557	310	867	43.99
6–10	423	119	542	27.50
11–15	111	27	138	7.00
16–20	39	9	48	2.44
21–25	41	4	45	2.28
26–30	30	11	41	2.08
31–35	22	13	35	1.78
36–40	25	13	38	1.93
41–45	21	17	38	1.93
46–50	20	17	37	1.88
51–55	18	22	40	2.03
56–60	5	25	30	1.52
61–65	3	13	16	0.81
66–70	5	18	23	1.17
71–75	1	15	16	0.81
76–80	2	6	8	0.41
81–85	1	3	4	0.20
≥86	2	3	5	0.25
Total	1,326	645	1,971	100.00

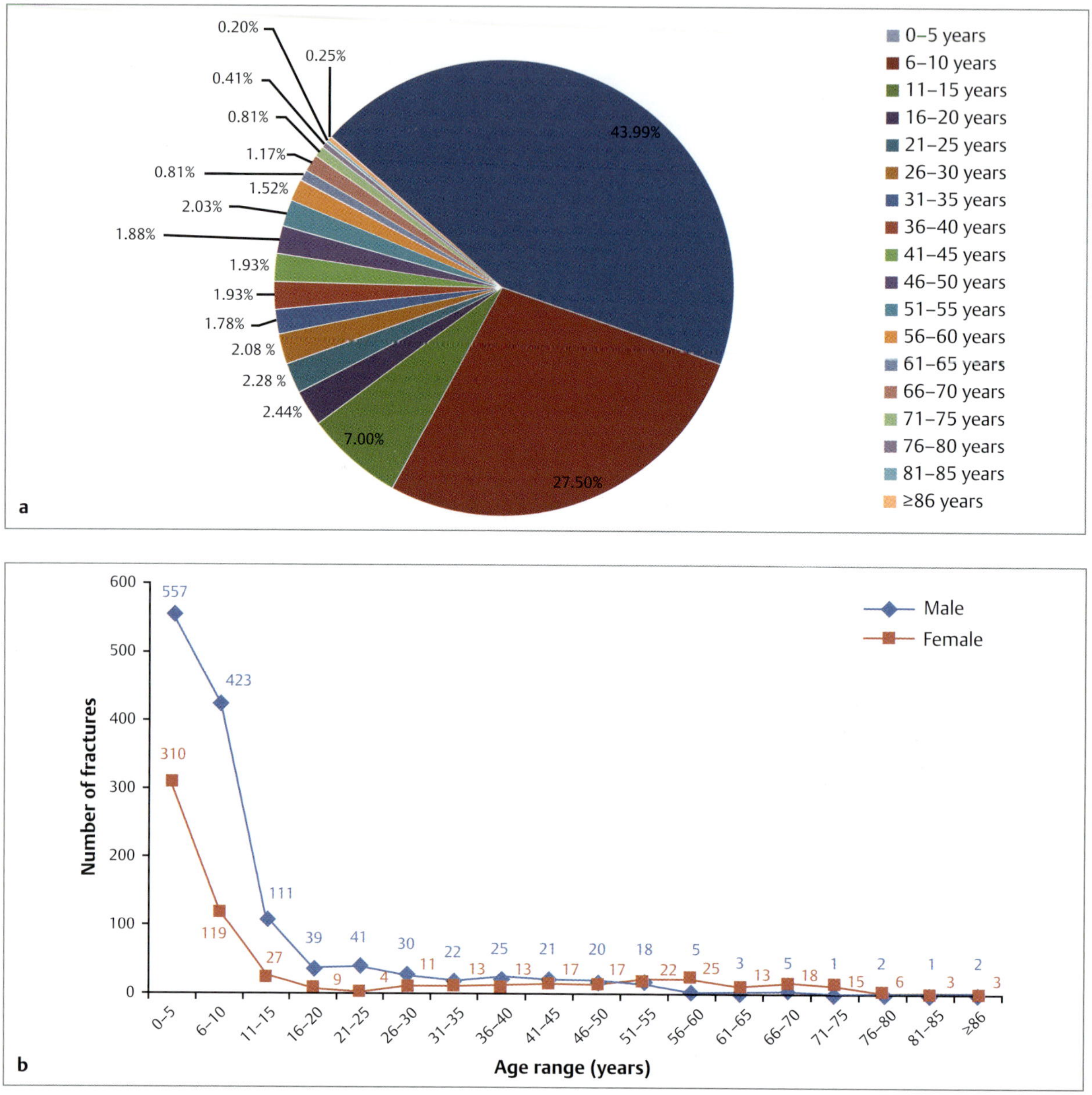

Fig. 2.25 **(a)** Age distribution of 1,971 lateral condylar fractures of the humerus.
(b) Age and sex distribution of 1,971 lateral condylar fractures of the humerus.

Medial Humeral Condylar Fractures

Overview

The true mechanism of injury for medial condylar fracture of the humerus remains unclear. It is likely to occur when violent force transmits to or directly acts on the elbow. In effect, the trochlear (semilunar) notch of the ulna strikes on the medial condyle and leads to fracture of the medial condyle.

Depending on the course of the fracture line and the displacement of medial condylar fragment, medial humeral condylar fracture is classified into three types (**Plates 2.46–2.50**):

- *Type I*: with minimal or no displacement between fragments. The fracture line runs obliquely downward and outward from the medial epicondyle up to the trochlear articulation surface.
- *Type II*: similar fracture line course as in type I, but the fragment is displaced either laterally or slightly upward, with no rotation.
- *Type III*: the fracture line is the same as seen in type II; however, here the fragment is displaced ulnarly or anteriorly, with rotary dislocation.

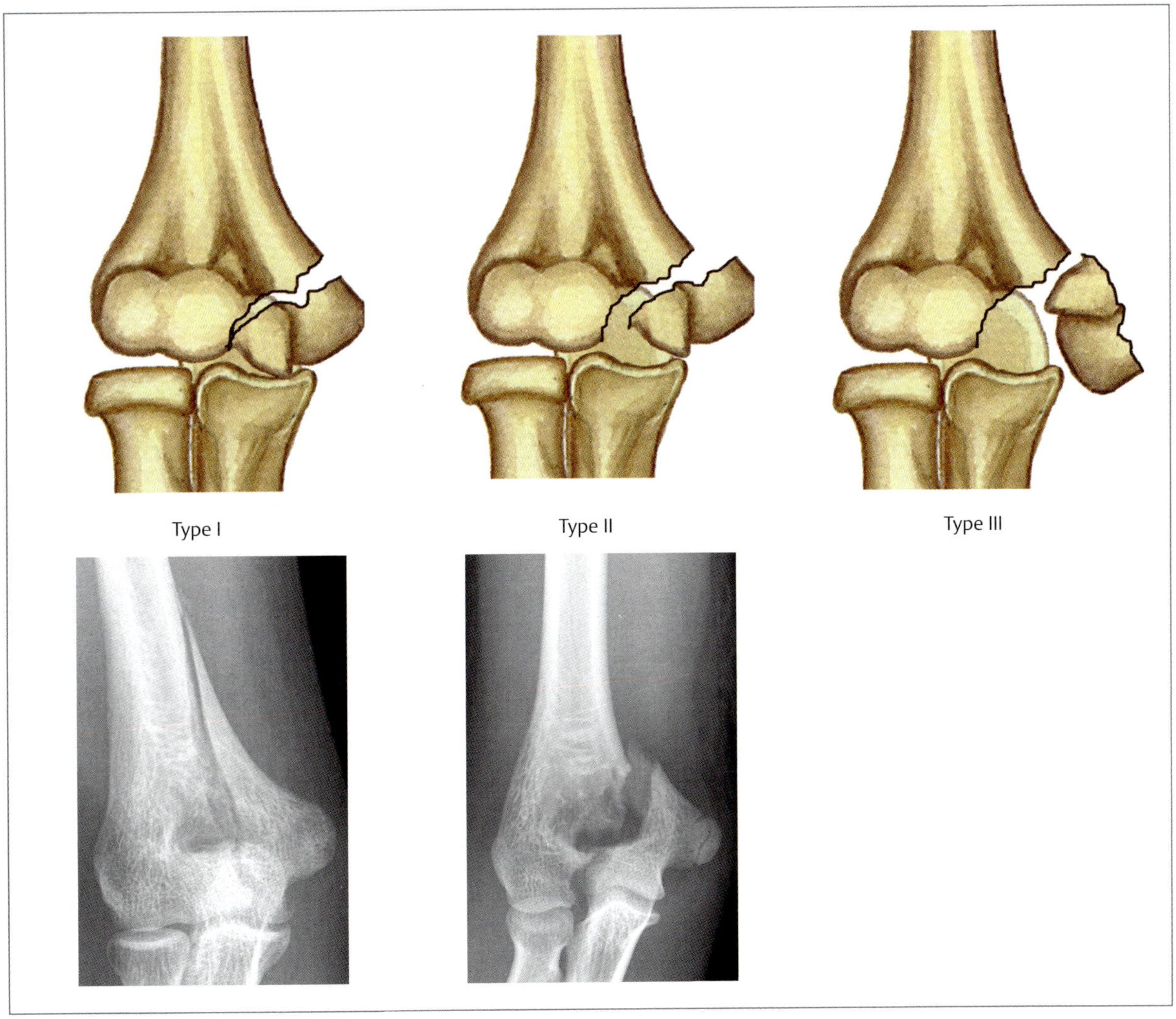

Plates 2.46–2.50

Clinical Epidemiologic Features of Medial Humeral Condylar Fractures

A total of 895 medial humeral condylar fractures were treated in 83 hospitals in China over a 2-year period from 2010 to 2011; the fractures accounted for 2.50% of all humeral fractures. The epidemiologic features are as follows:

- More males than females
- The high risk age group is 0–5 years and 6–10 years.

Medial Humeral Condylar Fractures by Sex

Table 2.26 Sex distribution of 895 medial condylar fractures of the humerus

Sex	Number of fractures	Percentage (%)
Male	560	62.57
Female	335	37.43
Total	895	100.00

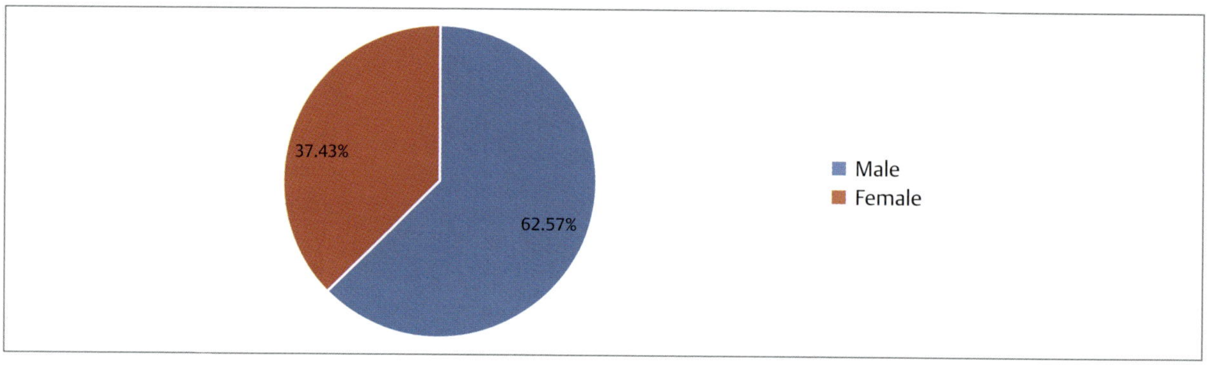

Fig. 2.26 Sex distribution of 895 medial condylar fractures of the humerus.

Medial Humeral Condylar Fractures by Age Group

Table 2.27 Age and sex distribution of 895 medial condylar fractures of the humerus

Age group (years)	Male	Female	Number of fractures	Percentage (%)
0–5	212	113	325	36.31
6–10	114	64	178	19.89
11–15	67	23	90	10.06
16–20	39	12	51	5.70
21–25	12	11	23	2.57
26–30	19	8	27	3.02
31–35	14	7	21	2.35
36–40	14	10	24	2.68
41–45	23	8	31	3.46
46–50	17	8	25	2.79
51–55	8	9	17	1.90
56–60	7	17	24	2.68
61–65	0	12	12	1.34
66–70	4	9	13	1.45
71–75	2	8	10	1.12
76–80	7	7	14	1.56
81–85	1	4	5	0.56
≥86	0	5	5	0.56
Total	560	335	895	100.00

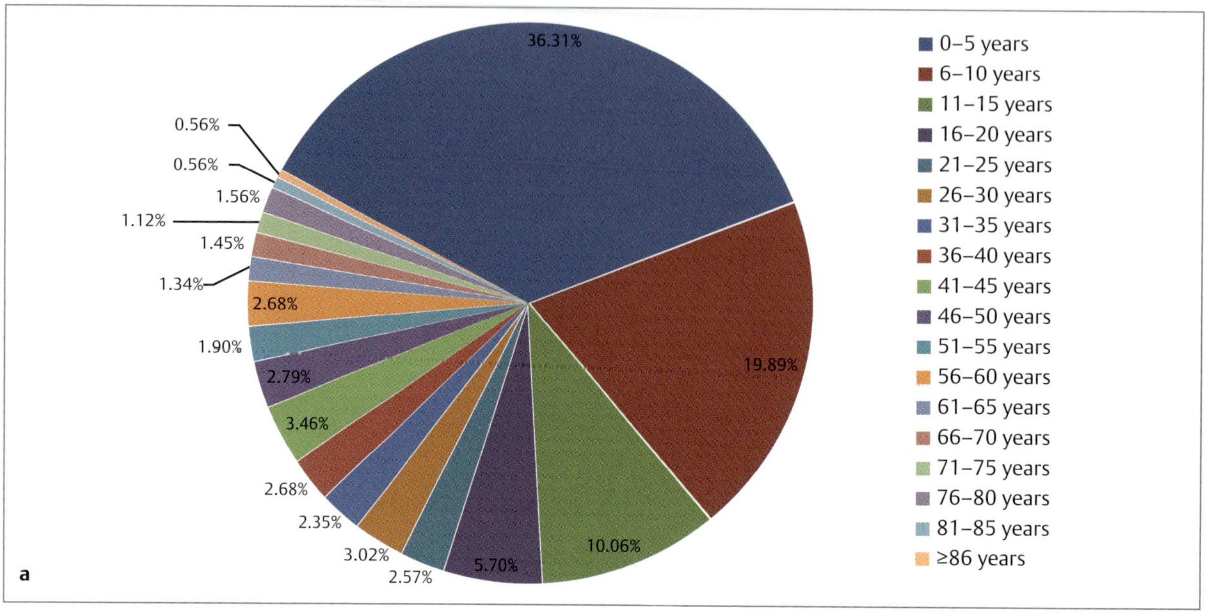

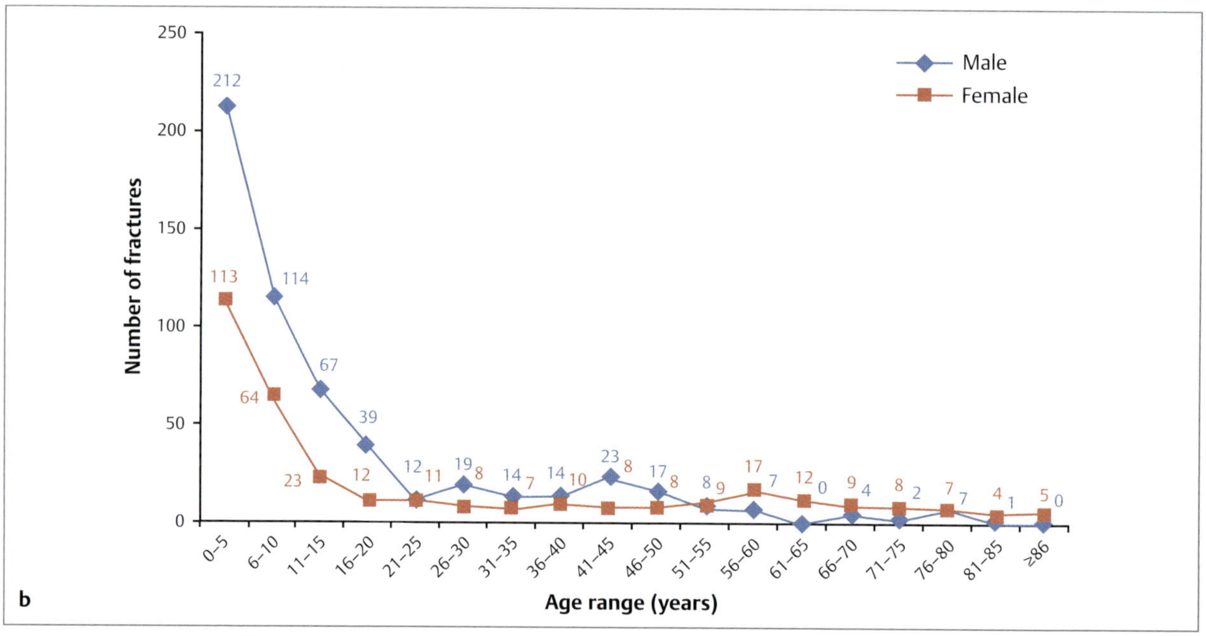

Fig. 2.27 **(a)** Age distribution of 895 medial condylar fractures of the humerus.
(b) Age and sex distribution of 895 medial condylar fractures of humerus.

Lateral Humeral Epicondyle Fractures

Overview

This type of injury is often seen as an avulsion fracture due to violent contraction of the extensor muscle; the mechanism involves a fall on an outstretched hand with the forearm in excessive pronation and adduction. Fragments may be slightly displaced or may have 60 to 180 degrees of rotary dislocation (**Plates 2.51–2.56**).

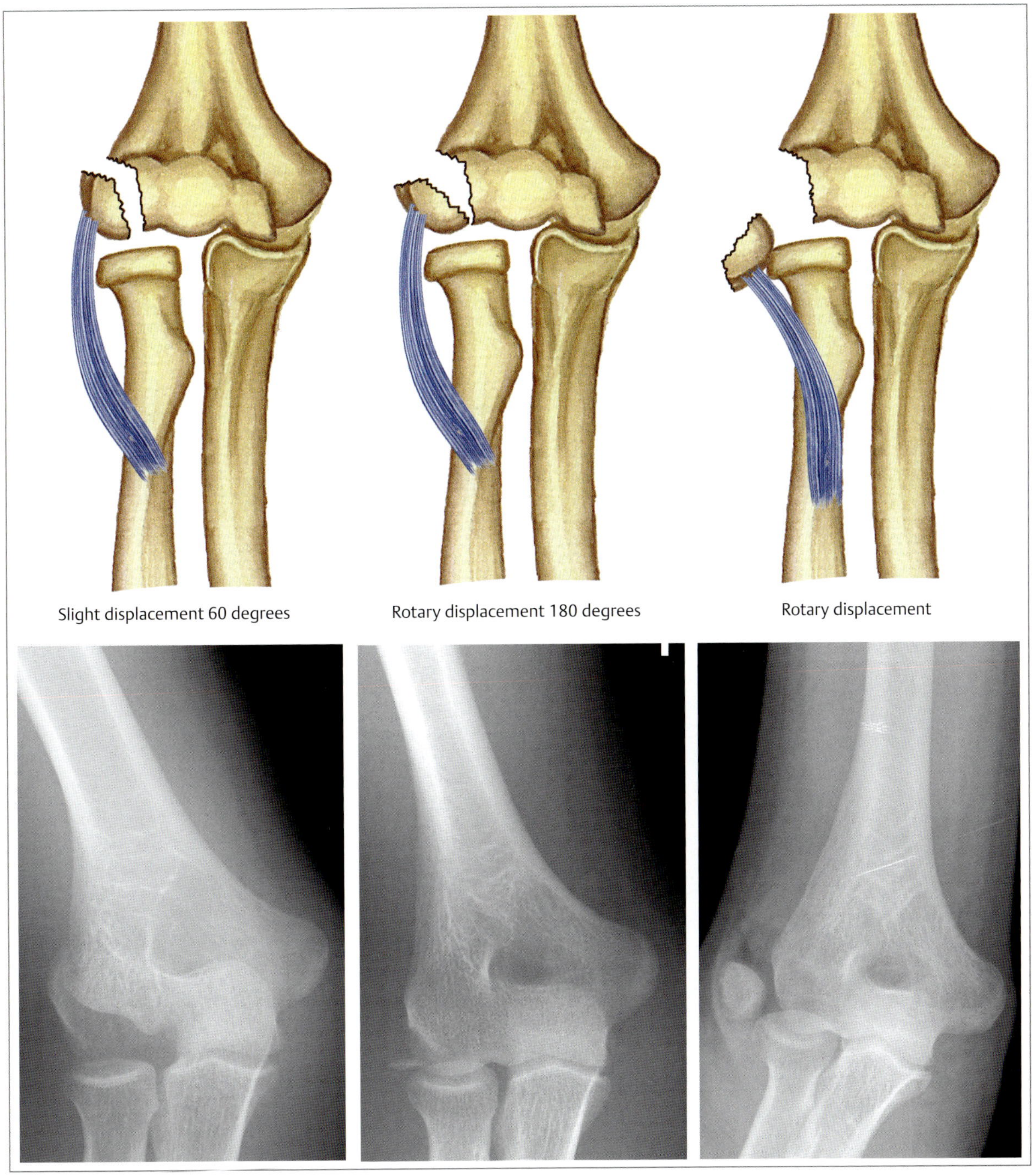

Plate 2.51–2.56

Clinical Epidemiologic Features of Lateral Humeral Epicondyle Fractures

A total of 756 lateral humeral epicondyle fractures were treated in 83 hospitals in China over a 2- year period from 2010 to 2011. All cases were reviewed and statistically studied; the fractures accounted for 2.11% of all humeral fractures. Their epidemiologic features are as follows:
- More males than females
- The high-risk age group is 0–5 years and 6–10 years.

Lateral Humeral Epicondyle Fractures by Sex

Table 2.28 Sex distribution of 756 lateral epicondyle fractures of the humerus

Sex	Number of fractures	Percentage (%)
Male	481	63.62
Female	275	36.38
Total	756	100.00

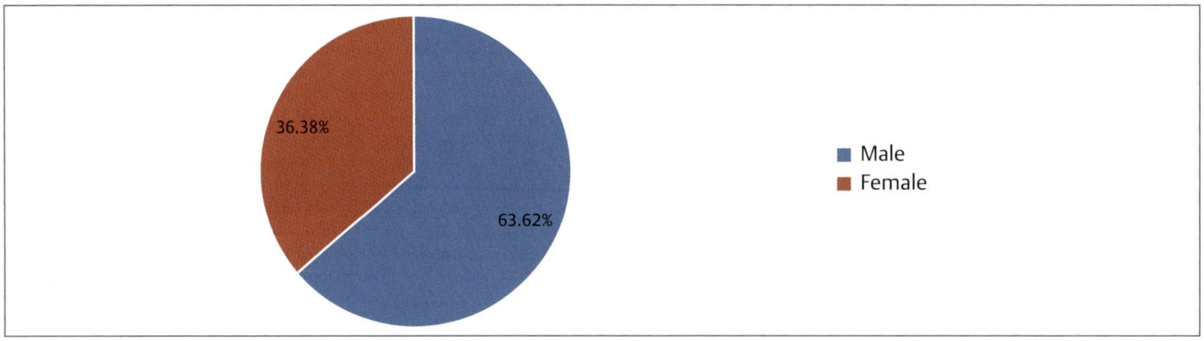

Fig. 2.28 Sex distribution of 756 lateral epicondyle fractures of the humerus.

Lateral Humeral Epicondyle Fractures by Age Group

Table 2.29 Age and sex distribution of 756 lateral epicondyle fractures of the humerus

Age group (years)	Male	Female	Number of fractures	Percentage (%)
0–5	80	43	123	16.27
6–10	72	31	103	13.62
11–15	47	20	67	8.86
16–20	47	22	69	9.13
21–25	56	16	72	9.52
26–30	47	3	50	6.61
31–35	23	15	38	5.03
36–40	41	14	55	7.28
41–45	18	10	28	3.70
46–50	13	15	28	3.70
51–55	10	20	30	3.97
56–60	12	22	34	4.50
61–65	5	8	13	1.72
66–70	4	18	22	2.91
71–75	4	5	9	1.19
76–80	0	6	6	0.79
81–85	1	6	7	0.93
≥86	1	1	2	0.26
Total	481	275	756	100.00

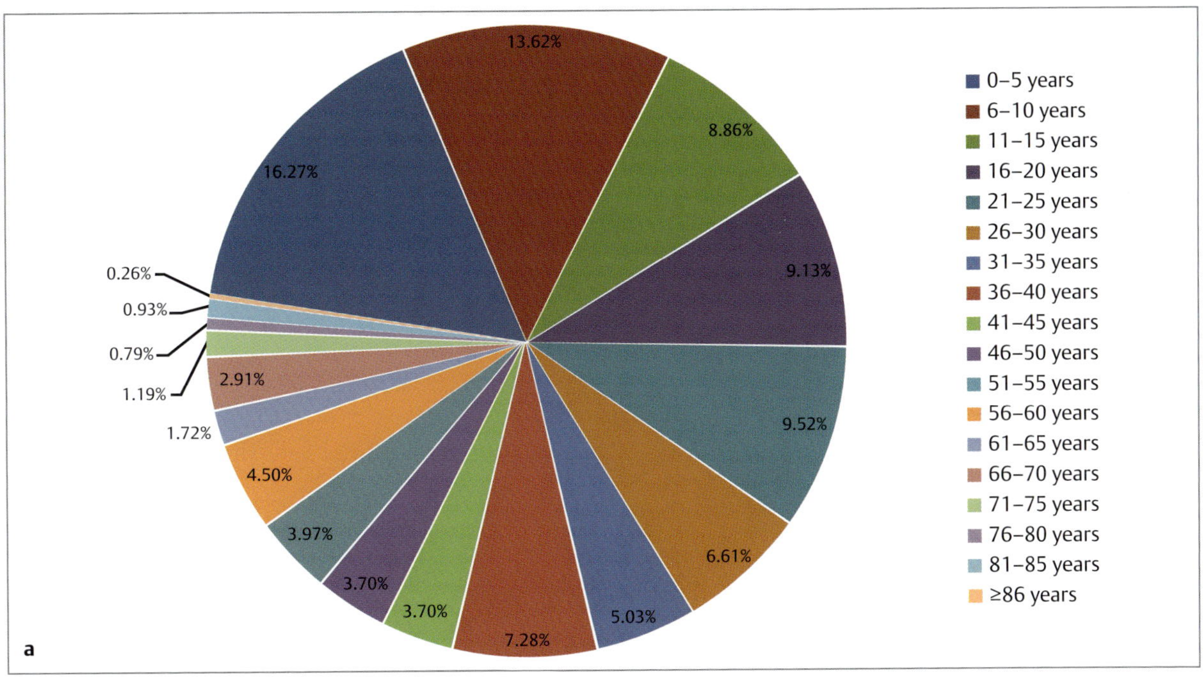

Fig. 2.29 **(a)** Age distribution of 756 lateral epicondyle fractures of the humerus. (*Continued*)

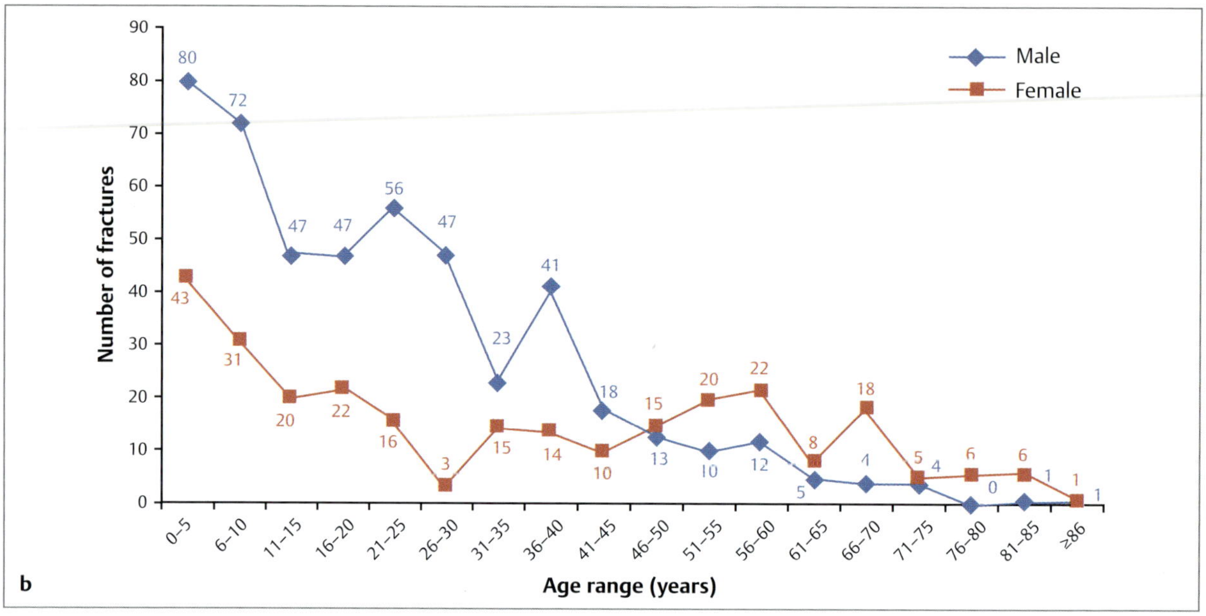

Fig. 2.29 (*continued*) **(b)** Age and sex distribution of 756 lateral epicondyle fractures of the humerus.

Medial Humeral Epicondyle Fractures

Overview

This type of injury is often caused by a fall on flat ground or a sports-related injury such as throwing a ball. It produces a muscular avulsion fracture secondary to contraction of the forearm flexor musculature, due to a fall with the forearm in backward extension and abduction. The avulsion fragment displaces anteriorly and distally, and with possible rotation.

Based on the degree of fragment displacement and the alteration in the elbow joint, medial epicondyle humeral fracture is classified into four types (**Plates 2.57–2.64**):

- *Type I*: with minimal fragment displacement.
- *Type II*: the fragment is markedly displaced by traction of the muscle, and may reach the same level as the elbow joint, with possible rotation (< 30 degrees).
- *Type III*: the fragment is detached and stuck within the elbow joint space, with the elbow in semi-dislocation.
- *Type IV*: the fragment is detached and stuck within the articulation site, with posterior or posterolateral elbow dislocation.

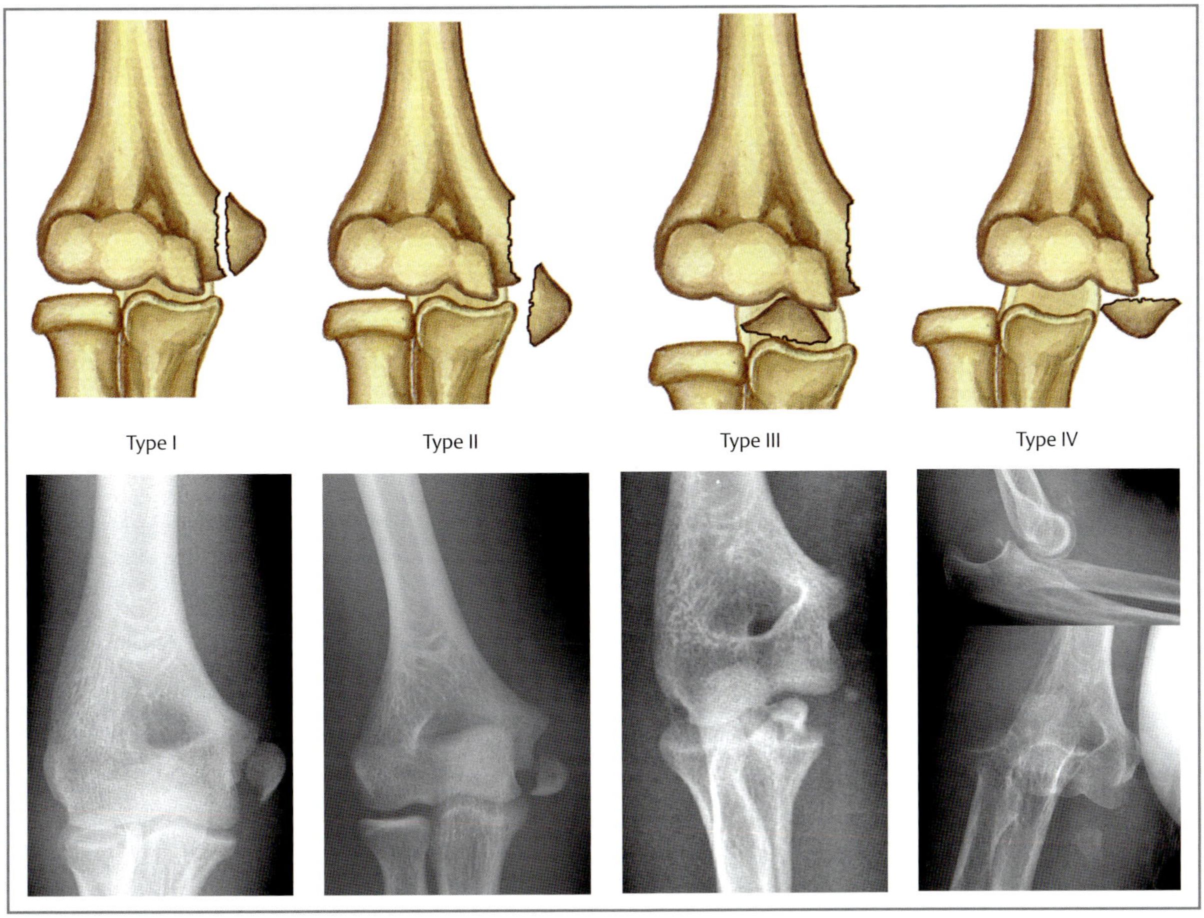

Plates 2.57–2.64

Clinical Epidemiologic Features of Medial Epicondyle Fractures

A total of 865 medial epicondyle humeral fractures were treated in 83 hospitals in China over a 2-year period from 2010 to 2011. All cases were reviewed and statistically studied; the fractures accounted for 2.42% of all humeral fractures. The epidemiologic features are as follows:

- More males than females
- The high-risk age group is 11–15 years.

Medial Humeral Epicondyle Fractures by Sex

Table 2.30 Sex distribution of 865 medial epicondyle fractures of the humerus

Sex	Number of fractures	Percentage (%)
Male	568	65.66
Female	297	34.34
Total	865	100.00

2

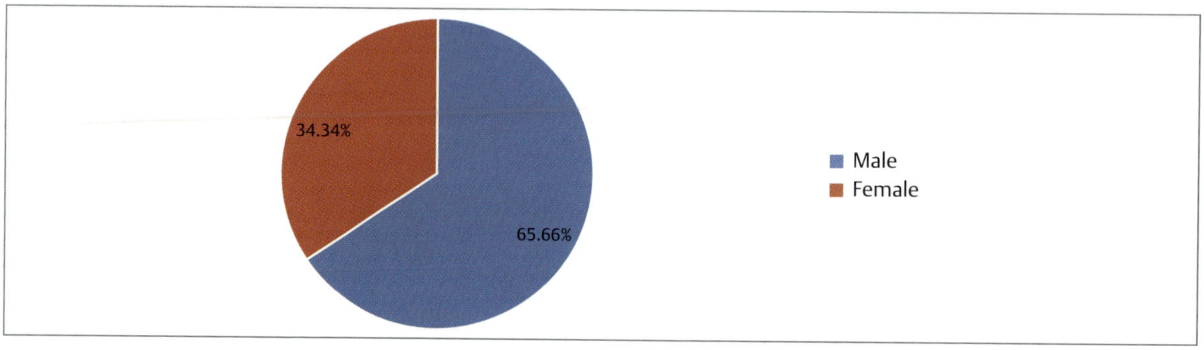

Fig. 2.30 Sex distribution of 865 medial epicondyle fractures of the humerus.

Medial Humeral Epicondyle Fractures by Age Group

Table 2.31 Age and sex distribution of 865 medial epicondyle fractures of the humerus

Age group (years)	Male	Female	Number of fractures	Percentage (%)
0–5	42	40	82	9.48
6–10	73	54	127	14.68
11–15	117	52	169	19.54
16–20	98	12	110	12.72
21–25	58	8	66	7.63
26–30	30	9	39	4.51
31–35	28	13	41	4.74
36–40	25	15	40	4.62
41–45	19	16	35	4.05
46–50	15	13	28	3.24
51–55	20	16	36	4.16
56–60	18	15	33	3.82
61–65	8	11	19	2.20
66–70	6	8	14	1.62
71–75	5	10	15	1.73
76–80	5	2	7	0.81
81–85	1	2	3	0.35
≥86	0	1	1	0.12
Total	568	297	865	100.00

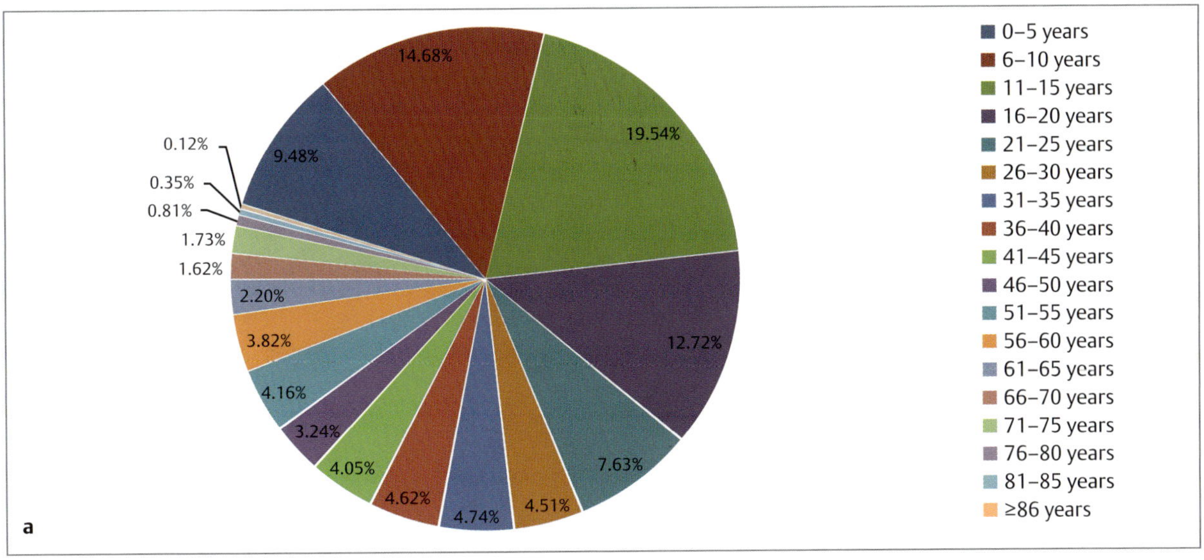

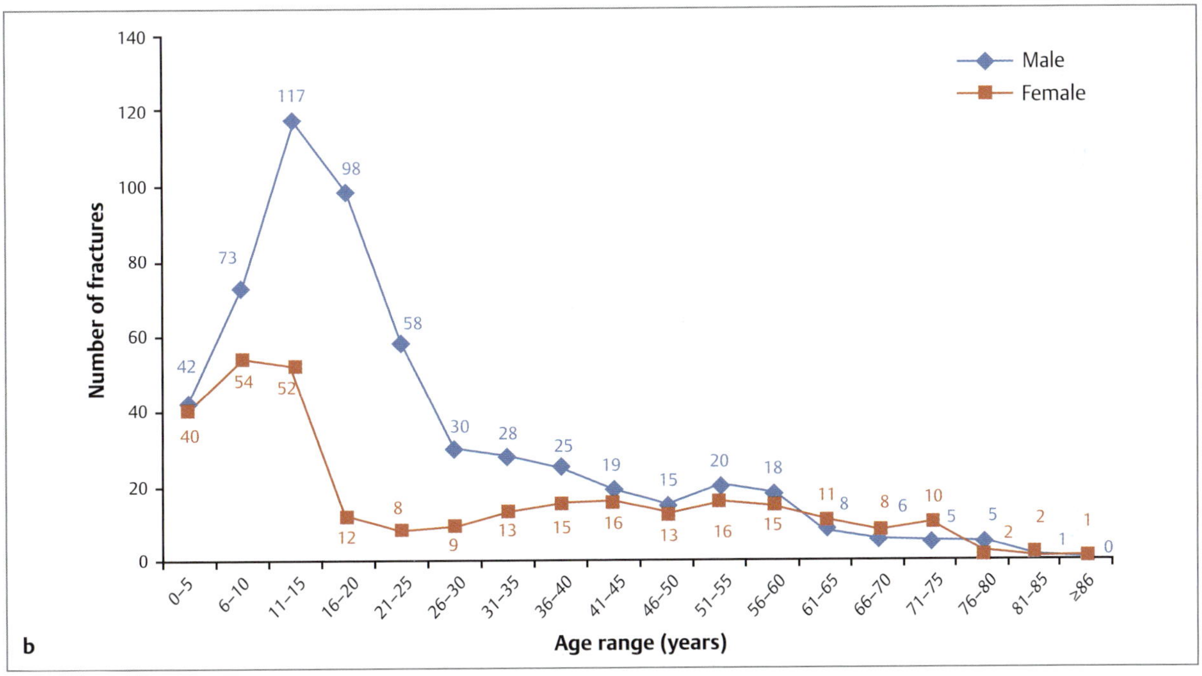

Fig. 2.31 **(a)** Age distribution of 865 medial epicondyle fractures of the humerus. **(b)** Age and sex distribution of 865 medial epicondyle fractures of the humerus.

Humeral Capitellum Fractures

Overview

The most frequently reported mechanism of injury to the humeral capitellum is a fall on an outstretched hand, with axial compression and the elbow in slight flexion. The resulting axial force shears the capitellum from the distal humerus through the radial head.

Based on the size of the fracture fragment and extent of the fracture line, capitellum fracture can be classified into three types (**Plates 2.65–2.70**):

- *Type I (Hahn-Steinthal fracture)*: complete fracture with fragments containing capitellum and the adjacent lip of the trochlea.
- *Type II (Kocher-Lorenz fracture)*: simple complete capitellum fracture with minimal fragmentation, which is difficult to detect on X-ray film.
- *Type III*: the capitellum is comminuted with separate trochlear fragments.

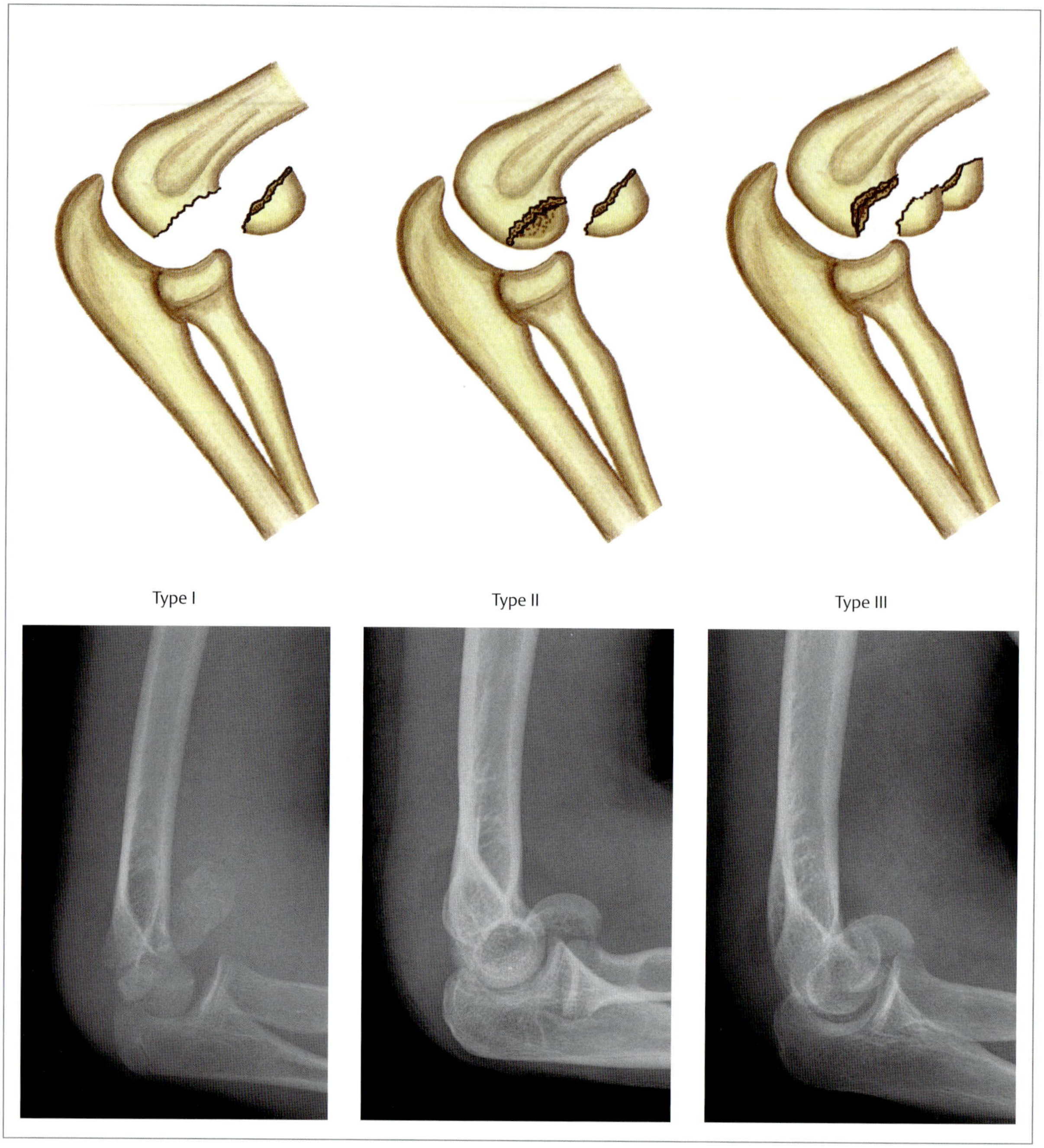

Plates 2.65–2.70

Clinical Epidemiologic Features of Humeral Capitellum Fractures

A total of 196 capitellum fractures were treated in 83 hospitals in China over a 2-year period from 2010 to 2011. All cases were reviewed and statistically studied; the fractures accounted for 0.55% of all humeral fractures. The epidemiologic features are as follows:

- More males than females
- The high-risk age group is 6–10 years.

Humeral Capitellum Fractures by Sex

Table 2.32 Sex distribution of 196 capitellum fractures of the humerus

Sex	Number of fractures	Percentage (%)
Male	122	62.24
Female	74	37.76
Total	196	100.00

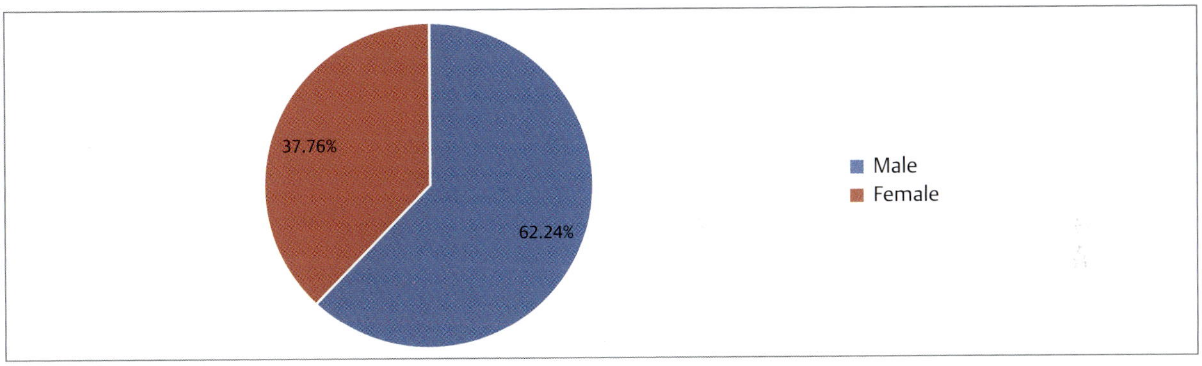

Fig. 2.32 Sex distribution of 196 capitellum fractures of the humerus.

Humeral Capitellum Fractures by Age Group

Table 2.33 Age and sex distribution of 196 capitellum fractures of the humerus

Age group (years)	Male	Female	Number of fractures	Percentage (%)
0–5	18	8	26	13.27
6–10	21	14	35	17.86
11–15	8	2	10	5.10
16–20	15	6	21	10.71
21–25	11	8	19	9.69
26–30	8	2	10	5.10
31–35	12	3	15	7.65
36–40	6	3	9	4.59
41–45	5	5	10	5.10
46–50	4	4	8	4.08
51–55	5	4	9	4.59
56–60	1	4	5	2.55
61–65	2	4	6	3.06
66–70	1	0	1	0.51
71–75	3	3	6	3.06
76–80	1	3	4	2.04
81–85	1	1	2	1.02
≥86	0	0	0	0.00
Total	122	74	196	100.00

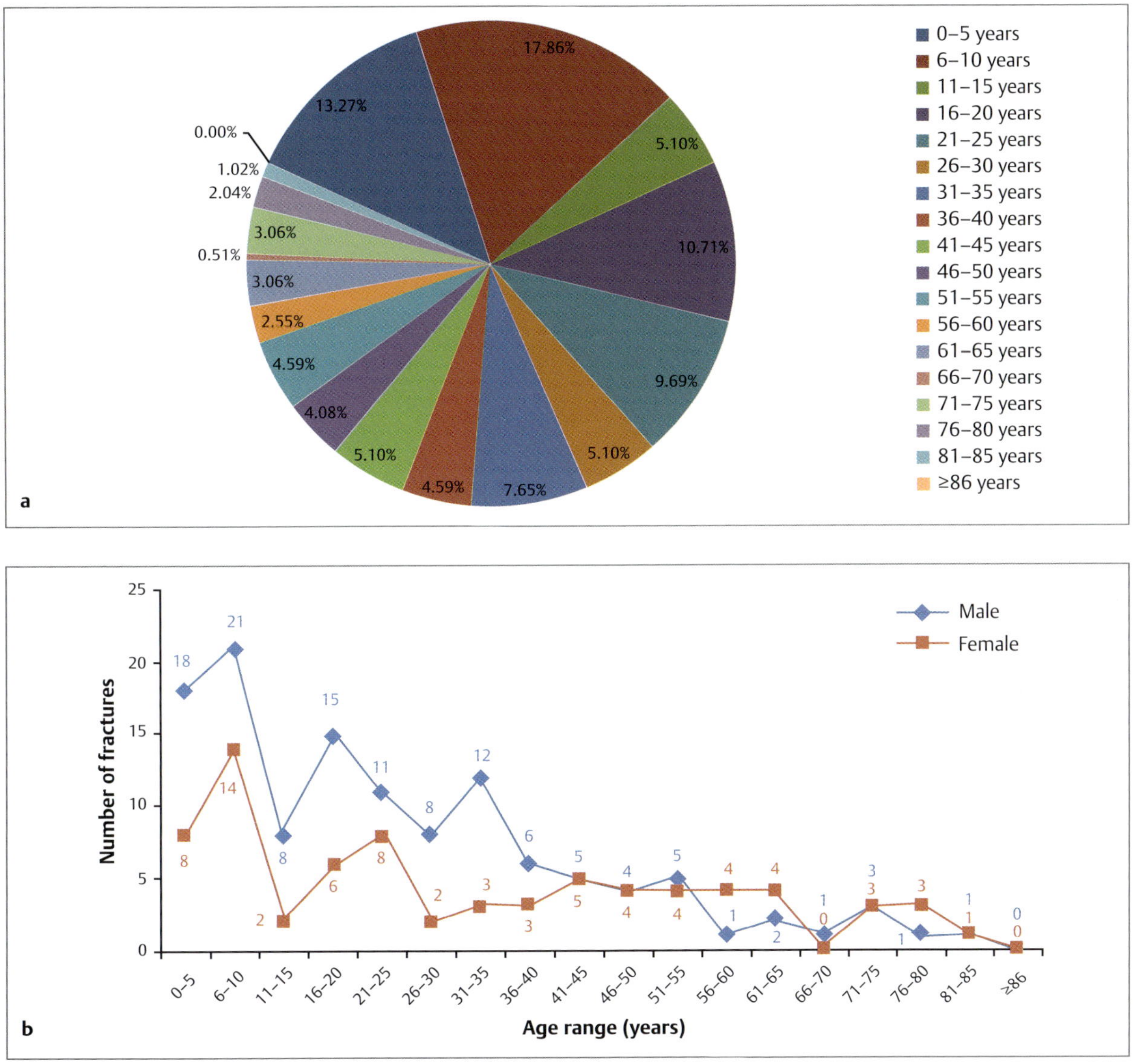

Fig. 2.33 **(a)** Age distribution of 196 capitellum fractures of the humerus.
(b) Age and sex distribution of 196 capitellum fractures of the humerus.

3 Fractures of the Ulna and Radius

Overview

Anatomical Features

The ulna and radius are the bony structures of the forearm that form the elbow joint proximally with the humerus and the wrist joint distally with the carpals. The radius and ulna are joined by the proximal and distal radioulnar joints and by the interosseous membrane (IOM). The radioulnar joints are pivot joints where movements of supination and pronation take place. If one bone shows a fracture with displacement or angulation, usually the other bone will also have a fracture or displacement. Both the radius and ulna are long bones, prismatic in form, and lie roughly parallel to each other when the forearm is supinated. The ulna is relatively straight whereas the radius is slightly curved longitudinally (**Plate 3.1**).

AO Classification and Coding System for Fractures of the Ulna and Radius

Based on the AO classification, the ulna/radius should be considered as one unit of bone, with the location coding number 2. The anatomical delineation of the segments, proximal, shaft, and distal is performed according to the Heim's square, with assigned numbers of 21, 22, and 23, respectively (**Plates 3.2** and **3.3**).

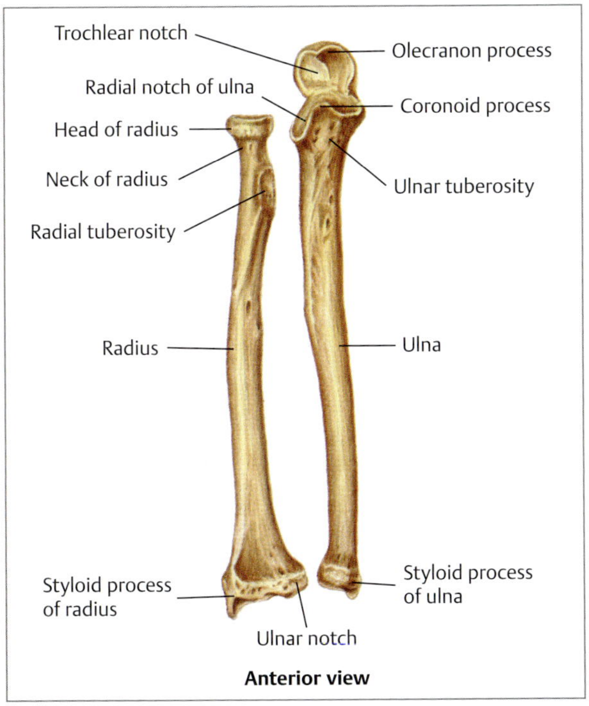

Plate 3.1

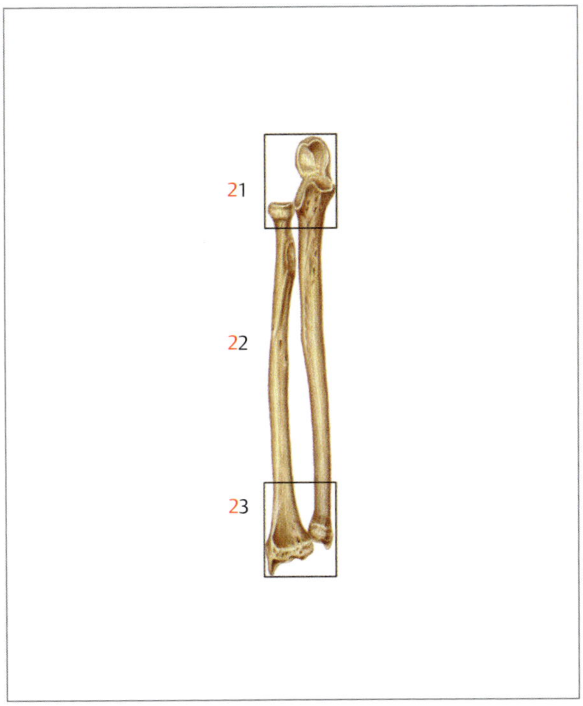

Plate 3.2

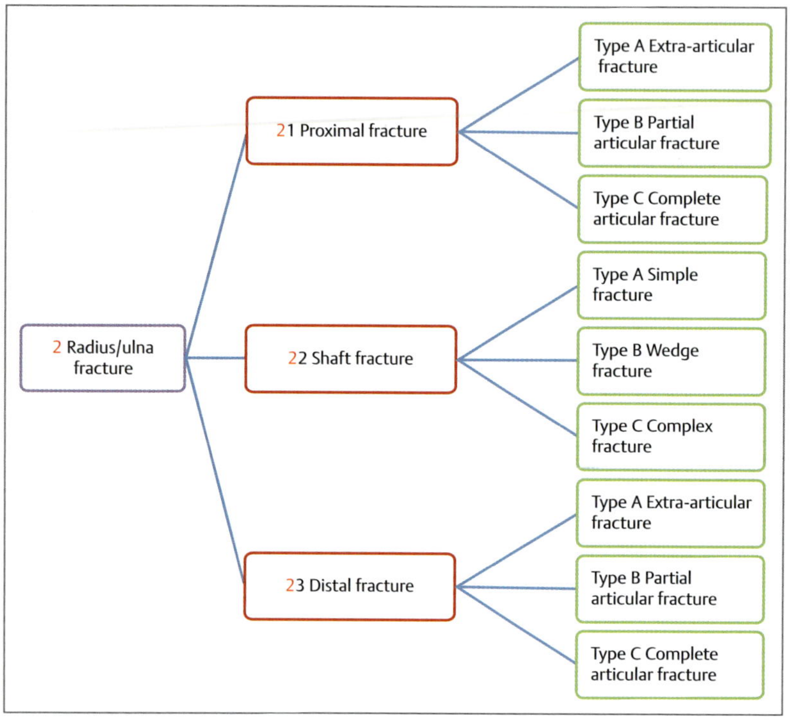

Plate 3.3

Clinical Epidemiologic Features of Radius/Ulna Fractures

A total of 75,850 patients with 76,550 radius/ulna fractures were treated in 83 hospitals in China over a 2-year period from 2010 to 2011. All cases were reviewed and statistically studied; the fractures accounted for 18.28% of all patients with fractures and 17.73% of all types of fractures, respectively. Among these 75,850 patients, 18,274 were children with 18,334 fractures, and 57,576 were adults with 58,216 fractures.

Epidemiologic features of radius/ulna fractures are as follows:

- More males than females
- More left sides involved than right sides
- The highest risk age group is 11–15 years. The most affected female age group includes ages 56–60, while males between the ages of 11 and 15 years have the highest risk.
- Distal fracture of the radius/ulna is the most common forearm fracture.

3

Radius/Ulna Fractures by Sex

Table 3.1 Sex distribution of 75,850 patients with radius/ulna fractures

Sex	Number of patients	Percentage (%)
Male	41,592	54.83
Female	34,258	45.17
Total	75,850	100.00

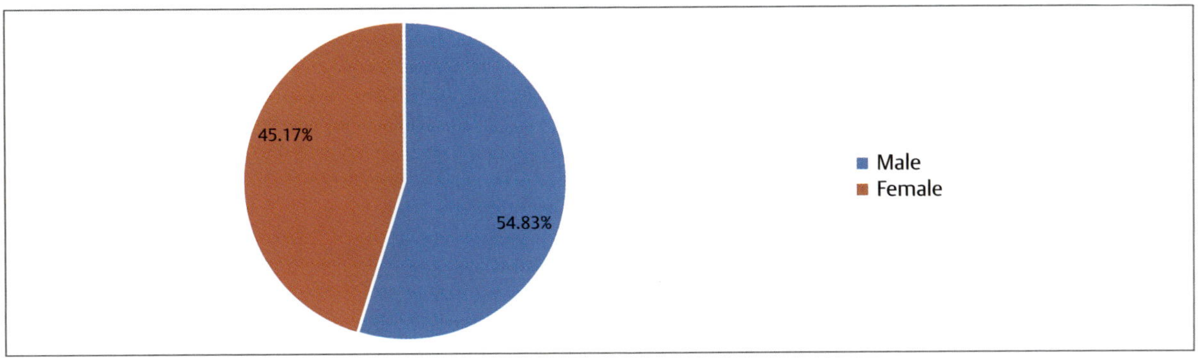

Fig. 3.1 Sex distribution of 75,850 patients with radius/ulna fractures.

Radius/Ulna Fractures by Injured Side

Table 3.2 Injury side distribution of 75,850 patients with radius/ulna fractures

Injury Side	Number of patients	Percentage (%)
Left	40,576	53.50
Right	34,936	46.06
Bilateral	338	0.45
Total	75,850	100.00

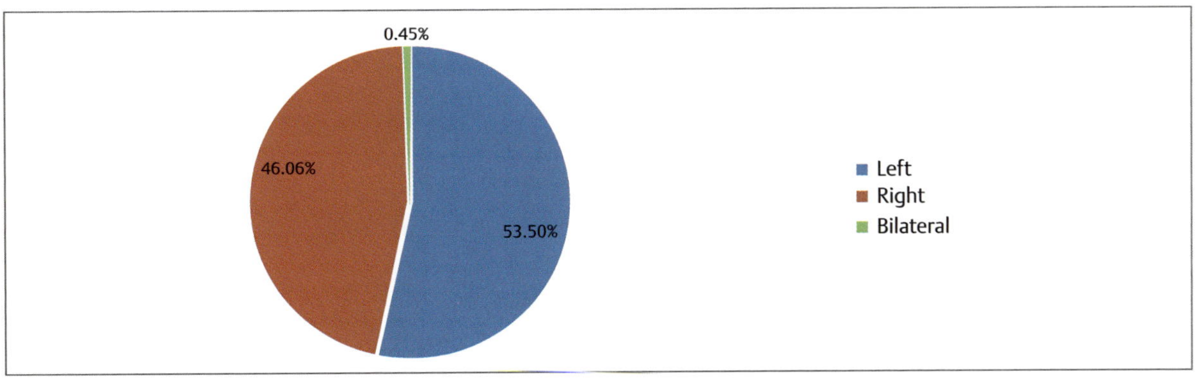

Fig. 3.2 Injury side distribution of 75,850 patients with radius/ulna fractures.

Radius/Ulna Fractures by Age Group

Table 3.3 Age and sex distribution of 75,850 patients with radius/ulna fractures

Age Group (years)	Male	Female	Number of patients	Percentage (%)
0–5	2,742	1,552	4,294	5.66
6–10	4,789	1,764	6,553	8.64
11–15	6,306	1,121	7,427	9.79
16–20	3,508	820	4,328	5.71
21–25	3,258	1,047	4,305	5.68
26–30	2,679	1,036	3,715	4.90
31–35	2,363	1,167	3,530	4.65
36–40	3,023	1,562	4,585	6.04
41–45	2,958	1,800	4,758	6.27
46–50	2,950	2,854	5,804	7.65
51–55	2,039	3,685	5,724	7.55
56–60	1,835	4,853	6,688	8.82
61–65	1,096	3,205	4,301	5.67
66–70	723	2,635	3,358	4.43
71–75	529	2,088	2,617	3.45
76–80	426	1,720	2,146	2.83
81–85	243	889	1,132	1.49
≥86	125	460	585	0.77
Total	41,592	34,258	75,850	100.00

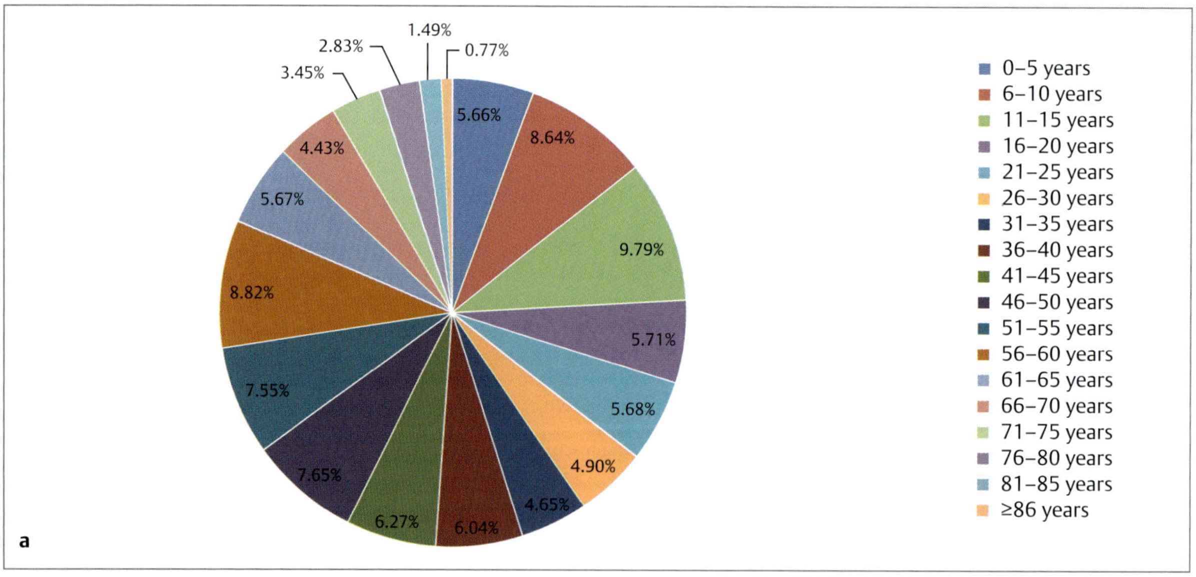

Fig. 3.3 **(a)** Age distribution of 75,850 patients with radius/ulna fractures.

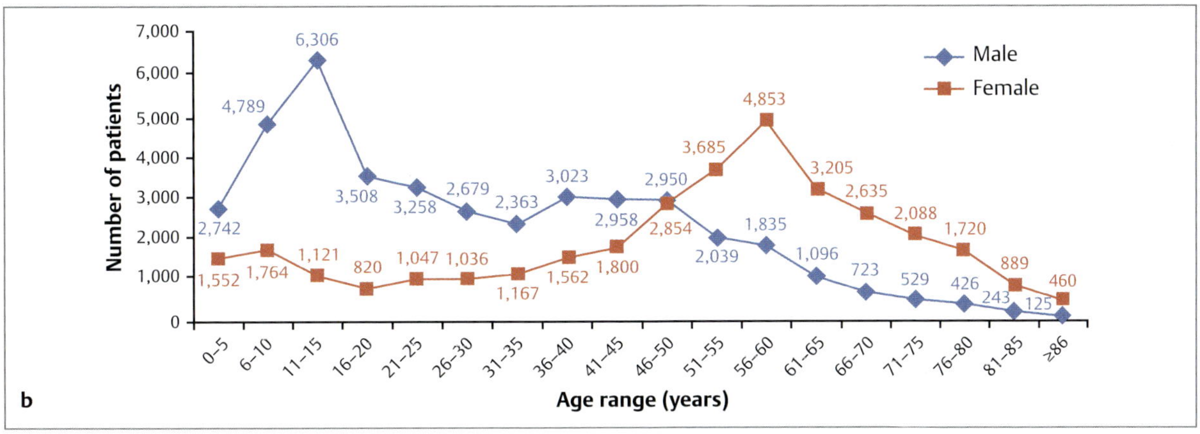

Fig. 3.3 (*continued*) **(b)** Age and sex distribution of 75,850 patients with radius/ulna fractures.

Radius/Ulna Fractures by Location

Radius/Ulna Fractures in Adults by Segment Based on AO Classification

Table 3.4 Segment distribution of 58,216 radius/ulna fractures in adults based on AO classification

Segment	Number of fractures	Percentage (%)
21	7,202	12.37
22	7,594	13.04
23	43,420	74.58
Total	58,216	100.00

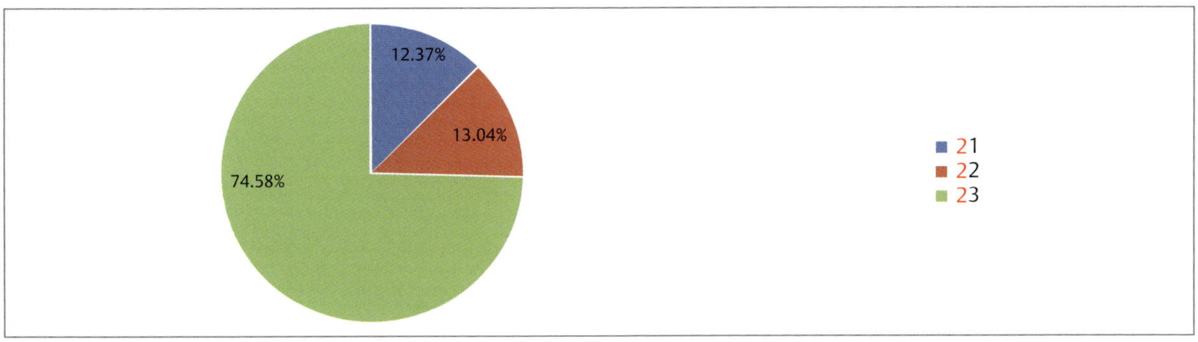

Fig. 3.4 Segment distribution of 58,216 radius/ulna fractures in adults based on AO classification.

Radius/Ulna Fractures in Children by Segment

Table 3.5 Segment distribution of 18,334 radius/ulna fractures in children

Segment	Number of fractures	Percentage (%)
Proximal	3,427	18.69
Diaphysis	6,113	33.34
Distal	8,794	47.97
Total	18,334	100.00

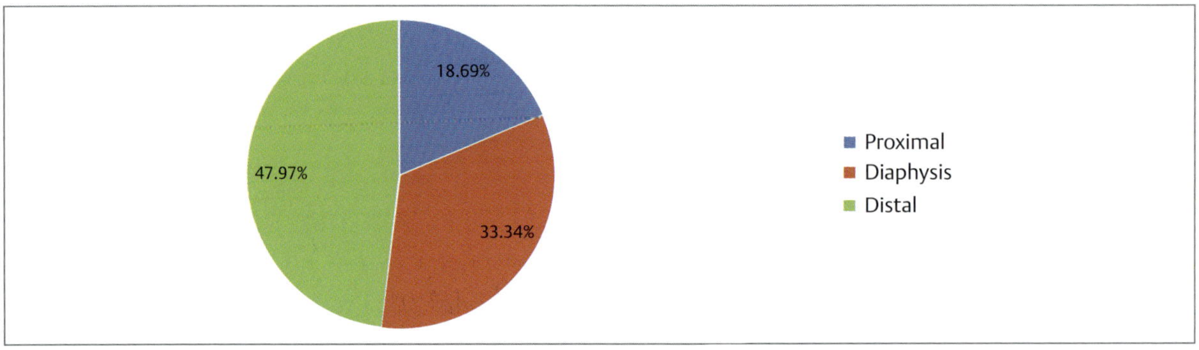

Fig. 3.5 Segment distribution of 18,334 radius/ulna fractures in children.

Proximal Fractures of the Radius and Ulna (Segment 21)

Anatomical Features

The bony structures of the proximal part of the radius/ulna consist of the olecranon, coronoid process, radial head, radial neck, and part of the metaphysis. The bony surfaces of the humeroradial joint constitute an enarthrosis or ball and socket joint, between the radial head and the capitulum of the humerus, while the proximal radioulnar joint is a trochoid or pivot joint between the radial head and the ring formed by the radial notch of the ulna and the annular ligament. These two joints play an important role in the complex action of turning the forearm over as in pronation or supination. The humeroradial joint is considered similar to a lateral column that provides stability to the elbow joint during its motion in flexion or extension.

The articular surfaces of the elbow joint are connected by a capsule that is attached to the radial neck, 1.5 cm distal to the humeroradial joint. The radial tuberosity, also known as the bicipital tuberosity, is the main insertion of the biceps brachii muscle.

The olecranon and the coronoid process form a large depression called the semilunar notch that serves as an articulation site with the trochlea of the humerus. The humeroulnar joint is a simple hinge joint that allows for flexion and extension. The tendon of the triceps brachii muscle inserts into the posterior portion of the upper surface of the olecranon, while the ulnar nerve winds along the olecranon or epicondylar groove.

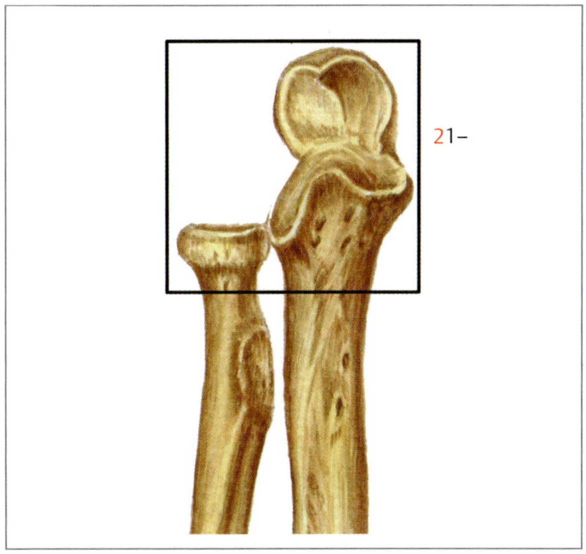

Plate 3.4

AO Classification of Proximal Radial/Ulnar Fractures

Based on the AO classification, the delineation of the proximal radius/ulna is illustrated by a square whose lateral sides are parallel to the axis of the bone and their length equal to the maximum width of the epiphysis. According to this formula, the proximal radius/ulna is coded as the number 21 (**Plate 3.4**). On the basis of articular surface involvement, the radial/ulnar fracture is further divided into three types: 21-A, extra-articular fracture; 21-B, partial articular fracture; and 21-C, complex articular fracture (**Plate 3.5**).

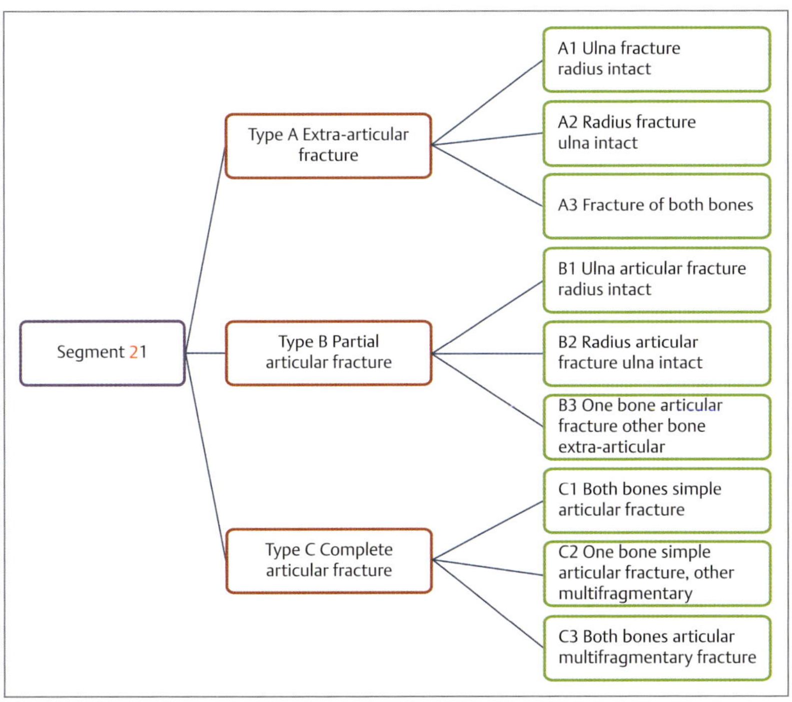

Plate 3.5

Clinical Epidemiologic Features of the Proximal Radius /Ulna Fractures (Segment 21)

A total of 7,202 adult proximal radius/ulna fractures (segment 21) were treated in 83 hospitals in China over a 2-year period from 2010 to 2011. All cases were reviewed and statistically studied; the fractures accounted for 12.37% of all fractures of the radius/ulna in adults. Their epidemiologic features are as follows:

- More males than females
- The high-risk age group is 21–25 years; the same age group for males, while the most affected female age group is age 46–50.
- The most common fracture type among segment 21 fractures is type 21-B; the same fracture type for both males and females.
- The most common fracture group among segment 21 fractures is group 21-B1; the same fracture group for both males and females.

Fractures of Segment 21 by Sex

Table 3.6 Sex distribution of 7,202 fractures of segment 21

Sex	Number of fractures	Percentage (%)
Male	4,526	62.84
Female	2,676	37.16
Total	7,202	100.00

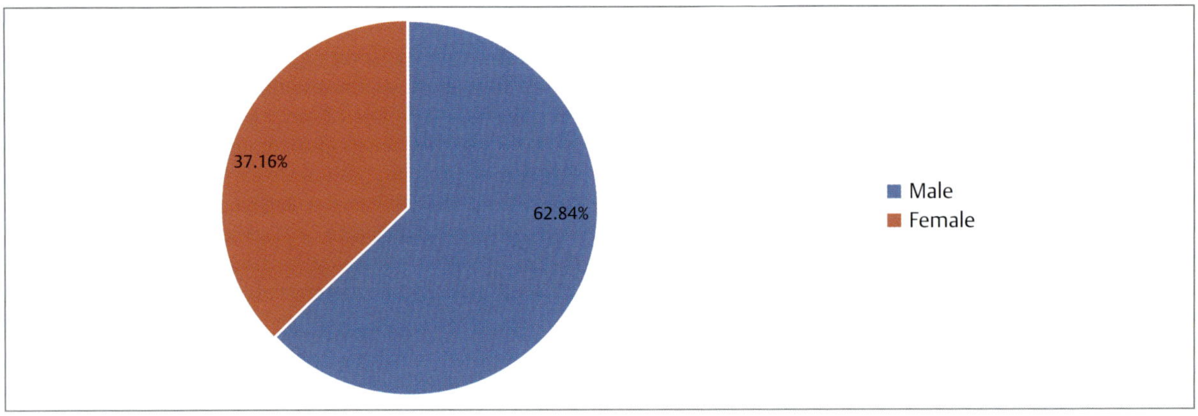

Fig. 3.6 Sex distribution of 7,202 fractures of segment 21.

Fractures of Segment 21 by Age Group

Table 3.7 Age and sex distribution of 7,202 fractures of segment 21

Age Group (years)	Male	Female	Number of fractures	Percentage (%)
16–20	521	133	654	9.08
21–25	667	240	907	12.59
26–30	602	202	804	11.16
31–35	520	173	693	9.62
36–40	602	233	835	11.59
41–45	501	292	793	11.01
46–50	402	317	719	9.98
51–55	232	289	521	7.23
56–60	193	258	451	6.26
61–65	103	164	267	3.71
66–70	57	137	194	2.69
71–75	53	93	146	2.03
76–80	45	73	118	1.64
81–85	21	55	76	1.06
≥86	7	17	24	0.33
Total	4,526	2,676	7,202	100.00

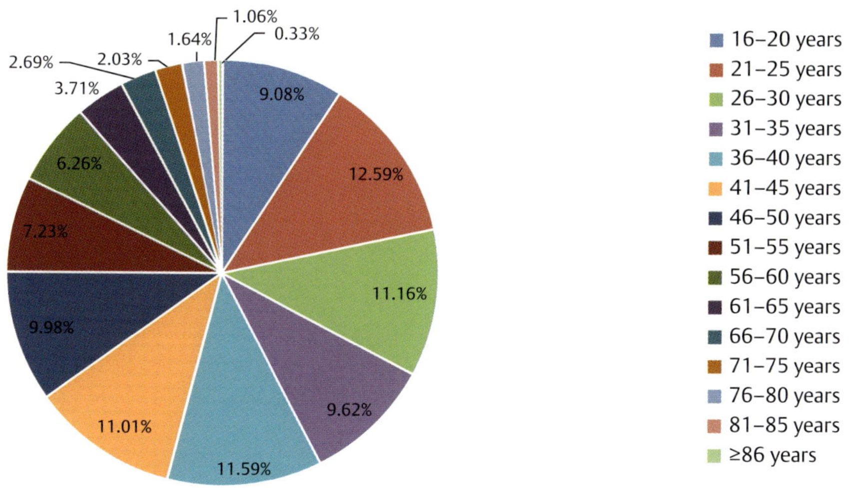

a

Fig. 3.7 **(a)** Age distribution of 7,202 fractures of segment 21. (*Continued*)

b

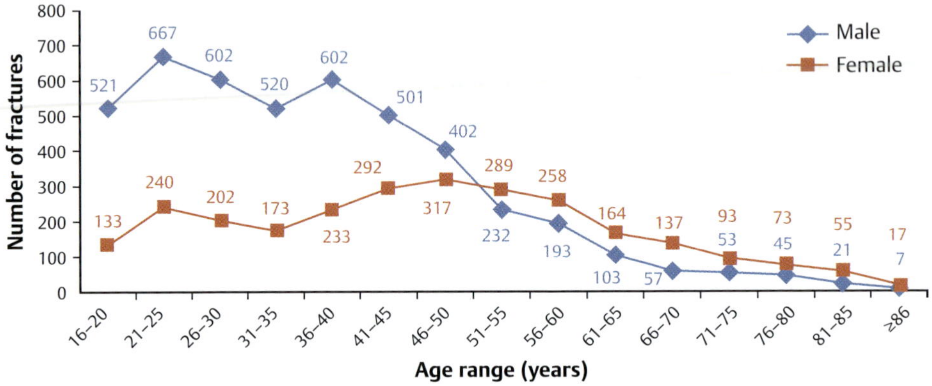

Fig. 3.7 (*continued*) **(b)** Age and sex distribution of 7,202 fractures of segment 21.

Fractures of Segment 21 by Fracture Type

Table 3.8 Sex and fracture type distribution of 7,202 fractures of segment 21

Fracture Type	Male	Female	Number of fractures	Percentage (%)
21-A	972	678	1,650	22.91
21-B	3,364	1,903	5,267	73.13
21-C	190	95	285	3.96
Total	4,526	2,676	7,202	100.00

a

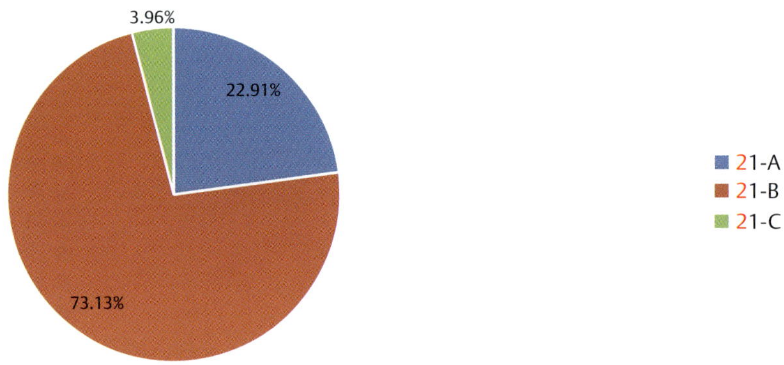

Fig. 3.8 **(a)** Fracture type distribution of 7,202 fractures of segment 21.

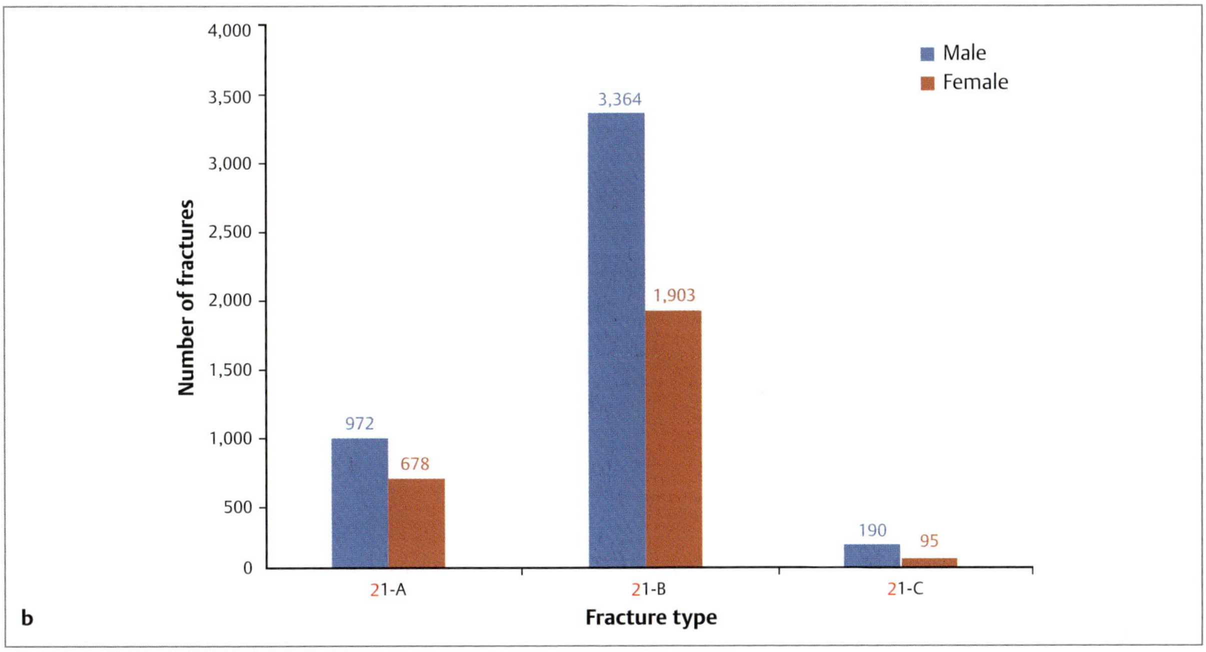

Fig. 3.8 (*continued*) **(b)** Sex and fracture type distribution of 7,202 fractures of segment 21.

Table 3.9 Sex and fracture group distribution of 7,202 fractures of segment 21

Fracture group	Male	Female	Number of fractures	Percentage of segment 21 fractures (%)	Percentage of radius/ulna fractures (%)
21-A1	521	256	777	10.79	1.33
21-A2	412	394	806	11.19	1.38
21-A3	39	28	67	0.93	0.12
21-B1	1,809	964	2,773	38.50	4.76
21-B2	1,426	866	2,292	31.82	3.94
21-B3	129	73	202	2.80	0.35
21-C1	76	49	125	1.74	0.21
21-C2	66	24	90	1.25	0.15
21-C3	48	22	70	0.97	0.12
Total	4,526	2,676	7,202	100.00	12.37

3

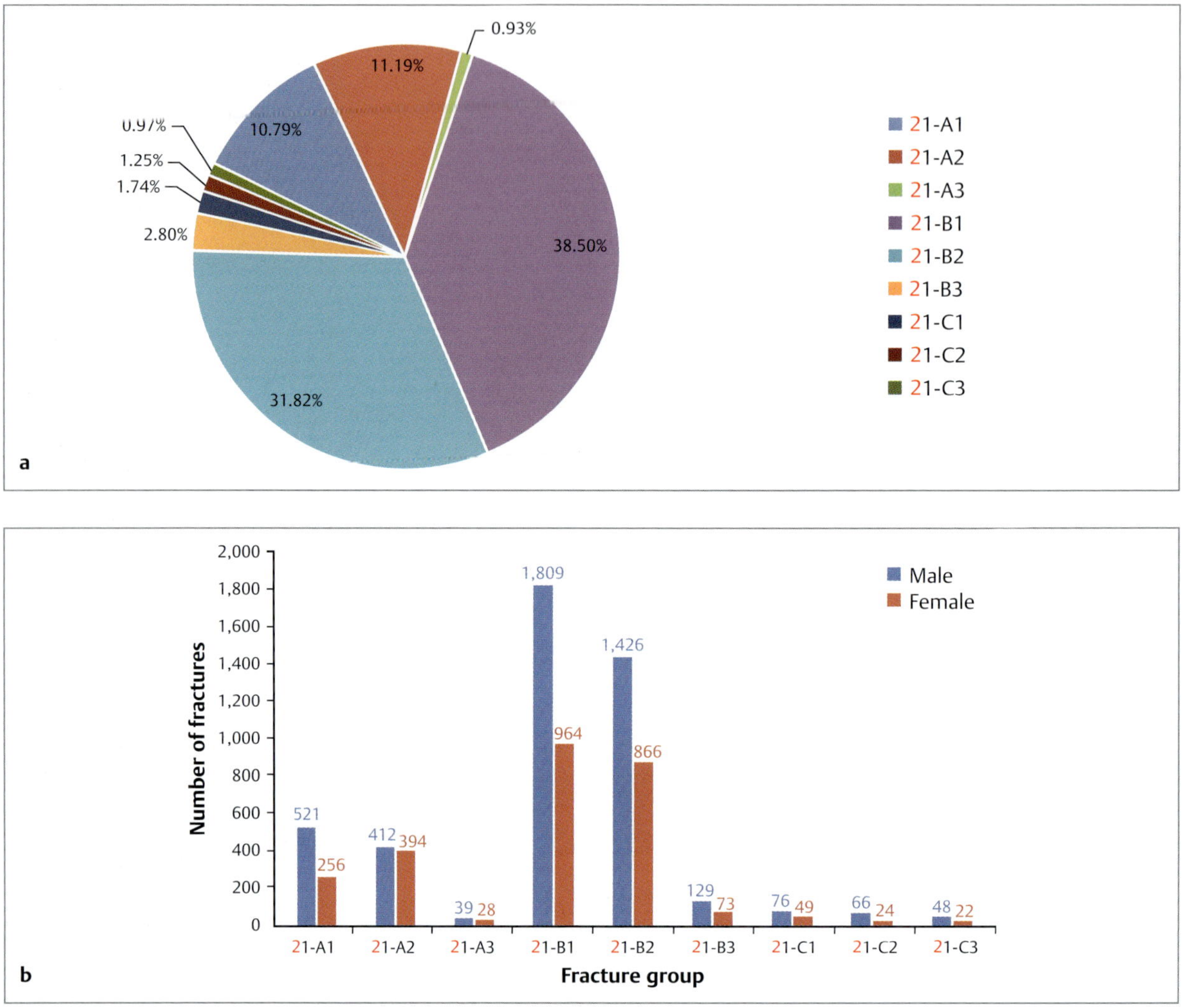

Fig. 3.9 **(a)** Fracture group distribution of 7,202 fractures of segment 21.
(b) Sex and fracture group distribution of 7,202 fractures of segment 21.

21-A Radius/ulna, proximal extra-articular fractures

21-A1
Ulna,
radius intact
777 fractures
M: 521 (67.05%)
F: 256 (32.95%)
0.21% of total adult fractures
1.33% of adult radius/ulna
10.79% of segment 21
47.09% of type 21-A

21-A1.1

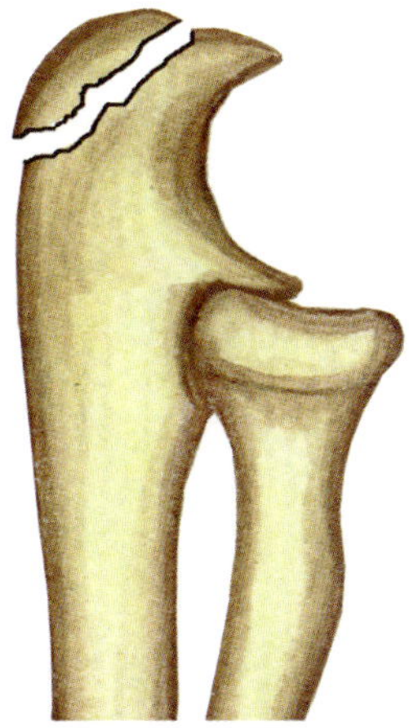

Avulsion of triceps insertion from the olecranon

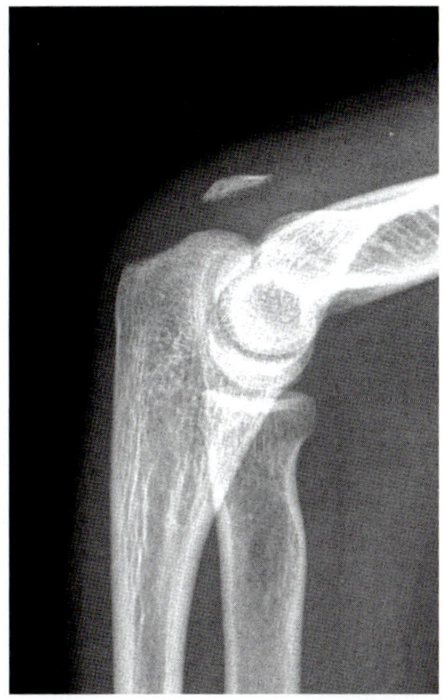

21-A1.2

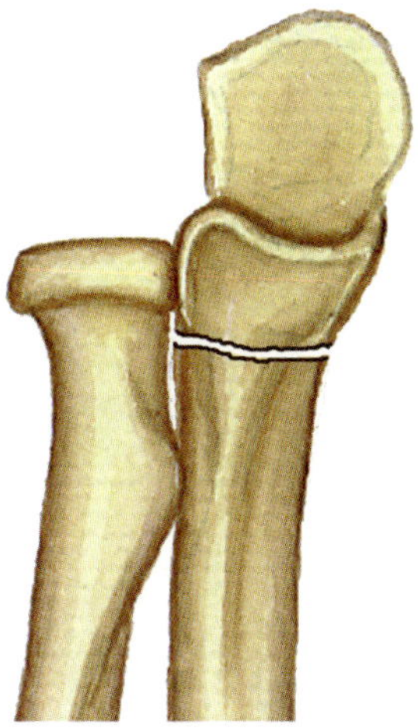

Metaphyseal simple fracture

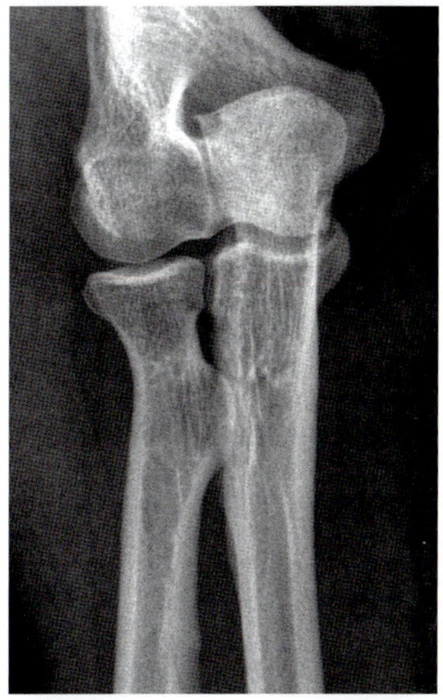

21-A1.3

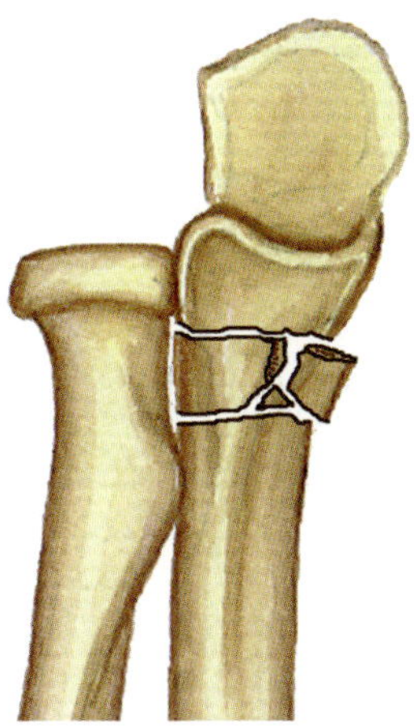

Metaphyseal multifragmentary fracture

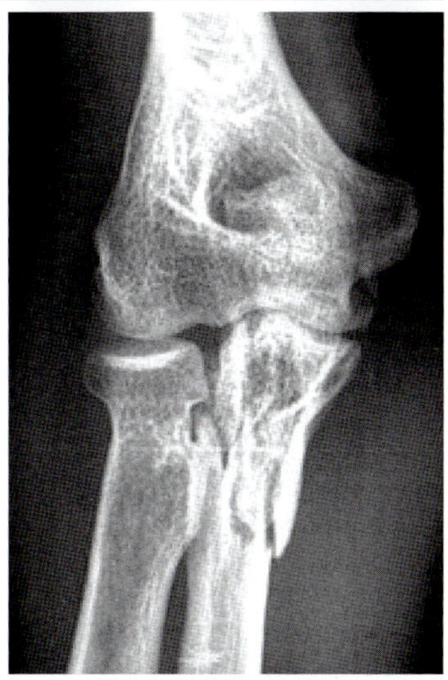

21-A Radius/ulna, proximal extra-articular fractures

21-A2
Radius,
ulna intact
806 fractures
M: 412 (51.12%)
F: 394 (48.88%)
0.22% of total adult fractures
1.38% of adult radius/ulna
11.19% of segment 21
48.85% of type 21-A

21-A2.1

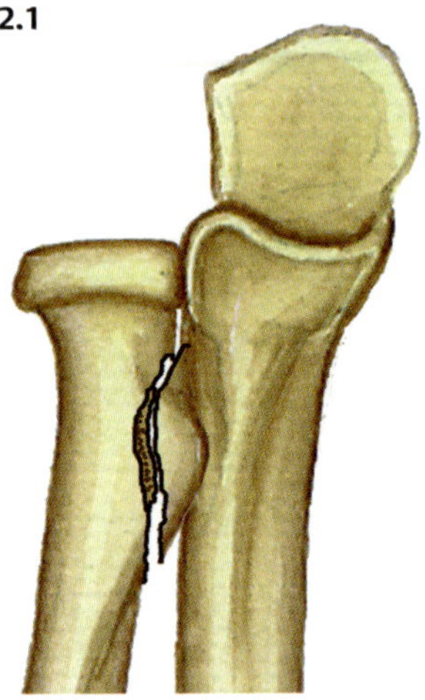

Avulsion of biceps insertion from the radial tuberosity

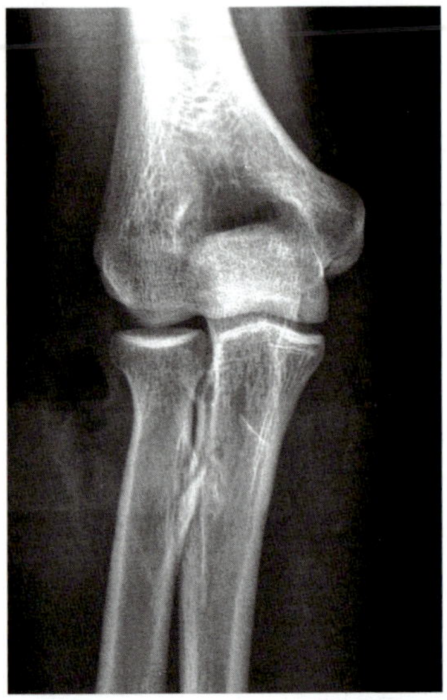

21-A2.2

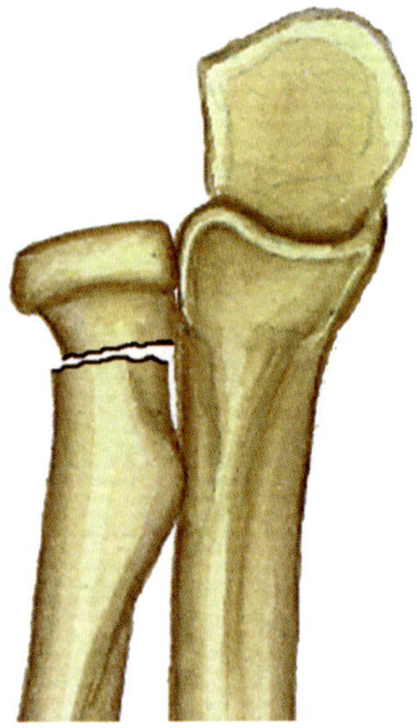

Radial neck simple fracture

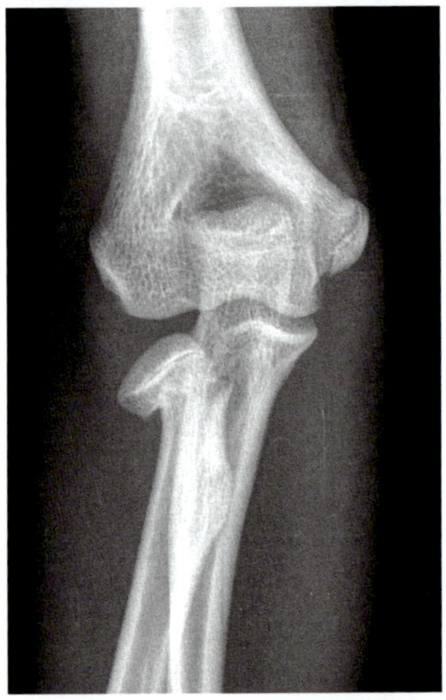

21-A2.3

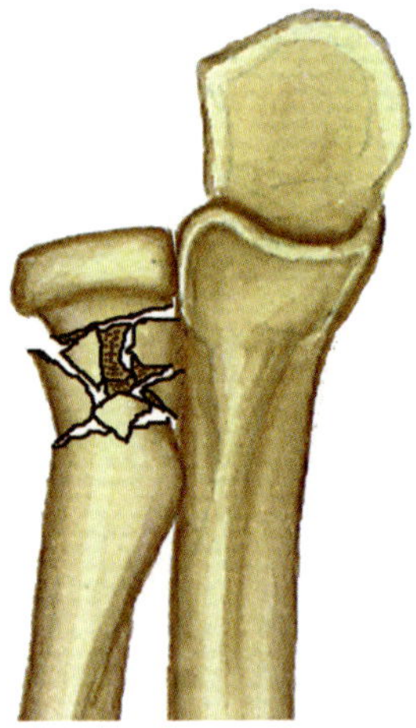

Radial neck multifragmentary fracture

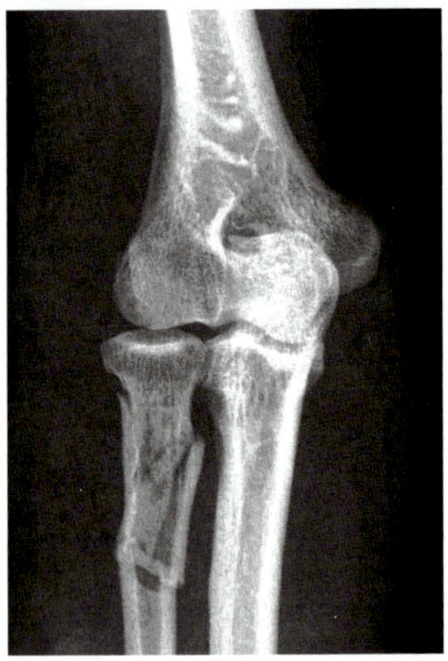

21-A Radius/ulna, proximal extra-articular fractures

21-A3
Both bones
67 fractures
M: 39 (58.21%)
F: 28 (41.79%)
0.02% of total adult fractures
0.12% of adult radius/ulna
0.93% of segment 21
4.06% of type 21-A

21-A3.1

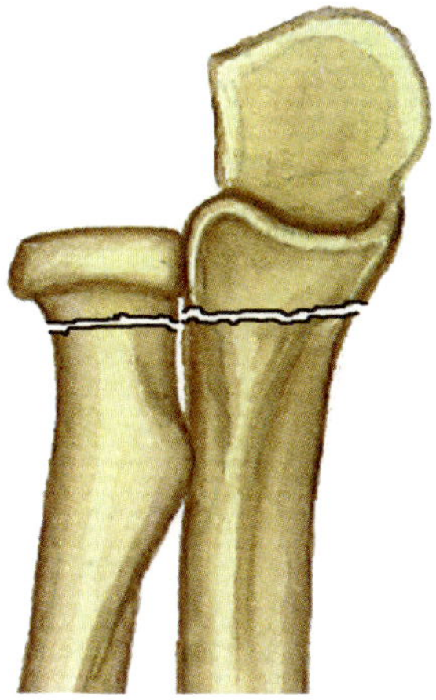

Both bones simple fracture

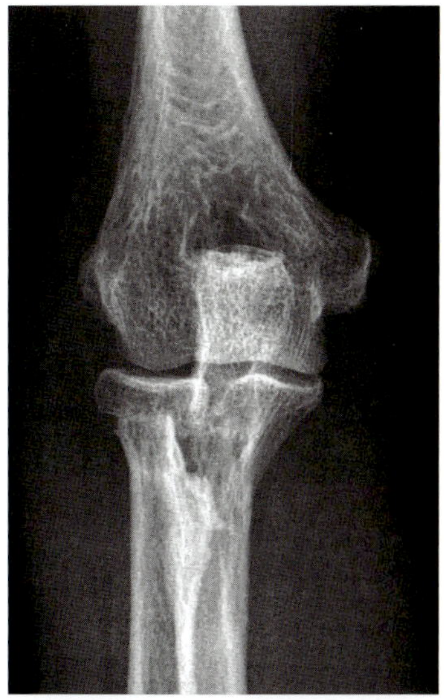

21-A3.2

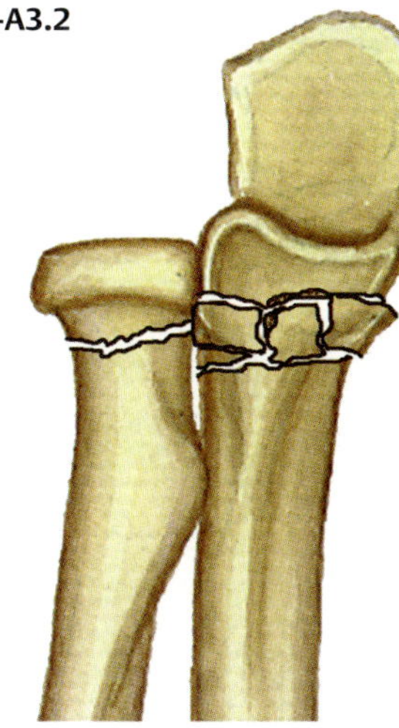

One bone simple fracture, other bone multifragmentary fracture

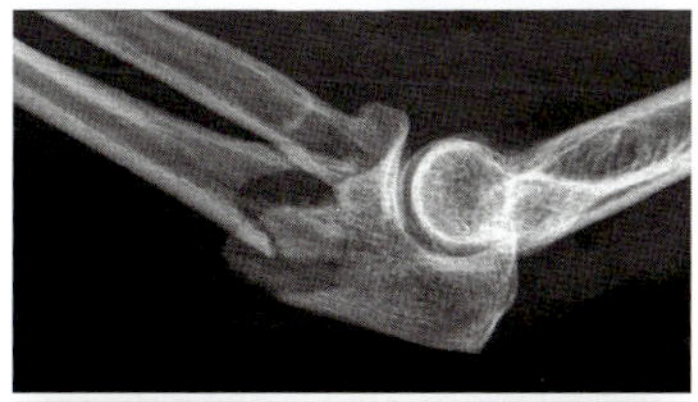

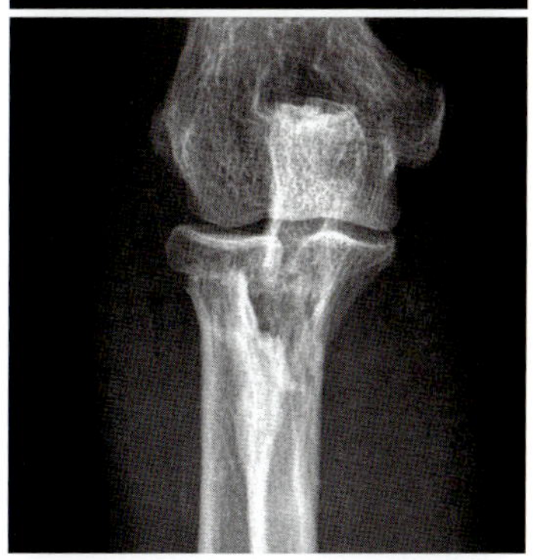

21-A3.3

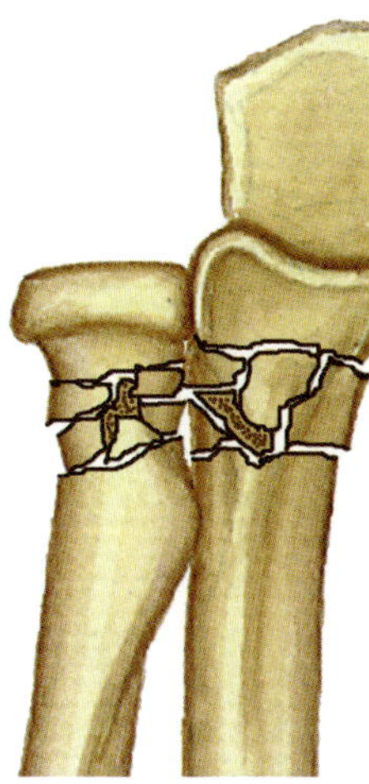

Both bones multifragmentary

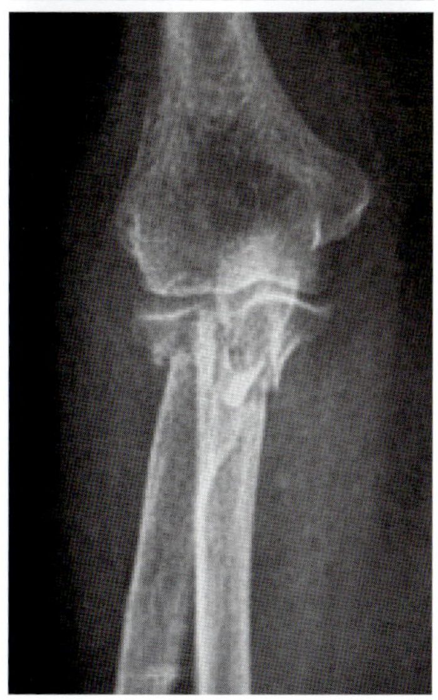

21-B Radius/ulna, proximal partial articular fractures

21-B1
Ulna,
radius intact
2,773 fractures
M: 1,809 (65.24%)
F: 964 (34.76%)
0.74% of total adult fractures
4.76% of adult radius/ulna
38.50% of segment 21
52.65% of type 21-B

21-B1.1

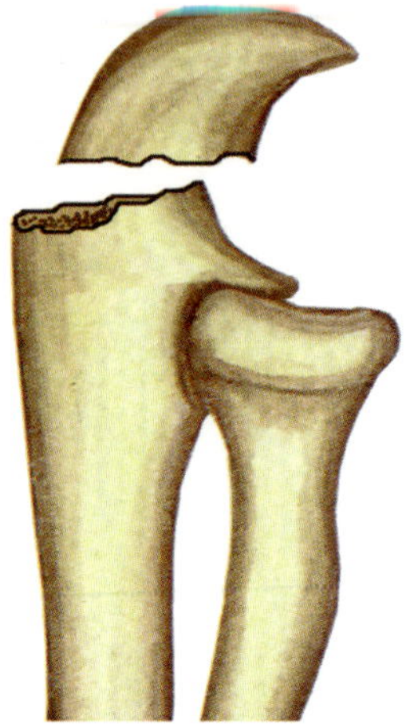

Unifocal simple fracture

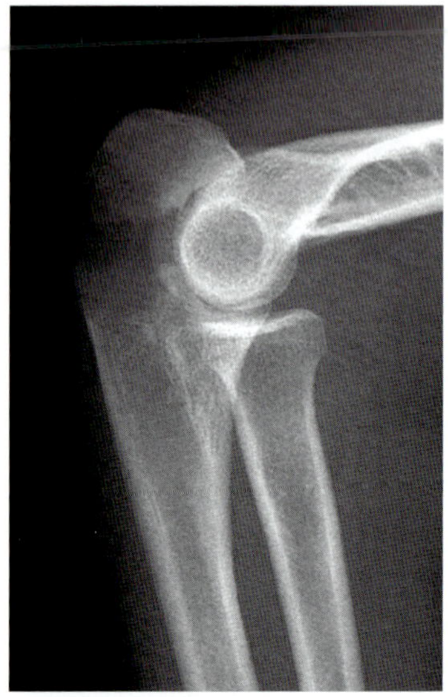

21-B1.2

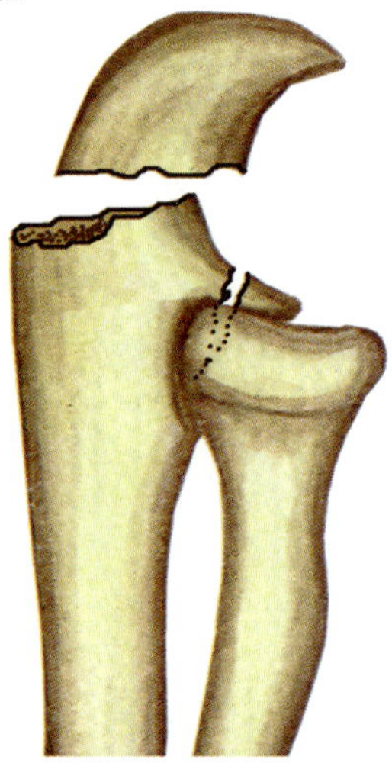

Bifocal simple fracture

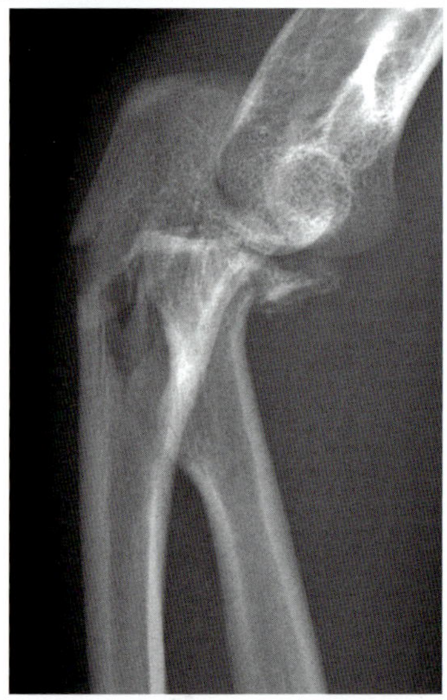

21-B1.3

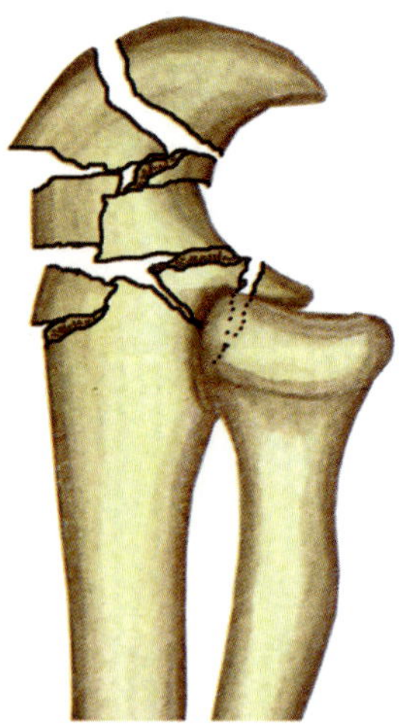

Bifocal multifragmentary

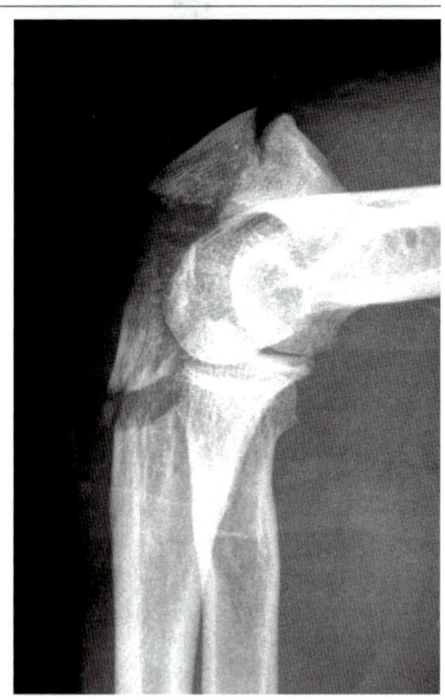

21-B Radius/ulna, proximal partial articular fractures

21-B2
Radius,
ulna intact
2,292 fractures
M: 1,426 (62.22%)
F: 866 (37.78%)
0.61% of total adult fractures
3.94% of adult radius/ulna
31.82% of segment 21
43.52% of type 21-B

21-B2.1

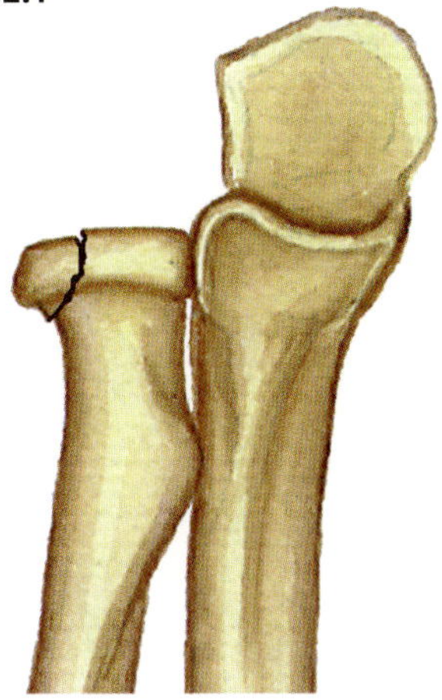

Simple fracture with minimal or no displacement

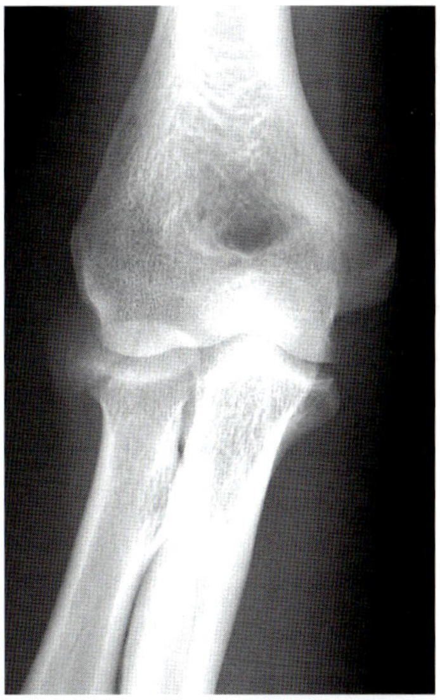

21-B2.2

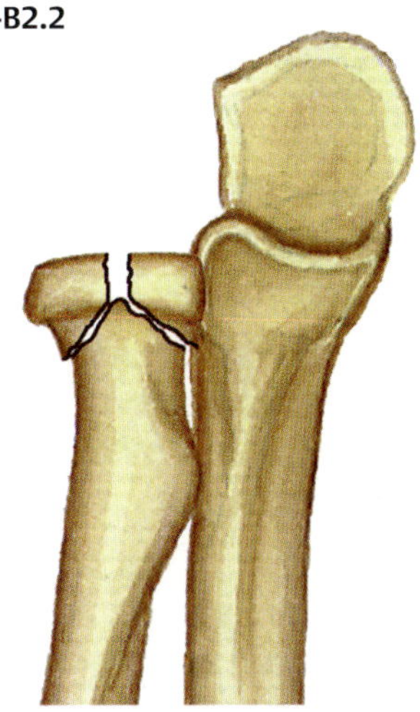

Multifragmentary without depression

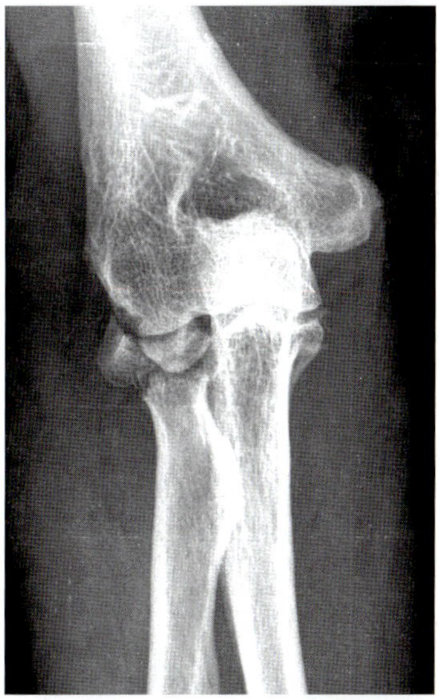

21-B2.3

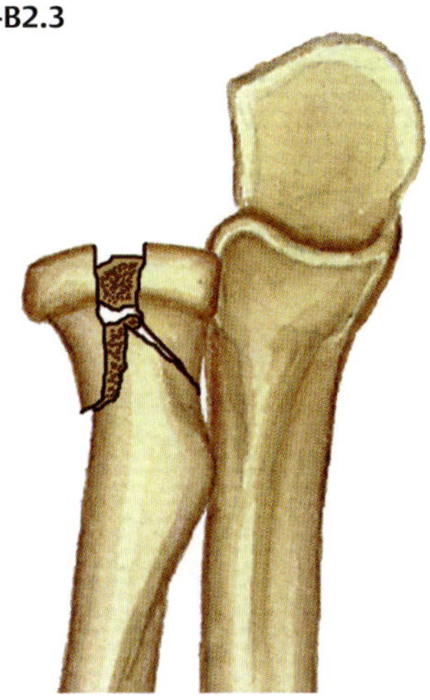

Multifragmentary with depression

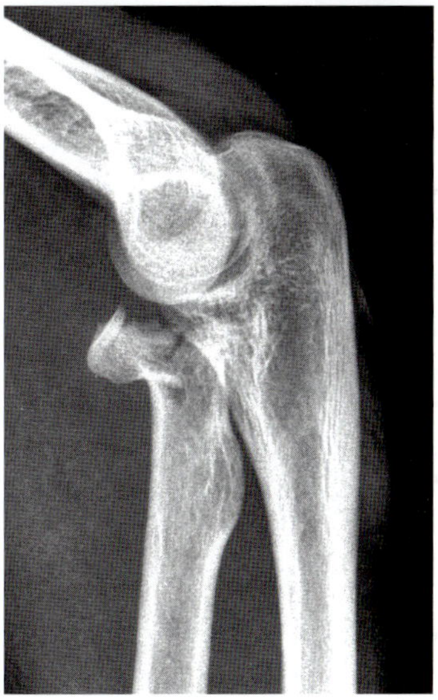

21-B Radius/ulna, proximal partial articular fractures

21-B3
One bone articular, other bone extra-articular

202 fractures
M: 129 (63.86%)
F: 73 (36.14%)
0.05% of total adult fractures
0.35% of adult radius/ulna
2.80% of segment 21
3.84% of type 21-B

21-B3.1

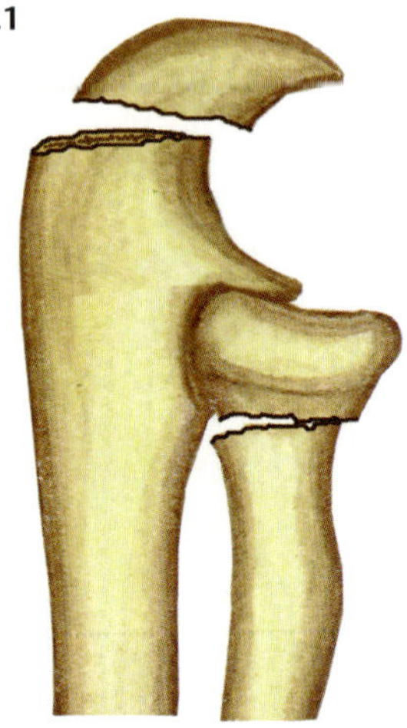

Ulna articular simple, radius extra-articular fracture

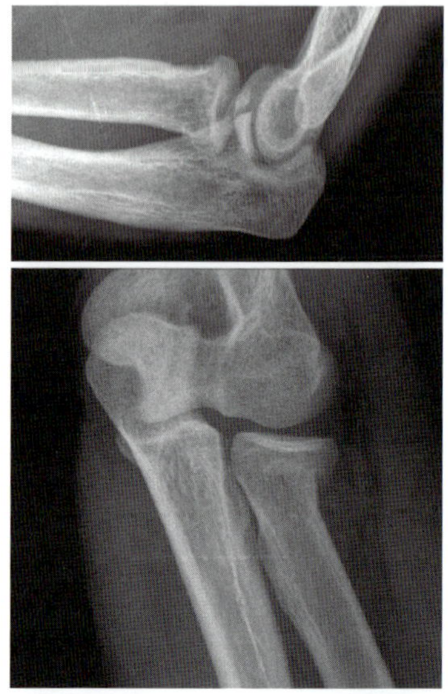

21-B3.2

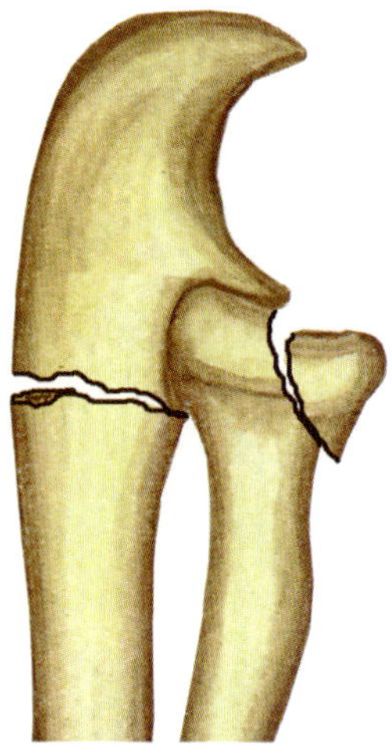

Radius articular simple, ulna extra-articular fracture

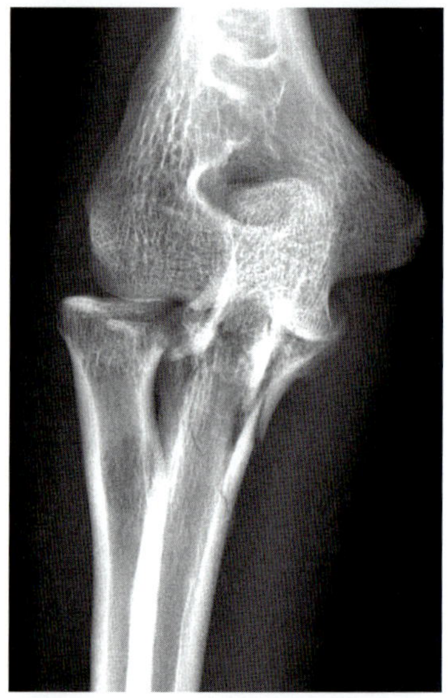

21-B3.3

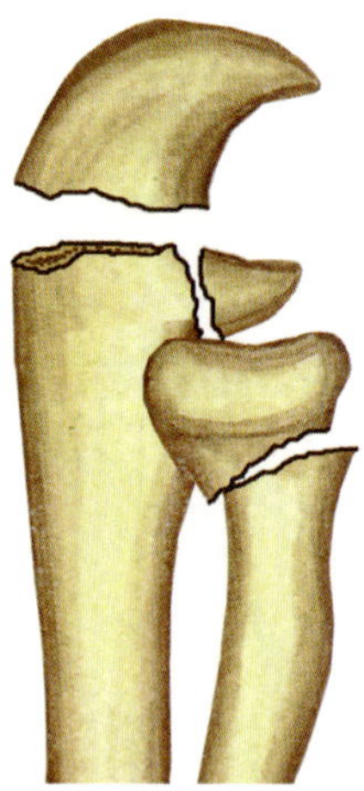

One bone articular multifragmentary, other bone extra-articular fracture

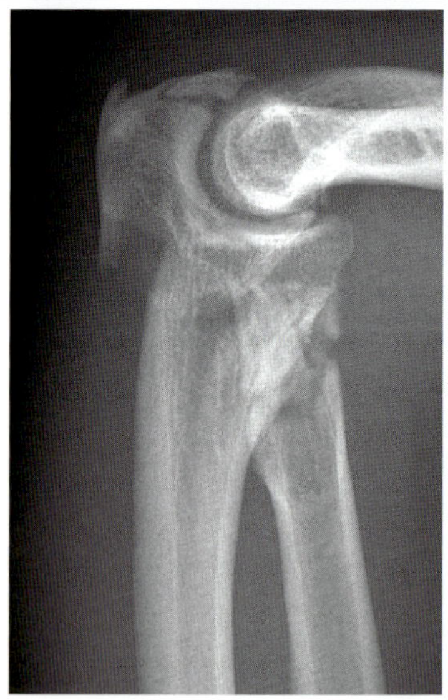

21-C Radius/ulna, proximal complete articular fractures

21-C1
Both bones, simple fracture
125 fractures
M: 76 (60.80%)
F: 49 (39.20%)
0.03% of total adult fractures
0.21% of adult radius/ulna
1.74% of segment 21
43.86% of type 21-C

21-C1.1

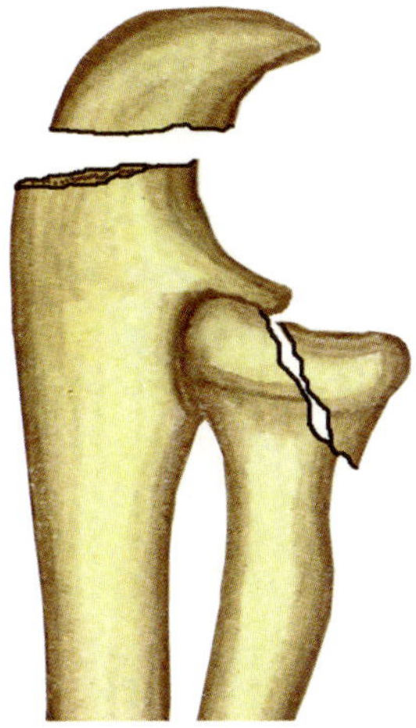

Olecranon and radial head

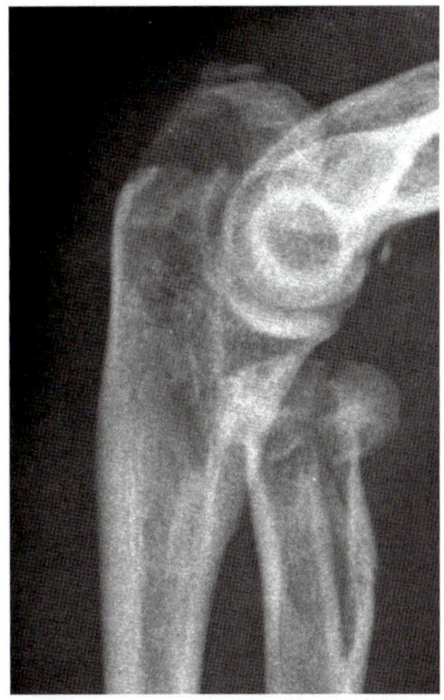

21-C1.2

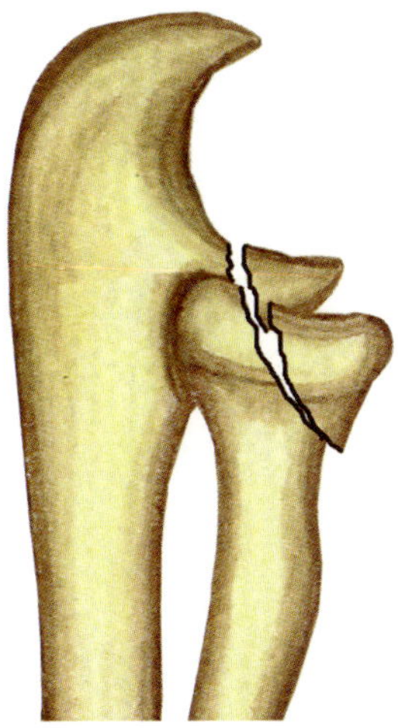

Coronoid process and radial head

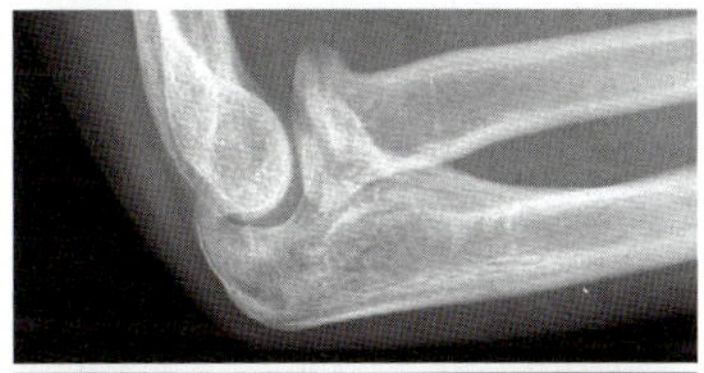

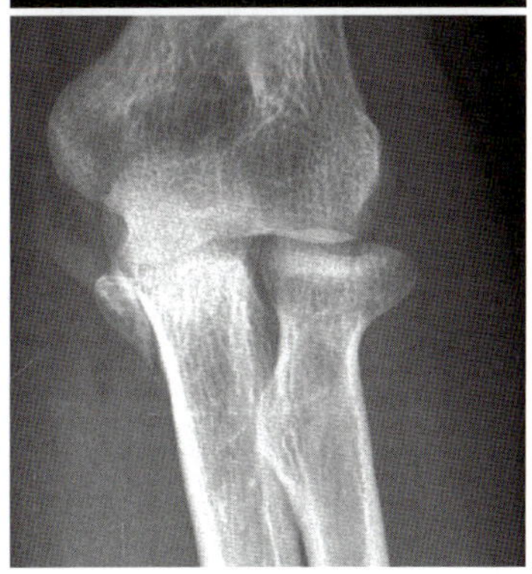

21-C Radius/ulna, proximal complete articular fractures

21-C2

Both bones, one articular simple, the other articular multifragmentary

90 fractures
M: 66 (73.33%)
F: 24 (26.67%)
0.02% of total adult fractures
0.15% of adult radius/ulna
1.25% of segment 21
31.58% of type 21-C

21-C2.1

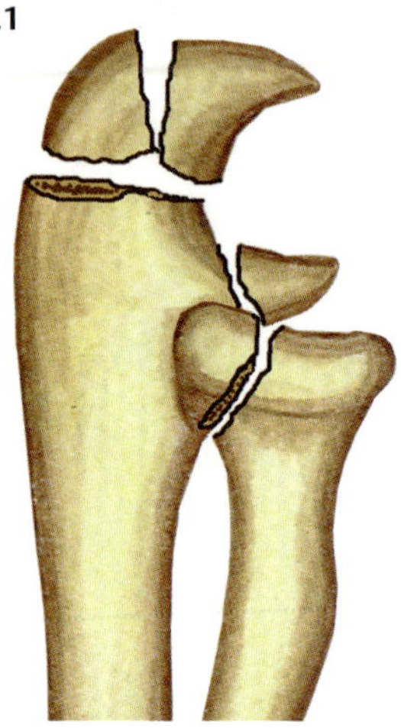

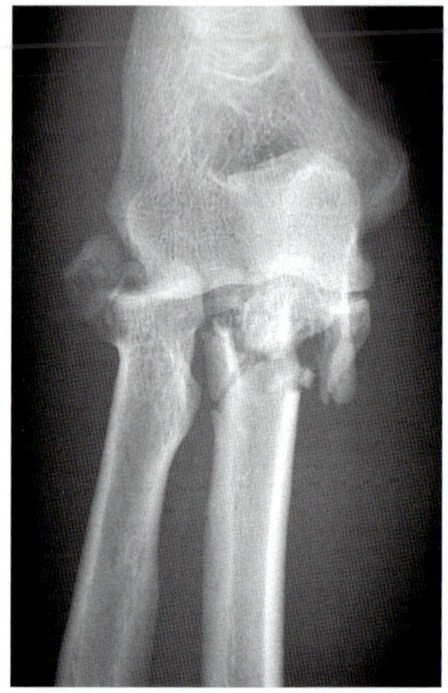

Olecranon multifragmentary, radial head simple split

21-C2.2

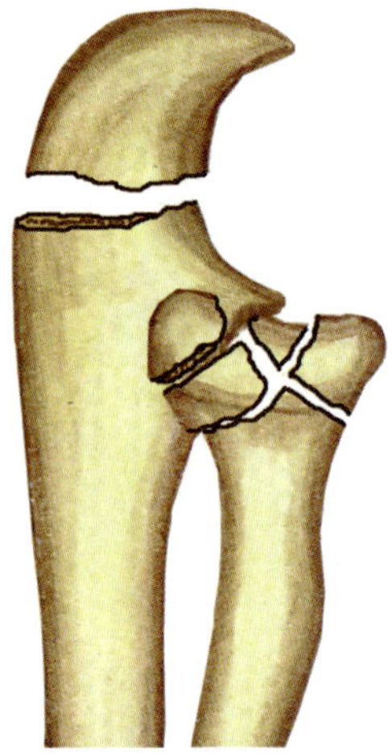

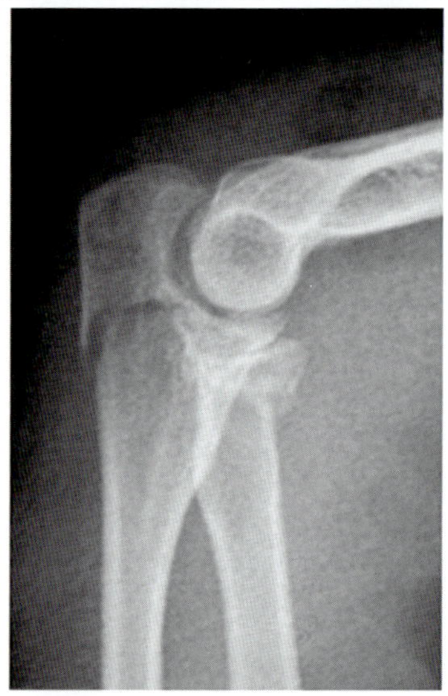

Olecranon simple, radial head multifragmentary

21-C2.3

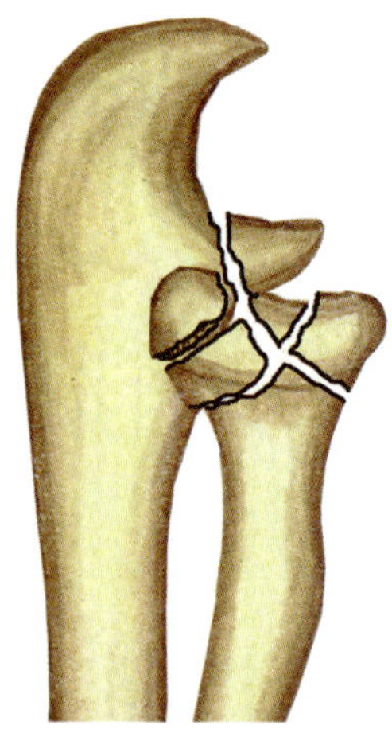

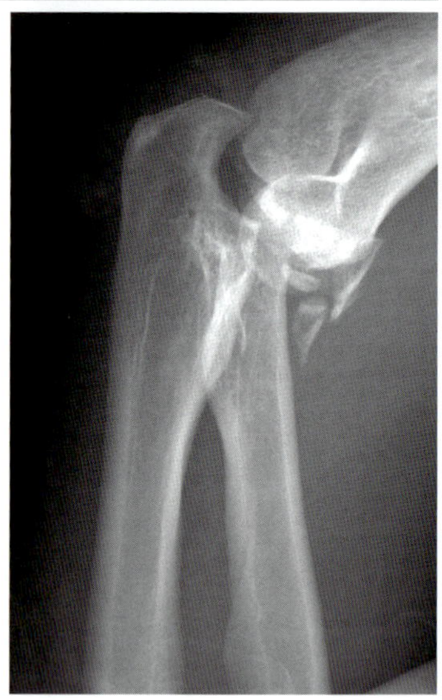

Coronoid process simple, radial head multifragmentary

21-C Radius/ulna, proximal complete articular fractures

21-C3
Both bones articular multifragmentary
70 fractures
M: 48 (68.57%)
F: 22 (31.43%)
0.02% of total adult fractures
0.12% of adult radius/ulna
0.97% of segment 21
24.56% of type 21-C

21-C3.1

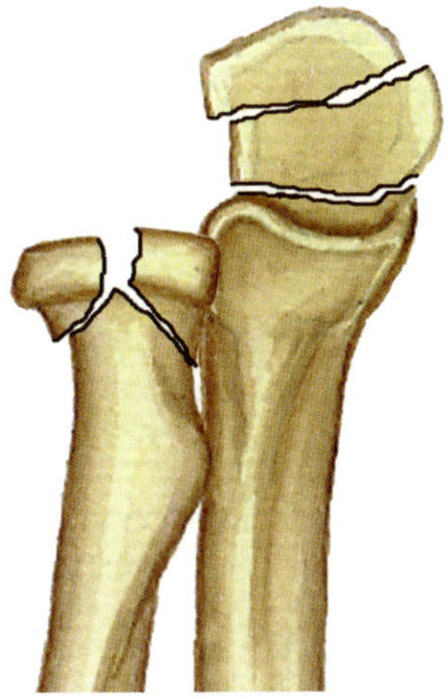

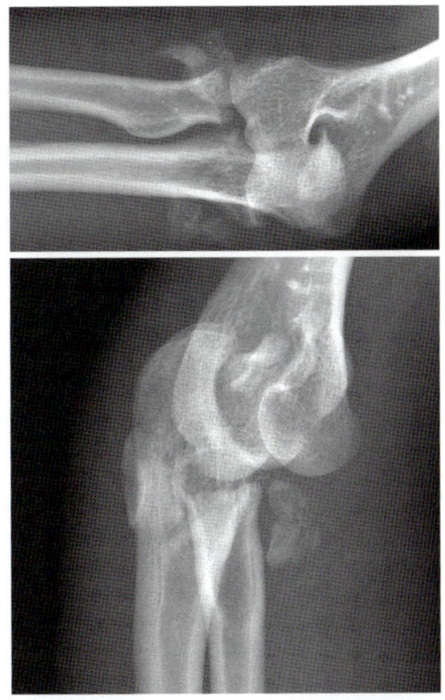

Three fragments each bone

21-C3.2

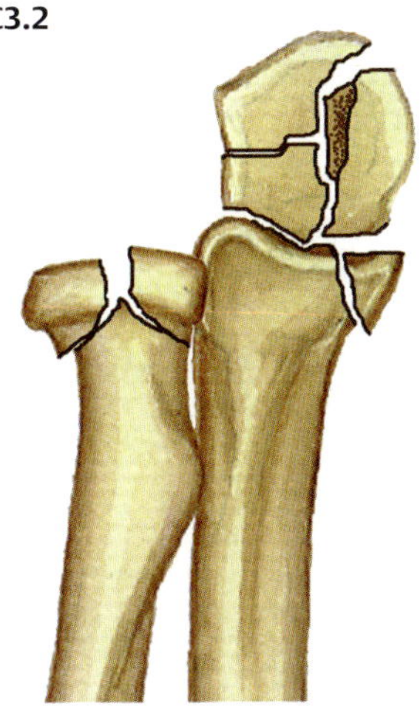

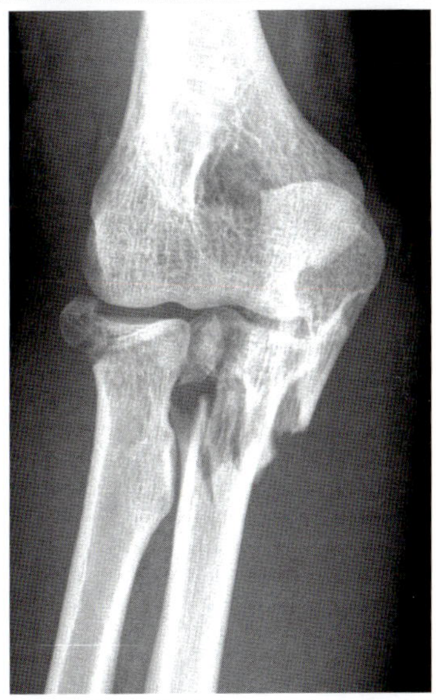

Ulna more than three fragments, radius three or more fragments

21-C3.3

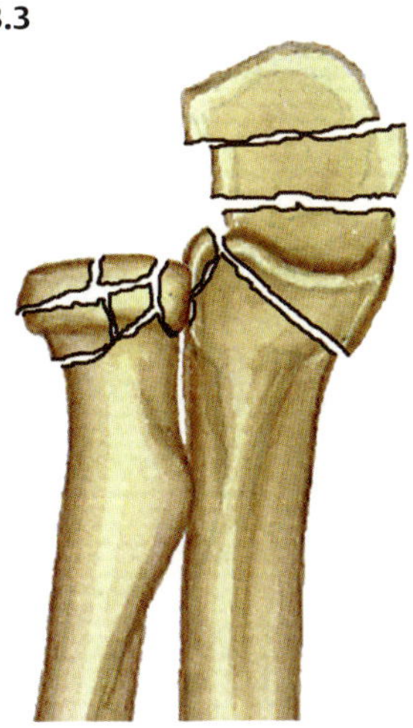

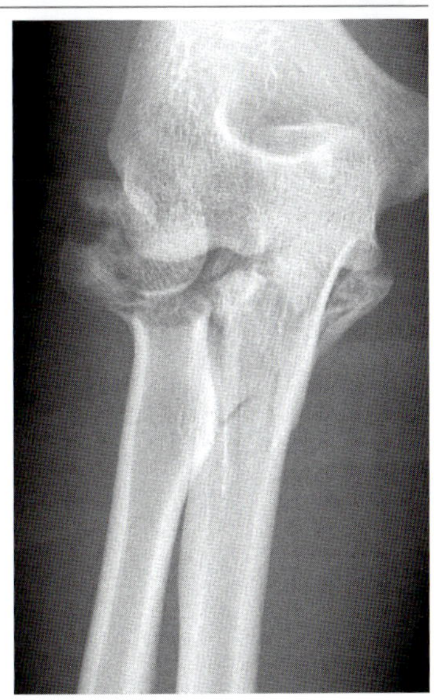

Radius more than three fragments, ulna three or more fragments

Injury Mechanism

Olecranon Fractures

Olecranon multifragmentary fracture can be caused by direct trauma, as in falls on or blows to the point of the elbow. Such types of fractures also occur during a fall on the semiflexed supinated forearm with the hand striking the ground, and the pull of the triceps muscle leading to a transverse or wedge fracture of the olecranon.

Fractures of Radial Head or Neck of the Radius

This type of injury is usually from a fall on an outstretched arm with the force of impact transmitted up the hand through the forearm to the radial head, which is forced to the capitellum and often causes fractures in the anterolateral aspect of the radial head or neck of the radius. Multifragmentary fractures or dislocation may occur by high-energy trauma.

Coronoid Fractures

Coronoid fracture, rarely seen in isolation, usually occurs in combination with olecranon fracture; this type of fracture results from an avulsion fracture of the bony structure of the coronoid, by contraction of the joint capsule with the elbow in hyperextension.

Diagnosis

The insertion of the triceps muscle on the olecranon is usually compromised when olecranon fractures occur. In most cases, patients cannot fully straighten their arms due to the pain and are unable to overcome any resistance. The movement of supination aggravates the pain from fractures in the radial head or neck of the radius and limits the range of motion.

The radiographic examination should include anteroposterior (AP) and lateral views of the elbow. If the patient has marked physical signs but inconclusive X-rays, computed tomography (CT) or magnetic resonance imaging (MRI) may be required to clarify the nature and extent of the injury. Note that the individual will be unable to fully extend the forearm when taking the AP view of the elbow, so the beam must be placed perpendicularly to the radial head (the *left* figure shows the correct projection position, while the wrong one commonly seen in practice is shown on the *right*) (**Plate 3.6**).

Treatment

Olecranon fractures are unstable fractures, usually requiring surgical intervention. Plate fixation, tension band wiring, and other internal fixators can be utilized in stabilizing the fracture, depending on the fracture type.

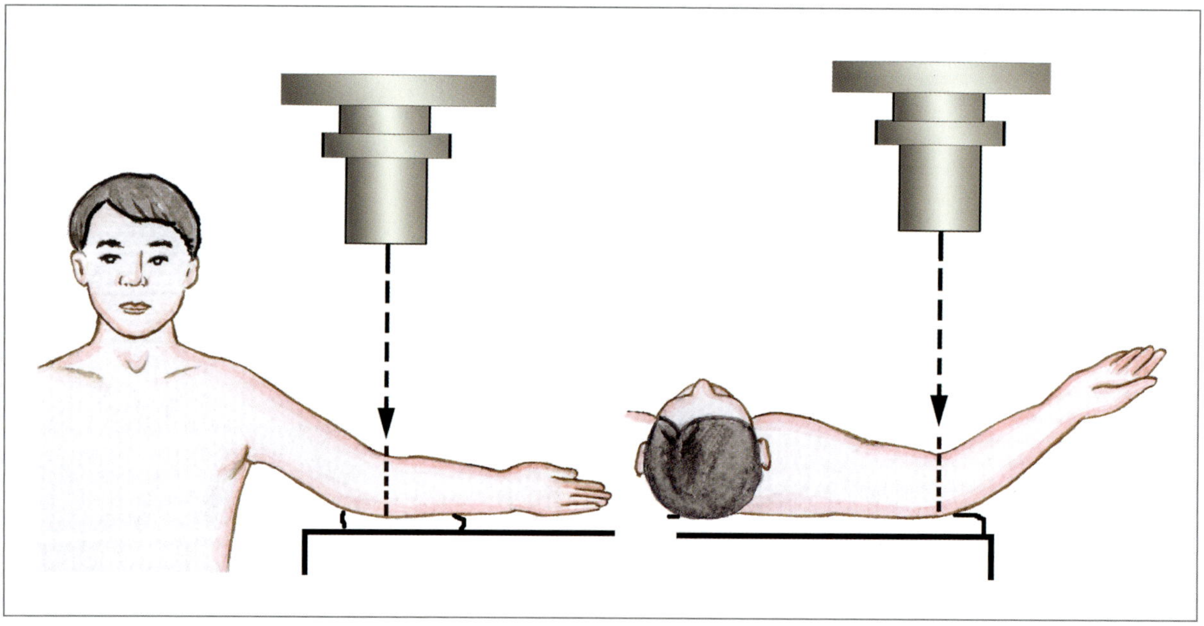

Plate 3.6

Stable fractures of the radial head or the neck of the radius with no displacement can be managed nonsurgically, but with close monitoring of fracture progression for 4 weeks. Minimal invasive internal fixation is preferable for fractures with dislocation or when nonsurgical treatment fails. Based on fracture type, patient age, and general condition, various internal fixators can be selected, including screws, absorbable screws, and Kirschner wires (K-wires). Anatomical reduction to the utmost, rigid fixation, and early mobilization are applied even for complex fractures. Excision of the radial head and replacement with a prosthesis should be considered only as a last resort.

Fractures of the Radial/Ulnar Shaft (Segment 22)

Anatomical Features

The ulna is relatively straight whereas the radius is slightly curved. In the anatomical position, the width of the space between the ulna and radius is variable, with a maximum width of 1.5–2 cm. The IOM, which connects the radius and ulna along their entire length, bears loads with the forearm in a neutral position and is slackened when the forearm is in pronated position. The fibers of the IOM run obliquely upward and lateral from the interosseous crest of the ulna to that of the radius. When one of the bones is fractured, energy is transmitted along the IOM, causing fractures on the other bone in a different plane and a dislocated proximal radioulnar joint. Many muscles are attached to the radius and ulna with their insertion points spread around their shafts. Consequently, complex fractures with marked displacement usually occur due to contraction of multiple muscles, which make the reduction very difficult.

AO Classification of Fractures of Radial/Ulnar Shaft

The numeric code for shaft of the radius and ulna is 22 based on the AO classification (**Plate 3.7**). Fracture of the radial/ulnar shaft is divided into three types: 22-A, simple fracture; 22-B, wedge fracture; and 22-C, complex fracture (**Plate 3.8**).

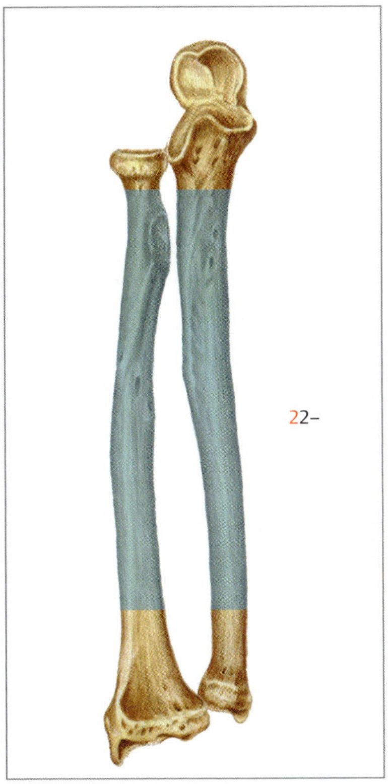

Plate 3.7

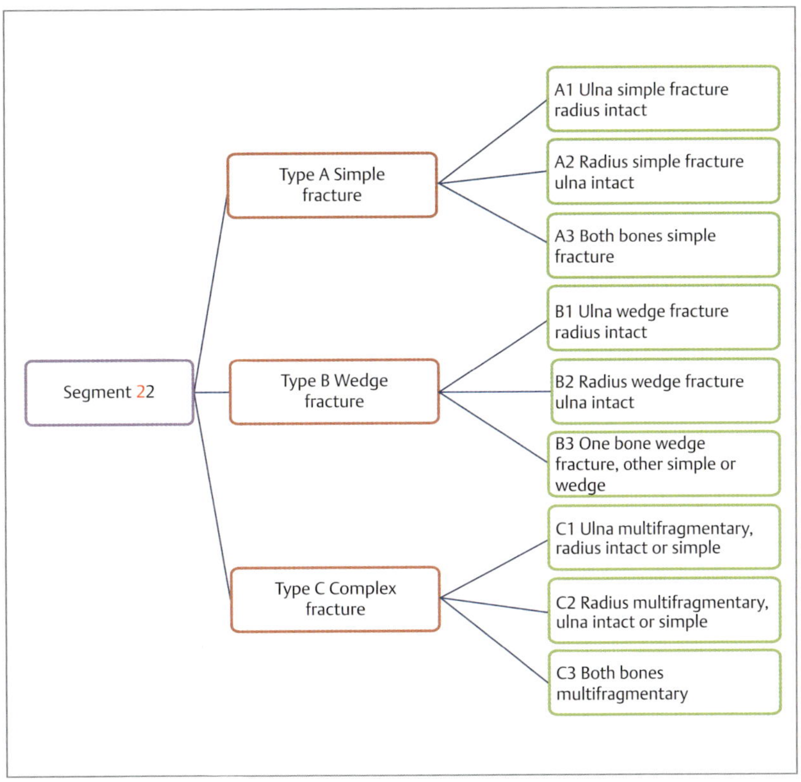

Plate 3.8

Clinical Epidemiologic Features of the Radial/Ulnar Shaft Fractures (Segment 22)

A total of 7,594 adult radial/ulnar shaft fractures (segment 22) were treated in 83 hospitals in China over a 2-year period from 2010 to 2011. All cases were reviewed and statistically studied; the fractures accounted for 13.04% of all adult fractures of the radius/ulna. Their epidemiologic features are as follows:

- More males than females
- The high-risk age group includes the ages 21–25 years; the age group 21–25 years is the highest risk group for males, for females it is 36–40 years
- The most common fracture type among segment 22 fractures is type 22-A; the same fracture type for both males and females.
- The most common fracture group among segment 22 fractures is group 22-A1; the same fracture group for both males and females.

Fractures of Segment 22 by Sex

Table 3.10 Sex distribution of 7,594 fractures of segment 22

Sex	Number of fractures	Percentage (%)
Male	5,709	75.18
Female	1,885	24.82
Total	7,594	100.00

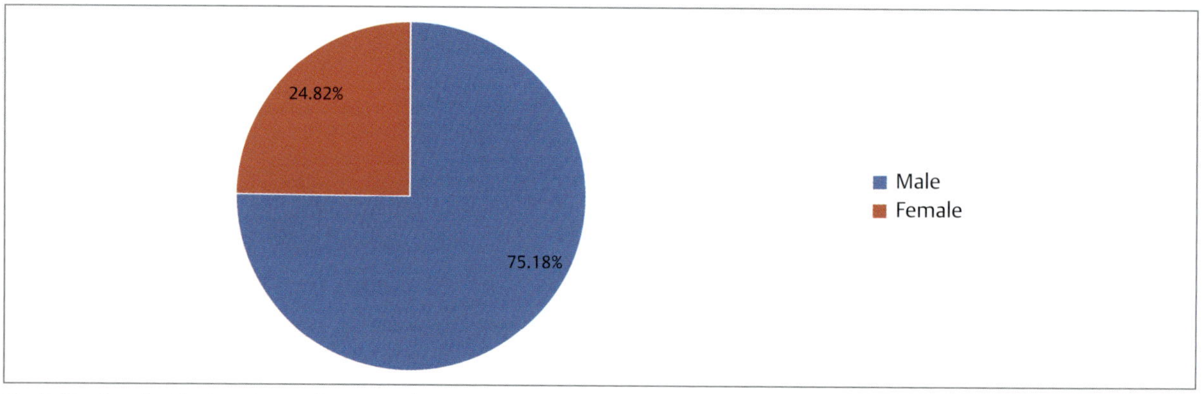

Fig. 3.10 Sex distribution of 7,594 fractures of segment 22.

Fractures of Segment 22 by Age Group

Table 3.11 Age and sex distribution of 7,594 fractures of segment 22

Age group (years)	Male	Female	Number of fractures	Percentage (%)
16–20	826	148	974	12.83
21–25	865	161	1,026	13.51
26–30	683	182	865	11.39
31–35	528	175	703	9.26
36–40	674	257	931	12.26
41–45	623	227	850	11.19
46–50	587	242	829	10.92
51–55	346	122	468	6.16
56–60	272	86	358	4.71
61–65	147	88	235	3.09
66–70	70	66	136	1.79
71–75	30	56	86	1.13
76–80	34	47	81	1.07
81–85	14	19	33	0.43
≥86	10	9	19	0.25
Total	5,709	1,885	7,594	100.00

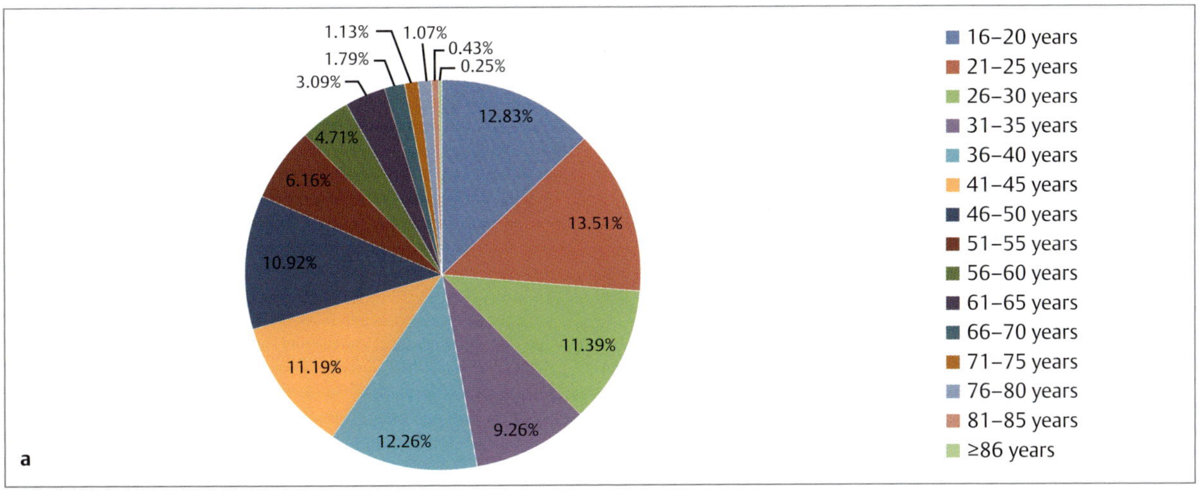

Fig. 3.11 **(a)** Age distribution of 7,594 fractures of segment 22. (*Continued*)

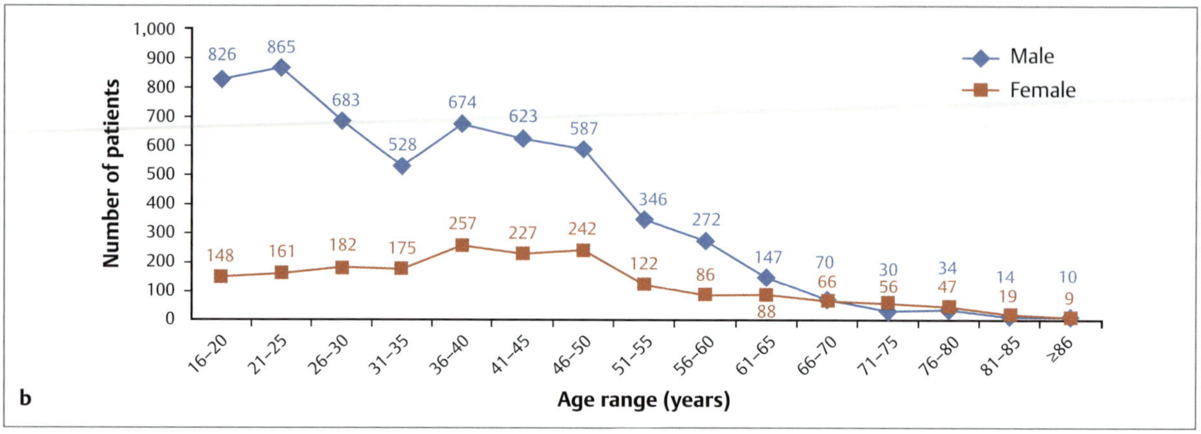

Fig. 3.11 (*continued*) **(b)** Age and sex distribution of 7,594 fractures of segment 22.

Fractures of Segment 22 by Fracture Type

Table 3.12 Sex and fracture type distribution of 7,594 fractures of segment 22

Fracture type	Male	Female	Number of fractures	Percentage of radius/ ulna fractures (%)
22-A	3,456	1,201	4,657	61.32
22-B	1,785	538	2,323	30.59
22-C	468	146	614	8.09
Total	5,709	1,885	7,594	100.00

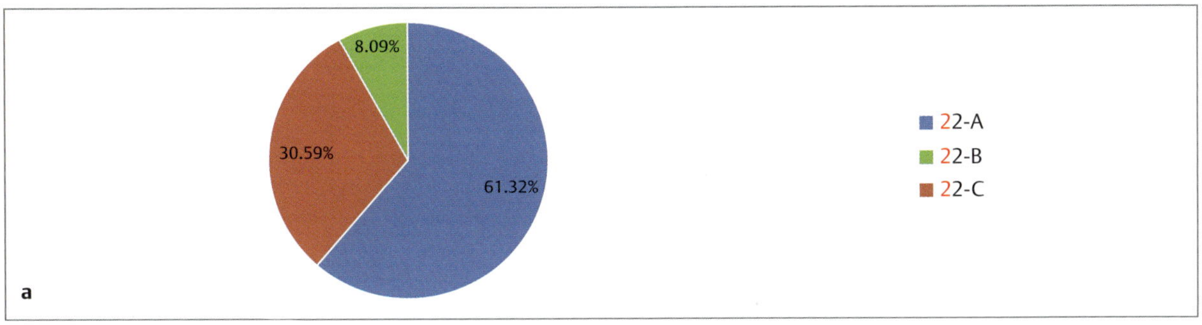

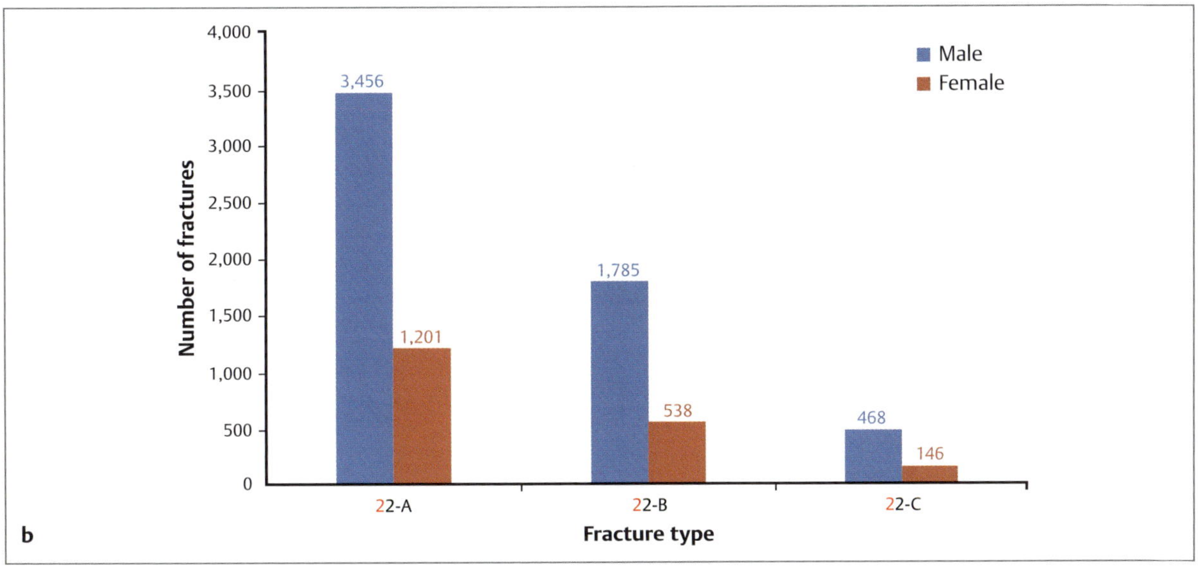

Fig. 3.12 **(a)** Fracture type distribution of 7,594 fractures of segment 22.
(b) Sex and fracture type distribution of 7,594 fractures of segment 22.

Table 3.13 Sex and fracture group distribution of 7,594 fractures of segment 22

Fracture group	Male	Female	Number of fractures	Percentage of segment 22 fractures (%)	Percentage of radius/ulna fractures (%)
22-A1	1,268	463	1,731	22.79	2.97
22-A2	1,188	367	1,555	20.48	2.67
22-A3	1,000	371	1,371	18.05	2.36
22-B1	694	156	850	11.19	1.46
22-B2	469	133	602	7.93	1.03
22-B3	622	249	871	11.47	1.50
22-C1	178	55	233	3.07	0.40
22-C2	154	48	202	2.66	0.35
22-C3	136	43	179	2.36	0.31
Total	5,709	1,885	7,594	100.00	13.04

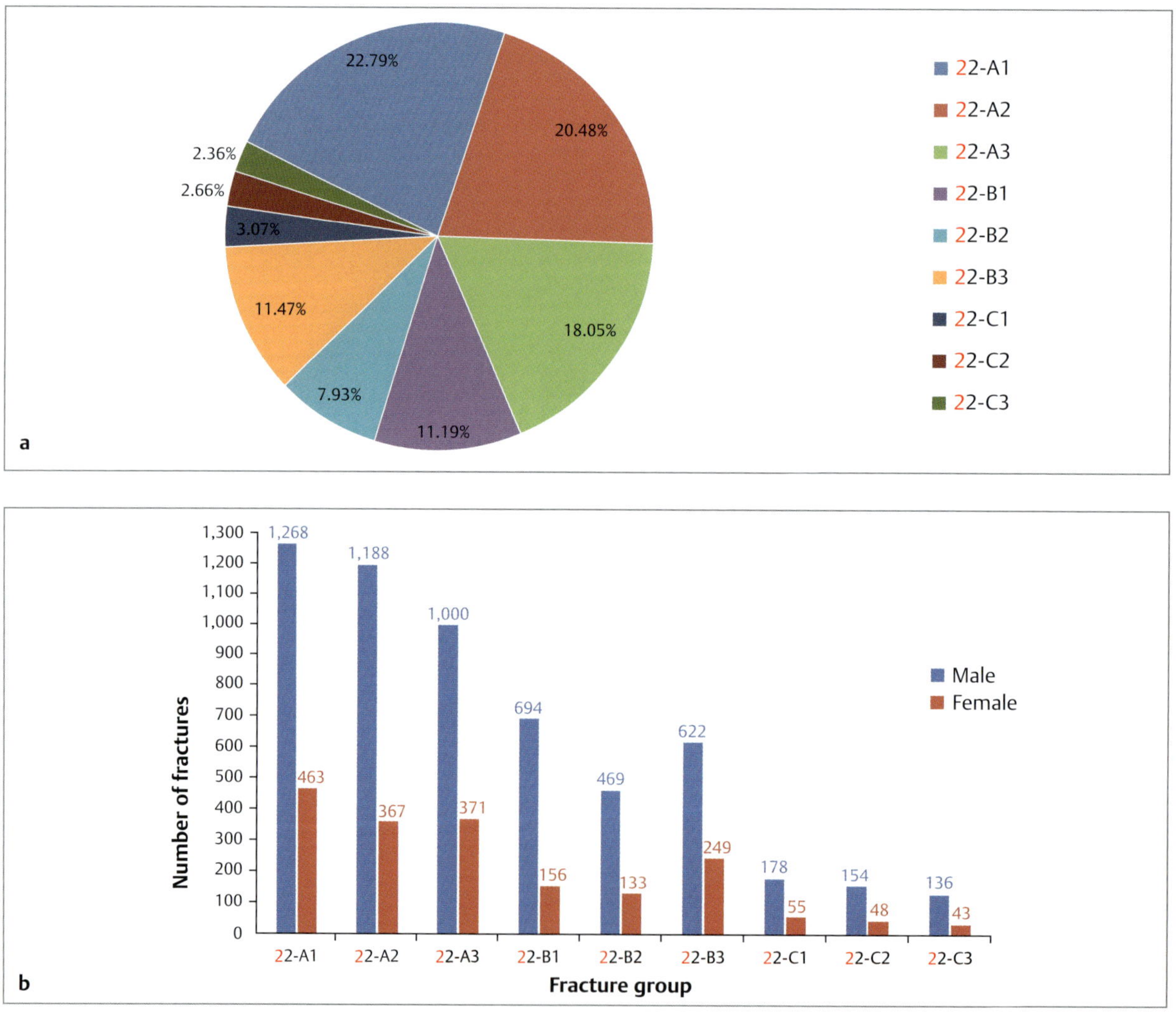

Fig. 3.13 **(a)** Fracture group distribution of 7,594 fractures of segment 22.
(b) Sex and fracture group distribution of 7,594 fractures of segment 22.

22-A Radius/ulna shaft simple fractures

22-A1
Ulna,
radius intact
1,731 fractures
M: 1,268 (73.25%)
F: 463 (26.75%)
0.46% of total adult fractures
2.97% of adult radius/ulna
22.79% of segment 22
37.17% of type 22-A

22-A1.1

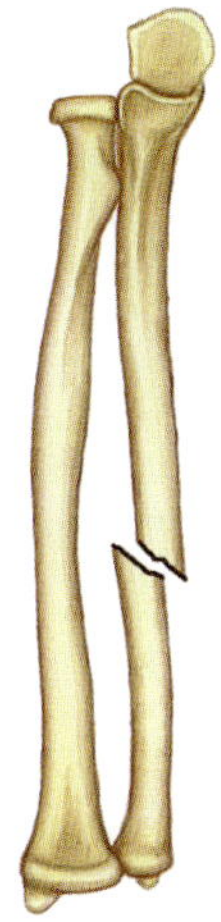

Oblique

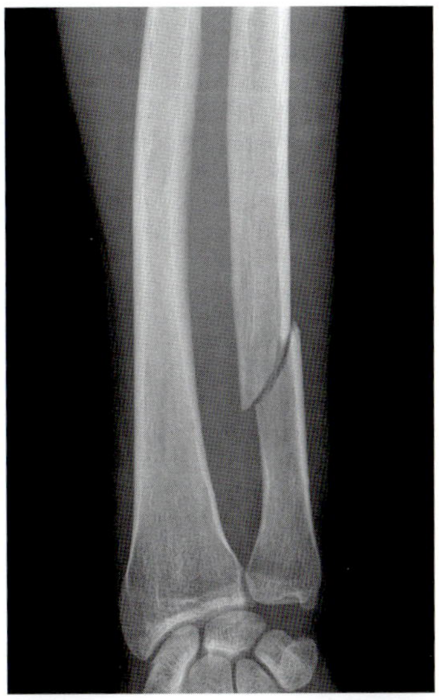

22-A1.2

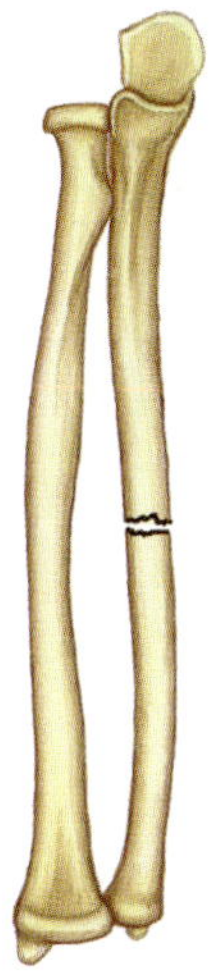

Transverse

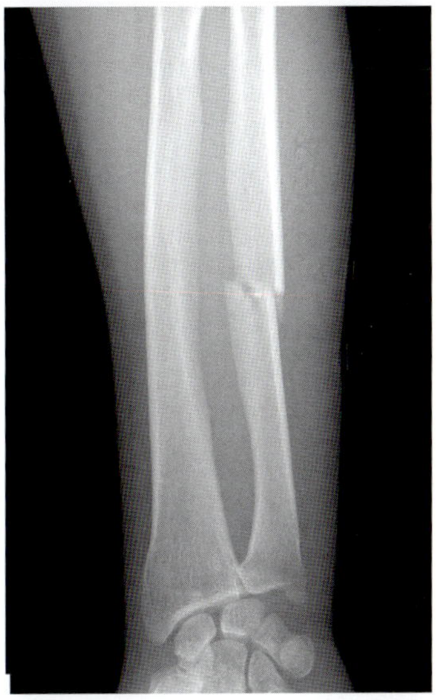

22-A1.3

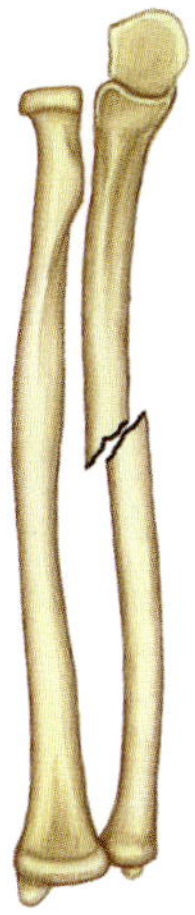

With radial head dislocation (Monteggia)

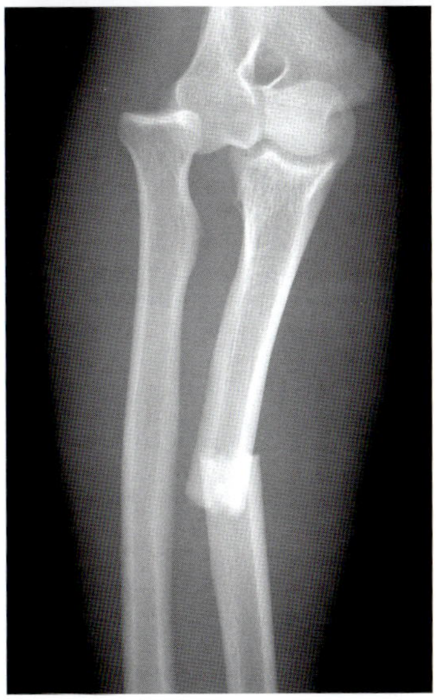

22-A Radius/ulna shaft simple fractures

22-A2
Radius,
ulna intact
1,555 fractures
M: 1,188 (76.40%)
F: 367 (23.60%)
0.42% of total adult fractures
2.67% of adult radius/ulna
20.48% of segment 22
33.39% of type 22-A

22-A2.1

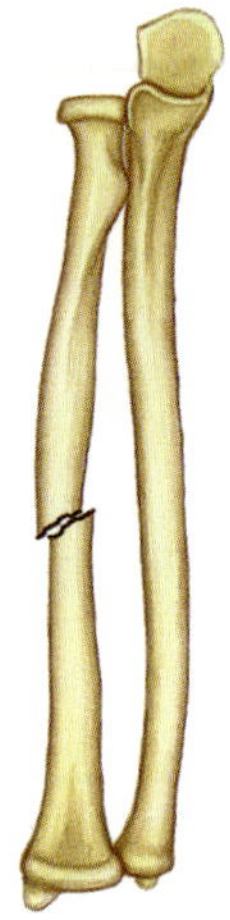

Oblique

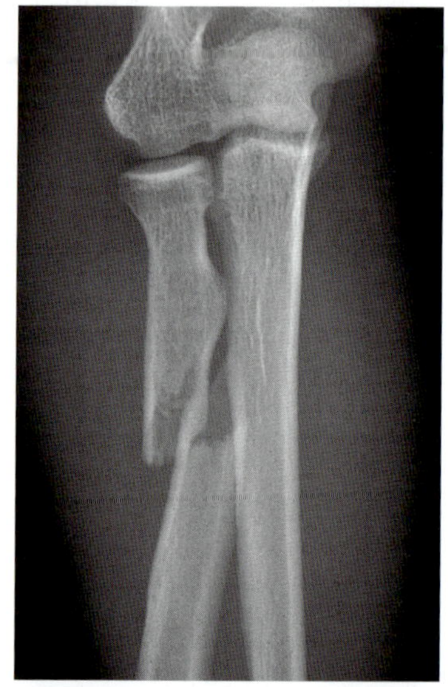

22-A2.2

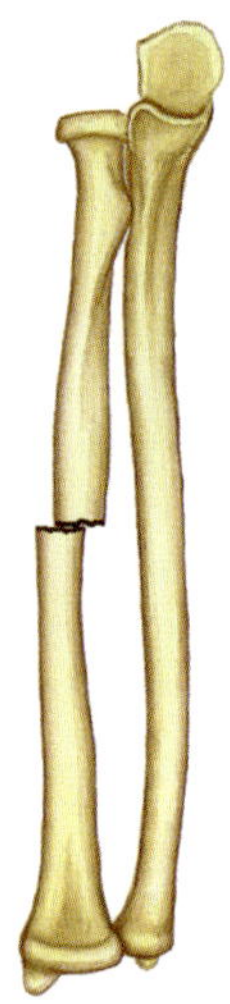

Transverse

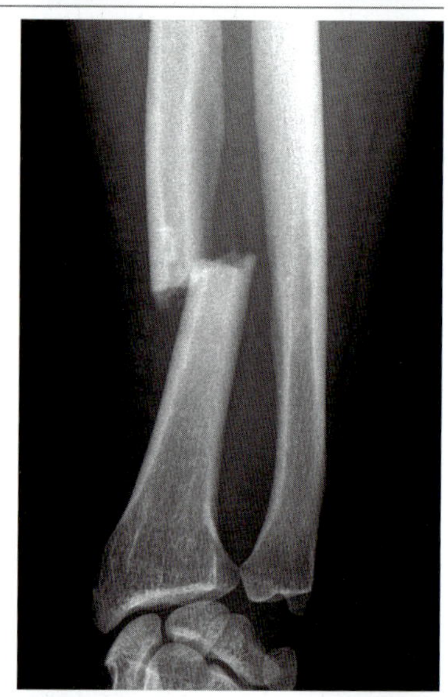

22-A2.3

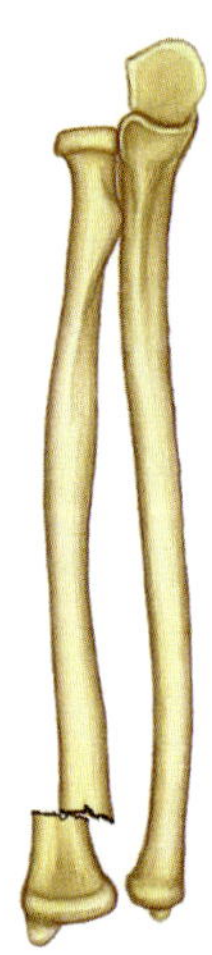

With distal radioulnar
joint dislocation (Galeazzi)

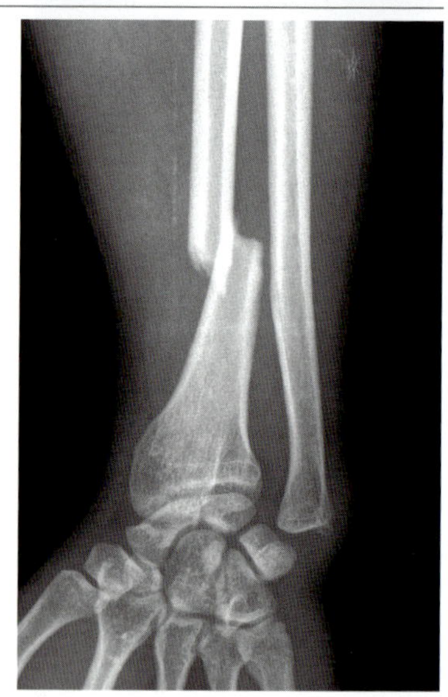

22-A Radius/ulna shaft simple fractures

22-A3
Both bones
1,371 fractures
M: 1,000 (72.94%)
F: 371 (27.06%)
0.37% of total adult fractures
2.36% of adult radius/ulna
18.05% of segment 22
29.44% of type 22-A

22-A3.1

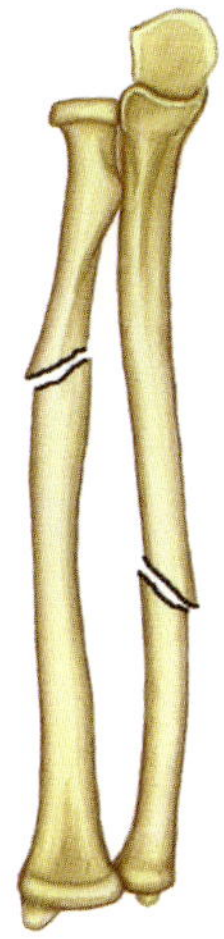

Radius, proximal section

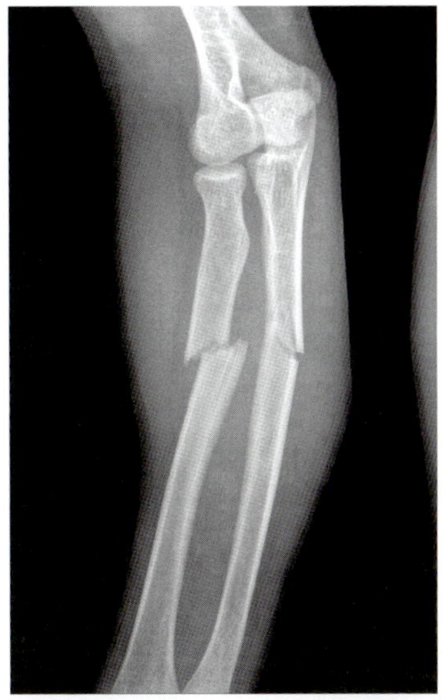

22-A3.2

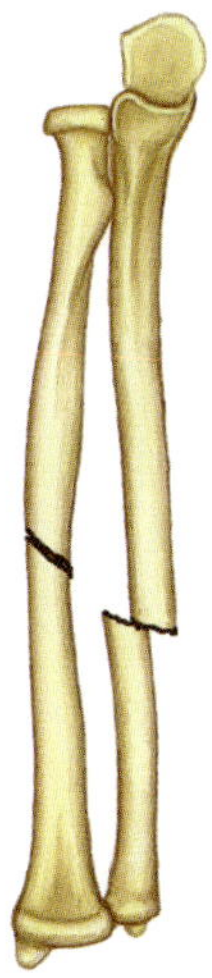

Radius, middle section

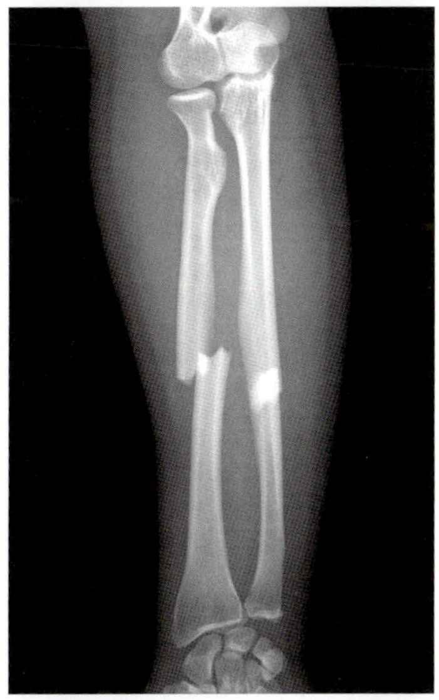

22-A3.3

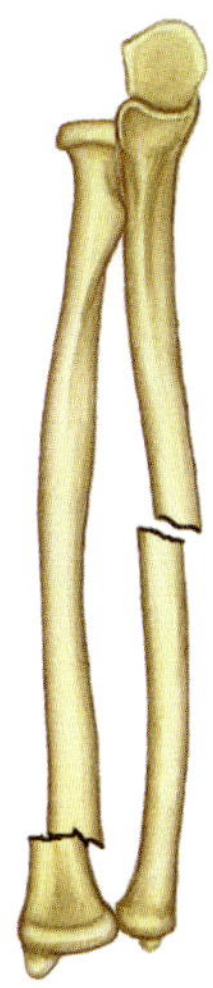

Radius, distal section

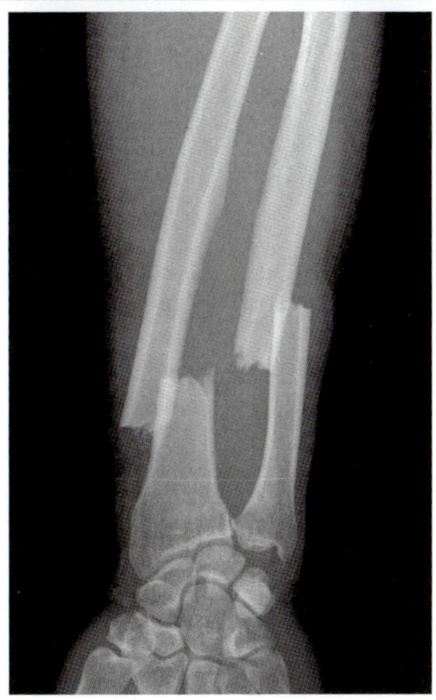

22-B Radius/ulna shaft wedge fractures

22-B1
Ulna,
radius intact
850 fractures
M: 694 (81.65%)
F: 156 (18.35%)
0.23% of total adult fractures
1.46% of adult radius/ulna
11.19% of segment 22
36.59% of type 22-B

22-B1.1

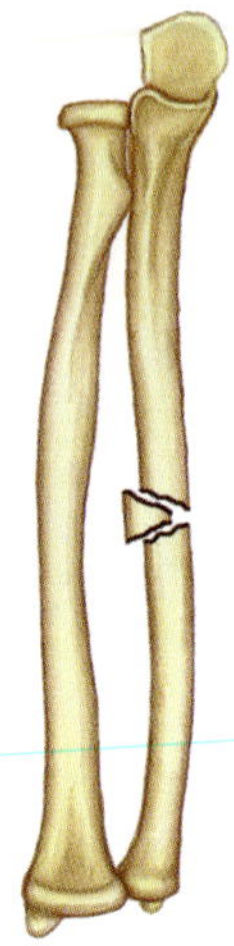

Intact wedge

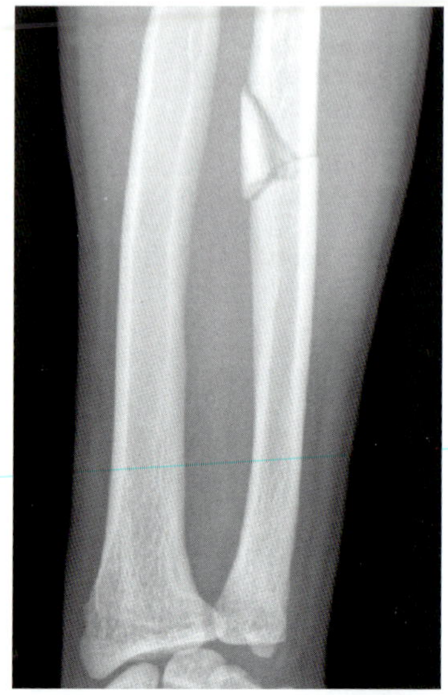

22-B1.2

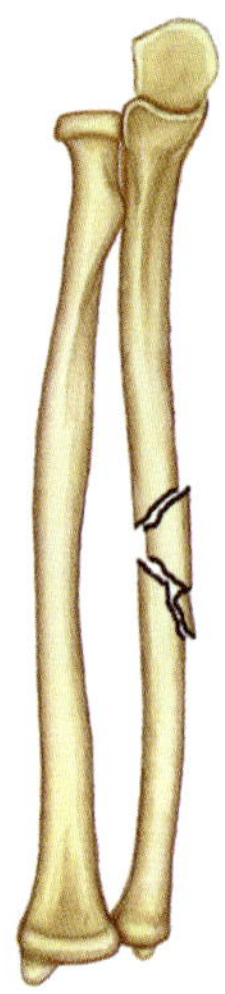

Fragmented wedge

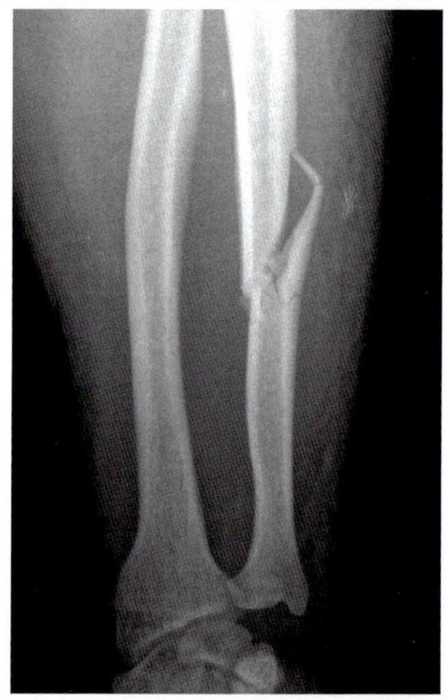

22-B1.3

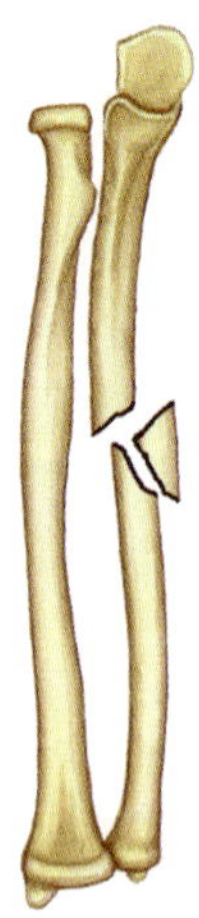

With radial head dislocation (Monteggia)

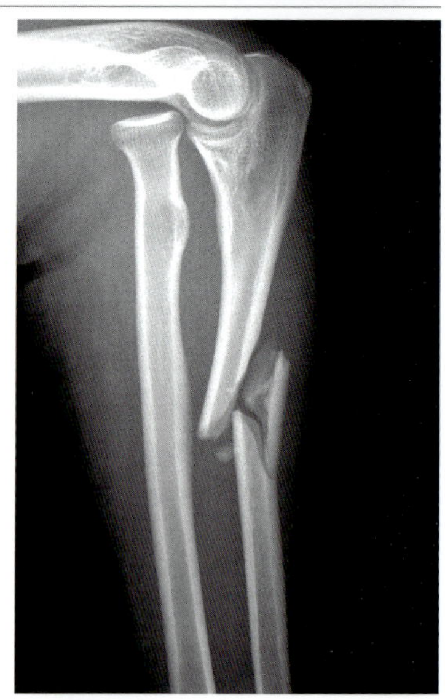

3

22-B Radius/ulna shaft wedge fractures

22-B2
Radius,
ulna intact
602 fractures
M: 469 (77.91%)
F: 133 (22.09%)
0.16% of total adult fractures
1.03% of adult radius/ulna
7.93% of segment 22
25.91% of type 22-B

22-B2.1

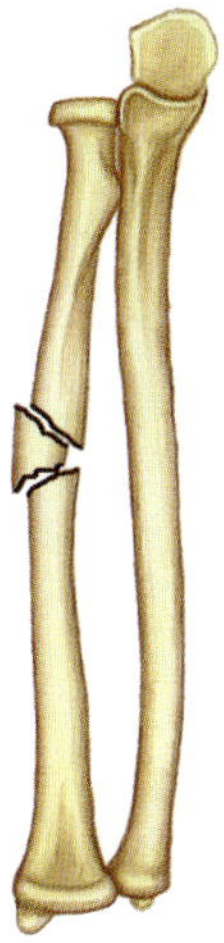

Intact wedge

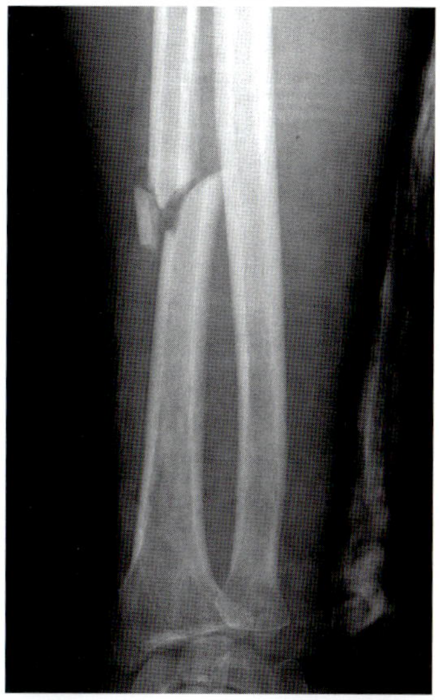

22-B2.2

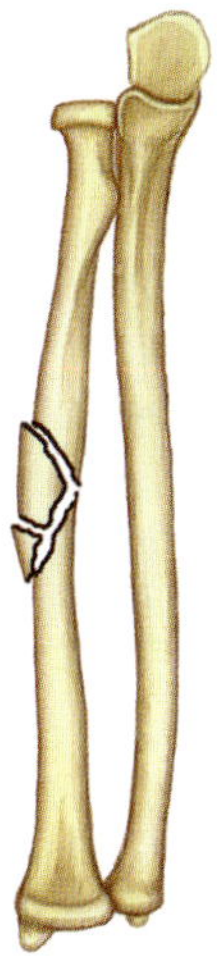

Fragmented wedge

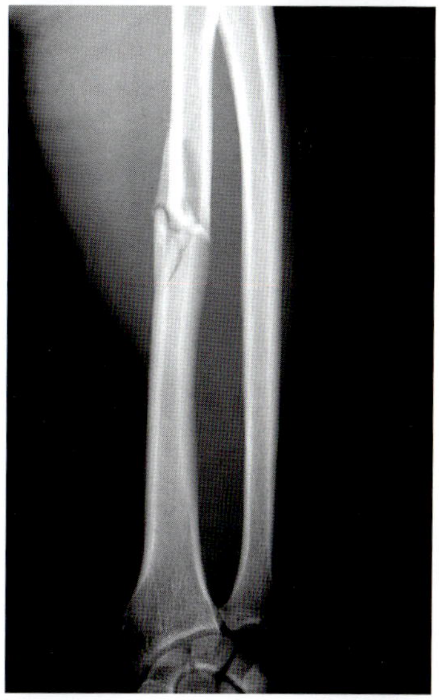

22-B2.3

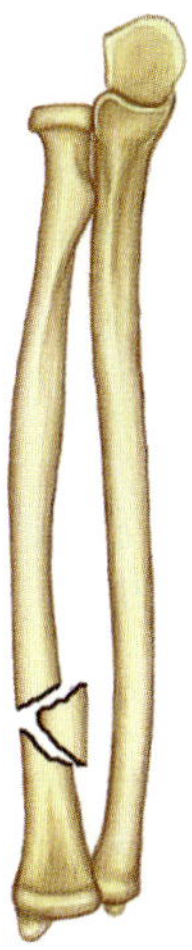

With distal radioulnar joint dislocation (Galeazzi)

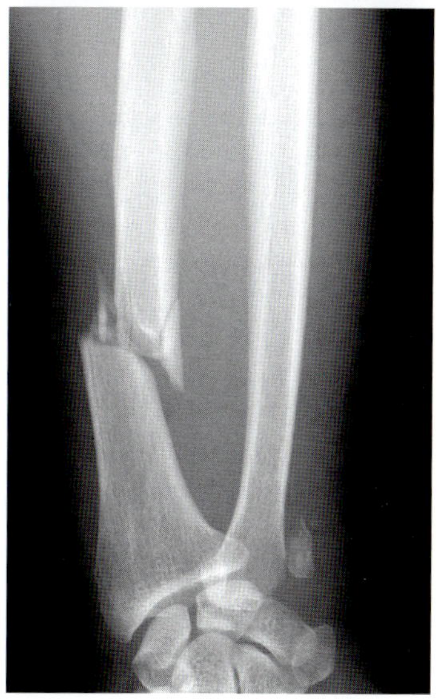

22-B Radius/ulna shaft wedge fractures

22-B3
One bone wedge, the other simple or wedge
871 fractures
M: 622 (71.41%)
F: 249 (28.59%)
0.23% of total adult fractures
1.50% of adult radius/ulna
11.47% of segment 22
37.49% of type 22-B

22-B3.1

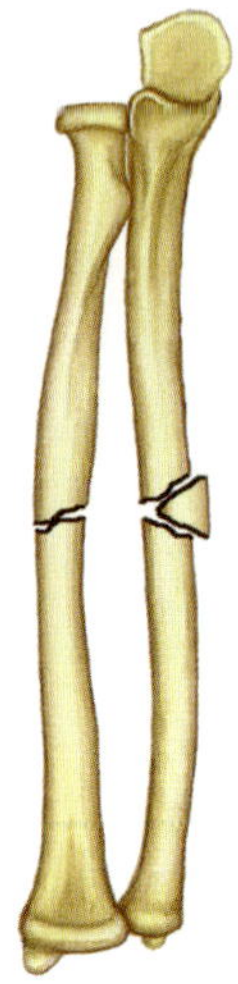

Ulna wedge, radius simple

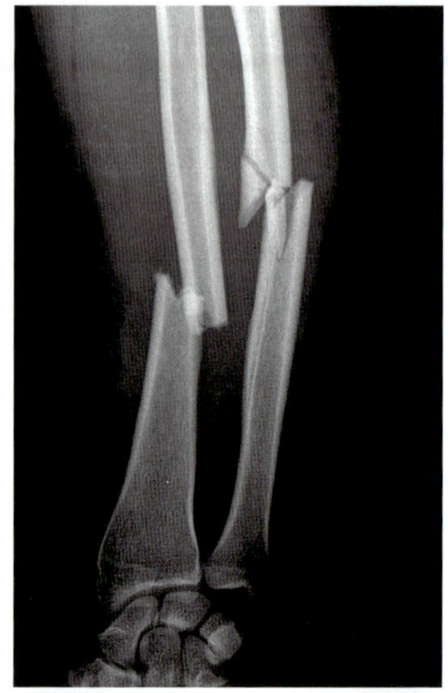

22-B3.2

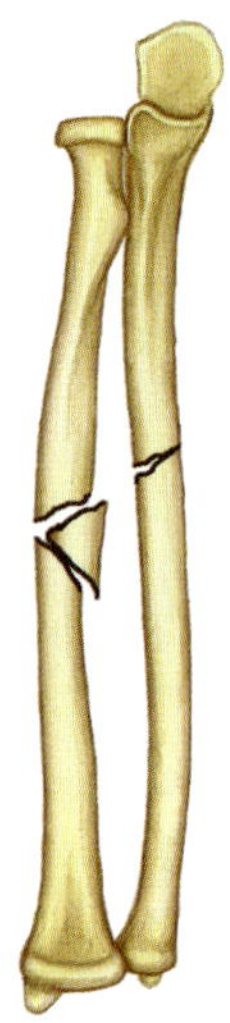

Radius wedge, ulna simple

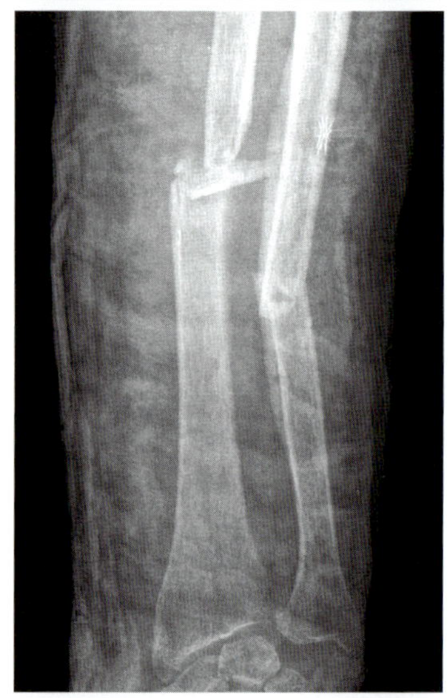

22-B3.3

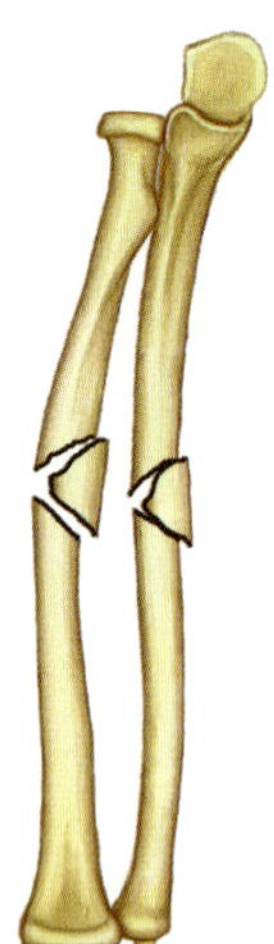

Both bones wedge

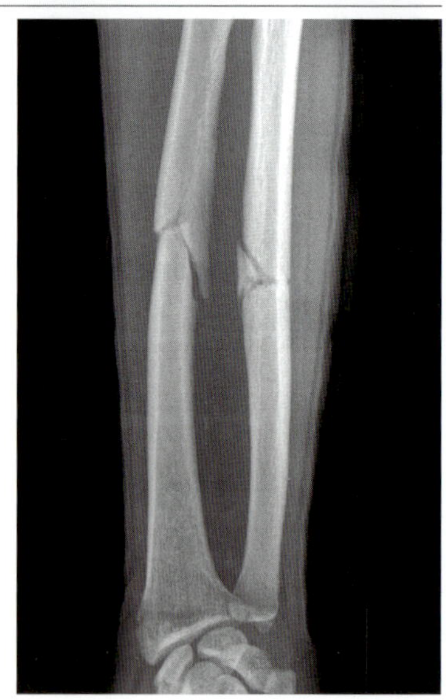

22-C Radius/ulna shaft complex fractures

22-C1
Ulna multifragmentary, radius intact or simple
233 fractures
M: 178 (76.39%)
F: 55 (23.61%)
0.06% of total adult fractures
0.40% of adult radius/ulna
3.07% of segment 22
37.95% of type 22-C

22-C1.1

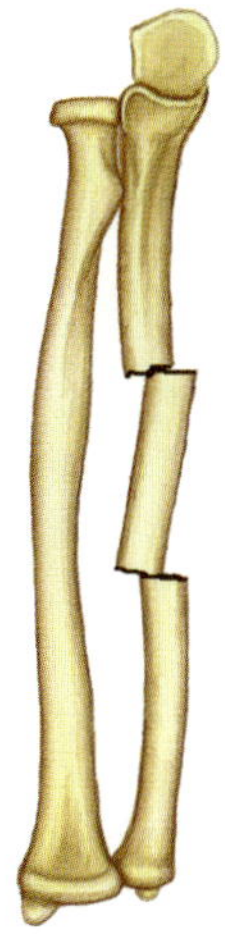

Ulna segmental, radius intact or dislocation

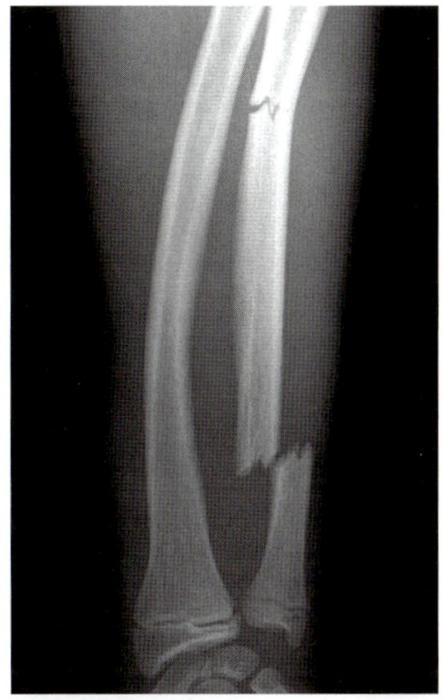

22-C1.2

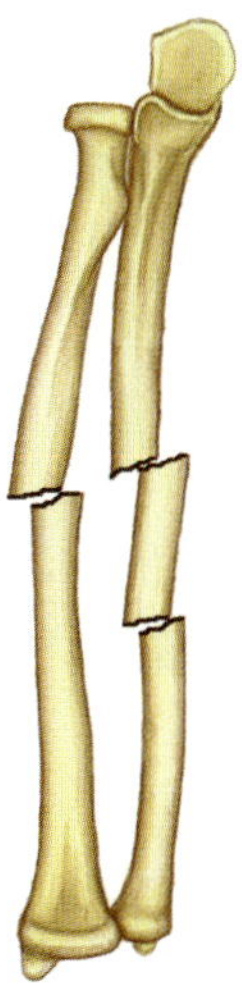

Ulna segmental, radius simple or wedge

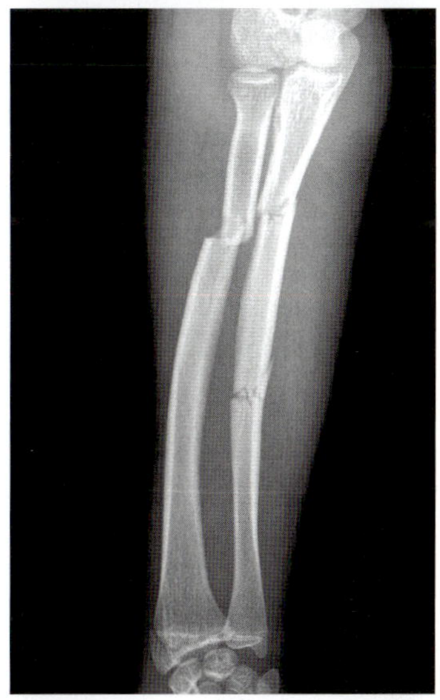

22-C1.3

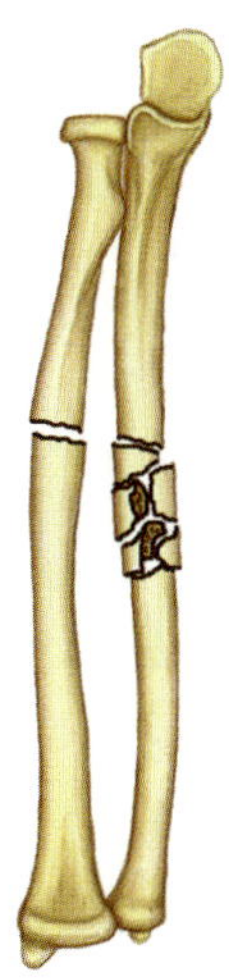

Ulna complex, radius intact, simple or wedge

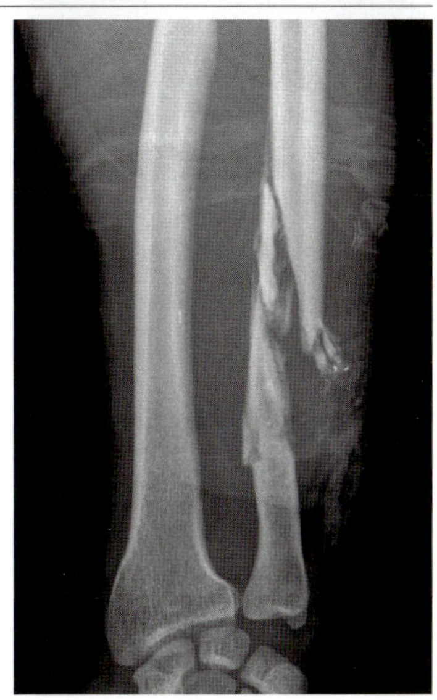

22-C Radius/ulna shaft complex fractures

22-C2
Radius multifragmentary, ulna intact or simple
202 fractures
M: 154 (76.24%)
F: 48 (23.76%)
0.05% of total adult fractures
0.35% of adult radius/ulna
2.66% of segment 22
32.90% of type 22-C

22-C2.1

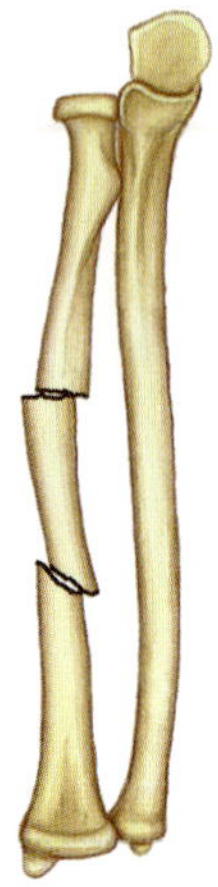

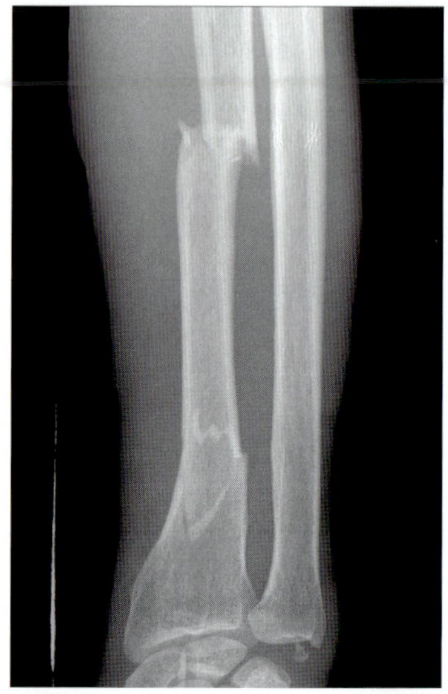

Radius segmental, ulna intact without dislocation or with dislocation of distal radioulnar joint (Galeazzi)

22-C2.2

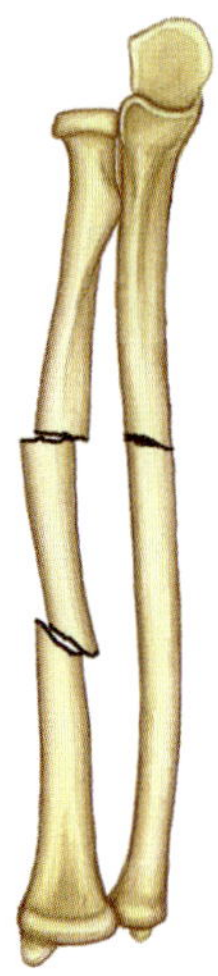

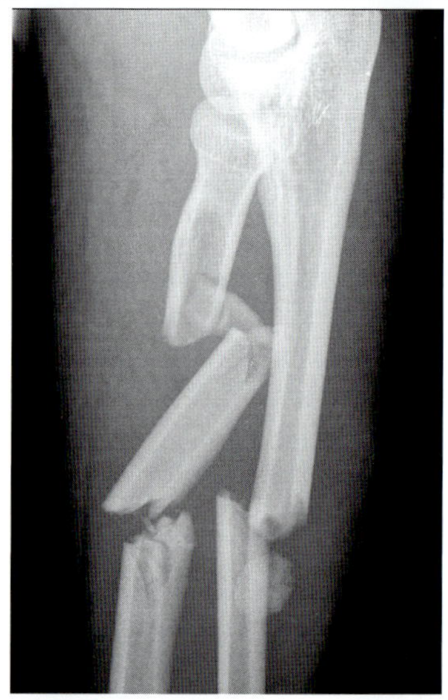

Radius segmental, simple or wedge ulna fracture

22-C2.3

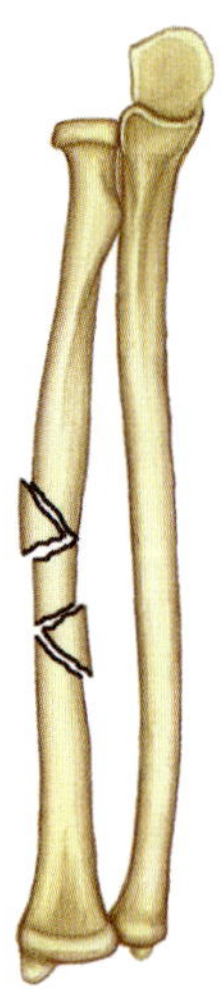

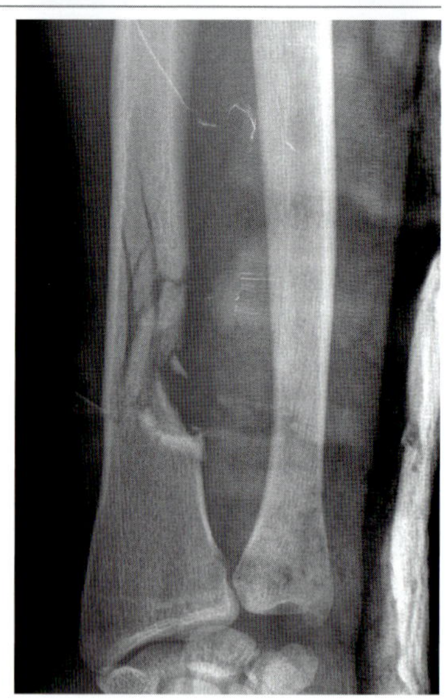

Radius complex, ulna intact or simple

22-C Radius/ulna shaft complex fractures

22-C3
Both bones multifragmentary
179 fractures
M: 136 (75.98%)
F: 43 (24.02%)
0.05% of total adult fractures
0.31% of adult radius/ulna
2.36% of segment 22
29.15% of type 22-C

22-C3.1

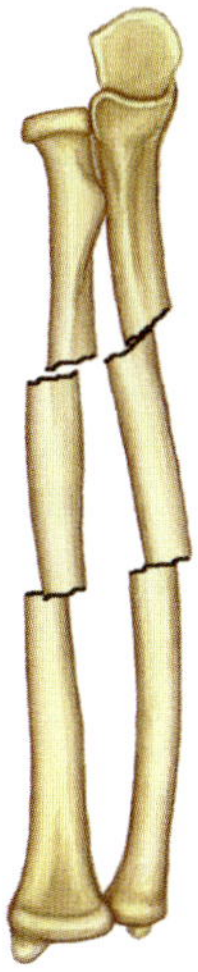

Both bones segmental

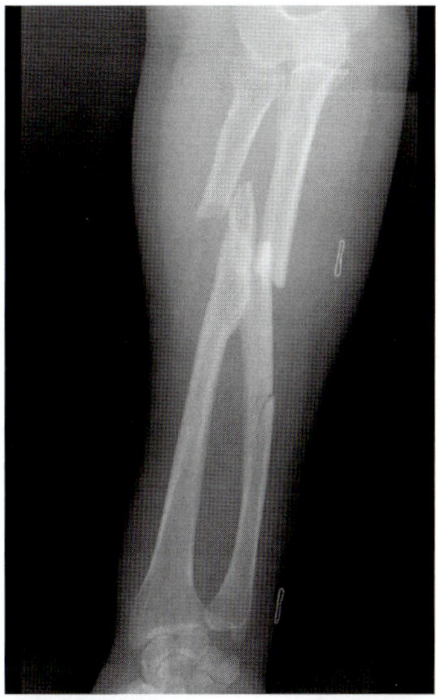

22-C3.2

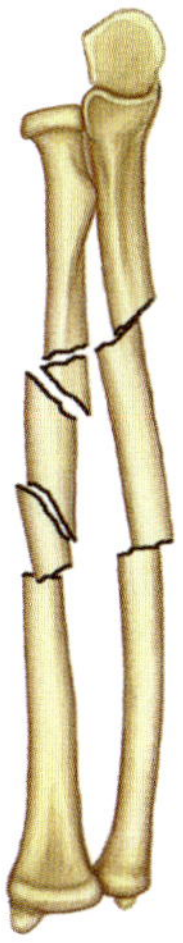

One bone segmental,
the other complex

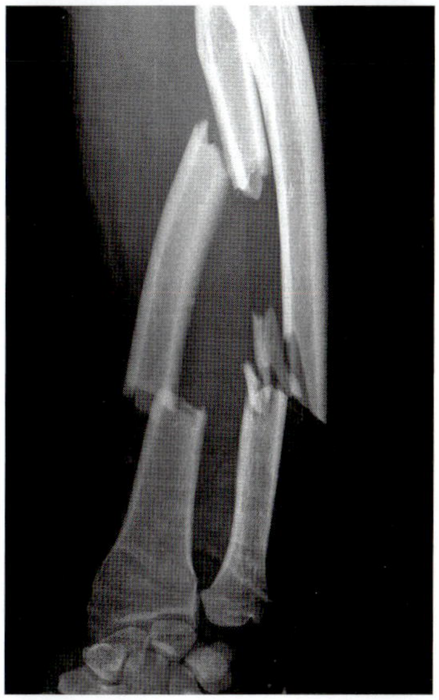

22-C3.3

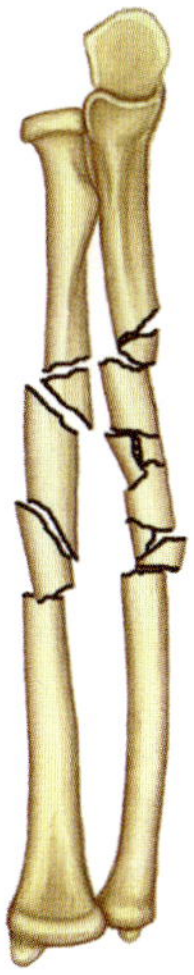

Both bones complex

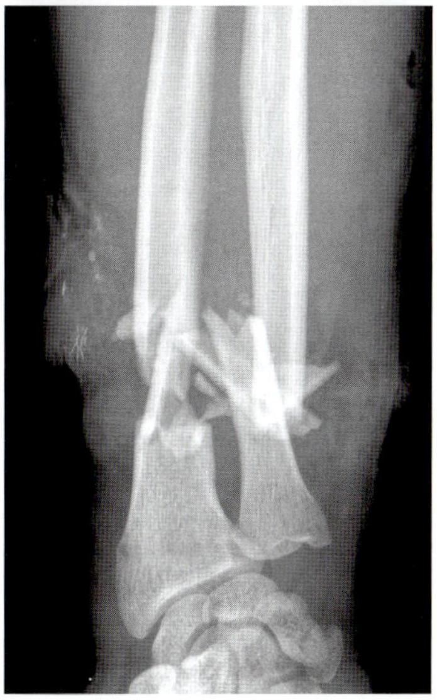

Injury Mechanism

Radial Shaft Fractures

This type of injury is usually caused by a direct blow on the forearm.

Ulnar Shaft Fractures

This fracture type most commonly occurs from direct trauma along its subcutaneous border, classically described as a nightstick fracture, when the forearm is used to block a blow. The fracture may also be caused by indirect force with the forearm in hypersupination or hyperpronation.

Fractures of the Shaft of the Radius and Ulna

This type of injury commonly results from a direct blow, such as in a fall from a height with the axial force transmitted through the ulna and radius.

Diagnosis

Patients with isolated fractures of the ulna or radius usually do not present with marked deformity, but the rotation of the forearm may be limited or partially limited. Physical examination reveals fracture pain that is aggravated by palpation over the injury region or when an increased axial load is applied. When both bones fracture, diagnosis is easily made based on physical signs like obvious deformity, bony crepitus, and limited rotation of the forearm. In patients with fractures of the radius and ulna or with semi-dislocation or dislocation of the proximal or distal radioulnar joint, physical examination indicates focal tenderness to palpation and limited or partially limited rotational function of the forearm.

The radiographic examination must include an AP view of the elbow or wrist depending upon the clinical indication. An oblique view may be required if there is suspected articular involvement or an inconclusive AP view.

It should be noted that fractures of the proximal third of the ulna often accompany radial head dislocation (Monteggia), while fractures of the distal third of the radius are often associated with a distal radioulnar joint (DRUJ) dislocation (Galeazzi).

Treatment

Ulnar shaft fractures can usually be managed by nonsurgical treatment, and should be immobilized with the forearm in a neutral position to minimize the contracture of the IOM between the radius and ulna. Radial shaft fractures often require surgical intervention. Monteggia and Galeazzi fractures include not only bony fractures but also joint dislocations, and consequently should be managed by surgical treatment. Fractures of both bones in the middle third of the forearm in an adult should be treated by the surgical approach. In this scenario, the surgeon should avoid managing both bone fractures from the same incision to minimize the chance of osseous bridge formation after the operation.

Distal Fractures of the Radius and Ulna (Segment 23)

Anatomical Features

The bony structures of the distal radius and ulna include the articular surface of the distal radius, DRUJ, and styloid process of the radius and ulna.

The area where bony substance changes from cancellous bone to compact bone in the distal end of the radius and ulna is an anatomically weak spot, and often a seat of fracture occurrence.

The slope of the dorsal to palmar surface of the distal radius and the slope volarly from the radius to the ulna form a palmar tilt angle and a radial inclination angle, respectively.

The distal radioulnar articulation, formed between the head of the ulna and the ulnar notch on the distal radius, is the anatomical foundation for the rotation of the forearm. The radial styloid process is 1–1.5 cm below the styloid process of the ulna.

The radiocarpal joint or wrist joint is an ellipsoid joint, formed by the distal portion of the radius and the proximal portion of the carpal bone. The proximal articular surface of the scaphoid, lunate, and triquetrum forms a smooth convex surface, which rests in the concavity formed by the articular surface of the radius and the undersurface of the articular disk. The capsule of the wrist joint, which is lax and unbranched, is strengthened by numerous ligaments anteroposteriorly and laterally.

AO Classification of Distal Fractures of the Radius and Ulna

Based on the AO classification, the delineation of the distal radius/ulna is illustrated by a square whose lateral sides are parallel to the axis of the bone and their length equal to the maximum width of the epiphysis. According to this formula, the distal radius/ulna is coded as 23 (**Plate 3.9**). On the basis of articular surface involvement, the distal radial/ulnar fracture (23) is further divided into three types: 23-A, extra-articular fracture; 23-B, partial articular fracture; and 23-C, complex articular fracture (**Plate 3.10**).

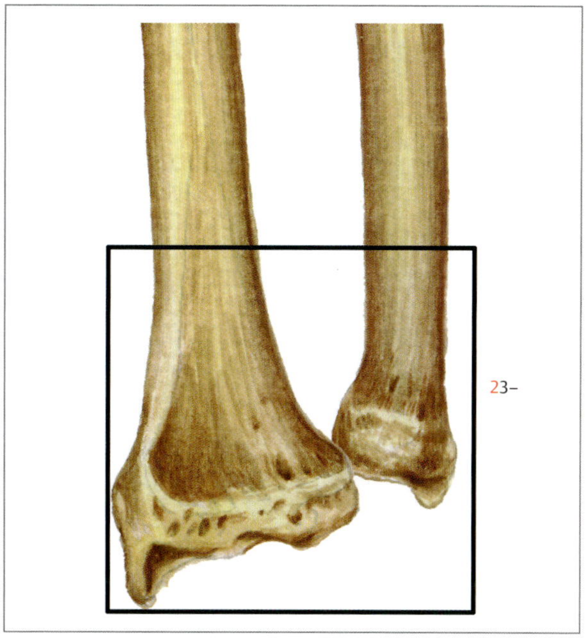

Plate 3.9

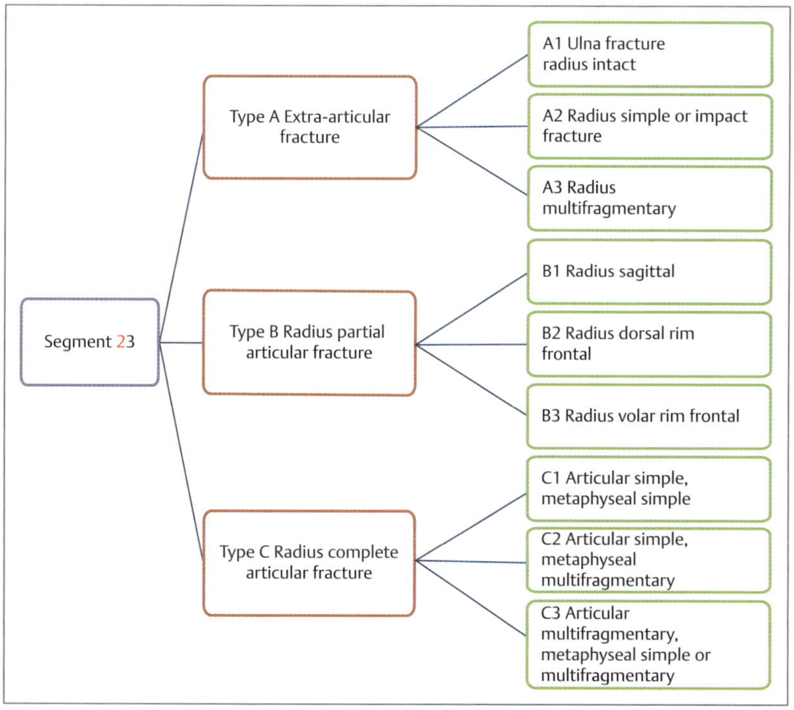

Plate 3.10

Clinical Epidemiologic Features of Distal Fractures of the Radius and Ulna (Segment 23)

A total of 43,420 adult distal radius/ulna fractures (segment 23) were treated in 83 hospitals in China over a 2-year period from 2010 to 2011. All cases were reviewed and statistically studied; the fractures accounted for 74.58% of all fractures of the radius/ulna in adults. Their epidemiologic features are as follows:

- More females than males
- The high-risk age group is 56–60 years; females are in this same age group, while males between the ages of 16 and 20 are most affected.
- The most common fracture type among segment 23 fractures is type 23-A; the same fracture type for both males and females.
- The most common fracture group among segment 23 fractures is group 23-A2; the same fracture group for both males and females.

Fractures of segment 23 by Sex

Table 3.14 Sex distribution of 43,420 fractures of segment 23

Sex	Number of fractures	Percentage (%)
Male	18,009	41.48
Female	25,411	58.52
Total	43,420	100.00

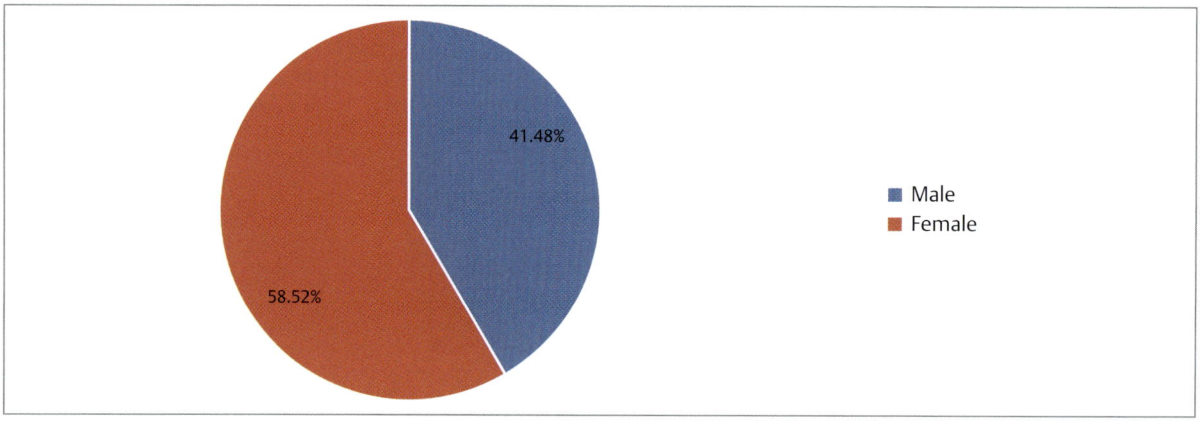

Fig. 3.14 Sex distribution of 43,420 fractures of segment 23.

Fractures of Segment 23 by Age Group

Table 3.15 Age and sex distribution of 43,420 fractures of segment 23

Age group (years)	Male	Female	Number of fractures	Percentage (%)
16–20	2,216	533	2,749	6.33
21–25	1,791	656	2,447	5.64
26–30	1,450	660	2,110	4.86
31–35	1,364	822	2,186	5.03
36–40	1,808	1,082	2,890	6.66
41–45	1,914	1,301	3,215	7.40
46–50	2,005	2,310	4,315	9.94
51–55	1,490	3,286	4,776	11.00
56–60	1,390	4,539	5,929	13.65
61–65	863	2,964	3,827	8.81
66–70	602	2,443	3,045	7.01
71–75	447	1,951	2,398	5.52
76–80	352	1,610	1,962	4.52
81–85	209	818	1,027	2.37
≥86	108	436	544	1.25
Total	18,009	25,411	43,420	100.00

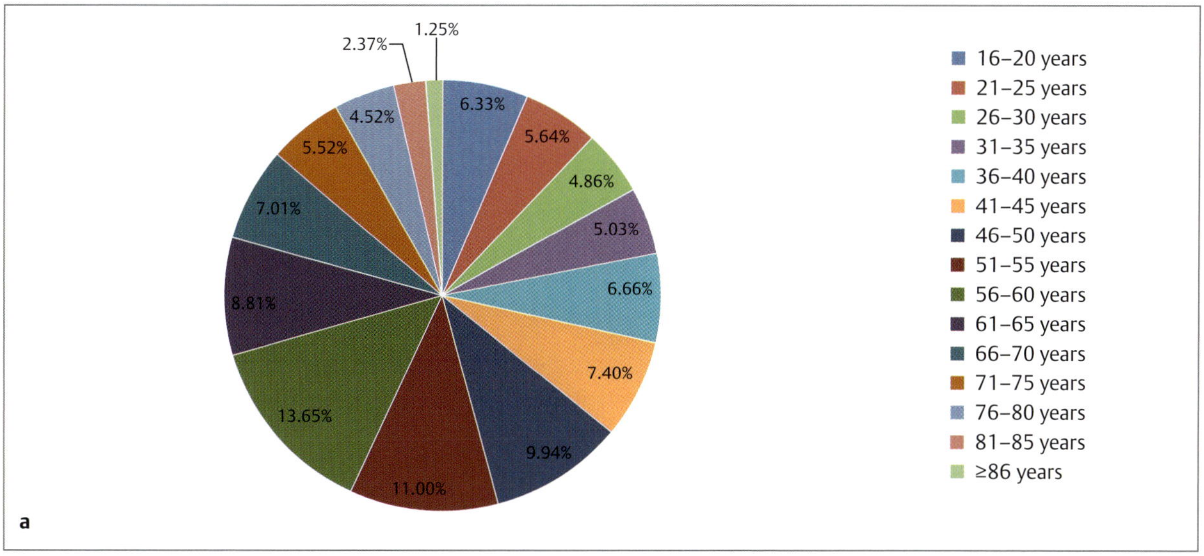

Fig. 3.15 **(a)** Age distribution of 43,420 fractures of segment 23. (*Continued*)

3

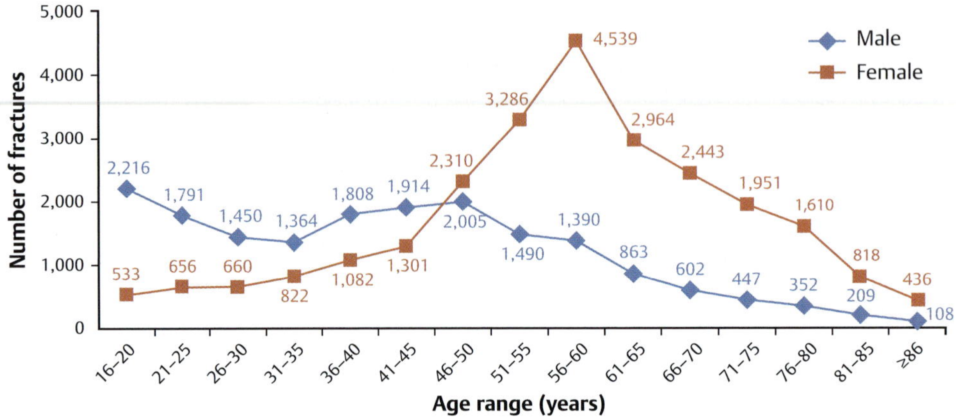

b

Fig. 3.15 (*continued*) **(b)** Age and sex distribution of 43,420 fractures of segment 23.

Fractures of Segment 23 by Fracture Type

Table 3.16 Sex and fracture type distributions of 43,420 fractures of segment 23

Fracture type	Male	Female	Number of fractures	Percentage (%)
23-A	9,423	16,148	25,571	58.89
23-B	4,246	3,527	7,773	17.90
23-C	4,340	5,736	10,076	23.21
Total	18,009	25,411	43,420	100.00

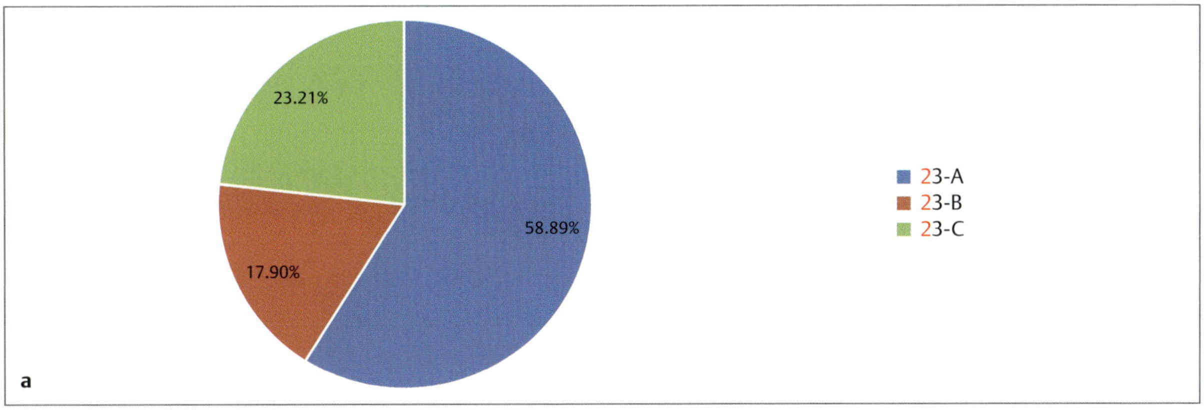

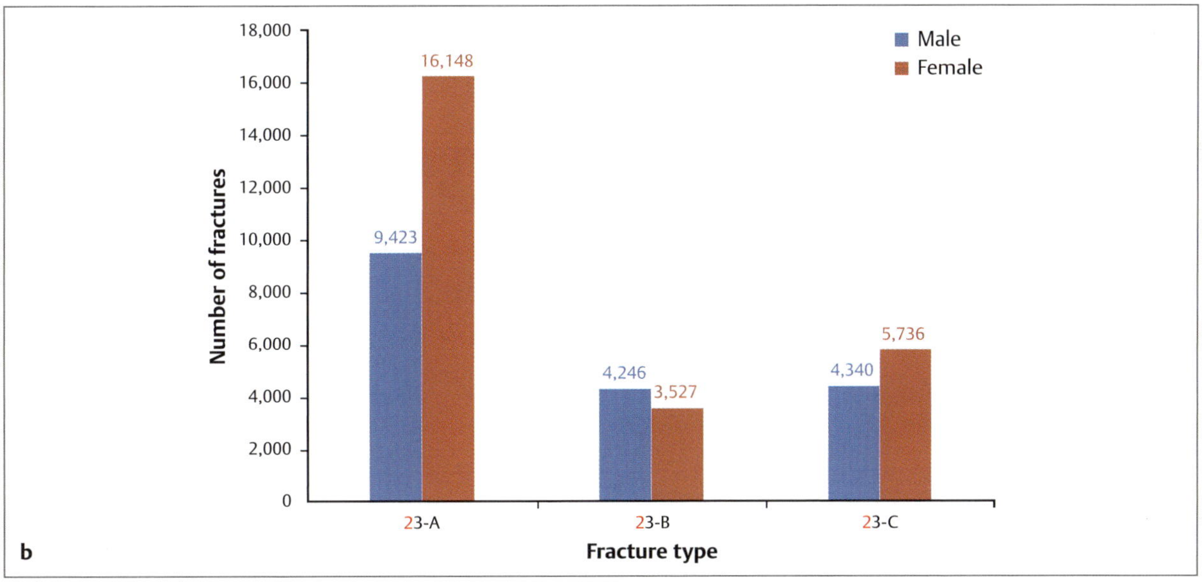

Fig. 3.16 **(a)** Fracture type distribution of 43,420 fractures of segment 23.
(b) Sex and fracture type distribution of 43,420 fractures of segment 23.

Table 3.17 Sex and fracture group distribution of 43,420 fractures of segment 23

Fracture group	Male	Female	Number of fractures	Percentage of segment 23 fractures (%)	Percentage of radius/ulna fractures (%)
23-A1	1,598	852	2,450	5.64	4.21
23-A2	6,038	11,706	17,744	40.87	30.48
23-A3	1,787	3,590	5,377	12.38	9.24
23-B1	2,929	2,072	5,001	11.52	8.59
23-B2	662	759	1,421	3.27	2.44
23-B3	655	696	1,351	3.11	2.32
23-C1	1,997	2,958	4,955	11.41	8.51
23-C2	978	1,226	2,204	5.08	3.79
23-C3	1,365	1,552	2,917	6.72	5.01
Total	18,009	25,411	43,420	100.00	74.58

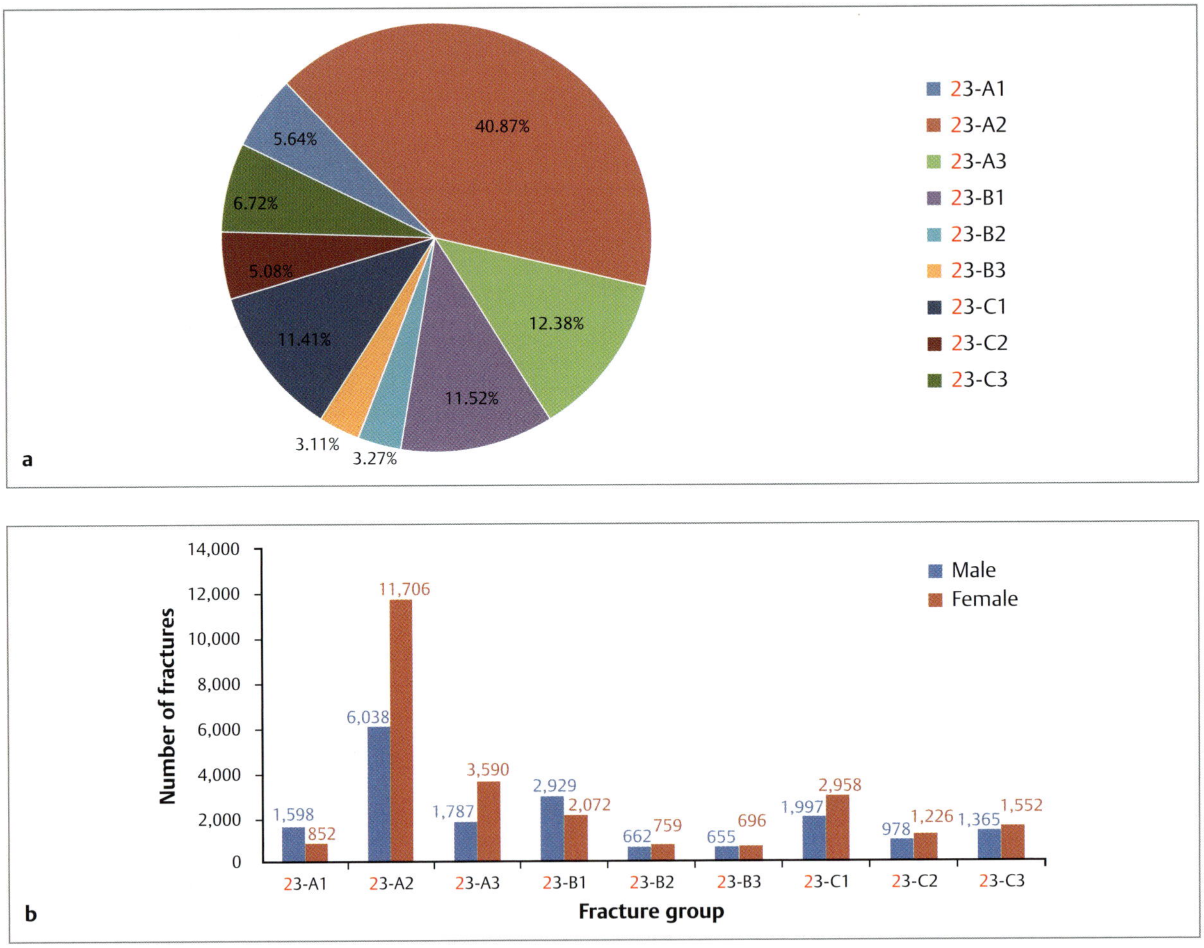

Fig. 3.17 **(a)** Fracture group distribution of 43,420 fractures of segment 23.
(b) Sex and fracture group distribution of 43,420 fractures of segment 23.

23-A Radius/ulna, distal, extra-articular fractures

23-A1
Ulna,
radius intact
2,450 fractures
M: 1,598 (65.22%)
F: 852 (34.78%)
0.65% of total adult fractures
4.21% of adult radius/ulna
5.64% of segment 23
9.58% of type 23-A

23-A1.1

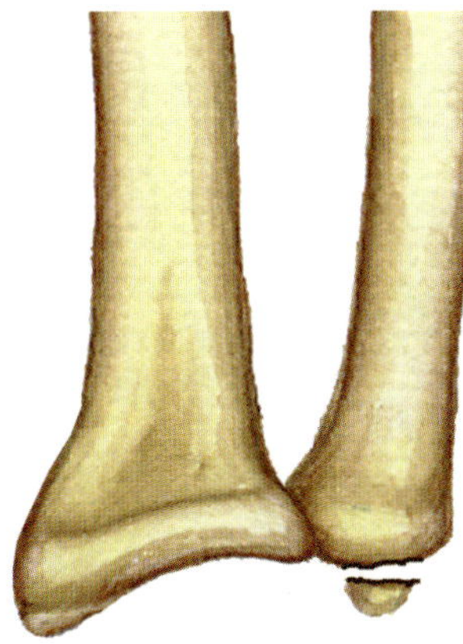

Styloid process

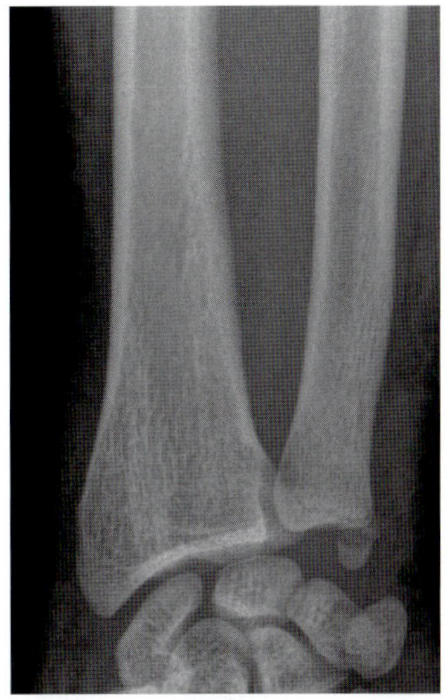

23-A1.2

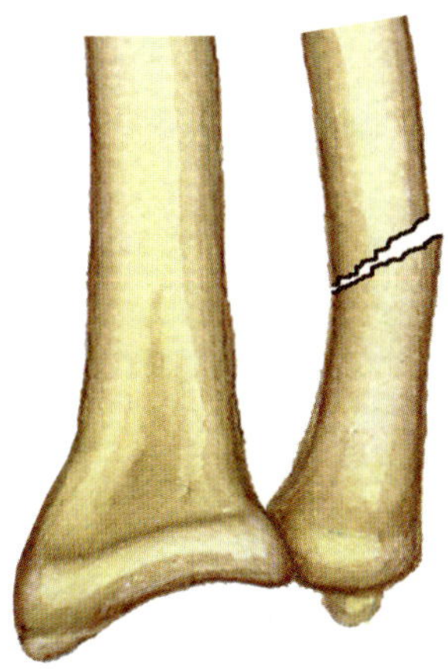

Metaphyseal simple

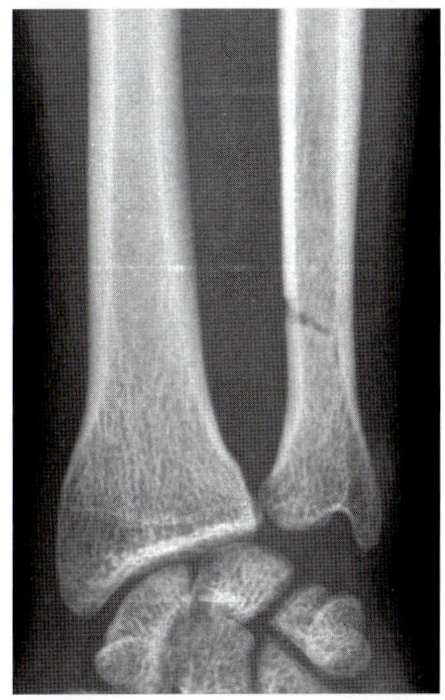

23-A1.3

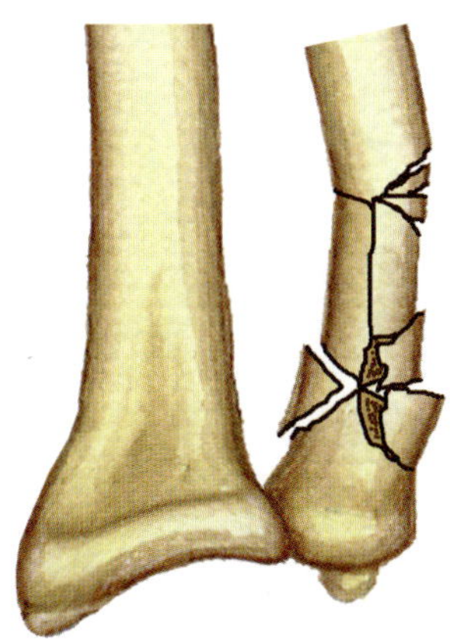

Metaphyseal multifragmentary

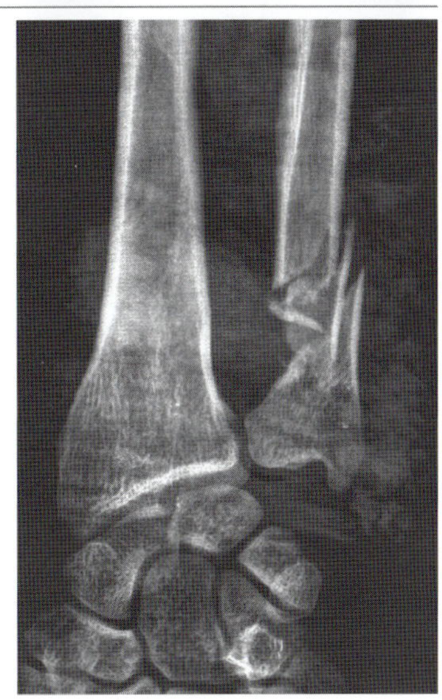

23-A Radius/ulna, distal, extra-articular fractures

23-A2
Radius simple or impact
17,744 fractures
M: 6,038 (34.03%)
F: 11,706 (65.97%)
4.74% of total adult fractures
30.48% of adult radius/ulna
40.87% of segment 23
69.39% of type 23-A

23-A2.1

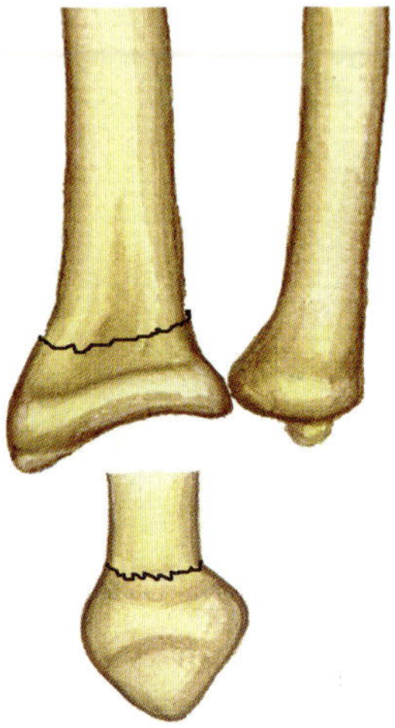

Without displacement

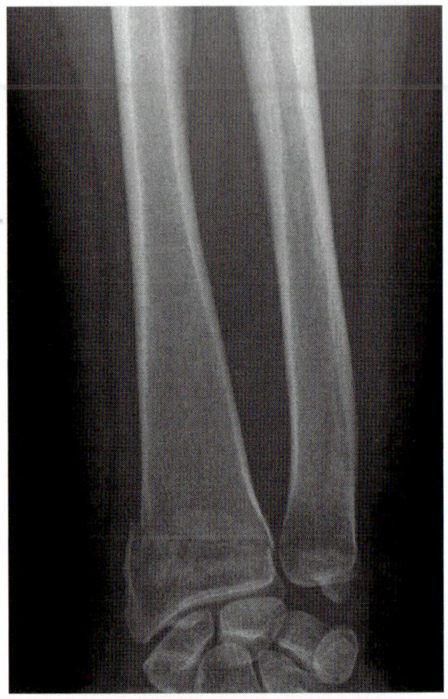

23-A2.2

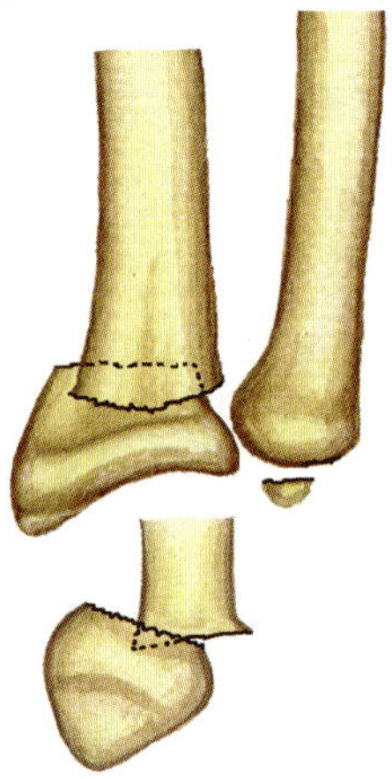

With dorsal displacement
(Colles fracture)

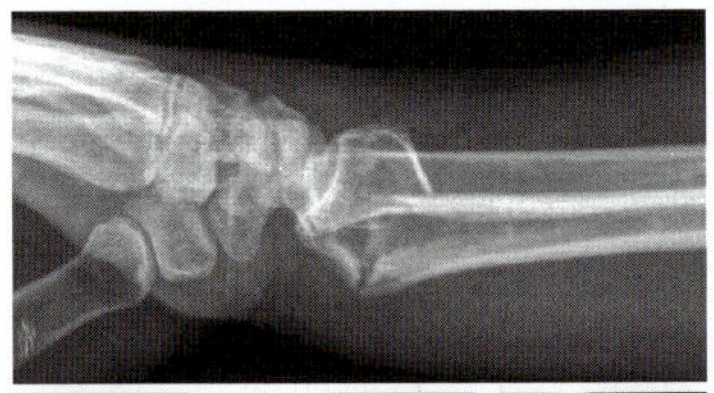

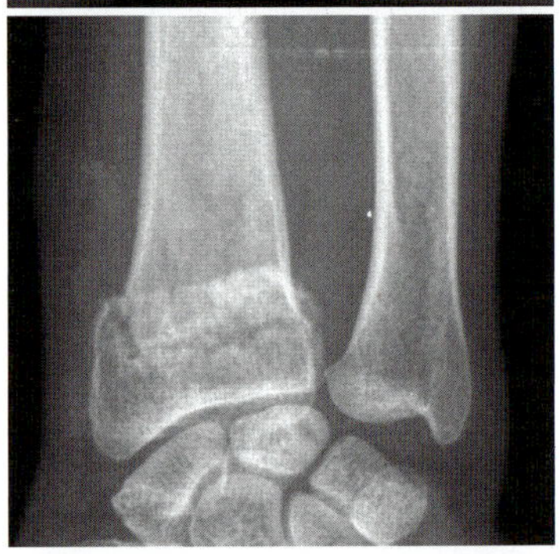

23-A2.3

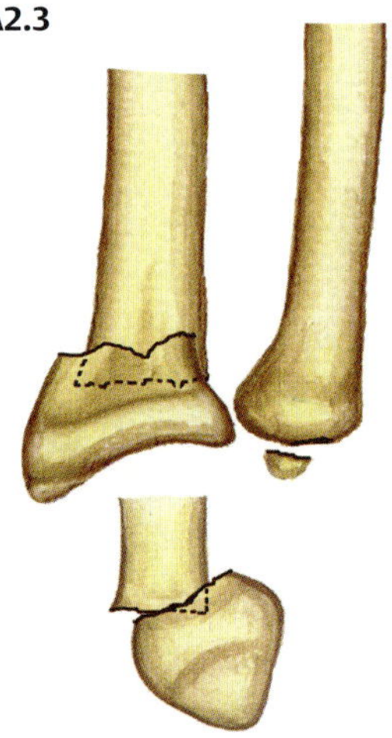

With volar displacement
(Smith fracture)

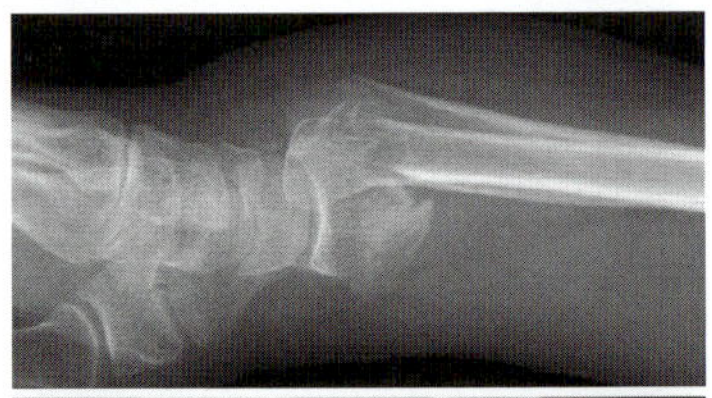

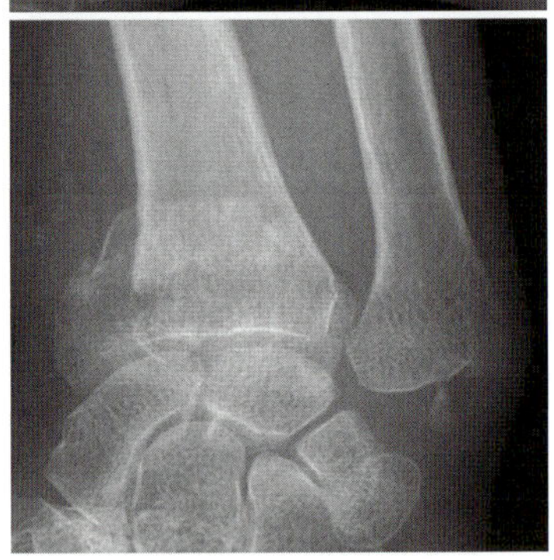

23-A Radius/ulna, distal, extra-articular fractures

23-A3
Radius multifragmentary
5,377 fractures
M: 1,787 (33.23%)
F: 3,590 (66.77%)
1.44% of total adult fractures
9.24% of adult radius/ulna
12.38% of segment 23
21.03% of type 23-A

23-A3.1

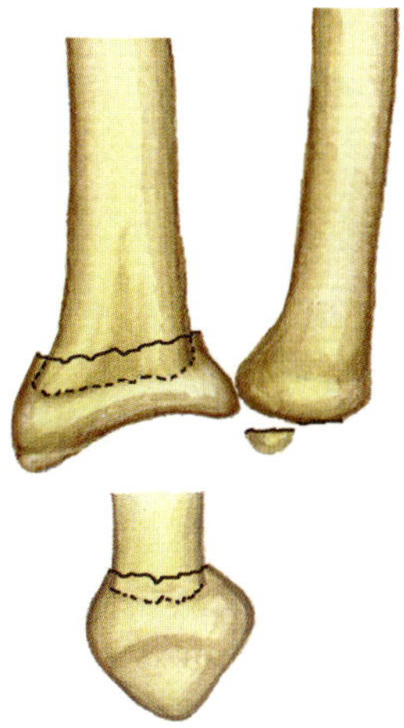

Impacted with axial shortening

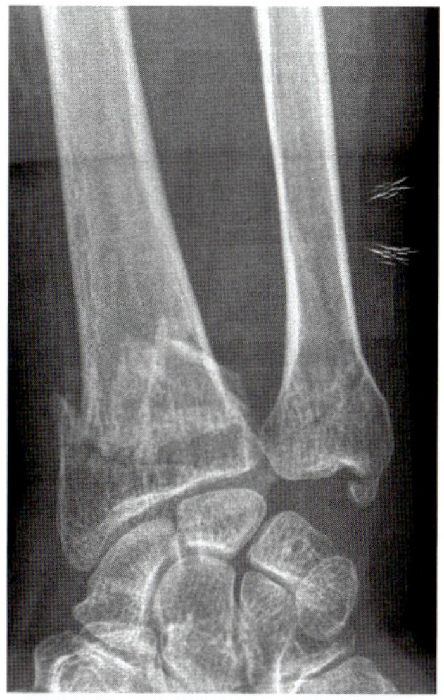

23-A3.2

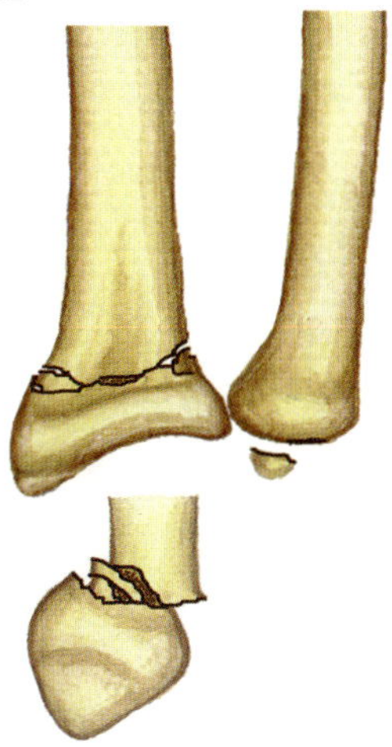

Impacted with wedge fragments

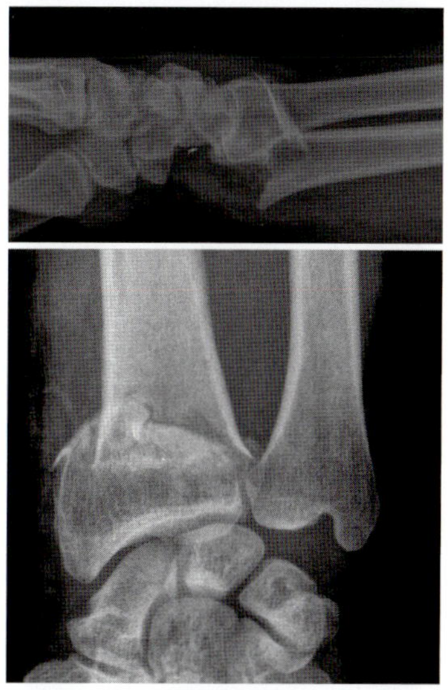

23-A3.3

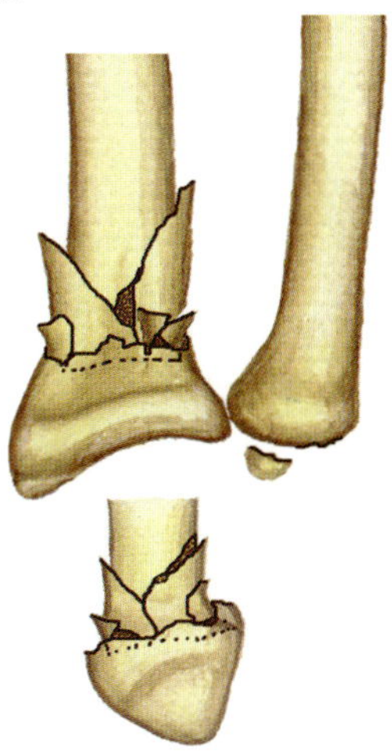

Complex

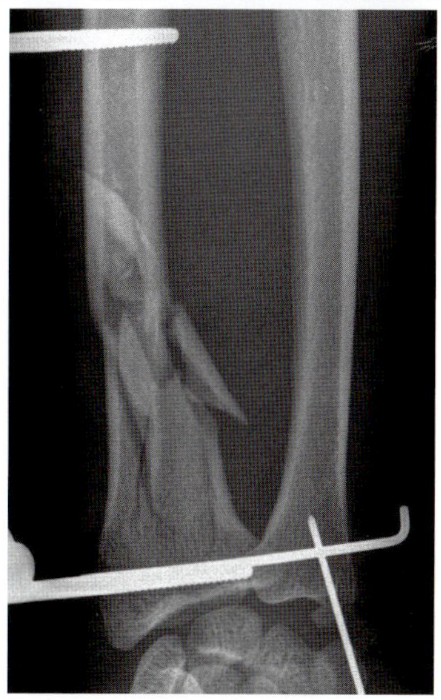

23-B Radius/ulna, distal, partial articular fractures

23-B1
Radius, sagittal
5,001 fractures
M: 2,929 (58.57%)
F: 2,072 (41.43%)
1.34% of total adult fractures
8.59% of adult radius/ulna
11.52% of segment 23
64.34% of type 23-B

23-B1.1

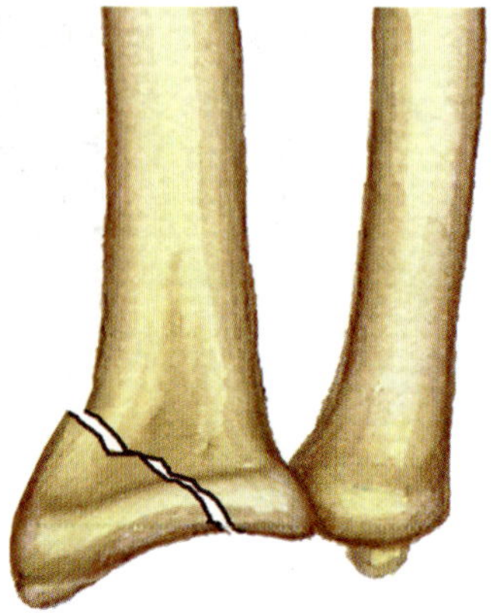

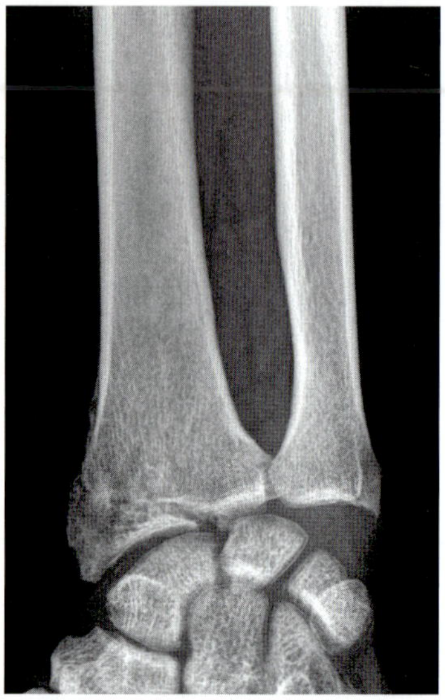

Lateral simple

23-B1.2

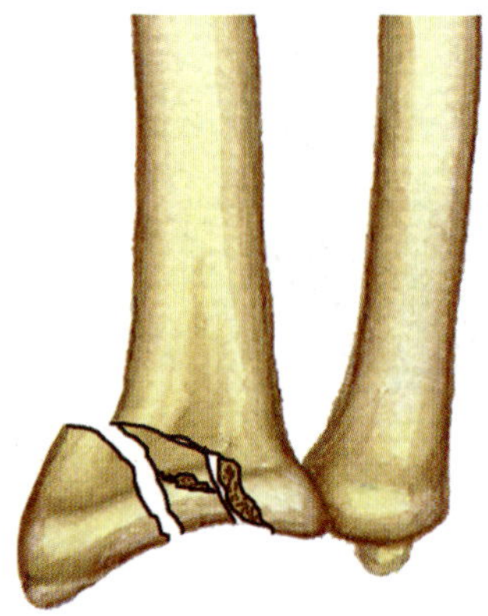

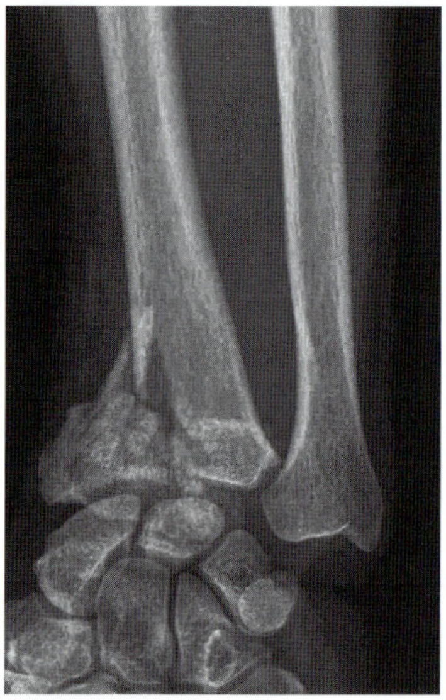

Lateral multifragmentary

23-B1.3

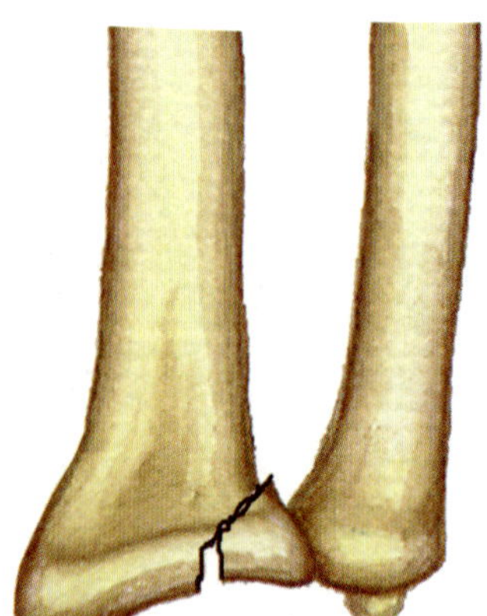

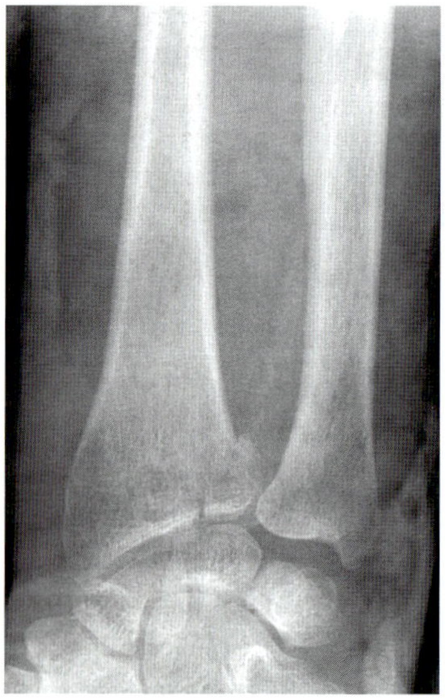

Medial

23-B Radius/ulna, distal, partial articular fractures

23-B2
Radius dorsal rim frontal
1,421 fractures
M: 662 (46.59%)
F: 759 (53.41%)
0.38% of total adult fractures
2.44% of adult radius/ulna
3.27% of segment 23
18.28% of type 23-B

23-B2.1

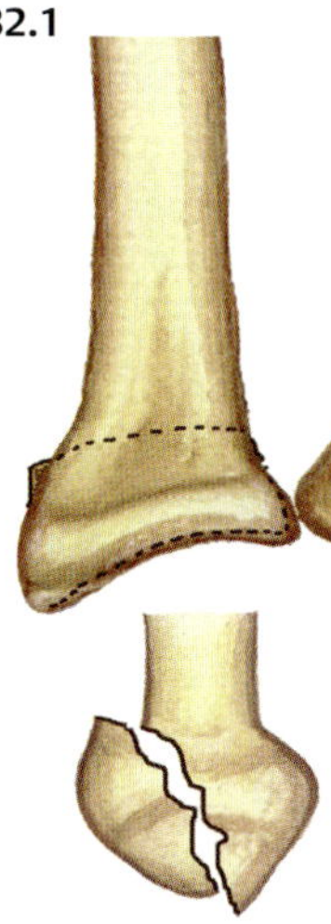

Simple

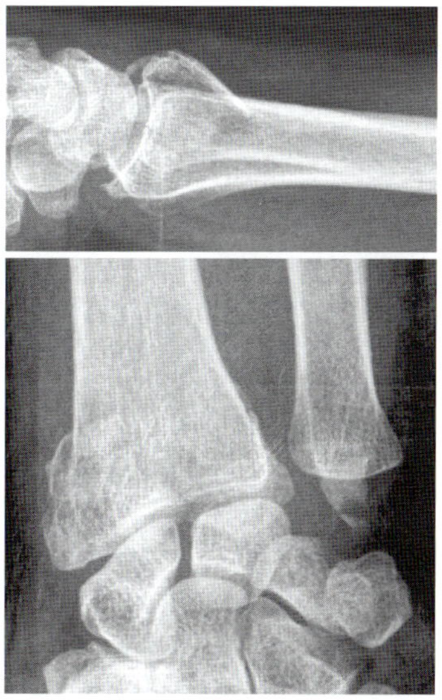

23-B2.2

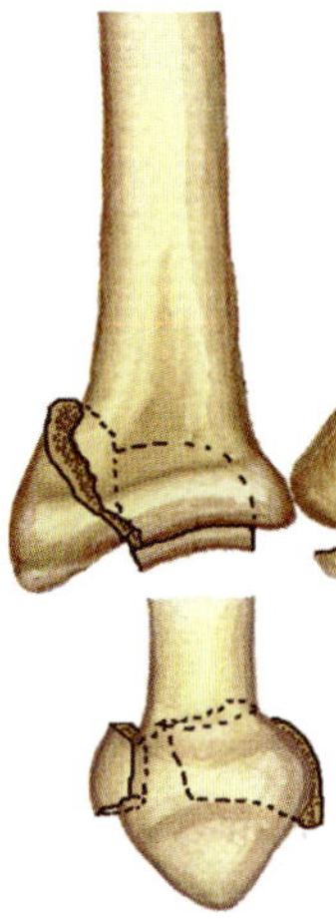

With lateral sagittal fracture line

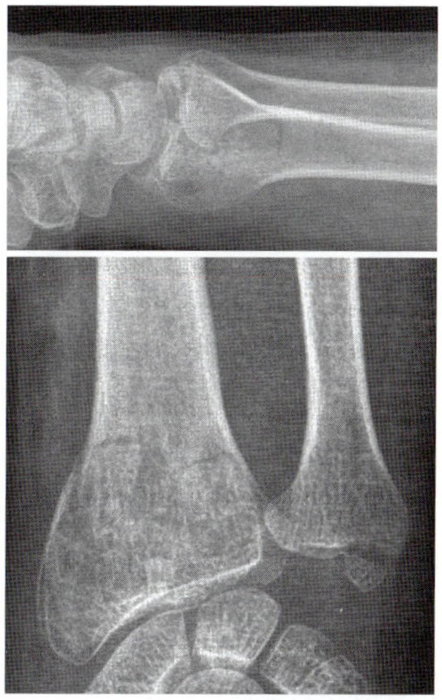

23-B2.3

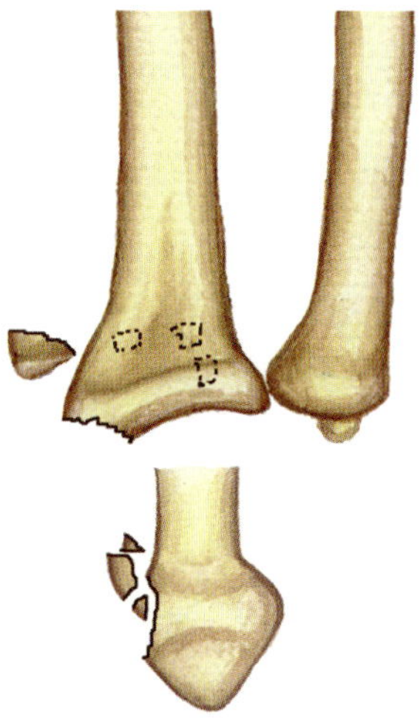

With dorsal displacement of carpus

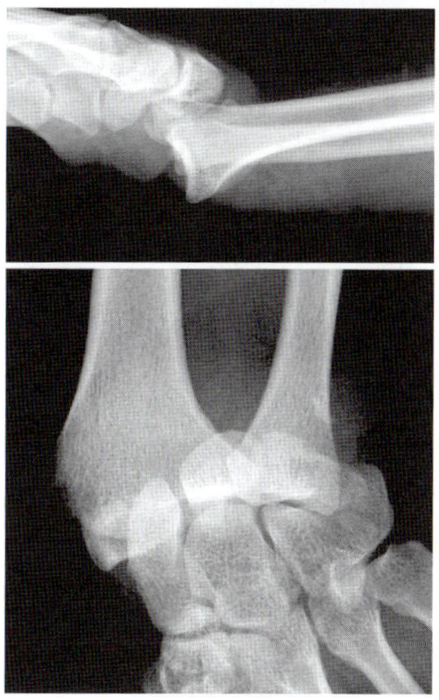

23-B Radius/ulna, distal, partial articular fractures

23-B3
Radius volar rim frontal
1,351 fractures
M: 655 (48.48%)
F: 696 (51.52%)
0.36% of total adult fractures
2.32% of adult radius/ulna
3.11% of segment 23
17.38% of type 23-B

23-B3.1

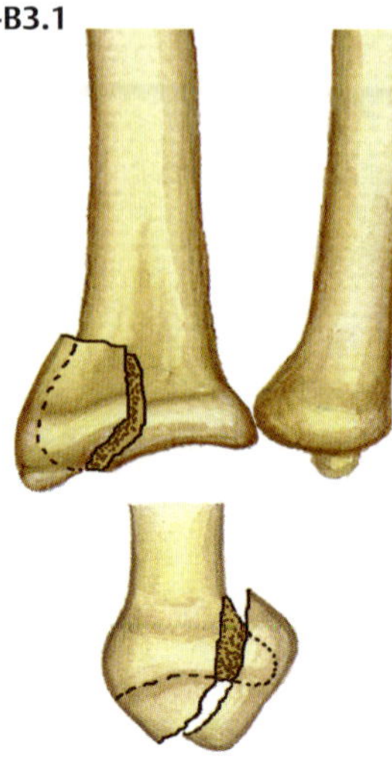

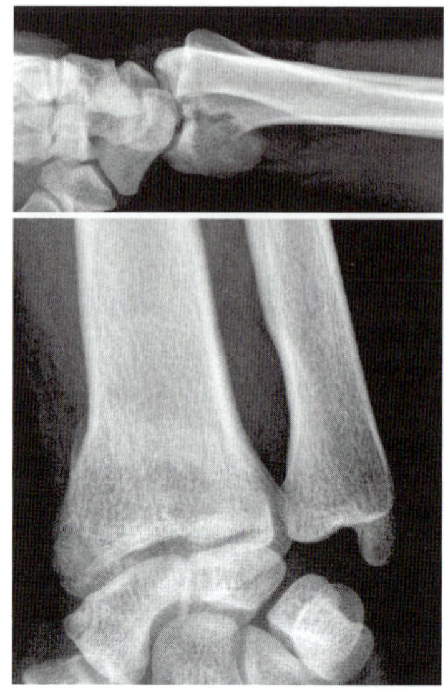

Simple with small fragment

23-B3.2

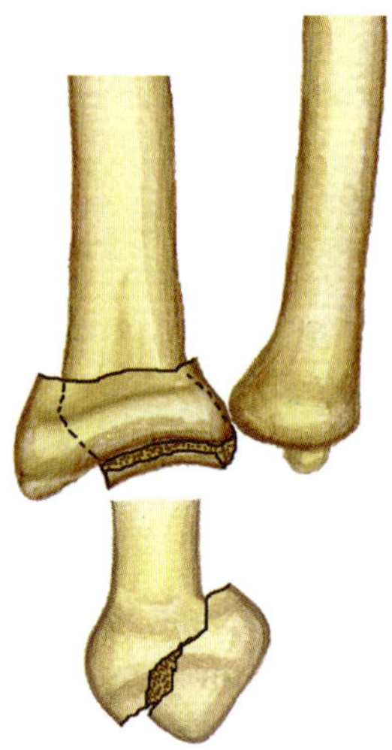

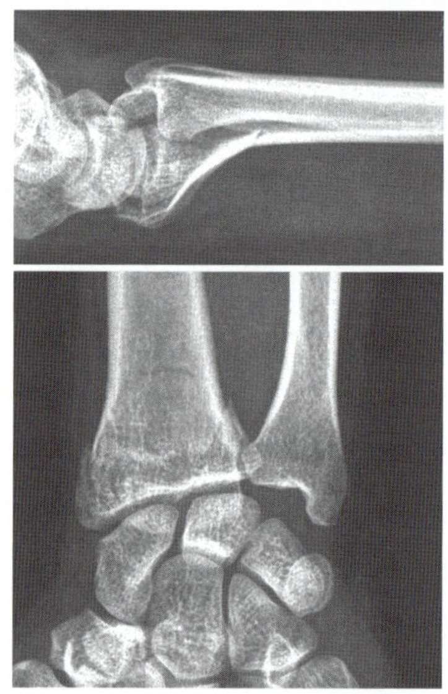

Simple with large fragment

23-B3.3

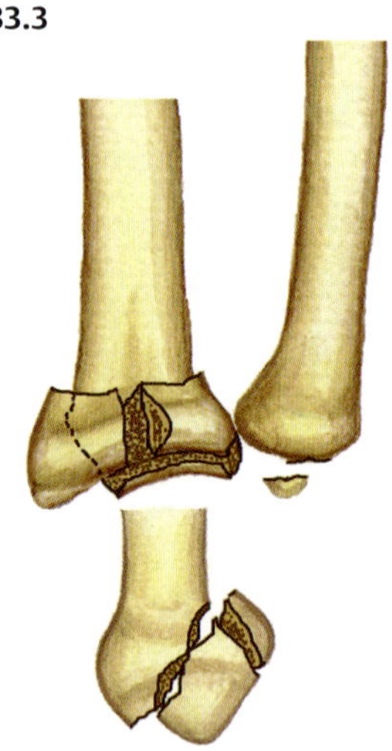

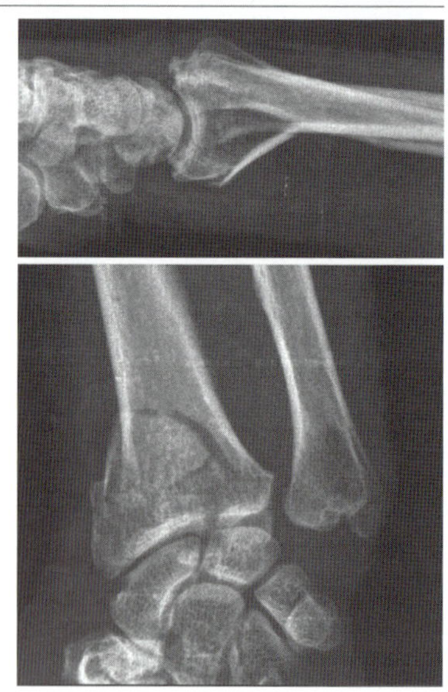

Multifragmentary

23-C Radius/ulna, distal, complete articular fractures

23-C1
Radius articular simple, metaphyseal simple
4,955 fractures
M: 1,997 (40.30%)
F: 2,958 (59.70%)
1.32% of total adult fractures
8.51% of adult radius/ulna
11.41% of segment 23
49.18% of type 23-C

23-C1.1

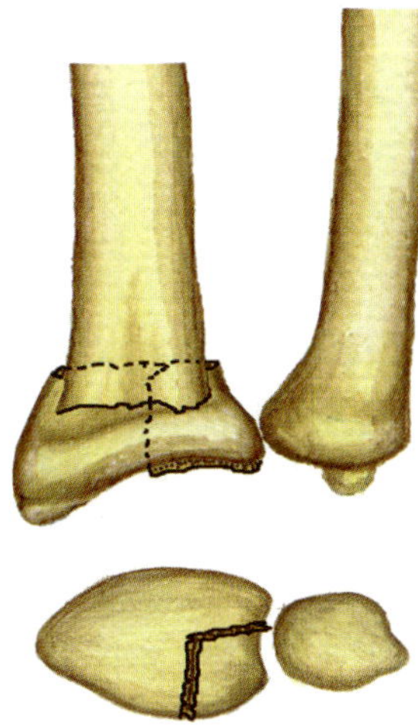

Posteromedial articular fragment

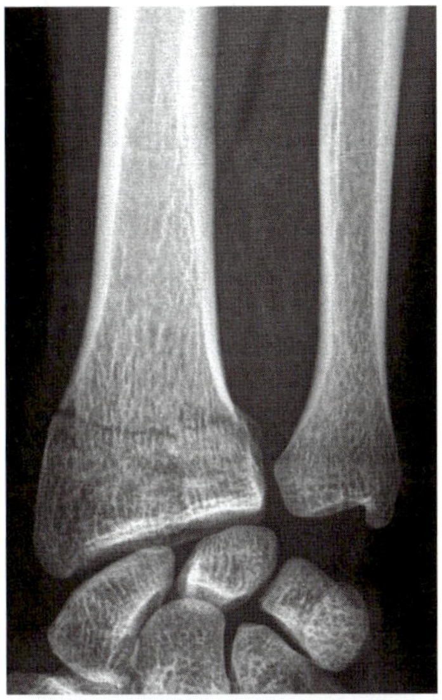

23-C1.2

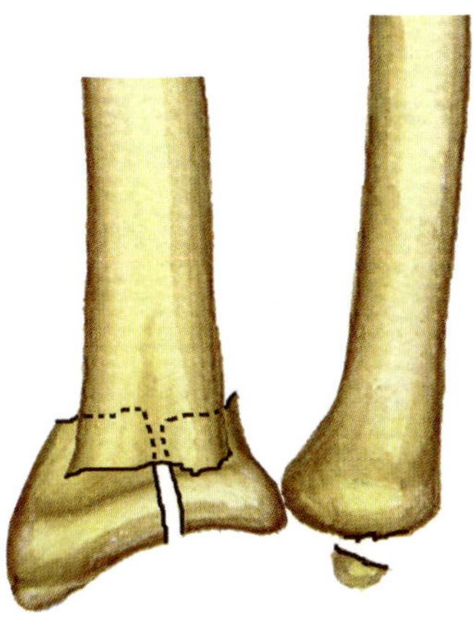

With sagittal articular fracture line

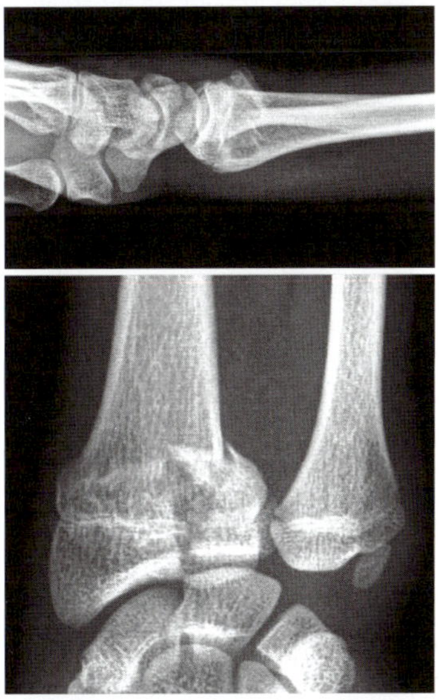

23-C1.3

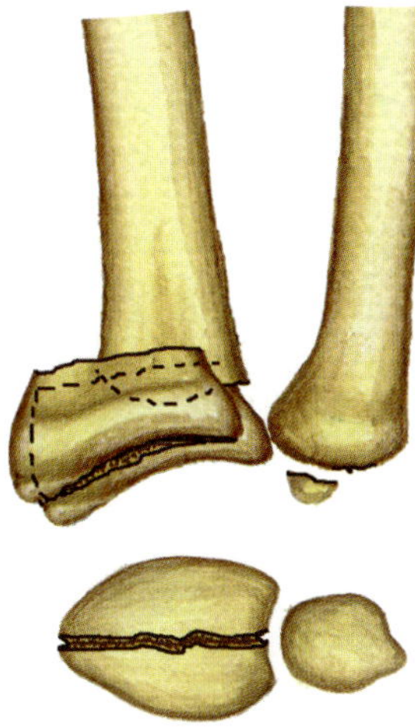

With frontal articular fracture line

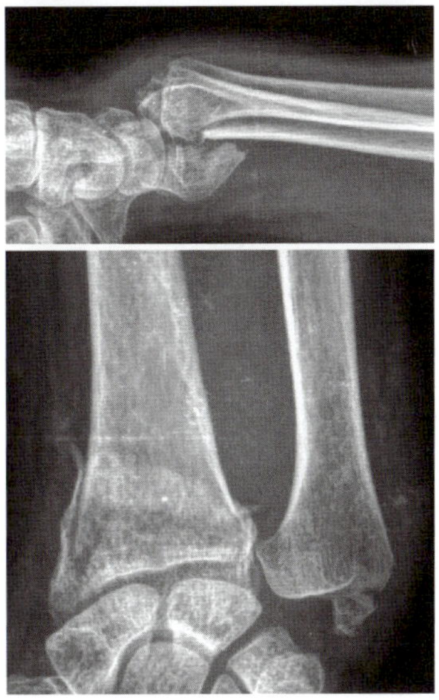

23-C Radius/ulna, distal, complete articular fractures

23-C2
Radius articular simple, metaphyseal multifragmentary
2,204 fractures
M: 978 (44.37%)
F: 1,226 (55.63%)
0.59% of total adult fractures
3.79% of adult radius/ulna
5.08% of segment 23
21.87% of type 23-C

23-C2.1

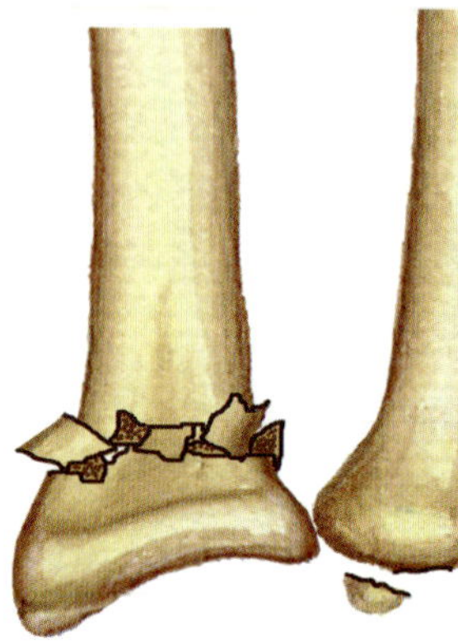
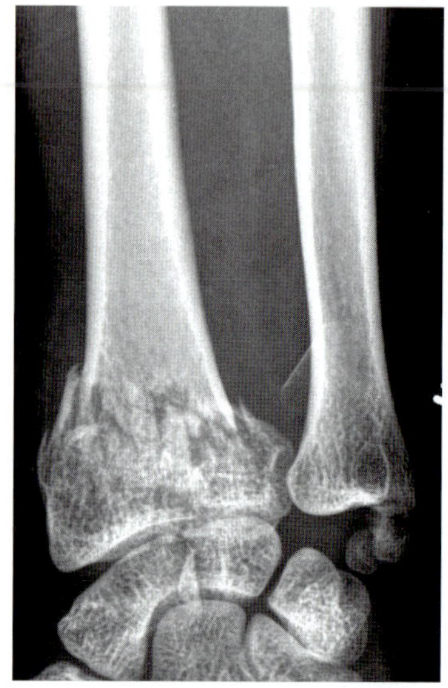

With sagittal articular fracture line

23-C2.2

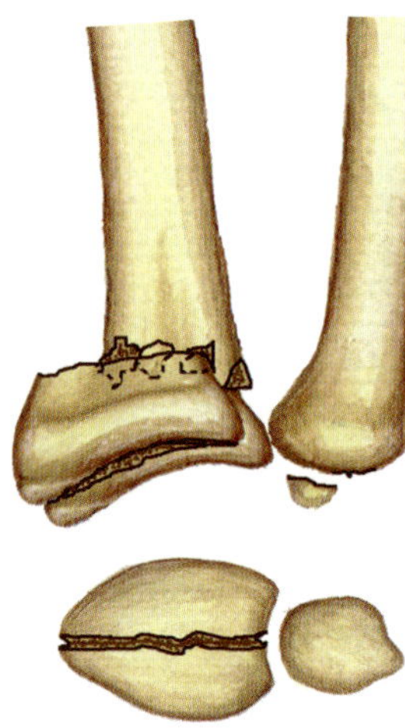
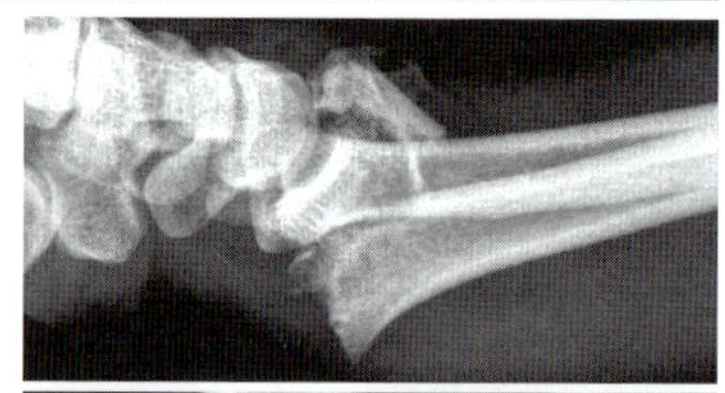
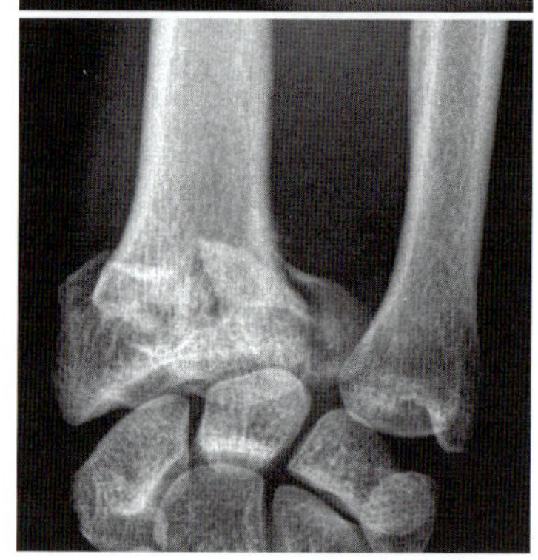

With frontal articular fracture line

23-C2.3

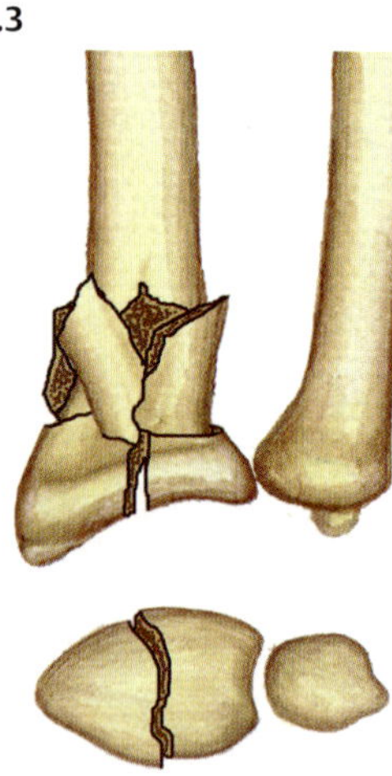
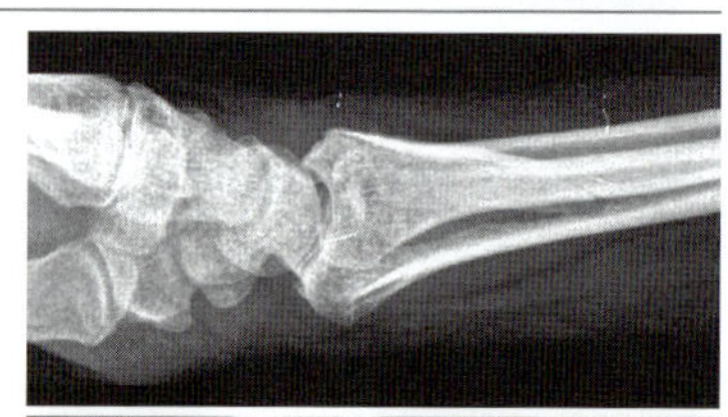
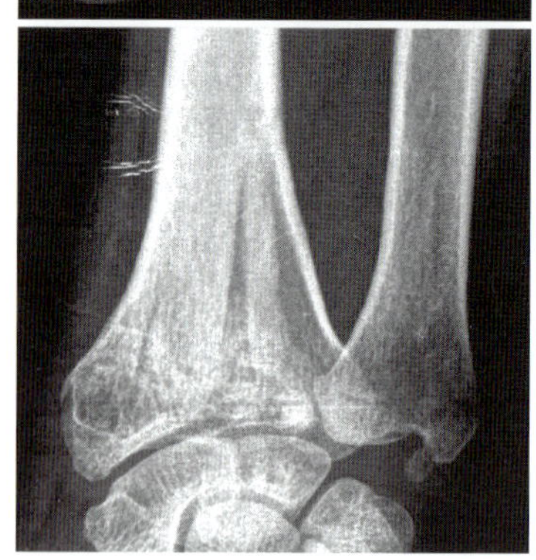

Fracture line extending from articulation into the diaphysis

23-C Radius/ulna, distal, complete articular fractures

23-C3
Radius articular multifragmentary, metaphyseal simple or multifragmentary
2,917 fractures
M: 1,365 (46.79%)
F: 1,552 (53.21%)
0.78% of total adult fractures
5.01% of adult radius/ulna
6.72% of segment 23
28.95% of type 23-C

23-C3.1

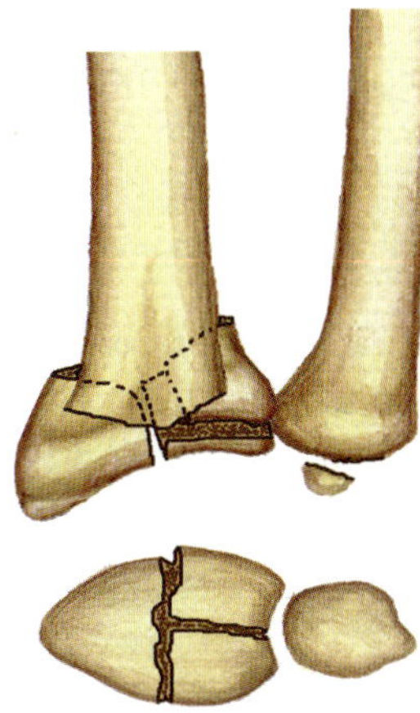

Metaphyseal simple

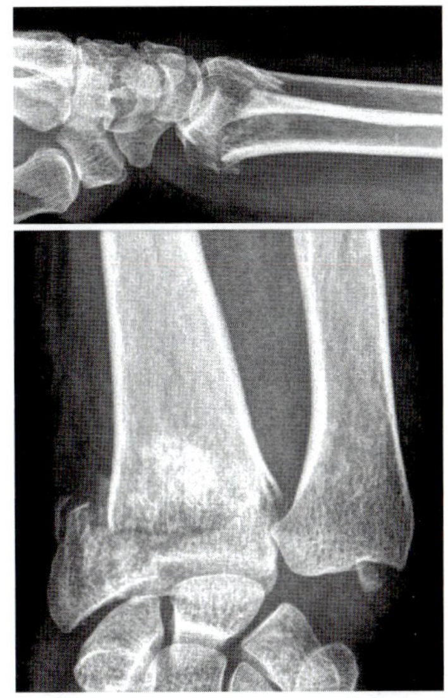

23-C3.2

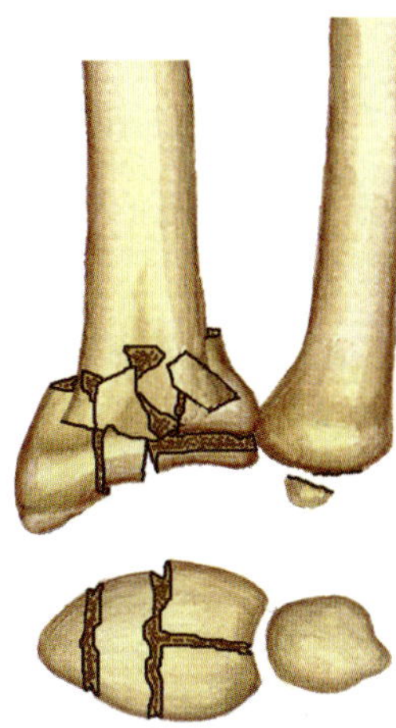

Metaphyseal multifragmentary

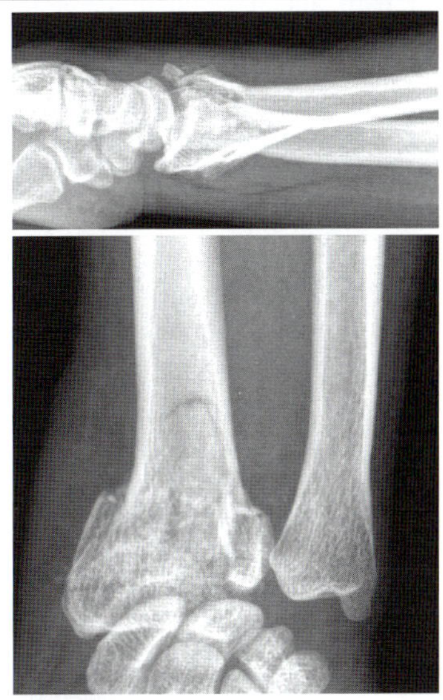

23-C3.3

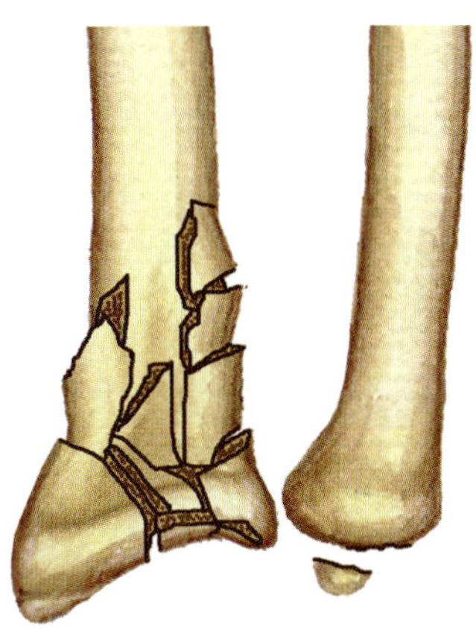

Fracture line extending from articulation into the diaphysis

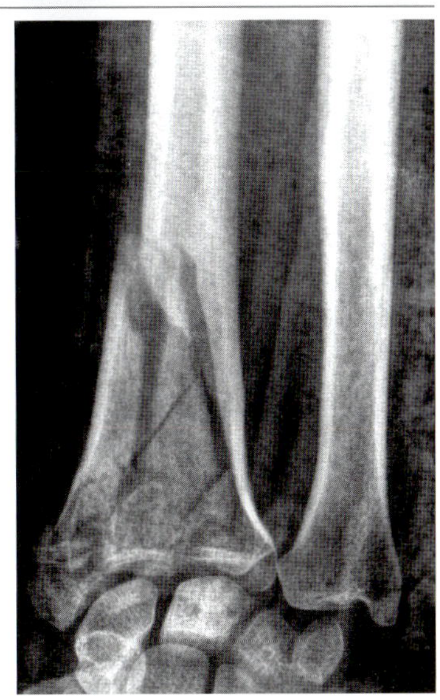

Injury Mechanism

Distal radius/ulna fracture results from force transmitted through the hand and wrist to the distal radius/ulna, which often occurs from a fall on an outstretched hand. Fractures of the distal radius/ulna can be further divided into extension fractures, flexion fractures, and intra-articular fractures, associated with a dislocation of the wrist joint depending on different injury mechanisms. Extension fractures result from a fall on an outstretched pronated hand with impact on the palm and subsequent forced dorsiflexion and hyperextension. A fall onto the back of the hand with the hand and carpus in hyperflexion can result in flexion fractures.

Diagnosis

Patients with fractures of the distal radius/ulna may present with pain and a swollen distal forearm with localized tenderness. If fractures are accompanied by significant displacement or angulation, a typical deformity will appear, such as a "dinner fork" deformity of the wrist. A detailed neurovascular examination is imperative.

Imaging studies should include an AP and lateral view of the wrist joint, which are both helpful in assessing the fracture type of the distal forearm and the degree of the displacement. A CT scan may be required to provide better visualization for complex or intra-articular fractures, or when the initial X-ray fails to indicate the position of the fragment.

3

Treatment

Intra- or extra-articular fractures with minimal or no displacement and stable, impacted fractures with minimal or no shortening can be managed by closed reduction and cast or splint immobilization. Surgical fixation should be considered in patients with unstable fractures of the distal radius/ulna and intra-articular fractures with marked displacement.

Other Classifications of Fractures of the Radius and Ulna

Monteggia Fractures

Overview

The Monteggia fracture is a fracture of the proximal third of the ulna with dislocation of the radial head. It is named after Giovanni Monteggia, who first described this injury in 1814. In 1967, Bado further divided Monteggia fractures into four types depending on displacement of the radial head. The types of Monteggia fractures (Bado type) and their injury mechanisms include:

- *Type I*: anterior dislocation of the radial head with associated anteriorly angulated fracture of the ulna, which usually occurs with the hand in forced pronation.
- *Type II:* posterior/posterolateral dislocation of the radial head with associated posteriorly angulated fracture of the ulnar shaft. This typically occurs from axial loading of the forearm with a flexed elbow.
- *Type III:* lateral/anterolateral dislocation of the radial head with fracture of the ulnar metaphysis. This typically occurs from forced abduction of the elbow. The radial head will dislocate posterolaterally if the hand is in forced supination, or anterolaterally if the hand is in forced pronation.
- *Type IV:* anterior dislocation of the radial head with fractures of both the radius and ulna within the proximal third at the same level. This typically occurs from a mechanism similar to type I but combined with a radial shaft fracture.

Monteggia Fractures

Type I: anterior dislocation of the radial head with associated anteriorly angulated fracture of the ulnar shaft
450 fractures
M: 297 (66%)
F: 153 (34%)
0.10% of total fractures
0.59% of radius/ulna
47.87% of Monteggia fractures

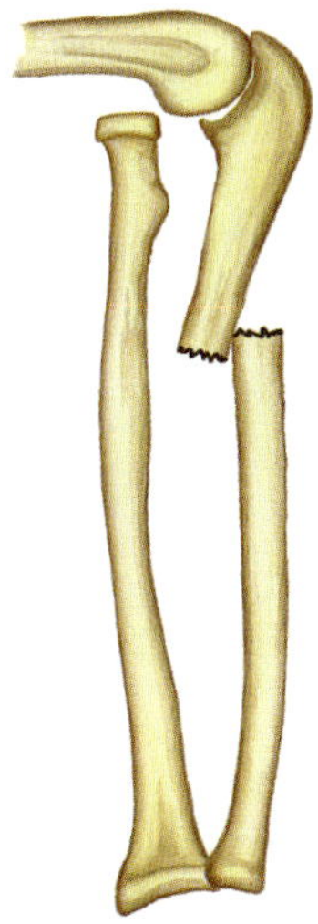

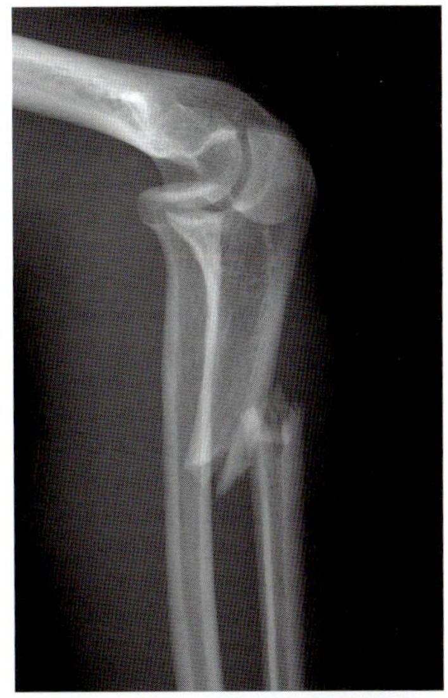

Type II: posterolateral dislocation of the radial head with associated posteriorly angulated fracture of the ulnar shaft
129 fractures
M: 90 (69.77%)
F: 39 (30.23%)
0.03% of total fractures
0.17% of radius/ulna
13.72% of Monteggia fractures

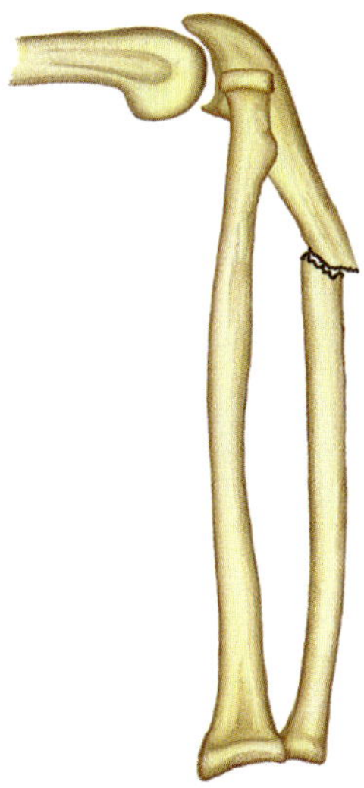

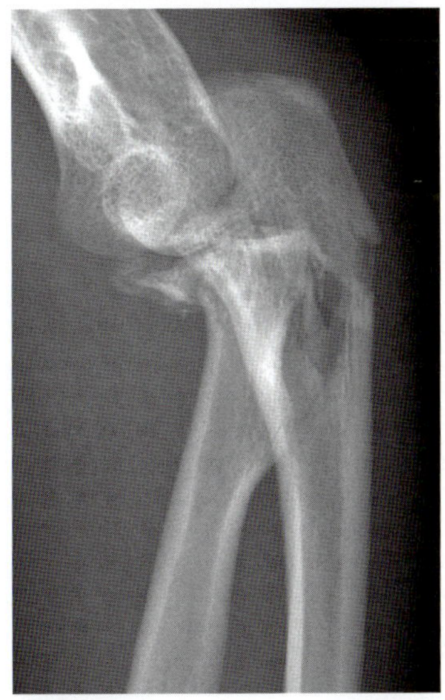

Type III: lateral/anterolateral dislocation of the radial head with fracture of ulnar metaphysis
276 fractures
M: 215 (77.9%)
F: 61 (22.1%)
0.06% of total fractures
0.36% of radius/ulna
29.36% of Monteggia fractures

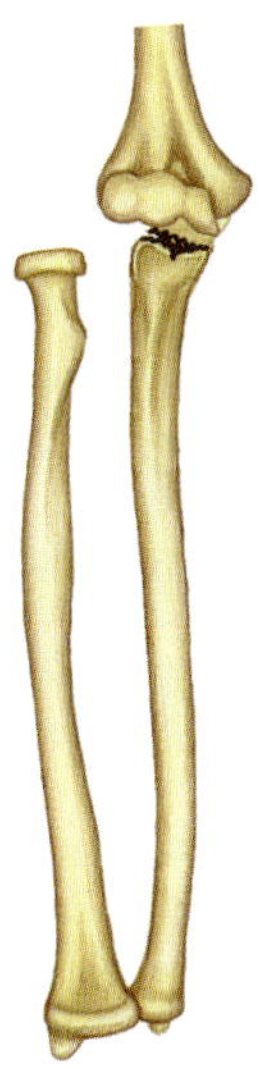

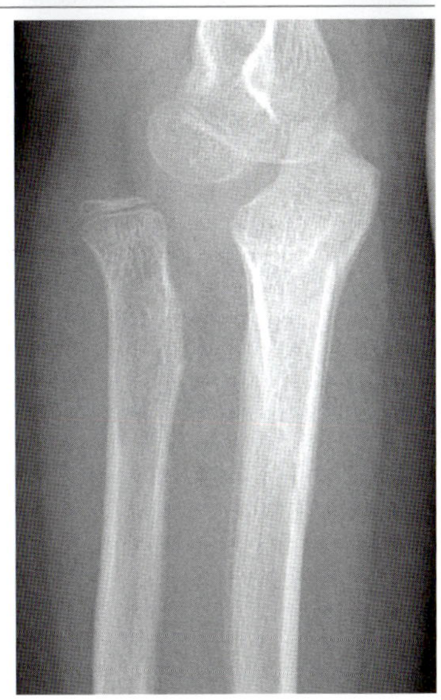

Monteggia Fractures

Type IV: anterior dislocation of radial head with fractures of both the radius and ulna within proximal third at the same level
85 fractures
M: 66 (77.65%)
F: 19 (22.35%)
0.02% of total fractures
0.11% of radius/ulna
9.04% of Monteggia fractures

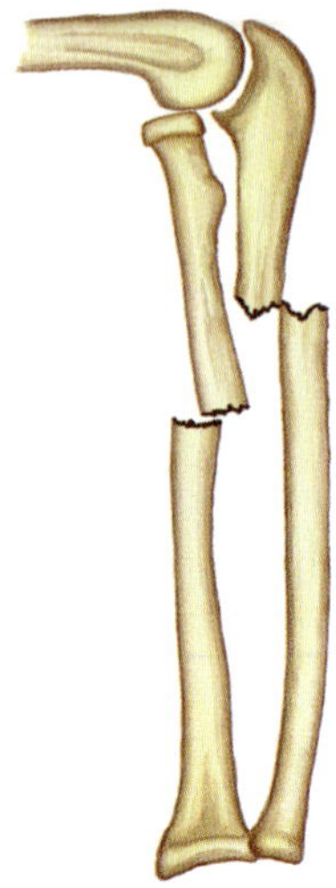

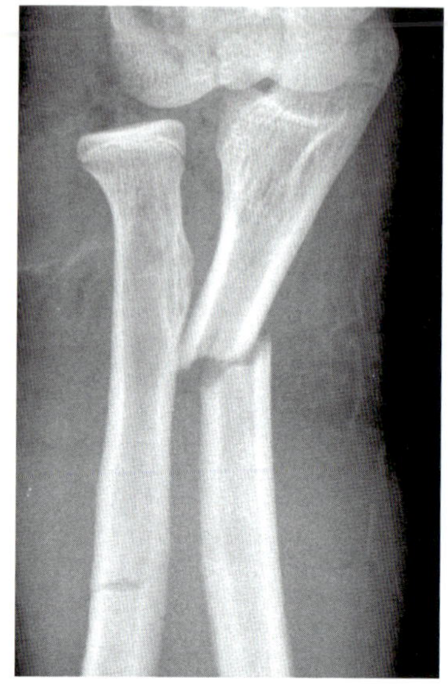

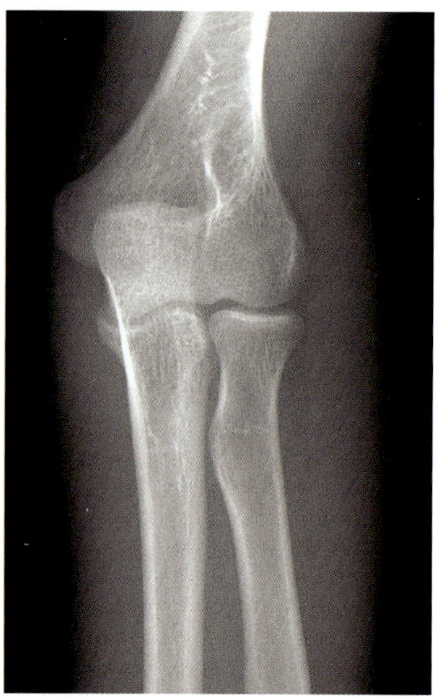

Plate 3.11

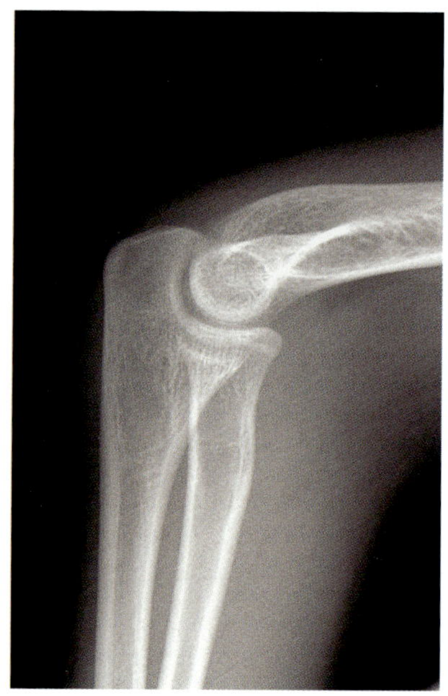

Plate 3.12

The typical presentation for a Monteggia fracture is a painful, swollen, and deformed elbow with bony crepitus and an abnormal range of motion of the injured area. Particular attention should be paid to the posterior interosseous branch of the radial nerve, which courses around the radial neck, and is especially at risk in Monteggia fractures. Imaging studies must include AP and lateral views of the elbow joint. Determining whether or not the extension of the long axis of the radius points directly at the capitellum can be helpful in assessing the radiocapitellar joint, which can be better visualized on the lateral projection of the elbow (**Plates 3.11** and **3.12**).

Compared with other fracture types of the forearm, Monteggia fractures are more likely to cause unstable fractures and stiffness of the elbow joint. Most pediatric fracture patterns can be managed conservatively with closed reduction and casting, but may require open reduction if the closed reduction fails due to an impacted or torn annular ligament. However, most adult fractures require surgical treatment. Fractures with radial nerve injuries should be treated with open reduction and internal fixation, and exploration of the radial nerve should be performed as well.

Clinical Epidemiologic Features of Monteggia Fractures

A total of 940 Monteggia fractures were treated in 83 hospitals in China over a 2-year period from 2010 to 2011. All cases were reviewed and statistically studied; the fractures accounted for 0.22% of all fractures and 1.23% of fractures of the radius/ulna. The epidemiologic features of Monteggia fracture are as follows:

- More males than females
- The high-risk age group is 6–10 years
- The most common Monteggia fracture type by Bado classification is type I.

Monteggia Fractures by Sex

Table 3.18 Sex distribution of 940 Monteggia fractures

Sex	Number of fractures	Percentage (%)
Male	668	71.06
Female	272	28.94
Total	940	100.00

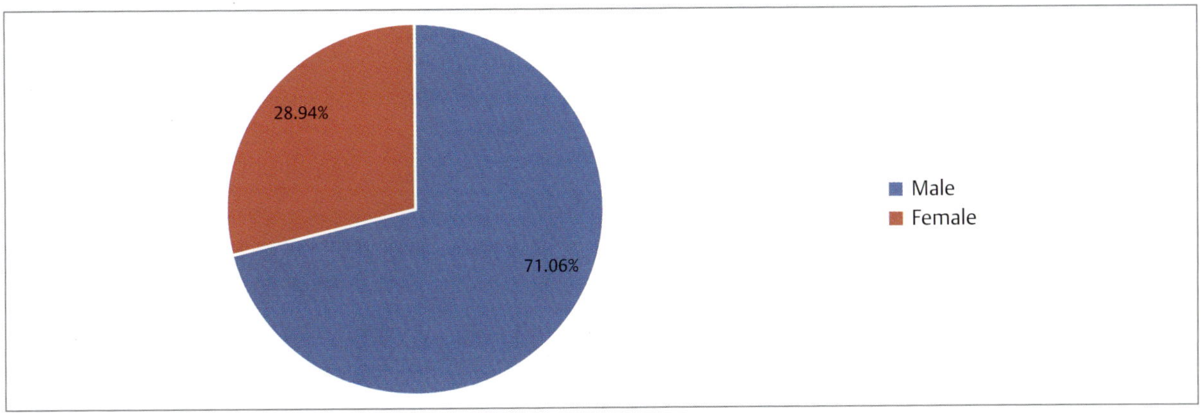

Fig. 3.18 Sex distribution of 940 Monteggia fractures.

Monteggia Fractures by Age Group

Table 3.19 Age and sex distribution of 940 Monteggia fractures

Age group (years)	Male	Female	Number of fractures	Percentage (%)
0–5	92	62	154	16.38
6–10	110	55	165	17.55
11–15	55	5	60	6.38
16–20	45	13	58	6.17
21–25	51	22	73	7.77
26–30	49	16	65	6.91
31–35	61	24	85	9.04
36–40	57	7	64	6.81
41–45	56	20	76	8.09
46–50	40	17	57	6.06
51–55	23	9	32	3.40
56–60	15	5	20	2.13
61–65	10	3	13	1.38
66–70	3	4	7	0.74
71–75	0	8	8	0.85
76–80	0	1	1	0.11
81–85	1	1	2	0.21
≥86	0	0	0	0.00
Total	668	272	940	100.00

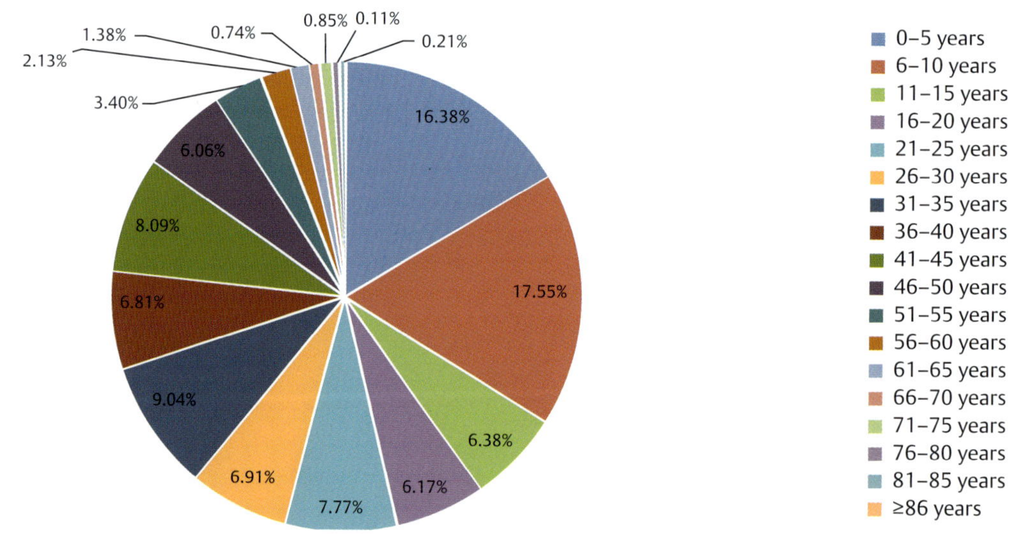

a

Fig. 3.19 **(a)** Age distribution of 940 Monteggia fractures.

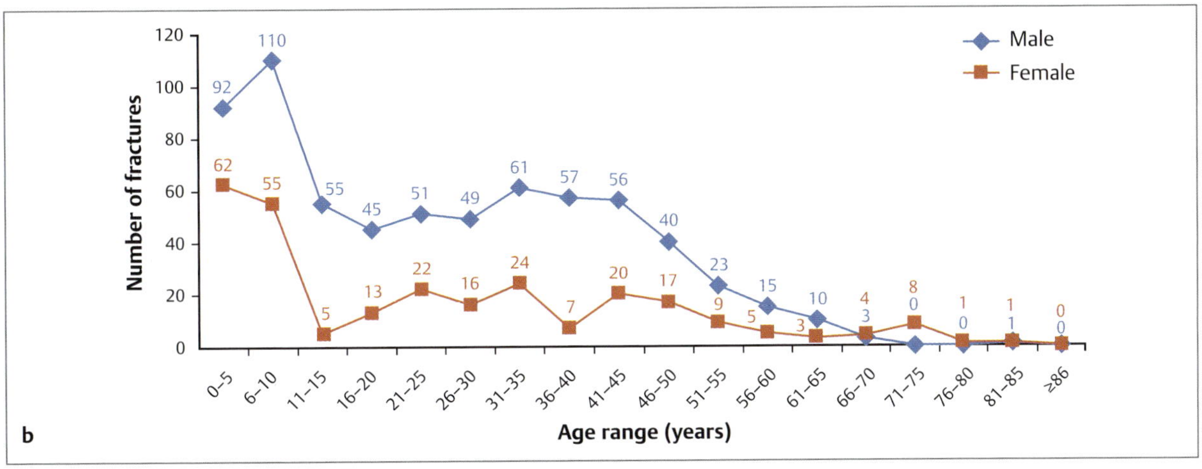

Fig. 3.19 (*continued*) **(b)** Age and sex distribution of 940 Monteggia fractures.

Monteggia Fractures by Type

Table 3.20 Sex and fracture type distribution of 940 Monteggia fractures

Fracture type	Male	Female	Number of fractures	Percentage (%)
I	297	153	450	47.87
II	90	39	129	13.72
III	215	61	276	29.36
IV	66	19	85	9.04
Total	668	272	940	100.00

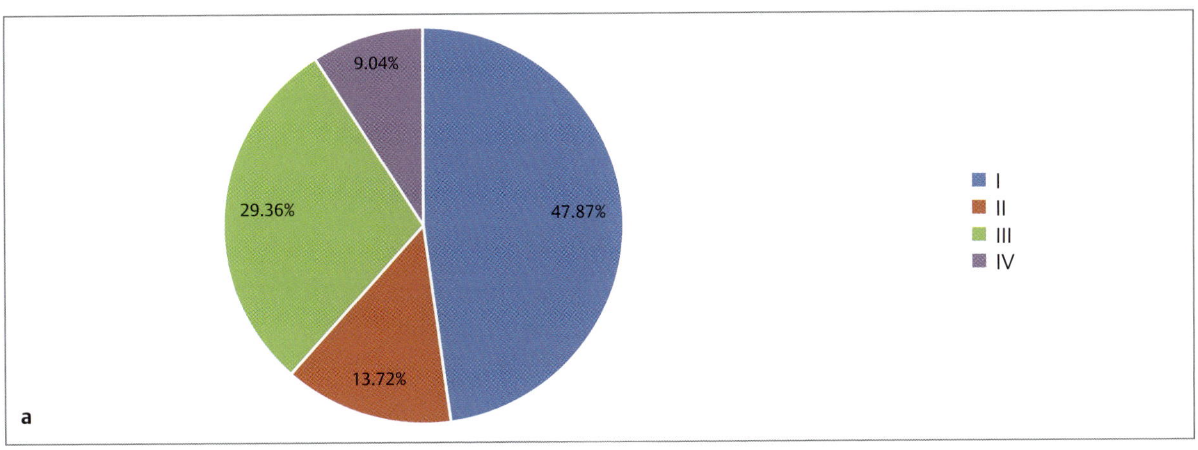

Fig. 3.20 **(a)** Fracture type distribution of 940 Monteggia fractures. (*Continued*)

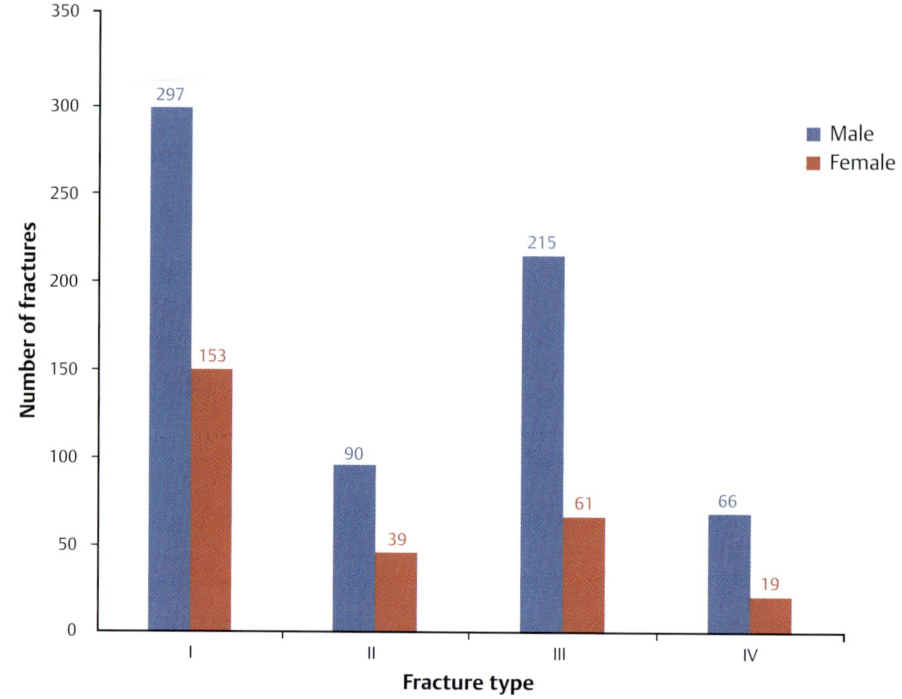

b

Fig. 3.20 (*continued*) **(b)** Sex and fracture type distribution of 940 Monteggia fractures.

Galeazzi Fractures

Overview

The Galeazzi fracture is an injury pattern involving a fracture of the distal third of the radial shaft with associated subluxation or dislocation of the DRUJ (**Plates 3.13** and **3.14**).

Galeazzi fractures usually occur from a fall on the outstretched hand, causing an axial load on the hyperpronated forearm. This type of injury can also result from a direct blow on the wrist joint or dorsal rim of the distal third of the radial shaft, or from a manufacturing injury.

In a fracture of the radial shaft with marked displacement, the radius will be shortened and angulated in relation to the ulna, with associated dorsal displacement of the ulnar head. Physical examination reveals tenderness to palpation over the DRUJ. Radiographic examination often shows dorsal angulation of the radial fracture with dorsal displacement of ulnar head. The injury of the DRUJ may occur as a purely ligamentous injury, or may be associated with an avulsion fracture of the ulnar styloid process.

Galeazzi fractures are easily misdiagnosed, and closed reduction and cast application have led to unsatisfactory results. Open reduction and stable internal fixation of the radial fracture can usually reduce the DRUJ to a normal anatomical position. If the DRUJ is reducible but unstable, stabilization of the DRUJ in supination should be attempted by placing a K-wire from the ulna into the radius, just proximal to the articular surface, for 6 weeks after surgery.

Clinical Epidemiologic Features of Galeazzi Fractures

A total of 796 Galeazzi fractures were treated in 83 hospitals in China over a 2-year period from 2010 to 2011. All cases were reviewed and statistically studied; the fractures accounted for 0.18% of all fractures and 1.04% of fractures of the radius/ulna. Their epidemiologic features are as follows:

- More males than females
- The high-risk age group is between ages 11 and 15; the most affected female age group includes ages 6–10, while males between the ages of 11 and 15 have the highest risk.

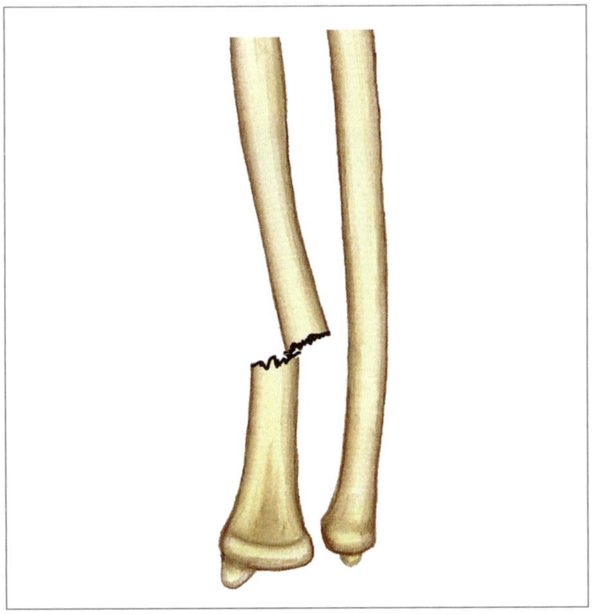

Plate 3.13

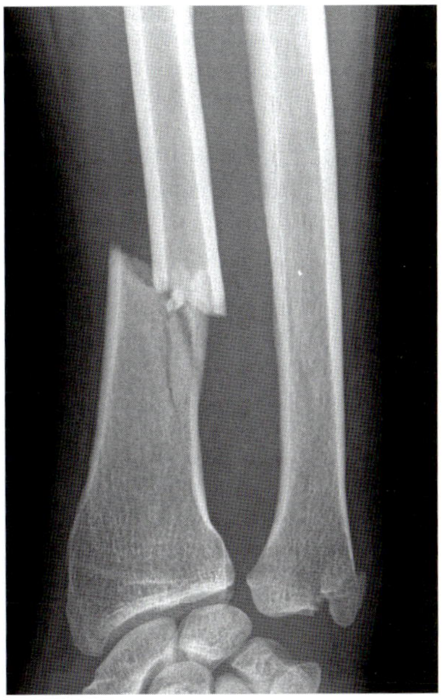

Plate 3.14

Galeazzi Fractures by Sex

Table 3.21 Sex distribution of 796 Galeazzi fractures

Sex	Number of fractures	Percentage (%)
Male	571	71.73
Female	225	28.27
Total	796	100.00

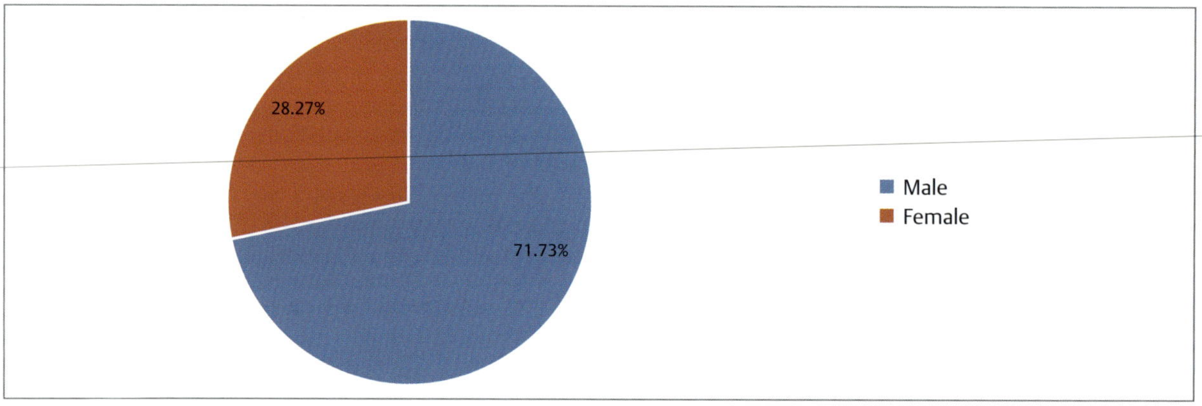

Fig. 3.21 Sex distribution of 796 Galeazzi fractures.

Galeazzi Fractures by Age Group

Table 3.22 Age and sex distribution of 796 Galeazzi fractures

Age group (years)	Male	Female	Number of fractures	Percentage (%)
0–5	27	23	50	6.28
6–10	85	29	114	14.32
11–15	113	13	126	15.83
16–20	52	8	60	7.54
21–25	57	8	65	8.17
26–30	57	11	68	8.54
31–35	31	9	40	5.03
36–40	42	23	65	8.17
41–45	30	23	53	6.66
46–50	25	15	40	5.03
51–55	16	17	33	4.15
56–60	18	13	31	3.89
61–65	8	9	17	2.14
66–70	3	9	12	1.51
71–75	3	4	7	0.88
76–80	2	7	9	1.13
81–85	2	2	4	0.50
≥86	0	2	2	0.25
Total	571	225	796	100.00

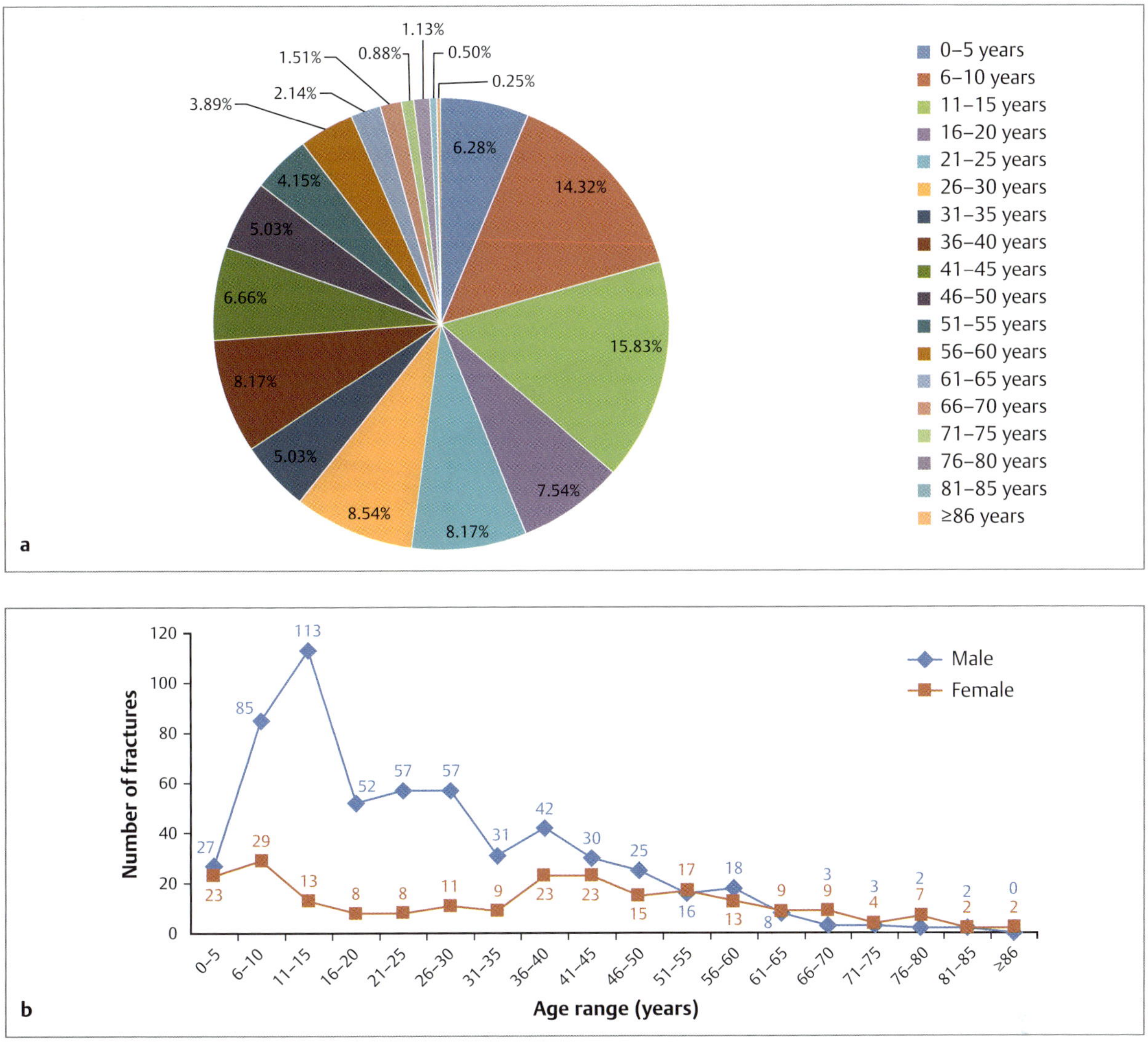

Fig. 3.22 **(a)** Age distribution of 796 Galeazzi fractures.
(b) Age and sex distribution of 796 Galeazzi fractures.

Colles Fractures

Overview

Colles fracture describes a fracture through the distal metaphysis, ~ 2–3 cm proximal to the articular surface of the radius, with dorsal displacement of the distal fragment, and may be associated with an avulsion fracture of the ulnar styloid process (**Plates 3.15, 3.16,** and **3.17**). Characteristic findings in a Colles fracture are a "dinner fork" deformity from the lateral view and a bayonet-shaped deformity from the anterior view. Typical plain film findings include dorsal displacement of the distal radial fragment, dorsal tilt, radial shortening, ulnar angulation of the wrist, loss of radial inclination, and comminution at the fracture site. The wrist joint and DRUJ can be involved separately or in conjunction with each other.

The fracture is most commonly caused by falling forward on an outstretched hand with the wrist in extension. Treatment depends on the severity of the fracture; however, most Colles fractures can be managed by closed reduction and casting application and they rarely require surgical intervention.

Clinical Epidemiologic Features of Colles Fractures

A total of 14,790 Colles fractures were treated in 83 hospitals in China over a 2-year period from 2010 to 2011. All cases were reviewed and statistically studied; they accounted for 3.43% of all fractures and 19.32% of fractures of the radius/ulna. Their epidemiologic features are as follows:

- More females than males
- The high-risk age group is 56–60 years; males between the ages of 11 and 15 years and females between the ages of 56 and 60 years have the highest risk.

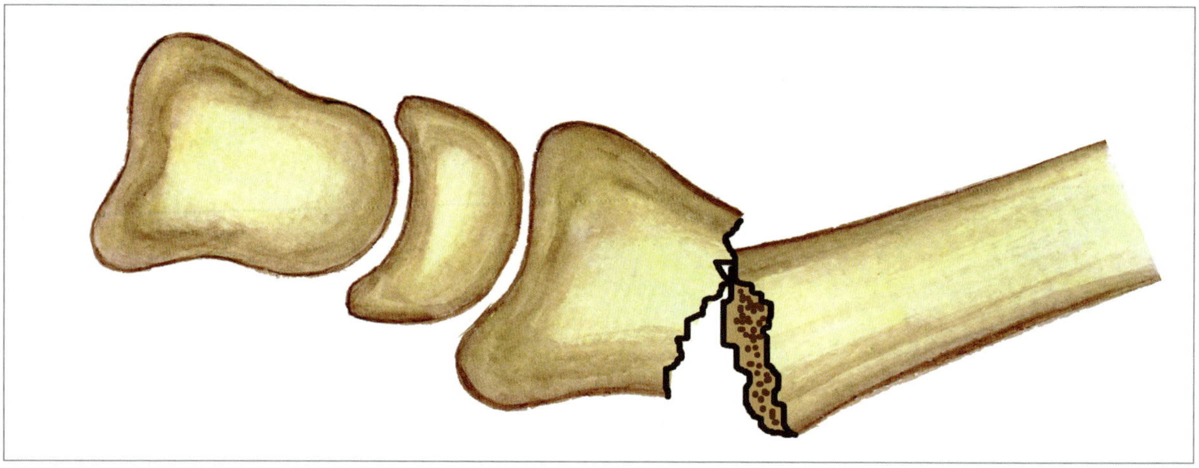

Plate 3.15

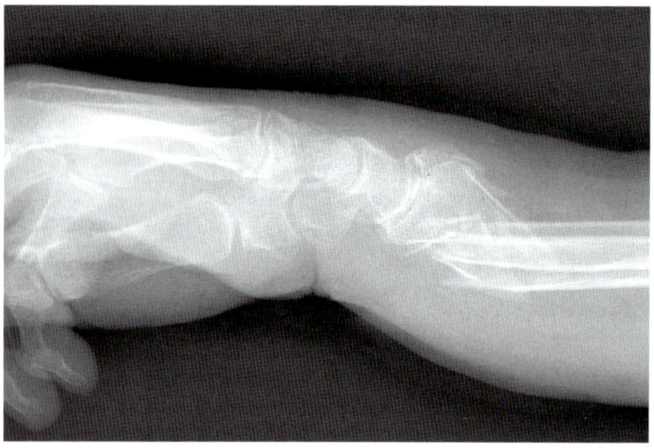

Plate 3.16

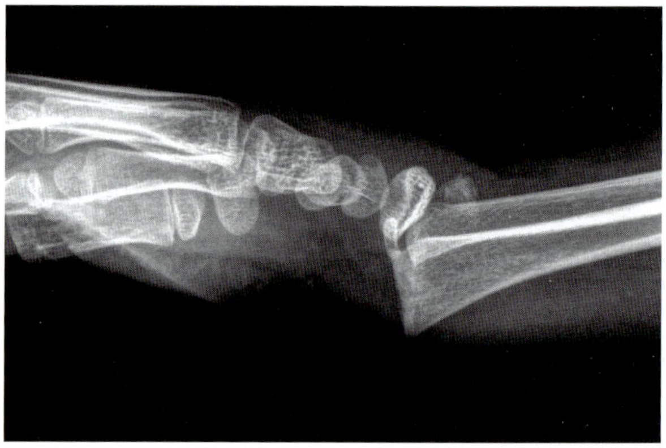

Plate 3.17

Colles Fractures by Sex

Table 3.23 Sex distribution of 14,790 Colles fractures

Sex	Number of fractures	Percentage (%)
Male	6,842	46.26
Female	7,948	53.74
Total	14,790	100.00

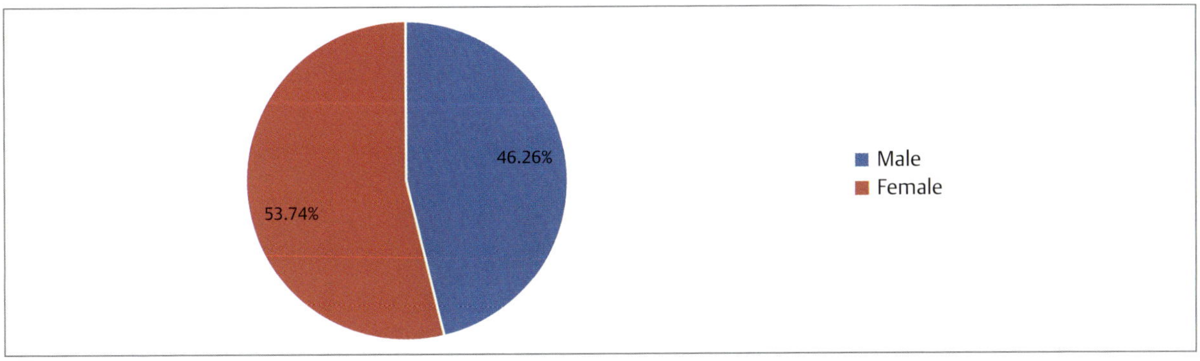

Fig. 3.23 Sex distribution of 14,790 Colles fractures.

Colles Fractures by Age Group

Table 3.24 Age and sex distribution of 14,970 Colles fractures

Age group (years)	Male	Female	Number of fractures	Percentage (%)
0–5	280	130	410	2.77
6–10	954	272	1,226	8.29
11–15	1,327	199	1,526	10.32
16–20	654	124	778	5.26
21–25	429	158	587	3.97
26–30	308	165	473	3.20
31–35	306	207	513	3.47
36–40	362	274	636	4.30
41–45	389	359	748	5.06
46–50	413	618	1,031	6.97
51–55	376	927	1,303	8.81
56–60	329	1,335	1,664	11.25
61–65	227	830	1,057	7.15
66–70	182	736	918	6.21
71–75	112	658	770	5.21
76–80	107	531	638	4.31
81–85	56	278	334	2.26
≥86	31	147	178	1.20
Total	6,842	7,948	14,790	100.00

3

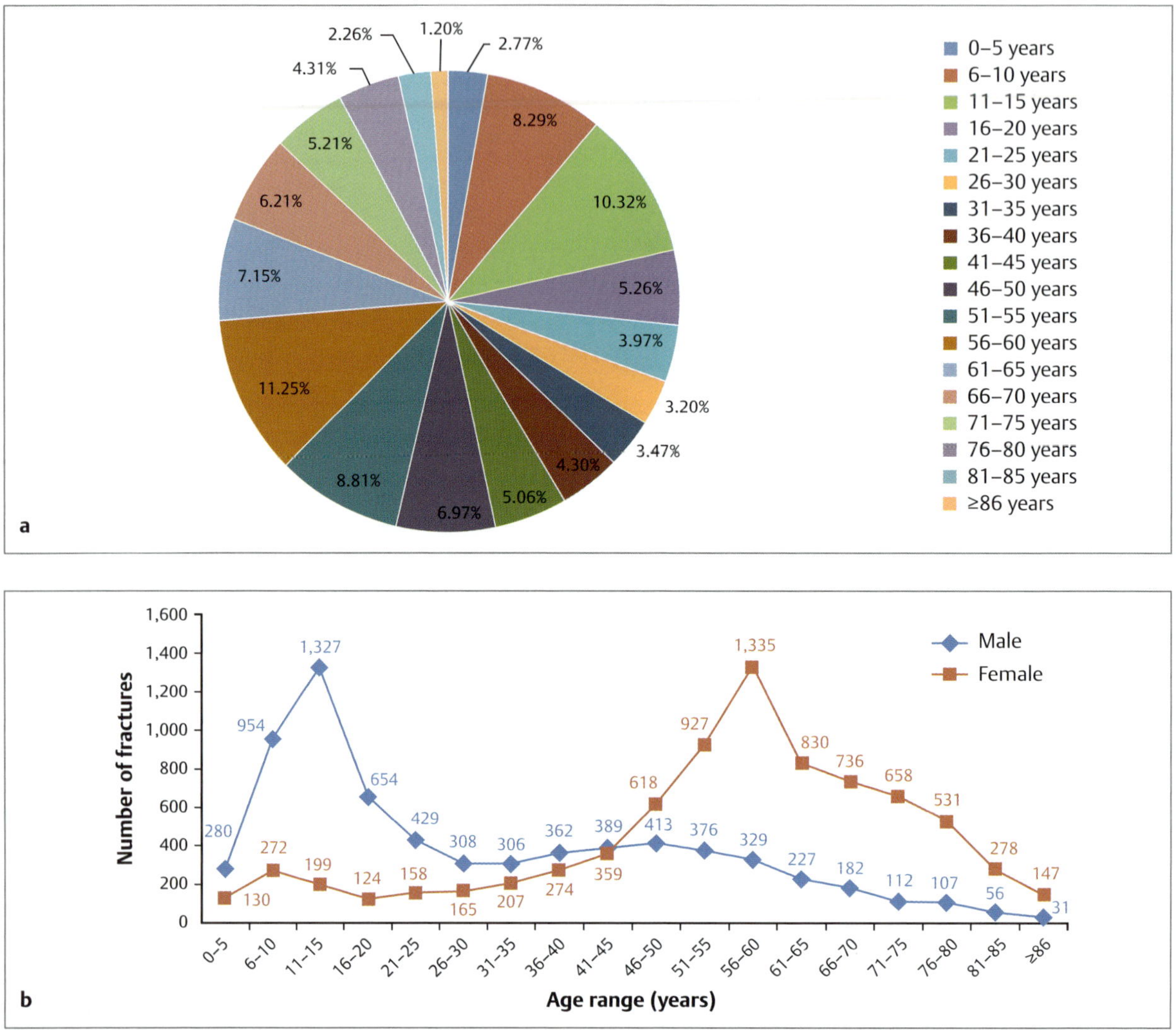

Fig. 3.24 **(a)** Age distribution of 14,790 Colles fractures.
(b) Age and sex distribution of 14,790 Colles fractures.

Smith Fractures

Overview

A Smith fracture, also known as a reverse Colles fracture because it shares the same fracture location, is a fracture of the distal radius with associated volar displacement of the distal fragment. The injury usually occurs from falling on the back of the hand with the wrists in flexion, or from a direct blow to the dorsal wrist.

The classic finding in Smith fractures is a garden spade deformity resulting from volar angulation of the fracture. The subsequent compression on the carpal tunnel by the displaced fracture will cause carpal tunnel syndrome. Typical X-ray findings include volar displacement of the distal fragment, volar and radial angulation, comminution of volar cortex at the fracture site, fragment rotation, and radial shortening.

According to Thomas, Smith fractures can be classified into three types (**Plates 3.18, 3.19, 3.20,** and **3.21**).

- *Type I:* extra-articular fracture of the distal radius with dorsal angulation and volar displacement.
- *Type II:* intra-articular oblique fracture of the distal radius into the radiocarpal joint with volar displacement of the distal fragment with the carpal bones—equivalent to the volar type of Barton fractures.
- *Type III:* oblique juxta-articular fracture of the distal radius with volar displacement of the distal fragment with the carpal bones.

Treatment of Smith fractures depends on the severity of the fracture. A Smith fracture usually can be treated by closed reduction, splinting, or cast application. If the fracture is reducible but still unstable, the fracture should be stabilized by an external fixator. Significant angulation and displacement may require open reduction and internal fixation with a plate or K-wire.

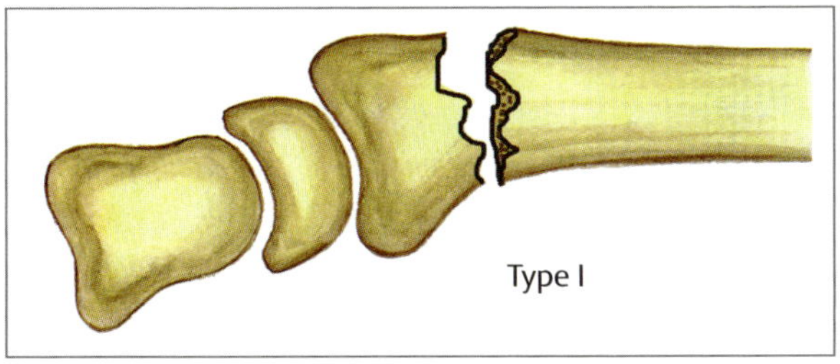

Plate 3.18

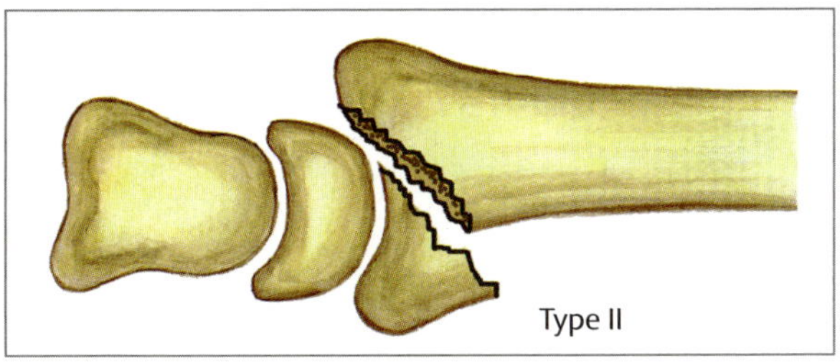

Plate 3.19

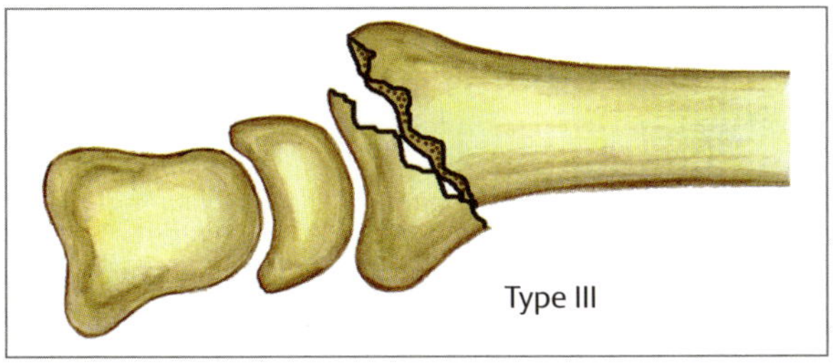

Plate 3.20

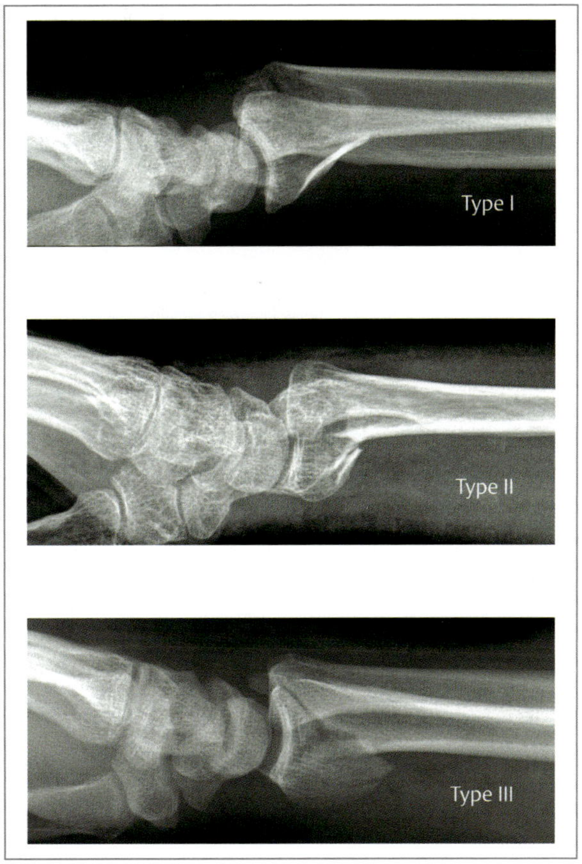

Plate 3.21

Clinical Epidemiologic Features of Smith Fractures

A total of 3,237 Smith fractures were treated in 83 hospitals in China over a 2-year period from 2010 to 2011. All cases were reviewed and statistically studied; the fractures accounted for 4.23% of all fractures and 6.20% of fractures of the radius/ulna. Their epidemiologic features are as follows:

- More males than females
- The high-risk age group is 11–15 years; males belong to the aforementioned age group, while females between the ages of 61 and 65 years have the highest risk.
- The most common fracture type is type I.

Smith Fractures by Sex

Table 3.25 Sex distribution of 3,237 Smith fractures

Sex	Number of fractures	Percentage (%)
Male	1,728	53.38
Female	1,509	46.62
Total	3,237	100.00

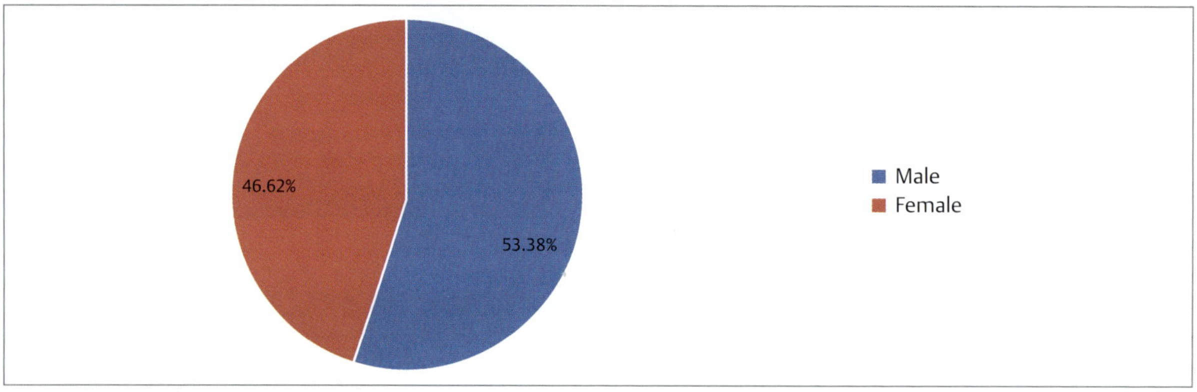

Fig. 3.25 Sex distribution of 3,237 Smith fractures.

3

Smith Fractures by Age Group

Table 3.26 Age and sex distribution of 3,237 Smith fractures

Age group (years)	Male	Female	Number of fractures	Percentage (%)
0–5	55	29	84	2.59
6–10	205	99	304	9.39
11–15	487	113	600	18.54
16–20	157	29	186	5.75
21–25	95	37	132	4.08
26–30	80	47	127	3.92
31–35	72	50	122	3.77
36–40	80	63	143	4.42
41–45	107	64	171	5.28
46–50	117	117	234	7.23
51–55	79	155	234	7.23
56–60	55	158	213	6.58
61–65	52	162	214	6.61
66–70	34	125	159	4.91
71–75	28	125	153	4.73
76–80	15	72	87	2.69
81–85	4	41	45	1.39
≥86	6	23	29	0.90
Total	1,728	1,509	3,237	100.00

3

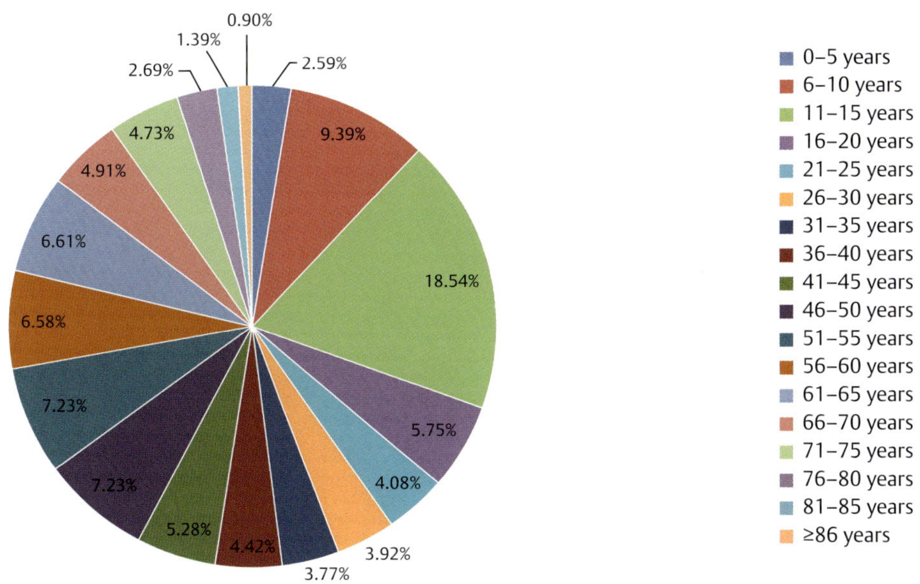

a

Fig. 3.26 **(a)** Age distribution of 3,237 Smith fractures. (*Continued*)

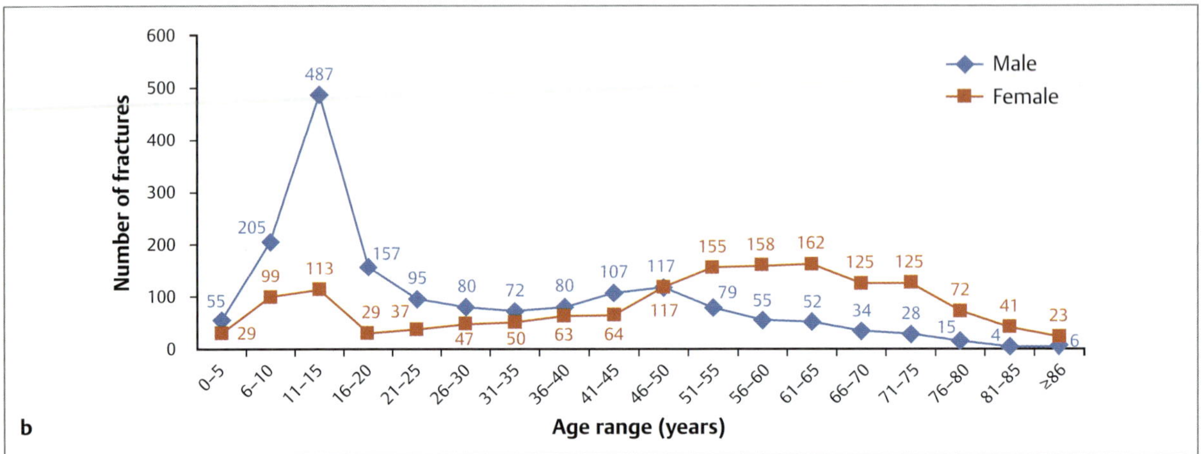

Fig. 3.26 (*continued*) **(b)** Age and sex distribution of 3,237 Smith fractures.

Smith Fractures by Fracture Type

Table 3.27 Sex and fracture type distribution of 3,237 Smith fractures

Fracture type	Male	Female	Number of fractures	Percentage (%)	Percentage of radius/ulna fractures (%)	Percentage of total (%)
I	1,223	1,043	2,266	70.00	2.96	0.52
II	436	421	857	26.48	1.12	0.20
III	69	45	114	3.52	0.15	0.03
Total	1,728	1,509	3,237	100.00	4.23	0.75

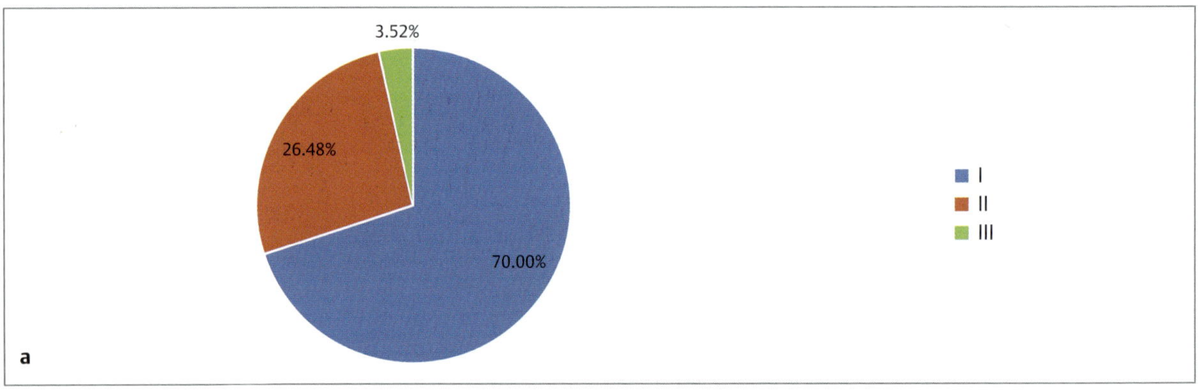

Fig. 3.27 **(a)** Fracture type distribution of 3,237 Smith fractures.

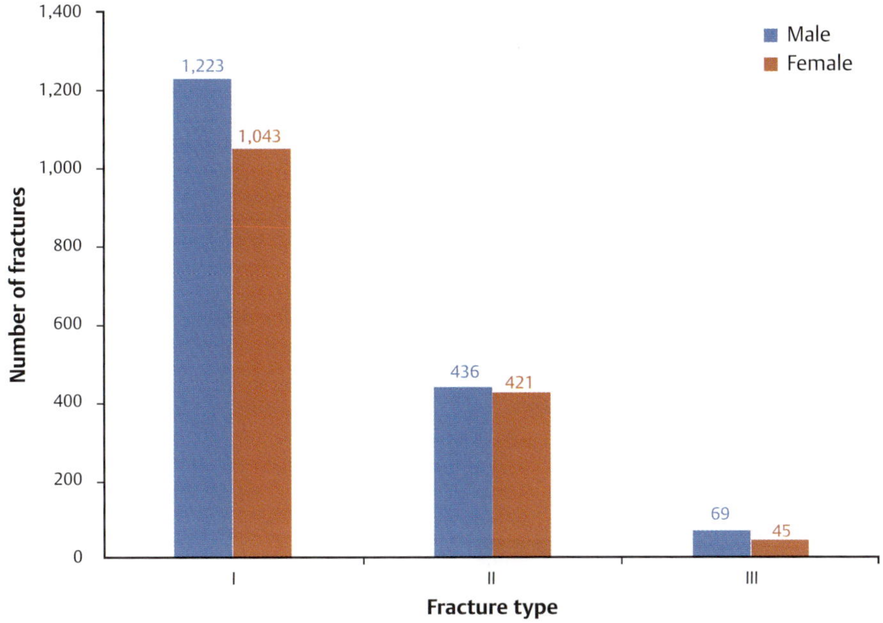

b

Fig. 3.27 (*continued*) **(b)** Sex and fracture type distribution of 3,237 Smith fractures.

Barton Fractures

Overview

A Barton fracture is an intra-articular fracture of the distal radius with dislocation of the radiocarpal joint. The fracture cleft extends proximally and obliquely in the coronal plane, and involves a single-wedged fragment of either the dorsal or palmar lip of the radius. As such, there are two types of Barton fracture, dorsal and palmar, the latter being more common.

The palmar type of Barton fracture has a similar injury mechanism to the Smith fracture (**Plate 3.22**).

The dorsal type of Barton fracture usually results from a fall on an extended hand with wrists in forced pronation (**Plate 3.23**).

A Barton fracture, being exclusively an intra-articular fracture, does not have characteristic deformities such as those seen in Colles and Smith fractures. Typical X-ray findings reveal an intra-articular fracture of the dorsal or palmar rim of the distal radius, with displacement of the carpal bones. If the fragment is small, it may be associated with an avulsion fracture. If the fragment is large, it is usually subluxed toward the palmar direction, or dorsally along with the carpal bones. Subluxation or dislocation of the wrist joint can also result from severely damaged ligaments, even with a small-sized fragment.

Treatment for both types of injuries should first be attempted with a manipulative method, splinting, or a casting application. If the fracture is reducible but unstable, open reduction and internal fixation with a plate or K-wire may be indicated.

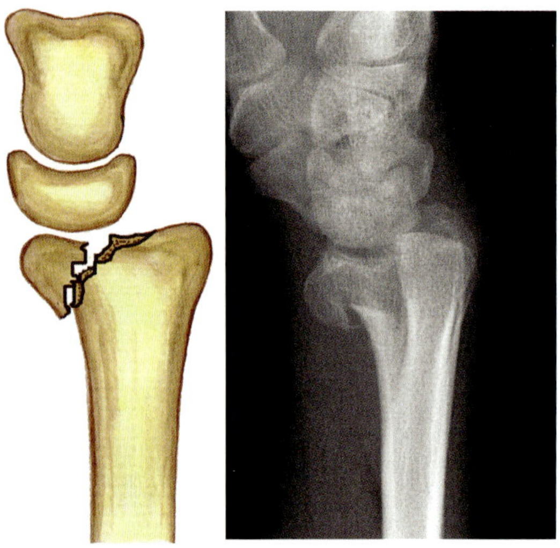

Palmar-type Barton fracture

Plate 3.22

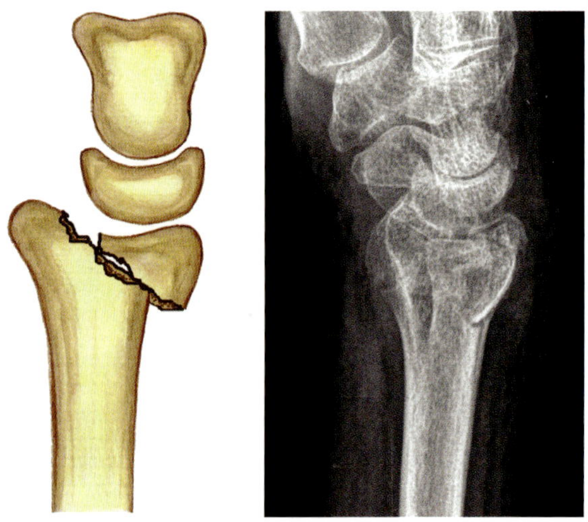

Dorsal-type Barton fracture

Plate 3.23

Clinical Epidemiologic Features of Barton Fractures

A total of 2,012 Barton fractures were treated in 83 hospitals in China over a 2-year period from 2010 to 2011. All cases were reviewed and statistically studied; the fractures accounted for 0.47% of all fractures and 2.63% of fractures of the radius/ulna and 3.85% of fractures of the distal radius/ulna. Their epidemiologic features are as follows:

- Slightly more males than females
- The high-risk age group is between ages 56 and 60; males between ages 16 and 20, and 36 and 40, while females between ages 56 and 60 have the highest risk.
- The palmar type is more common than the dorsal type of Barton fracture.

Barton Fractures by Sex

Table 3.28 Sex distribution of 2,012 Barton fractures

Sex	Number of fractures	Percentage (%)
Male	982	48.81
Female	1,030	51.19
Total	2,012	100.00

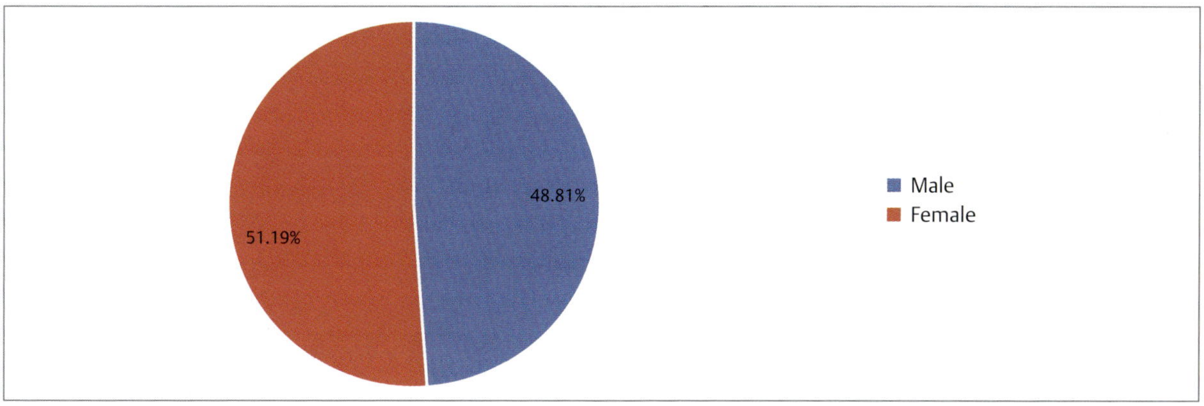

Fig. 3.28 Sex distribution of 2,012 Barton fractures.

3

Barton Fractures by Age Group

Table 3.29 Age and sex distribution of 2,012 Barton fractures

Age group (years)	Male	Female	Number of fractures	Percentage (%)
0–5	3	2	5	0.25
6–10	23	10	33	1.64
11–15	31	5	36	1.79
16–20	117	21	138	6.86
21–25	88	24	112	5.57
26–30	87	27	114	5.67
31–35	78	37	115	5.72
36–40	119	44	163	8.10
41–45	105	53	158	7.85
46–50	91	92	183	9.10
51–55	60	140	200	9.94
56–60	67	172	239	11.88
61–65	49	113	162	8.05
66–70	18	104	122	6.06
71–75	20	91	111	5.52
76–80	17	55	72	3.58
81–85	4	24	28	1.39
≥86	5	16	21	1.04
Total	982	1,030	2,012	100.00

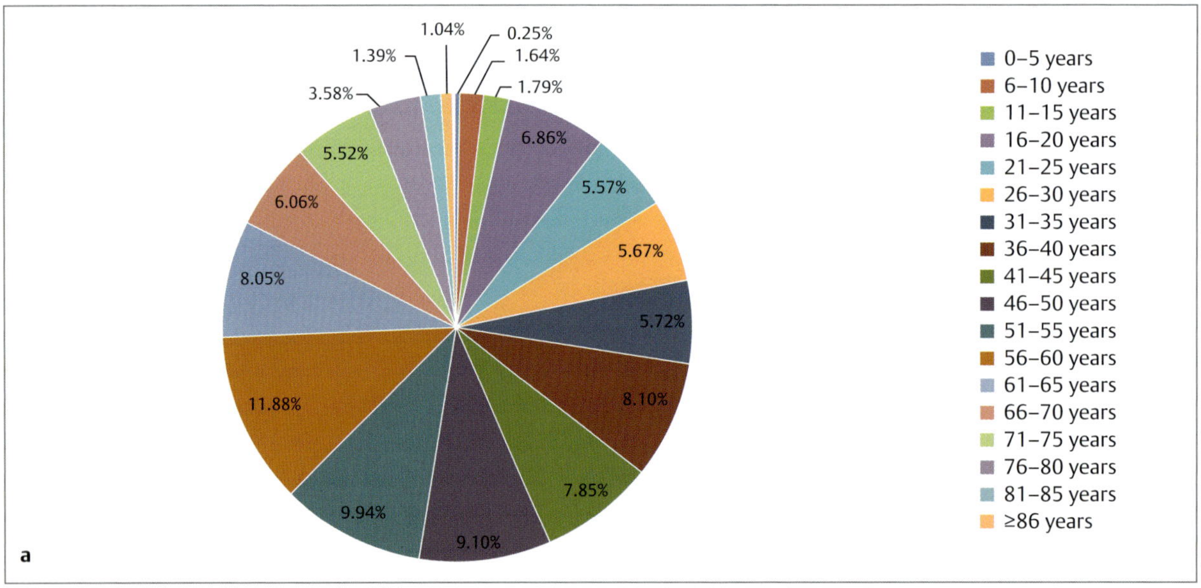

Fig. 3.29 **(a)** Age distribution of 2,012 Barton fractures.

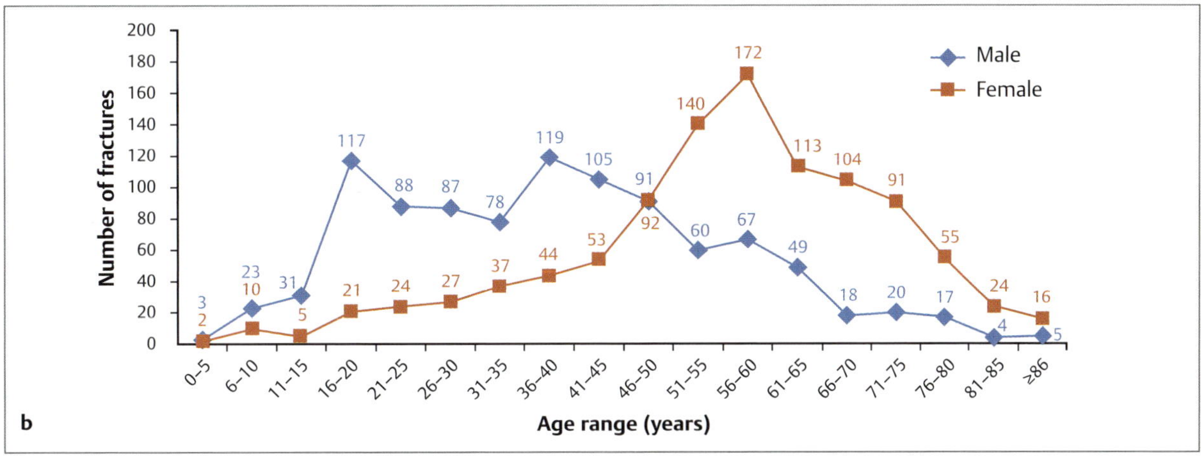

Fig. 3.29 (*continued*) **(b)** Age and sex distribution of 2012 Barton fractures.

Barton Fractures by Fracture Type

Table 3.30 Sex and fracture type distribution of 2,012 Barton fractures

Fracture type	Male	Female	Number of fractures	Percentage (%)
Palmar-type Barton fracture	642	637	1,279	63.57
Dorsal-type Barton fracture	340	393	733	36.43
Total	982	1,030	2,012	100.00

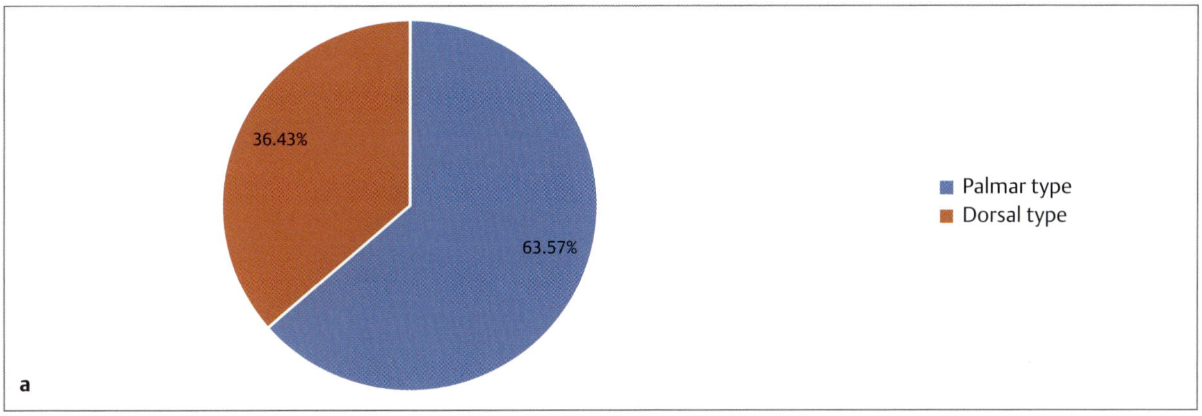

Fig. 3.30 **(a)** Fracture type distribution of 2,012 Barton fractures. (*Continued*)

3

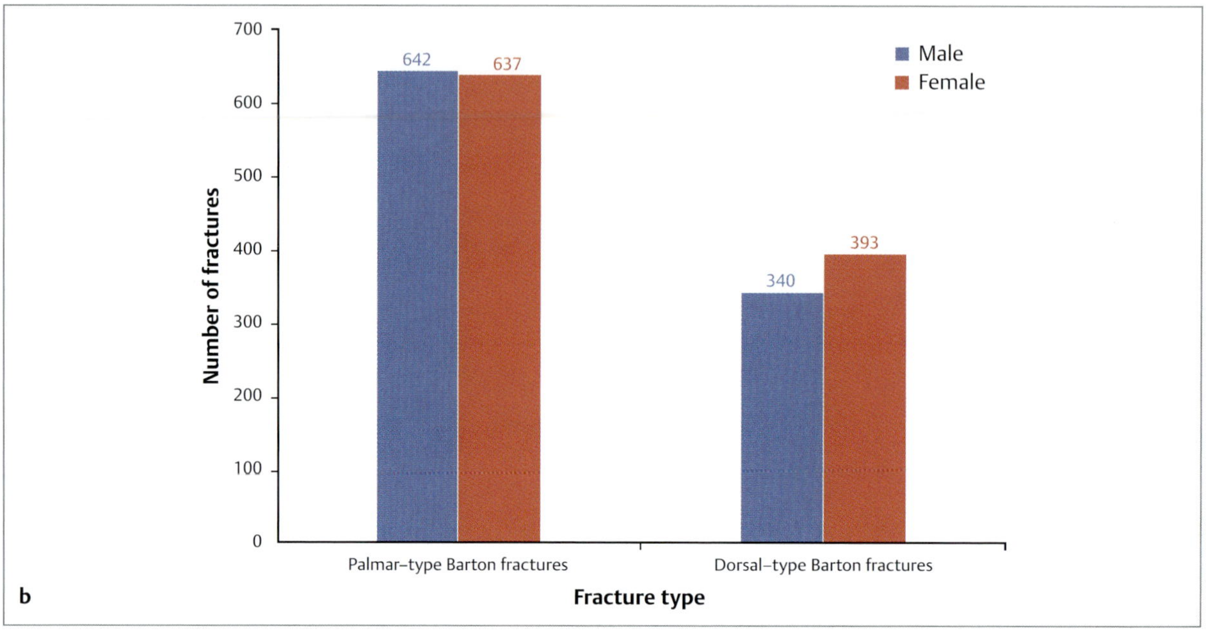

Fig. 3.30 (*continued*) **(b)** Sex and fracture type distribution of 2,012 Barton fractures.

3

4 Fractures of the Femur

Overview

Anatomical Features

The femur is the longest and largest tubular bone in the human skeleton; the average length of an adult femur is 42.48 cm on the left side and 42.39 cm on the right side. The femur is cylindric in the upper third of its length, with the pectineal line running through the posteromedial surface of the femur, up to the base of the lesser trochanter. The pectineal line then continues with the intertrochanteric line, and down to the medial lip of the linea aspera. The gluteal tuberosity lies on the posterolateral aspect of the femur, up to the base of the greater trochanter and down to the lateral lip of the linea aspera. The middle part of the femur is slightly twisted and curved, with an anterior convexity that is 30 degrees rotated from the superolateral to inferomedial part of the femur. The lower third of the femur becomes flattened and widened anteroposteriorly. The linea aspera on the dorsal side of middle third has two lips that diverge and turn into the medial and lateral supracondylar ridges, respectively. The rough impression above the medial epicondyle gives origin to the medial head of the gastrocnemius, while the plantaris arises in the impression above and to the medial side of the lateral epicondyle (**Plate 4.1**).

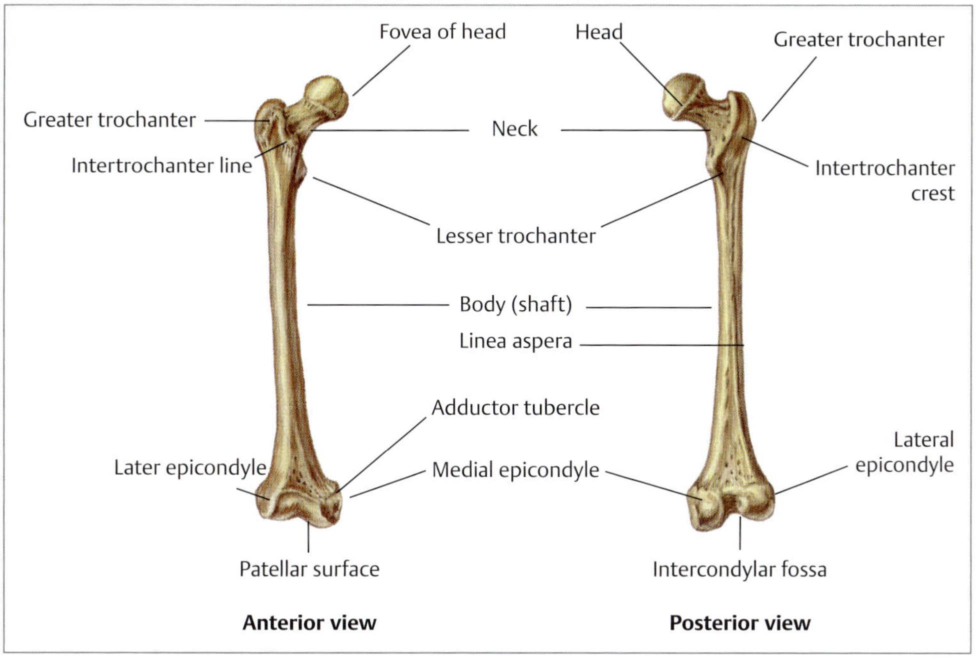

Plate 4.1

AO Classification and Coding System for Femoral Fractures

Based on the AO classification, the femur fracture is coded as number 3. According to Heim's square, the anatomical delineation of the proximal and distal shaft are numbers 31, 32, and 33, respectively (**Plates 4.2** and **4.3**).

Clinical Epidemiologic Features of Femoral Fractures

A total of 42,377 patients with 42,978 femoral fractures were treated in 83 hospitals in China over a 2-year period from 2010 to 2011. All cases were reviewed and statistically studied, accounting for 10.21% of all patients with fractures and 9.95% of all types of fractures, respectively. Among these 42,377 patients, 3,243 are children with 3,282 fractures and 39,134 are adults with 39,696 fractures.

Epidemiologic features of femur fractures are as follows:

- More males than females
- More left-side injuries than right-side injuries
- The highest risk age group is 76–80 years. The most affected male age group is 41–45 years, while females aged 76–80 years have the highest risk
- The proximal femoral fracture is the most common femoral fracture in adults. The diaphyseal femoral fracture is the most common femoral fracture in children.

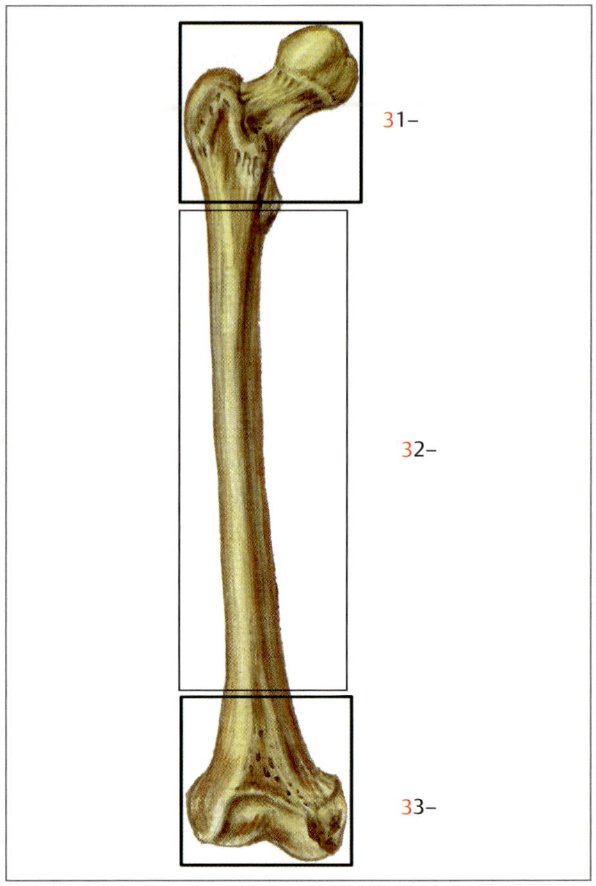

Plate 4.2

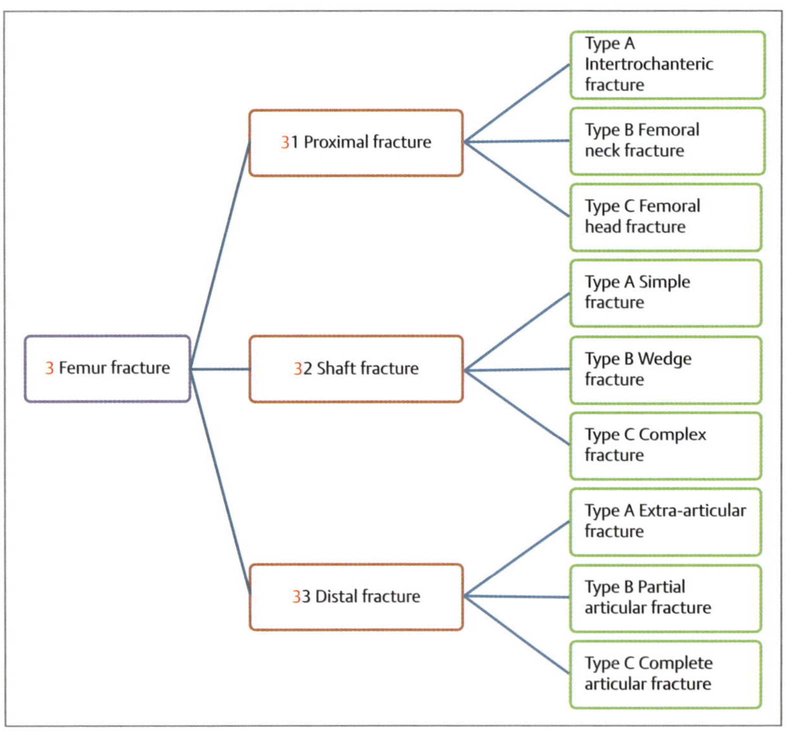

Plate 4.3

Femoral Fractures by Sex

Table 4.1 Sex distribution of 42,377 patients with femoral fractures

Sex	Number of patients	Percentage (%)
Male	23,234	54.83
Female	19,143	45.17
Total	42,377	100.00

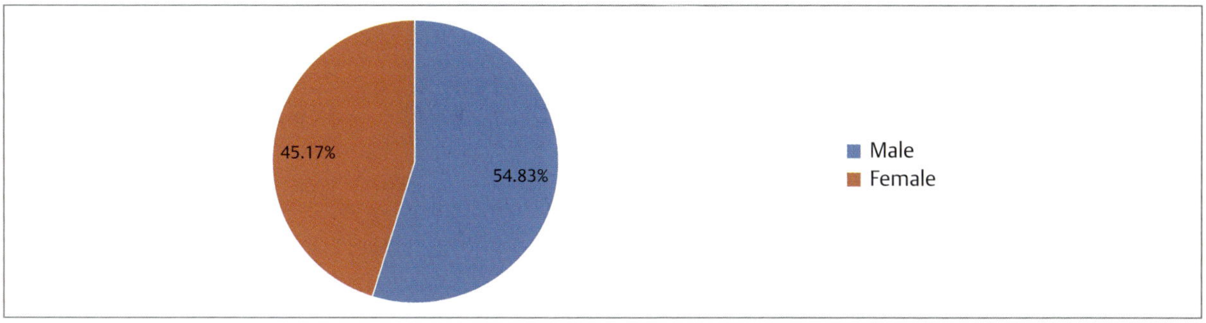

Fig. 4.1 Sex distribution of 42,377 patients with femoral fractures.

Femoral Fractures by Injury Side

Table 4.2 Injury side distribution of 42,377 patients with femoral fractures

Injured side	Number of patients	Percentage (%)
Left	21,931	51.75
Right	20,287	47.87
Bilateral	159	0.38
Total	42,377	100.00

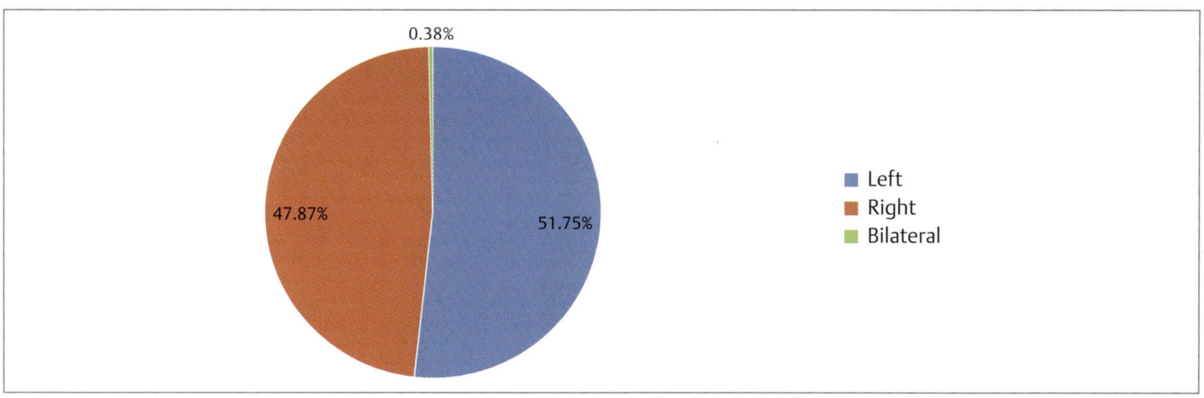

Fig. 4.2 Injury side distribution of 42,377 patients with femoral fractures.

Femoral Fractures by Age Group

Table 4.3 Age and sex distribution of 42,377 patients with femoral fractures

Age group (years)	Male	Female	Number of patients	Percentage (%)
0–5	958	585	1,543	3.64
6–10	583	343	926	2.19
11–15	552	222	774	1.83
16–20	1,105	264	1,369	3.23
21–25	1,503	403	1,906	4.50
26–30	1,354	322	1,676	3.95
31–35	1,431	404	1,835	4.33
36–40	1,718	493	2,211	5.22
41–45	1,889	578	2,467	5.82
46–50	1,617	670	2,287	5.40
51–55	1,567	1,051	2,618	6.18
56–60	1,525	1,386	2,911	6.87
61–65	1,176	1,377	2,553	6.02
66–70	1,085	1,654	2,739	6.46
71–75	1,437	2,382	3,819	9.01
76–80	1,572	2,840	4,412	10.41
81–85	1,252	2,330	3,582	8.45
≥86	910	1,839	2,749	6.49
Total	23,234	19,143	42,377	100.00

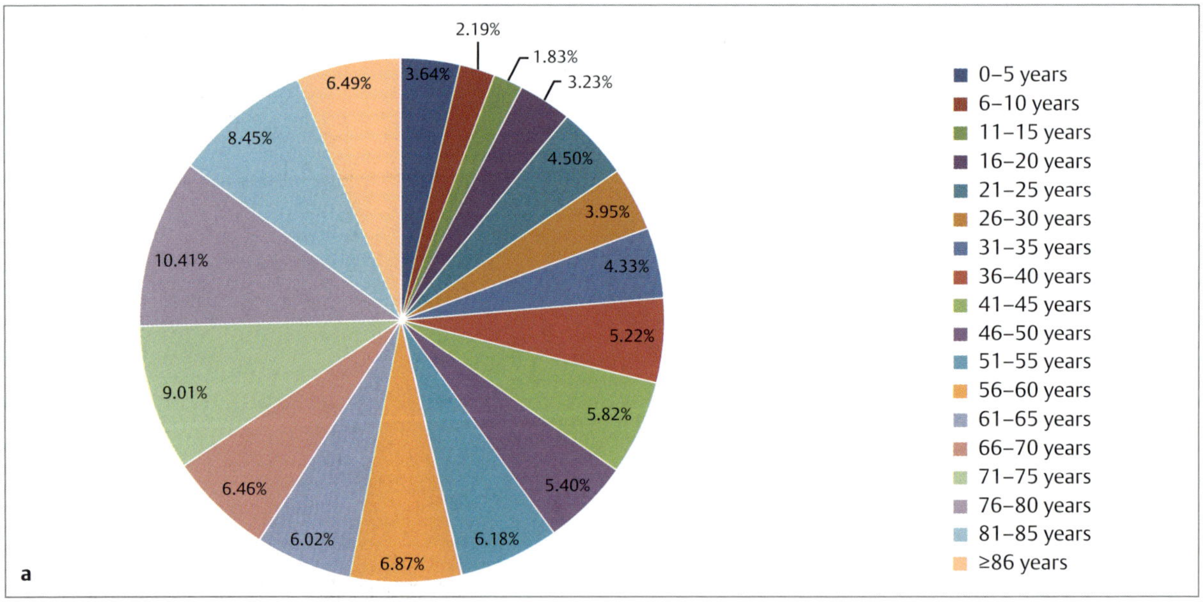

Fig. 4.3 **(a)** Age distribution of 42,377 patients with femoral fractures.

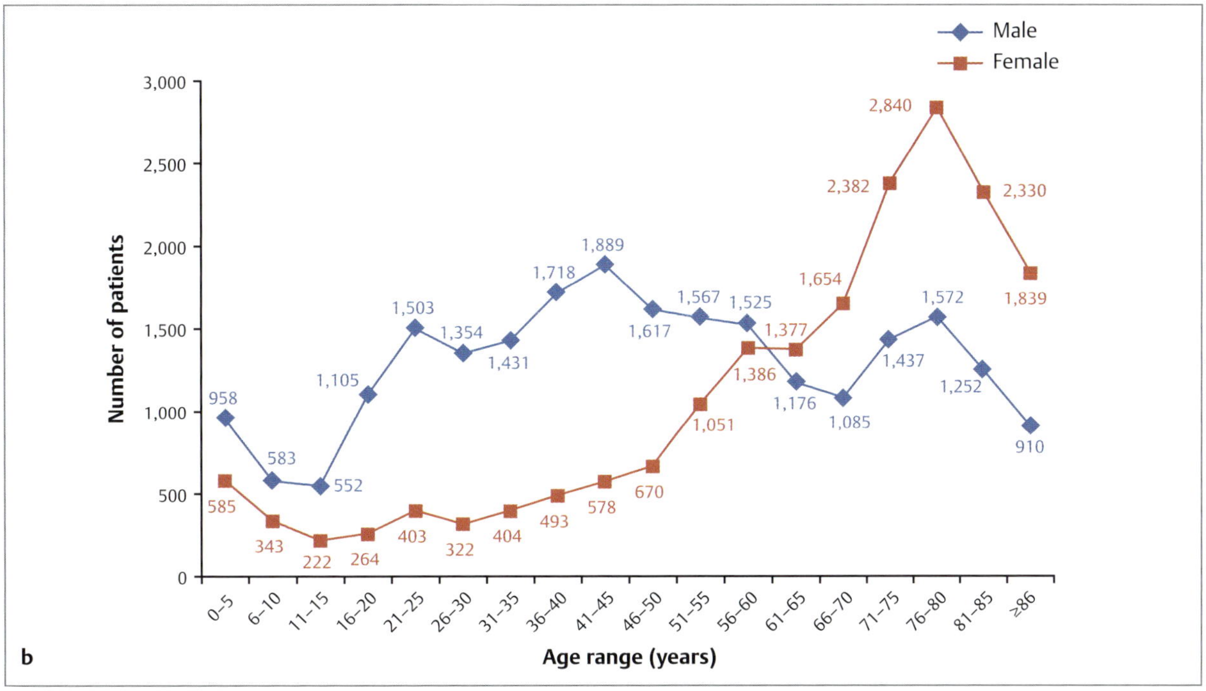

Fig. 4.3 (*continued*) **(b)** Age and sex distribution of 42,377 patients with femoral fractures.

Femoral Fractures by Fracture Segment

Segment Distribution of Femoral Fractures in Adults Based on AO Classification

Table 4.4 Fracture segment distribution of 39,696 femoral fractures in adults based on AO classification

Segment	Number of fractures	Percentage (%)
31 (proximal)	28,027	70.60
32 (diaphysis)	8,235	20.75
33 (distal)	3,434	8.65
Total	39,696	100.00

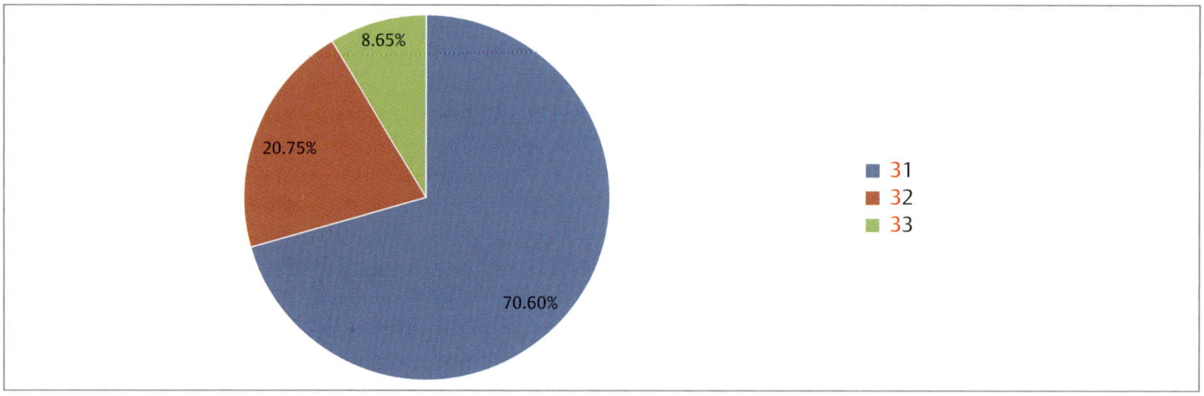

Fig. 4.4 Segment distribution of 39,696 adult femoral fractures based on AO classification.

Segment Distribution of Femoral Fractures in Children

Table 4.5 Segment distribution of 3,282 femoral fractures in children

Segment	Number of fractures	Percentage (%)
Proximal	717	21.85
Diaphysis	2,183	66.51
Distal	382	11.64
Total	3,282	100.00

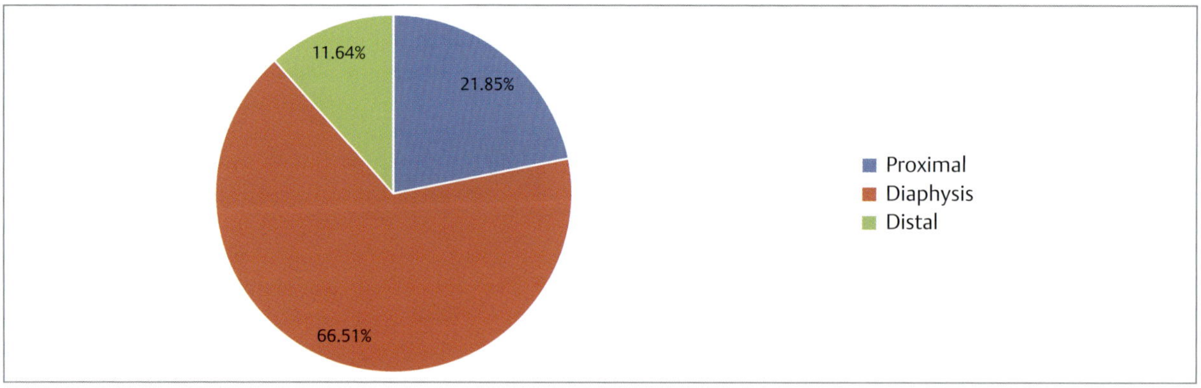

Fig. 4.5 Segment distribution of 3,282 femoral fractures in children.

4

Proximal Femoral Fractures (Segment 31)

Anatomical Features

The head of the femur is globular in shape and forms about two-thirds of a sphere (**Plate 4.4**). The neck projects forward to some extent, with an average anterior projection of 10–15 degrees. Flattened posteriorly, the neck is contracted in the middle, which is often the site of fractures. In adults, the neck forms an angle of ~ 120–130 degrees with the body. At the junction of the neck with the upper part of the body, there is a large eminence called the greater trochanter. A smaller eminence projecting from the lower and posterior part of the base of the neck is called the lesser trochanter. Running obliquely downward and medial from the tubercle is the intertrochanteric line, while the intertrochanteric crest courses obliquely downward and medially from the summit of the greater trochanter on the posterior surface of the neck.

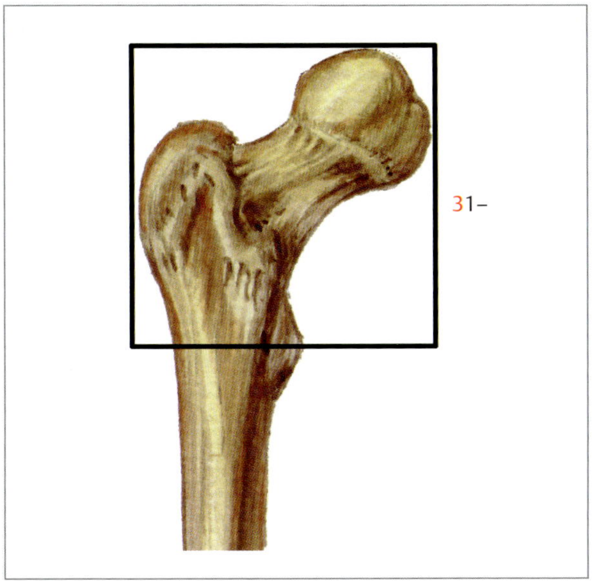

Plate 4.4

AO Classification of Proximal Femoral Fractures

Based on the AO classification, the proximal femur is coded as the number 31. It is further divided into three types: 31-A, trochanteric fractures (extra-articular); 32-B, femoral neck fractures (articular); 33-C, femoral head fractures (intra-articular) (**Plate 4.5**).

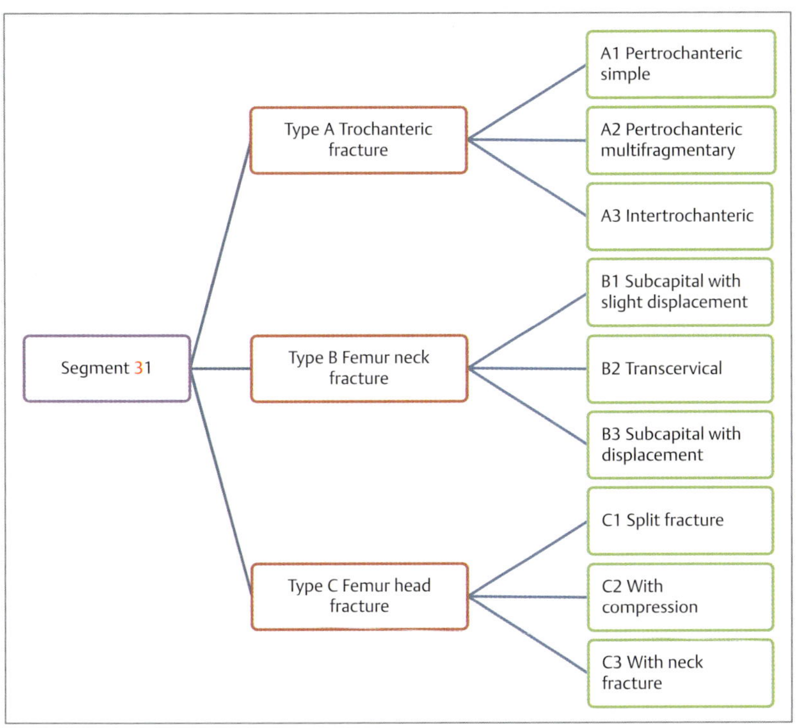

Plate 4.5

Clinical Epidemiologic Features of Proximal Femoral Fractures (Segment 31)

A total of 28,027 proximal femoral fractures were treated in 83 hospitals in China over a 2-year period from 2010 to 2011. All cases were reviewed and statistically studied; the fractures accounted for 70.60% of femur fractures in adults. Their epidemiologic features are as follows:

- More males than females
- The highest risk age group for both sexes is 76–80 years
- The most common fracture type among segment 31 fractures is type 31-B; however, 31-A is more common in males while 31-B is more common in females
- The most common fracture group among segment 31 fractures is group 31-A2; the same fracture group in both males and females

Fractures of Segment 31 by Sex

Table 4.6 Sex distribution of 28,027 fractures of segment 31

Sex	Number of fractures	Percentage (%)
Male	13,154	46.93
Female	14,873	53.07
Total	28,027	100.00

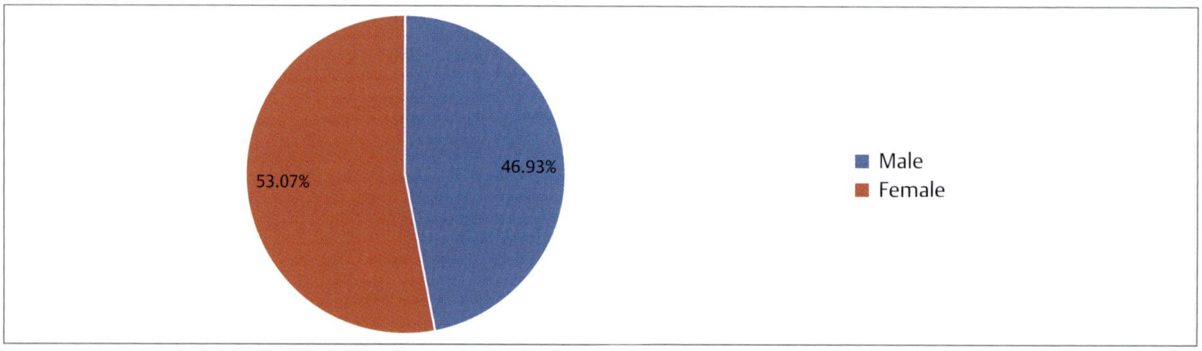

Fig. 4.6 Sex distribution of 28,027 fractures of segment 31.

Fractures of Segment 31 by Age Group

Table 4.7 Age and sex distribution of 28,027 fractures of segment 31

Age group (years)	Male	Female	Number of fractures	Percentage (%)
16–20	306	100	406	1.45
21–25	453	171	624	2.23
26–30	465	153	618	2.21
31–35	655	217	872	3.11
36–40	814	258	1,072	3.82
41–45	888	343	1,231	4.39
46–50	893	433	1,326	4.73
51–55	981	785	1,766	6.30
56–60	1,026	1,069	2,095	7.47
61–65	901	1,156	2,057	7.34
66–70	927	1,433	2,360	8.42
71–75	1,311	2,180	3,491	12.46
76–80	1,472	2,626	4,098	14.62
81–85	1,193	2,200	3,393	12.11
≥86	869	1,749	2,618	9.34
Total	13,154	14,873	28,027	100.00

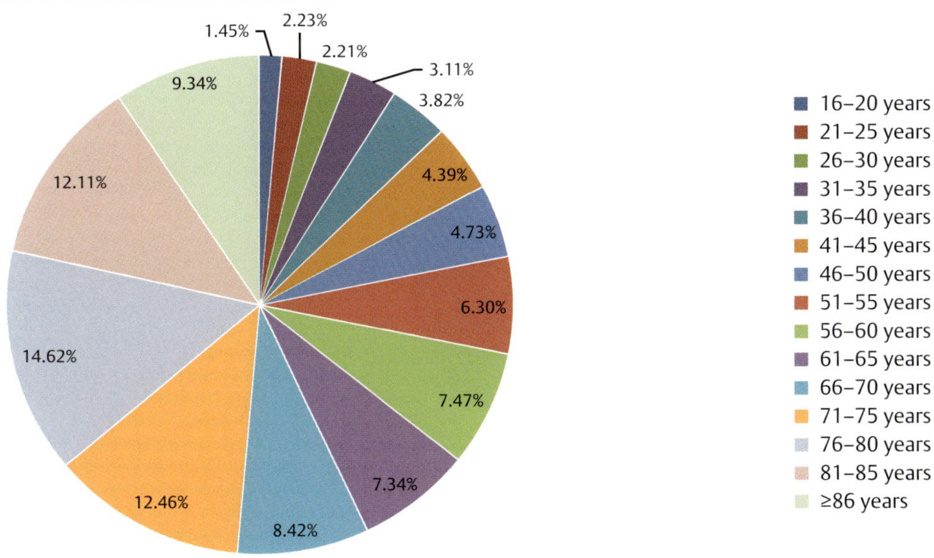

a

Fig. 4.7 **(a)** Age distribution of 28,027 fractures of segment 31. (*Continued*)

4

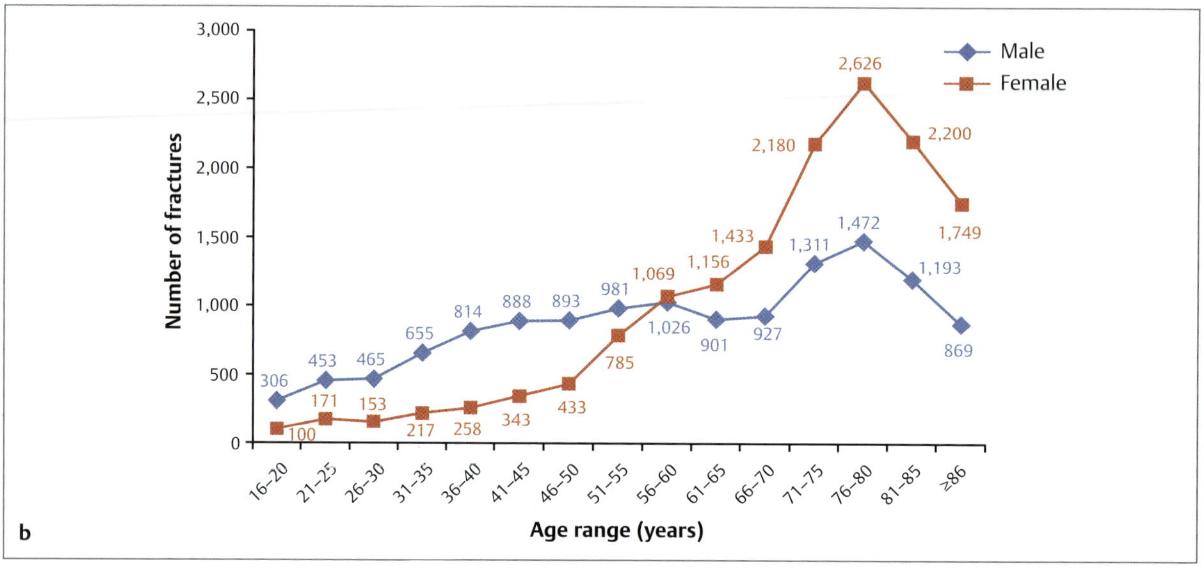

Fig. 4.7 (*continued*) **(b)** Age and sex distribution of 28,027 fractures of segment 31.

Fractures of Segment 31 by Fracture Type

Table 4.8 Sex and fracture type distribution of 28,027 fractures of segment 31

Fracture type	Male	Female	Number of fractures	Percentage (%)
31-A	6,480	6,263	12,743	45.47
31-B	5,635	7,881	13,516	48.22
31-C	1,039	729	1,768	6.31
Total	13,154	14,873	28,027	100.00

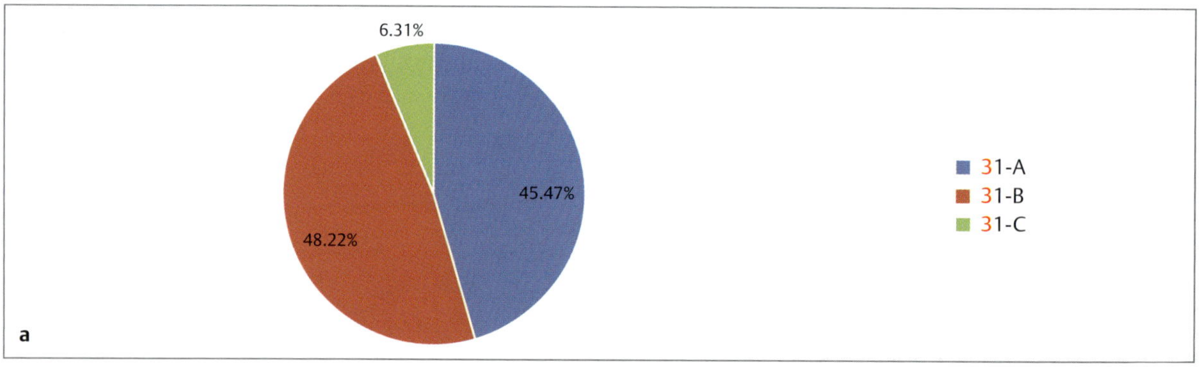

Fig. 4.8 **(a)** Fracture type distribution of 28,027 fractures of segment 31.

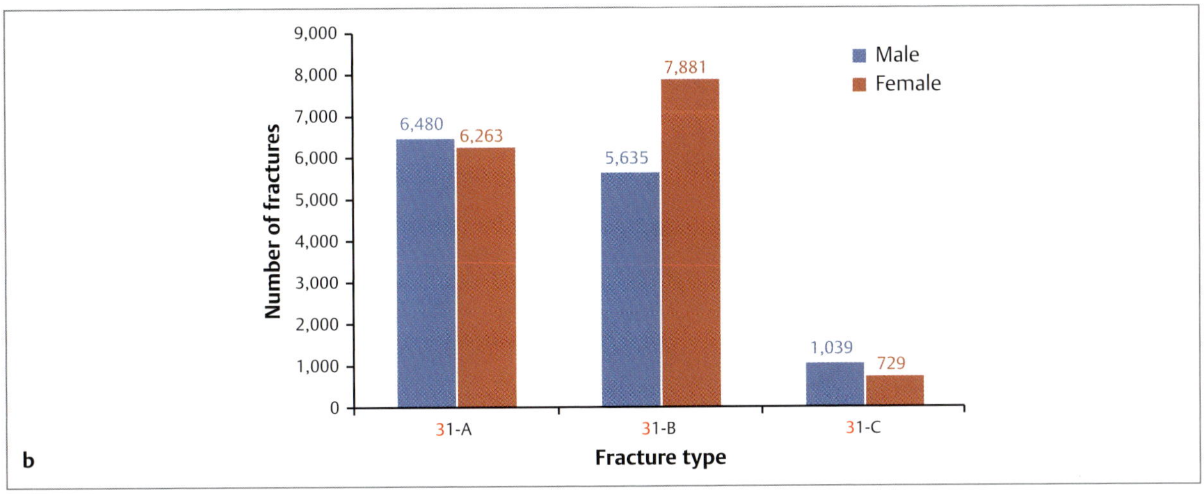

Fig. 4.8 (*continued*) **(b)** Sex and fracture type distribution of 28,027 fractures of segment 31.

Fractures of Segment 31 by Fracture Group

Table 4.9 Sex and fracture group distribution of 28,027 fractures of segment 31

Fracture group	Male	Female	Number of fractures	Percentage of segment 31 fractures (%)	Percentage of femur fractures (%)
31-A1	1,719	1,609	3,328	11.87	8.38
31-A2	3,542	3,866	7,408	26.43	18.66
31-A3	1,219	788	2,007	7.16	5.06
31-B1	1,234	1,711	2,945	10.51	7.42
31-B2	3,070	3,800	6,870	24.51	17.31
31-B3	1,331	2,370	3,701	13.21	9.32
31-C1	493	309	802	2.86	2.02
31-C2	348	269	617	2.20	1.55
31-C3	198	151	349	1.25	0.88
Total	13,154	14,873	28,027	100.00	70.60

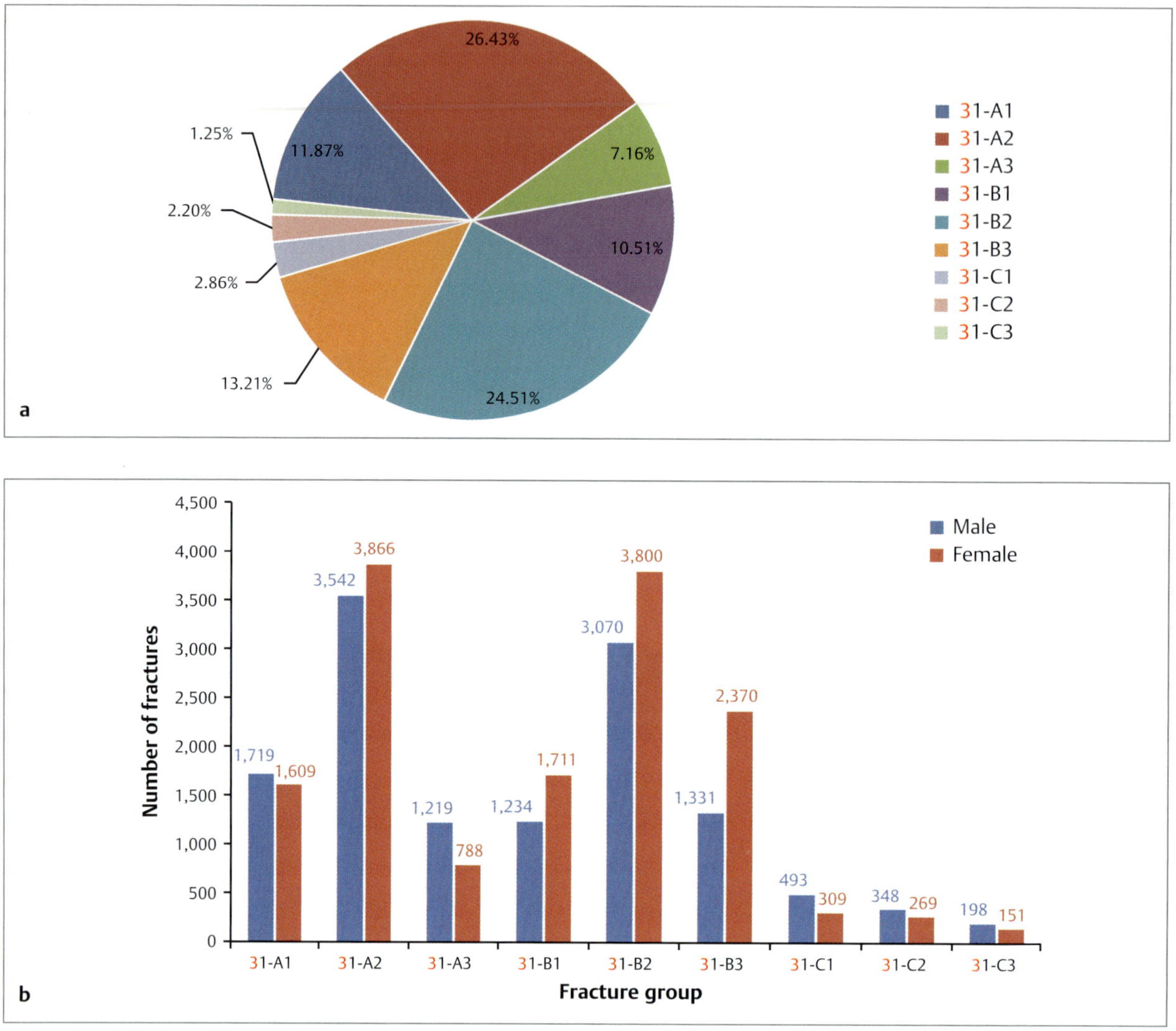

Fig. 4.9 **(a)** Fracture group distribution of 28,027 fractures of segment 31.
(b) Sex and fracture group distribution of 28,027 fractures of segment 31.

31-A Femur proximal extra-articular trochanteric fractures

31-A1
Pertrochanteric simple
3,328 fractures
M: 1,719 (51.65%)
F: 1,609 (48.35%)
0.89% of total adult fractures
8.38% of adult femur fractures
11.87% of segment 31
26.12% of type 31-A

31-A1.1

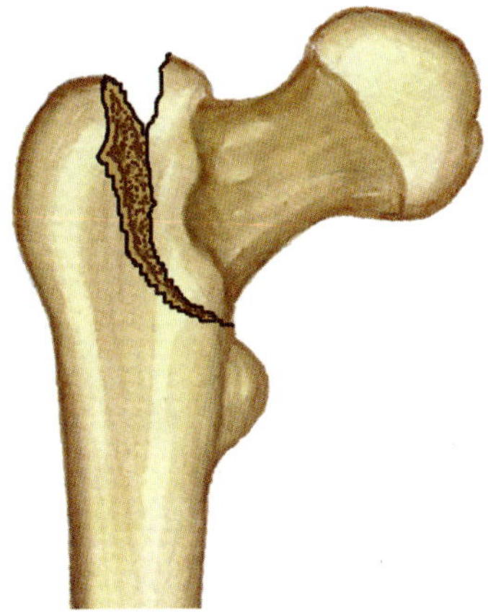

Along the intertrochanteric line

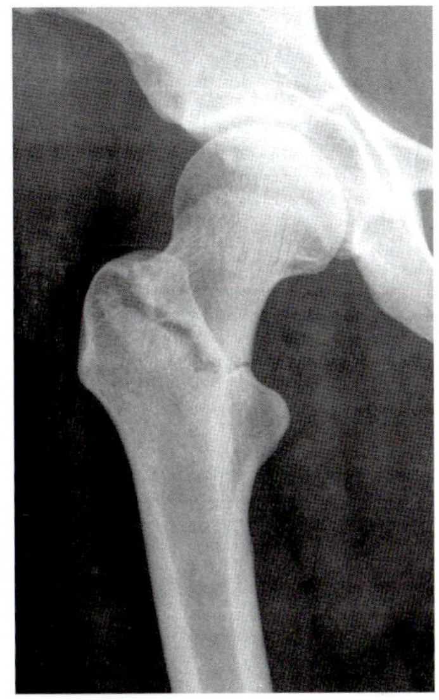

31-A1.2

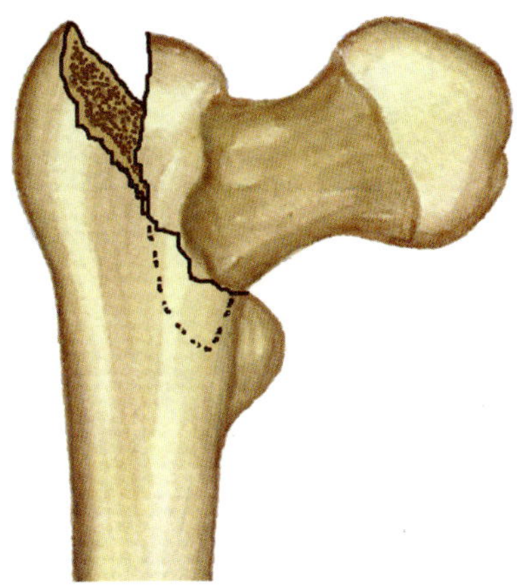

Through the greater trochanter

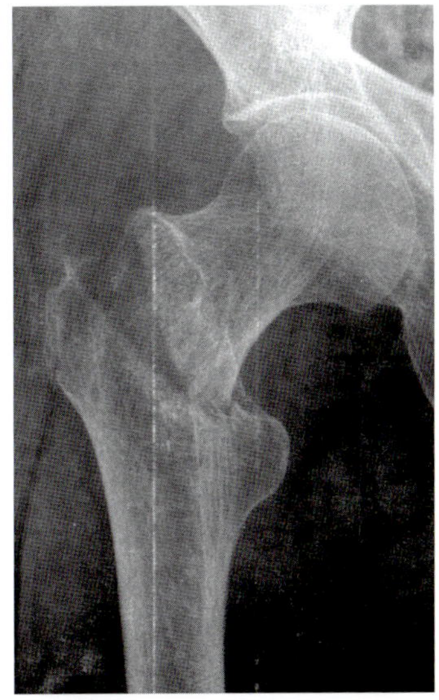

31-A1.3

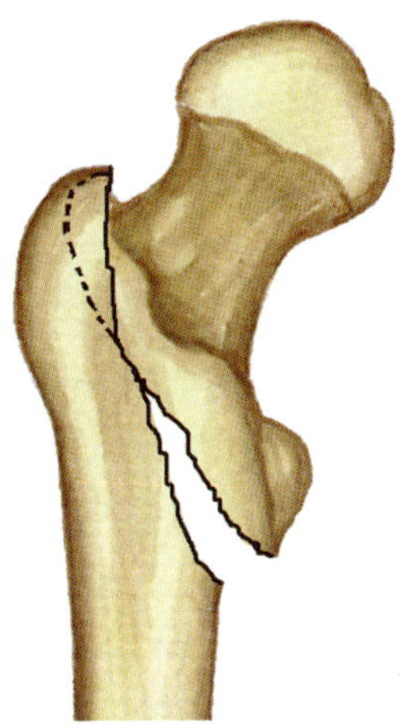

Below the lesser trochanter

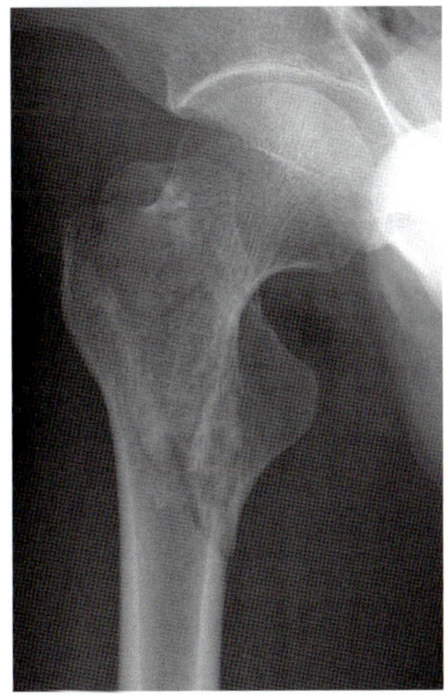

31-A Femur proximal extra-articular, trochanteric fractures

31-A2
Pertrochanteric multifragmentary
7,408 fractures
M: 3,542 (47.81%)
F: 3,866 (52.19%)
1.98% of total adult fractures
18.66% of adult femur fractures
26.43% of segment 31
58.13% of type 31-A

31-A2.1

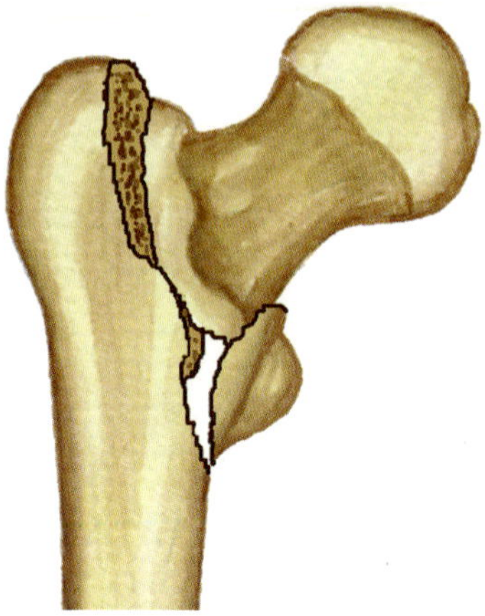

With one intermediate fragment

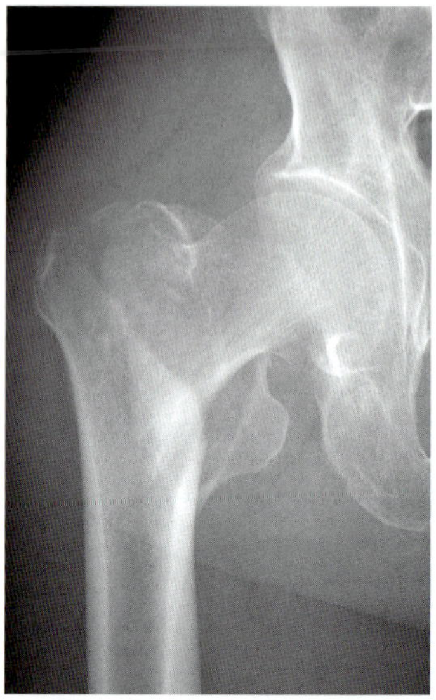

31-A2.2

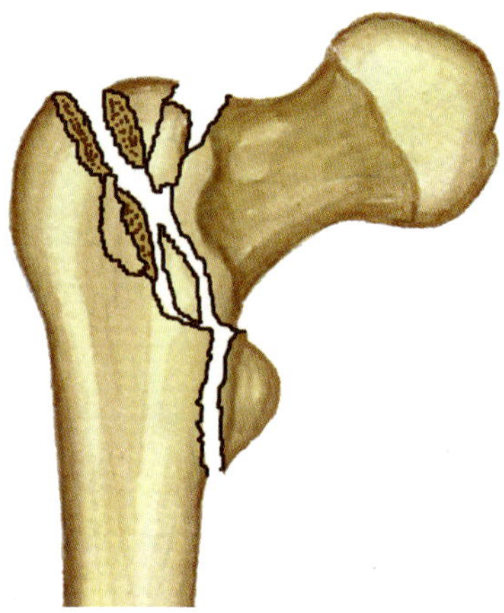

With several intermediate fragments

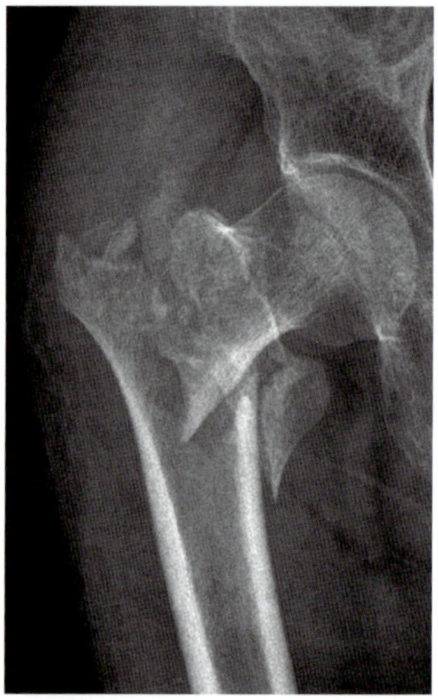

31-A2.3

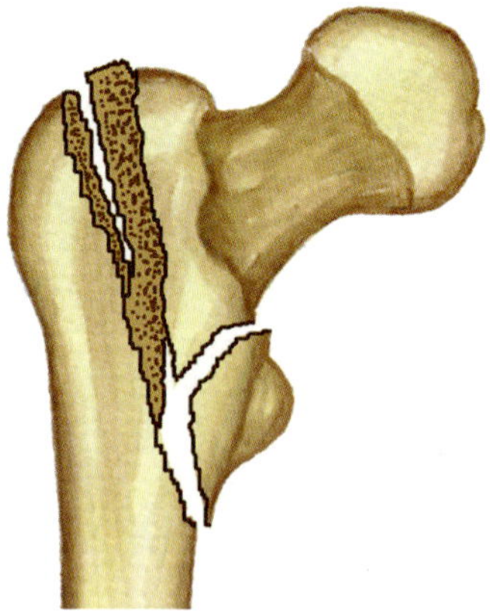

Extending more than 1 cm below the lesser trochanter

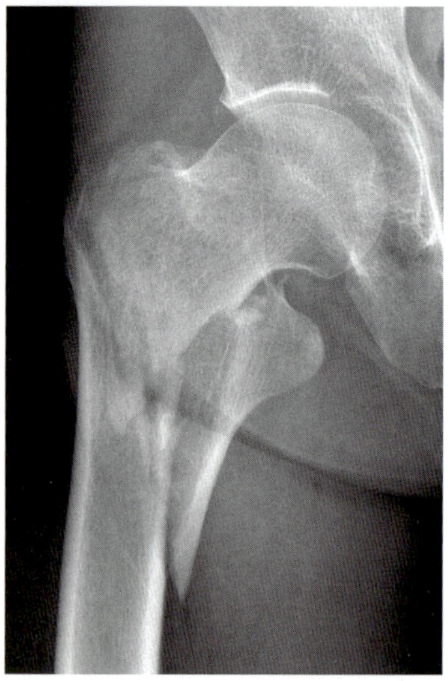

31-A Femur proximal extra-articular, trochanteric fractures

31-A3
Intertrochanteric
2,007 fractures
M: 1,219 (60.74%)
F: 788 (39.26%)
0.54% of total adult fractures
5.06% of adult femur fractures
7.16% of segment 31
15.75% of type 31-A

31-A3.1

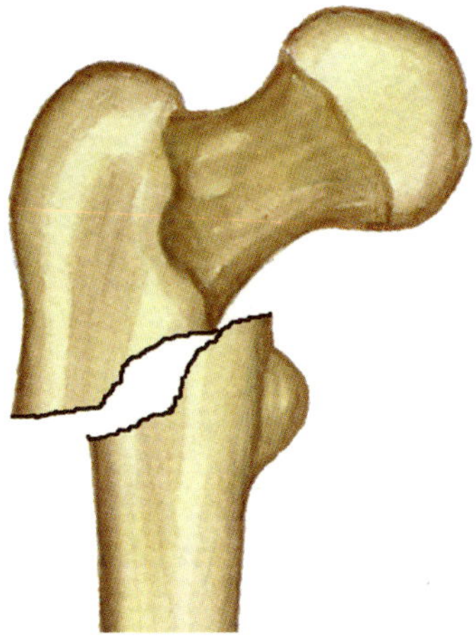

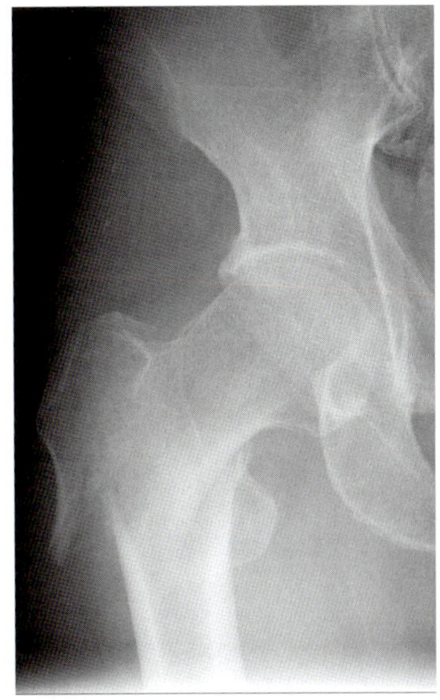

Simple oblique

31-A3.2

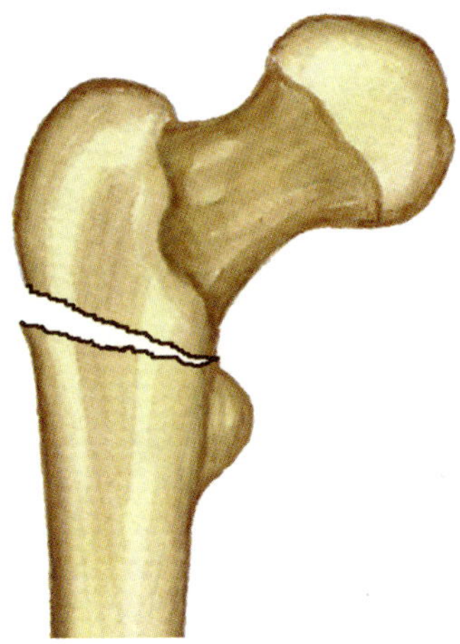

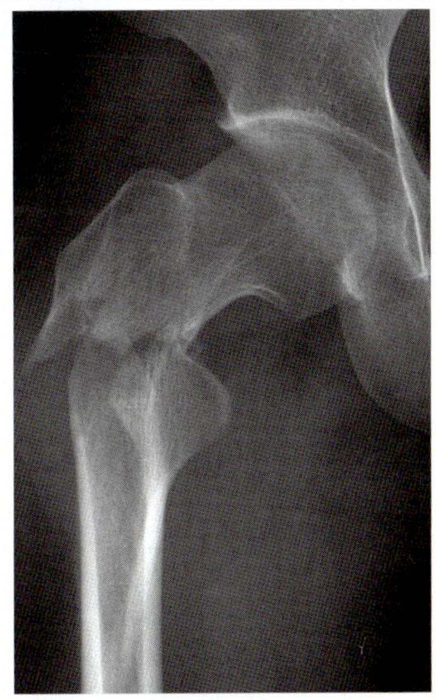

Simple transverse

31-A3.3

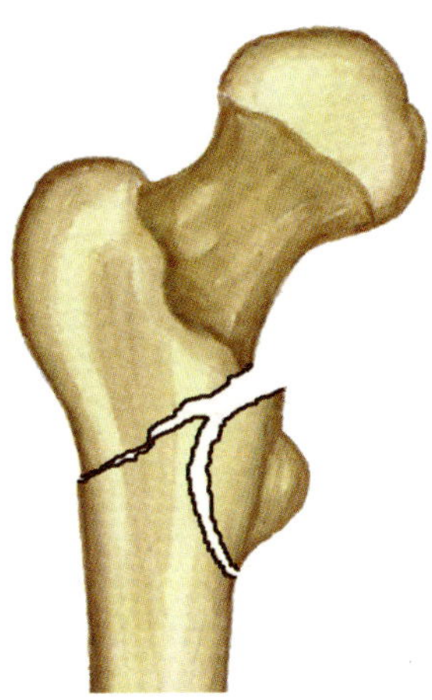

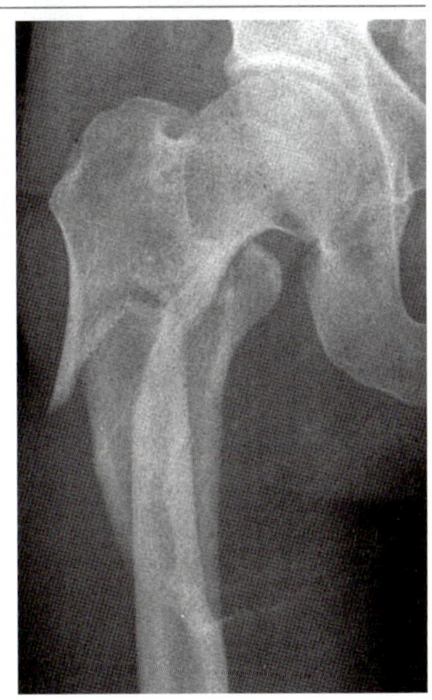

Multifragmentary, fracture line extending into the diaphysis

31-B Femur proximal intra-articular, neck fractures

31-B1
Subcapital, with slight or no displacement

2,945 fractures
M: 1,234 (41.90%)
F: 1,711 (58.10%)
0.79% of total adult fractures
7.42% of adult femur fractures
10.51% of segment 31
21.79% of type 31-B

31-B1.1

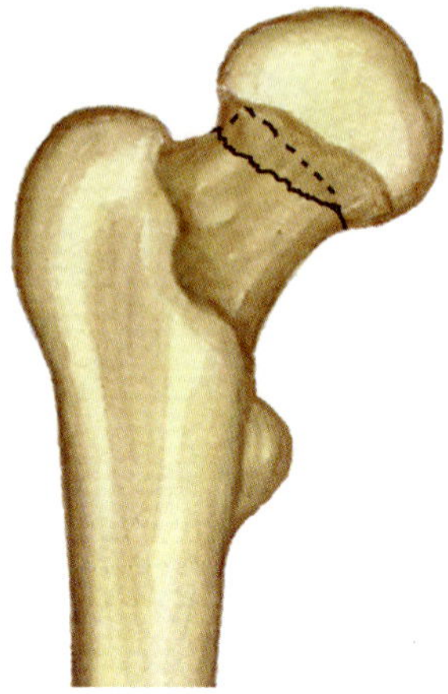

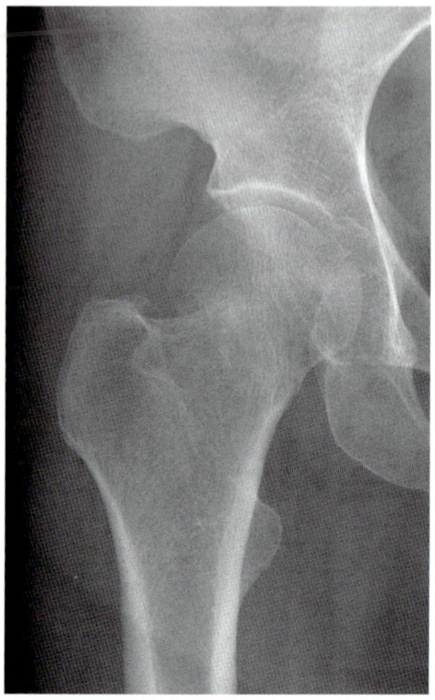

Impacted with valgus displacement ≥ 15 degrees

31-B1.2

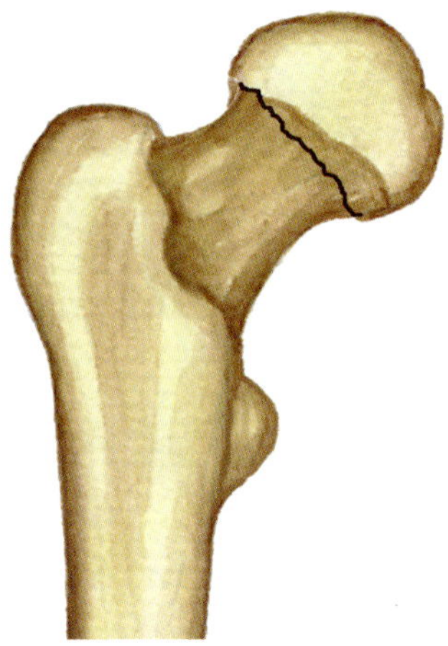

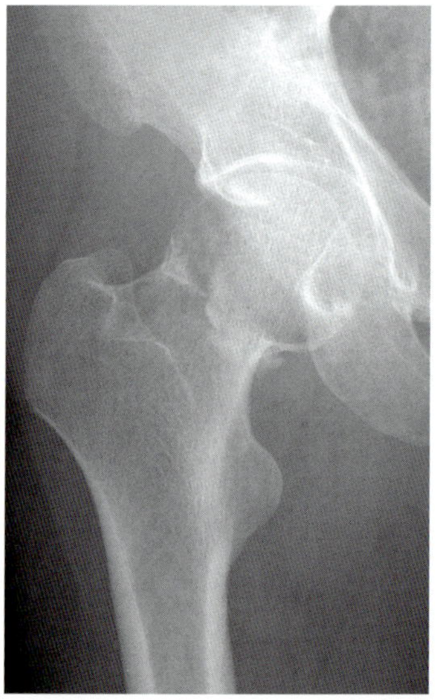

Impacted with valgus displacement ≤ 15 degrees

31-B1.3

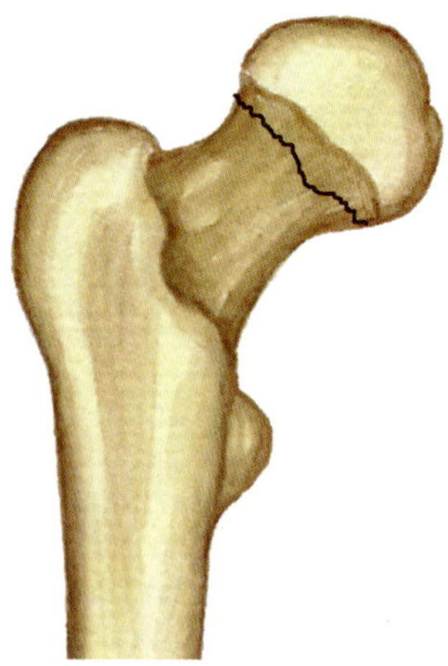

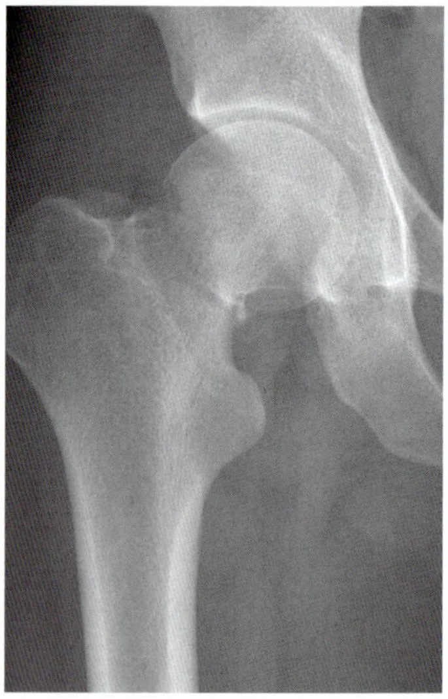

Non-impacted

31-B Femur proximal intra-articular, neck fractures

31-B2
Transcervical, with minimal displacement
6,870 fractures
M: 3,070 (44.69%)
F: 3,800 (55.31%)
1.83% of total adult fractures
17.31% of adult femur fractures
24.51% of segment 31
50.83% of type 31-B

31-B2.1

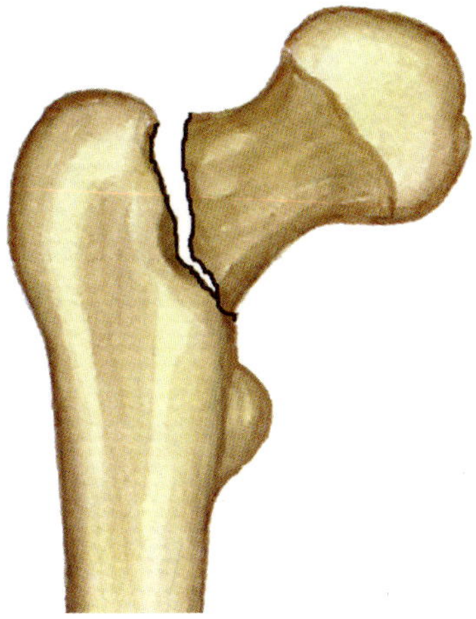

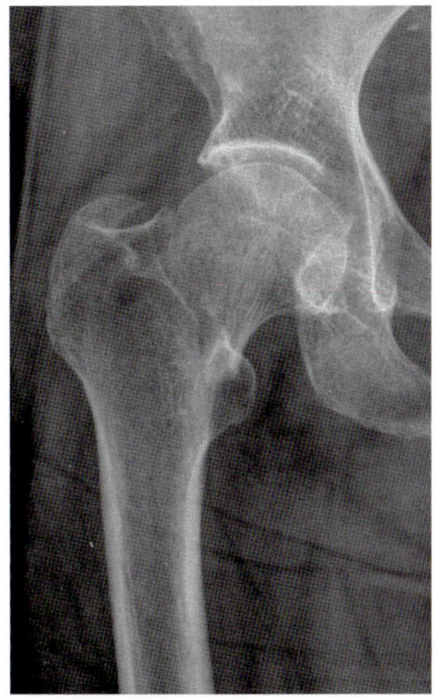

Basicervical

31-B2.2

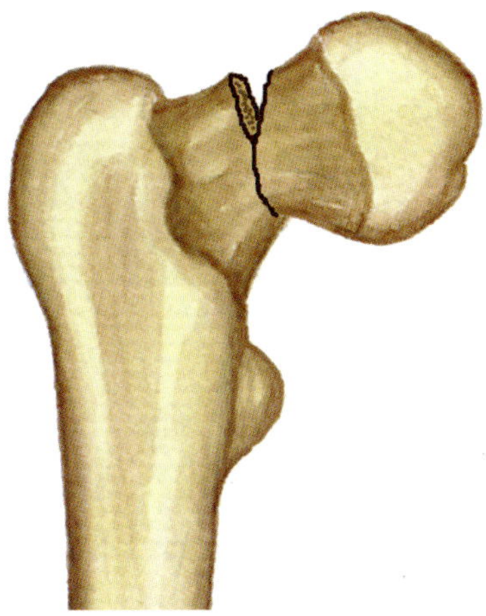

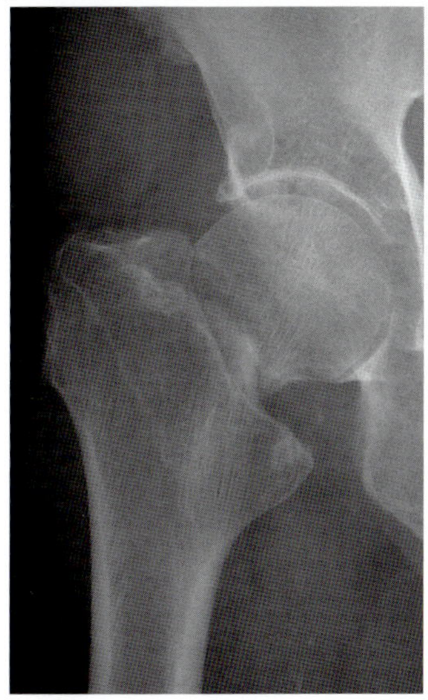

Midcervical adduction

31-B2.3

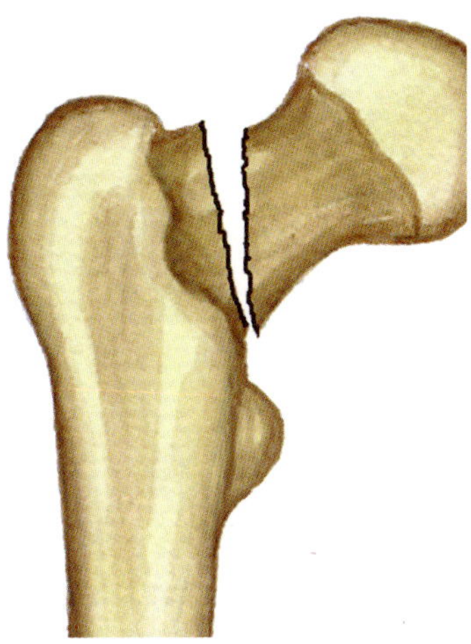

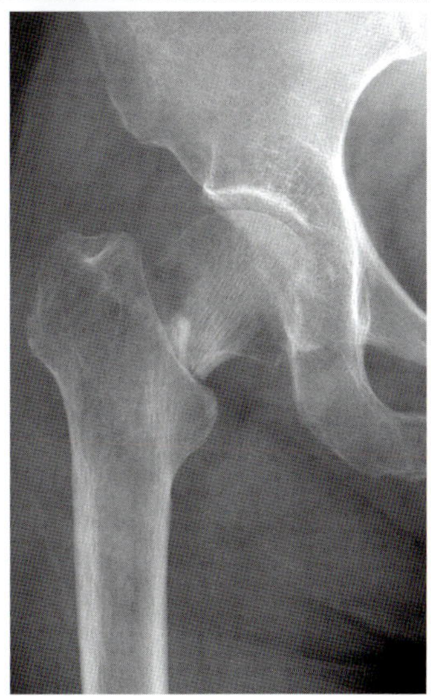

Cervical shear

31-B Femur proximal intra-articular, neck fractures

31-B3

Subcapital, displaced without impaction

3,701 fractures
M: 1,331 (35.96%)
F: 2,370 (64.04%)
0.99% of total adult fractures
9.32% of adult femur fractures
13.21% of segment 31
27.38% of type 31-B

31-B3.1

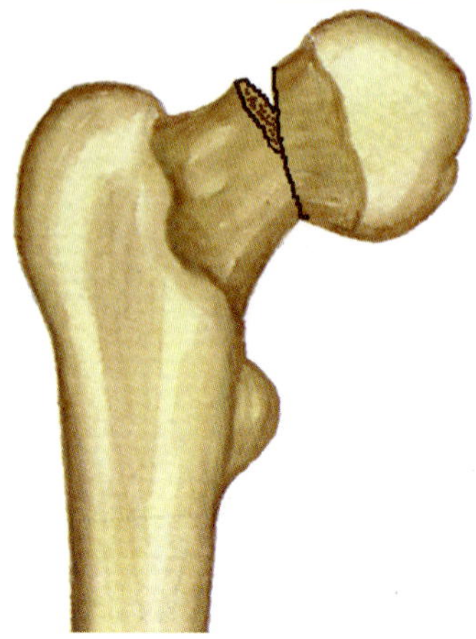

Moderate displacement in varus and external rotation

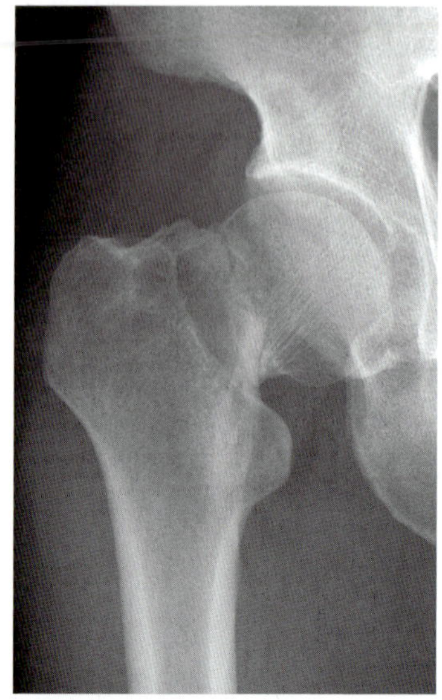

31-B3.2

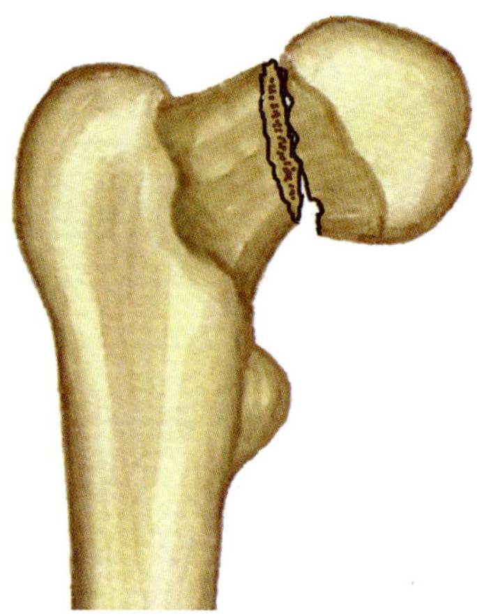

Moderate displacement in vertical translation and external rotation

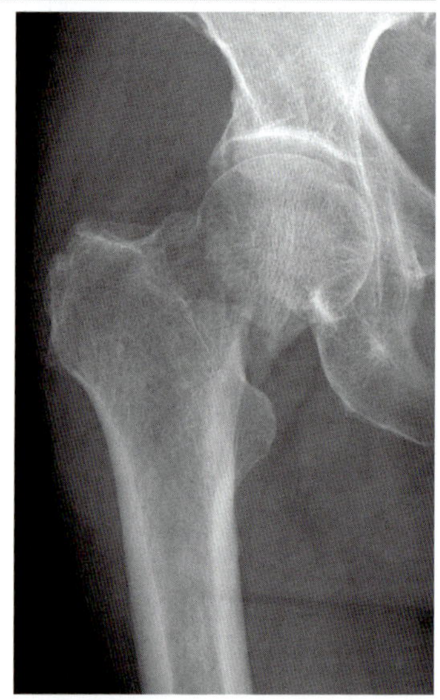

31-B3.3

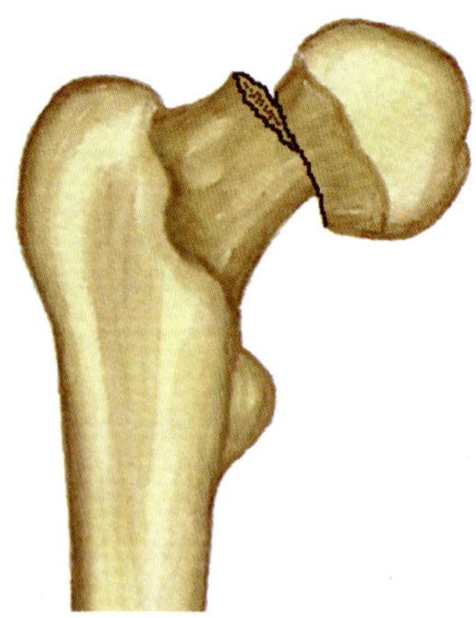

Marked displacement in varus or vertical translation

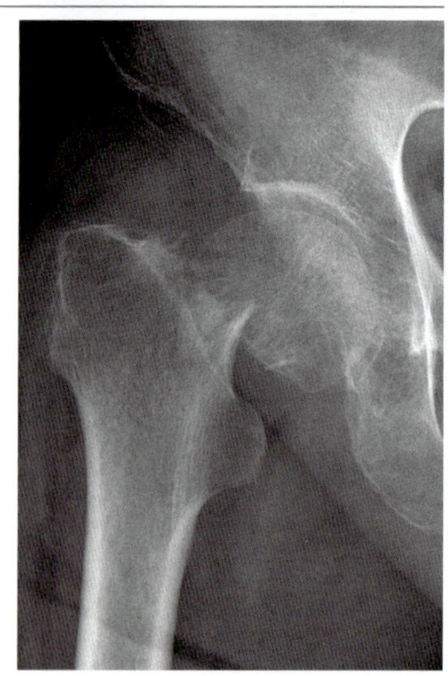

31-C Femur proximal intra-articular, head fractures

31-C1
Split
802 fractures
M: 493 (61.47%)
F: 309 (38.53%)
0.21% of total adult fractures
2.02% of adult femur fractures
2.86% of segment 31
45.36% of type 31-C

31-C1.1

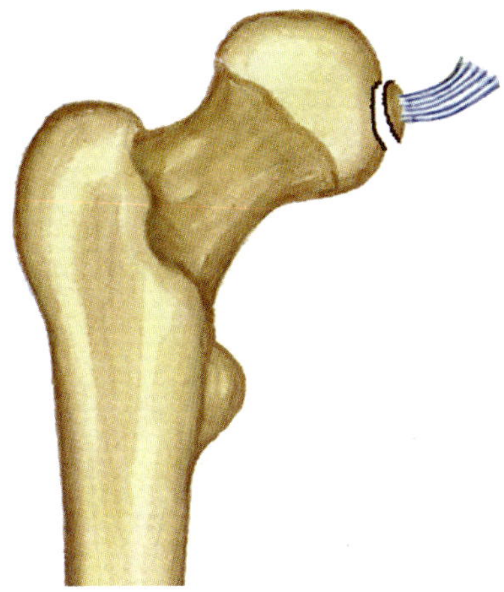

Avulsion of the round ligament

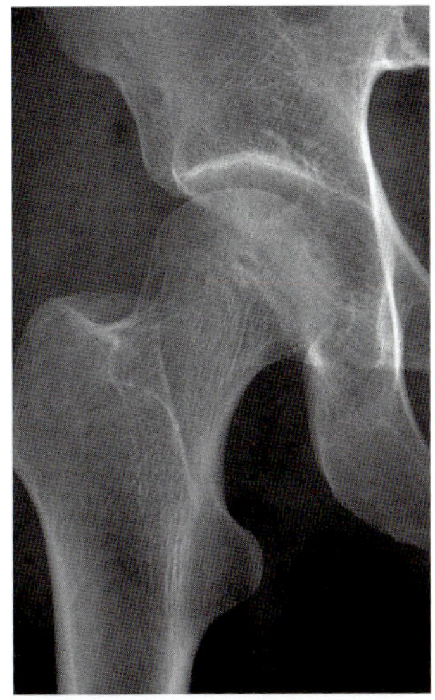

31-C1.2

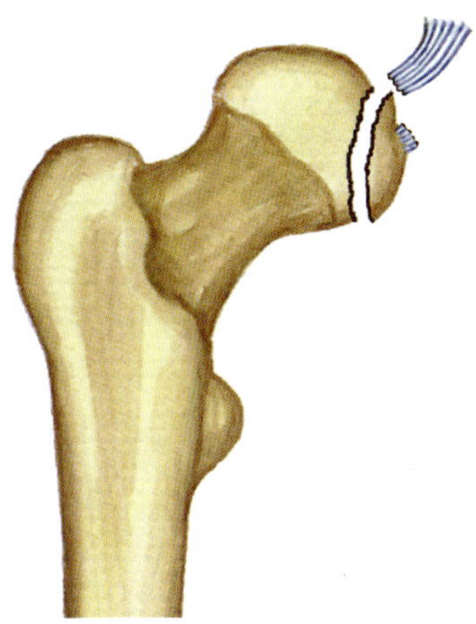

Fracture with rupture of the round ligament

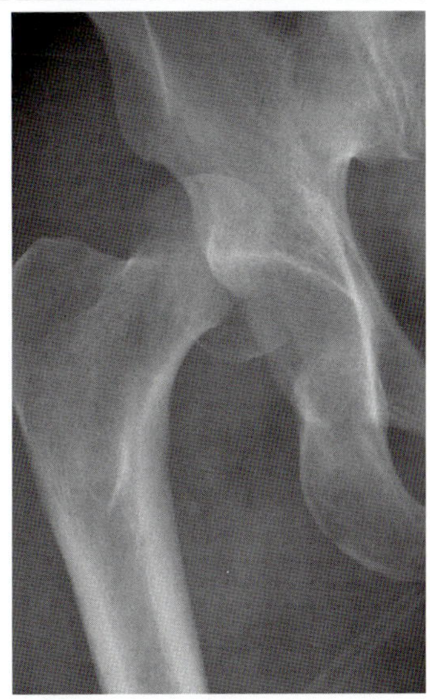

31-C1.3

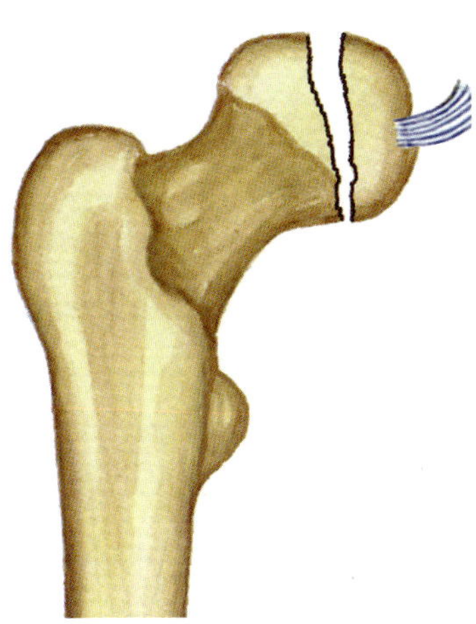

With a large fragment

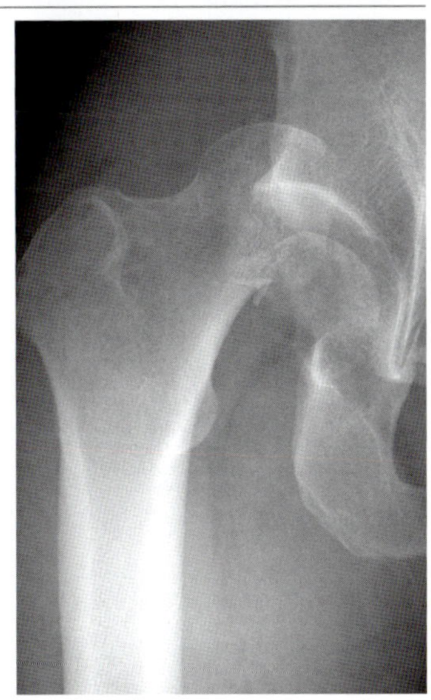

4

31-C Femur proximal intra-articular, head fractures

31-C2
Compressed
617 fractures
M: 348 (56.40%)
F: 269 (43.60%)
0.16% of total adult fractures
1.55% of adult femur fractures
2.2% of segment 31
34.9% of type 31-C

31-C2.1

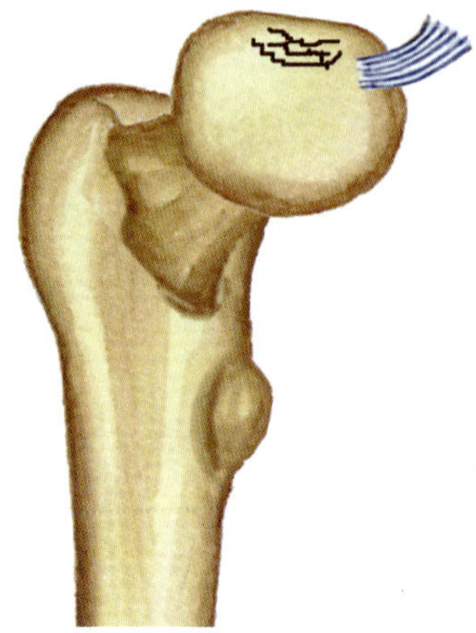

Posterior and superior

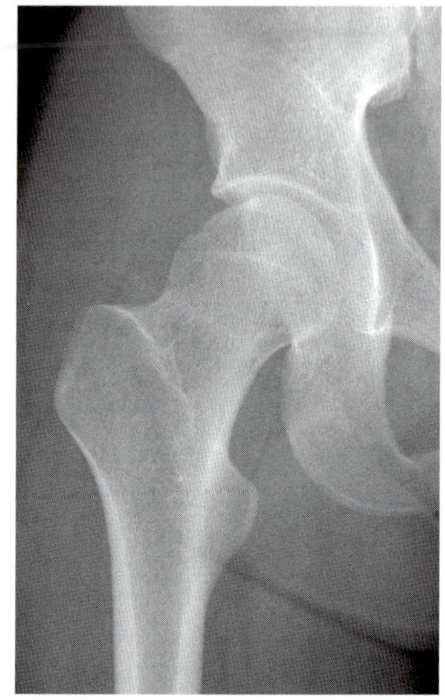

31-C2.2

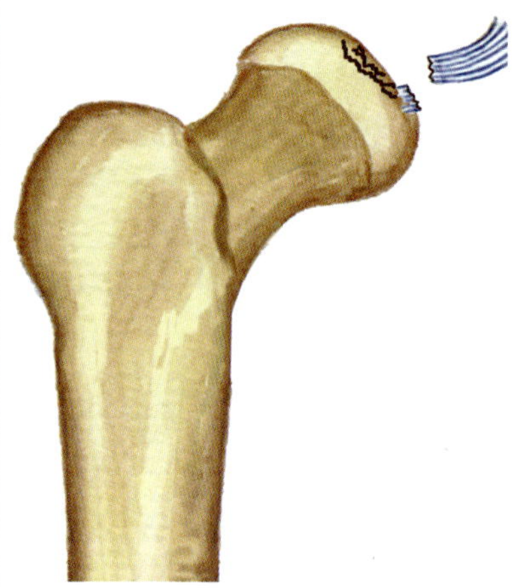

Anterior and superior

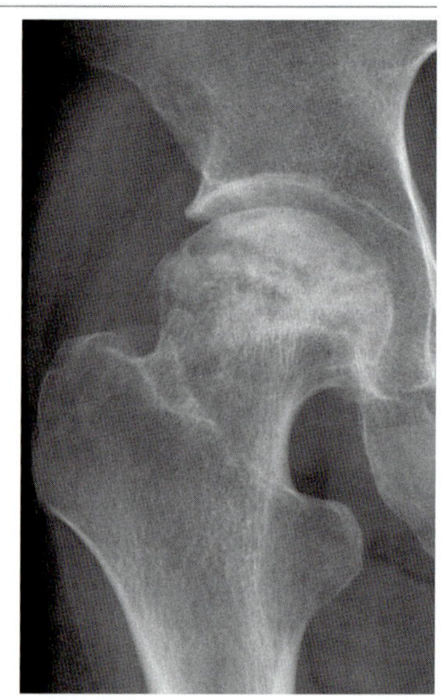

31-C2.3

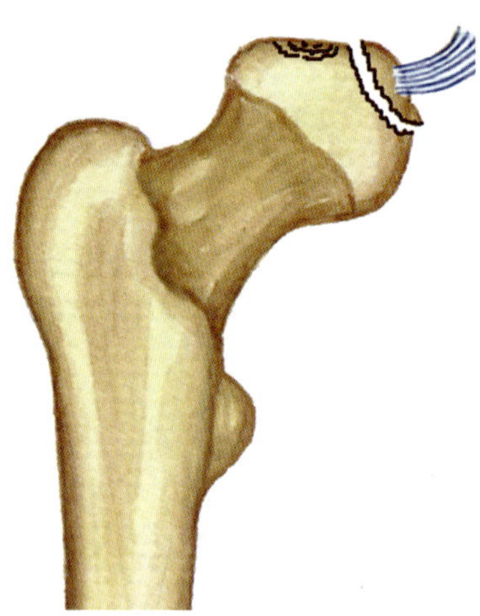

Split and compressed

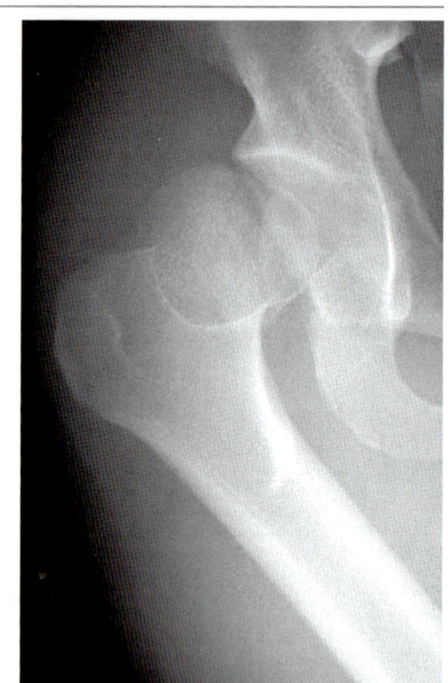

31-C Femur proximal intra-articular, head fractures

31-C3
With neck fracture
349 fractures
M: 198 (56.73%)
F: 151 (43.27%)
0.09% of total adult fractures
0.88% of adult femur fractures
1.25% of segment 31
19.74% of type 31-C

31-C3.1

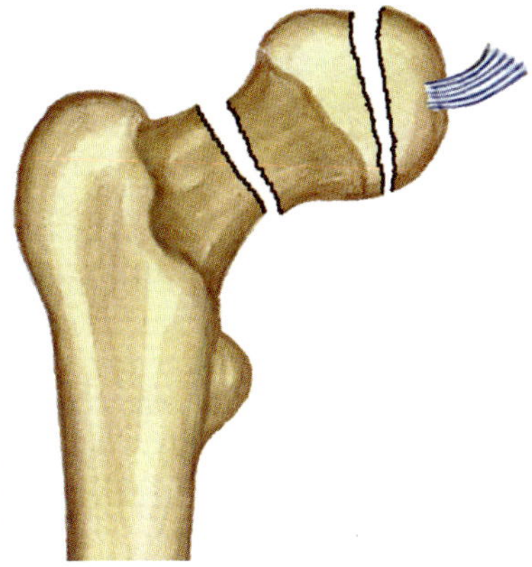

Head split and neck fractured in transcervical region

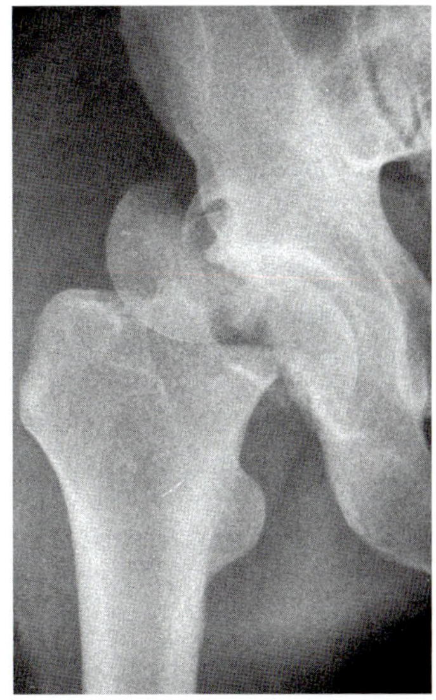

31-C3.2

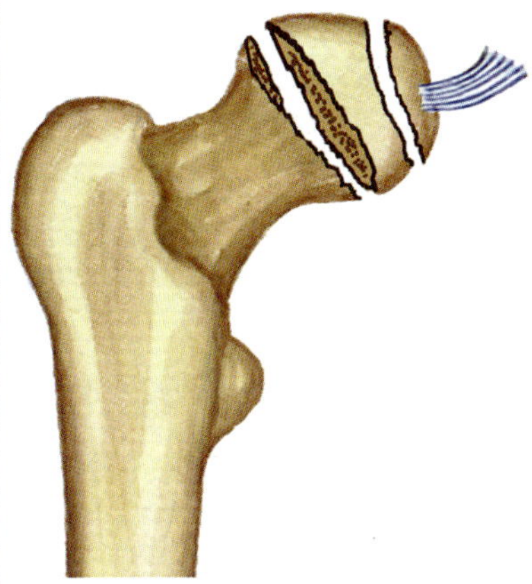

Head split and neck fractured in subcapital region

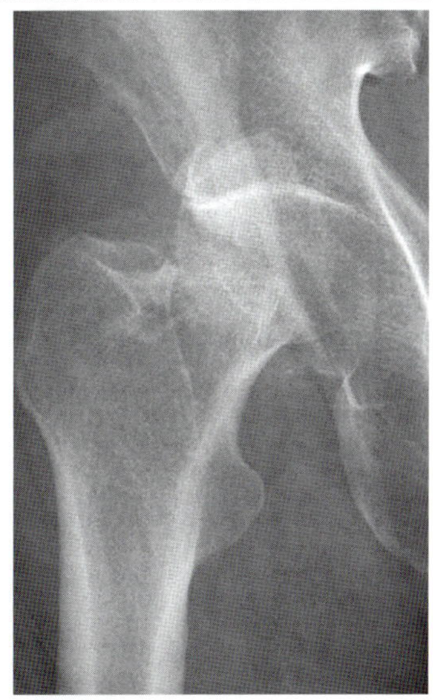

31-C3.3

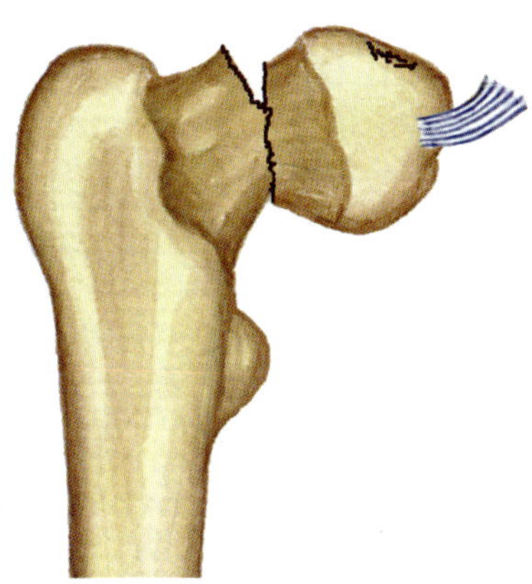

Head compressed and neck fractured

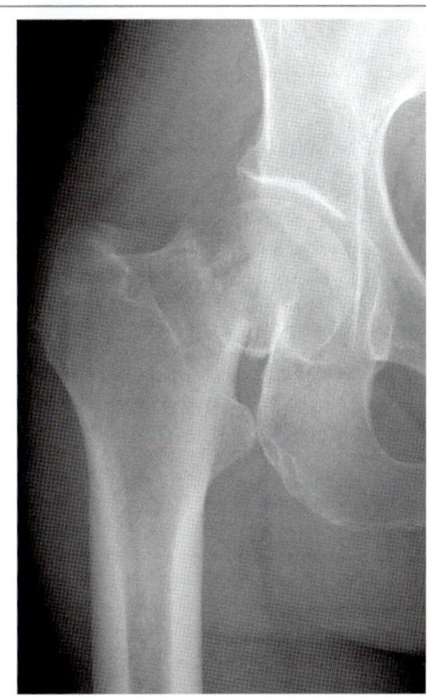

Injury Mechanism

Intertrochanteric fracture can be caused by a direct force applied perpendicularly to the trochanteric area, or an indirect varus force transmitted to the intertrochanteric area through the hip. The forceful contraction of the gluteus medius and gluteus minimus muscles, or having the lower limb in hyperadduction, may lead to an avulsion fracture of the greater trochanter, while the pull of the iliopsoas muscle may result in avulsion of the lesser trochanter. Intertrochanteric fractures often occur in the elderly, mostly caused by falls. Since elderly patients often have osteoporotic bones, the resulting fractures are frequently complex fractures.

Femoral neck fractures can be caused by two types of force. Fractures may result from violent rotation of the hip as a result of falling onto the lateral aspect of the hip. This type of injury can also be caused by an indirect force transmitted to the neck through the greater trochanter, as seen in falls onto one's side from a height or a standing position. With decreased muscle tone in the hip area and increased bone fragility resulting from osteoporosis, elderly patients can sustain femoral neck fractures from minimal forces like a fall from a bed, sudden movements, or twisting of the leg. In young people, fractures of the femoral neck occur more frequently from high-energy trauma like car accidents or falls from a significant height. Avascular necrosis of the femoral head often occurs as a result of vascular disruption after fracture of the femoral neck.

Femoral head fractures usually result from a major force to a flexed knee and hip; the resulting force transmits to the hip joint through the axis of the femur and often leads to a posterior dislocation of the hip joint. When the fracture occurs with the hip flexed, abducted, and externally rotated, an anterior dislocation of hip joint usually follows.

4

Diagnosis

Intertrochanteric Fracture

If there is minimal or no displacement, patients may present with pain on palpation and percussive pain along the axis of the femur. If there is marked displacement, a typical presentation may include pain, deformity, abnormal range of movement, bony crepitus, and shortening of the involved limb. Imaging examinations must include standard anteroposterior (AP) and lateral views of the fracture site. A comparison AP view of the pelvis with the uninjured side is helpful in detecting fracture displacement, if the displacement is minimal. Computed tomography (CT) scanning might be indicated. For subtrochanteric fractures, radiographs should be taken to include the whole length of the diaphysis, to rule out diaphyseal fractures of the femur.

Femoral Neck Fractures

Femoral neck fractures are intracapsular; therefore, patients may not present with much swelling. Physical examination reveals local pain to palpation and percussive pain along the axis of the femur. A standard hip radiographic series, including AP and lateral views of the affected hip, or a comparison AP view of the pelvis with the unaffected side, should be considered if neck fracture is suspected. Measurement of the Pauwel angle will be helpful in assessing the degree of fracture stability. If indicated, a CT scan of the hip joint should be carried out, which should include views of the acetabulum, the neck of the femur, the head of the femur, and the greater and lesser trochanter. A thin-slice CT scan or two-dimensional or three-dimensional CT reconstruction may also be required. CT is exquisitely useful for imaging abnormalities of the bone itself, such as in the disruption of the cortical bone and trabecula, and especially in detecting incomplete fractures without trabecula displacement. CT is the most useful test for evaluating bony injury, assessing the type of fracture and the degree of the displacement, and detecting the number and the location of the fragments.

The Garden classification is the most commonly used standard to assess the severity of femoral neck fracture in clinical cases. Garden type I femoral neck fractures are defined as incomplete fractures of the neck of the femur as seen on the AP radiograph of the injured hip. Zhang et al confirmed that incomplete femoral neck fractures identified on X-ray films are actually complete fractures on CT through a prospective study.

Femoral Head Fractures

The clinical presentation of femoral head fractures is atypical if the fractures are not displaced. Patients with femoral neck fractures usually present with different levels of pain to palpation over the hip joint, and percussive pain along the axis of the femur. If the fractures are displaced, physical examination reveals bony crepitus, or a limited range of movement of the hip joint. Imaging examinations should include AP and lateral views of the hip joint and an AP view of the pelvis. A CT scan should be considered if X-ray films are equivocal. CT scans are not only useful in diagnosing but can also provide guidance in treatment. Plain radiographic findings on pediatric slipped capital femoral epiphysis and traumatic femoral head epiphysiolysis include a widening of the epiphyseal line, widening and irregularity of the growth plate, separation and displacement of the epiphyseal line from the metaphyses, and inferomedial displacement of the epiphysis. CT and magnetic resonance imaging (MRI) should be considered under such circumstances. Femoral head fractures in adults are more commonly fractures of the apex of the femoral head, and the resulting fragments often lie within the capsule. Radiographic images reveal the femoral head defect or irregularity. If there is fracture displacement, the fracture of the superior rim of the acetabulum usually accompanies the fracture. If the X-ray film cannot point to a clear diagnosis of a femoral head fracture when the head of the femur is intact, MRI is required to further assess the nature of the fracture, or the location and the course of the fracture line. When fractures involve subchondral bones, MRI can clearly reveal the extent of the fracture.

Treatment

Intertrochanteric Fractures

Intramedullary nails, like the Gamma nail and proximal femoral nail (PFN), are usually used for internal fixation of proximal femur fractures. Intramedullary nails have the biomechanical properties of internal fixators, and offer the advantage of small incisions and short operation times. Gamma nail fixation requires the affected limb to be slightly adducted, and traction for anatomical reduction. Radiographic measurement of femoral canal diameters and the shape of the femur diaphysis must be done before the surgery. PFNs should not be used in patients with marked anterior bowing of the femur. Other internal fixators often used for fixation of proximal femoral fractures include dynamic hip screw/dynamic condylar screw (DHS/DCS), and DHS trochanter stabilizing plates, which provide double fixation by performing compression and a sliding motion leading to dynamic compression at the fracture site.

Femoral Neck Fractures

Subcapital fractures of the femoral neck have a high incidence of avascular necrosis of the femoral head. In young patients with good preservation of bone stock, one should consider artificial femoral head replacement or biological fixation of a total hip prosthesis. For elderly patients with osteoporotic bones, a self-centering bipolar head or total hip replacement is recommended. Transcervical femoral neck fractures can be fixed by screws, usually by three cancellous screws, which offer the advantages of providing significant compression to the fracture site, avoiding rotation, and causing minimal bone damage. The Anchor nail, developed by a group of talented orthopaedic surgeons at our hospital, combines the beauty of the Trifin nail and compression screw, which has the advantages of providing compression and antirotation at the fracture site with a simple procedure. A good clinical outcome has been observed after its application in treating femoral neck fractures in our hospital. Basicervical fractures can be treated surgically or conservatively, depending on the patient's medical condition. If complex basicervical fractures occur in patients with osteoporotic bones or with multifragmentary fractures of the cortical bone, management should involve DHS and angle plates. A screw can be added to the DHS proximally to restore the rotational stability of the bone and provide support and fixation.

Some femoral neck fractures make it difficult to achieve anatomical reduction with routine manipulative maneuvers, and they require open surgical intervention. This kind of irreducible femoral neck fracture is frequently complicated by avascular necrosis of the femoral head and nonunion of the fracture. Three-dimensional inter-reaction reduction was invented by Zhang et al to deal with those problems. Zhang et al designed a quantitative score system used in treatment of adult femoral neck fractures with high factors for nonunion (age > 50 years, females, displacement fracture, high energy injury, and American Society of Anesthesia [ASA] grade above III), which includes patient's age, fracture type, bone mineral density, activities of daily living, and medical comorbidities. This quantitative score system helps surgical decision making regarding the treatment choice for adult patients with femoral neck fractures. In order to prevent nonunion and femoral head necrosis of femoral neck fracture, adult fresh femoral neck fractures with high factors for nonunion require early intervention, which consists of free iliac bone graft transplanting with bilateral cortical bone and internal fixation.

Femoral Head Fractures

If the fracture occurs in a non-weight-bearing part of the femur, with small free-floating fragments sitting within the joint capsule, then the floating fragments should be taken out to avoid further damage to the joint. If the fracture occurs in a weight-bearing section of the femur, small lag screws or absorbable screws can be inserted from the non-weight-bearing section to fix the fracture, with the head of the nail just beneath subchondral bone. As more than two-thirds of femoral head fractures involve a split head with an associated neck fracture or acetabular fracture, a total hip replacement is usually the treatment of choice.

Diaphyseal Femoral Fractures (Segment 32)

Anatomical Features

Femoral shaft fractures occur in the region extending from the lesser trochanter to the flare of femoral condyles (**Plate 4.6**).

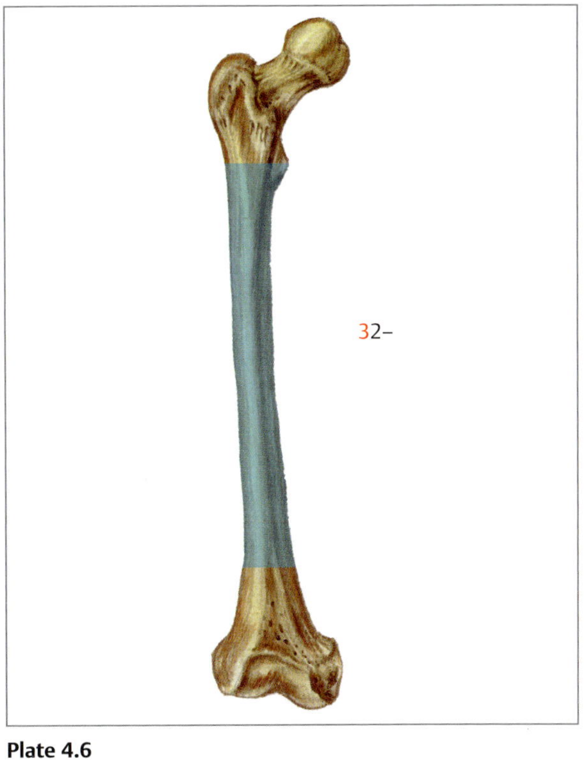

Plate 4.6

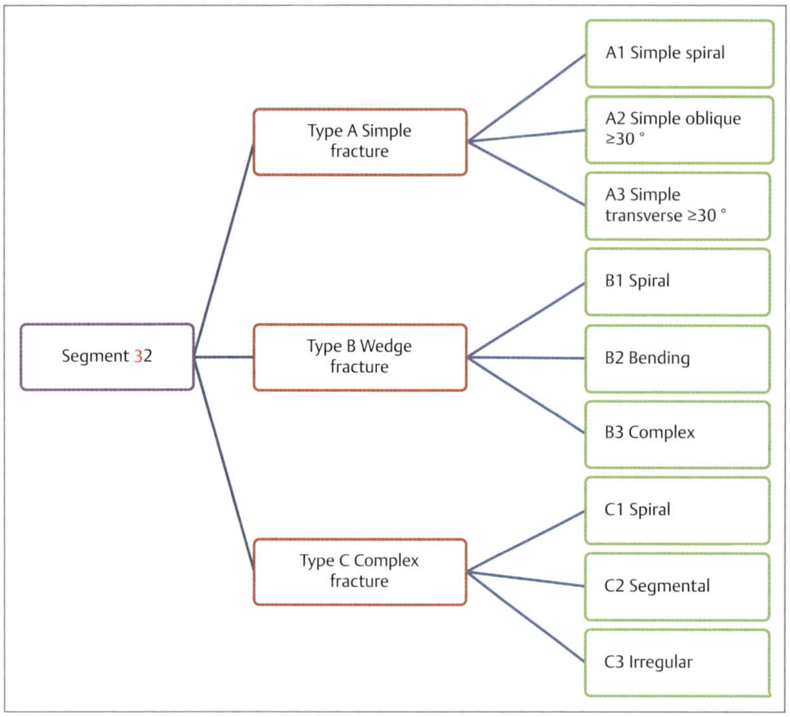

Plate 4.7

The body of the femur, almost cylindrical in form, is a little broader superiorly than in the center, and somewhat flattened and widened anteroposteriorly, especially at the lower end. It is slightly curved with a smooth convexity anteriorly, and strengthened posteriorly by a prominent longitudinal ridge, the linea aspera, which continues into the gluteal tuberosity superolaterally. The diameter of the femoral shaft and the thickness of the cortical layer of the shaft are associated with the weight bearing and the tension applied to the femur. As a result, the cortical layer of the shaft attenuates toward the proximal and distal ends of the femur.

AO Classification of Diaphyseal Femoral Fractures

Based on the AO classification, the diaphysis of the femur is coded as the number 32. It is further divided into three types depending on fracture patterns: 32-A, simple fracture; 32-B, wedge fracture; and 32-C, complex fracture (**Plate 4.7**).

Clinical Epidemiologic Features of Diaphyseal Femoral Fractures (Segment 32)

A total of 8,235 diaphyseal femoral fractures were treated in 83 hospitals in China over a 2-year period from 2010 to 2011. All cases were reviewed and statistically studied, accounting for 20.75% of femoral fractures in adults. Their epidemiologic features are as follows:

- More males than females
- The highest risk age group for both sexes is 21–25 years
- The most common fracture type among segment 32 fractures is type 32-A; the same fracture type in males and females.
- The most common fracture group among segment 32 fractures is group 32-A3; however, 32-A3 is most common in males while 32-A1 and 32-A3 are most common in females.

Fractures of Segment 32 by Sex

Table 4.10 Sex distribution of 8,235 fractures of segment 32

Sex	Number of fractures	Percentage (%)
Male	6,275	76.20
Female	1,960	23.80
Total	8,235	100.00

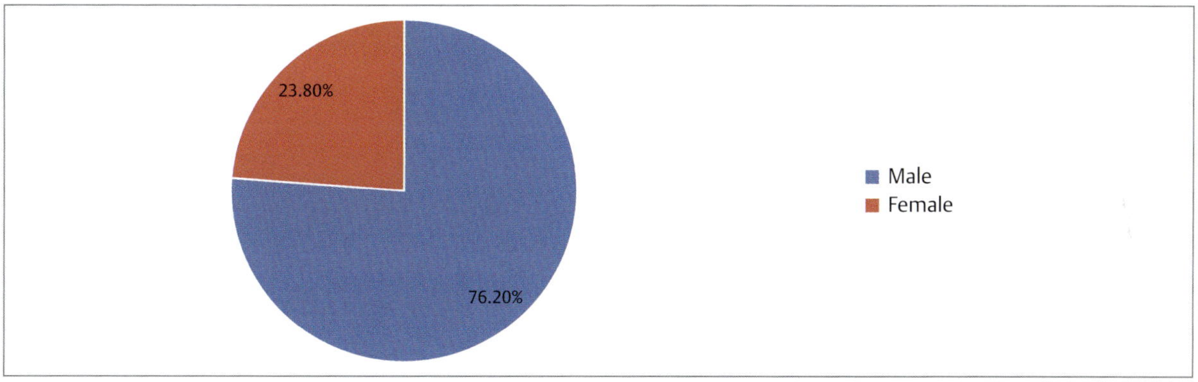

Fig. 4.10 Sex distribution of 8,235 fractures of segment 32.

Fractures of Segment 32 by Age Group

Table 4.11 Age and sex distribution of 8,235 fractures of segment 32

Age group (years)	Male	Female	Number of fractures	Percentage (%)
16–20	635	122	757	9.19
21–25	892	193	1,085	13.18
26–30	758	138	896	10.88
31–35	640	145	785	9.53
36–40	689	157	846	10.27
41–45	778	157	935	11.35
46–50	546	154	700	8.50
51–55	413	131	544	6.61
56–60	361	187	548	6.65
61–65	200	95	295	3.58
66–70	115	101	216	2.62
71–75	89	121	210	2.55
76–80	79	119	198	2.40
81–85	47	89	136	1.65
≥86	33	51	84	1.02
Total	6,275	1,960	8,235	100.00

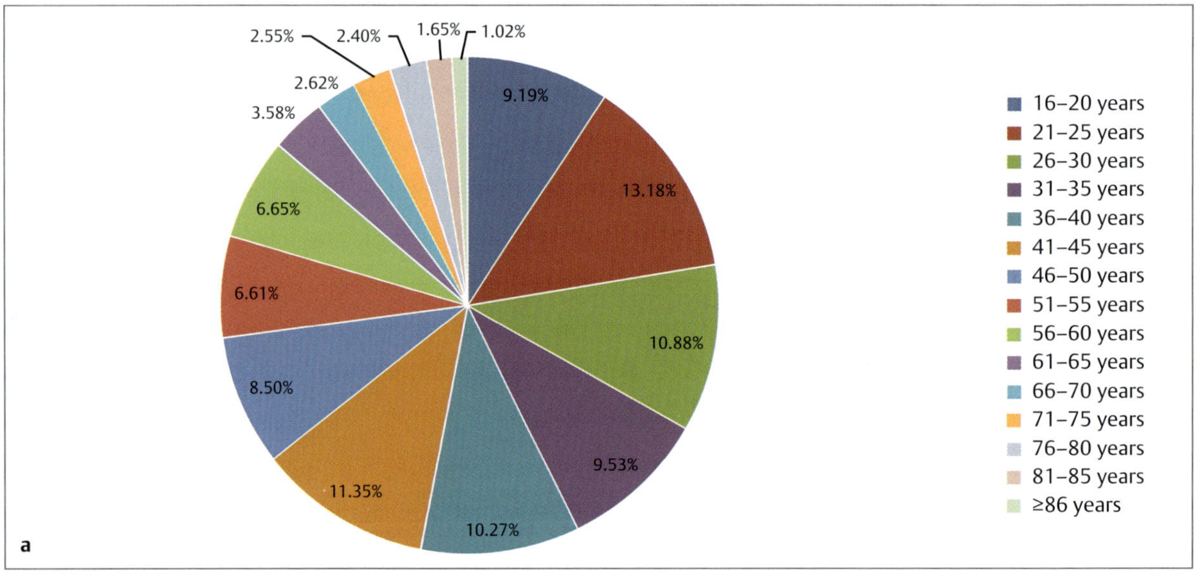

Fig. 4.11 **(a)** Age distribution of 8,235 fractures of segment 32.

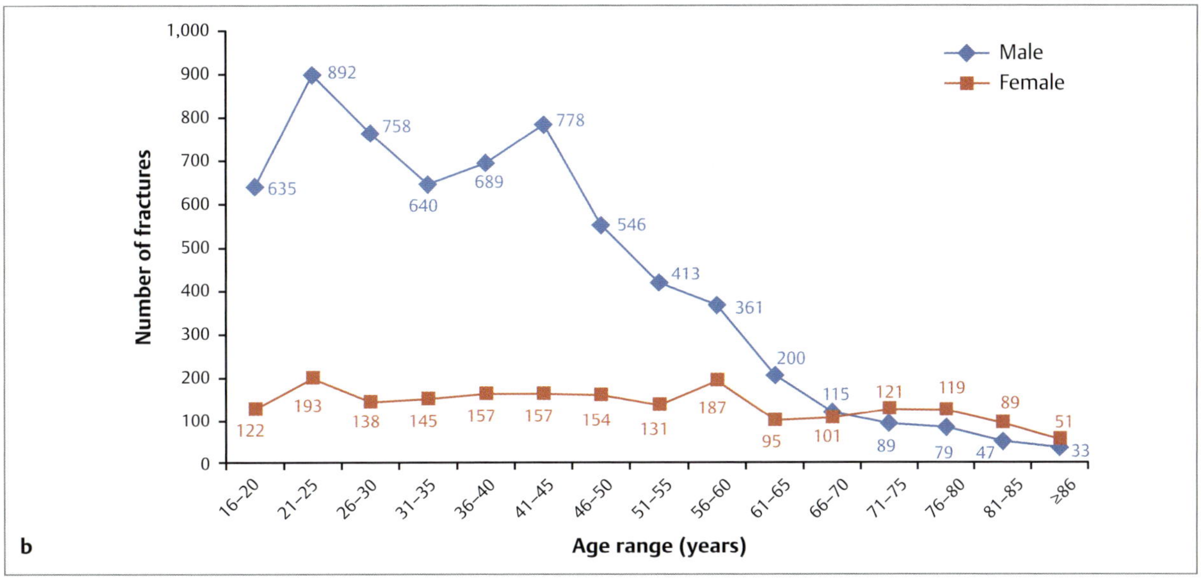

Fig. 4.11 (*continued*) **(b)** Age and sex distribution of 8,235 fractures of segment 32.

Fractures of Segment 32 by Fracture Type

Table 4.12 Sex and fracture type distribution of 8,235 fractures of segment 32

Fracture type	Male	Female	Number of fractures	Percentage (%)
32-A	3,027	1,093	4,120	50.03
32-B	2,303	611	2,914	35.39
32-C	945	256	1,201	14.58
Total	6,275	1,960	8,235	100.00

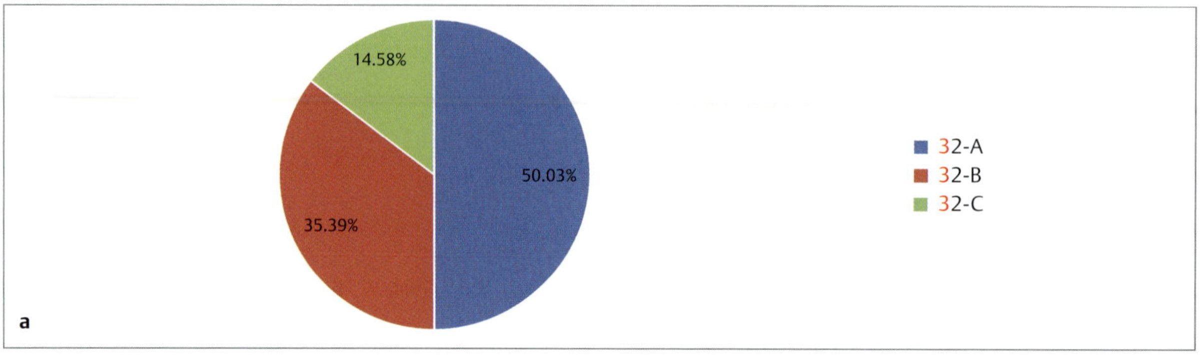

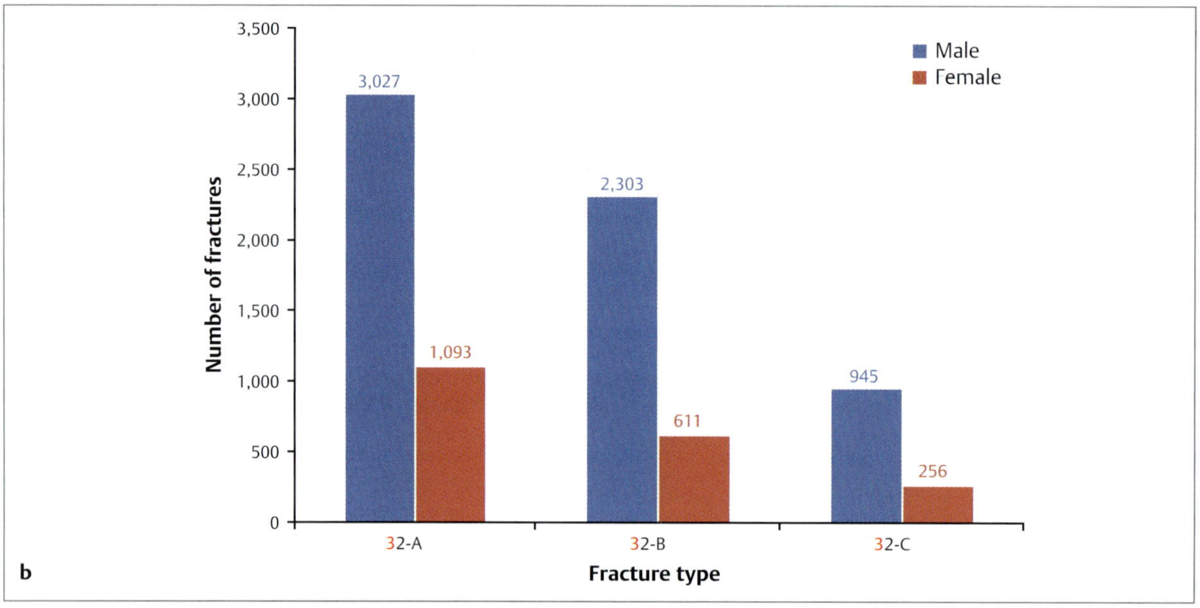

Fig. 4.12 **(a)** Fracture type distribution of 8,235 fractures of segment 32.
(b) Sex and fracture type distribution of 8,235 fractures of segment 32.

Fractures of Segment 32 by Fracture Group

Table 4.13 Sex and fracture group distribution of 8,235 fractures of segment 32

Fracture group	Male	Female	Number of fractures	Percentage of segment 32 fractures (%)	Percentage of femur fractures (%)
32-A1	704	388	1,092	13.26	2.75
32-A2	896	317	1,213	14.73	3.06
32-A3	1,427	388	1,815	22.04	4.57
32-B1	596	219	815	9.90	2.05
32-B2	1,098	280	1,378	16.73	3.47
32-B3	609	112	721	8.76	1.82
32-C1	260	74	334	4.06	0.84
32-C2	221	70	291	3.53	0.73
32-C3	464	112	576	6.99	1.45
Total	6,275	1,960	8,235	100.00	20.75

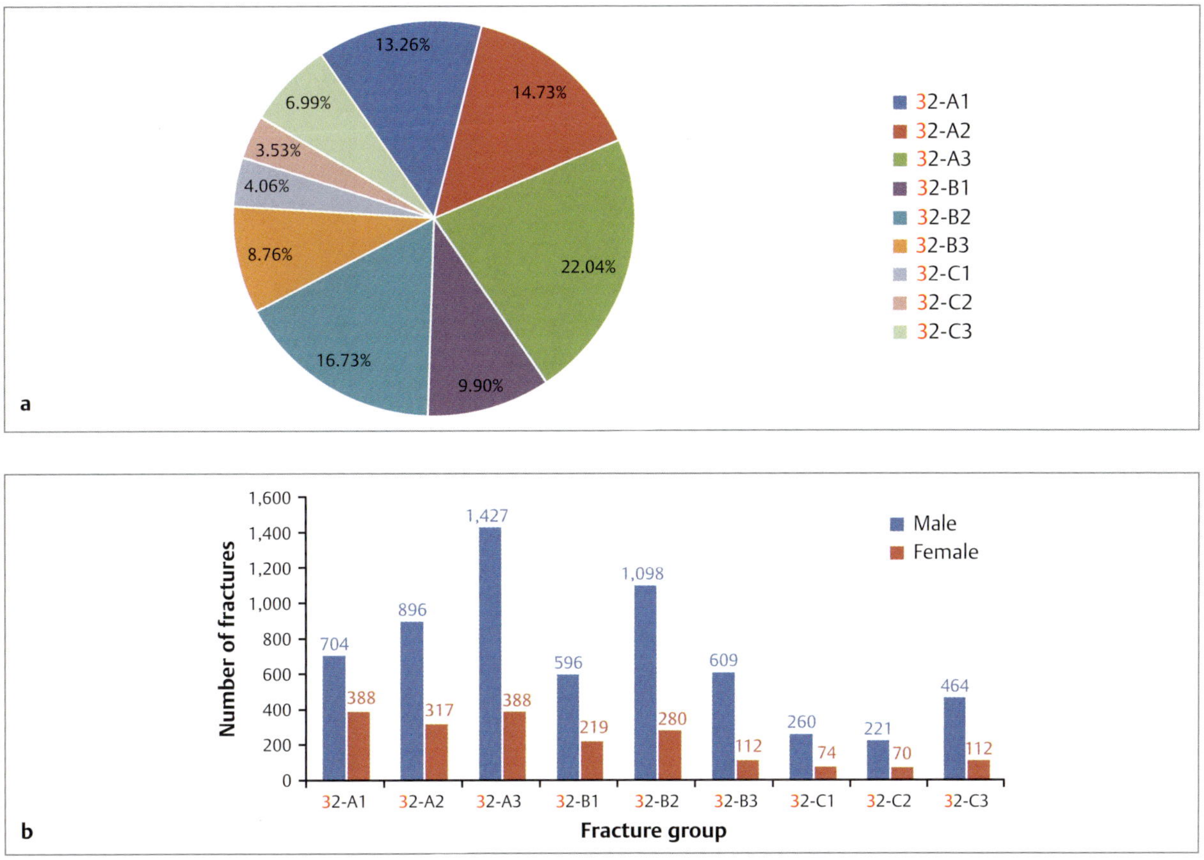

Fig. 4.13 **(a)** Fracture group distribution of 8,235 fractures of segment 32.
(b) Sex and fracture group distribution of 8,235 fractures of segment 32.

32-A Femur diaphysis, simple fractures

32-A1
Spiral
1,092 fractures
M: 704 (64.47%)
F: 388 (35.53%)
0.29% of total adult fractures
2.75% of adult femoral fractures
13.26% of segment 32
26.50% of type 32-A

32-A1.1

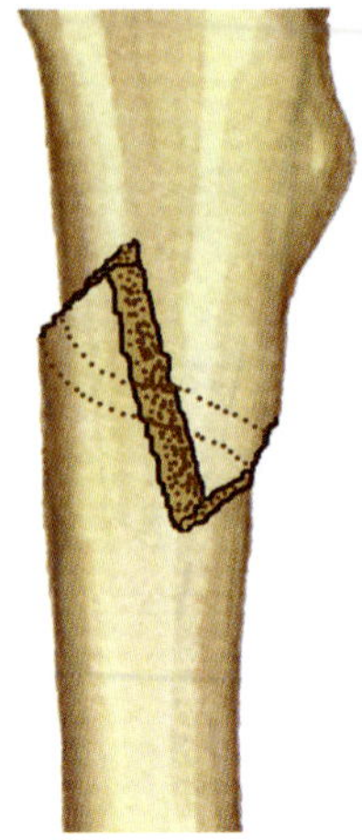

Subtrochanteric section

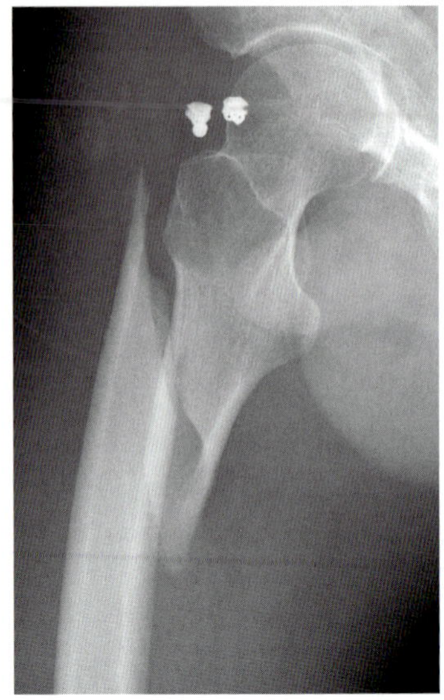

32-A1.2

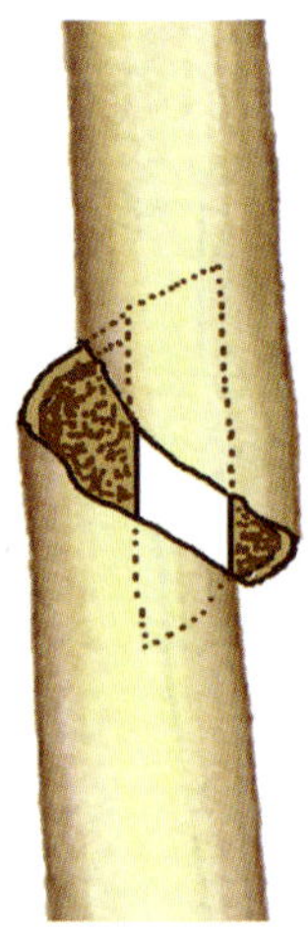

Middle section

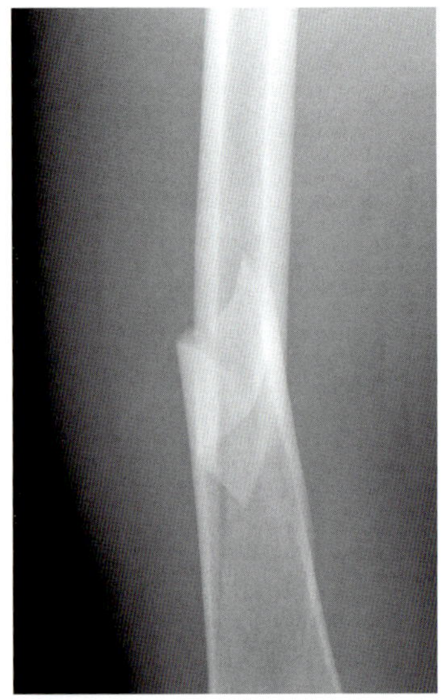

32-A1.3

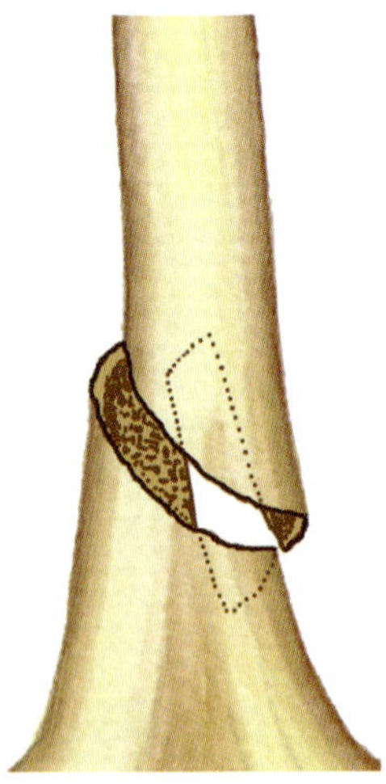

Distal section

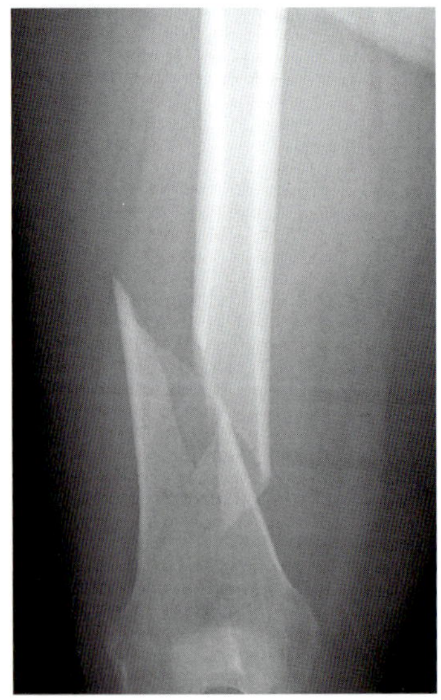

32-A Femur diaphysis, simple fractures

32-A2
Oblique (≥ 30 degrees)
1,213 fractures
M: 896 (73.87%)
F: 317 (26.13%)
0.32% of total adult fractures
3.06% of adult femoral fractures
14.73% of segment 32
29.44% of type 32-A

32-A2.1

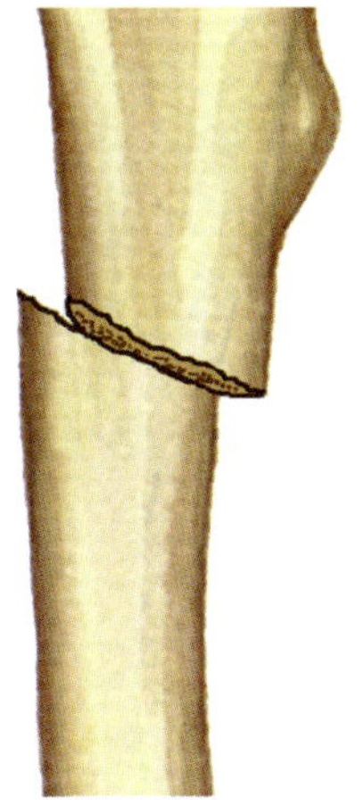

Subtrochanteric section

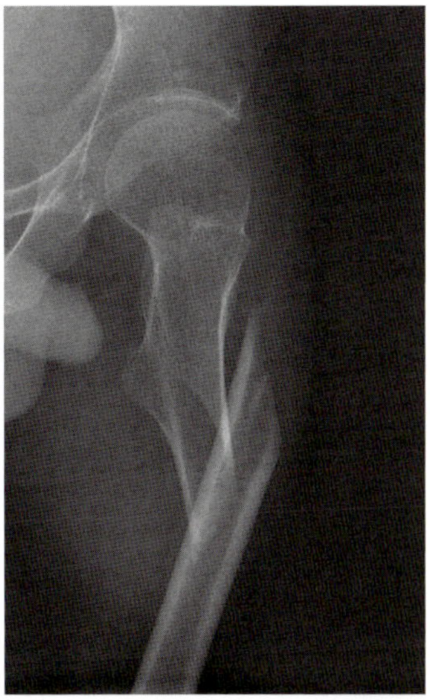

32-A2.2

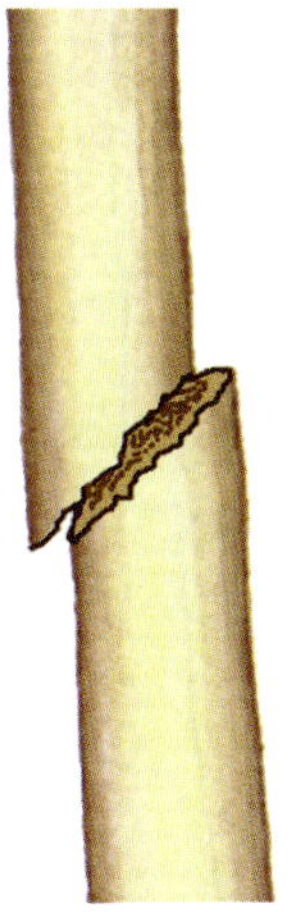

Middle section

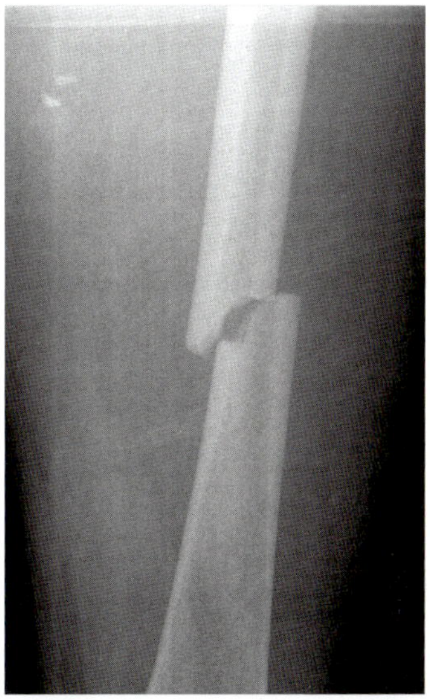

32-A2.3

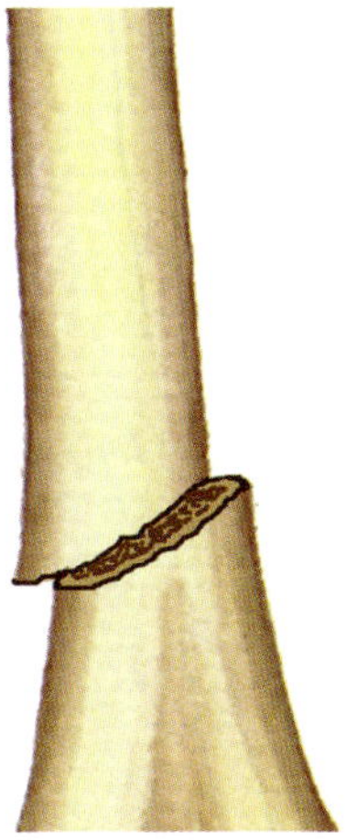

Distal section

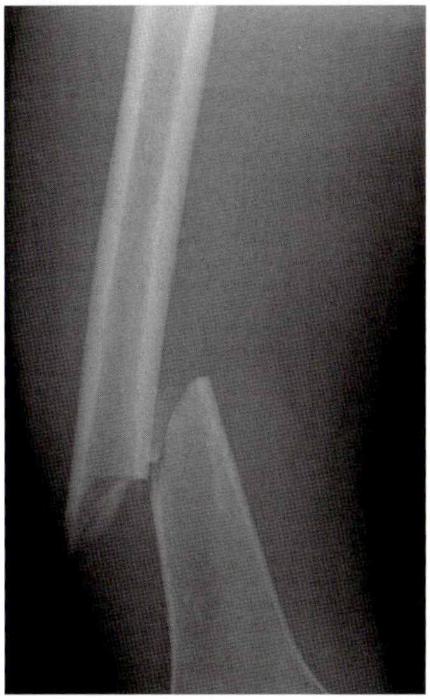

32-A Femur diaphysis, simple fractures

32-A3
Transverse (< 30 degrees)
1,815 fractures
M: 1,427 (78.62%)
F: 388 (21.38%)
0.48% of total adult fractures
4.57% of adult femoral fractures
22.04% of segment 32
44.05% of type 32-A

32-A3.1

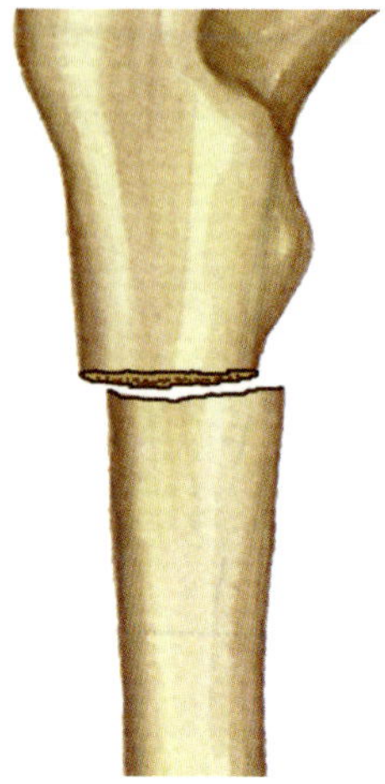

Subtrochanteric section

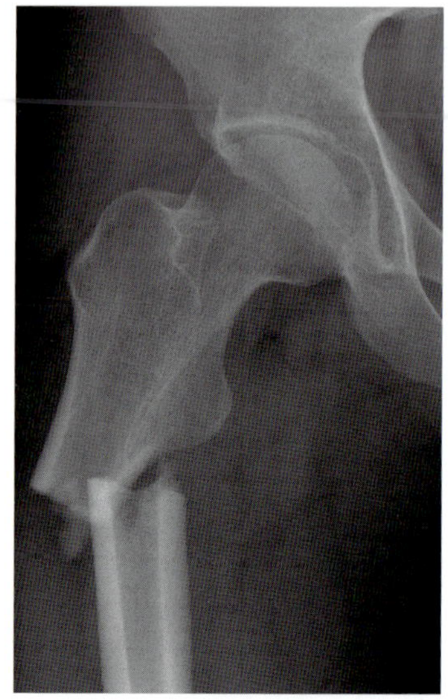

32-A3.2

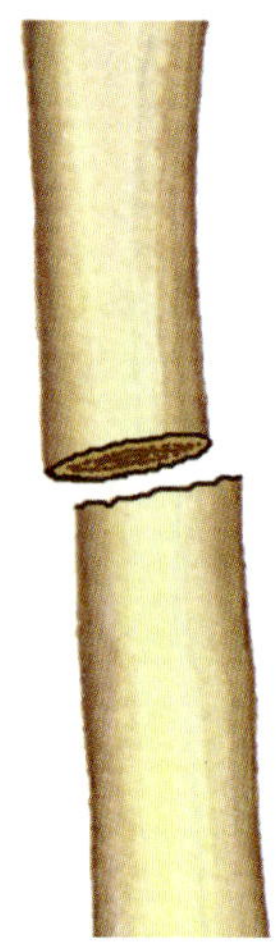

Middle section

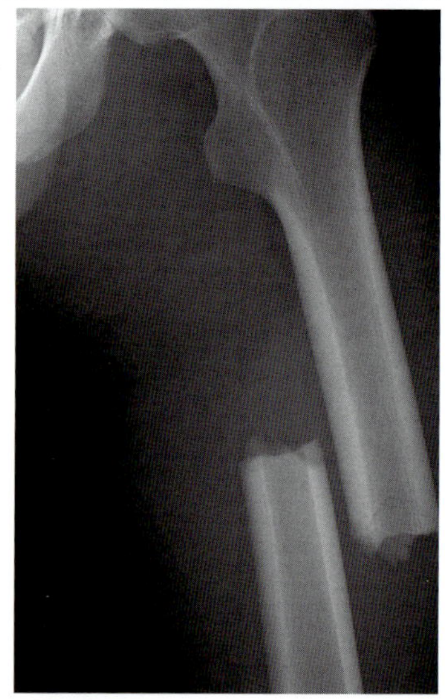

32-A3.3

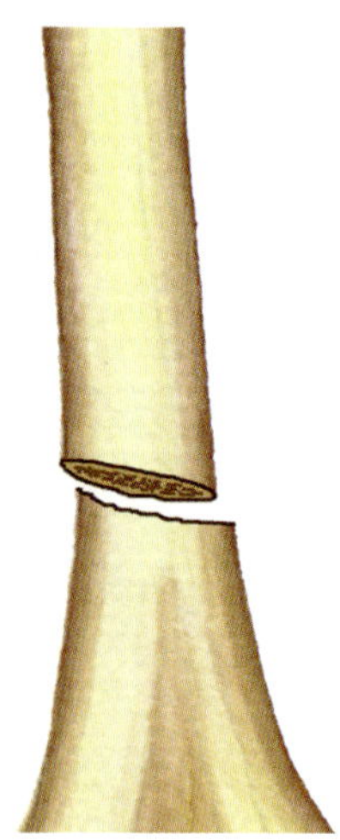

Distal section

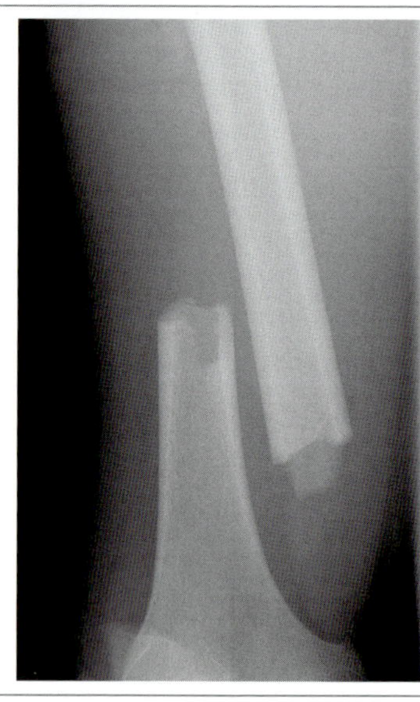

32-B Femur diaphysis, wedge fractures

32-B1
Spiral wedge
815 fractures
M: 596 (73.13%)
F: 219 (26.87%)
0.22% of total adult fractures
2.05% of adult femoral fractures
9.9% of segment 32
27.97% of type 32-B

32-B1.1

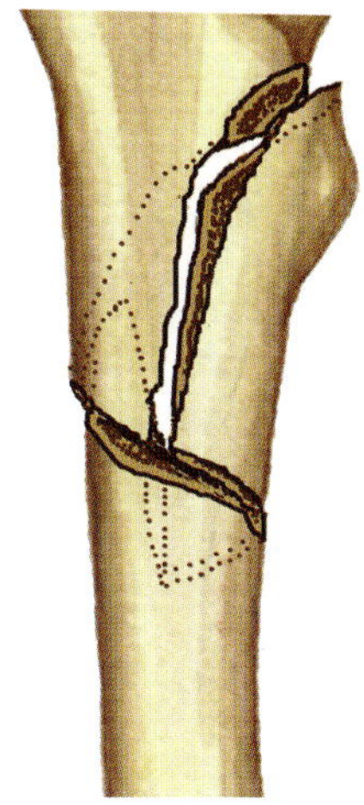

Subtrochanteric section

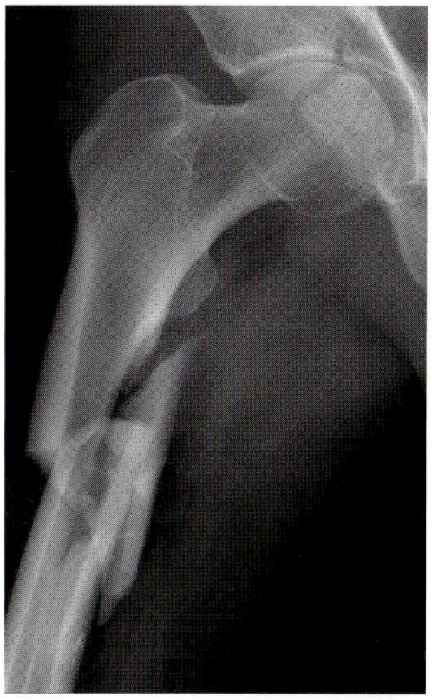

32-B1.2

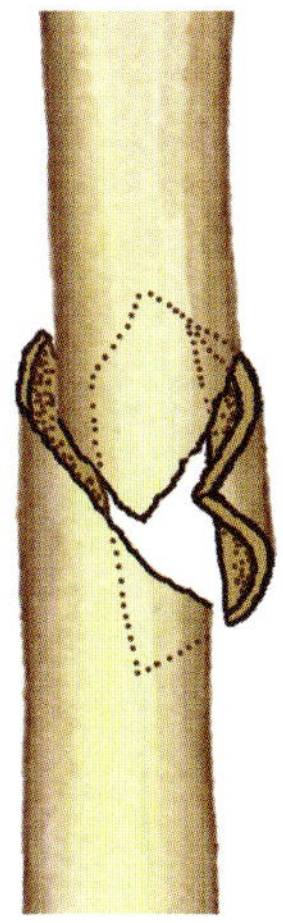

Middle section

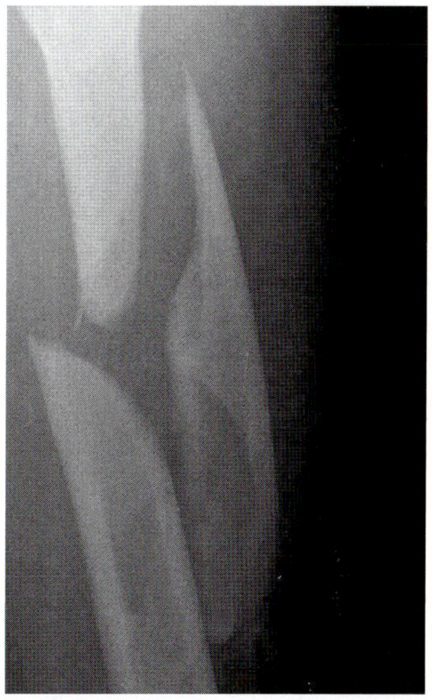

32-B1.3

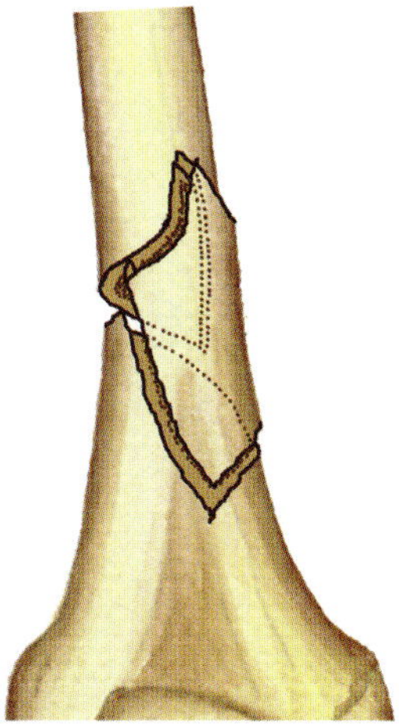

Distal section

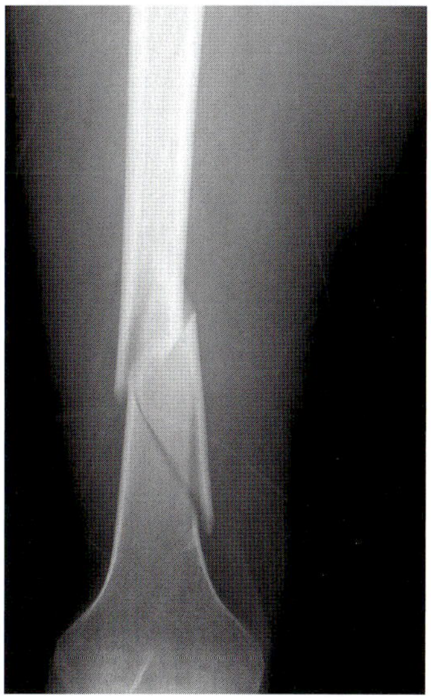

32-B Femur diaphysis, wedge fractures

32-B2
Bending wedge
1,378 fractures
M: 1,098 (79.68%)
F: 280 (20.32%)
0.37% of total adult fractures
3.47% of adult femoral fractures
16.73% of segment 32
47.29% of type 32-B

32-B2.1

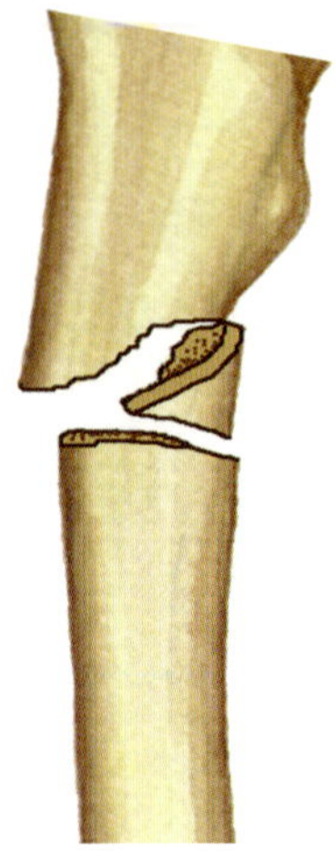

Subtrochanteric section

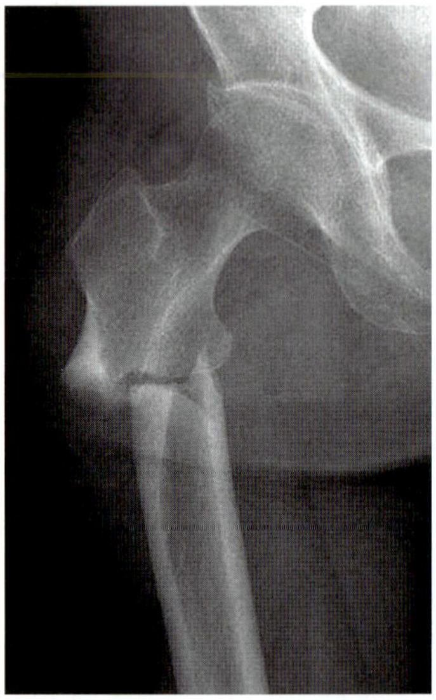

32-B2.2

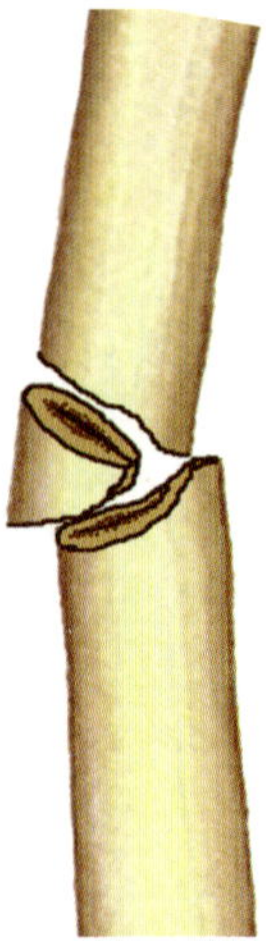

Middle section

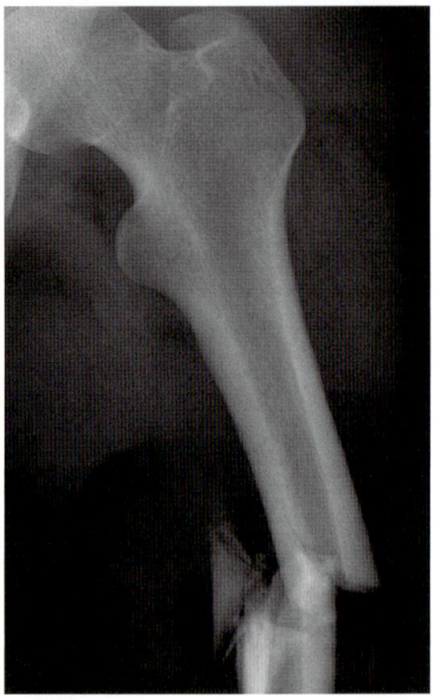

32-B2.3

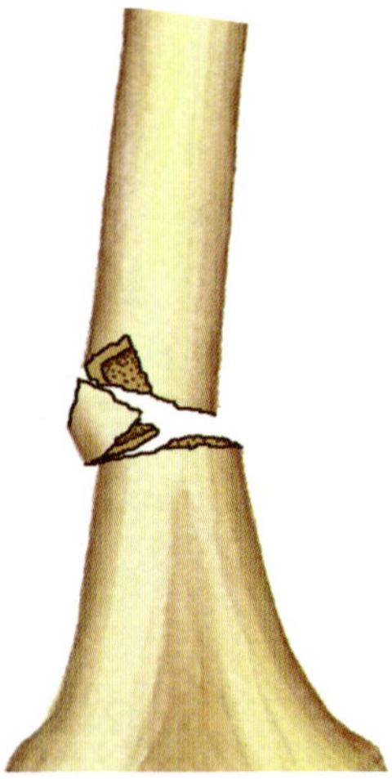

Distal section

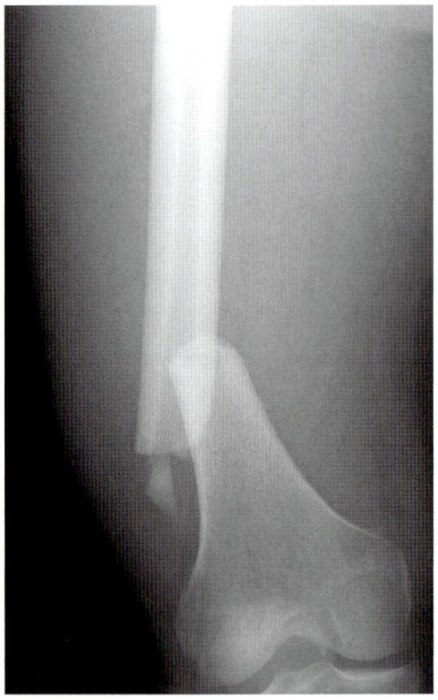

32-B Femur diaphysis, wedge fractures

32-B3
Complex
721 fractures
M: 609 (84.47%)
F: 112 (15.53%)
0.19% of total adult fractures
1.82% of adult femoral fractures
8.76% of segment 32
24.74% of type 32-B

32-B3.1

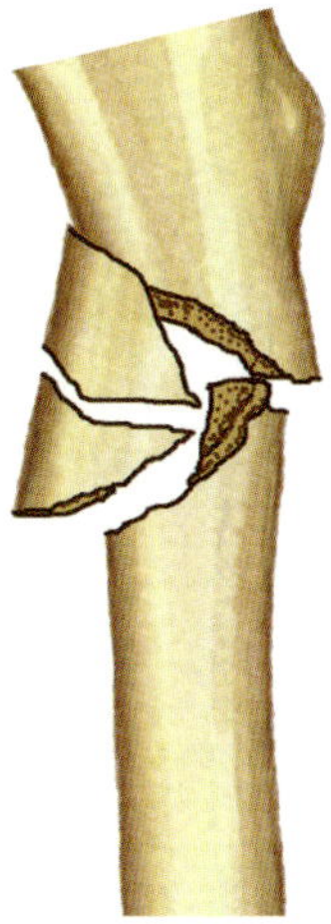

Subtrochanteric section

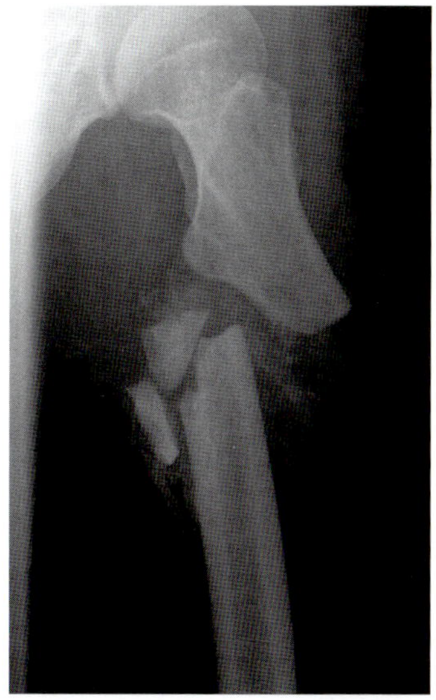

32-B3.2

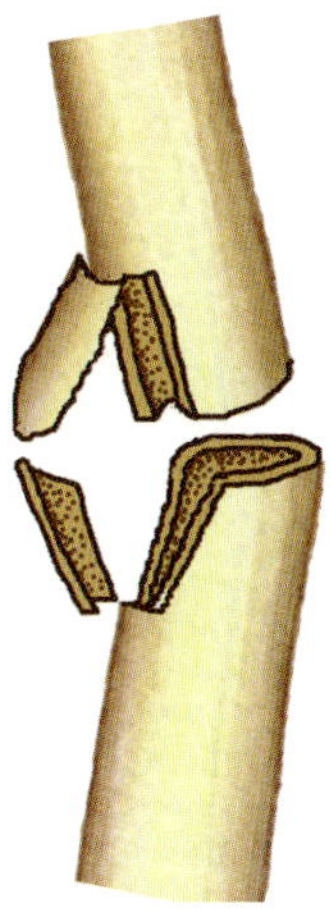

Middle section

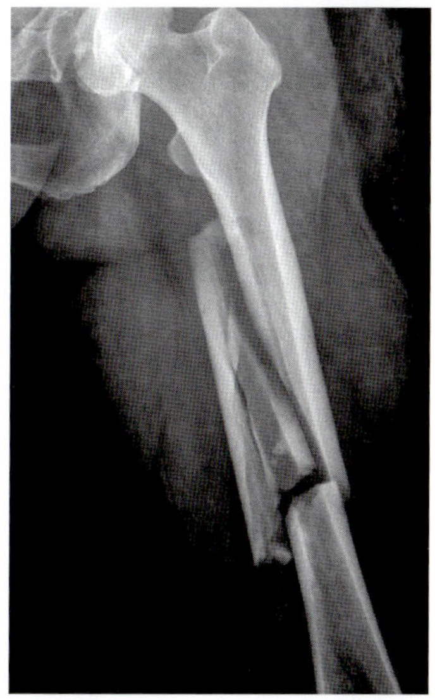

32-B3.3

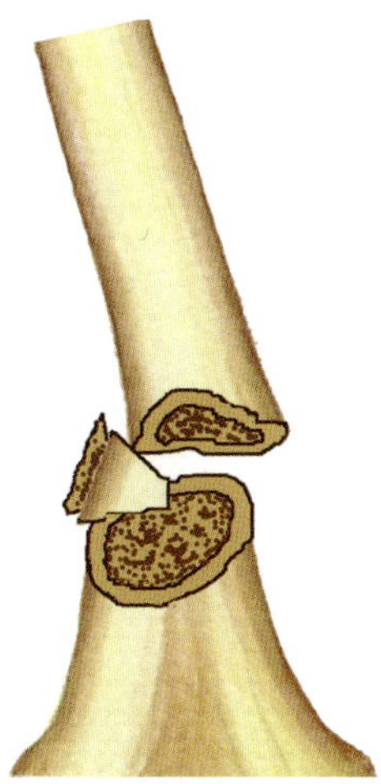

Distal section

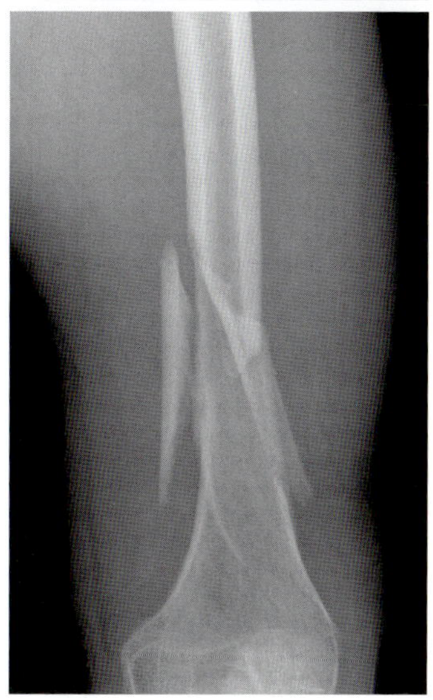

32-C Femur diaphysis, complex fractures

32-C1
Spiral
334 fractures
M: 260 (77.84%)
F: 74 (22.16%)
0.09% of total adult fractures
0.84% of adult femoral fractures
4.06% of segment 32
27.81% of type 32-C

32-C1.1

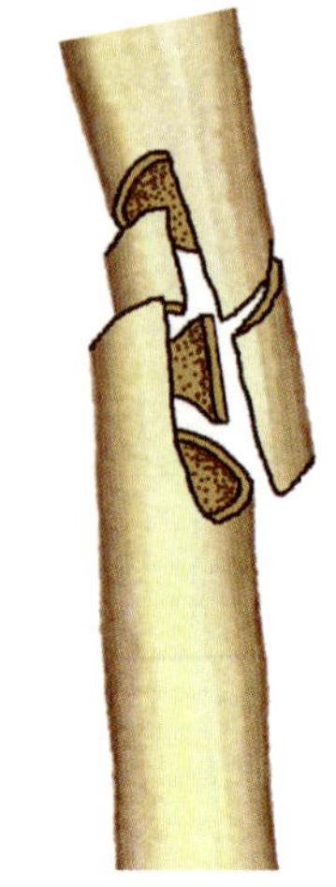

With two intermediate fragments

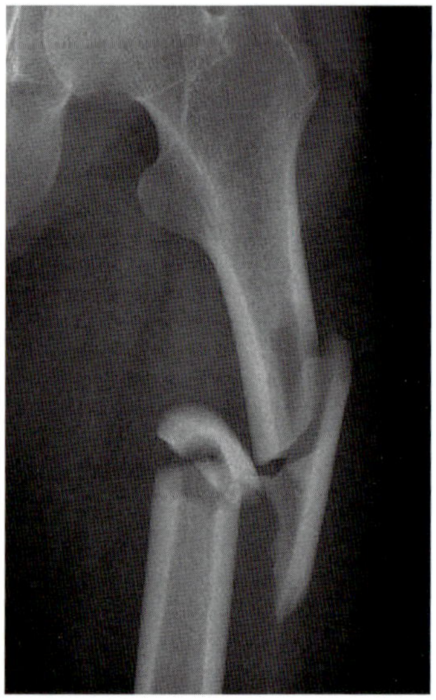

32-C1.2

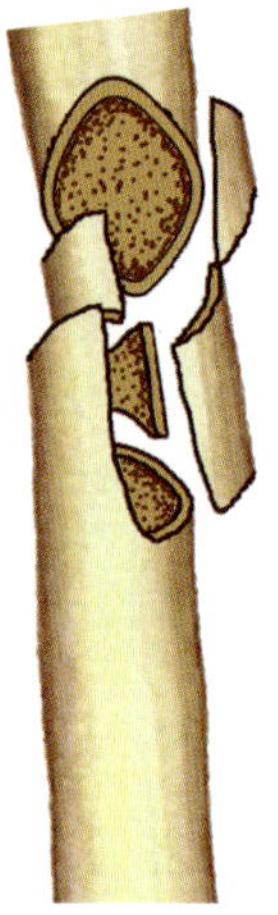

With three intermediate fragments

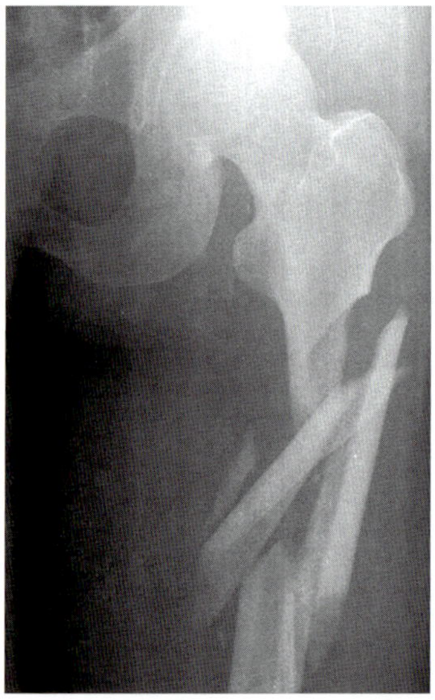

32-C1.3

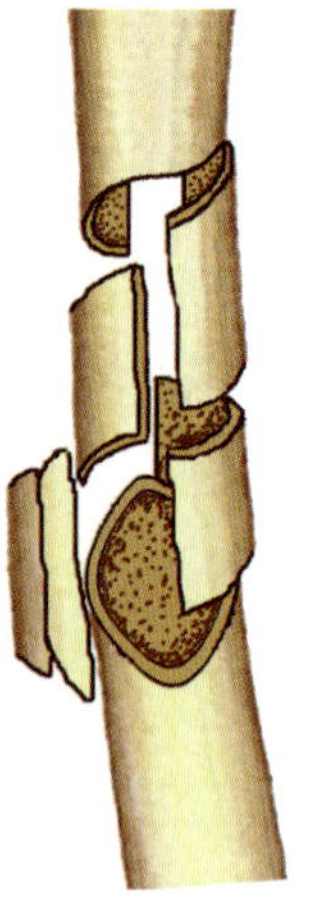

With more than three intermediate fragments

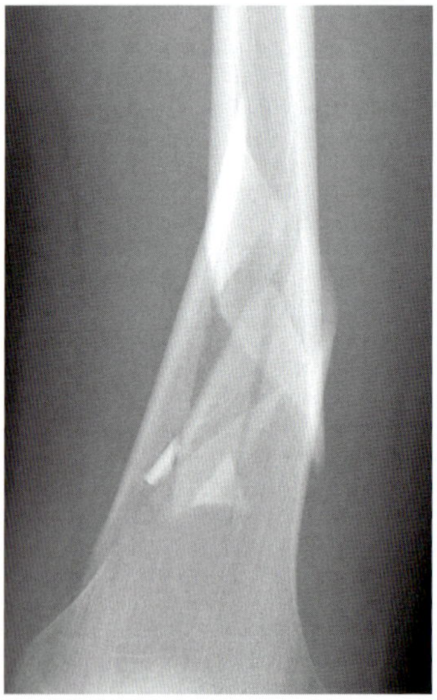

32-C Femur diaphysis, complex fractures

32-C2
Segmental
291 fractures
M: 221 (75.95%)
F: 70 (24.05%)
0.08% of total adult fractures
0.73% of adult femoral fractures
3.53% of segment 32
24.23% of type 32-C

32-C2.1

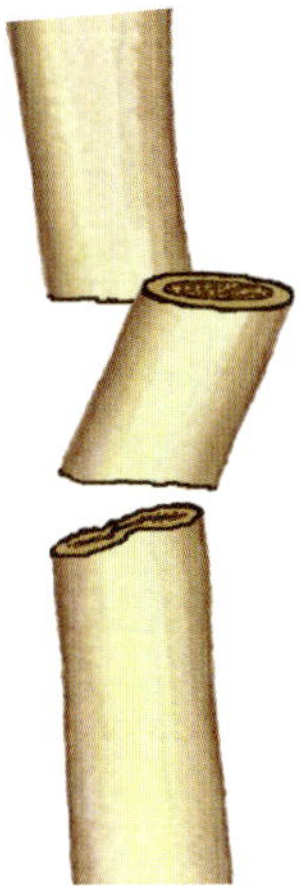

With one intermediate segmental fragment

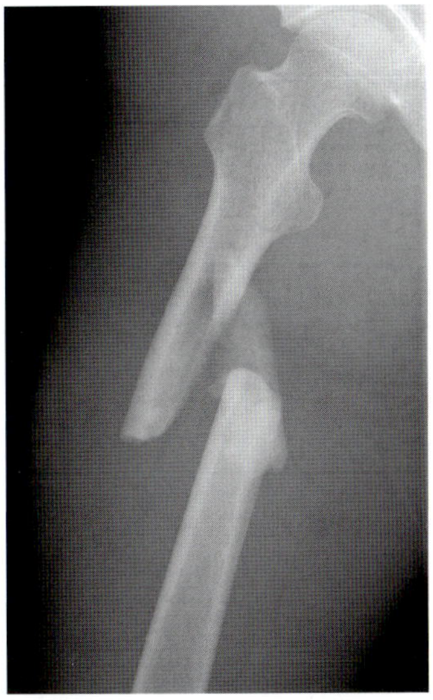

32-C2.2

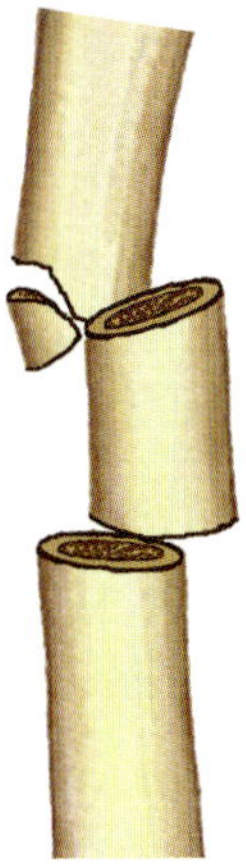

With one intermediate segmental fragment with an additional wedge fragment

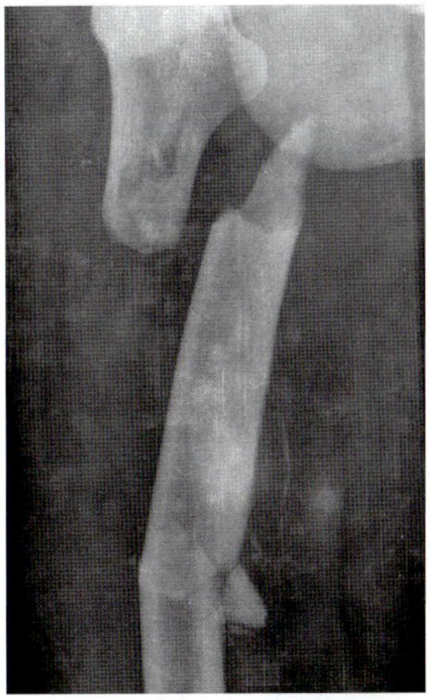

32-C2.3

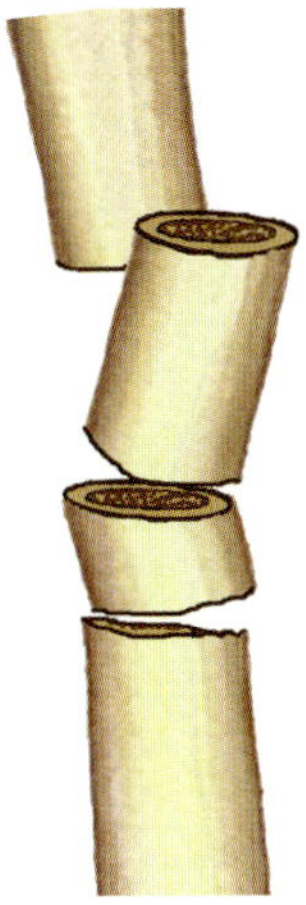

With two or more intermediate segmental fragments

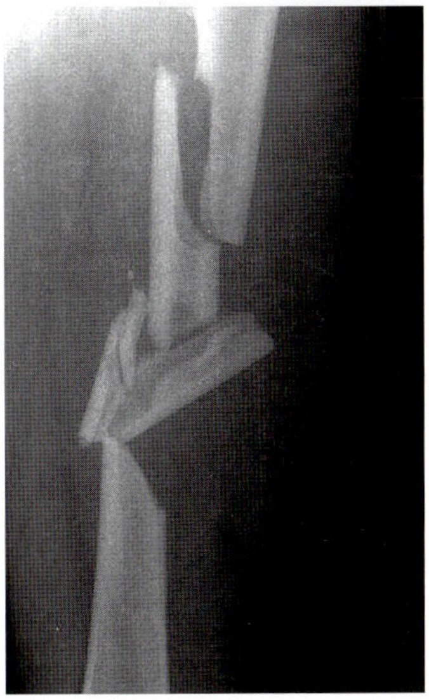

32-C Femur diaphysis, complex fractures

32-C3
Irregular
576 fractures
M: 464 (80.56%)
F: 112 (19.44%)
0.15% of total adult fractures
1.45% of adult femoral fractures
6.99% of segment 32
47.96% of type 32-C

32-C3.1

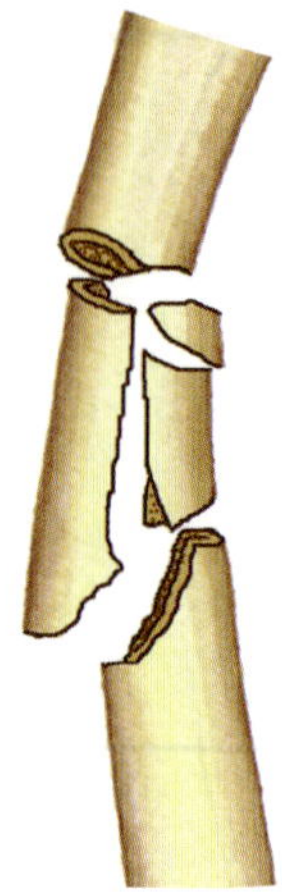

With two or three intermediate fragments

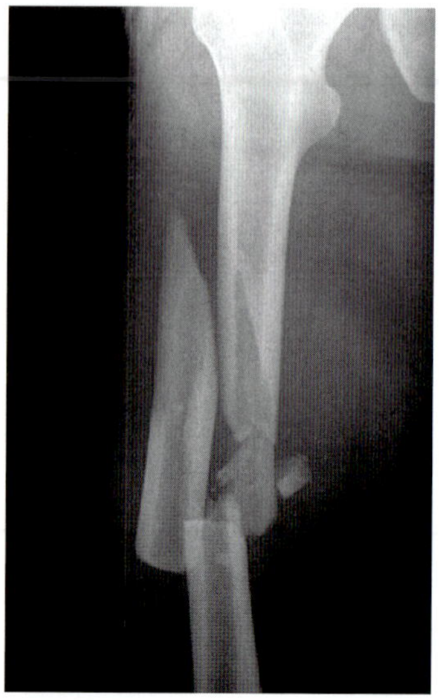

32-C3.2

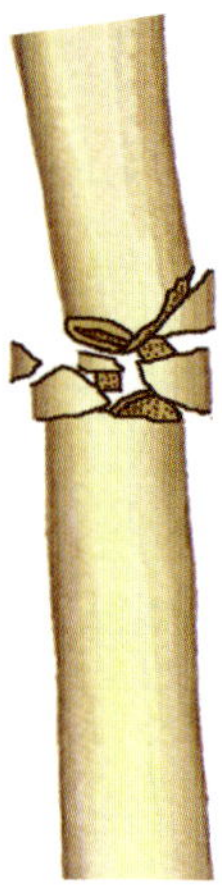

With limited shattering (< 5 cm)

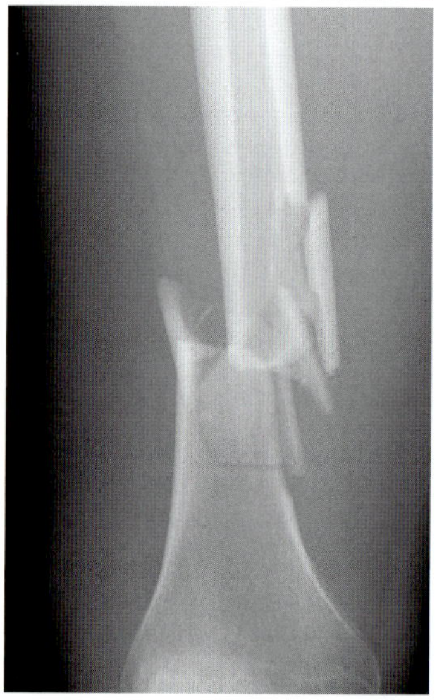

32-C3.3

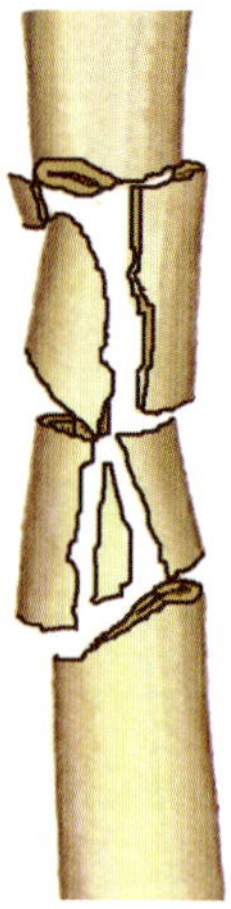

With extensive shattering (≥ 5 cm)

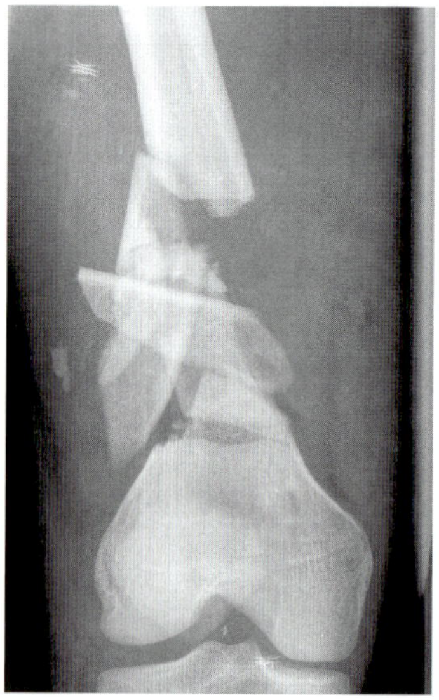

Injury Mechanism

Diaphyseal femoral fractures most often result from violent direct trauma, as seen in crush injuries or direct blows. A portion of fractures can be caused by indirect force, which involves leverage, twisting, or a fall from significant height. The direct trauma frequently leads to transverse or complex fractures, while oblique or spiral fractures may be the result of indirect force.

If fractures occur at the upper third of the femoral shaft, the distal segment of the fracture displaces superoposteriorly while the proximal segment is pulled into flexion, abduction, and external rotation by the activity of a group of muscles including the gluteus medius and minor, iliopsoas and short external rotators. Displacement of fractures of the middle third of the shaft has not been observed with much regularity. When fractures occur at the distal third of the femoral shaft, the proximal segment is usually pulled in adduction and displaces anteriorly and the distal segment displaces posteriorly due to traction from the gastrocnemius and the capsule, which may damage the popliteal artery, vein, and sciatic nerve.

Diagnosis

Patients with femoral shaft fractures usually present with pain, swelling, limb shortening, limited range of movement, and deformity of the affected limb. Radiographic examination should include an AP pelvic view, as well as AP and lateral views of the knee that show the entire femur, because fractures often involve both the hip and knee joint. The lateral view should include an extension view of the intertrochanteric fracture site to specifically detect the involvement of the anterior and posterior aspect of the sinus pyriformis. The diameter of the femoral canal, the shape of the shaft, the femoral neck angle, and the presence of prior deformity of the femur should be given special attention for proper choice of internal fixators.

Treatment

Early fixation of femoral shaft fractures can lead to satisfactory clinical outcomes, with better results in knee function and fewer complications. As such, these fractures in adults should be treated with surgical intervention. With the advancement of the interlocking intramedullary nail, it has become the preferred treatment of choice for fixation of femoral shaft fractures. The interlocking intramedullary nails provide fixation not only to fractures of the shaft, but also to fractures extending into the proximal and distal ends of the femur, especially to complex fractures of the femur. AO compression plates can be applied to treat transverse and short-oblique fractures of the upper middle third of the diaphysis. An angle plate with a wing is recommended for diaphyseal fractures of the distal third of the femur, especially when the intramedullary nail fails to provide stable fixation, and should be placed onto the femur laterally or anterolaterally. DHS and DCS plates are applied to both proximal and distal diaphyseal fractures. For various open fractures and closed femoral fractures in children, external fixators can be used to allow early mobilization and prompt recovery.

Distal Femoral Fractures (Segment 33)

Anatomical Features

The distal end of the femur extends laterally to form the medial and lateral condyles of the femur, with their anteroposterior diameter greater than their transverse diameter. The lateral condyle is the more prominent and is broader both in its anteroposterior and transverse diameters, but the medial condyle is longer and narrower. The location of the lateral condyle and its anterior projection protect the patella against lateral dislocation (**Plate 4.8**).

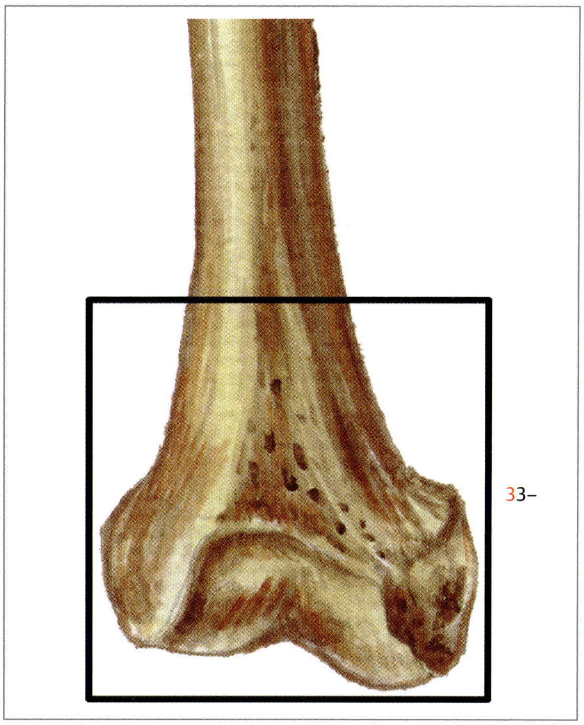

Plate 4.8

4

AO Classification of Distal Femoral Fractures

Based on the AO classification, distal femoral fractures are coded as the number 33. It is further divided into three types depending on fracture patterns: 33-A, extra-articular fracture; 33-B, partial articular fracture; and 33-C, complete articular fracture (**Plate 4.9**).

Clinical Epidemiologic Features of Distal Femoral Fractures (Segment 33)

A total of 3,434 distal femoral fractures were treated in 83 hospitals in China over a 2-year period from 2010 to 2011. All cases were reviewed and statistically studied, accounting for 8.65% of femoral fractures in adults. Their epidemiologic features are as follows:

- More males than females
- The high-risk age group is 41–45 years; the same high-risk age group for males, while females aged 51–55 years have highest risk
- The most common fracture type among segment 33 fractures is type 33-A; the same fracture type in both males and females
- The most common fracture group among segment 33 fractures is group 33-A1; the same fracture group in both males and females

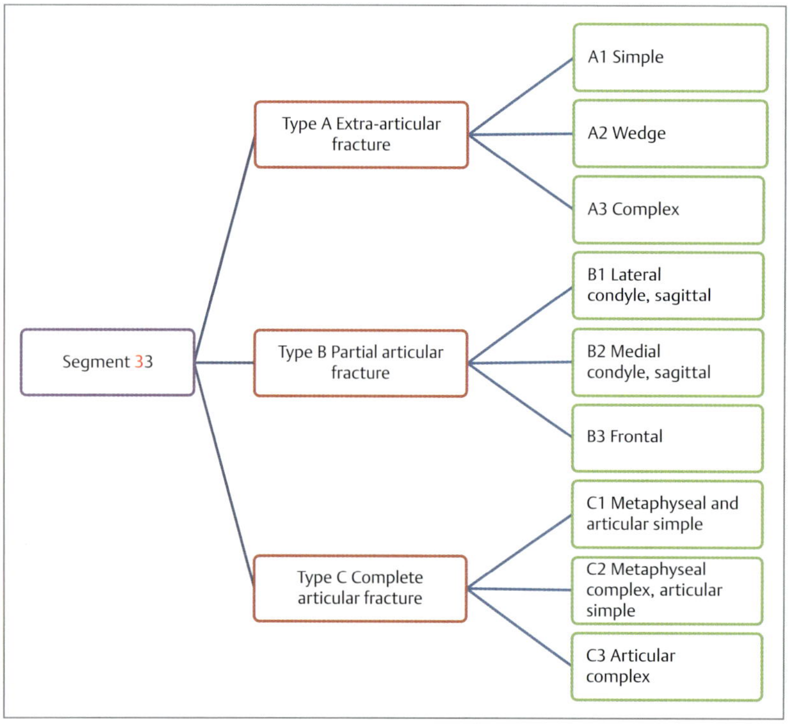

Plate 4.9

4

Fractures of Segment 33 by Sex

Table 4.14 Sex distribution of 3,434 fractures of segment 33

Sex	Number of fractures	Percentage (%)
Male	2,123	61.82
Female	1,311	38.18
Total	3,434	100.00

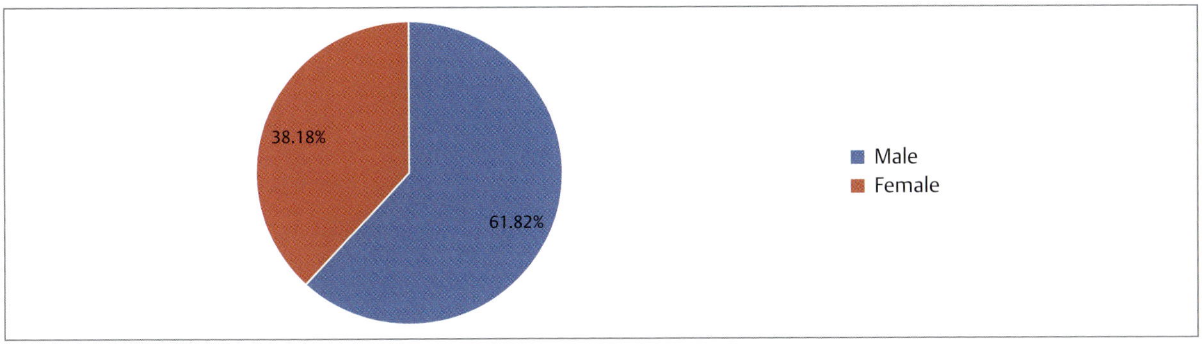

Fig. 4.14 Sex distribution of 3,434 fractures of segment 33.

Fractures of Segment 33 by Age Group

Table 4.15 Age and sex distribution of 3,434 fractures of segment 33

Age group (years)	Male	Female	Number of fractures	Percentage (%)
16–20	192	47	239	6.96
21–25	199	49	248	7.22
26–30	189	38	227	6.61
31–35	174	48	222	6.46
36–40	268	86	354	10.31
41–45	271	96	367	10.69
46–50	222	96	318	9.26
51–55	206	146	352	10.25
56–60	157	138	295	8.59
61–65	91	137	228	6.64
66–70	49	129	178	5.18
71–75	46	99	145	4.22
76–80	30	110	140	4.08
81–85	16	48	64	1.86
≥86	13	44	57	1.66
Total	2,123	1,311	3,434	100.00

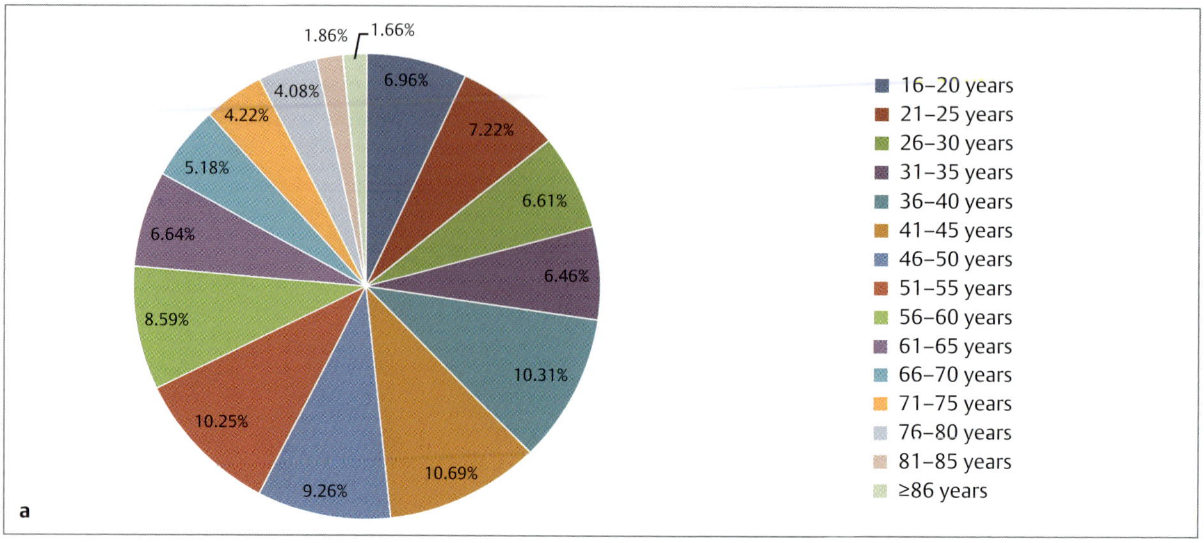

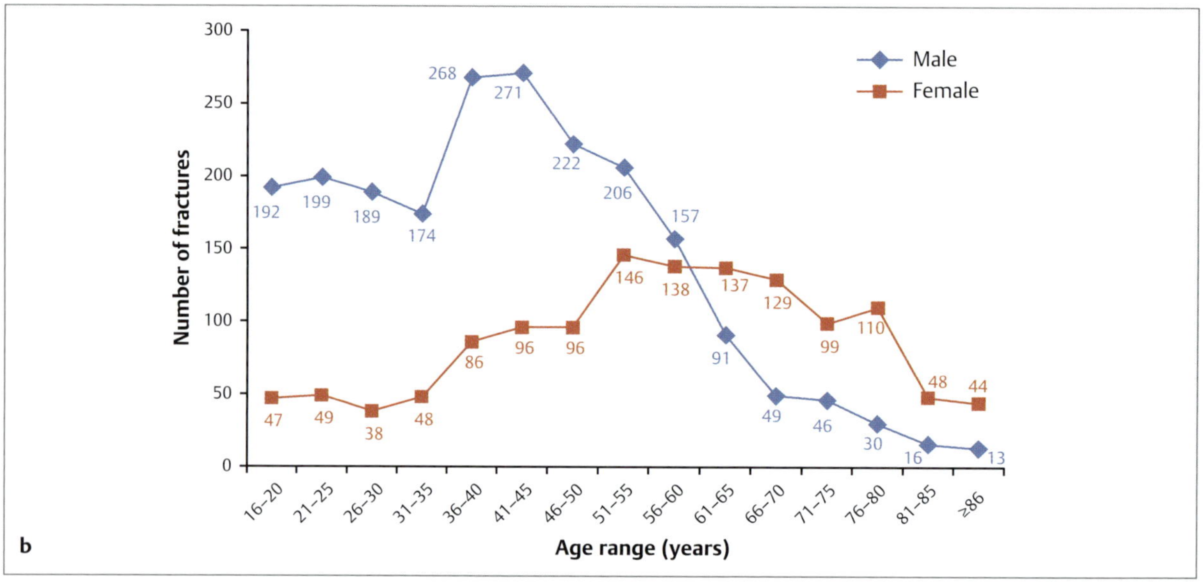

Fig. 4.15 (a) Age distributions of 3,434 fractures of segment 33.
(b) Age and sex distributions of 3,434 fractures of segment 33.

Fractures of Segment 33 by Fracture Type

Table 4.16 Sex and fracture type distribution of 3,434 fractures of segment 33

Fracture type	Male	Female	Number of fractures	Percentage (%)
33-A	967	752	1,719	50.06
33-B	406	236	642	18.70
33-C	750	323	1,073	31.25
Total	2,123	1,311	3,434	100.00

4

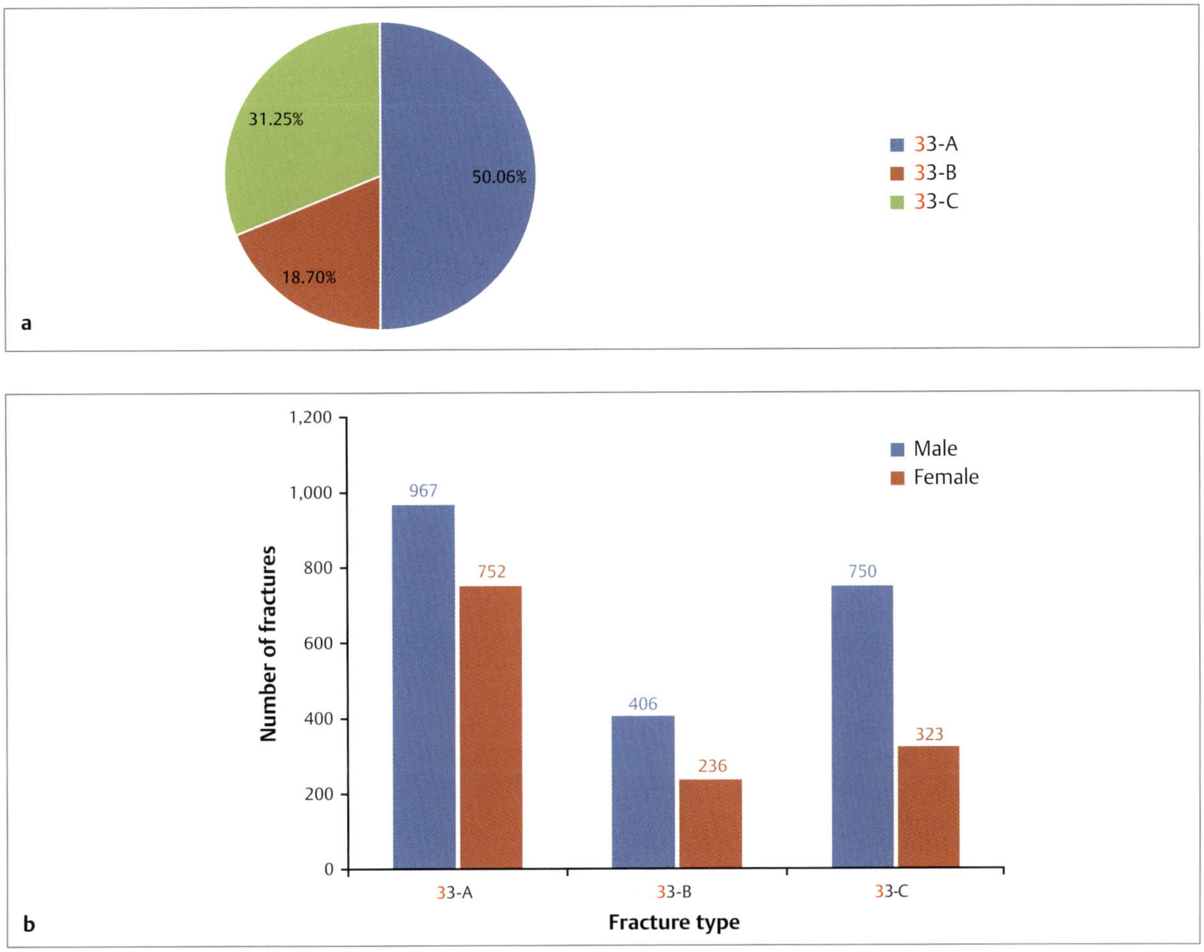

Fig. 4.16 **(a)** Fracture type distribution of 3,434 fractures of segment 33.
(b) Sex and fracture type distribution of 3,434 fractures of segment 33.

Fractures of Segment 33 by Fracture Group

Table 4.17 Sex and fracture group distribution of 3,434 fractures of segment 33

Fracture group	Male	Female	Number of fractures	Percentage of segment 33 fractures (%)	Percentage of femur fractures (%)
33-A1	506	407	913	26.59	2.30
33-A2	152	135	287	8.36	0.72
33-A3	309	210	519	15.11	1.31
33-B1	131	68	199	5.79	0.50
33-B2	172	90	262	7.63	0.66
33-B3	103	78	181	5.27	0.46
33-C1	103	76	179	5.21	0.45
33-C2	410	168	578	16.83	1.46
33-C3	237	79	316	9.20	0.80
Total	2,123	1,311	3,434	100.00	8.65

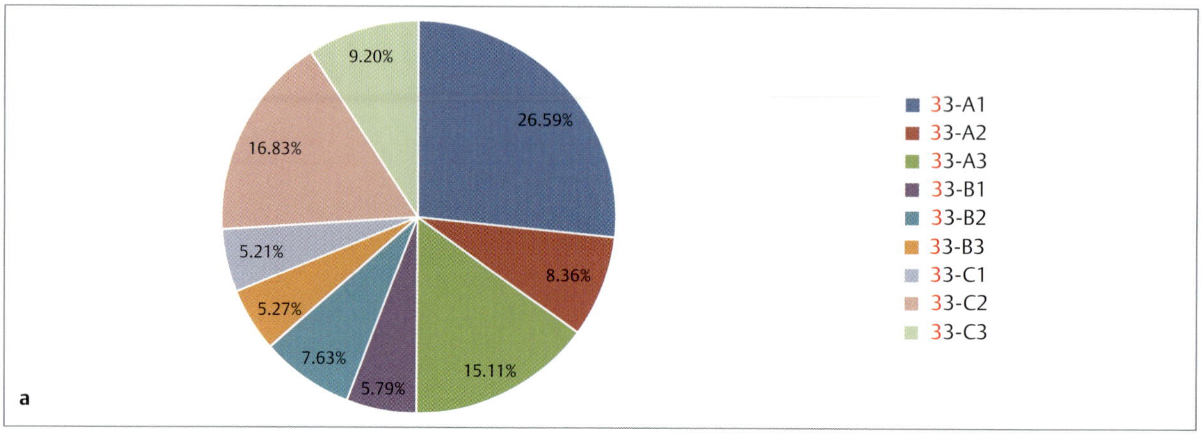

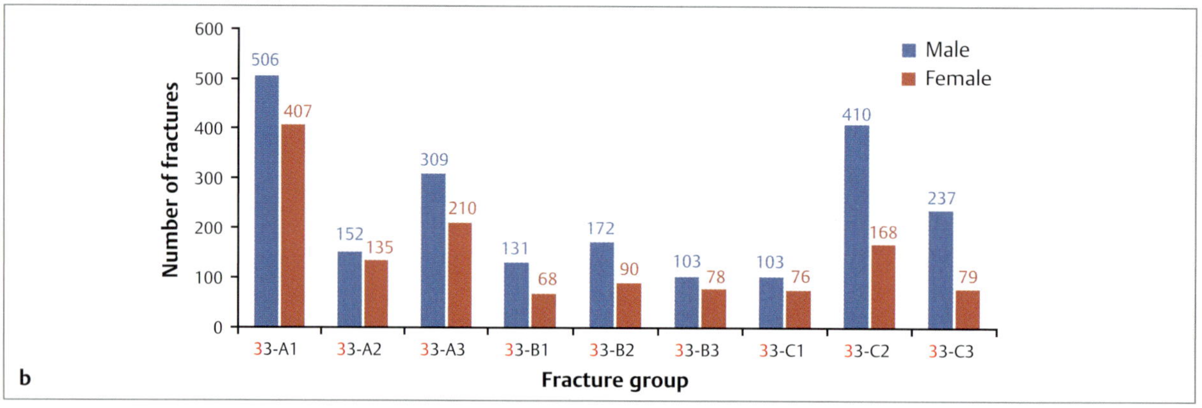

Fig. 4.17 **(a)** Fracture group distribution of 3,434 fractures of segment 33.
(b) Sex and fracture group distribution of 3,434 fractures of segment 33.

4

33-A Femur distal, extra-articular fractures

33-A1
Simple
913 fractures
M: 506 (55.42%)
F: 407 (44.58%)
0.24% of total adult fractures
2.30% of adult femoral fractures
26.59% of segment 33
53.11% of type 33-A

33-A1.1

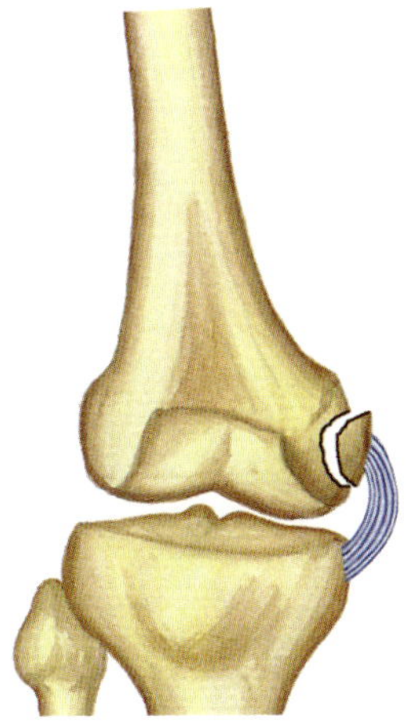

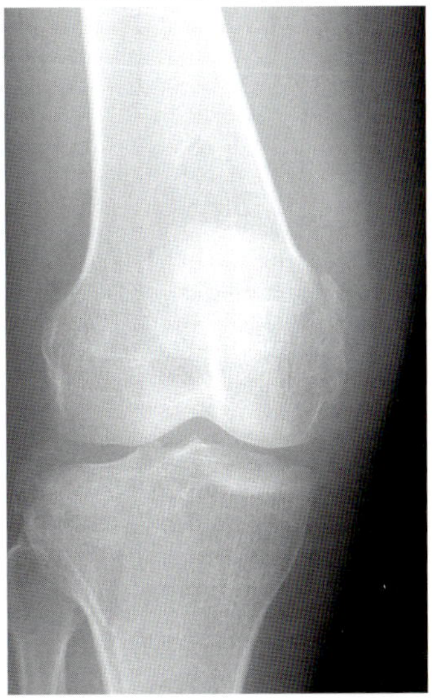

Apophyseal avulsion

33-A1.2

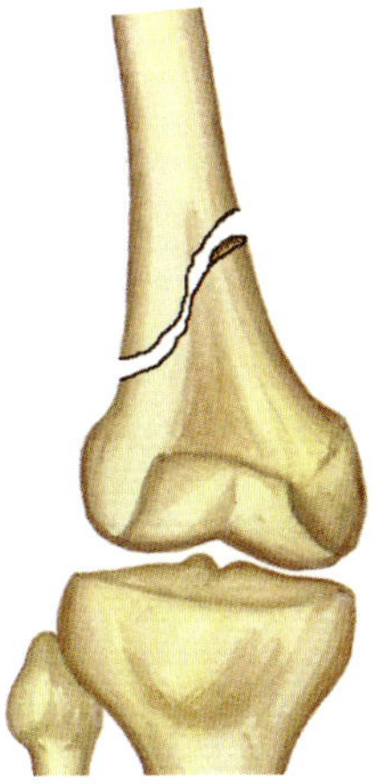

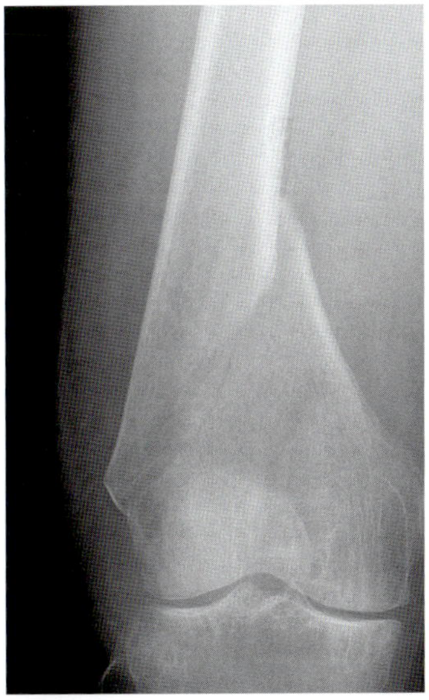

Oblique or spiral

33-A1.3

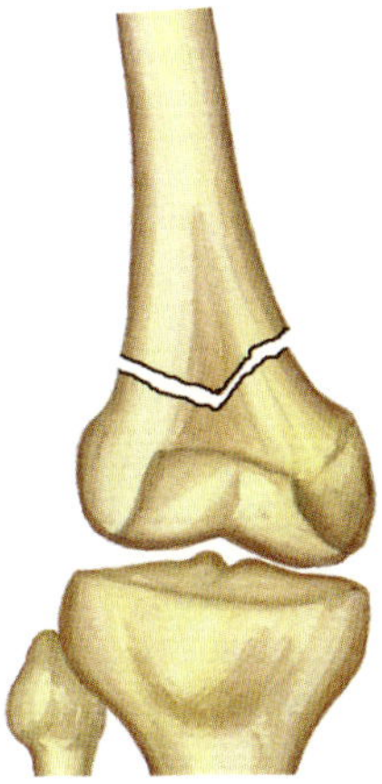

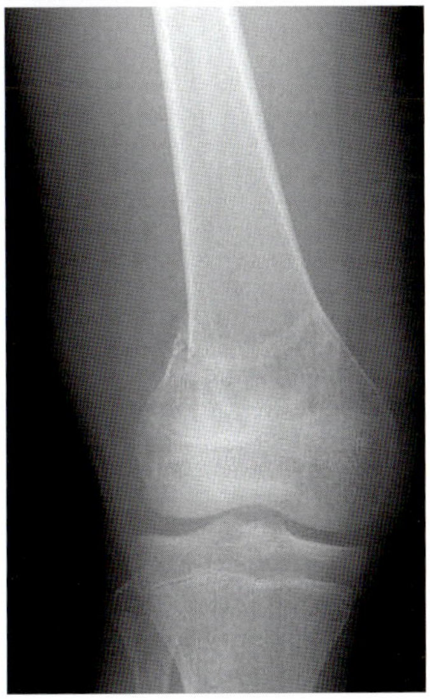

Transverse

33-A Femur distal, extra-articular fractures

33-A2
Wedge
287 fractures
M: 152 (52.96%)
F: 135 (47.04%)
0.08% of total adult fractures
0.72% of adult femoral fractures
8.36% of segment 33
16.70% of type 33-A

33-A2.1

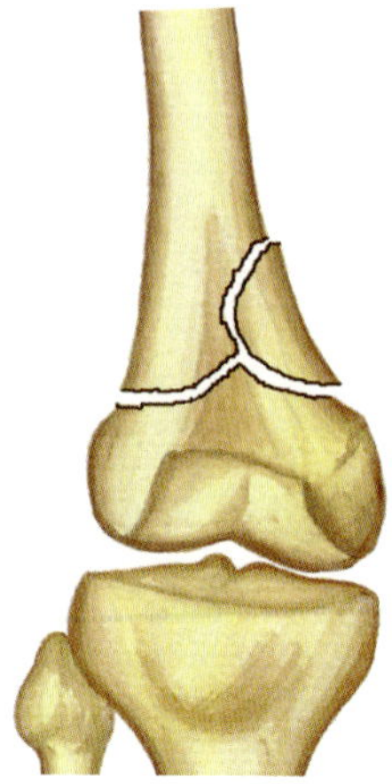

Intact

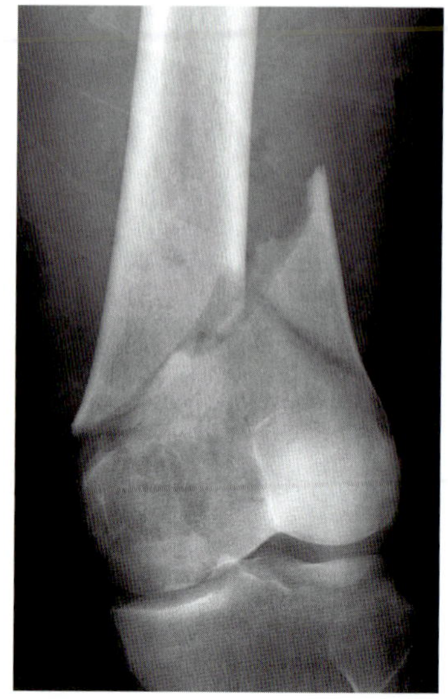

33-A2.2

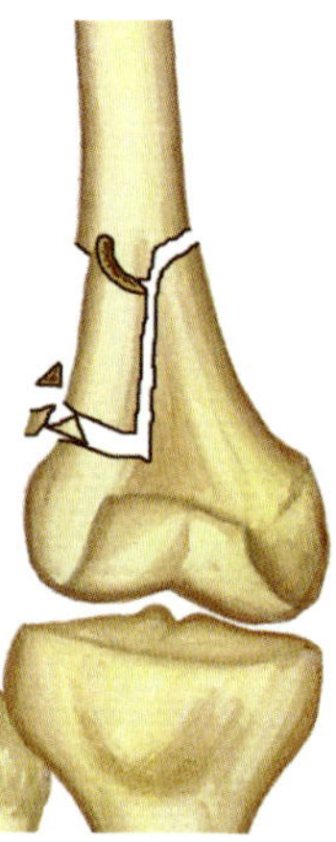

Lateral fragmented

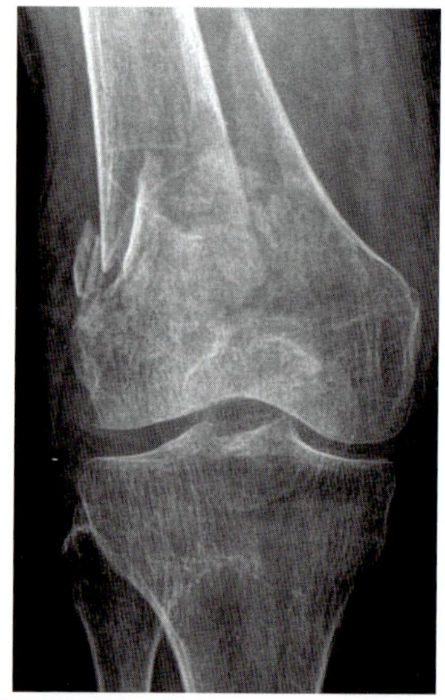

33-A2.3

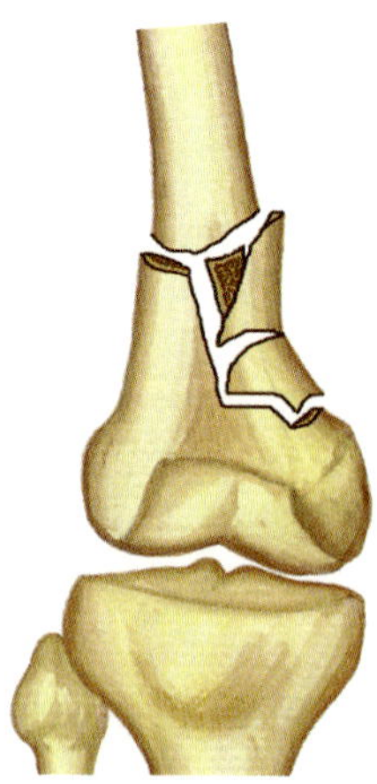

Medial fragmented

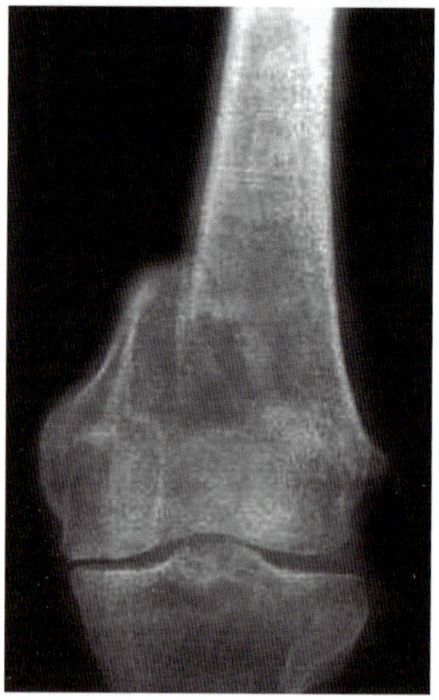

33-A Femur distal, extra-articular fractures

33-A3
Complex
519 fractures
M: 309 (59.54%)
F: 210 (40.46%)
0.14% of total adult fractures
1.31% of adult femoral fractures
15.11% of segment 33
30.19% of type 33-A

33-A3.1

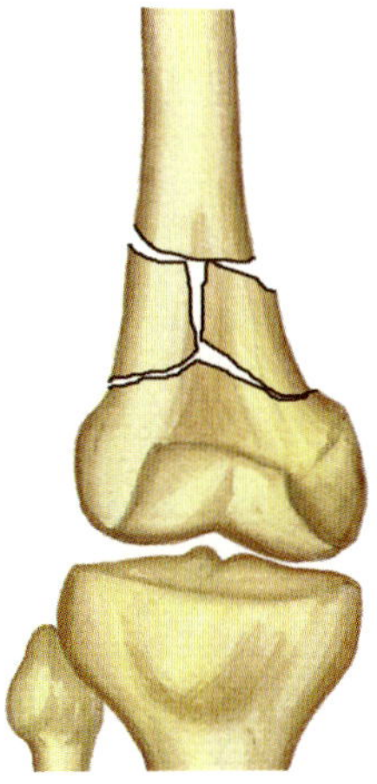

With an intermediate split fragment

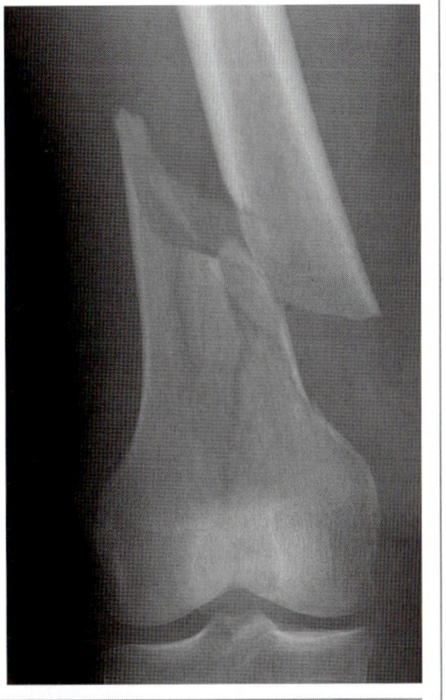

33-A3.2

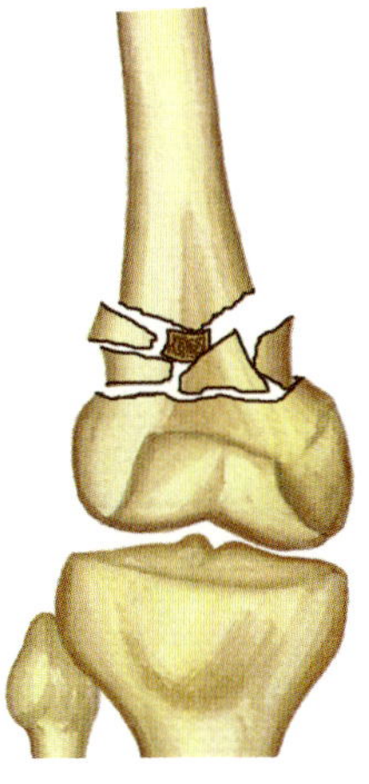

Irregular, limited to the metaphysis

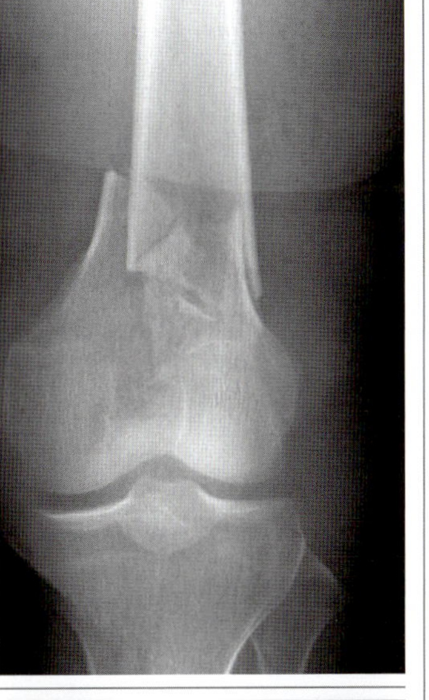

33-A3.3

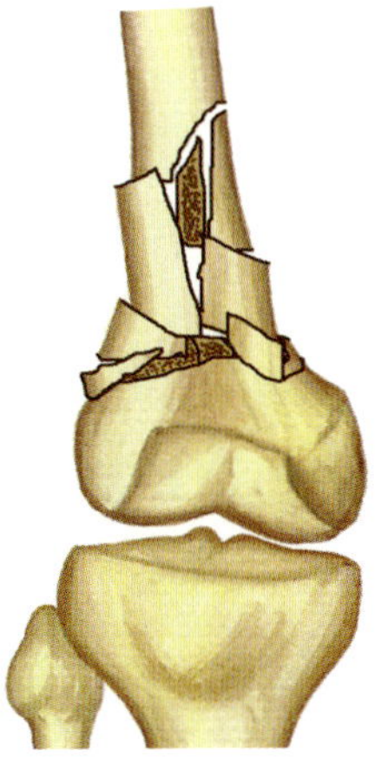

Irregular, extending into the diaphysis

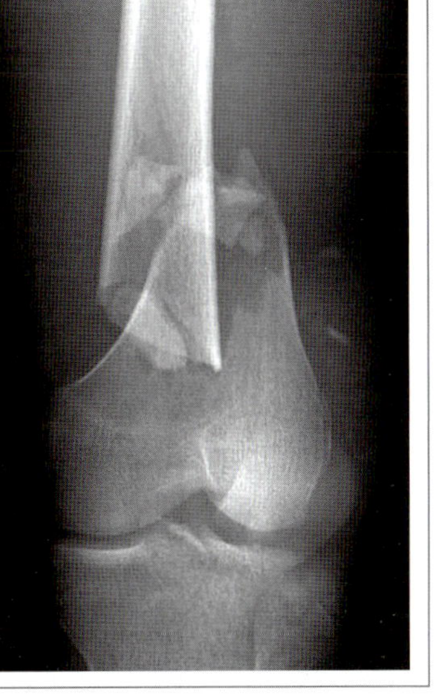

33-B Femur distal, partial-articular fractures

33-B1
Lateral condyle, sagittal
199 fractures
M: 131 (65.83%)
F: 68 (34.17%)
0.05% of total adult fractures
0.50% of adult femoral fractures
5.79% of segment 33
31.00% of type 33-B

33-B1.1

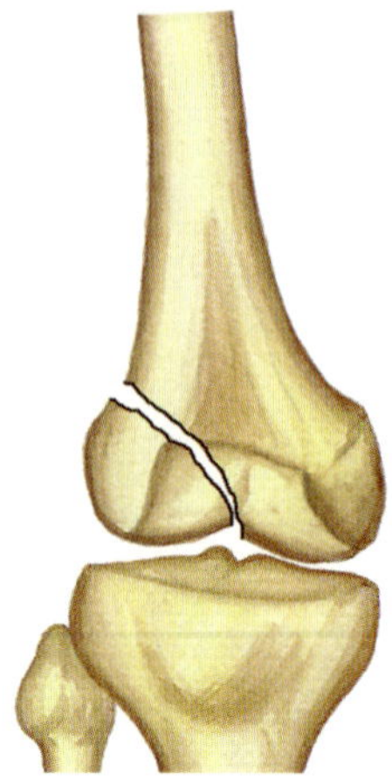

Simple, through the notch

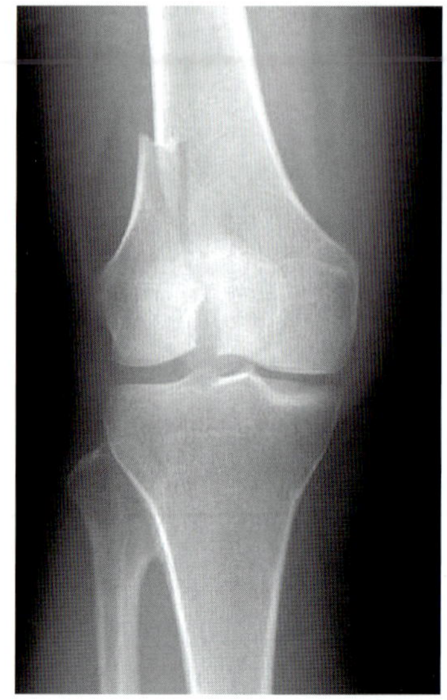

33-B1.2

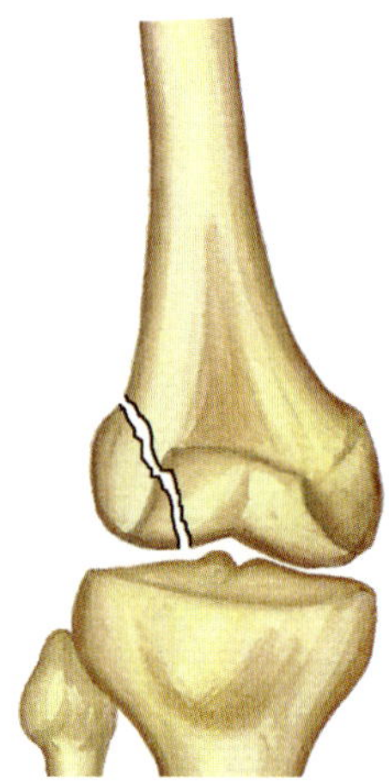

Simple, through the load-bearing surface

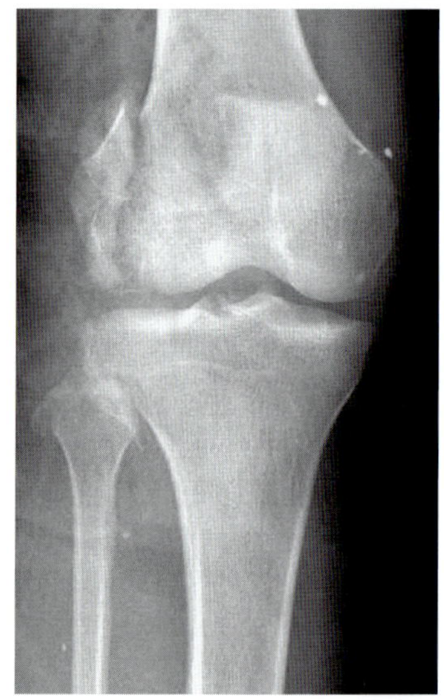

33-B1.3

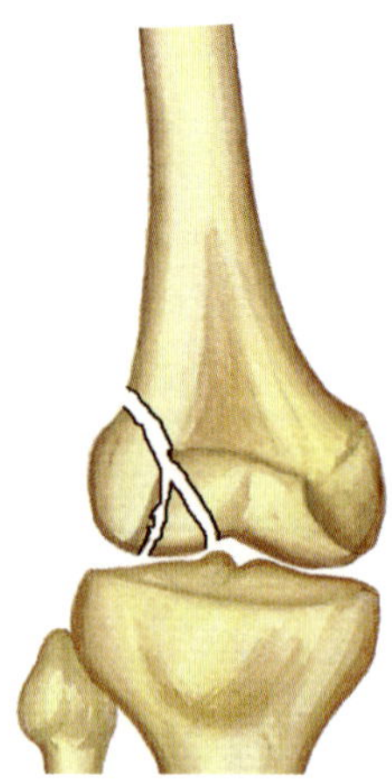

Complex, through the load-bearing surface

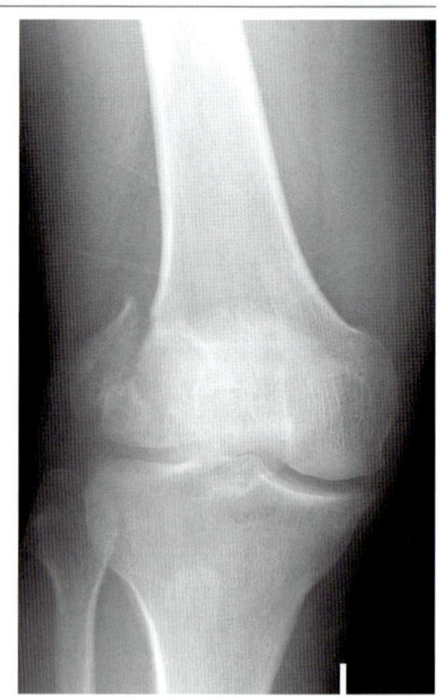

33-B Femur distal, partial-articular fractures

33-B2
Medial condyle, sagittal
262 fractures
M: 172 (65.65%)
F: 90 (34.35%)
0.07% of total adult fractures
0.66% of adult femoral fractures
7.63% of segment 33
40.81% of type 33-B

33-B2.1

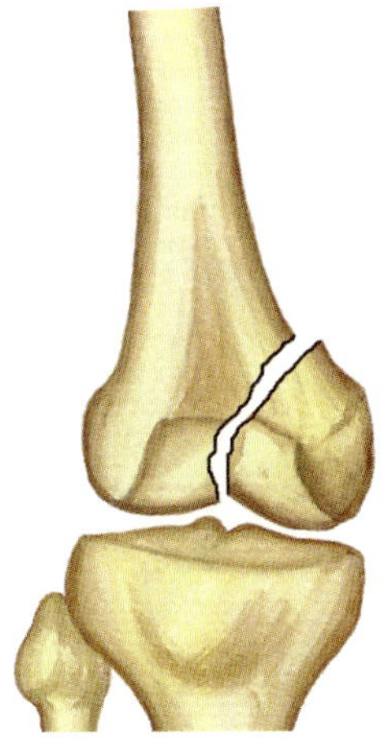

Simple, through the notch

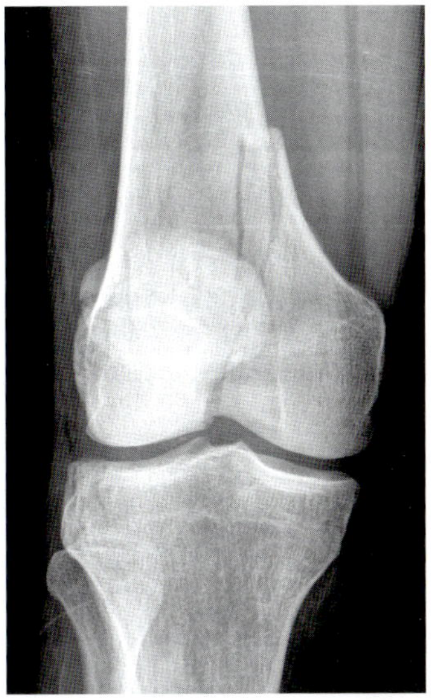

33-B2.2

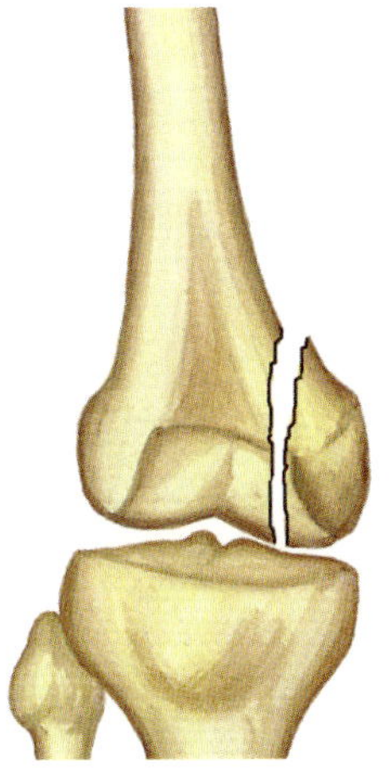

Simple, through the load-bearing surface

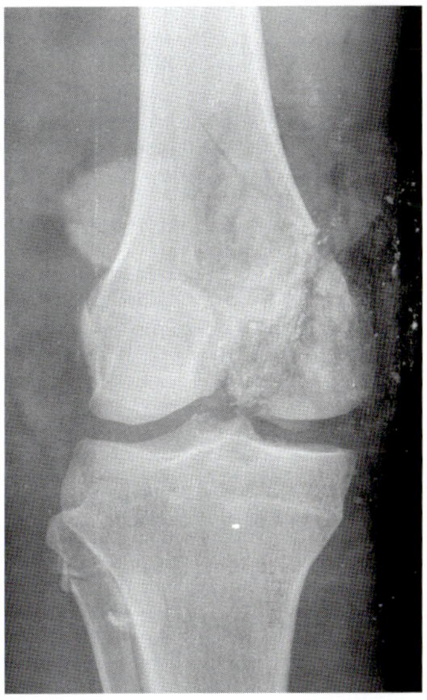

33-B2.3

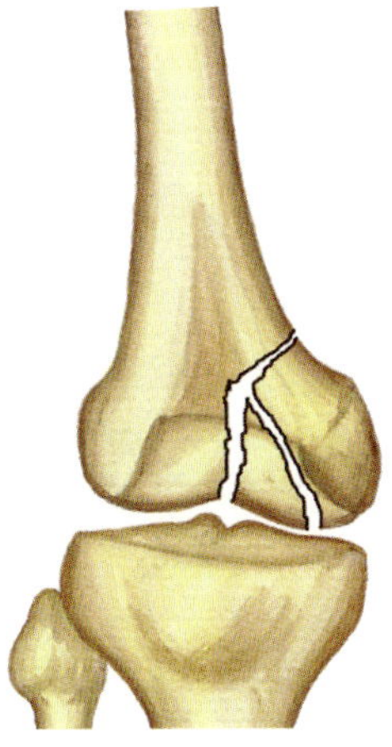

Complex, through the load-bearing surface

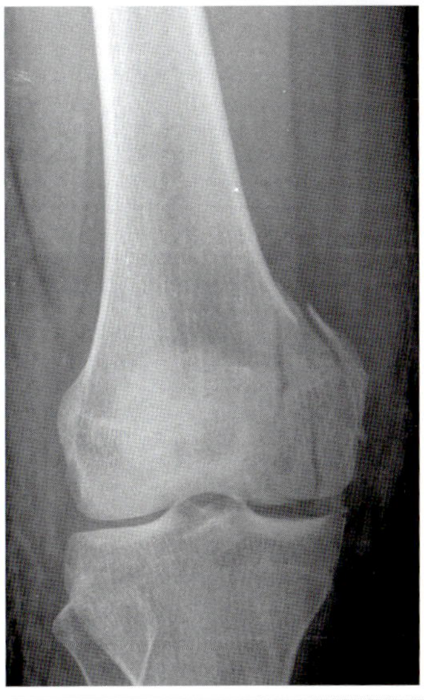

33-B Femur distal, partial-articular fractures

33-B3
Frontal
181 fractures
M: 103 (56.91%)
F: 78 (43.09%)
0.05% of total adult fractures
0.46% of adult femoral fractures
5.27% of segment 33
28.19% of type 33-B

33-B3.1

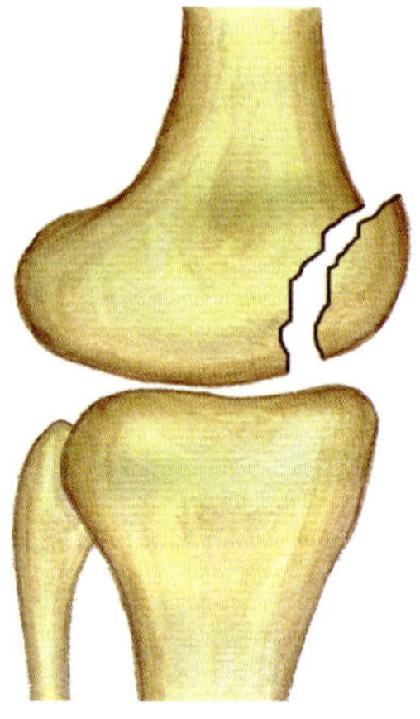

Anterior and lateral flake fracture

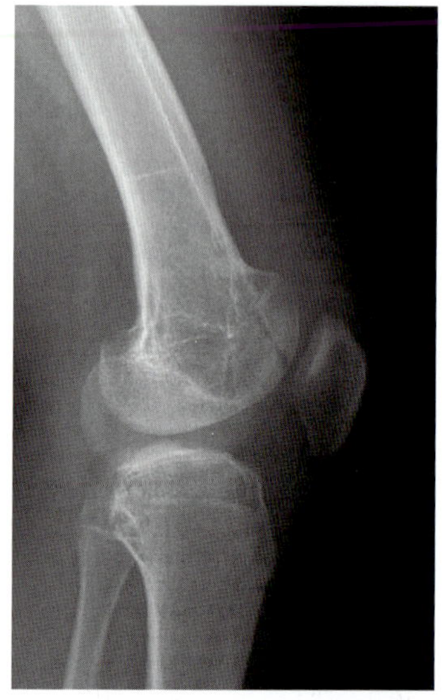

33-B3.2

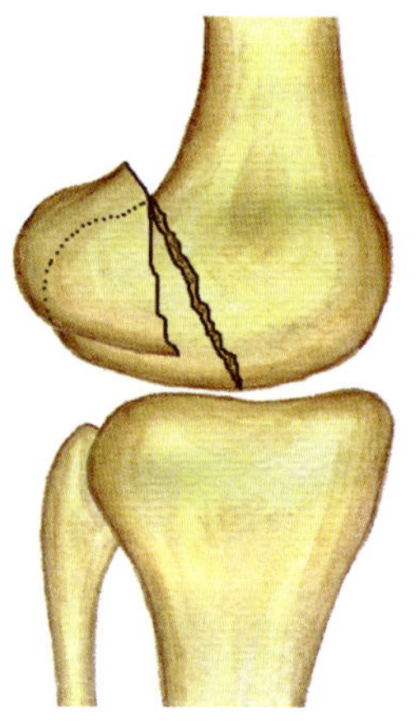

Unicondylar posterior

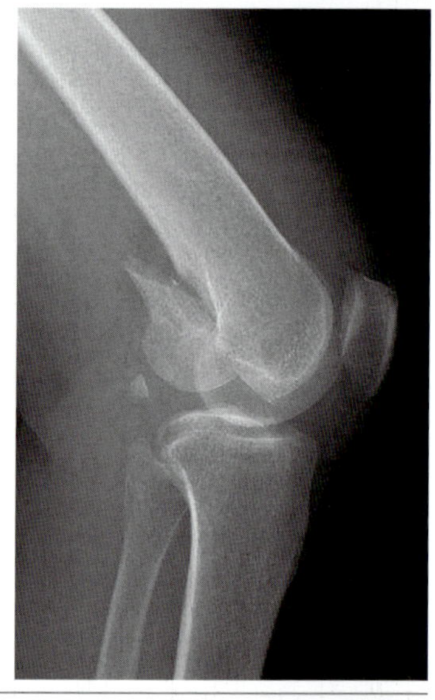

33-B3.3

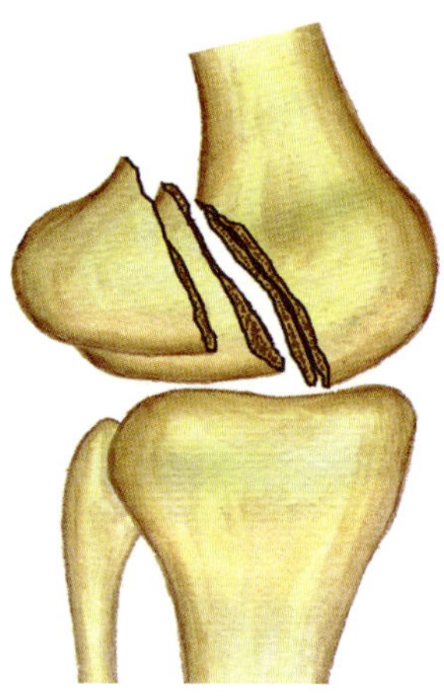

Bicondylar posterior

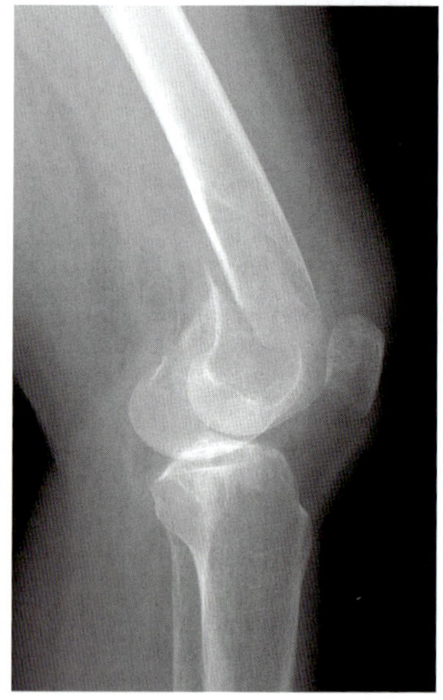

33-C Femur distal, complete-articular fractures

33-C1

Metaphyseal simple, articular simple

179 fractures
M: 103 (57.54%)
F: 76 (42.46%)
0.05% of total adult fractures
0.45% of adult femoral fractures
5.21% of segment 33
16.68% of type 33-C

33-C1.1

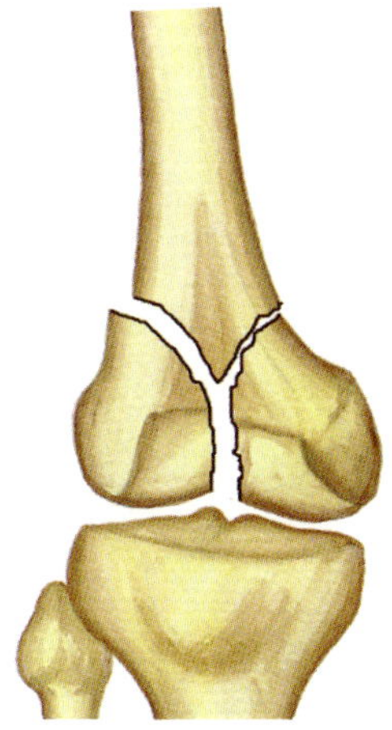

T- or Y-shaped fracture with slight displacement

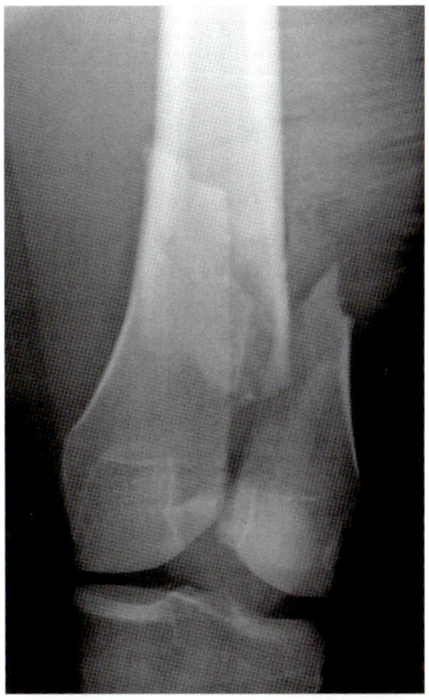

33-C1.2

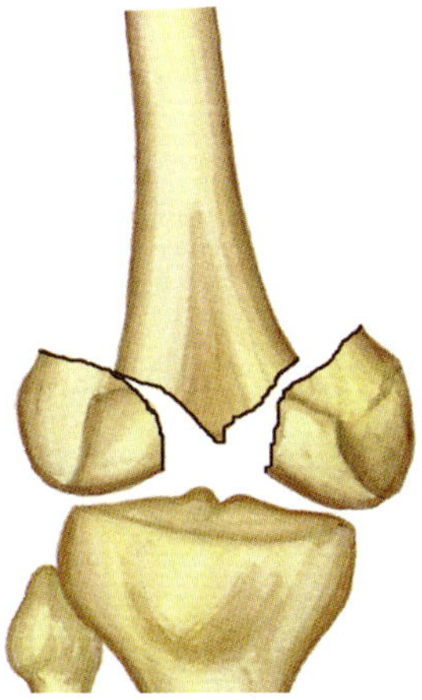

Y-shaped fracture with marked displacement

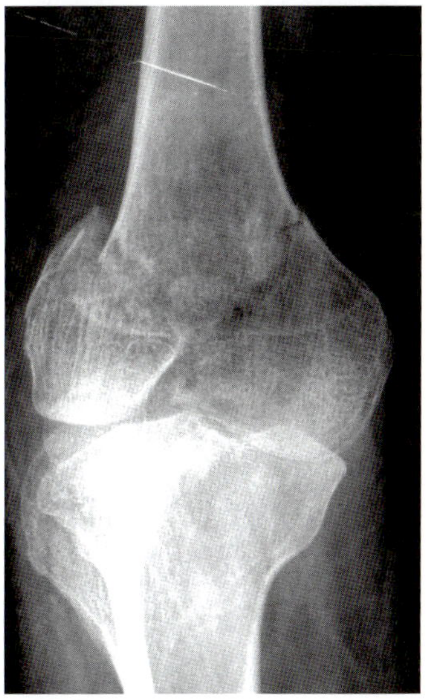

33-C1.3

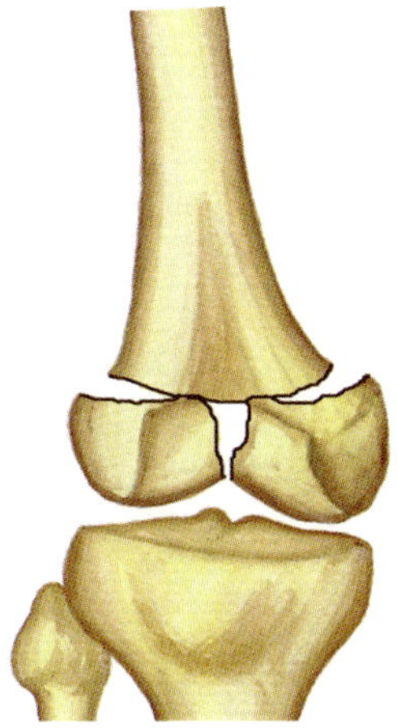

T-shaped fracture

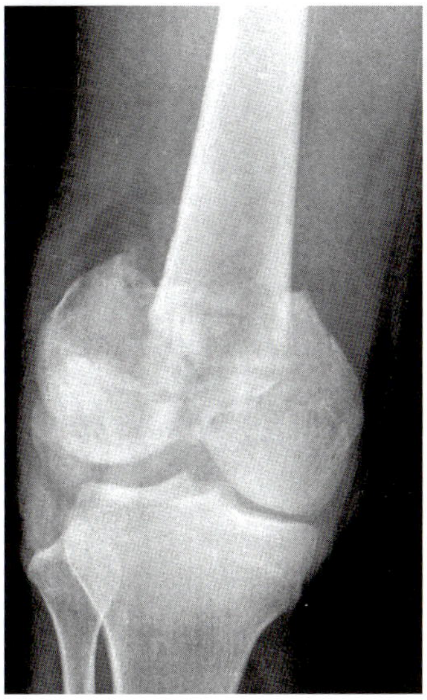

33-C Femur distal, complete-articular fractures

33-C2
Metaphyseal multifragmentary, articular simple
578 fractures
M: 410 (70.93%)
F: 168 (29.07%)
0.15% of total adult fractures
1.46% of adult femoral fractures
16.83% of segment 33
53.87% of type 33-C

33-C2.1

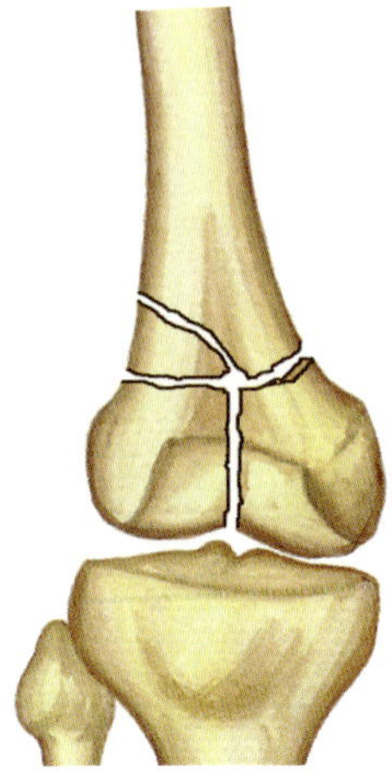

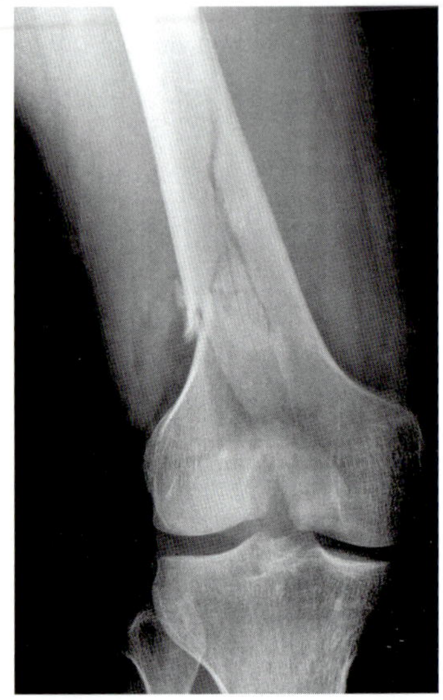

With an intact wedge fragment

33-C2.2

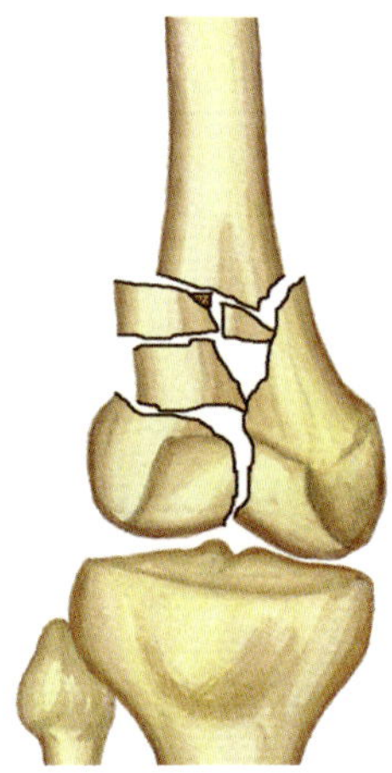

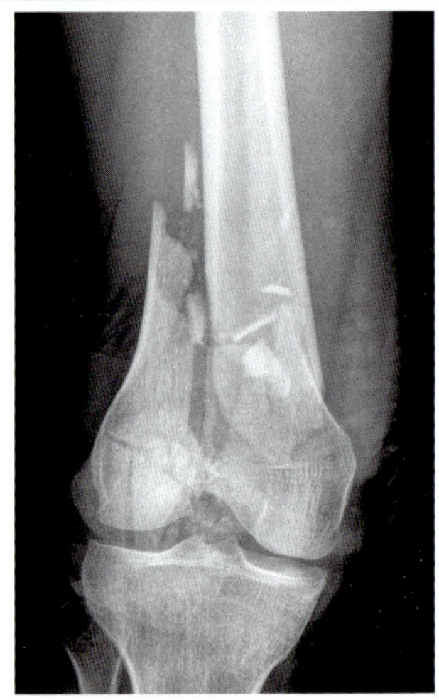

With a fragmented wedge

33-C2.3

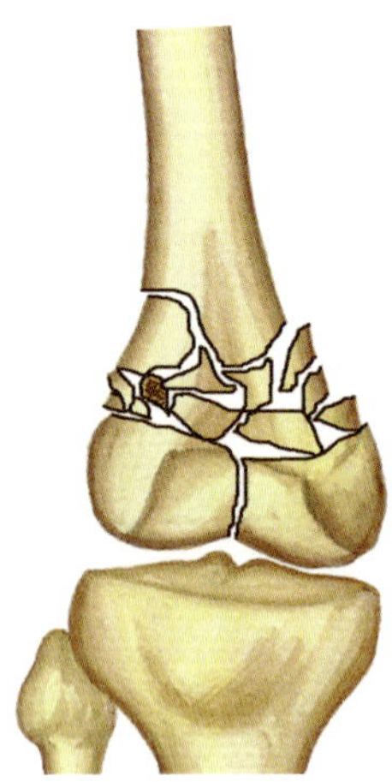

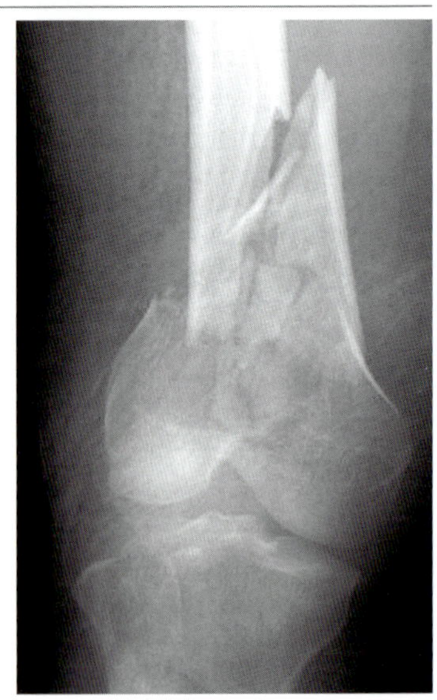

Metaphyseal complex

33-C Femur distal, complete-articular fractures

33-C3
Articular multifragmentary
316 fractures
M: 237 (75%)
F: 79 (25%)
0.08% of total adult fractures
0.80% of adult femoral fractures
9.20% of segment 33
29.45% of type 33-C

33-C3.1

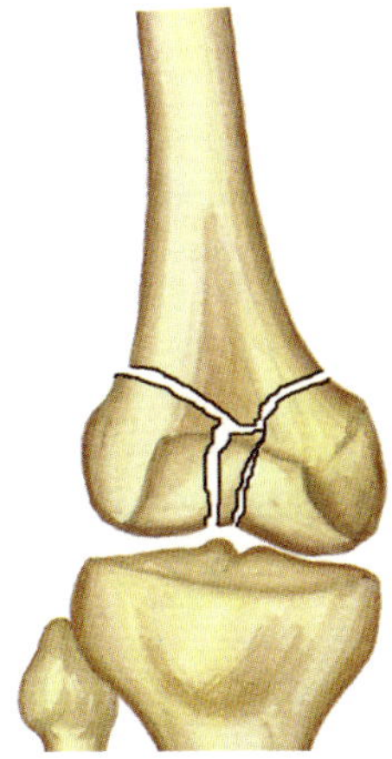

Metaphyseal simple, articular multifragmentary

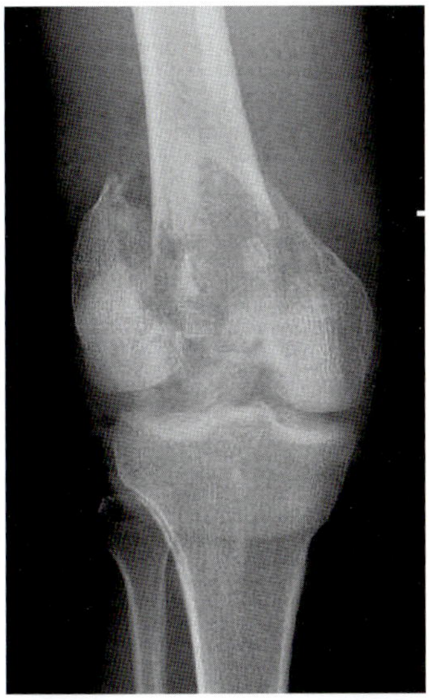

33-C3.2

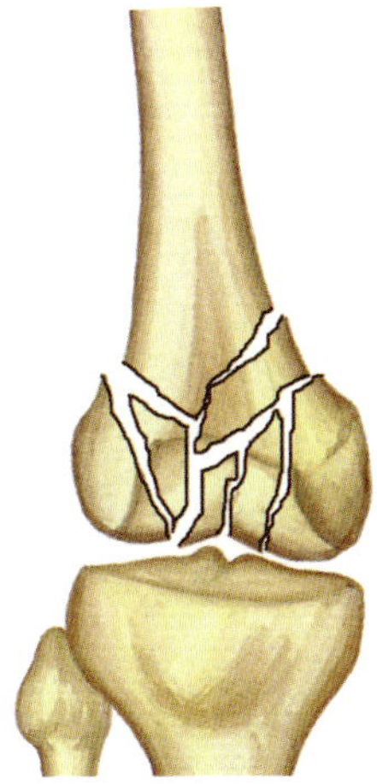

Metaphyseal multifragmentary, articular multifragmentary

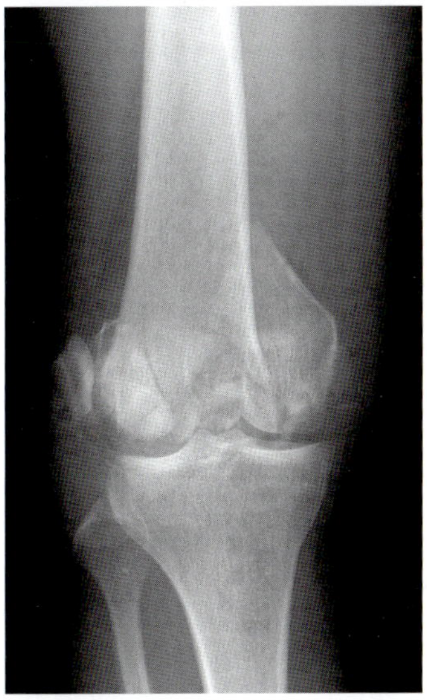

33-C3.3

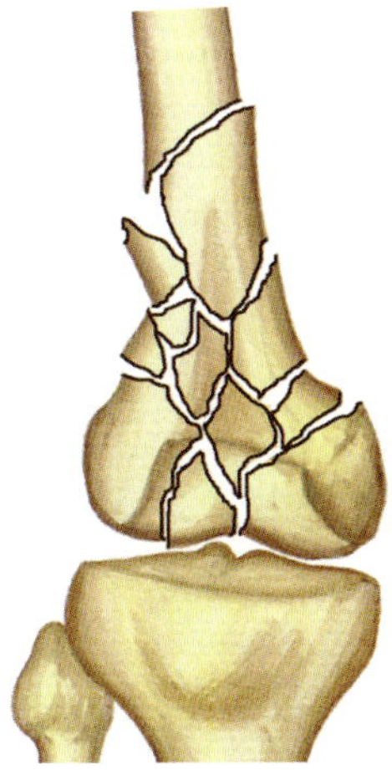

Metaphysio-diaphyseal multifragmentary

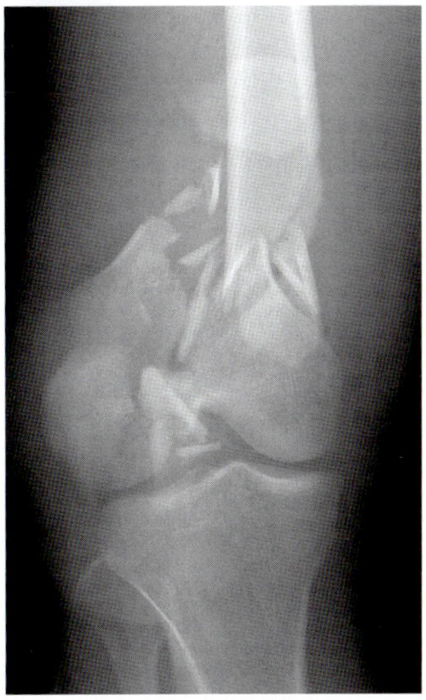

Injury Mechanism

Supracondylar Femoral Fractures

These types of fractures are usually found 2–4 cm superior to the insertion of the gastrocnemius and are caused by a direct blow to the femoral supracondyle or by indirect force, as seen in a fall from a significant height with the knee joint in flexion. Supracondylar fractures are generally transverse or oblique, and occasionally complex or associated with condylar fractures. When supracondylar fractures occur, the resulting posterior displacement of the distal fragment may injure the popliteal artery.

Femoral Condyle Fractures

Direct violent force on the femoral condyle frequently results in complex fractures, while V-, Y-, or T-shaped fractures can result from axial compression on the knee.

Diagnosis

The patient with a distal femoral fracture typically presents with pain, swelling, bony crepitus, decreased range of motion, and deformity of the affected limb. Hematoma of the knee joint may follow after intercondylar or condylar fractures. Radiographic examination for a fracture around the knee should include the standard AP, lateral, and oblique views. The 45-degree oblique views are useful in detecting fracture displacement if femoral condylar fracture is suspected. If distal femoral fractures occur in children, comparison views of the opposite extremity may be helpful in attempting to differentiate a fracture from a normal site. Femoral intercondylar fractures are severe intra-articular fractures, with a T- or Y-shaped fracture line, frequently accompanied by supracondylar fractures. A CT scan is useful in delineating the fracture, and detecting the severity of the fracture and the direction of the fracture displacement. If popliteal hematomas appear with weakened or absent pulsation in the dorsal artery of the foot following the supracondylar fracture, an angiogram should be considered to investigate popliteal artery injury.

4

Treatment

Appropriate internal fixators should be chosen for fixation of distal femoral fractures depending on the fracture patterns. The 95-degree condylar blade plate and DCS are classic internal fixators used to treat extra-articular complex and articular simple fractures. Femoral comminuted condylar fractures involving the frontal plane should be treated primarily with condylar buttress plates. The screw inserted into the condylar buttress plate provides enhanced fixation. Determination of the number of the screws is based on the individual circumstance. After the articular reduction under direct visualization, lag screws can be used to treat intra-articular fractures of the distal femur to provide compression between the fracture fragments. Retrograde intramedullary nails, locking compression plate (LCP), or less Invasive stabilization system (LISS) can be used for fixation of extra-articular and simple intra-articular fractures. Open fractures can be treated with external fixators.

Other Classification of Femoral Fractures

Evans' Classification for Trochanteric Fractures of the Femur

Evans presented his classification for trochanteric fractures of the femur based on the stability of the fracture. He proposed that the stability of proximal femoral fractures is dependent on posteromedial cortical continuity. In stable fracture patterns, the posteromedial cortex remains intact or has minimal fragmentation, while large posteromedial cortical fragments can be seen in unstable fracture patterns. If restoration of the posteromedial cortical continuity can be performed surgically, the unstable fracture can be reduced and stabilized. In addition, Evans described a fracture pattern called reversed obliquity fracture, which is inherently unstable. Evans' classification has the qualities of utility and ease of use, with emphasis on the difference between stable and unstable fractures.

A total of 12,743 trochanteric fractures of the femur were treated in 83 hospitals in China over a 2-year period from 2010 to 2011. All cases were reviewed and statistically studied.

Epidemiologic features of trochanteric femoral fractures are as follows:

- More males than females
- The most common fracture type based on Evans' classification is type I, the same fracture type in both males and females

Evans' classification of trochanteric femur fractures		
Type I 3,328 fractures M: 1,719 (51.65%) F: 1,609 (48.35%) 26.12% of adult trochanteric fractures	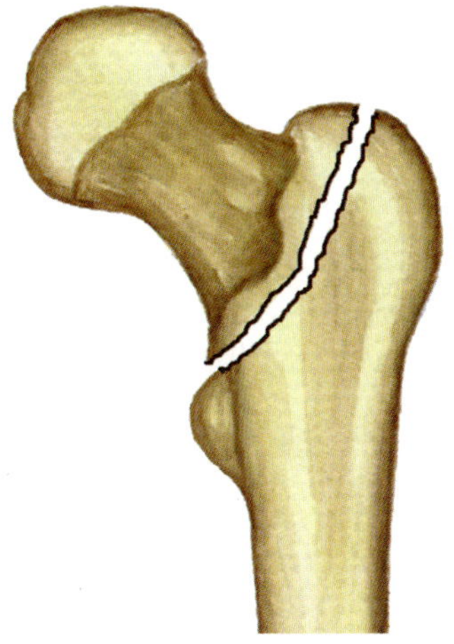 Nondisplaced two-fragment fracture Stable fracture	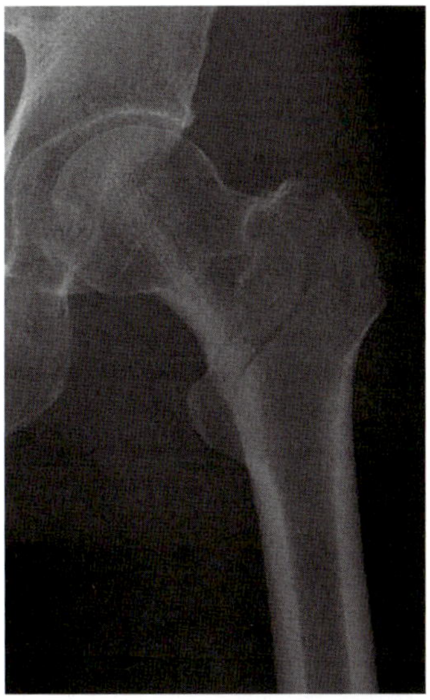
Type II 2,468 fractures M: 1,126 (45.62%) F: 1,342 (54.38%) 19.37% of adult trochanteric fractures	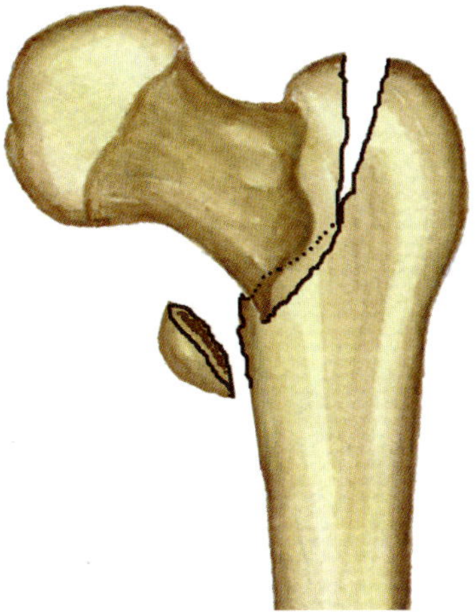 Lesser trochanter fracture with slight displacement Stable fracture	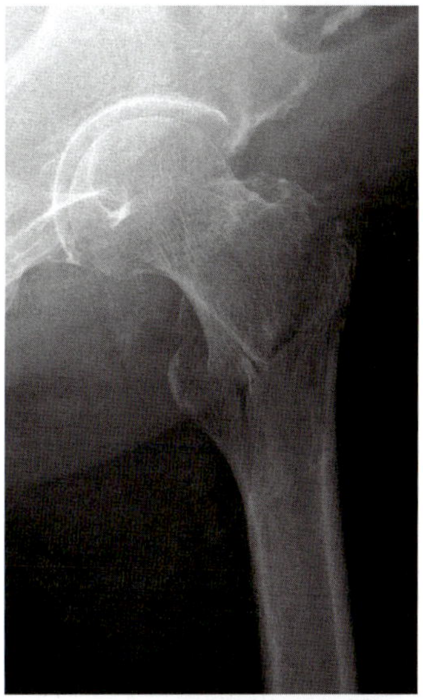
Type III 3,030 fractures M: 1,442 (47.59%) F: 1,588 (52.41%) 23.78% of adult trochanteric fractures	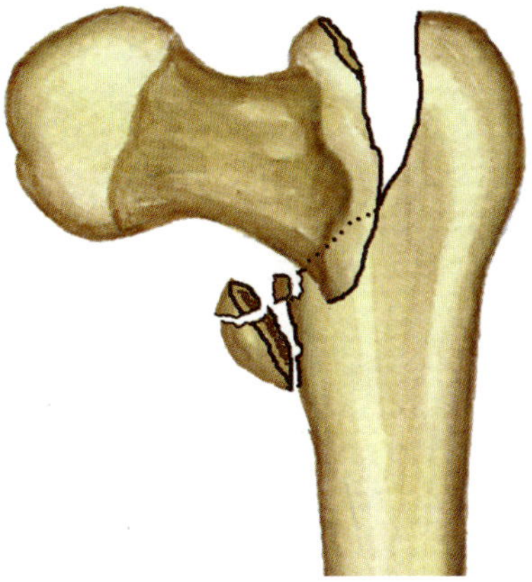 Lesser trochanter multifragmentary without posterolateral support	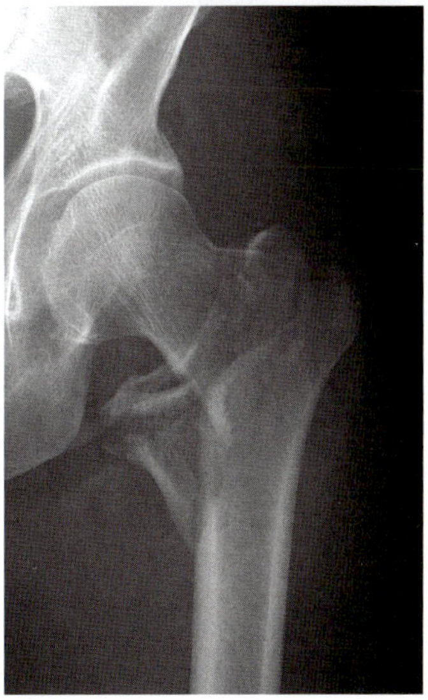

Type IV
1,910 fractures
M: 974 (50.99%)
F: 936 (49.01%)
14.99% of adult trochanteric fractures

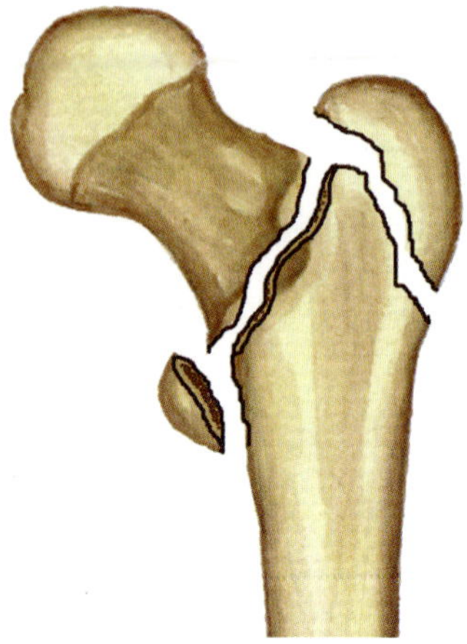

Type III + greater trochanter fracture
Unstable fracture

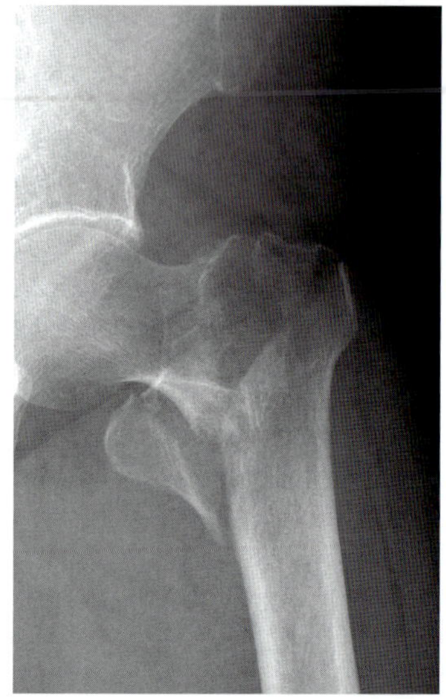

Type V
2,007 fractures
M: 1,219 (60.74%)
F: 788 (39.26%)
15.75% of adult trochanteric fractures

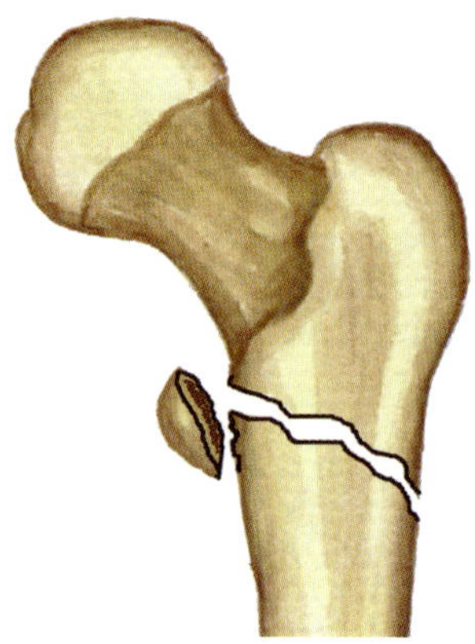

Reversed obliquity fracture with fracture line running upward and inward; extends above the lesser trochanter
Unstable fracture

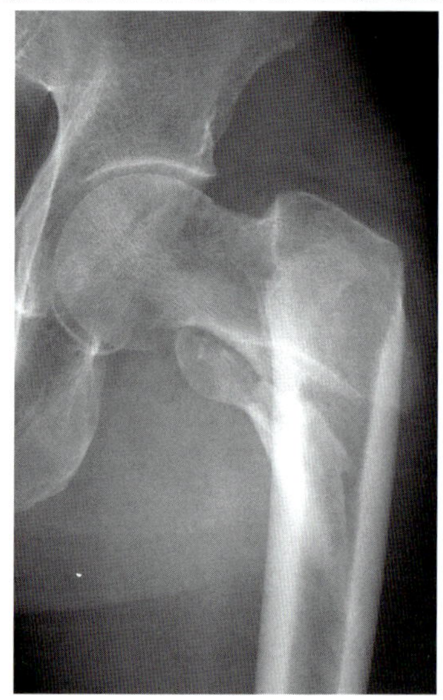

Table 4.18 Sex and fracture type distribution of 12,743 trochanteric fractures of the femur by Evans' classification

Fracture type	Male	Female	Number of fractures	Percentage (%)
I	1,719	1,609	3,328	26.12
II	1,126	1,342	2,468	19.37
III	1,442	1,588	3,030	23.78
IV	974	936	1,910	14.99
V	1,219	788	2,007	15.75
Total	6,480	6,263	12,743	100.00

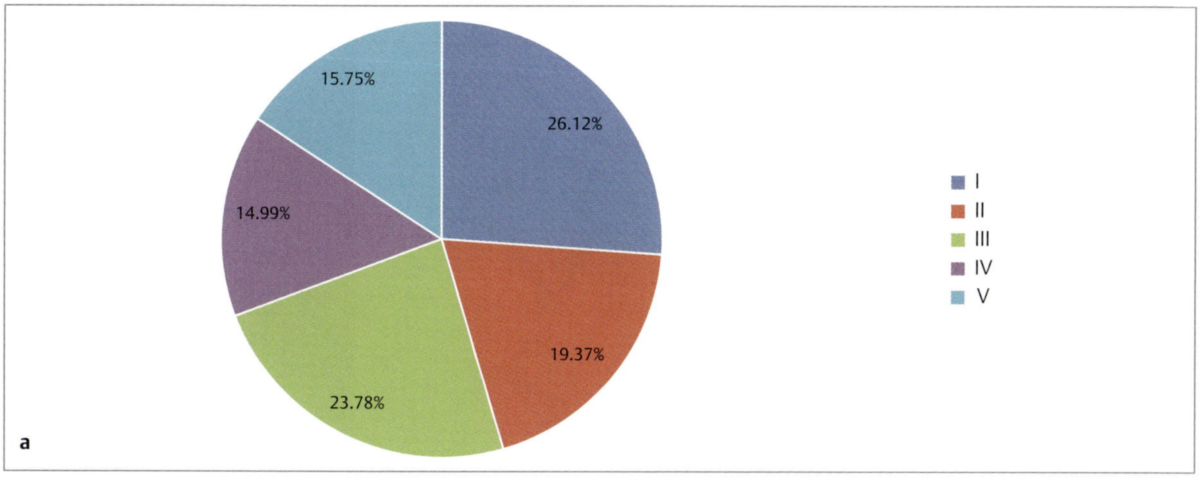

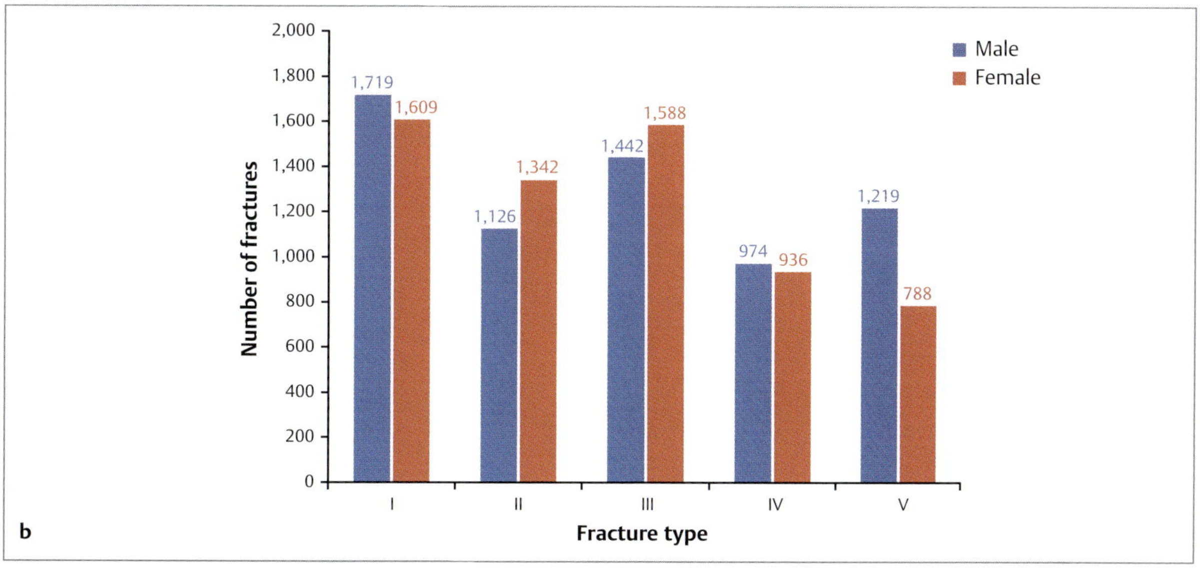

Fig. 4.18 **(a)** Fracture type distribution of 12,743 trochanteric fractures by Evans' classification.
(b) Sex and fracture type distribution of 12,743 trochanteric fractures by Evans' classification.

Garden Classification of Femoral Neck Fractures

Garden proposed a classification method for femoral neck fractures based on the degree of fracture displacement.

- *Type I*: incomplete or impacted fracture of the neck.
- *Type II*: complete fracture without displacement.
- *Type III*: complete fracture with marked displacement, and often accompanied by shortening and external rotation of the limb.
- *Type IV*: complete fracture with full displacement. The proximal fragment is not in contact with the distal part. Multifragmentation may occur.

A total of 13,516 femoral neck fractures were treated in 83 hospitals in China over a 2-year period from 2010 to 2011. All cases were reviewed and statistically studied. Epidemiologic features of femoral neck fractures are as follows:

- More females than males
- The most common fracture type based on the Garden classification is type III, the same fracture type in both males and females.

4

Garden classification of femoral neck fractures		
Type I 203 fractures M: 121 (59.61%) F: 82 (40.39%) 1.50% of adult femur neck	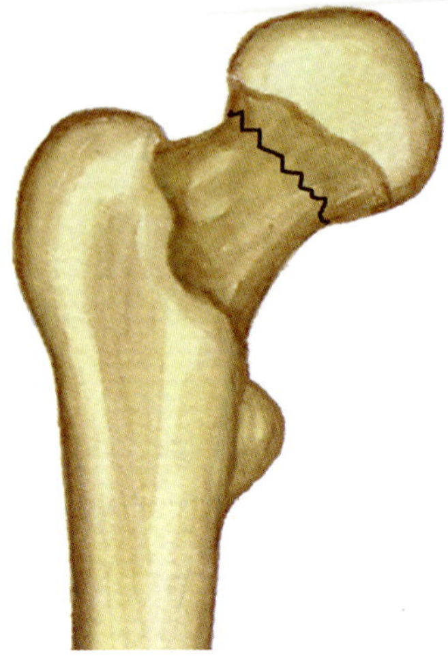 Incomplete fracture	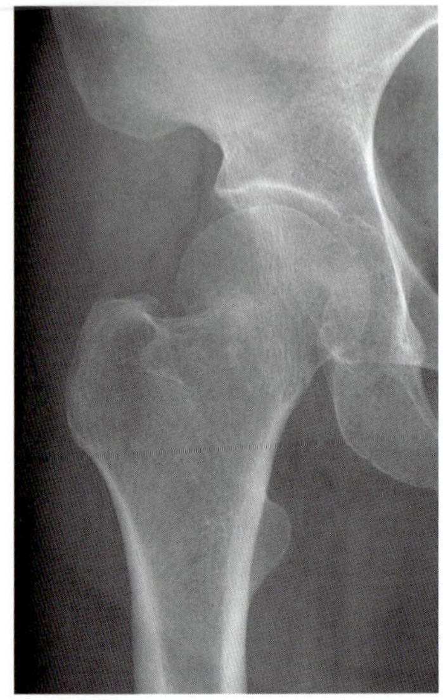
Type II 3,585 fractures M: 1,576 (43.96%) F: 2,009 (56.04%) 26.52% of adult femur neck	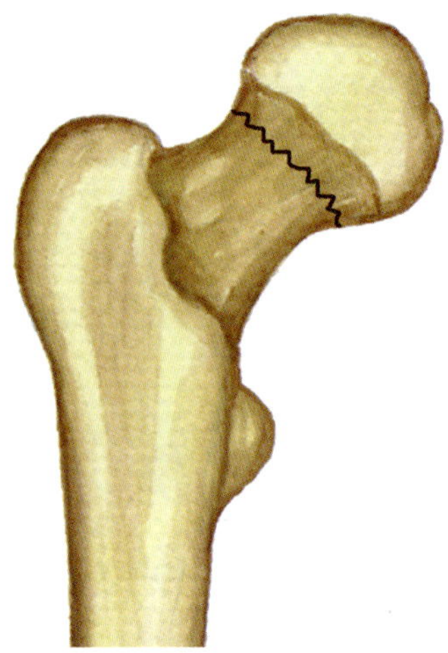 Complete fracture without displacement	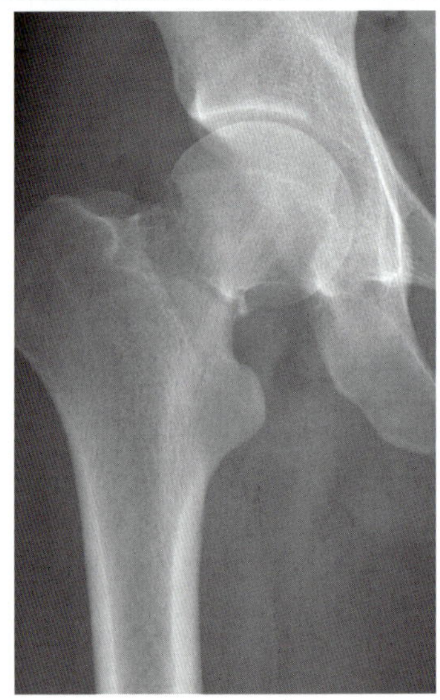

Garden classification of femoral neck fractures

Type III
8,457 fractures
M: 3,457 (40.88%)
F: 5,000 (59.12%)
62.57% of adult femur neck

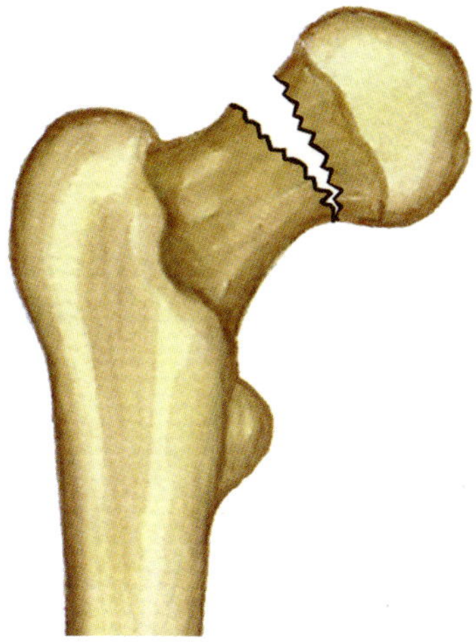

Complete fracture with displacement

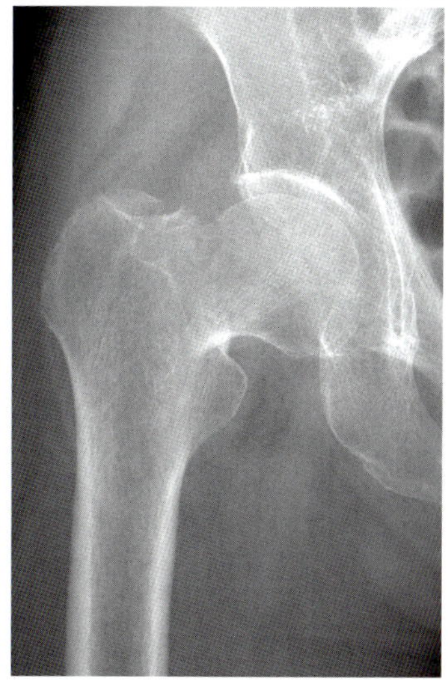

Type IV
1,271 fractures
M: 481 (37.84%)
F: 790 (62.16%)
9.40% of adult femur neck

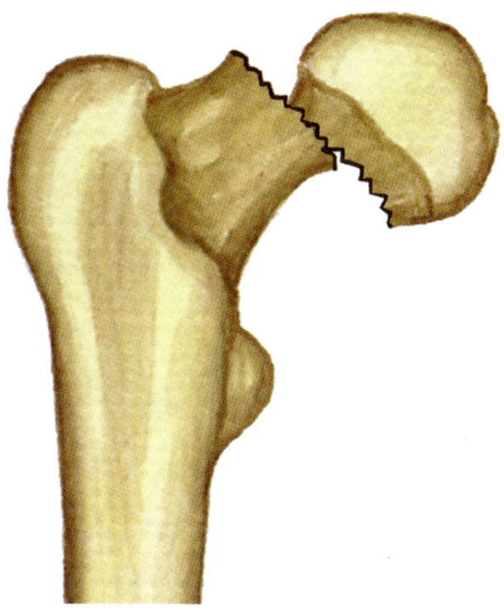

Complete fracture, multifragmentary

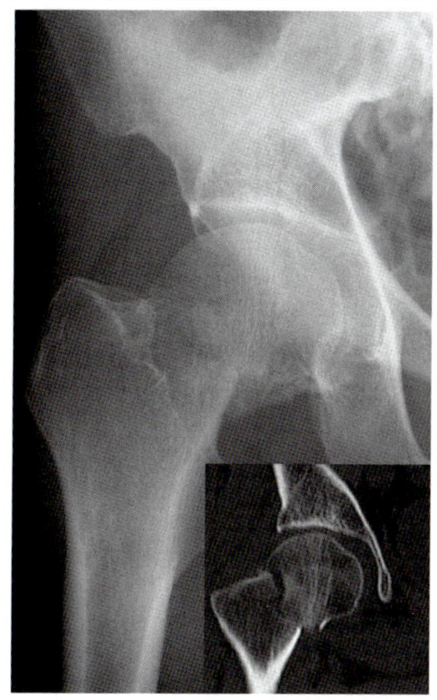

Table 4.19 Sex and fracture type distribution of 13,516 femoral neck fractures by Garden classification

Fracture type	Male	Female	Number of fractures	Percentage (%)
I	121	82	203	1.50
II	1,576	2,009	3,585	26.52
III	3,457	5,000	8,457	62.57
IV	481	790	1,271	9.40
Total	5,635	7,881	13,516	100.00

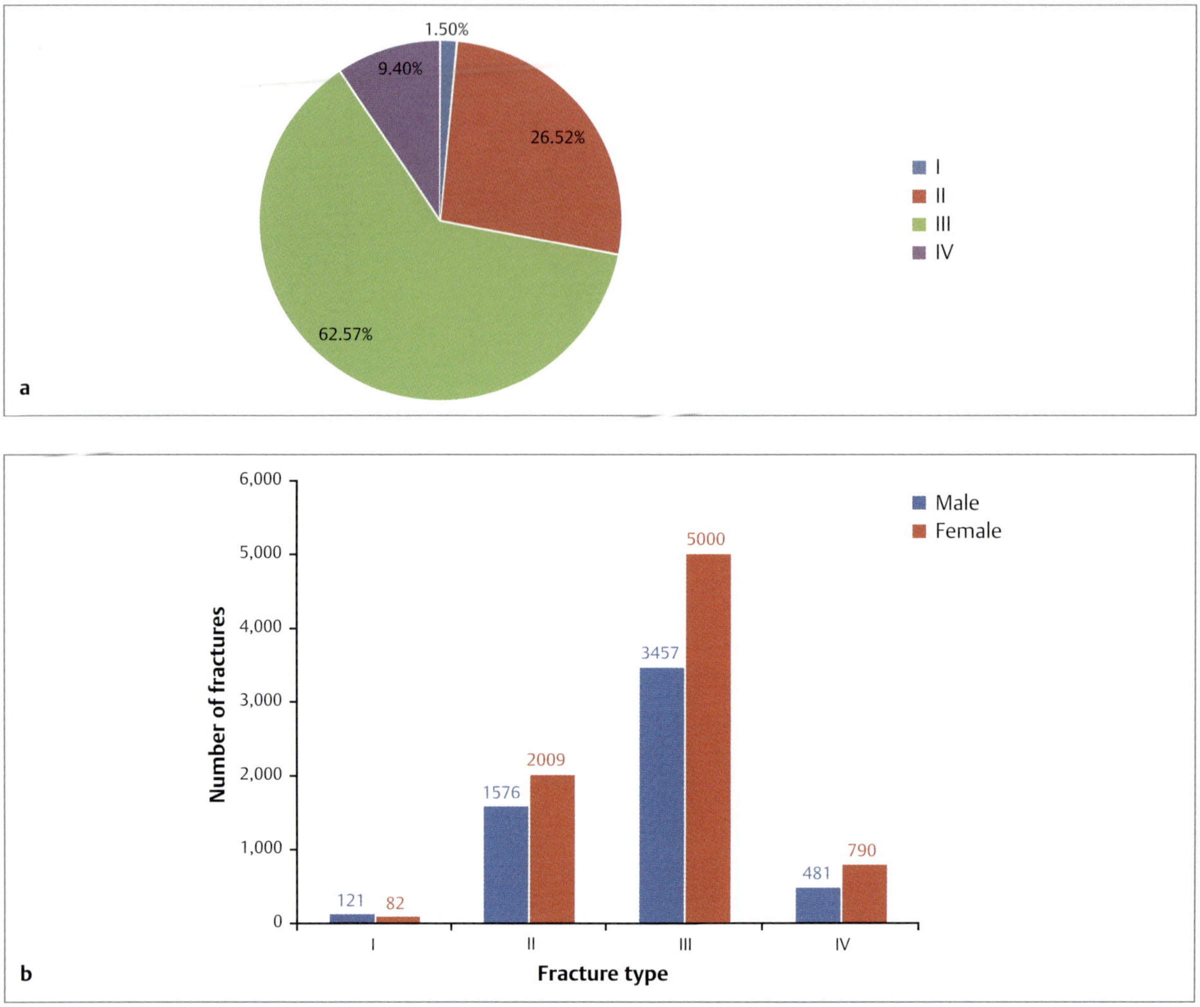

Fig. 4.19 **(a)** Fracture type distribution of 13,516 femoral neck fractures by Garden classification. **(b)** Sex and fracture type distribution of 13,516 femoral neck fractures by Garden classification.

Pipkin Classification of Femoral Head Fractures

Pipkin proposed a classification system for femoral head fractures in association with posterior dislocation of the hip that is very useful in guiding treatment and predicting prognosis. He divided femoral head fractures into four types.

- *Type I*: fracture of the femoral head inferior to the fovea centralis. Since the fracture is not within the weight-bearing area of the head, small, comminuted fragments can be excised without compromising outcome. If the fragment is large, absorbable screws can be used for fixation after the reduction.
- *Type II*: fracture of the femoral head superior to the fovea centralis. This fracture pattern involves the weight-bearing area of the head and requires anatomical reduction followed by absorbable screws for fixation. Each screw should be inserted perpendicular to the fracture line, with the head of the nail beneath the subchondral bone.
- *Type III*: similar to a type I or II injury but associated with fracture of the femoral neck. This injury is the most disruptive to the vascular supply of the femoral head, with high incidence of avascular necrosis and nonunion of the femoral head. For patients older than 65 years, total hip replacement should be recommended. In younger patients, anatomical reduction should be considered first.
- *Type IV*: similar to a type I or II injury but associated with fracture of the acetabular rim. Reconstruction plates can be used for fixation of the acetabular fracture after anatomical reduction of the femoral head.

A total of 1,768 femoral head fractures were treated at 83 hospitals in China over a 2-year period from 2010 to 2011. All cases were reviewed and statistically studied.

Epidemiologic features of femoral head fractures are as follows:

- More males than females
- The most common fracture type based on Pipkin classification is type II, the same fracture type in both males and females.

Pipkin classification of femoral head fractures		
Type I 455 fractures M: 257 (56.48%) F: 198 (43.52%) 25.74% of adult femoral head fractures	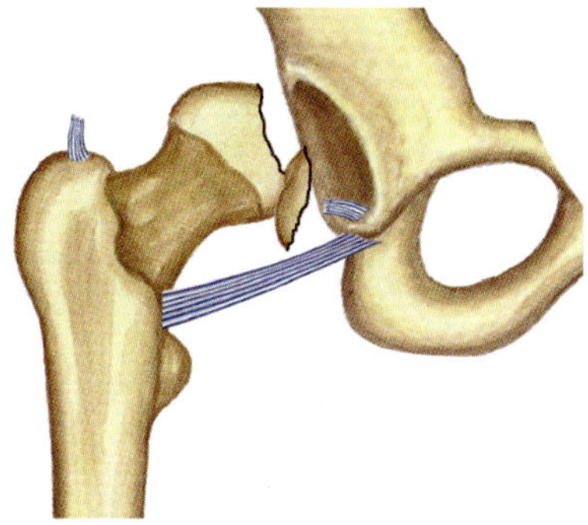 Fracture inferior to the fovea centralis	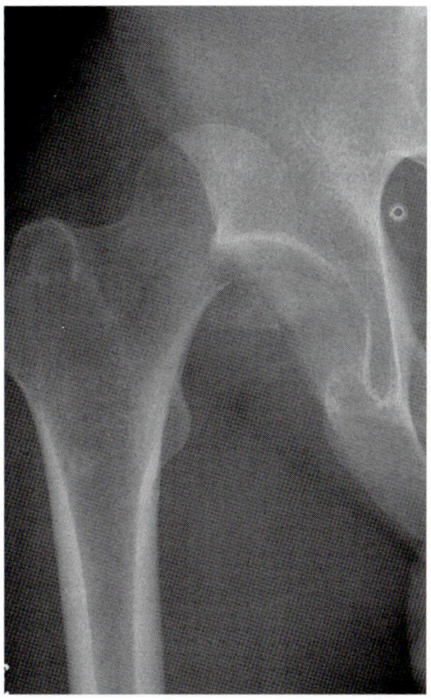
Type II 906 fractures M: 539 (59.49%) F: 367 (40.51%) 51.24% of adult femoral head fractures	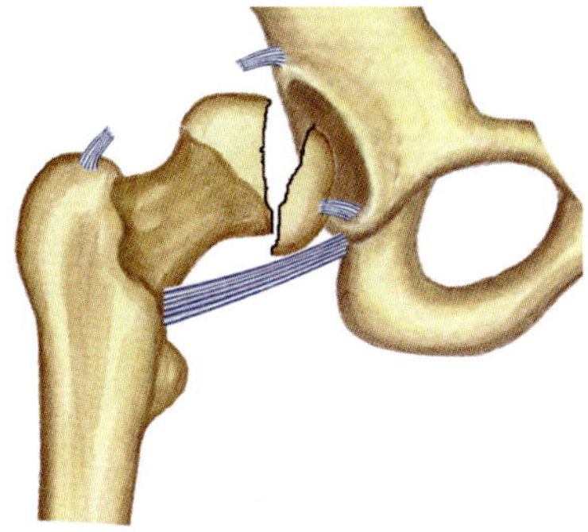 Fracture superior to the fovea centralis	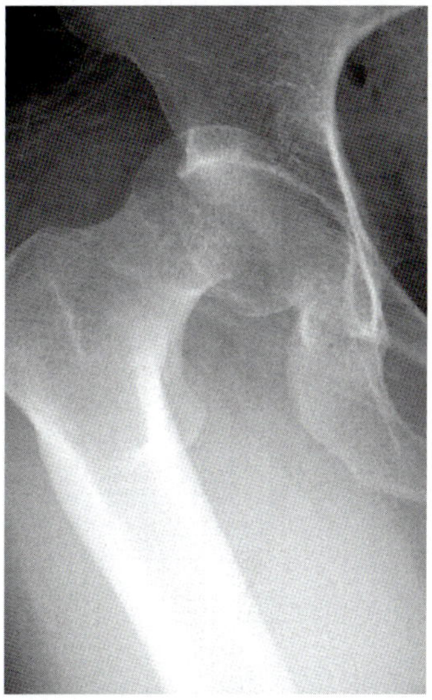
Type III 349 fractures M: 198 (56.73%) F: 151 (43.27%) 19.74% of adult femoral head fractures	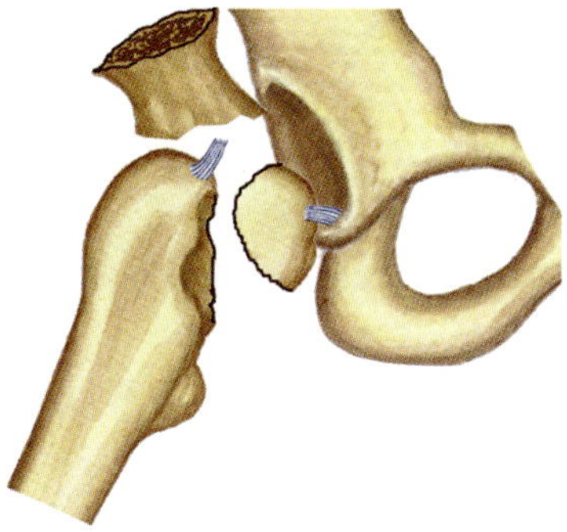 Type I or II associated with fracture of femoral neck	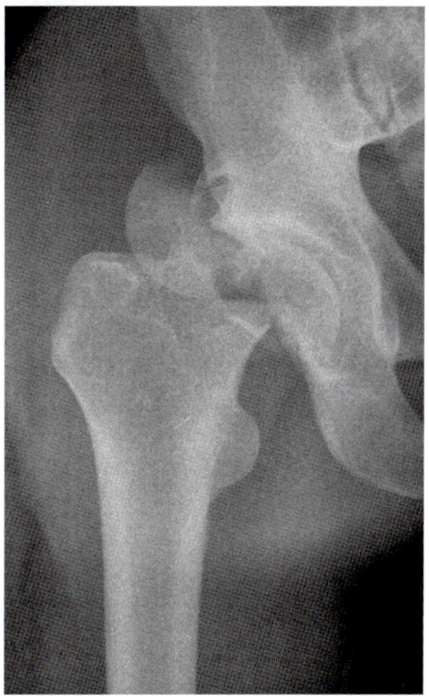

Type IV
58 fractures
M: 45 (77.59%)
F: 13 (22.41%)
3.28% of adult femoral head fractures

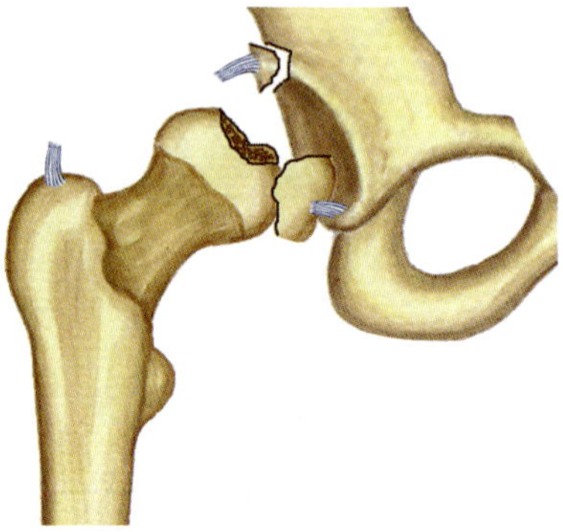

Type I or II associated with fracture of acetabular rim

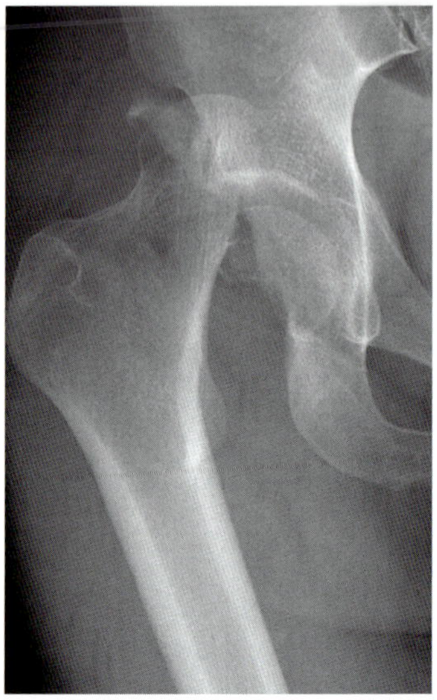

Table 4.20 Sex and fracture type distribution of 1,768 femoral head fractures by Pipkin classification

Fracture type	Male	Female	Number of fractures	Percentage (%)
I	257	198	455	25.74
II	539	367	906	51.24
III	198	151	349	19.74
IV	45	13	58	3.28
Total	1,039	729	1,768	100.00

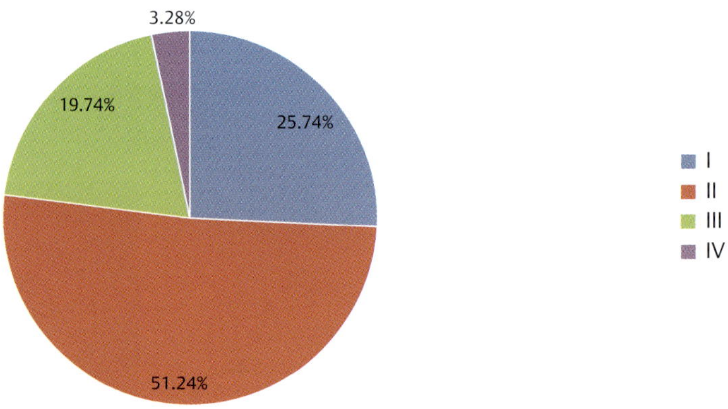

Fig. 4.20 **(a)** Fracture type distribution of 1,768 femoral head fractures by Pipkin classification.

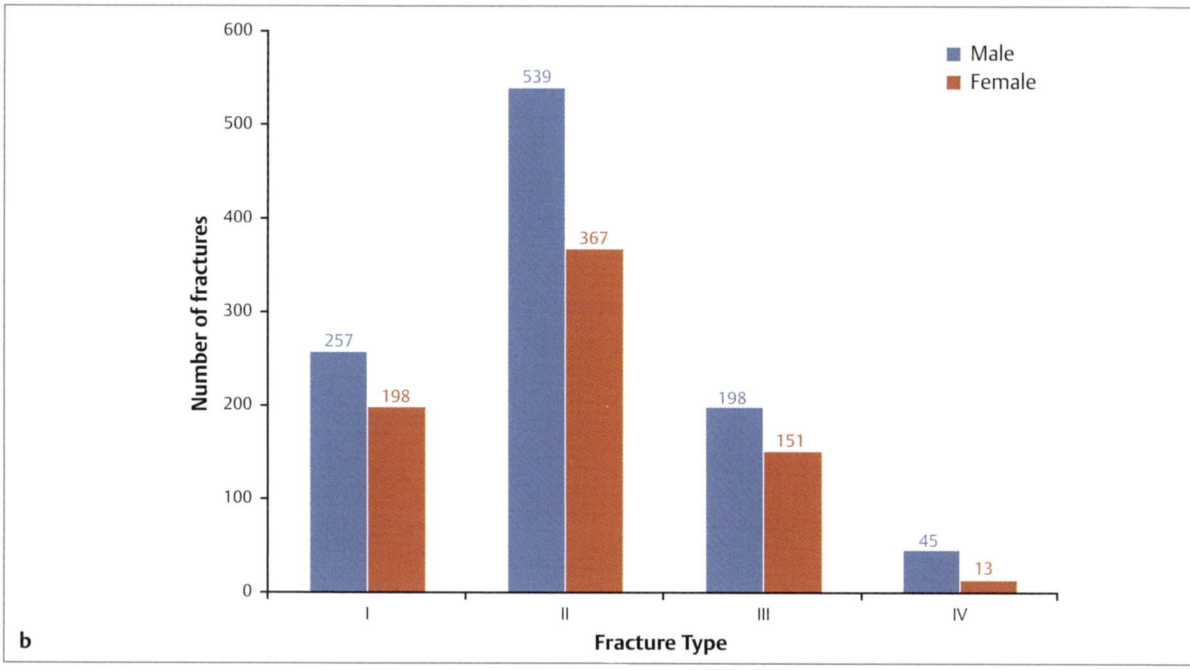

Fig. 4.20 (*continued*) **(b)** Sex and fracture type distribution of 1,768 femoral head fractures by Pipkin classification.

4

5 Fractures of the Tibia and Fibula

Overview

Anatomical Features

The tibia is a large weight-bearing bone, located on the anterior and medial side of the leg. The proximal end of the tibia extends laterally to form the medial and lateral tibial plateaus that articulate with the femoral condyles. Both plateaus slope posteriorly ~ 10 degrees. The medial plateau possesses higher mechanical strength and is better suited to withstand compression than the lateral plateau. The body of the tibia has three borders and three surfaces. It is sinuous and prominent in its upper two-thirds, but smooth and recessed below. The anterior border begins above at the tuberosity and ends below at the anterior margin of the medial malleolus. Tibia fractures are most often found at the junction of the middle and lower thirds of the bone, where tibial dimensions change. The fibula is situated on the lateral side of the tibia, to which it provides a small amount of support. The fibular head and distal third of the fibula are just beneath the skin surface, with the remaining parts attached by muscles and ligaments. The medial malleolus of the tibia and the distal end of the fibula, along with the talar articulations, form the ankle mortise. The continuity of the fibula is very important in maintaining the stability of the ankle mortise (**Plate 5.1**).

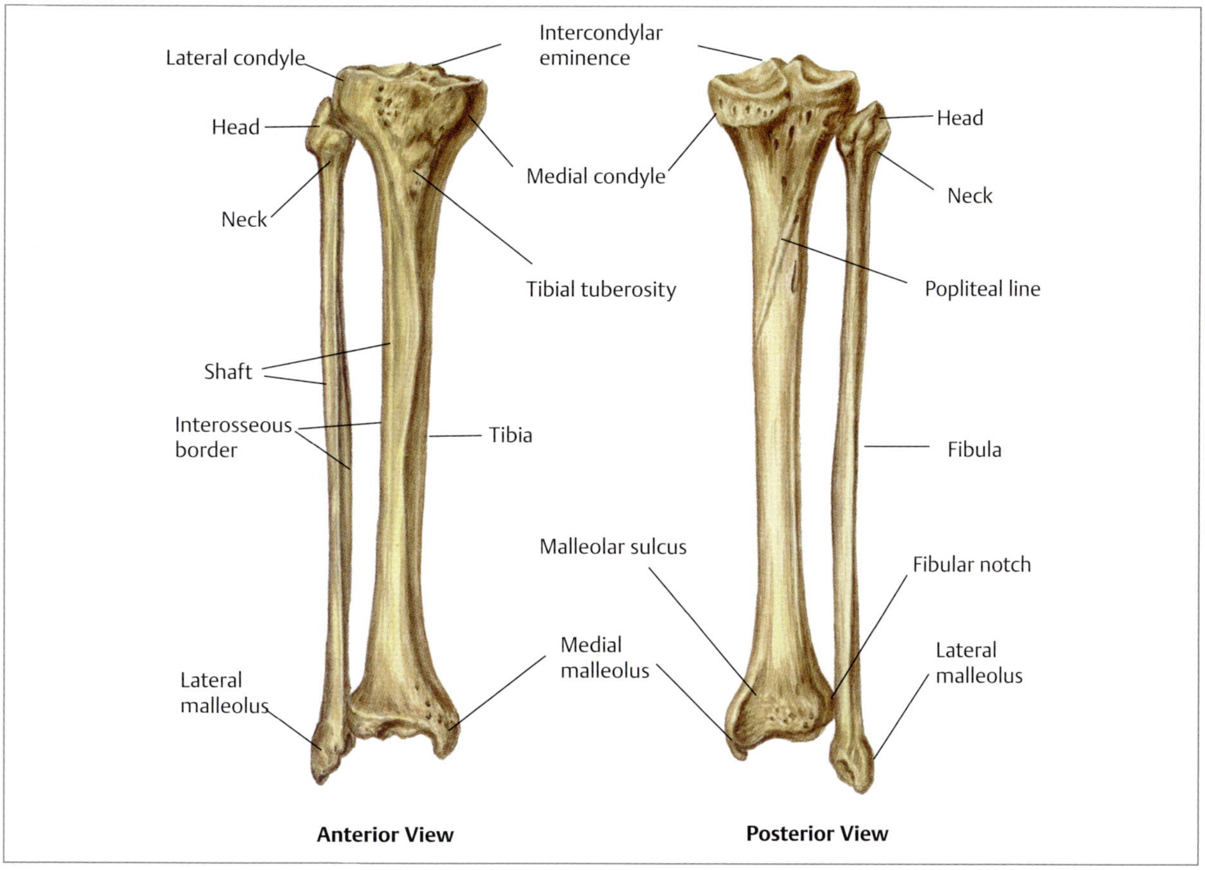

Plate 5.1

AO Classification and Coding System of Fractures of the Tibia and Fibula

Based on AO classification, the tibia and fibula can be considered as one unit, with the coding number 4. According to the Heim's square method, the anatomical assignment of the proximal, shaft, and distal portions are the numbers 41, 42, and 43, respectively. Malleolar fractures are the exception to the rule of dividing each long bone into three bony segments based on their anatomical characteristics. They are segment 44 of the tibial bone (**Plate 5.2**).

Clinical Epidemiologic Features of Fractures of the Tibia and Fibula

A total of 66,758 patients with 68,878 fractures of the tibia/fibula were treated in 83 hospitals in China over a 2-year period from 2010 to 2011. All cases were reviewed and statistically studied; the fractures accounted for 16.09% of all patients with fractures and 15.95% of all types of fractures, respectively. Among these 66,758 patients, 8,144 were children with 8,264 fractures, and 58,614 were adults with 60,614 fractures.

Epidemiologic features of tibia/fibula fractures are as follows:

- More males than females
- More left-side than right-side injuries
- The high-risk age group is 41–45 years. The most affected male age group is 41–45 years, while females aged 56–60 years have the highest risk.
- The malleolar injury is the most common tibia/fibula fracture.

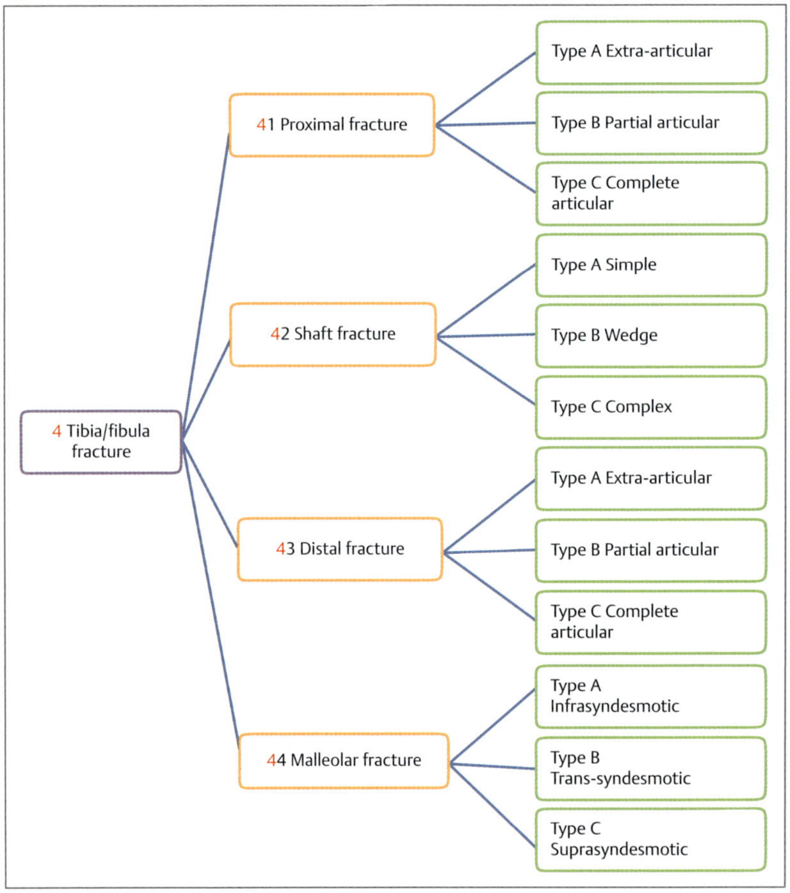

Plate 5.2

Tibia/Fibula Fractures by Sex

Table 5.1 Sex distribution of 66,758 patients with tibia/fibula fractures

Sex	Number of patients	Percentage (%)
Male	44,438	66.57
Female	22,320	33.43
Total	66,758	100.00

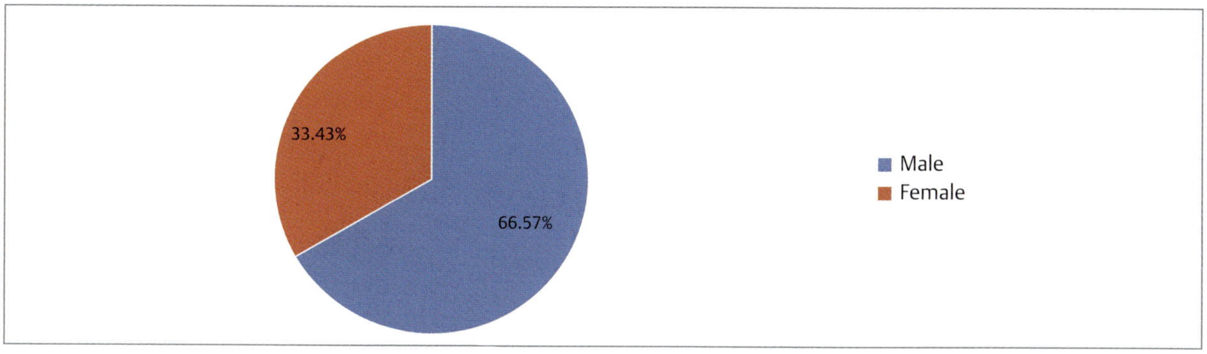

Fig. 5.1 Sex distribution of 66,758 patients with tibia/fibula fractures.

Tibia/Fibula Fractures by Injury Side

Table 5.2 Injury side distribution of 66,758 patients with tibia/fibula fractures

Injury side	Number of patients	Percentage (%)
Left	33,308	49.89
Right	32,700	48.98
Bilateral	750	1.12
Total	66,758	100.00

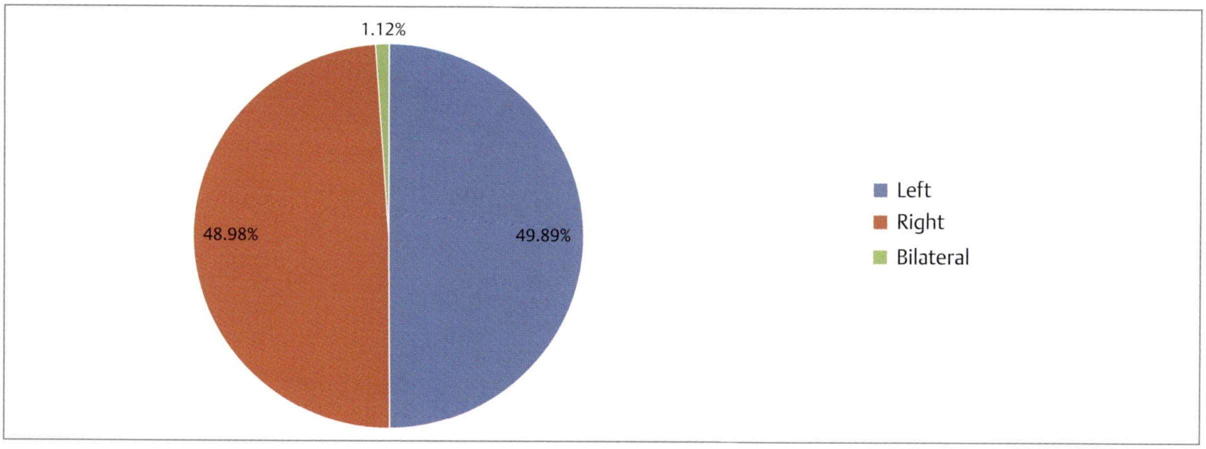

Fig. 5.2 Injury side distribution of 66,758 patients with tibia/fibula fractures.

Tibia/Fibula Fractures by Age Group

Table 5.3 Age and sex distribution of 66,758 patients with tibia/fibula fractures

Age group (years)	Male	Female	Number of patients	Percentage (%)
0–5	1,652	837	2,489	3.73
6–10	1,643	836	2,479	3.71
11–15	2,315	861	3,176	4.76
16–20	3,355	1,009	4,364	6.54
21–25	4,283	1,405	5,688	8.52
26–30	3,828	1,273	5,101	7.64
31–35	3,950	1,348	5,298	7.94
36–40	4,958	1,888	6,846	10.25
41–45	5,095	2,083	7,178	10.75
46–50	4,178	2,198	6,376	9.55
51–55	3,150	2,162	5,312	7.96
56–60	2,578	2,298	4,876	7.30
61–65	1,452	1,437	2,889	4.33
66–70	777	1,003	1,780	2.67
71–75	566	762	1,328	1.99
76–80	364	566	930	1.39
81–85	221	228	449	0.67
≥86	73	126	199	0.30
Total	44,438	22,320	66,758	100.00

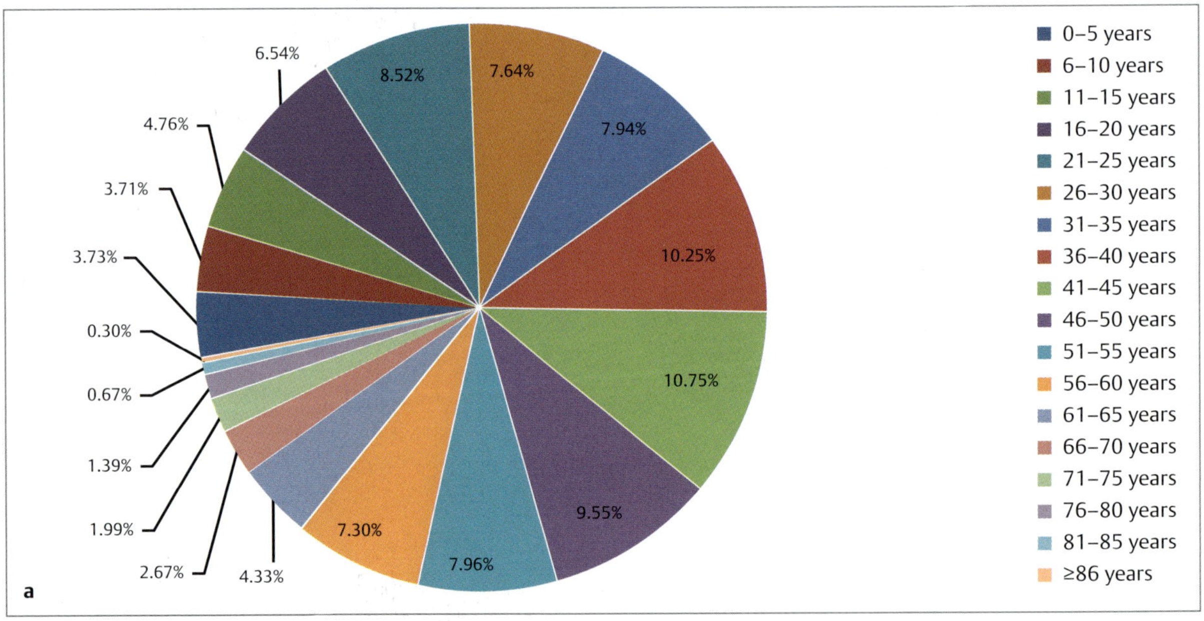

a

Fig. 5.3 **(a)** Age distribution of 66,758 patients with tibia/fibula fractures.

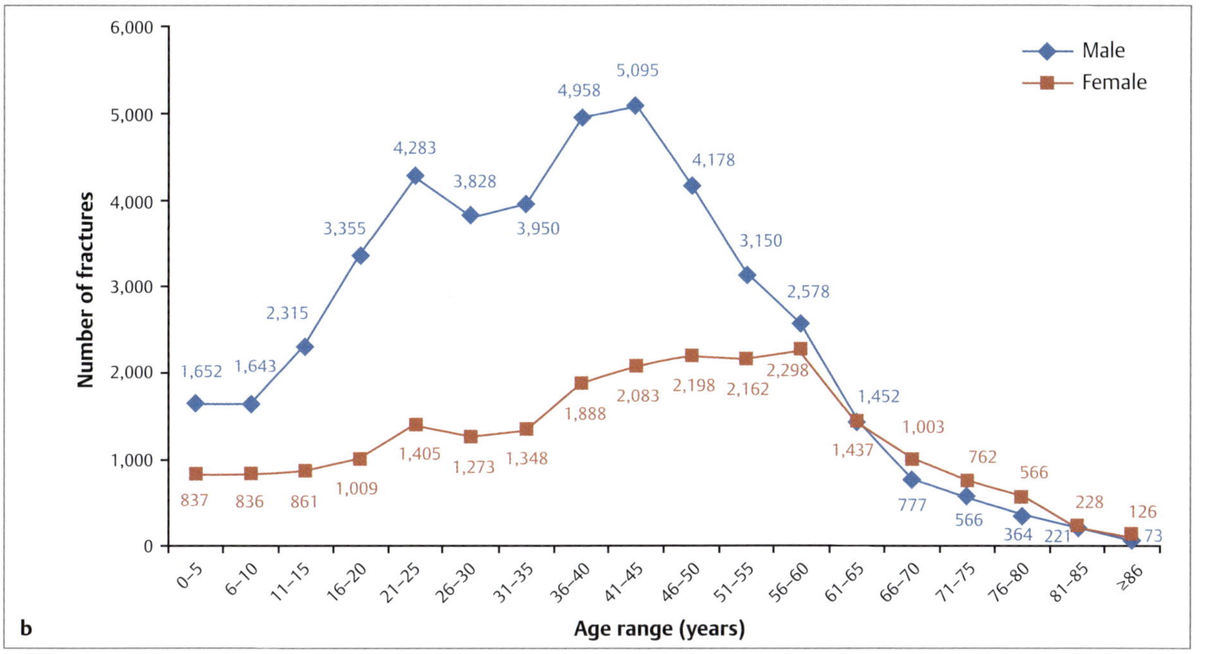

Fig. 5.3 (*continued*) **(b)** Age and sex distribution of 66,758 patients with tibia/fibula fractures.

Tibia/Fibula Fractures by Segment

Segment Distribution of Tibia/Fibula Fractures in Adults by AO Classification

Table 5.4 Segment distribution of 60,614 tibia/fibula fractures in adults based on AO classification

Segment	Number of fractures	Percentage (%)
41	10,944	18.06
42	15,000	24.75
43	6,391	10.54
44	28,279	46.65
Total	60,614	100.00

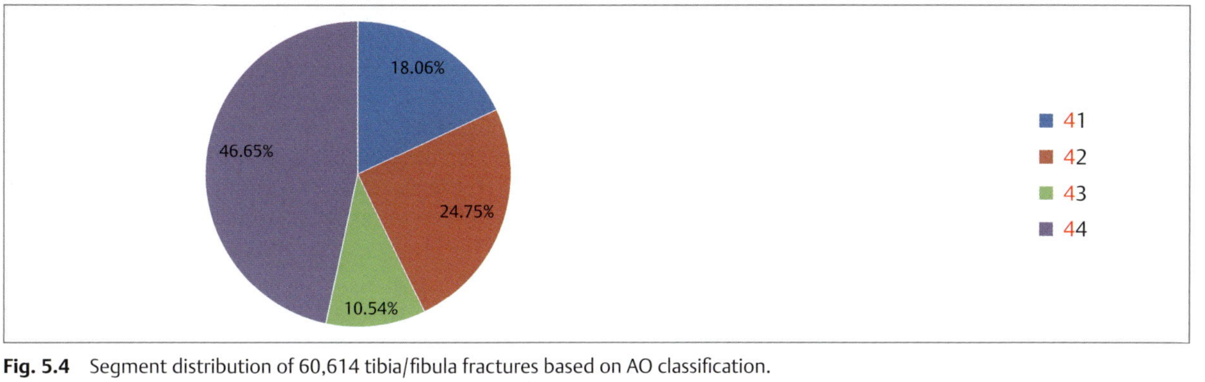

Fig. 5.4 Segment distribution of 60,614 tibia/fibula fractures based on AO classification.

Segment Distribution of Tibia/Fibula Fractures in Children

Table 5.5 Segment distribution of 8,264 tibia/fibula fractures in children

Segment	Number of fractures	Percentage (%)
Proximal	737	8.92
Diaphysis	4,079	49.36
Distal	1,469	17.78
Malleolus	1,979	23.95
Total	8,264	100.00

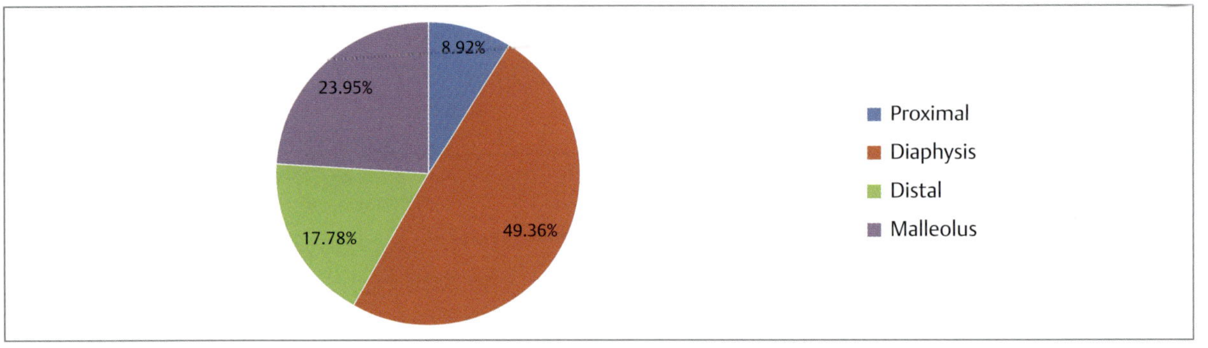

Fig. 5.5 Segment distribution of 8,264 tibia/fibula fractures in children.

Proximal Tibial Fractures (Segment 41)

Anatomical Features

The upper end of the tibia is large, and expands laterally into two ridges: the medial and lateral condyles. The medial and lateral tibial plateaus are the articular surfaces of the medial and lateral tibial condyles. These plateaus articulate with the medial and lateral femoral condyles, respectively. The tibial plateau is not perpendicular to the longitudinal axis of the tibial shaft, but slopes posteriorly at ~ 10 degrees. The bone comprising the tibial plateau is cancellous, as opposed to the thicker cortical bone of the tibial shaft. As a result, knee fractures often occur at the tibial plateau. The lateral plateau is smaller and higher than the medial plateau; thus, it decentralizes the shear load, which makes the lateral plateau more prone to fractures than the medial plateau. The outer portion of each plateau is covered by a semilunar fibrocartilaginous meniscus.

The two tibial plateaus are separated by the intercondyloid eminence, with its prominent medial and lateral tubercles, so-called tibial spines, where the anterior and posterior cruciate ligaments attach. The region of the tibial spines is extra-articular; therefore, there is no coverage by articular cartilage (**Plate 5.3**).

Between the lateral and medial condyles, on the proximal anterior surface of the tibia, lies a very large triangular prominence known as the tibial tuberosity. On the anterior side of the knee, running between the apex of the patella and tibial tuberosity, is the patellar ligament. The tibial attachment of the patellar ligament is 2.5–3 cm distal to the joint line on the anterior tibial crest. Between the patellar ligament and the tibia lies the deep infrapatellar bursa. A small prominence, located on the anterior aspect of the lateral condyle of the tibia, is known as the Gerdy tubercle, where the iliotibial band inserts. The fibula acts as a splint, or crutch, for the tibia but does not bear nearly as much weight of the body as the tibia. The head of fibula is the site for the insertion of the lateral collateral ligament and the tendon of the biceps femoris muscle.

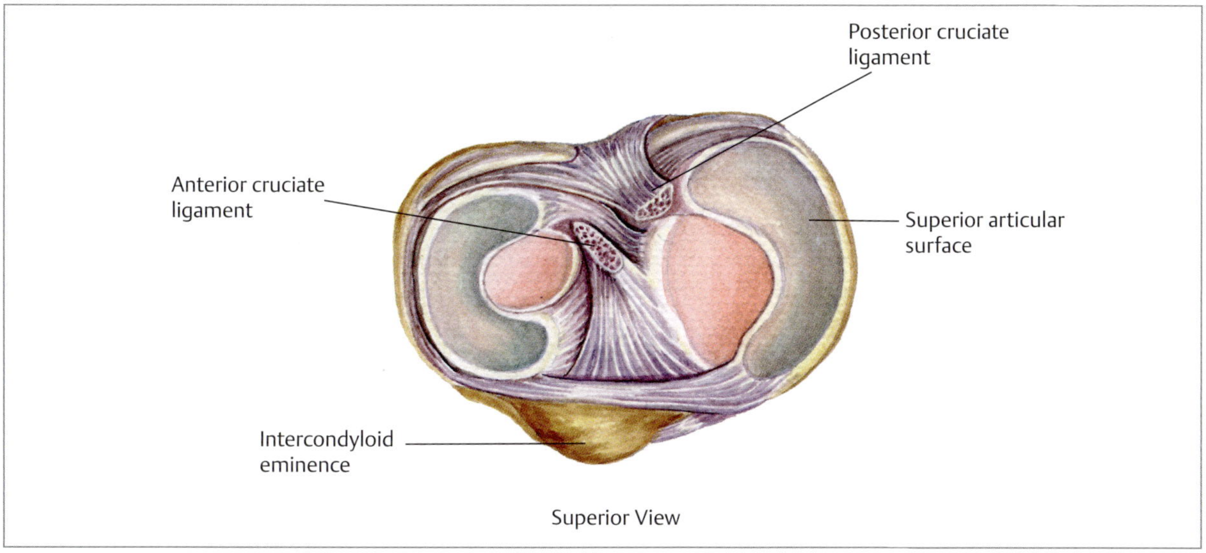

Plate 5.3

AO Classification of Proximal Tibial Fractures

Based on AO classification, the proximal tibia is coded as number 41 (**Plate 5.4**). Proximal tibial fractures can be divided into three types depending on articular involvement: 41-A, extra-articular fracture; 41-B, partial articular fracture; and 41-C, complete articular fracture (**Plate 5.5**).

Clinical Epidemiologic Features of Proximal Tibial Fractures (Segment 41)

A total of 10,944 adult fractures of the proximal tibia/fibula were treated in 83 hospitals in China over a 2-year period from 2010 to 2011. All cases were reviewed and statistically studied; the fractures accounted for 18.06% of all tibia/fibula fractures in adults. Their epidemiologic features are as follows:

- More males than females
- The high-risk age group is 41–45 years. The most affected male age group is 41–45 years, while females between 56 and 60 years have the highest risk.
- The most common fracture type among segment 41 fractures is type 41-A—the same fracture type for both males and females.
- The most common fracture group among segment 41 fractures is group 41-A1—the same fracture group for both males and females.

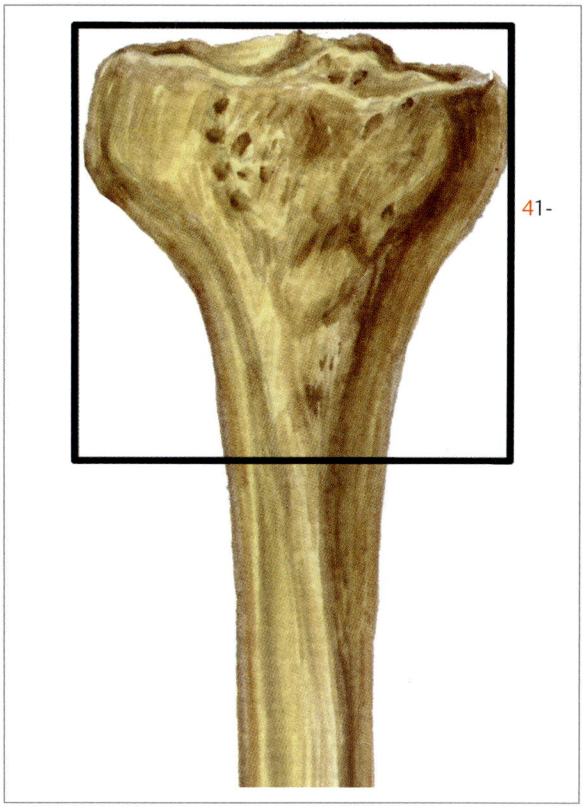

Plate 5.4

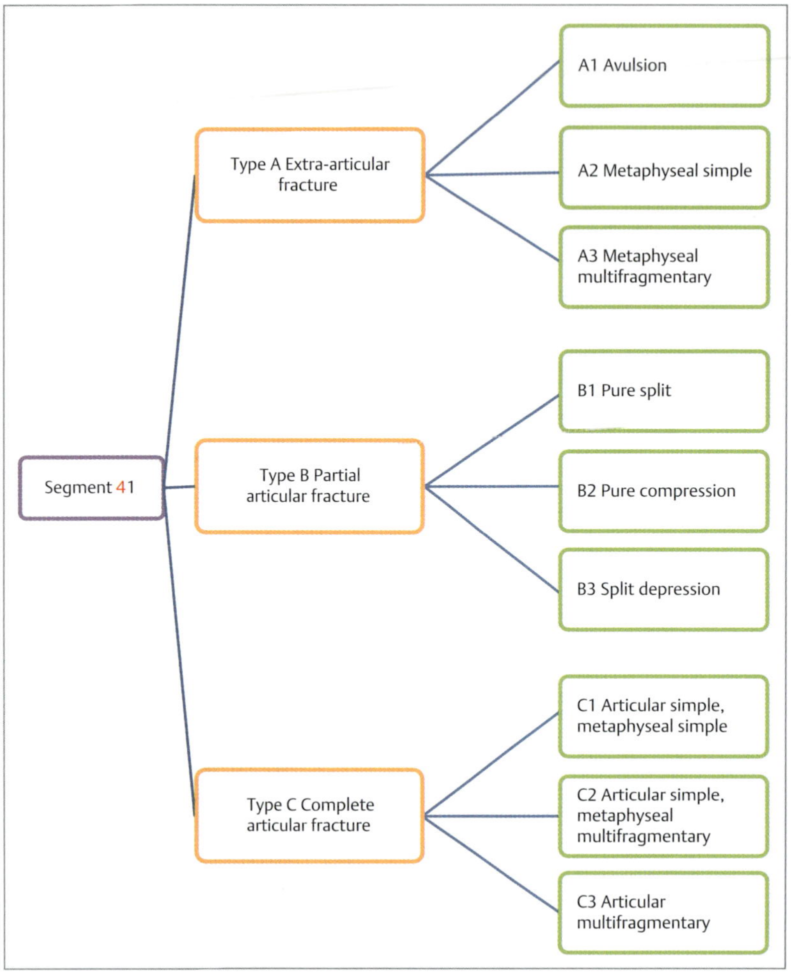

Plate 5.5

Fractures of Segment 41 by Sex

Table 5.6 Sex distribution of 10,944 fractures of segment 41

Sex	Number of fractures	Percentage (%)
Male	7,355	67.21
Female	3,589	32.79
Total	10,944	100.00

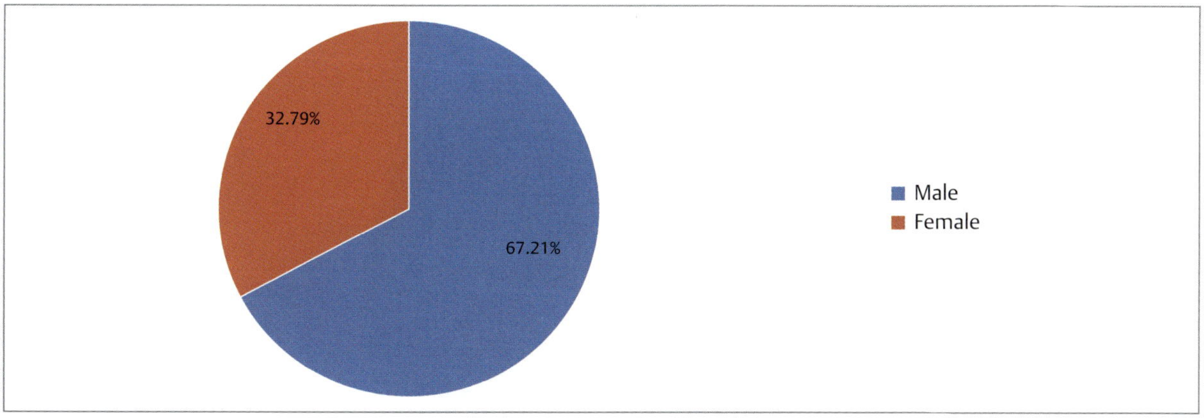

Fig. 5.6 Sex distribution of 10,944 fractures of segment 41.

Fractures of Segment 41 by Age Group

Table 5.7 Age and sex distribution of 10,944 fractures of segment 41

Age group (years)	Male	Female	Number of fractures	Percentage (%)
16–20	482	137	619	5.66
21–25	578	179	757	6.92
26–30	556	177	733	6.70
31–35	701	240	941	8.60
36–40	999	282	1,281	11.71
41–45	1,072	354	1,426	13.03
46–50	964	389	1,353	12.36
51–55	708	447	1,155	10.55
56–60	568	470	1,038	9.48
61–65	311	328	639	5.84
66–70	154	219	373	3.41
71–75	134	166	300	2.74
76–80	78	130	208	1.90
81–85	42	44	86	0.79
≥86	8	27	35	0.32
Total	7,355	3,589	10,944	100.00

5

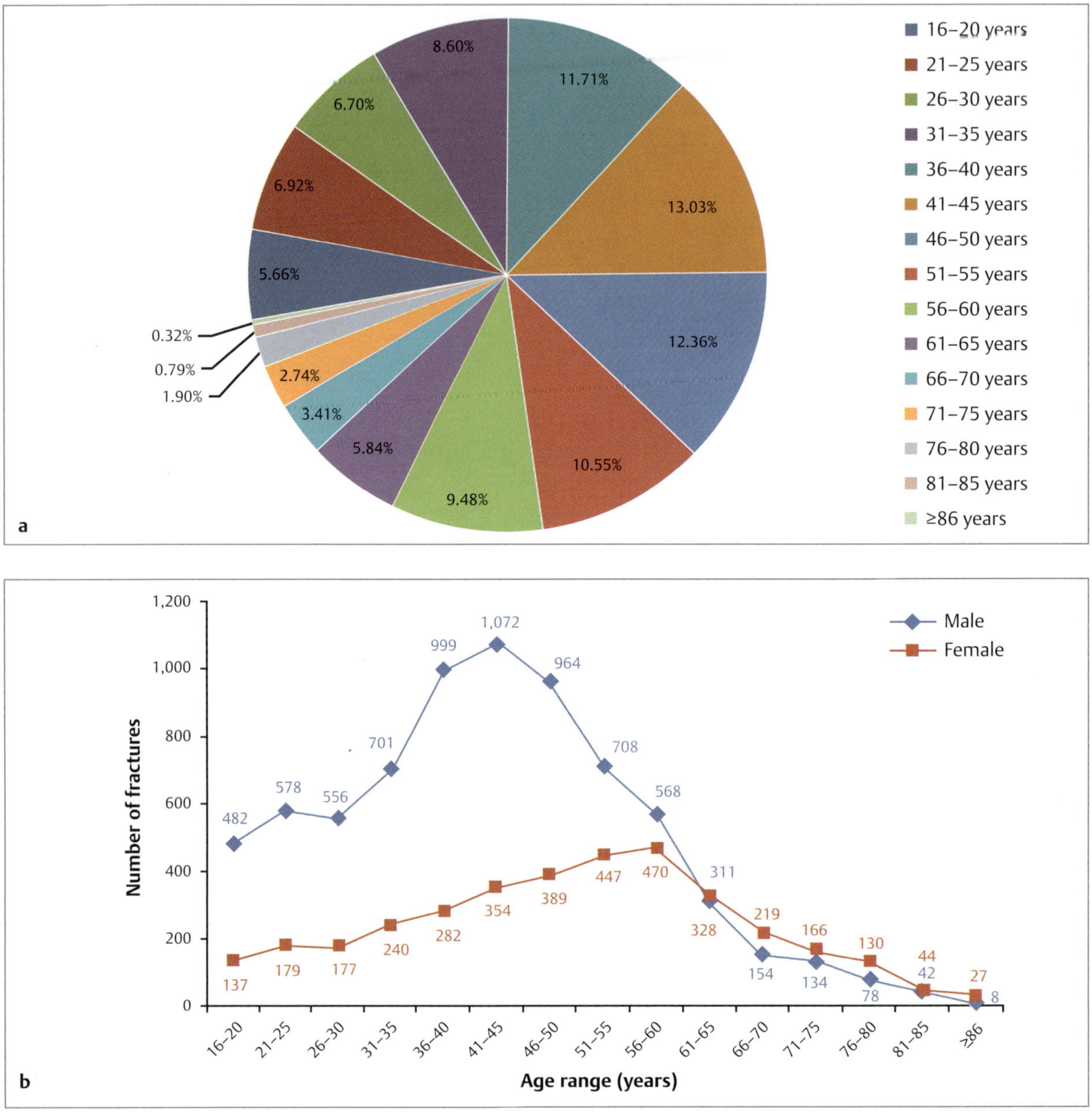

Fig. 5.7 **(a)** Age distribution of 10,944 fractures of segment 41.
(b) Age and sex distribution of 10,944 fractures of segment 41.

Fractures of Segment 41 by Fracture Type

Table 5.8 Sex and fracture type distribution of 10,944 fractures of segment 41

Fracture type	Male	Female	Number of fractures	Percentage (%)
41-A	3,080	1,637	4,717	43.10
41-B	2,529	1,469	3,998	36.53
41-C	1,746	483	2,229	20.37
Total	7,355	3,589	10,944	100.00

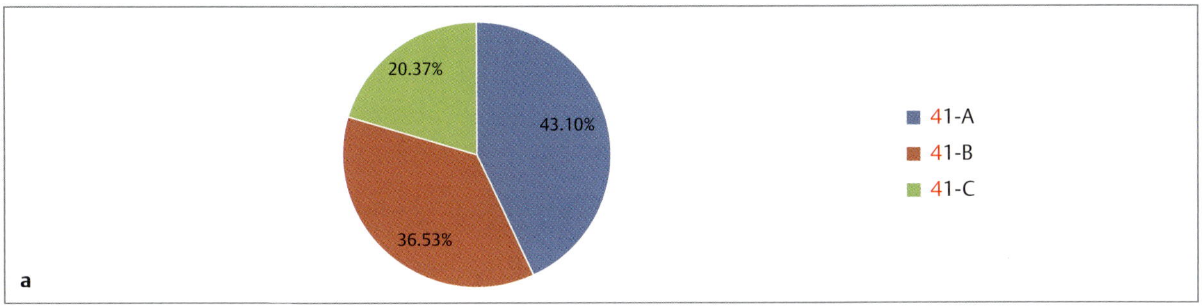

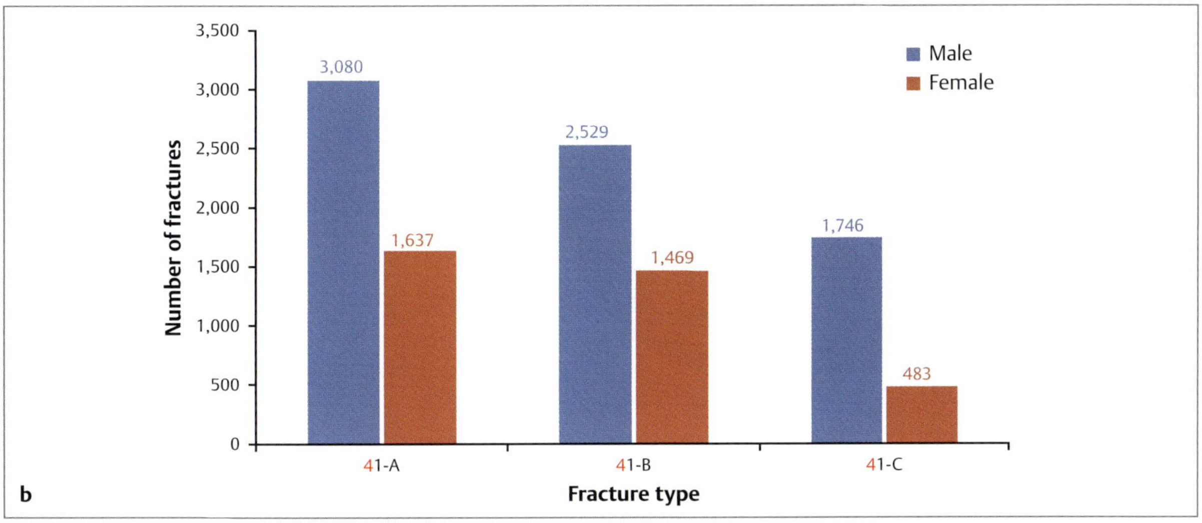

Fig. 5.8 **(a)** Fracture type distribution of 10,944 fractures of segment 41.
(b) Sex and fracture type distribution of 10,944 fractures of segment 41.

5

Table 5.9 Sex and fracture group distribution of 10,944 fractures of segment 41

Fracture group	Male	Female	Number of fractures	Percentage of segment 41 (%)	Percentage of tibia/fibula (%)
41-A1	2,069	1,354	3,423	31.28	5.65
41-A2	460	178	638	5.83	1.05
41-A3	551	105	656	5.99	1.08
41-B1	1,002	433	1,435	13.11	2.37
41-B2	731	626	1,357	12.40	2.24
41-B3	796	410	1,206	11.02	1.99
41-C1	440	155	595	5.44	0.98
41-C2	609	138	747	6.83	1.23
41-C3	697	190	887	8.10	1.46
Total	7,355	3,589	10,944	100.00	18.06

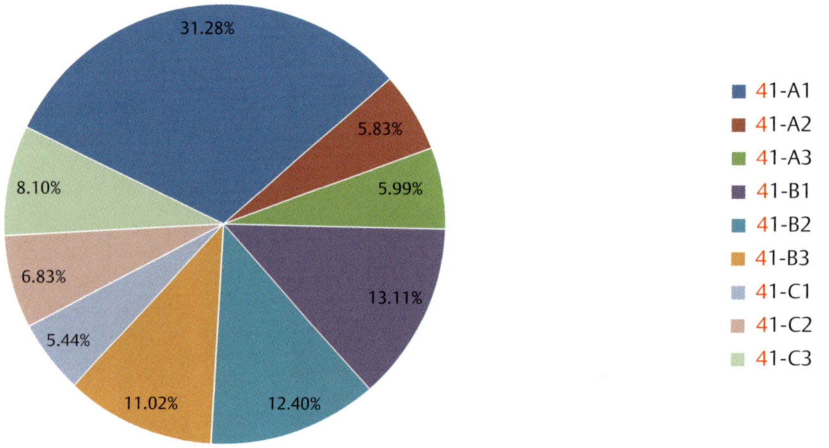

a

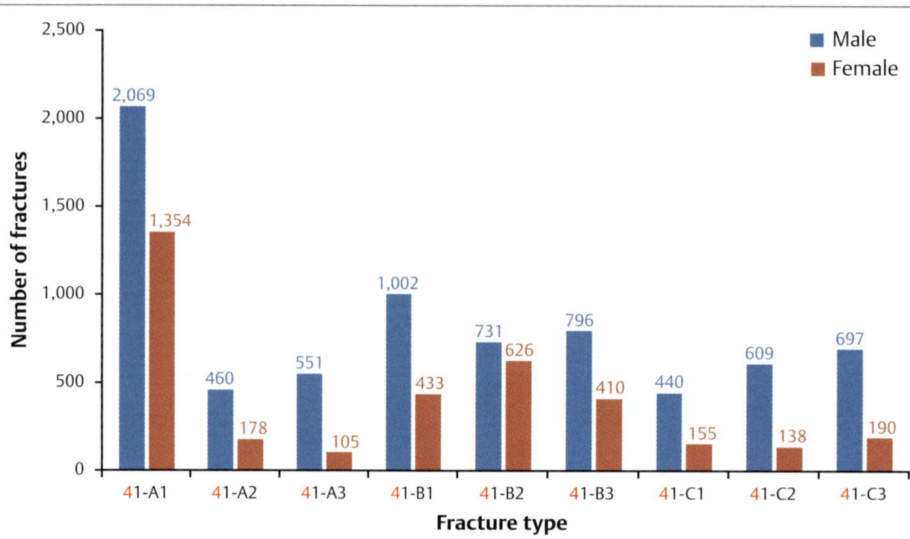

b

Fig.5.9 **(a)** Fracture group distribution of 10,944 fractures of segment 41.
(b) Sex and fracture group distribution of 10,944 fractures of segment 41.

41-A Tibia/fibula proximal, extra-articular fractures

41-A1
Avulsion
3,423 fractures
M: 2,069 (60.44%)
F: 1,354 (39.56%)
0.91% of total adult fractures
5.65%of adult tibia/fibula fractures
31.28% of segment 41
72.57% of type 41-A

41-A1.1

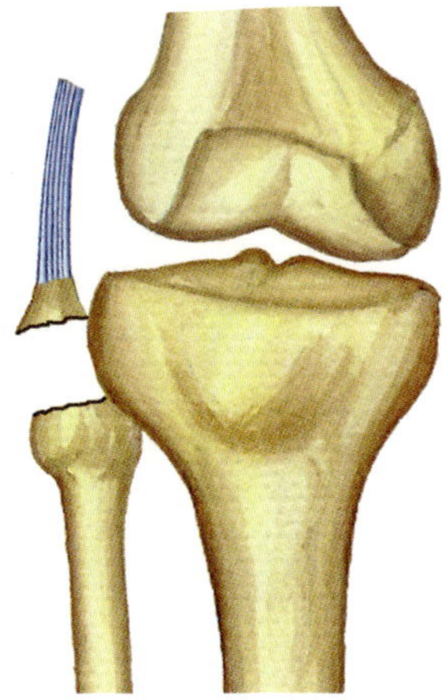

Of the fibular head

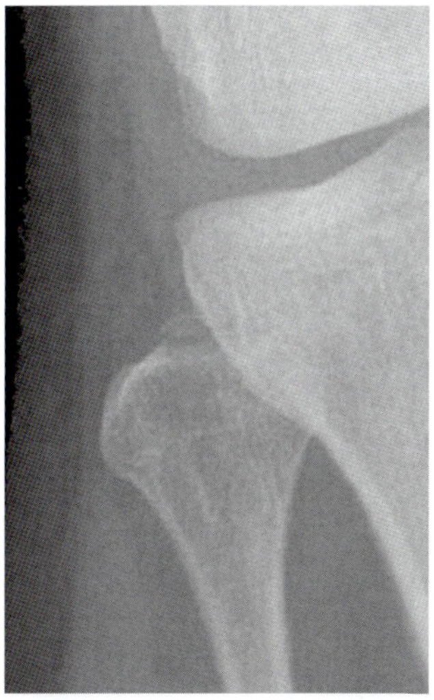

41-A1.2

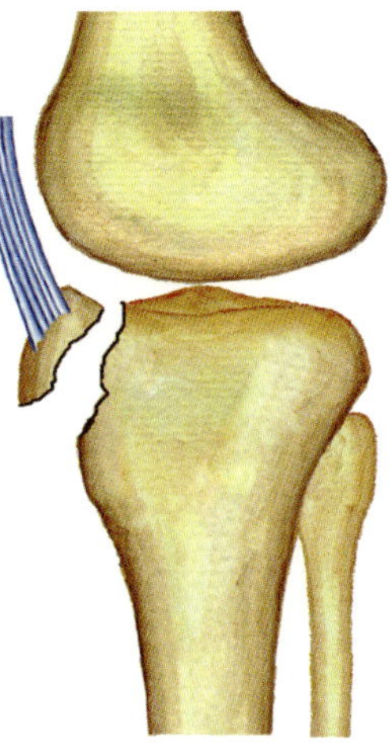

Of the tibial tuberosity

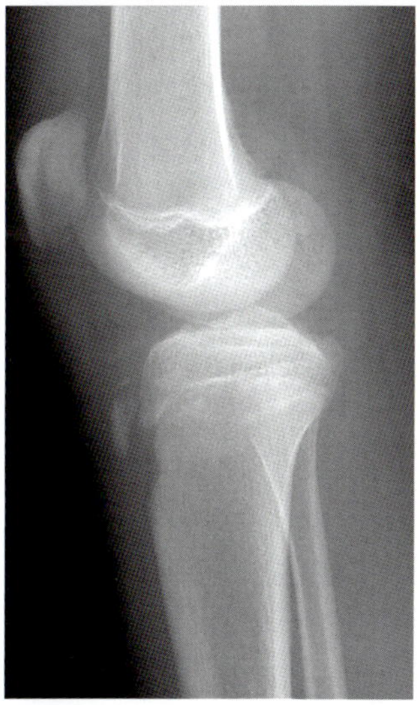

41-A1.3

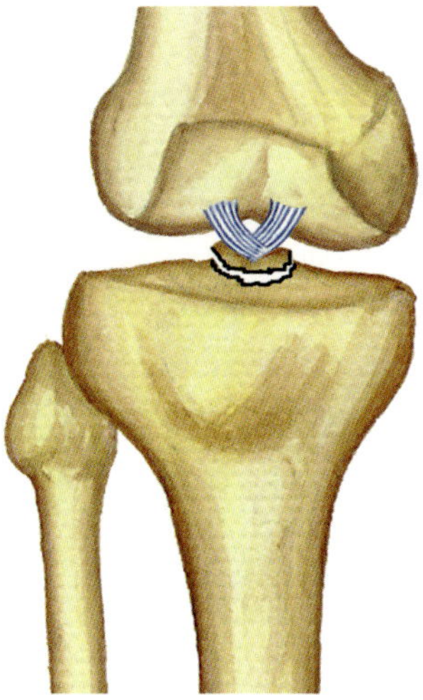

Of the cruciate insertion

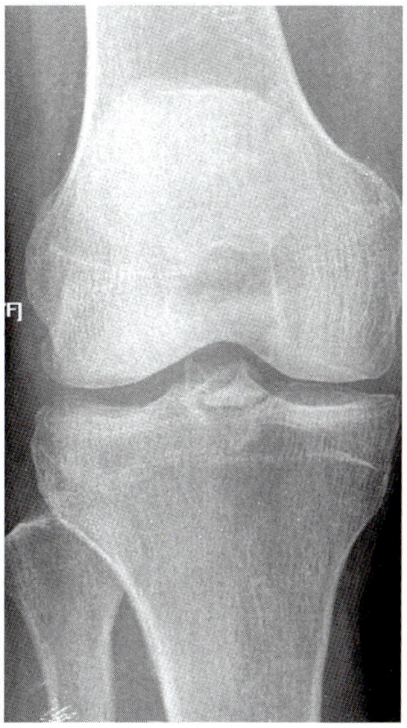

41-A Tibia/fibula proximal, extra-articular fractures

41-A2
Metaphyseal simple
638 fractures
M: 460 (72.10%)
F: 178 (27.90%)
0.17% of total adult fractures
1.05% of adult tibia/fibula fractures
5.83% of segment 41
13.53% of type 41-A

41-A2.1

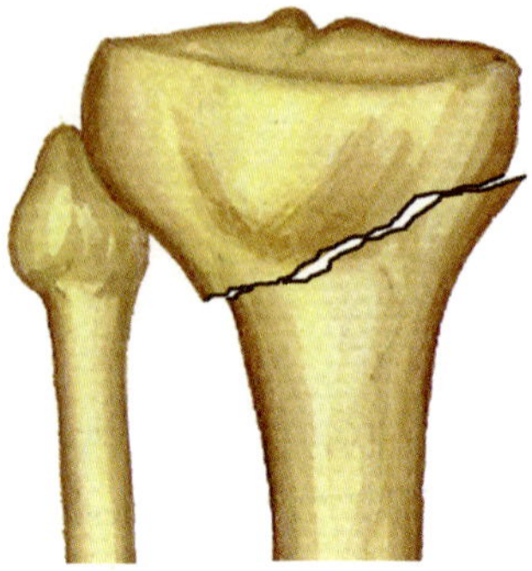

Oblique in the sagittal plane

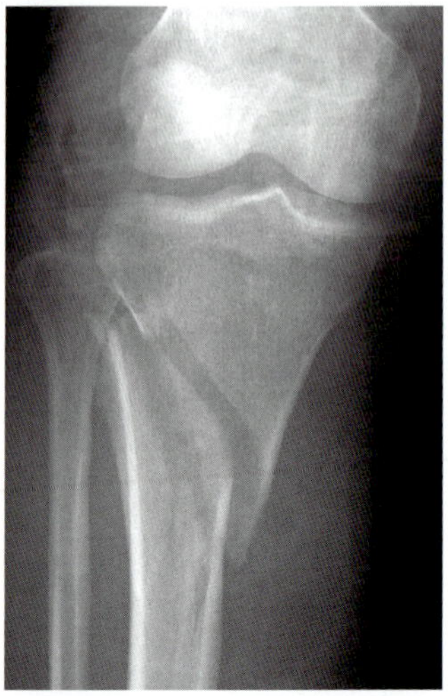

41-A2.2

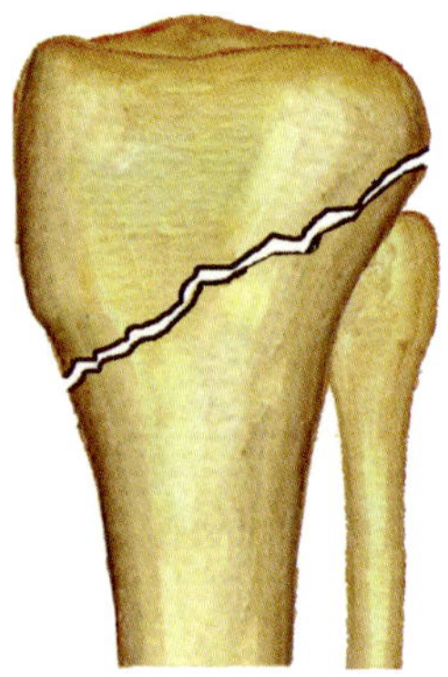

Oblique in the frontal plane

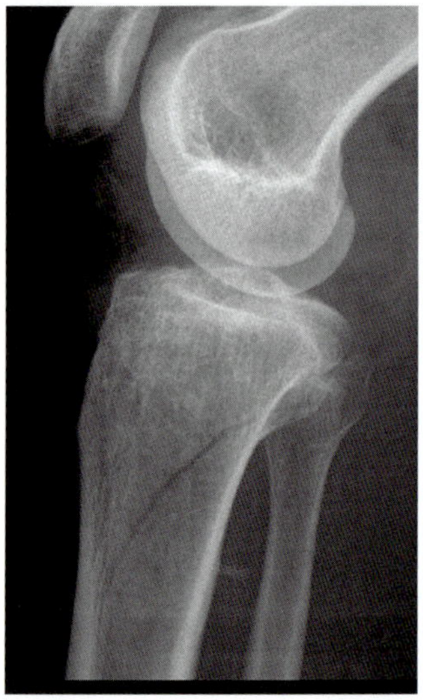

41-A2.3

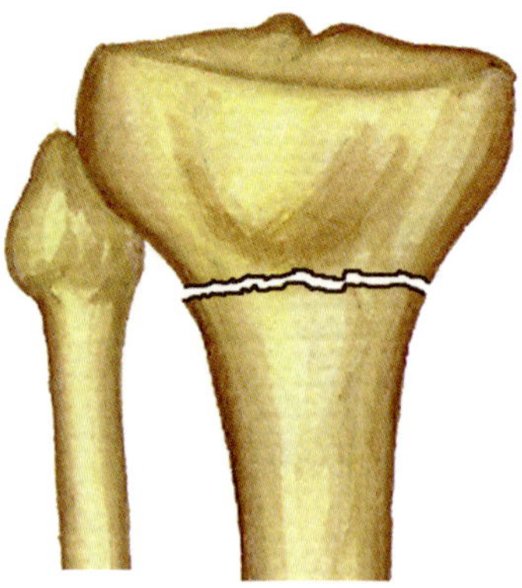

Transverse

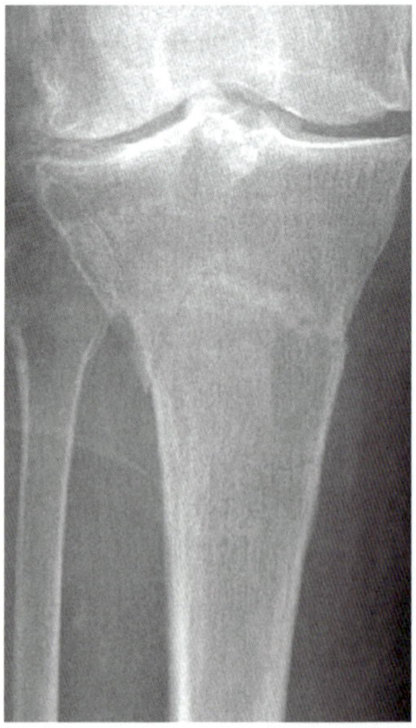

41-A Tibia/fibula proximal, extra-articular fractures

41-A3
Metaphyseal multifragmentary
656 fractures
M: 551 (83.99%)
F: 105 (16.01%)
0.18% of total adult fractures
1.08% of adult tibia/fibula fractures
5.99% of segment 41
13.91% of type 41-A

41-A3.1

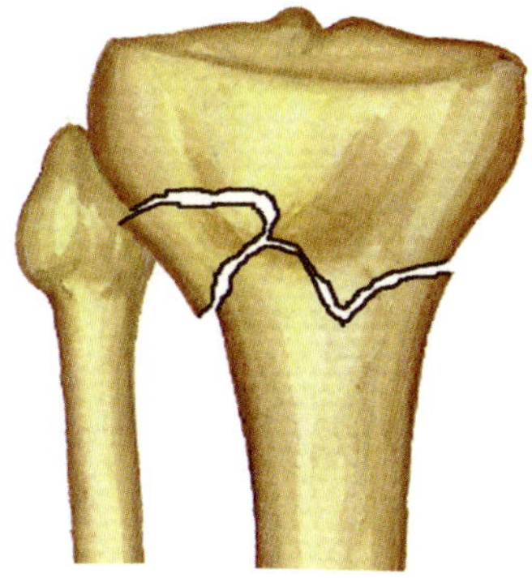

Intact wedge

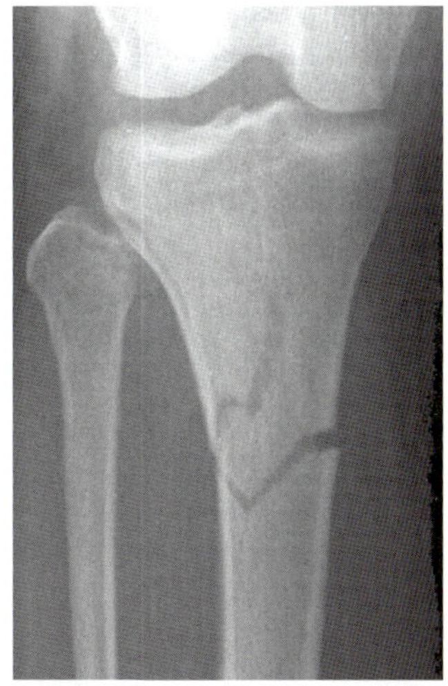

41-A3.2

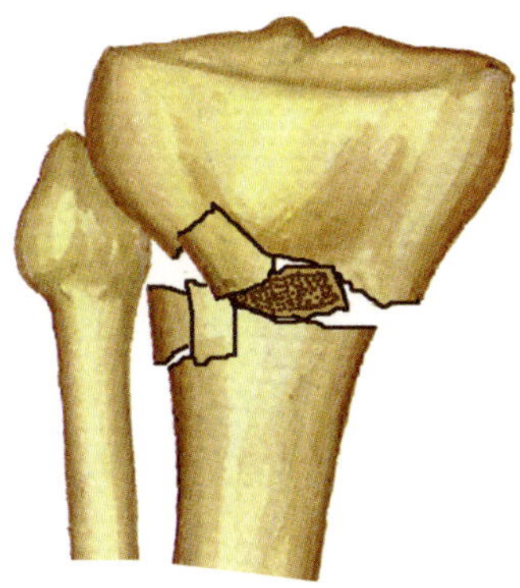

Fragmented wedge

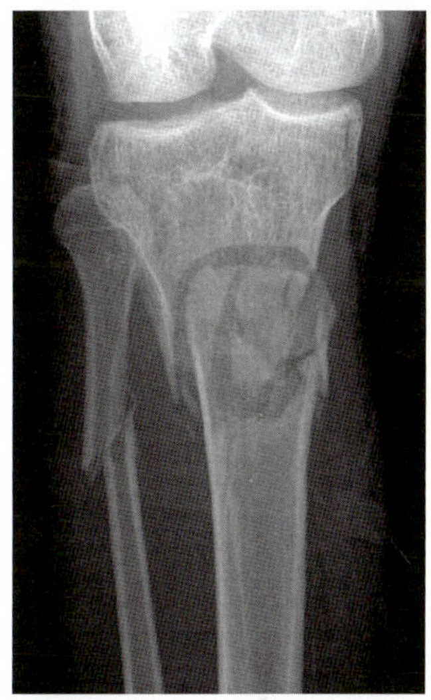

41-A3.3

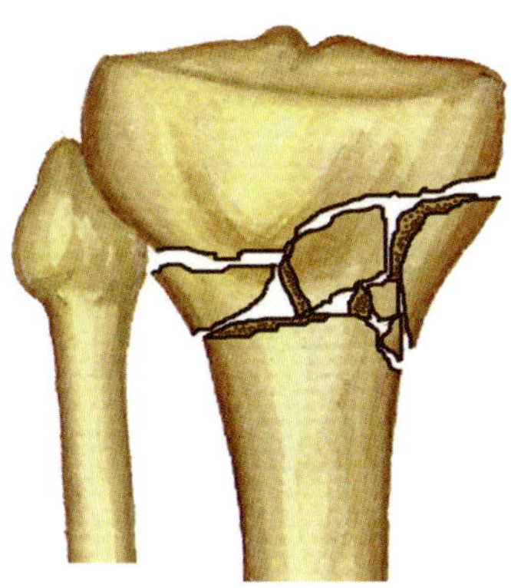

Multifragmentary

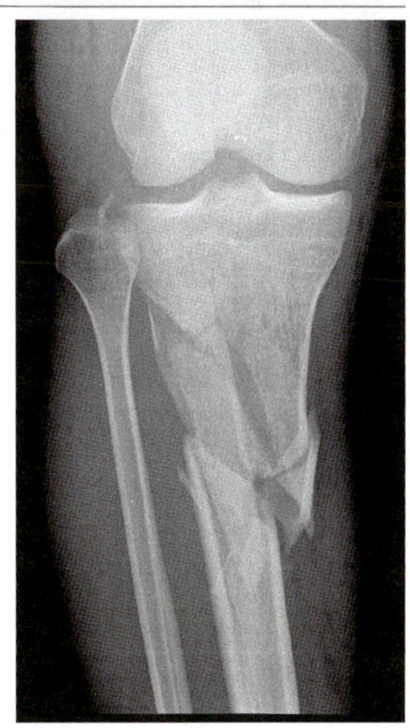

41-B Tibia/fibula proximal, partial articular fractures

41-B1
Split fracture involving the articular surface of one tibial plateau
1,435 fractures
M: 1,002 (69.83%)
F: 433 (30.17%)
0.38% of total adult fractures
2.37% of adult tibia/fibula fractures
13.11% of segment 41
35.89% of type 41-B

41-B1.1

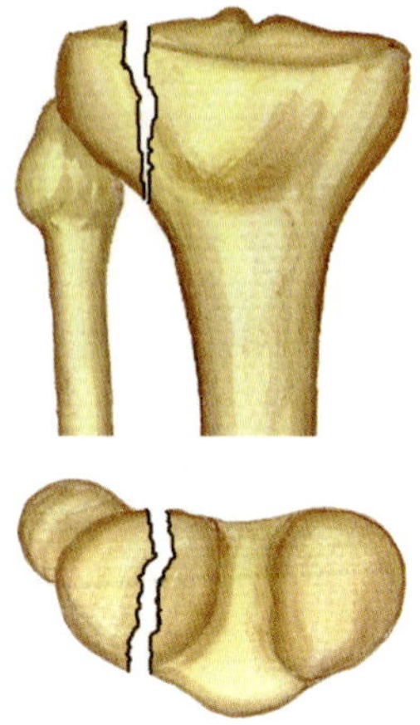

Of the lateral surface

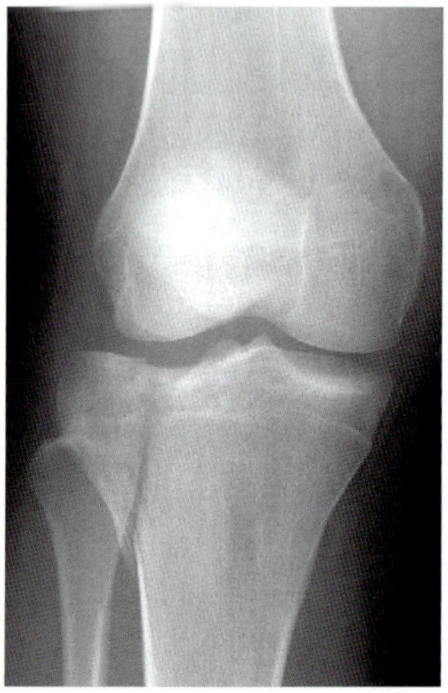

41-B1.2

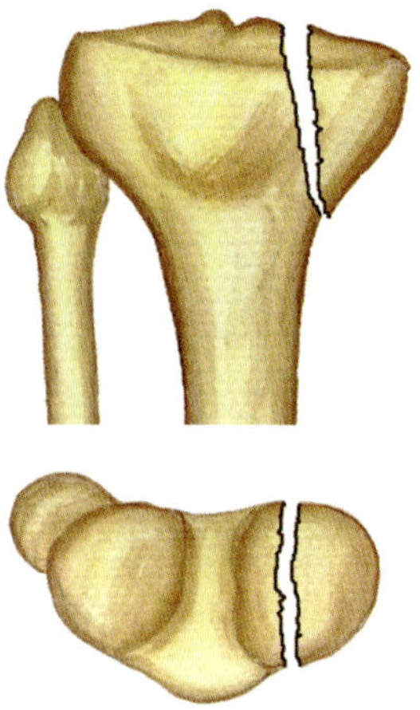

Of the medial surface

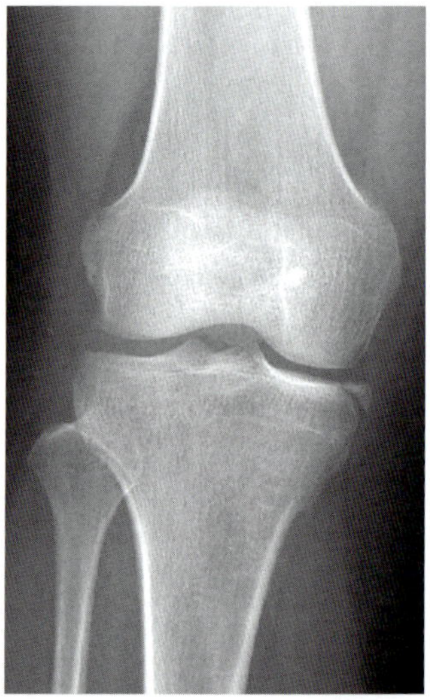

41-B1.3

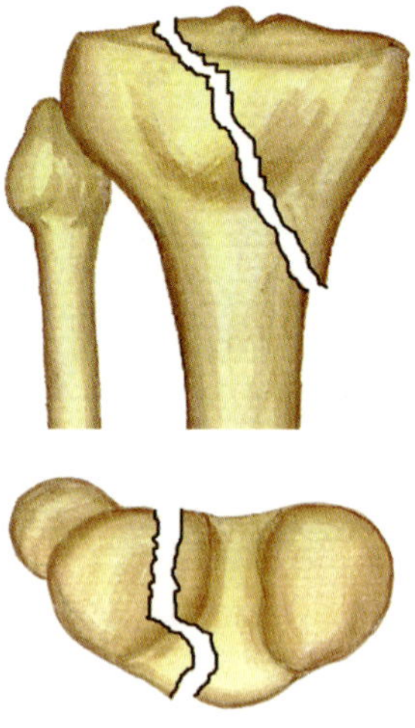

Oblique, involving the tibial spine and one of the plateaus

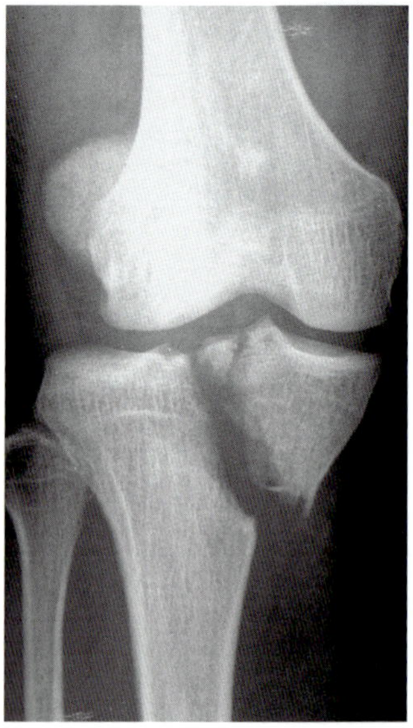

41-B Tibia/fibula proximal, partial articular fractures

41-B2

Depression fractures involving one tibial plateau

1,357 fractures
M: 731 (53.87%)
F: 626 (46.13%)
0.36% of total adult fractures
2.24% of adult tibia/fibula fractures
12.40% of segment 41
33.94% of type 41-B

41-B2.1

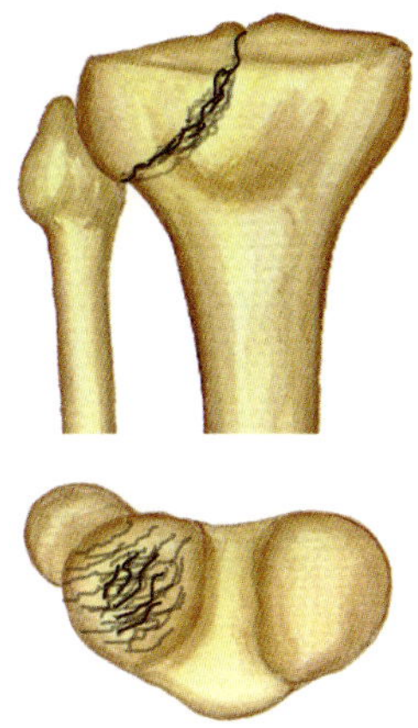

Lateral total

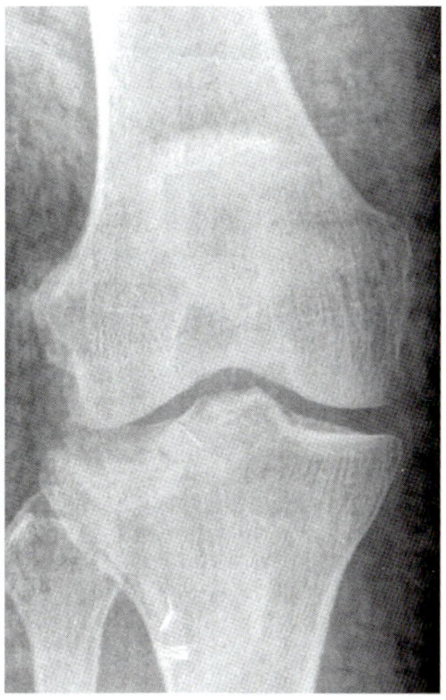

41-B2.2

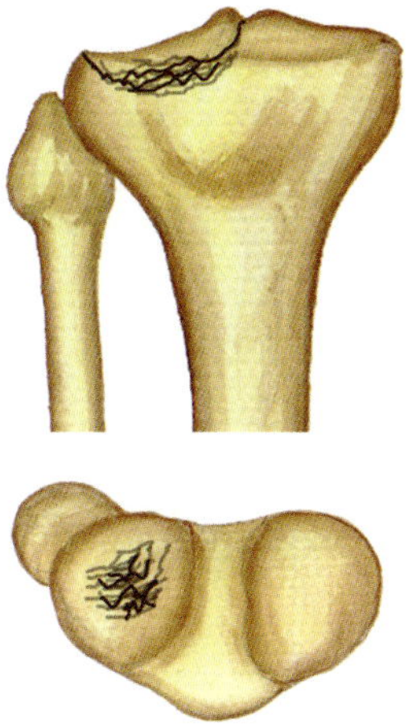

Lateral limited

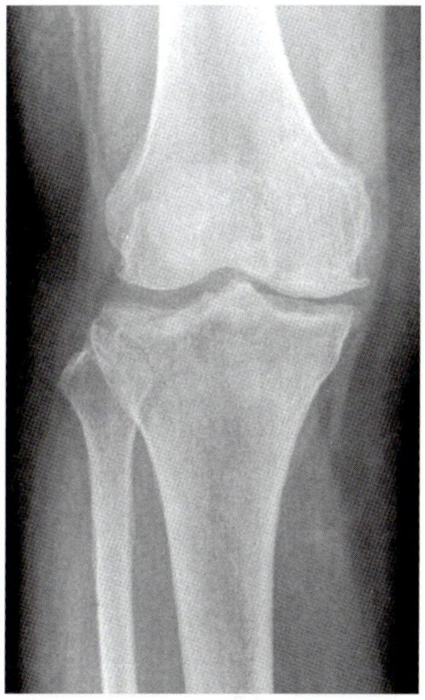

41-B2.3

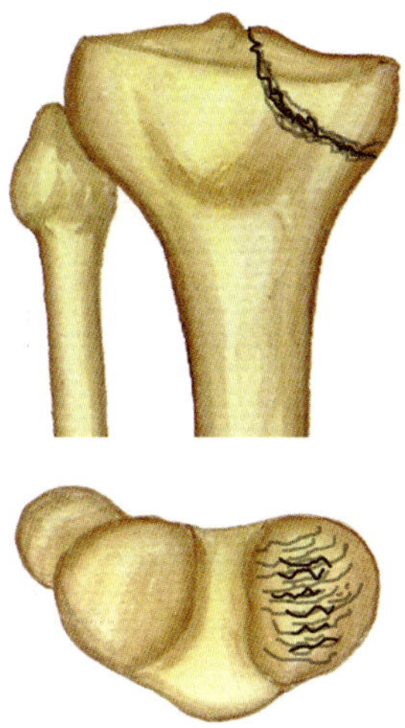

Medial

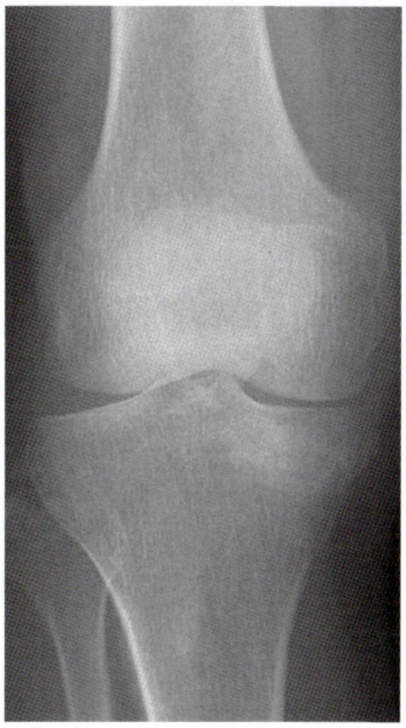

41-B Tibia/fibula proximal, partial articular fractures

41-B3

Split-depression, involving one tibial plateau

1,206 fractures
M: 796 (66.00%)
F: 410 (34.00%)
0.32% of total adult fractures
1.99% of adult tibia/fibula fractures
11.02% of segment 41
30.17% of type 41-B

41-B3.1

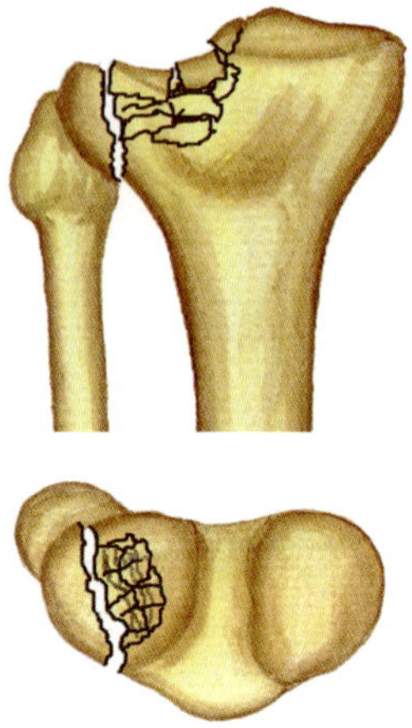

Lateral

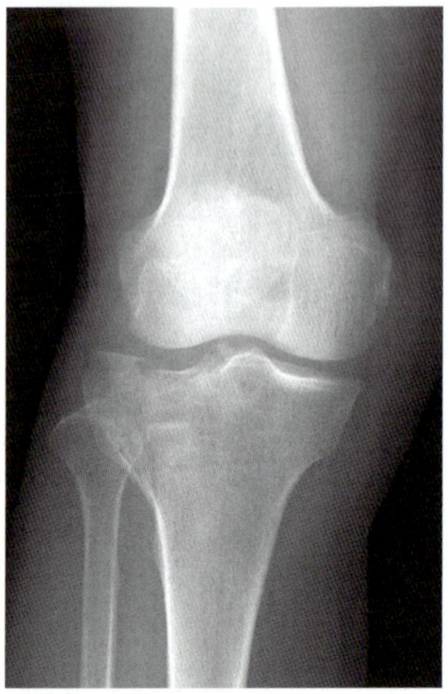

41-B3.2

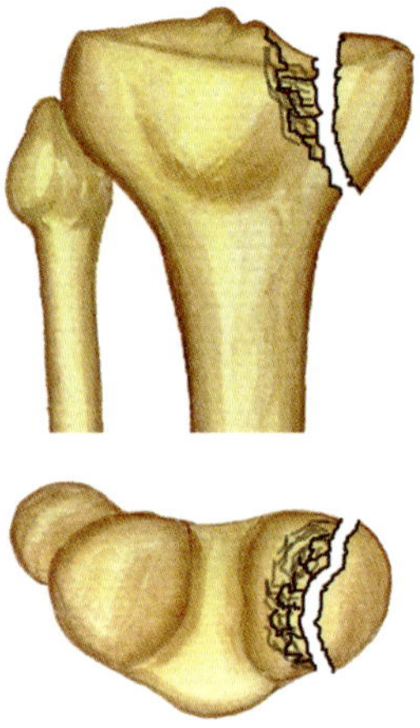

Medial

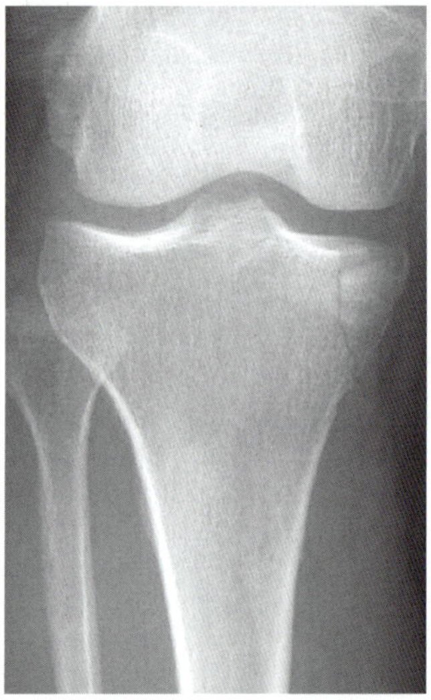

41-B3.3

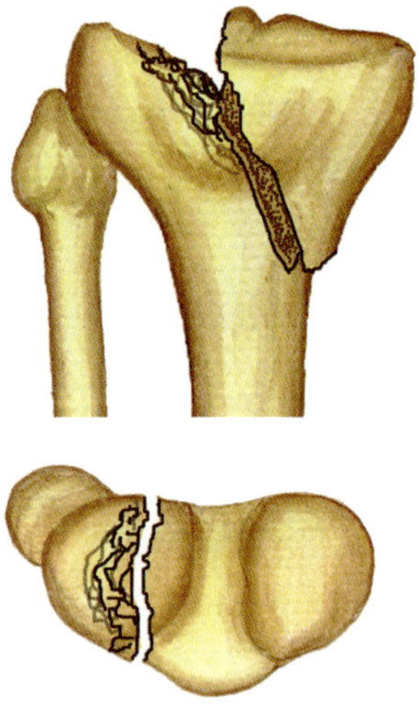

Oblique, involving the tibial spines and one of the plateaus

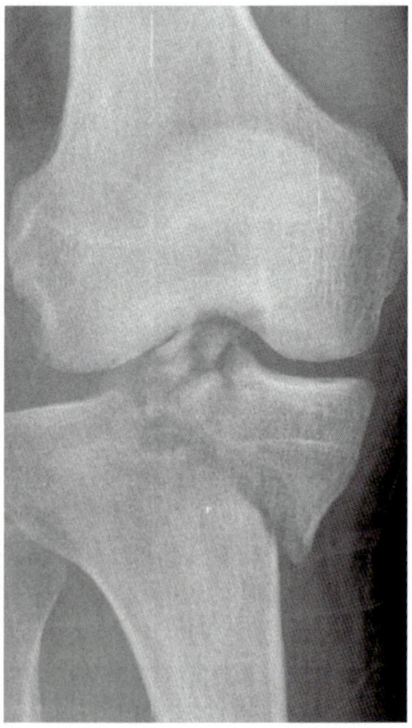

41-C Tibia/fibula proximal, complete-articular fractures

41-C1

Articular simple,
metaphyseal simple

595 fractures
M: 440 (73.95%)
F: 155 (26.05%)
0.16% of total adult fractures
0.98% of adult tibia/fibula fractures
5.44% of segment 41
26.69% of type 41-C

41-C1.1

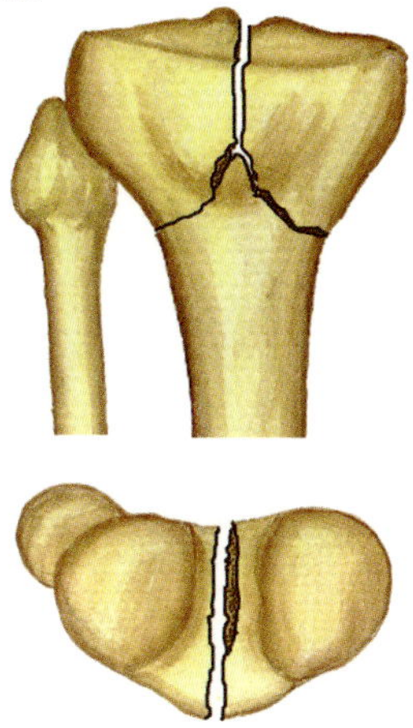

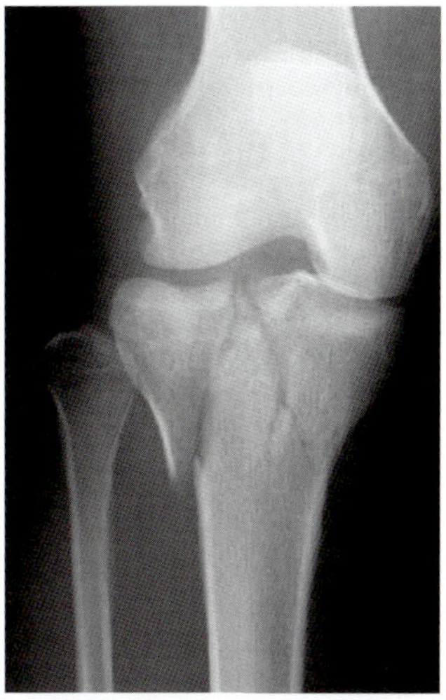

With minimal or no displacement

41-C1.2

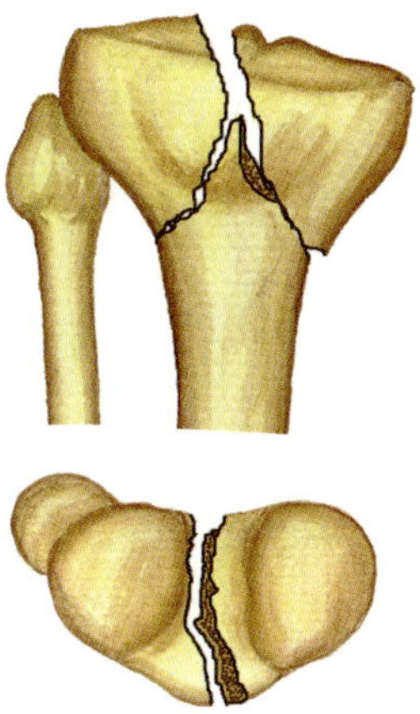

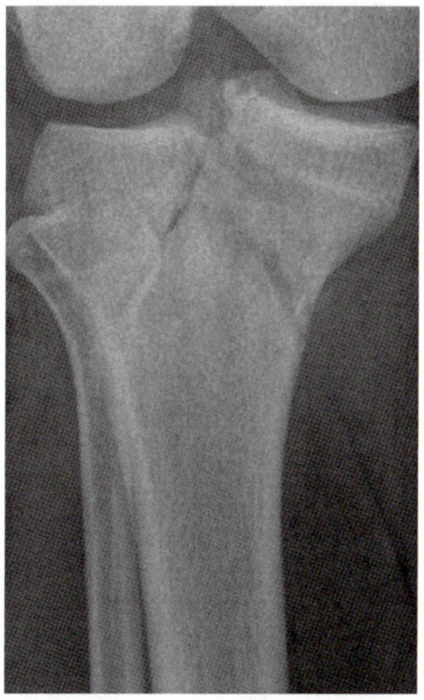

One plateau displaced

41-C1.3

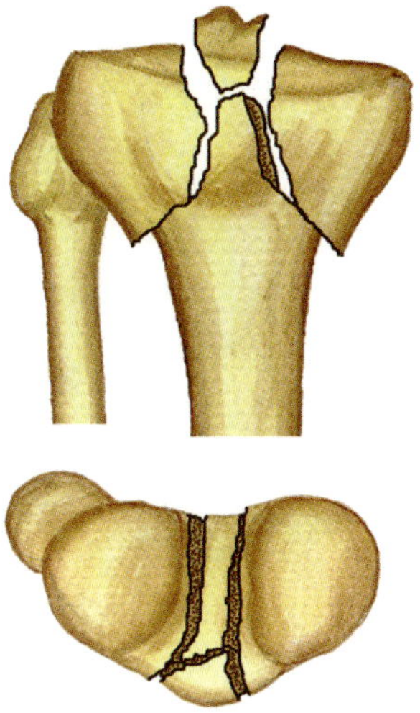

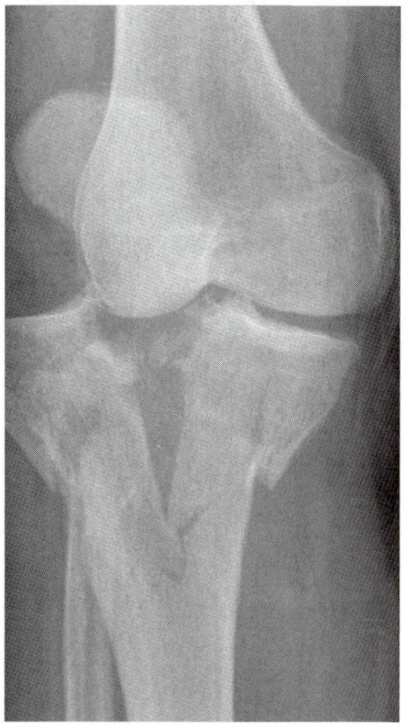

Both plateaus displaced

41-C Tibia/fibula proximal, complete-articular fractures

41-C2
Articular simple, metaphyseal multifragmentary
747 fractures
M: 609 (81.53%)
F: 138 (18.47%)
0.2% of total adult fractures
1.23% of adult tibia/fibula fractures
6.83% of segment 41
33.51% of type 41-C

41-C2.1

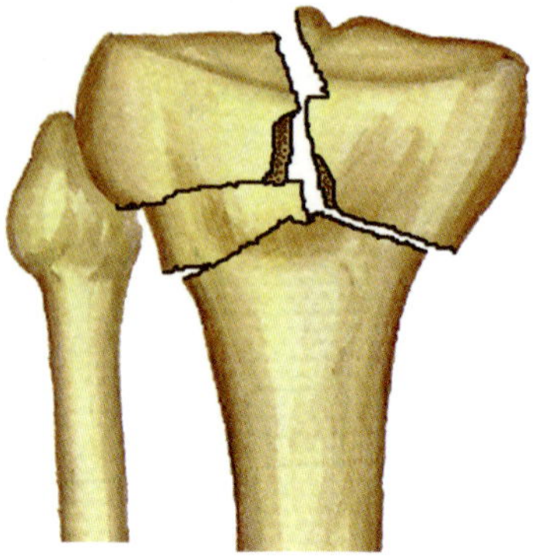

With intact wedge

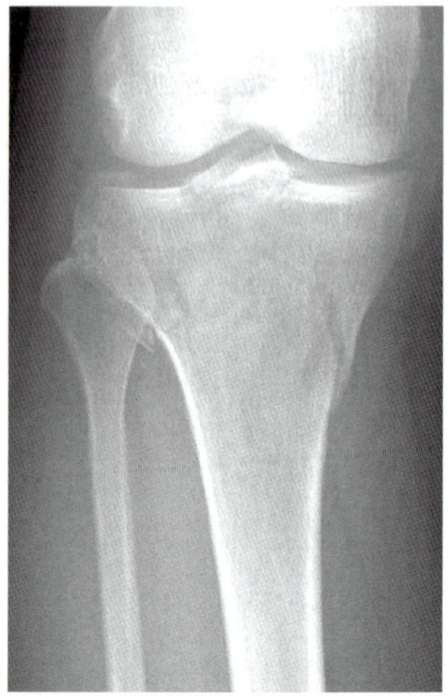

41-C2.2

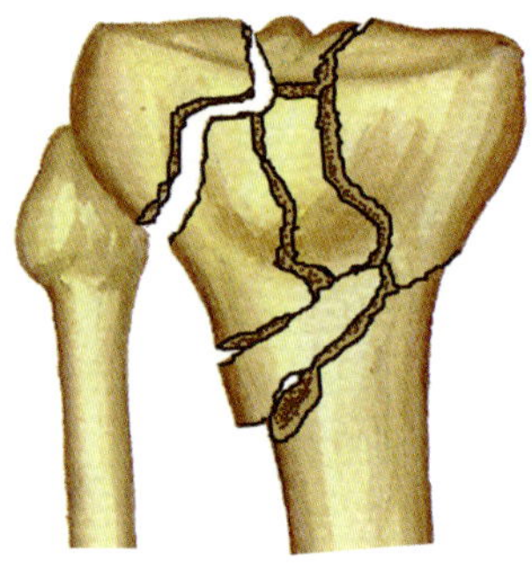

Fragmented wedge

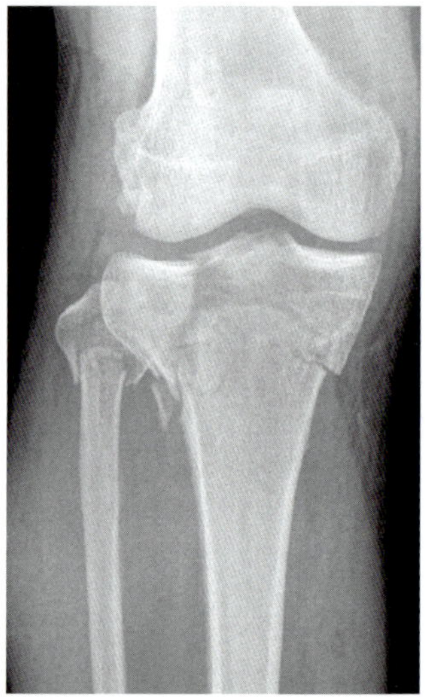

41-C2.3

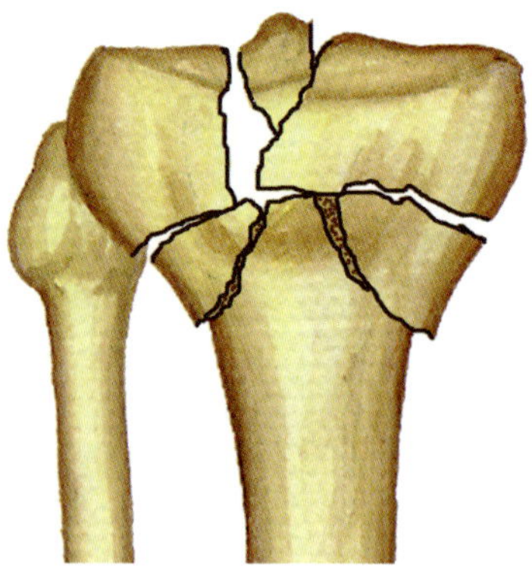

Complex

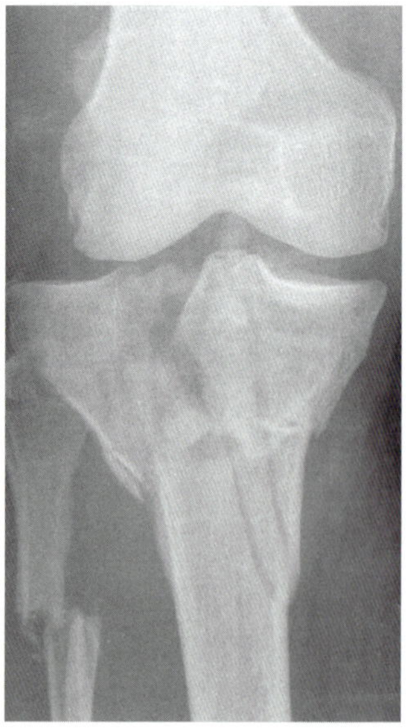

41-C Tibia/fibula proximal, complete-articular fractures

41-C3
Articular multifragmentary
887 fractures
M: 697 (78.58%)
F: 190 (21.42%)
0.24% of total adult fractures
1.46% of adult tibia/fibula fractures
8.10% of segment 41
39.79% of type 41-C

41-C3.1

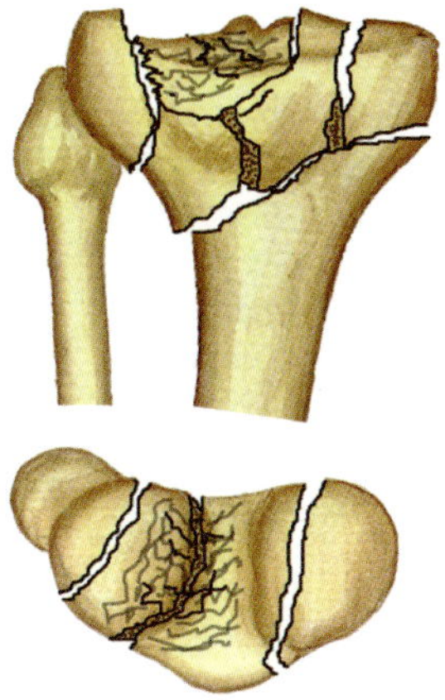

Lateral

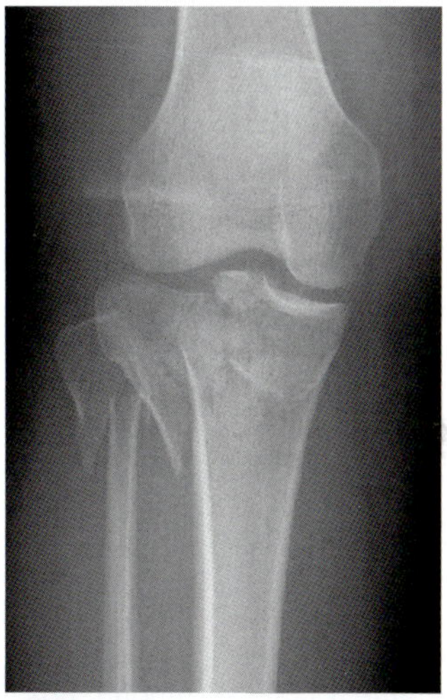

41-C3.2

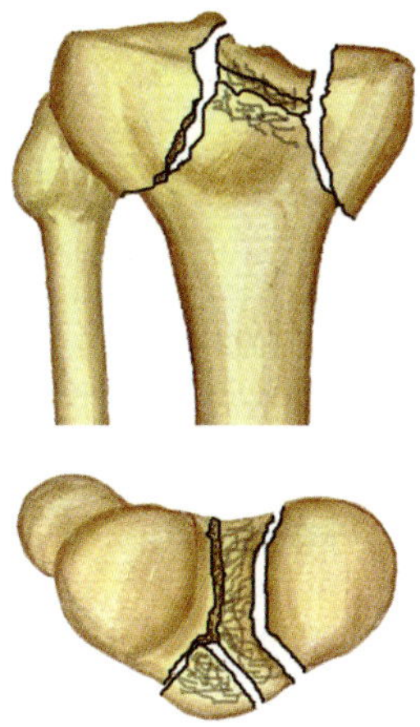

Medial

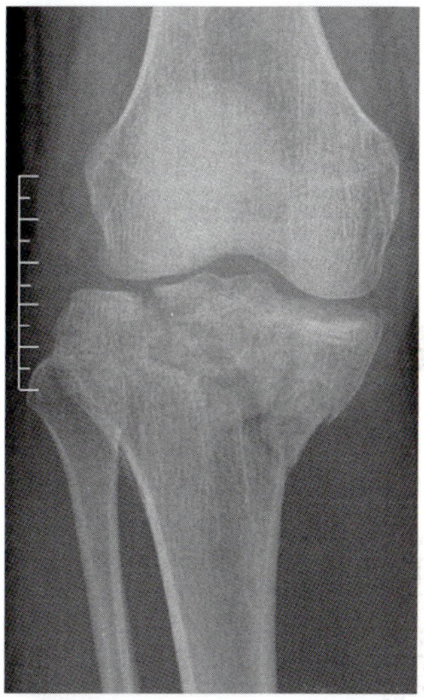

41-C3.3

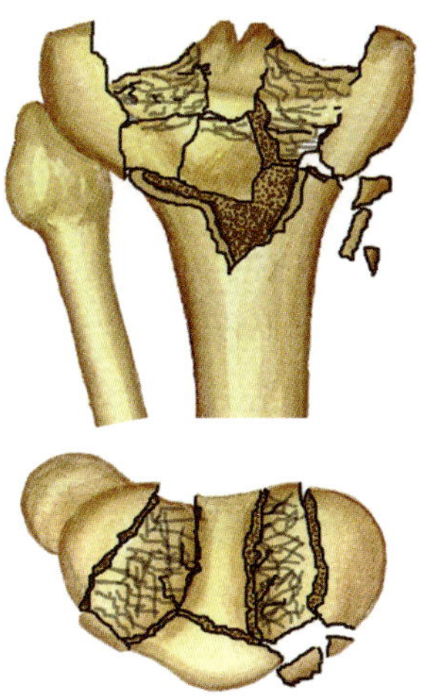

Lateral + medial

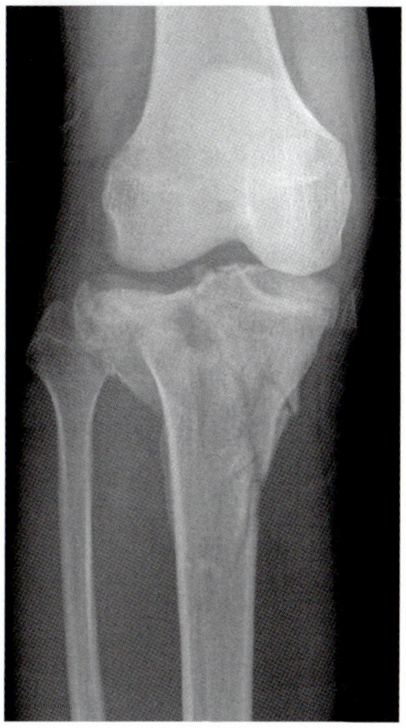

Injury Mechanism

The most common mechanism of injury involves axial loading and/or valgus or varus force, such as from a fall or automobile accident. The severity of the fracture is associated with the magnitude and duration of the force. The axial compression load resulting from a fall from a significant height can cause depression, splitting, or even comminuted fractures of the tibial plateau. Depression or avulsion of the lateral plateau is the most common trauma that results from valgus/varus or hyperflexion/ hyperextension forces, which also can cause avulsion of the tibial attachment of the anteroposterior cruciate ligaments.

Diagnosis

Patients with proximal tibia/fibula fractures may present with a knee effusion, pain, and stiffness, with a partial or limited range of motion. In severe fractures, a varus or valgus deformity of the affected limb may be present. If the injury resulted from high-energy trauma, a hypertonic blister, or compartment syndrome, rupture of ligaments, and disruption of the neurovascular supply may accompany the fractures. The neurovascular status of the extremity and the surrounding soft tissue must be carefully evaluated.

Most tibial plateau fractures are easy to identify on the standard anteroposterior (AP) and lateral projections of the knee. Traction views may be helpful in comminuted fractures that result from high-energy trauma, to identify the shape and location of the fracture fragments; 40-degree internal and external oblique films can be used in assessing fractures involved with both tibial plateau surfaces. An AP projection with a 15-degree backward inclination may be helpful in assessing the depression of the tibial plateau (**Plate 5.6**). Three-dimensional computed tomography (CT) reconstruction and magnetic resonance imaging (MRI) can be used to further characterize fractures of the tibial plateau, and assess the depression of the tibia and the degree of fragment splitting to plan for surgical intervention. MRI is excellent for illustrating ligamentous and meniscal injuries.

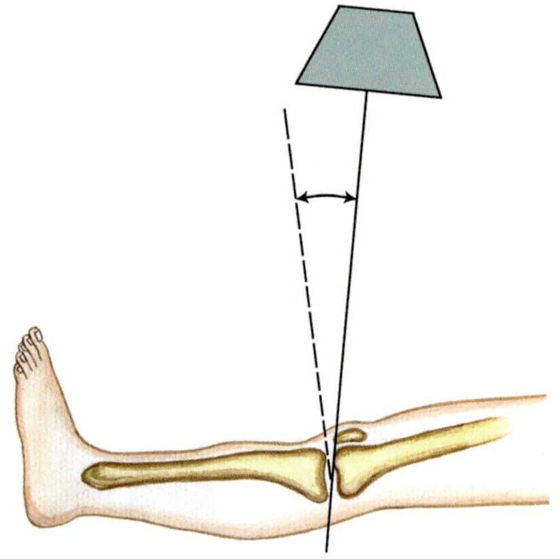

AP projection with 15-degree backward inclination

Plate 5.6

Treatment

Intra-articular fractures of the proximal tibia/fibula are always associated with unstable fragments. If the fracture involves the articular surface, surgical intervention must be considered, using the principles of anatomical reduction, large-volume bone grafting, rigid fixation, and early postoperative non-weight-bearing active mobilization, which can minimize joint adhesion and joint stiffness. Depending on the fracture healing stage, partial weight-bearing mobilization and exercise can be initiated under the supervision of an experienced therapist. Conservative methods such as casting or traction are inadequate in the treatment of such types of fractures, and should be applied cautiously even to treat fractures with minimal or no displacement.

Avulsion fractures of the fibular head are frequently associated with injuries of the lateral collateral ligament, and can be treated by casting, utilization of a joint–spanning external fixator, or internal fixation depending on the amount of fracture displacement and severity of ligamentous damage. The available internal fixators include a mini hook plate and Kirschner wire (K-wire), combined with a tension band wire. Tibial tuberosity fractures can be treated with lag screws, tension band wires, tension band wires combined with K-wires, or a mini hook plate, depending on the size of the fragments and amount of displacement. A few factors influence the treatment choice of either conservative or surgical intervention for fractures of the tibial spine, including the patient's age, size of the fragment, and amount of displacement. Surgical treatment usually can be performed by arthroscopic reduction and fixation by screws or K-wires.

Tibial Diaphyseal Fractures (Segment 42)

Anatomical Features

The tibia is triangular in cross-section, with proximal and distal flares. It has three surfaces, medial, lateral and posterior, separated by three borders, anterior, medial and lateral. This leg bone is thinnest in cross section at the junction of the middle and lower third, where fractures often occur. The anterior border, which begins at the tuberosity and ends below the anterior margin of the medial malleolus, is subcutaneous throughout its length. The tibial shaft bone is rigid, and can easily break through the skin to cause an open fracture if an injury occurs. As such, fractures of the tibia more commonly result in an open fracture than those of any other long bone. The intramedullary canal of the tibia is relatively straight longitudinally, and expands both proximally and distally. At the upper posterior surface of the tibia lies a prominent ridge, the soleal line, which extends obliquely from the superolateral to inferomedial. Although not able to withstand the weight of the body, the fibula functions as a splint or crutch to support the tibia (**Plate 5.7**).

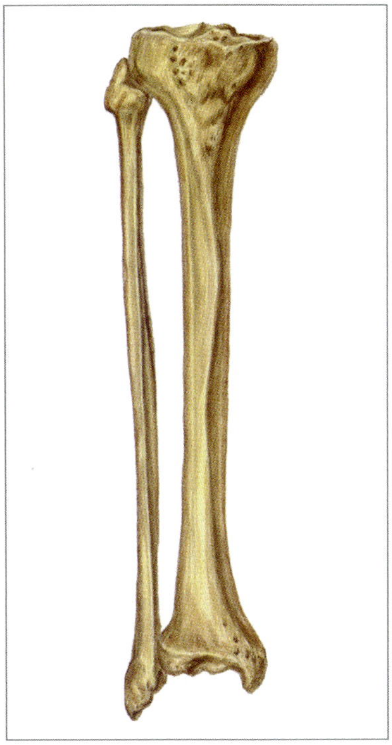

Plate 5.7

AO Classification of Tibial Diaphyseal Fractures

Based on AO classification, the tibial diaphysis is coded as the number 42 (**Plate 5.8**). Tibial diaphyseal fractures can be divided into three types based on individual fracture patterns: 42-A, simple fracture; 42-B, wedge fracture; and 42-C, complex fracture (**Plate 5.9**).

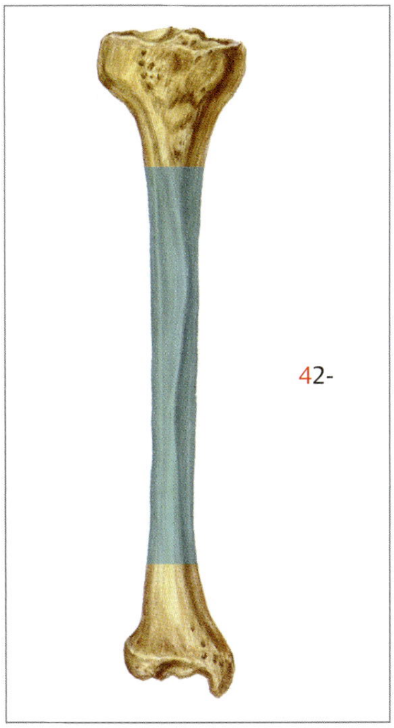

Plate 5.8

Clinical Epidemiologic Features of Tibial Diaphyseal Fractures (Segment 42)

A total of 15,000 adult tibial diaphyseal fractures were treated in 83 hospitals in China over a 2-year period from 2010 to 2011. All cases were reviewed and statistically studied; the fractures accounted for 24.75% of all tibia/fibula fractures in adults. Their epidemiologic features are as follows:

- More males than females
- The highest risk age group is 41–45 years. The most affected age group of both males and females is 41–45 years.
- The most common fracture type among segment 42 fractures is type 42-A—the same fracture type for both males and females.
- The most common fracture group among segment 42 fractures is group 42-A1; group 42-B2 in males and group 42-A1 in females.

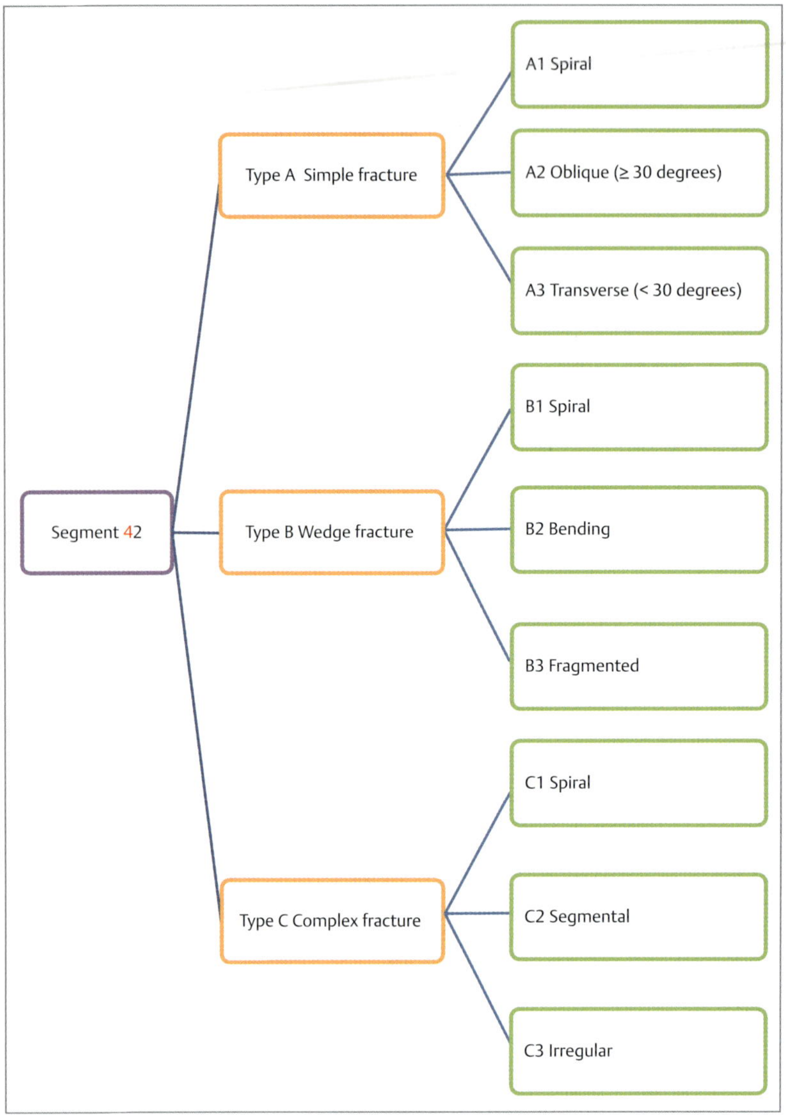

Plate 5.9

Fractures of Segment 42 by Sex

Table 5.10 Sex distribution of 15,000 fractures of segment 42

Sex	Number of fractures	Percentage (%)
Male	11,717	78.11
Female	3,283	21.89
Total	15,000	100.00

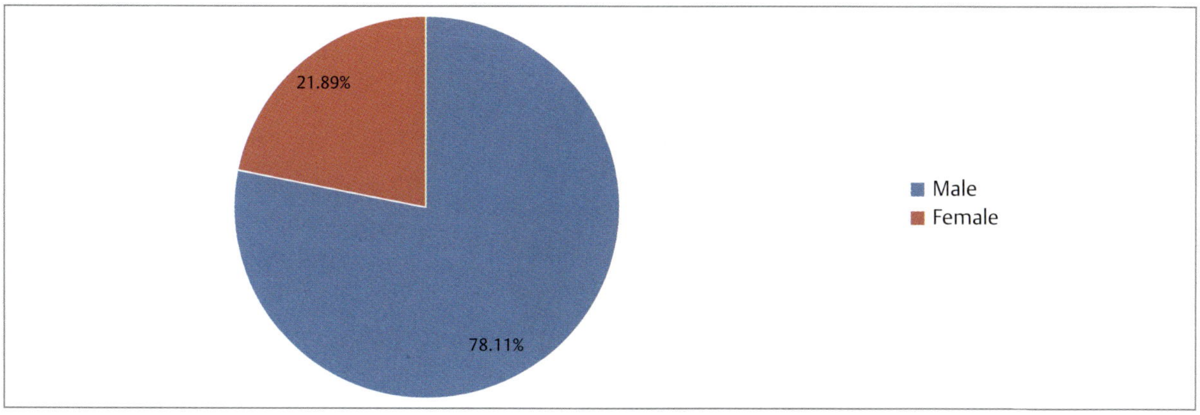

Fig. 5.10 Sex distribution of 15,000 fractures of segment 42.

Fractures of Segment 42 by Age Group

Table 5.11 Sex and age distribution of 15,000 fractures of segment 42

Age group (years)	Male	Female	Number of fractures	Percentage (%)
16–20	948	195	1,143	7.62
21–25	1,365	299	1,664	11.09
26–30	1,211	235	1,446	9.64
31–35	1,246	271	1,517	10.11
36–40	1,574	411	1,985	13.23
41–45	1,686	485	2,171	14.47
46–50	1,249	392	1,641	10.94
51–55	975	272	1,247	8.31
56–60	719	241	960	6.40
61–65	338	168	506	3.37
66–70	167	108	275	1.83
71–75	110	71	181	1.21
76–80	68	74	142	0.95
81–85	41	36	77	0.51
≥86	20	25	45	0.30
Total	11,717	3,283	15,000	100.00

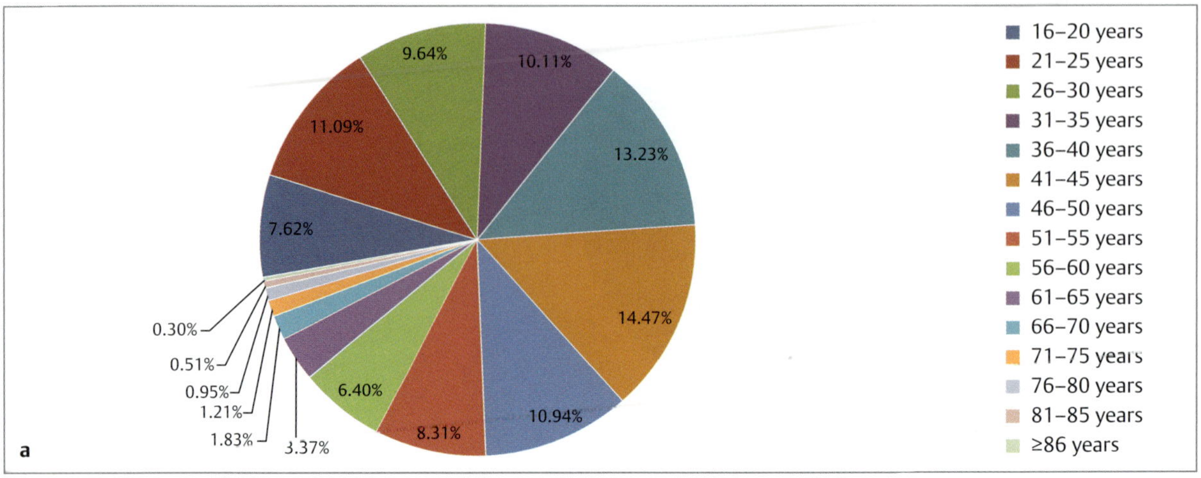

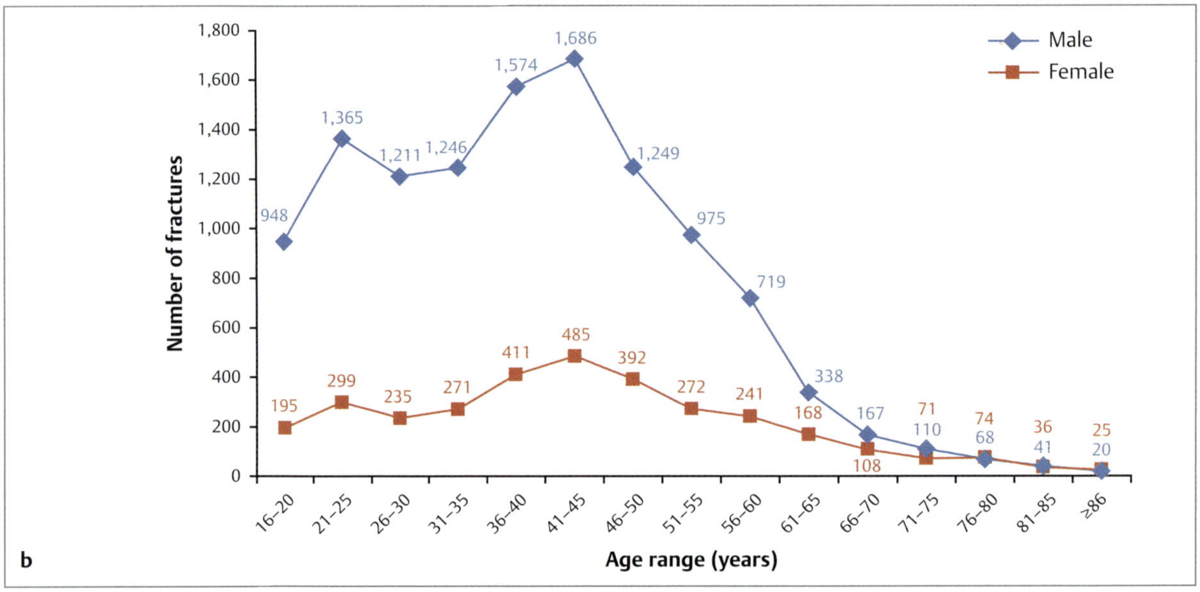

Fig. 5.11 **(a)** Age distribution of 15,000 fractures of segment 42.
(b) Age and sex distribution of 15,000 fractures of segment 42.

Fractures of Segment 42 by Fracture Type

Table 5.12 Sex and fracture type distribution of 15,000 fractures of segment 42

Fracture type	Male	Female	Number of fractures	Percentage (%)
42-A	5,176	1,744	6,920	46.13
42-B	4,209	1,114	5,323	35.49
42-C	2,332	425	2,757	18.38
Total	11,717	3,283	15,000	100.00

5

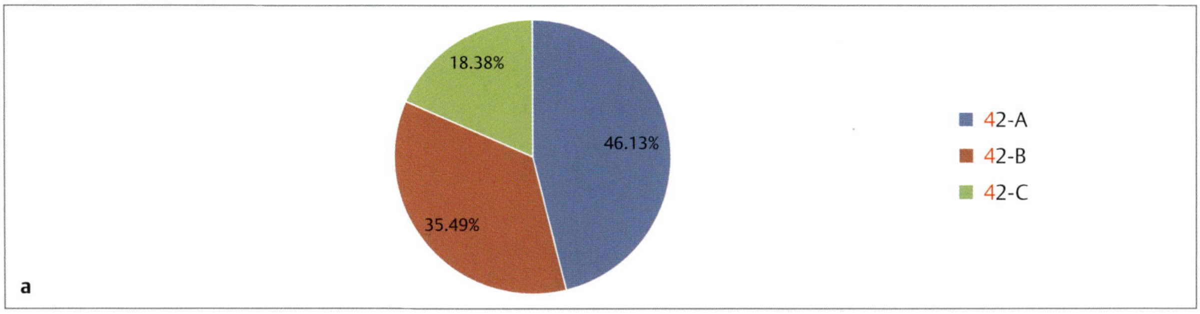

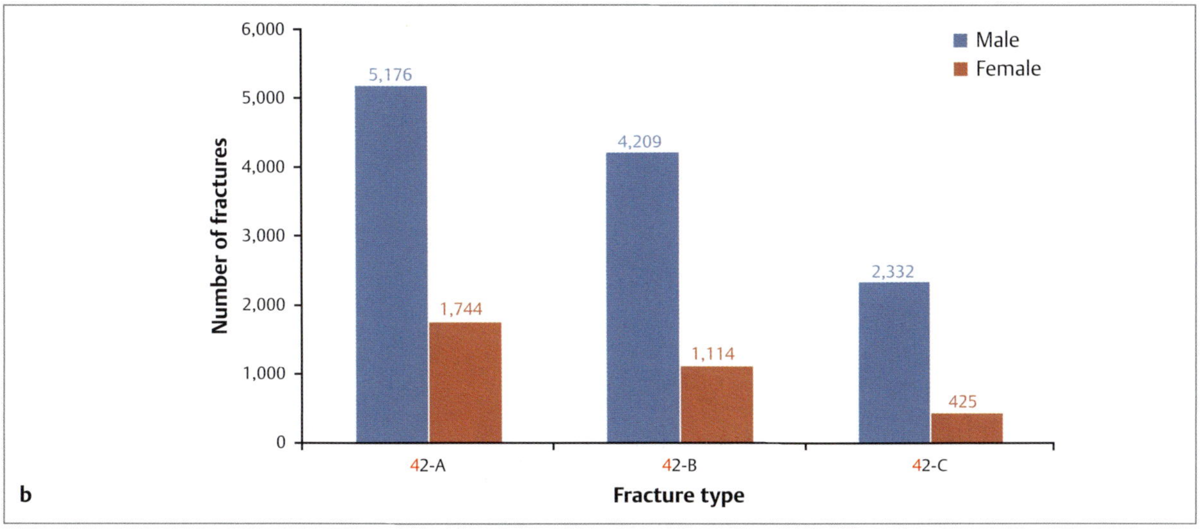

Fig. 5.12 **(a)** Fracture type distribution of 15,000 fractures of segment 42.
(b) Sex and fracture type distribution of 15,000 fractures of segment 42.

Table 5.13 Sex and fracture group distribution of 15,000 fractures of segment 42

Fracture group	Male	Female	Number of fractures	Percentage of segment 42 (%)	Percentage of tibia/fibula (%)
42-A1	1,881	889	2,770	18.47	4.57
42-A2	1,506	460	1,966	13.11	3.24
42-A3	1,789	395	2,184	14.56	3.60
42-B1	780	305	1,085	7.23	1.79
42-B2	2,072	542	2,614	17.43	4.31
42-B3	1,357	267	1,624	10.83	2.68
42-C1	404	89	493	3.29	0.81
42-C2	709	166	875	5.83	1.44
42-C3	1,219	170	1,389	9.26	2.29
Total	11,717	3,283	15,000	100.00	24.75

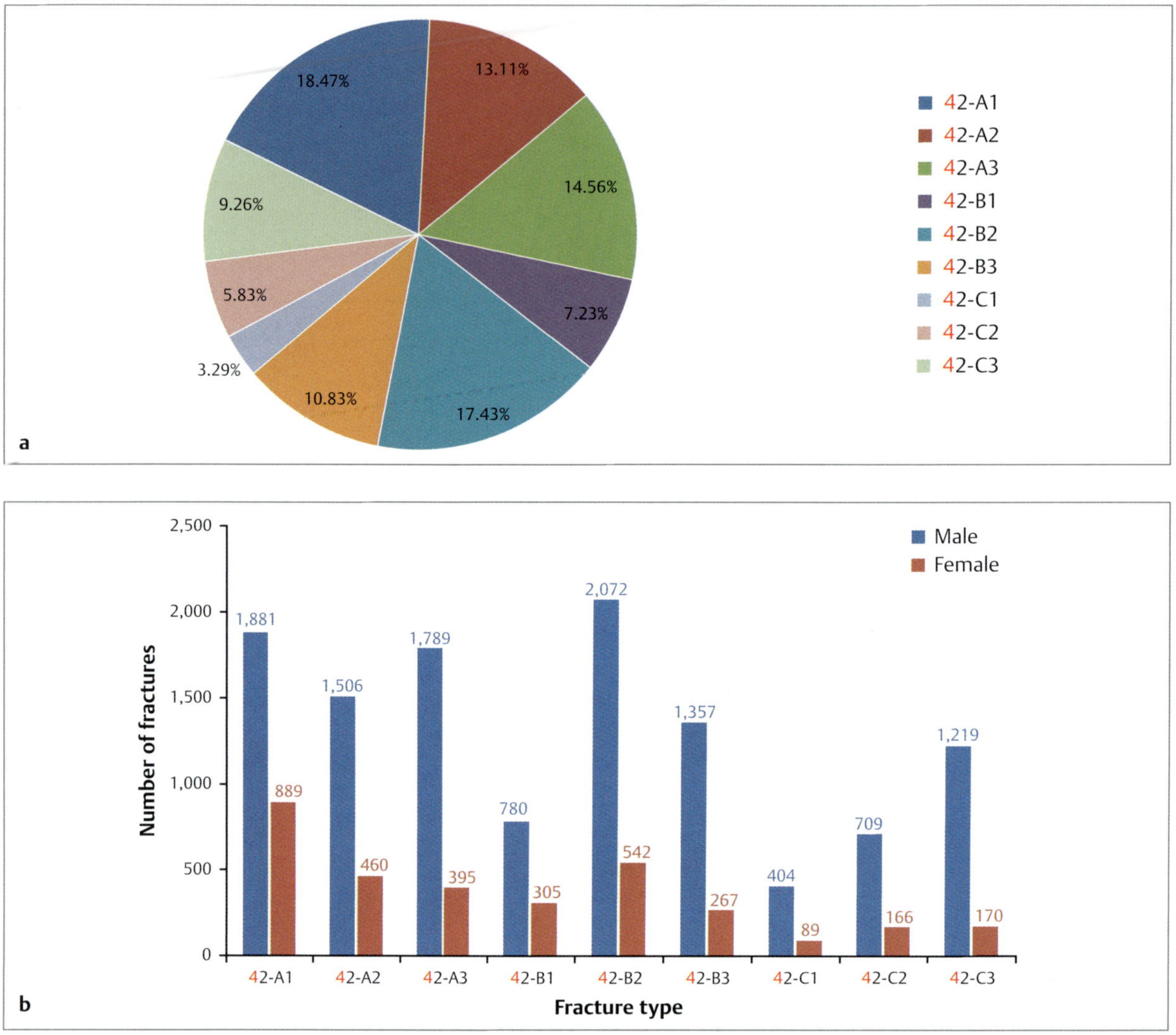

Fig. 5.13 **(a)** Fracture group distribution of 15,000 fractures of segment 42.
(b) Sex and fracture group distribution of 15,000 fractures of segment 42.

5

42-A Tibia/fibula diaphysis, simple fractures

42-A1
Spiral
2,770 fractures
M: 1,881 (67.91%)
F: 889 (32.09%)
0.74% of total adult fractures
4.57% of adult tibia/fibula fractures
18.47% of segment 42
40.03% of type 42A

42-A1.1

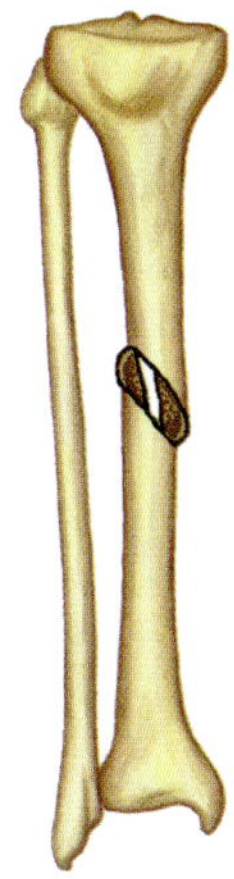

Fibula intact

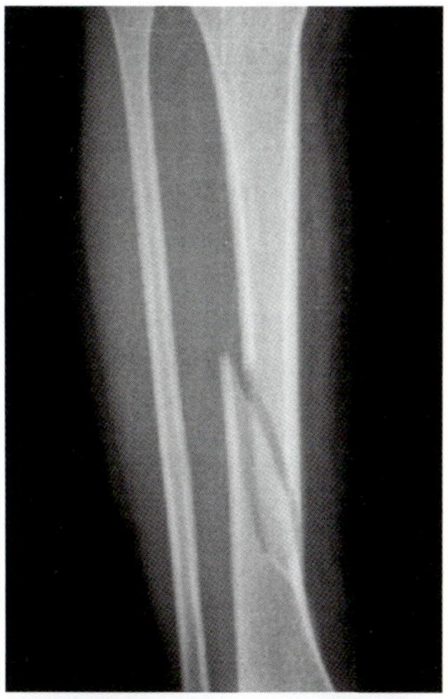

42-A1.2

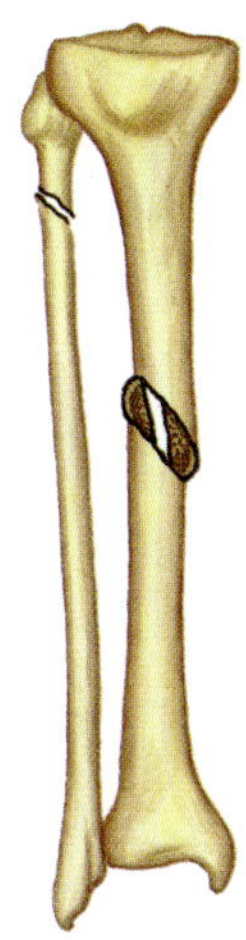

Tibia and fibula fractures at different level

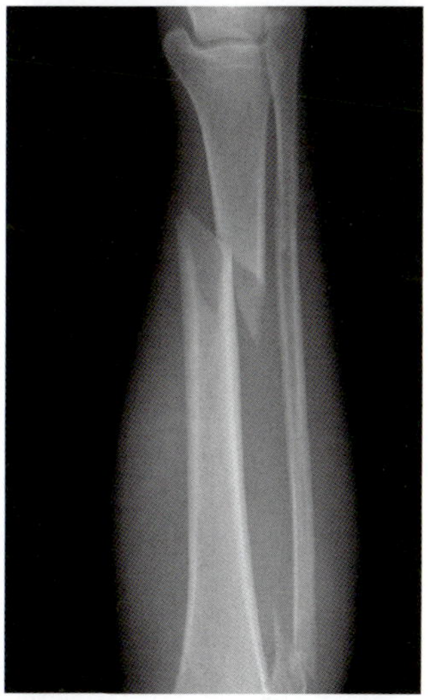

42-A1.3

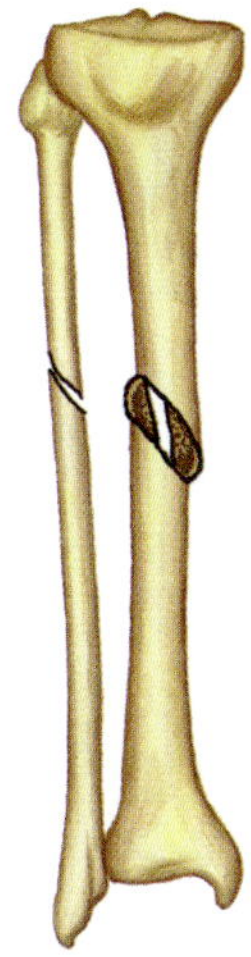

Tibia and fibula fractures at the same level

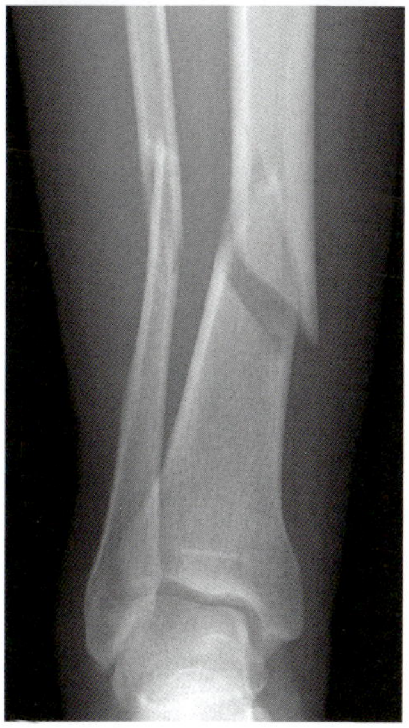

42-A Tibia/fibula diaphysis, simple fractures

42-A2
Oblique (≥ 30 degrees)
1,966 fractures
M: 1,506 (76.60%)
F: 460 (23.40%)
0.53% of total adult fractures
3.24% of adult tibia/fibula fractures
13.11% of segment 42
28.41% of type 42-A

42-A2.1

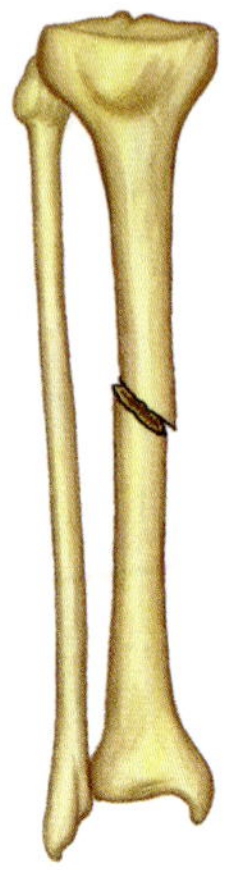

Fibula intact

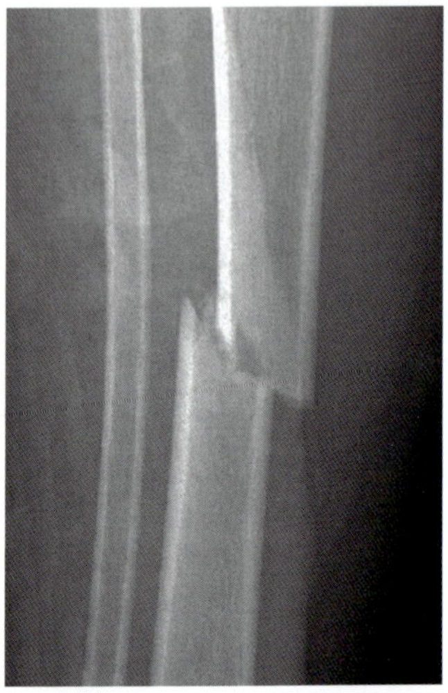

42-A2.2

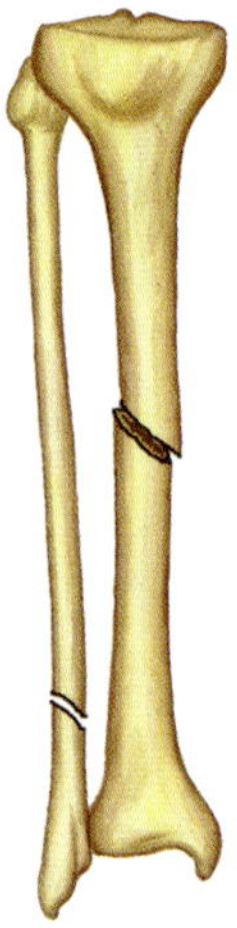

Tibia and fibula fractures at different levels

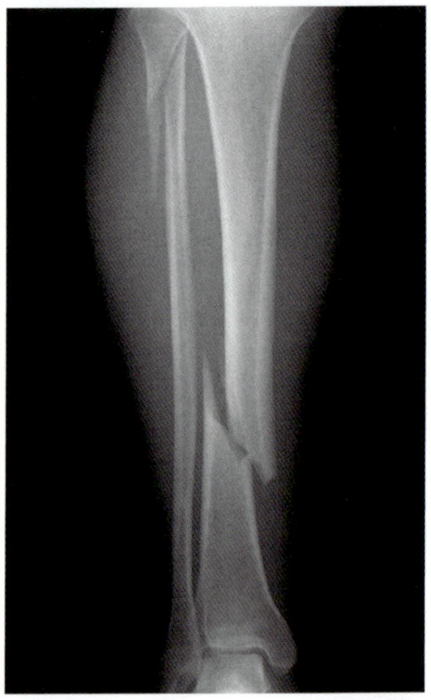

42-A2.3

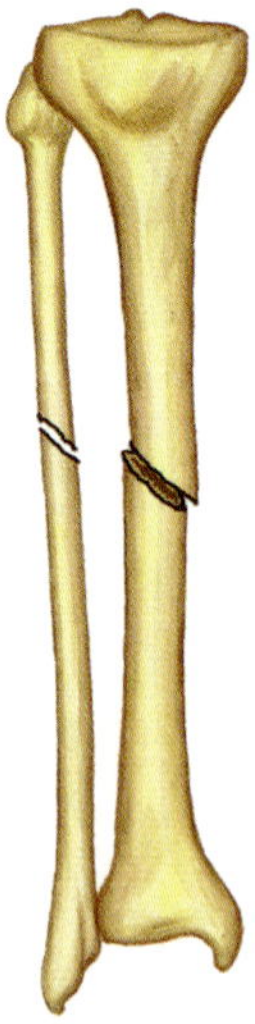

Tibia and fibula fractures at the same level

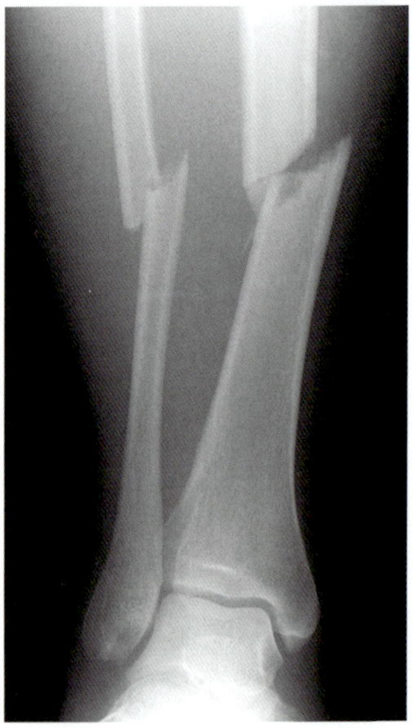

42-A Tibia/fibula diaphysis, simple fractures

42-A3

Transverse (< 30 degrees)

2,184 fractures
M: 1,789 (81.91%)
F: 395 (18.09%)
0.58% of total adult fractures
3.60% of adult tibia/fibula fractures
14.56% of segment 42
31.56% of type 42-A

42-A3.1

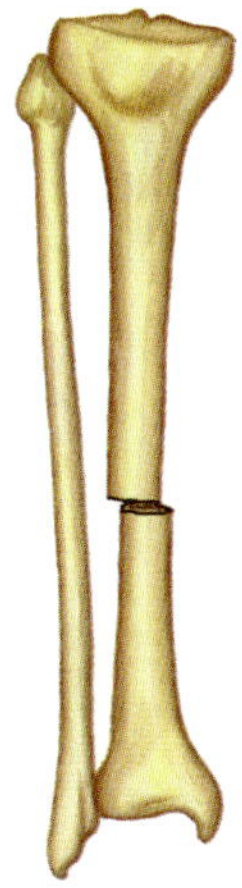

Fibula intact

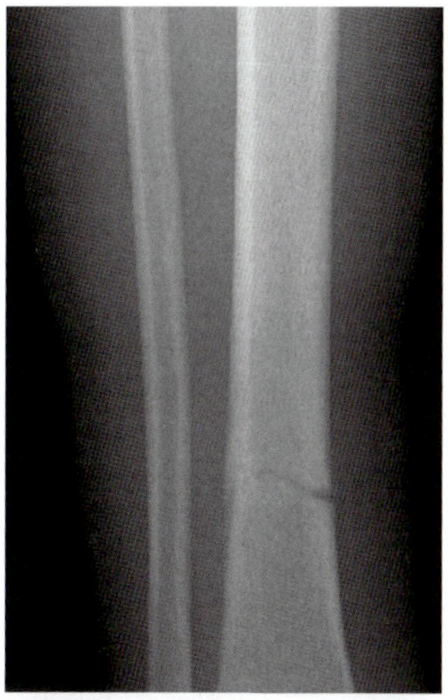

42-A3.2

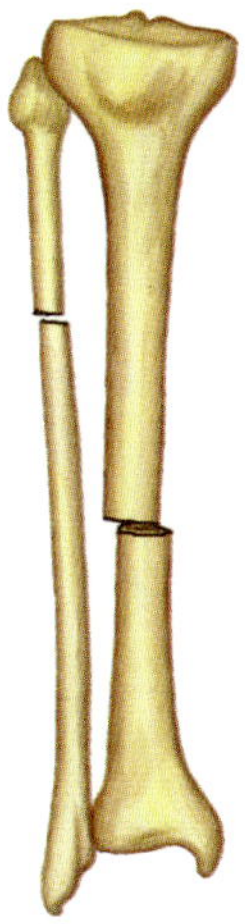

Tibia and fibula fractures at different levels

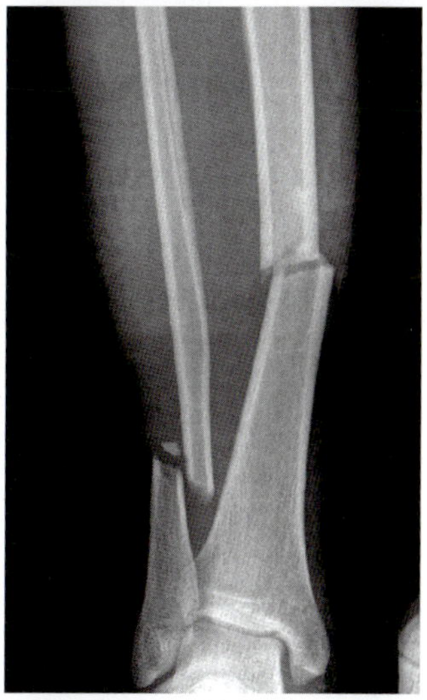

42-A3.3

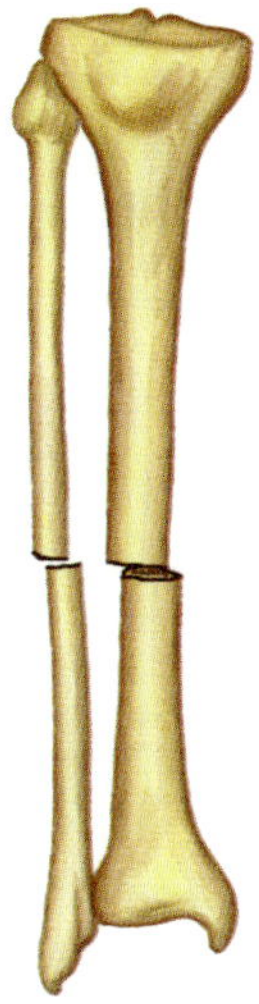

Tibia and fibula fractures at the same level

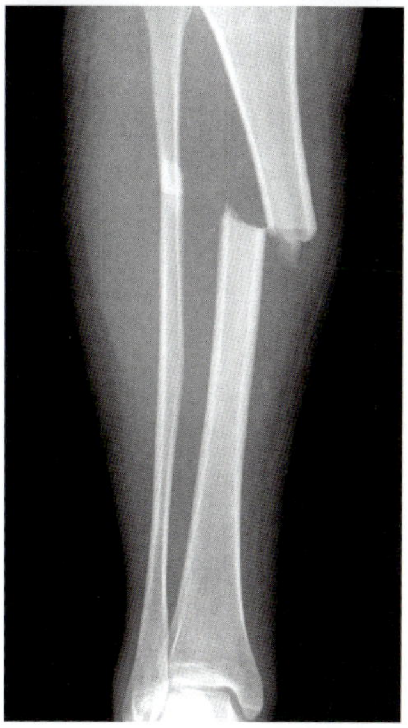

42-B Tibia/fibula diaphysis, wedge fractures

42-B1
Spiral
1,085 fractures
M: 780 (71.89%)
F: 305 (28.11%)
0.29% of total adult fractures
1.79% of adult tibia/fibula fractures
7.23% of segment 42
20.38% of type 42-B

42-B1.1

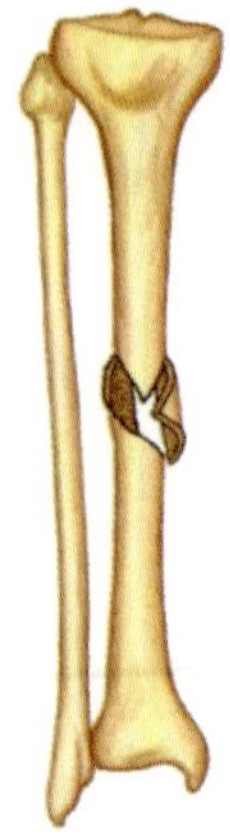

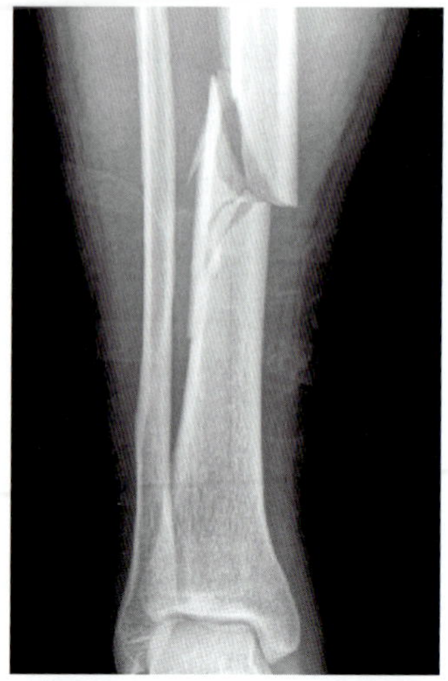

Fibula intact

42-B1.2

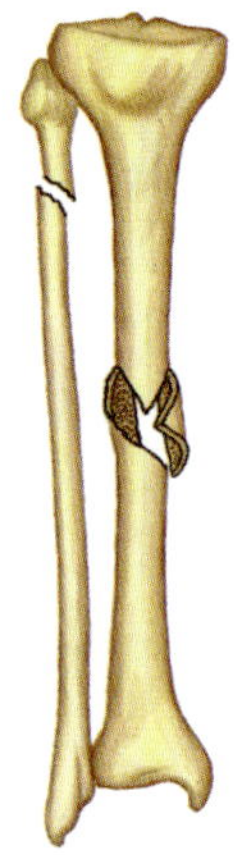

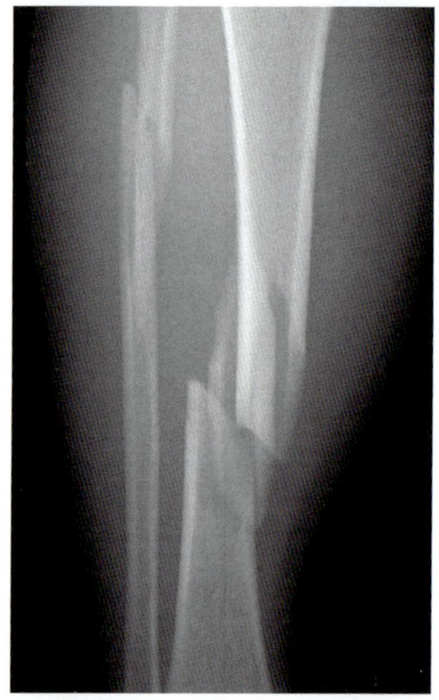

Tibia and fibula fractures at different levels

42-B1.3

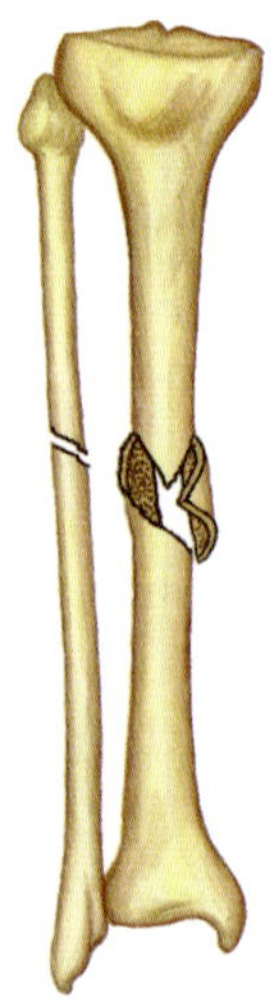

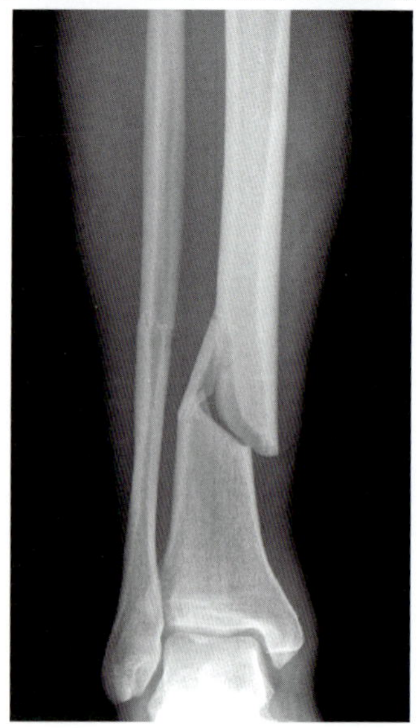

Tibia and fibula fractures at the same level

42-B Tibia/fibula diaphysis, wedge fractures

42-B2
Bending
2,614 fractures
M: 2,072 (79.27%)
F: 542 (20.73%)
0.7% of total adult fractures
4.31% of adult tibia/fibula fractures
17.43% of segment 42
49.11% of type 42-B

42-B2.1

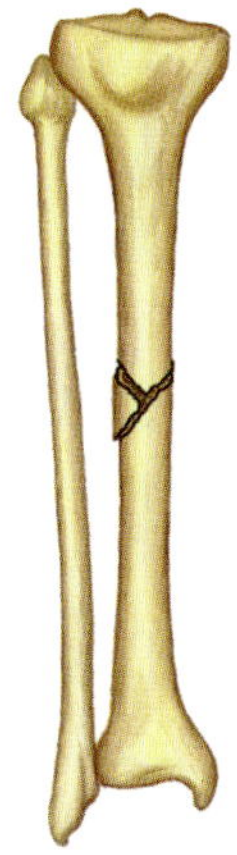

Fibula intact

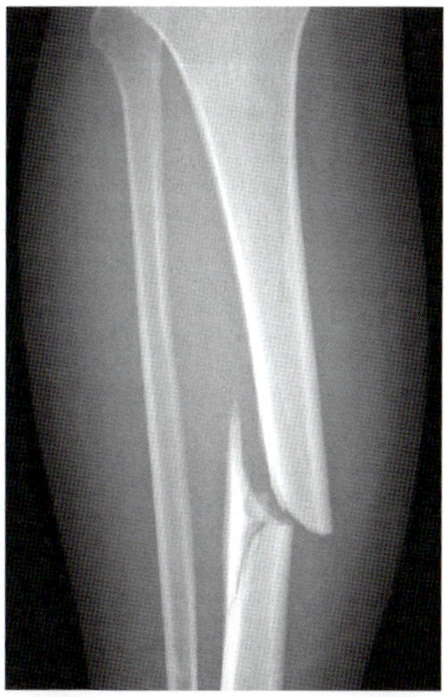

42-B2.2

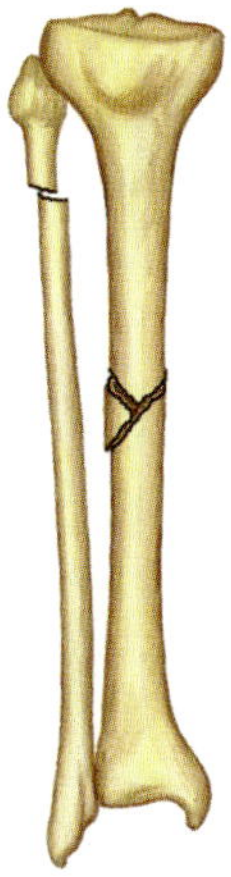

Tibia and fibula fractures at different levels

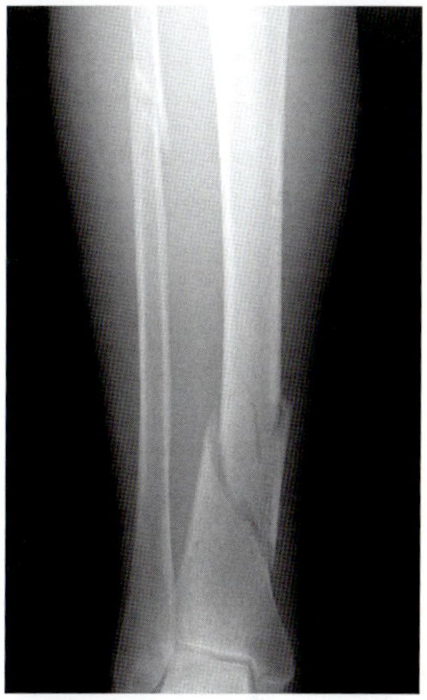

42-B2.3

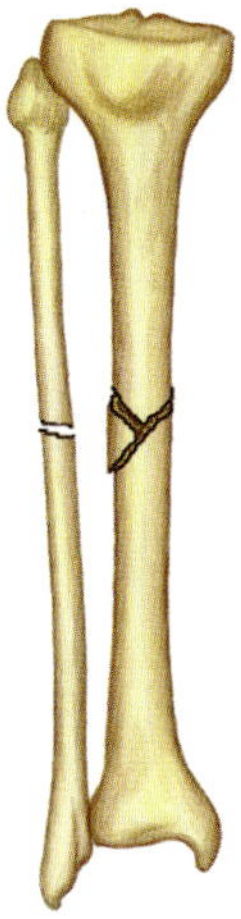

Tibia and fibula fractures at the same level

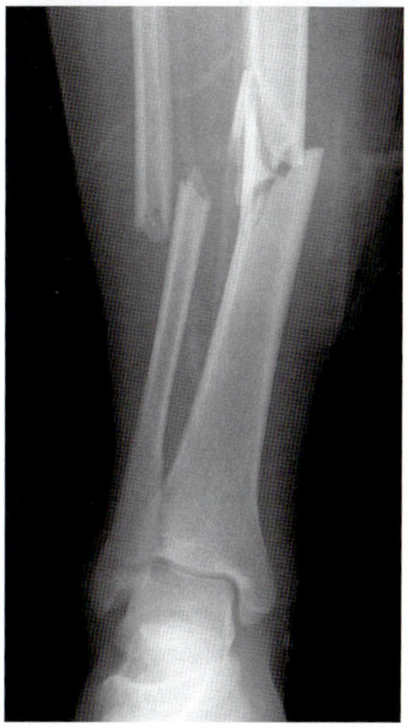

42-B Tibia/fibula diaphysis, wedge fractures

42-B3
Fragmented
1,624 fractures
M: 1,357 (83.56%)
F: 267 (16.44%)
0.43% of total adult fractures
2.68% of adult tibia/fibula fractures
10.83% of segment 42
30.51% of type 42-B

42-B3.1

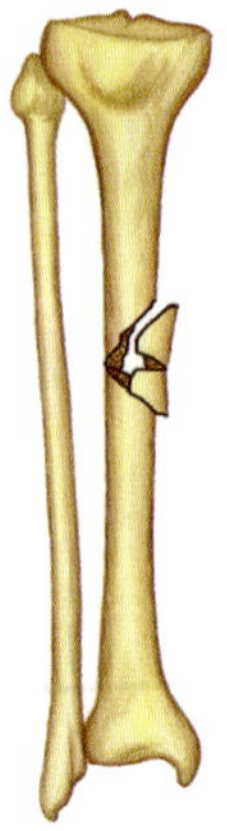

Fibula intact

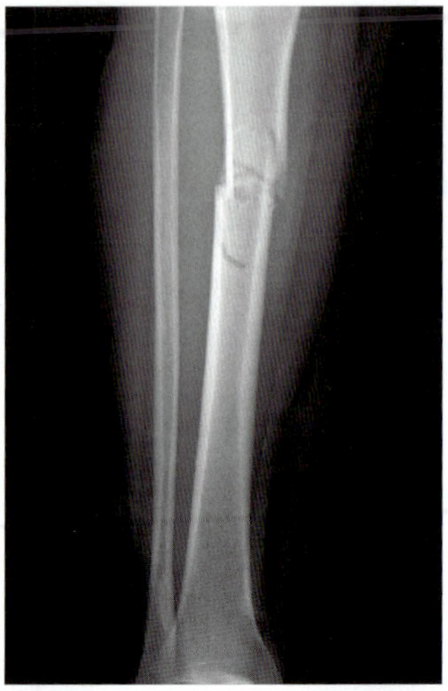

42-B3.2

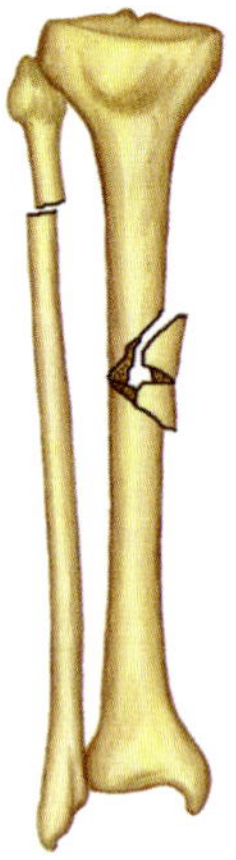

Tibia and fibula fractures at different levels

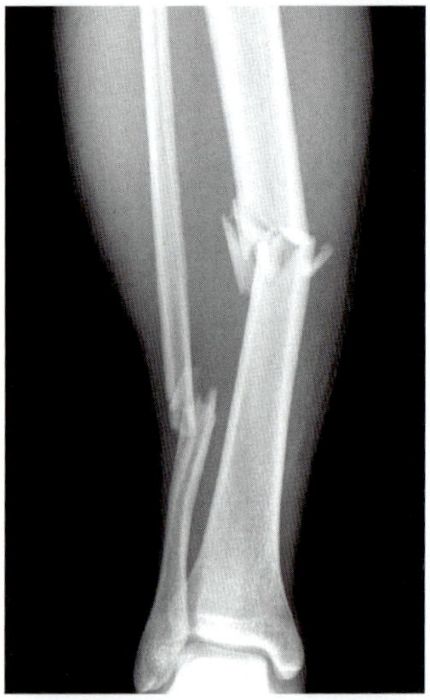

42-B3.3

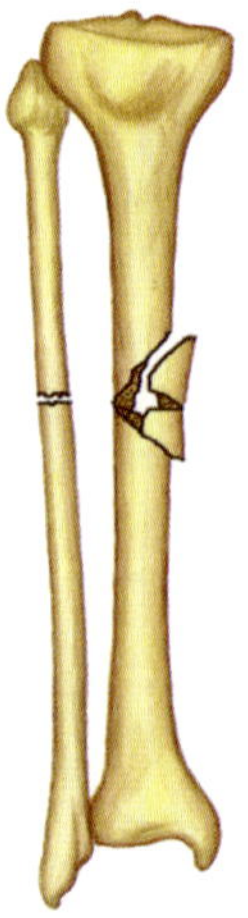

Tibia and fibula fractures at the same level

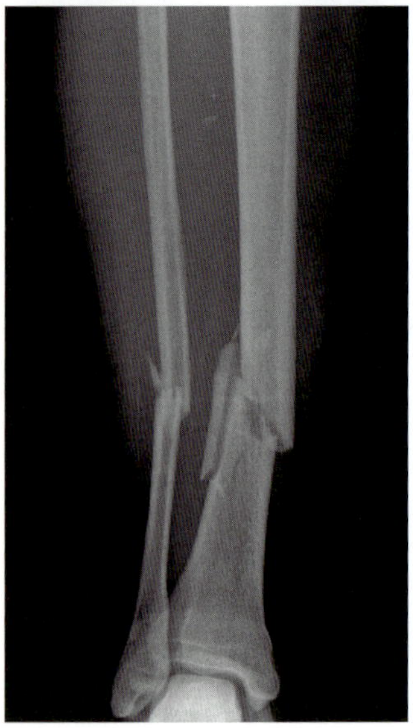

42-C Tibia/fibula diaphysis, complex fractures

42-C1
Spiral
493 fractures
M: 404 (81.95%)
F: 89 (18.05%)
0.13% of total adult fractures
0.81% of adult tibia/fibula fractures
3.29% of segment 42
17.88% of type 42-C

42-C1.1

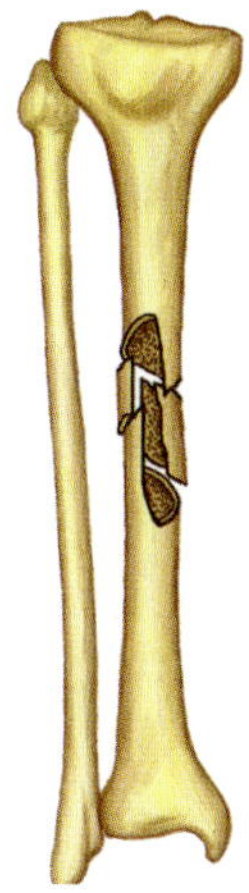

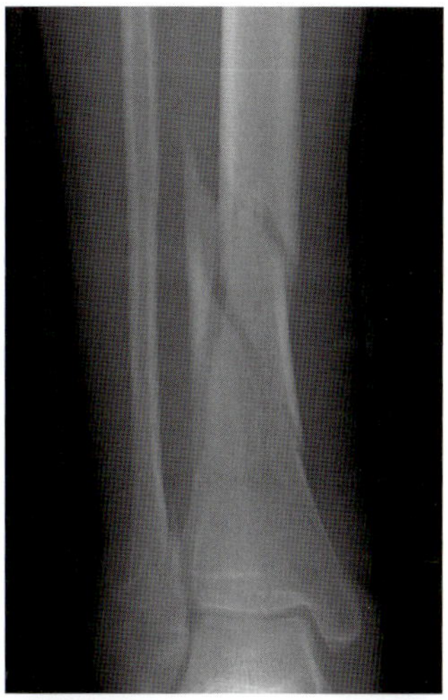

With two intermediate fragments

42-C1.2

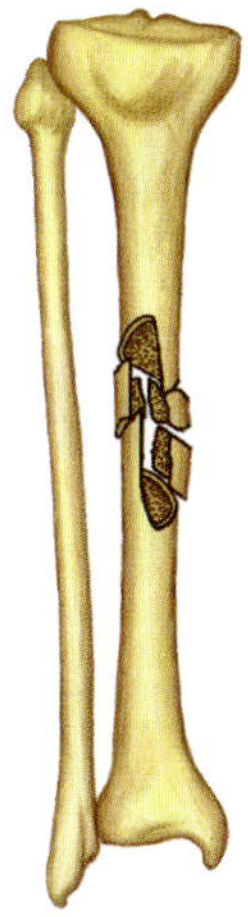

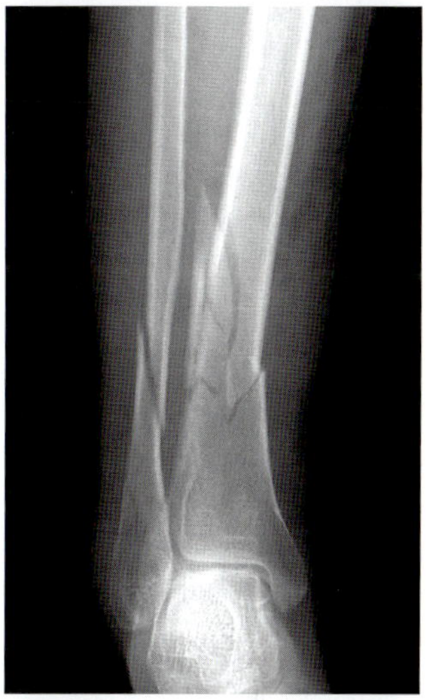

With three intermediate fragments

42-C1.3

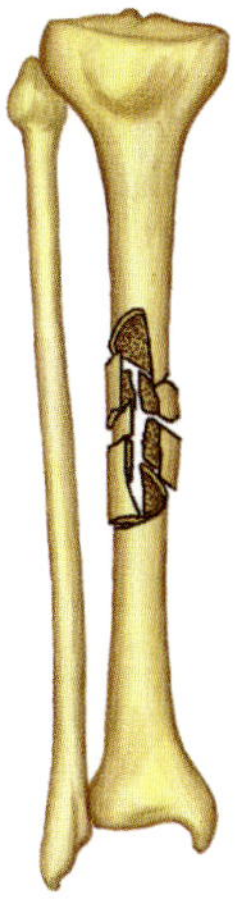

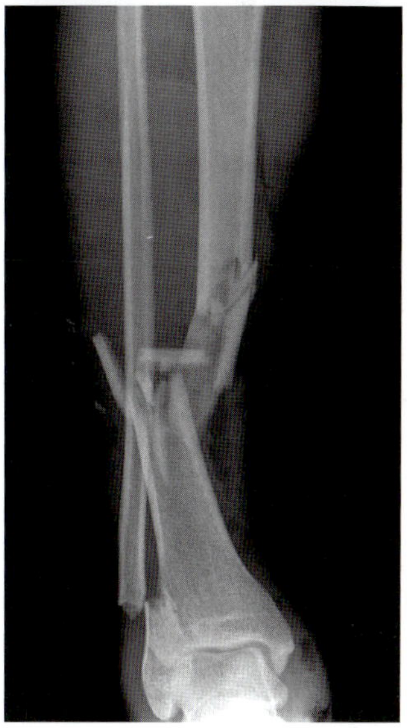

With more than three intermediate fragments

42-C Tibia/fibula diaphysis, complex fractures

42-C2
Segmental
875 fractures
M: 709 (81.03%)
F: 166 (18.97%)
0.23% of total adult fractures
1.44% of adult tibia/fibula fractures
5.83% of segment 42
31.74% of type 42-C

42-C2.1

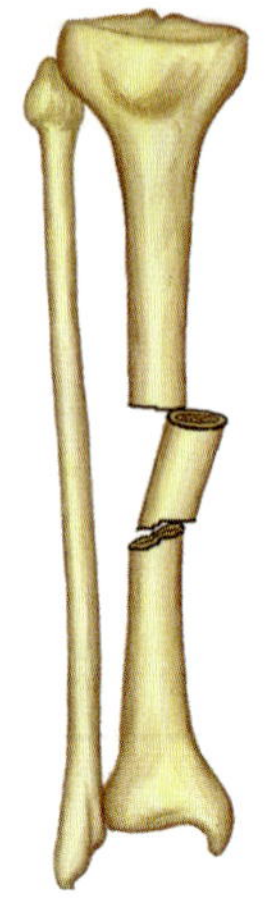

With one intermediate fragment

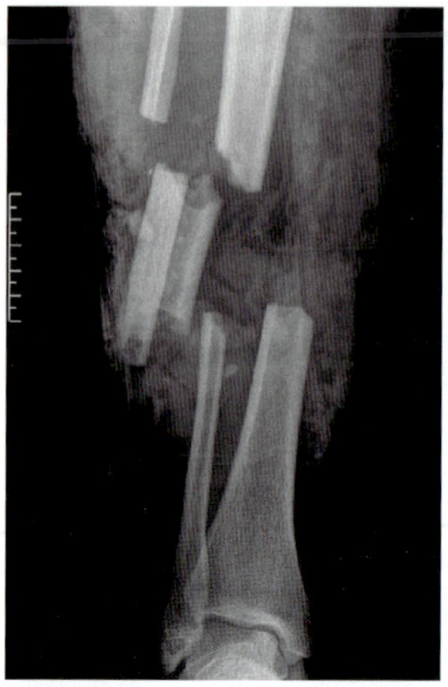

42-C2.2

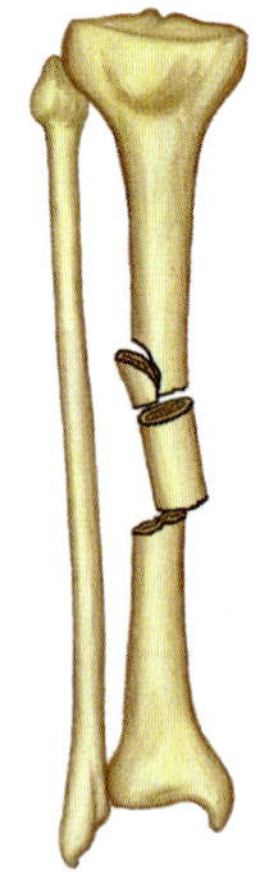

With one intermediate fragment and an additional wedge fragment

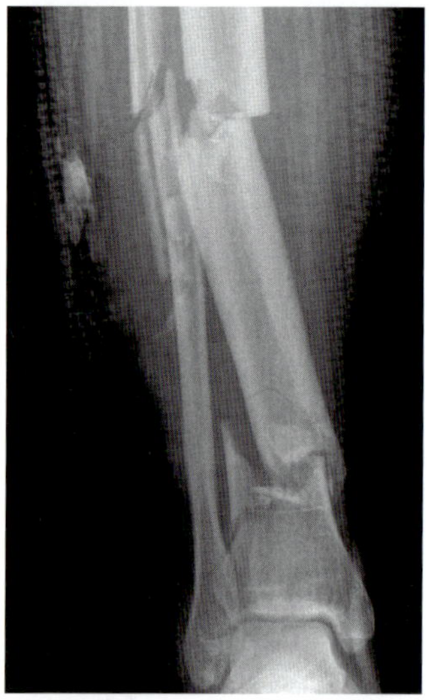

42-C2.3

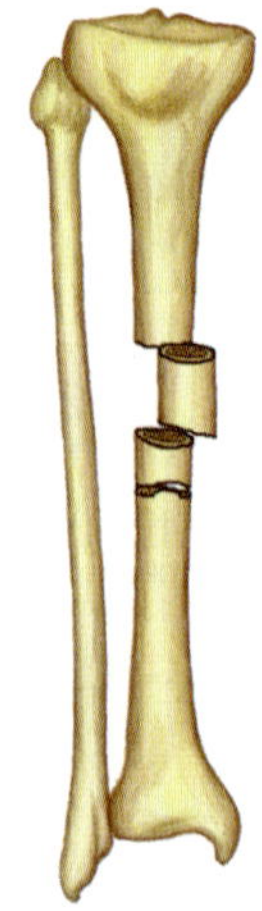

With two intermediate fragments

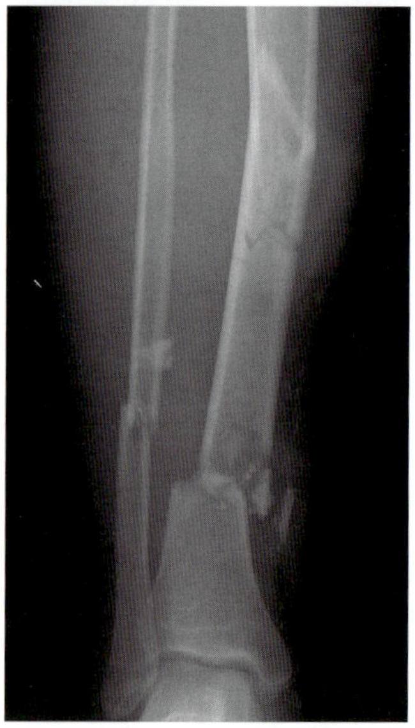

42-C Tibia/fibula diaphysis, complex fractures

42-C3
Irregular
1,389 fractures
M: 1,219 (87.76%)
F: 170 (12.24%)
0.37% of total adult fractures
2.29% of adult tibia/fibula fractures
9.26% of segment 42
50.38% of type 42-C

42-C3.1

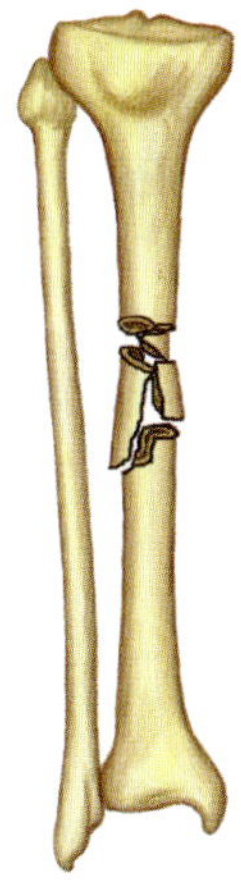

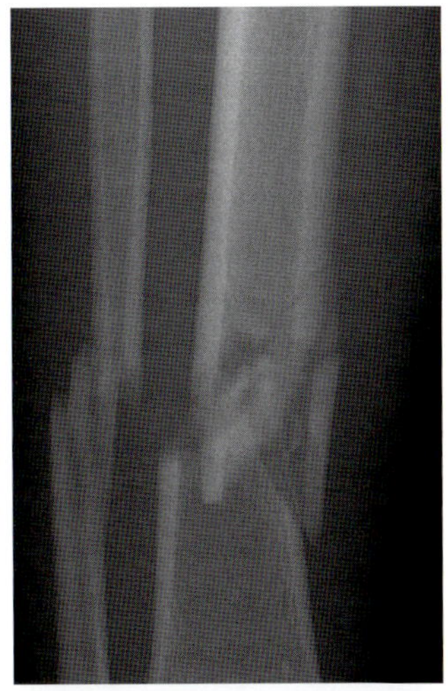

With two or three intermediate fragments

42-C3.2

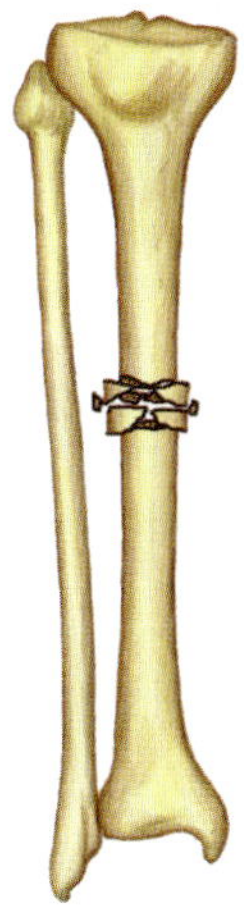

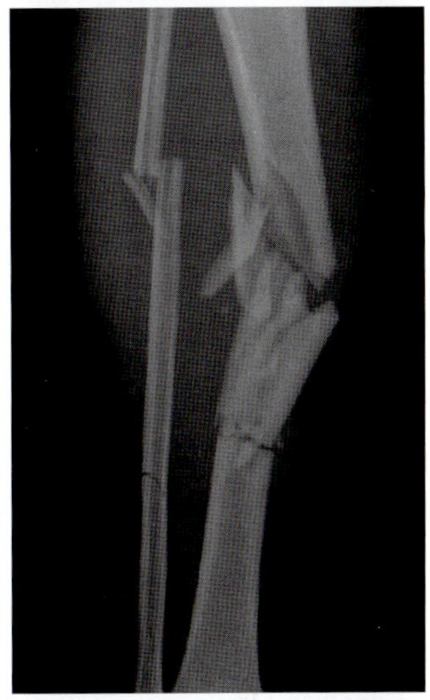

With limited shattering (< 4 cm)

42-C3.3

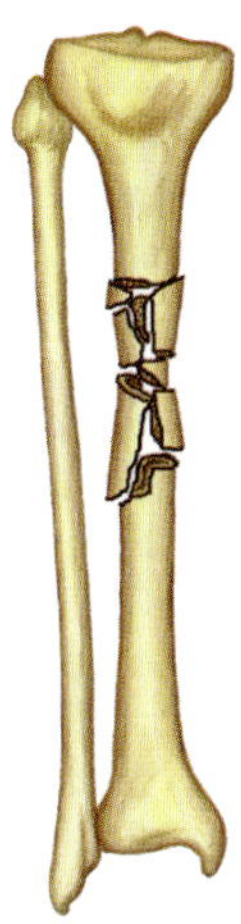

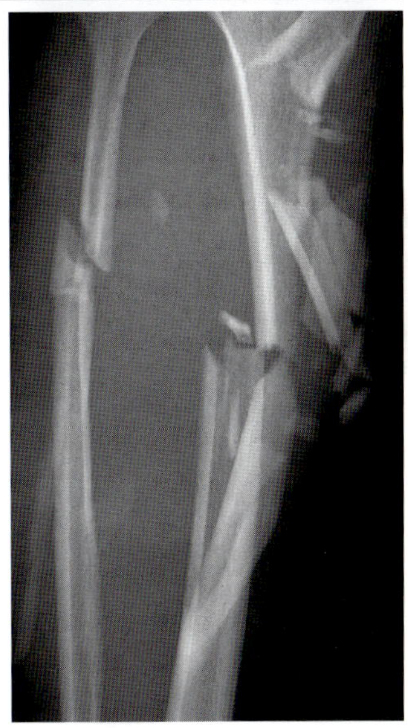

With extensive shattering (≥ 4 cm)

Injury Mechanism

The mechanism of a diaphyseal tibial fracture can be direct or indirect. Direct mechanisms of injury lead to high-energy fractures resulting from, for example, violent blows, motor vehicle crashes, being crushed by heavy objects, etc. High-energy insults produce transverse, short oblique, or comminuted displaced diaphyseal fractures with a high incidence of compound and soft tissue injuries. Indirect mechanisms lead to low-energy injuries, which produce spiral, nondisplaced, minimally comminuted fractures with minimal soft tissue damage.

Diagnosis

A thorough physical examination should be conducted to assess soft tissue damage, deformity of the affected limb, and stability of the fracture. Special attention should be given to assessment of neurovascular status and the presence of compartment syndrome. Standard AP and lateral views of the injured leg are invaluable in identifying the location and type of fracture. The ipsilateral knee and ankle are also often radiographically imaged because concomitant injury to one or both of these joints is common. Injury is especially likely when the deformity or point tenderness of the tibia and fibula are not at the same level, or if a fracture of the proximal fibula is suspected. Fractures of the distal third of the tibia are often associated with posterior malleolar fractures. If there is obvious point tenderness over the posterior malleolus but X-ray films are normal, CT or MRI should be considered to detect the evidence of fractures.

Treatment

The goals in treatment of diaphyseal tibial fractures are to correct angulation and deformity, and to restore normal alignment, length, and joint congruity. Closed fractures with minimal displacement or stable reduction may be treated nonoperatively with a long leg cast. Operative fixation is required when fractures are unstable. A few fixation methods are widely used, including intramedullary nailing, plating (locking compression plate or U-grooved locking compression plate), and external fixation—the choice of which is based on the fracture type and the severity of the soft tissue damage. When plating tibial shaft fractures, an anterolateral surgical incision should be used. The standard site for tibial plating is the lateral surface of the bone, due to the fact that skin lesions occur most frequently on the anteromedial side, because the medial surface is covered only with a layer of skin. Severe open tibial fractures should be treated primarily by external fixation, and converted to internal fixation only when the swelling of the soft tissue is diminished and the patient becomes stable. If there is a skin defect, a skin graft, or a free skin flap, a vascular pedicle flap can be used to cover the wound and reconstruct the defect. Since increased nonunion and healing times have been associated with tibial fractures, bone grafting, in addition to surgical reduction and internal fixation, is frequently used to augment the bone healing process.

Distal Tibial Fractures (Segment 43)

Anatomical Features

The lower end of the tibia expands and becomes quadrilateral-shaped. It has five surfaces: anterior, posterior, inferior, lateral, and medial. The anterior surface is smooth and covered by tendons of the extensor muscles; its lower margin presents a rough transverse depression for the attachment of the articular capsule of the ankle joint. The medial surface is convex and rough, and continues downward into a triangular process called the medial malleolus. On the posterior surface there are two grooves for passage of the flexor hallucis longus tendon. The lateral surface has a triangular rough depression, the lower part of which is called the fibular notch, where the tibia articulates with the fibula. The anterior and posterior margins of the fibular notch give attachment to the anterior and posterior tibiofibular ligaments, respectively. The inferior surface is four-sided, slightly concave, and smooth, for articulation with the talus. Its posterior margin, called the posterior malleolus, is slightly elevated to prevent posterior dislocation of the talus.

AO Classification of Distal Tibial Fractures

Based on AO classification, the distal tibia is coded as the number 43 (**Plate 5.10**). Distal tibia fractures can be divided into three types depending on articular involvement: 43-A, extra-articular fracture; 43-B, partial articular fracture; and 43-C, complete articular fracture (**Plate 5.11**).

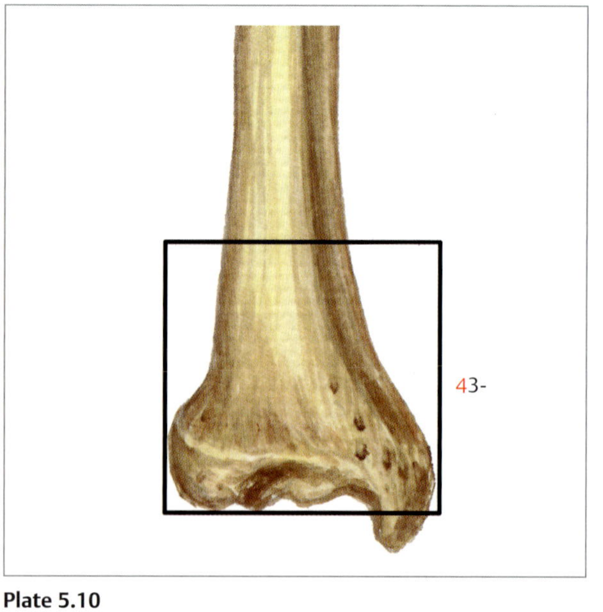

Plate 5.10

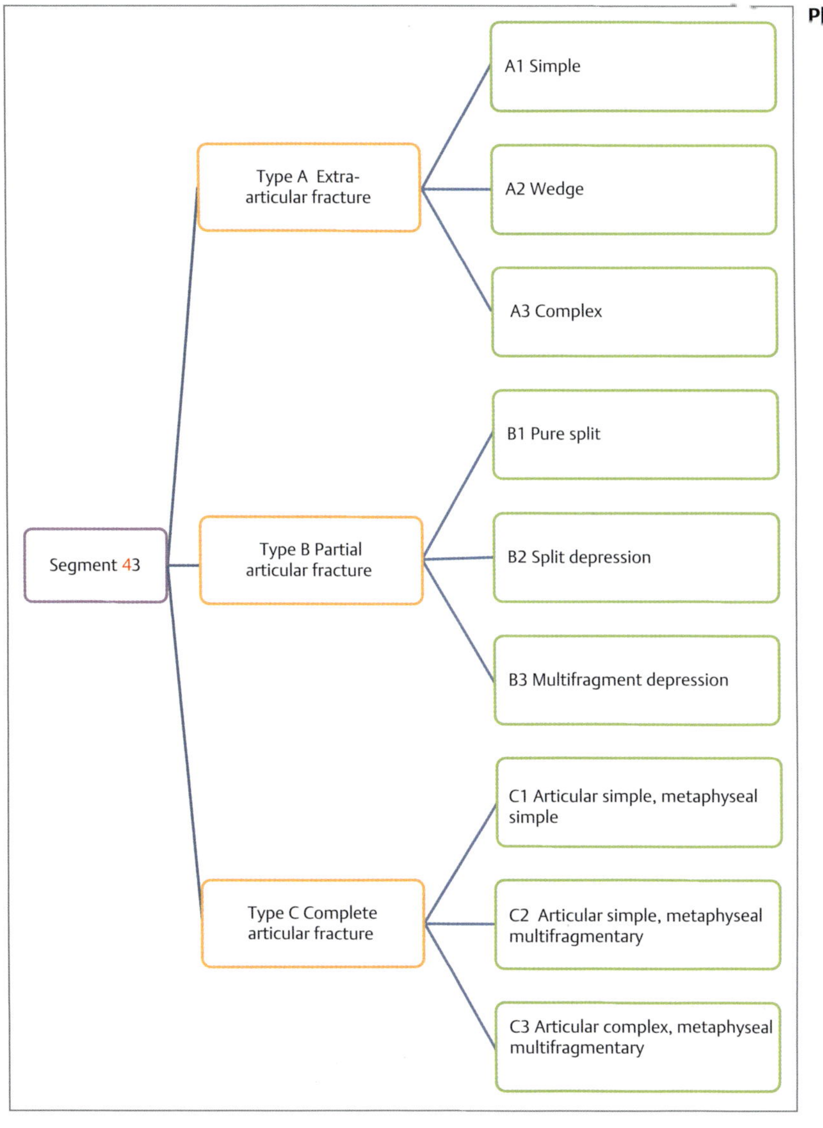

Plate 5.11

Clinical Epidemiologic Features of Distal Tibial Fractures (Segment 43)

A total of 6,391 distal tibial fractures were treated in 83 hospitals in China over a 2-year period from 2010 to 2011. All cases were reviewed and statistically studied; the fractures accounted for 10.54% of all tibia/fibula fractures in adults. Their epidemiologic features are as follows:

- More males than females
- The highest risk age group is 41–45 years. The most affected male age group is ages 41–45 years, while females of ages 56–60 years have the highest risk.
- The most common fracture type among segment 43 fractures is type 43-A—the same fracture type for both males and females.
- The most common fracture group among segment 43 fractures is group 43-A2—the same fracture group for both males and females.

ent 43 by Sex

ion of 6,391 fractures of segment 43

	Number of fractures	Percentage (%)
	4,445	69.55
	1,946	30.45
otal	6,391	100.00

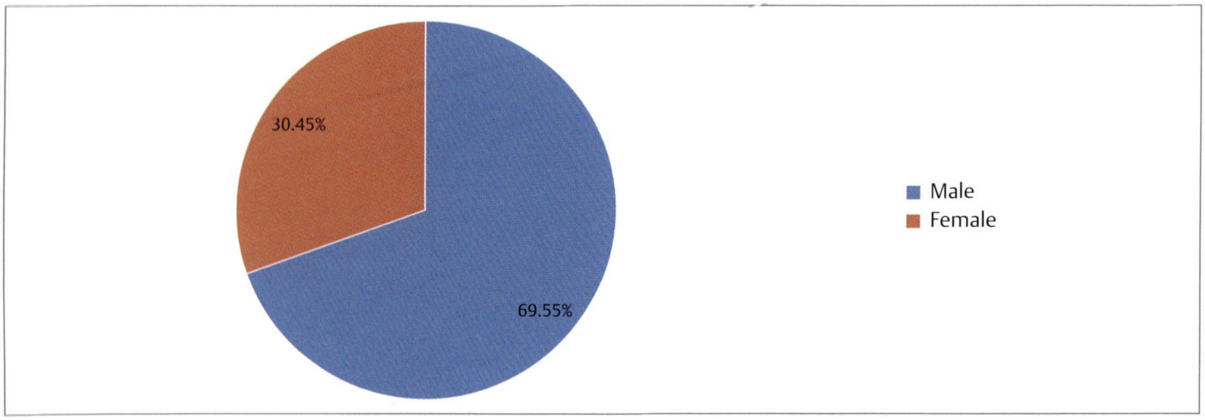

Fig.5.14 Sex distribution of 6,391 fractures of segment 43.

Fractures of Segment 43 by Age Group

Table 5.15 Age and sex distribution of 6,391 fractures of segment 43

Age group (years)	Male	Female	Number of fractures	Percentage (%)
16–20	265	47	312	4.88
21–25	320	104	424	6.63
26–30	403	120	523	8.18
31–35	491	127	618	9.67
36–40	631	200	831	13.00
41–45	713	213	926	14.49
46–50	527	213	740	11.58
51–55	384	213	597	9.34
56–60	296	226	522	8.17
61–65	190	138	328	5.13
66–70	83	122	205	3.21
71–75	64	81	145	2.27
76–80	39	60	99	1.55
81–85	27	49	76	1.19
≥86	12	33	45	0.70
Total	4,445	1,946	6,391	100.00

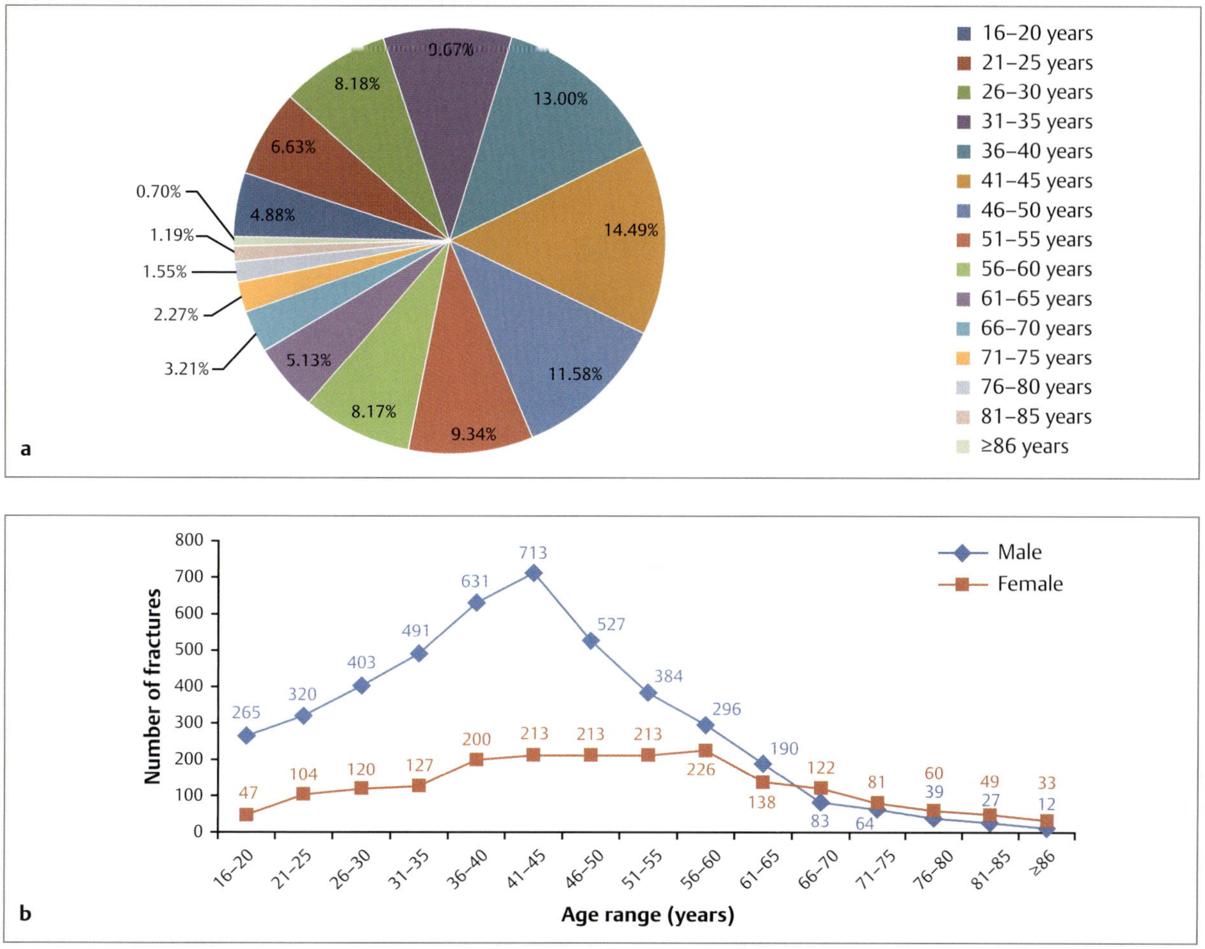

Fig. 5.15 **(a)** Age distribution of 6,391 fractures of segment 43.
(b) Age and sex distribution of 6,391 fractures of segment 43.

Fractures of Segment 43 by Fracture Type

Table 5.16 Sex and fracture type distribution of 6,391 fractures of segment 43

Fracture type	Male	Female	Number of fractures	Percentage (%)
43-A	1,731	796	2,527	39.54
43-B	1,264	732	1,996	31.23
43-C	1,450	418	1,868	29.23
Total	4,445	1,946	6,391	100.00

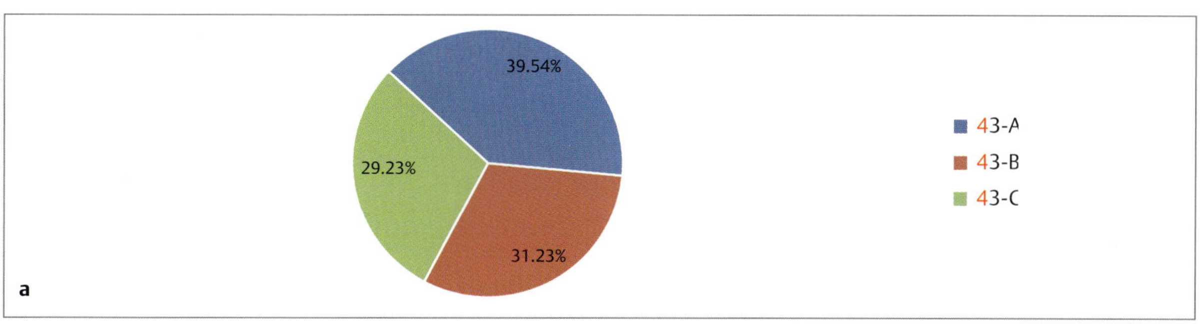

Fig. 5.16 **(a)** Fracture type distribution of 6,391 fractures of segment 43. *(Continued)*

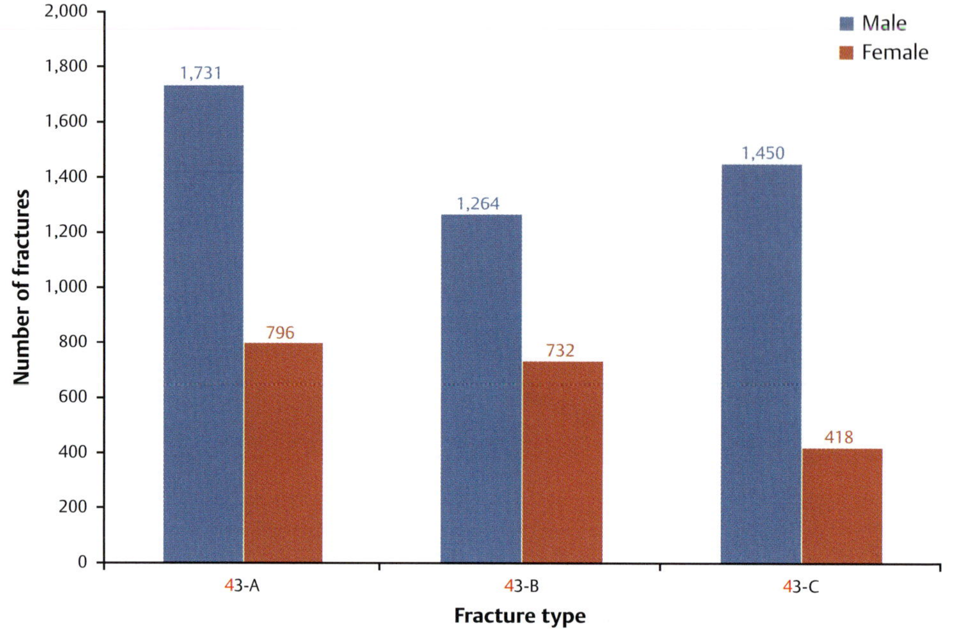

b

Fig. 5.16 (*continued*) **(b)** Sex and fracture type distribution of 6,391 fractures of segment 43.

Fractures of Segment 43 by Fracture Type

Table 5.17 Sex and fracture group distribution of 6,391 fractures of segment 43

Fracture type	Male	Female	Number of fractures	Percentage of segment 43 fractures (%)	Percentage of adult tibia/ fibula fractures (%)
43-A1	511	289	800	12.52	1.32
43-A2	541	259	800	12.52	1.32
43-A3	679	248	927	14.50	1.53
43-B1	827	519	1,346	21.06	2.22
43-B2	252	134	386	6.04	0.64
43-B3	185	79	264	4.13	0.44
43-C1	256	108	364	5.70	0.60
43-C2	521	150	671	10.50	1.11
43-C3	673	160	833	13.03	1.37
Total	4,445	1,946	6,391	100.00	10.54

5

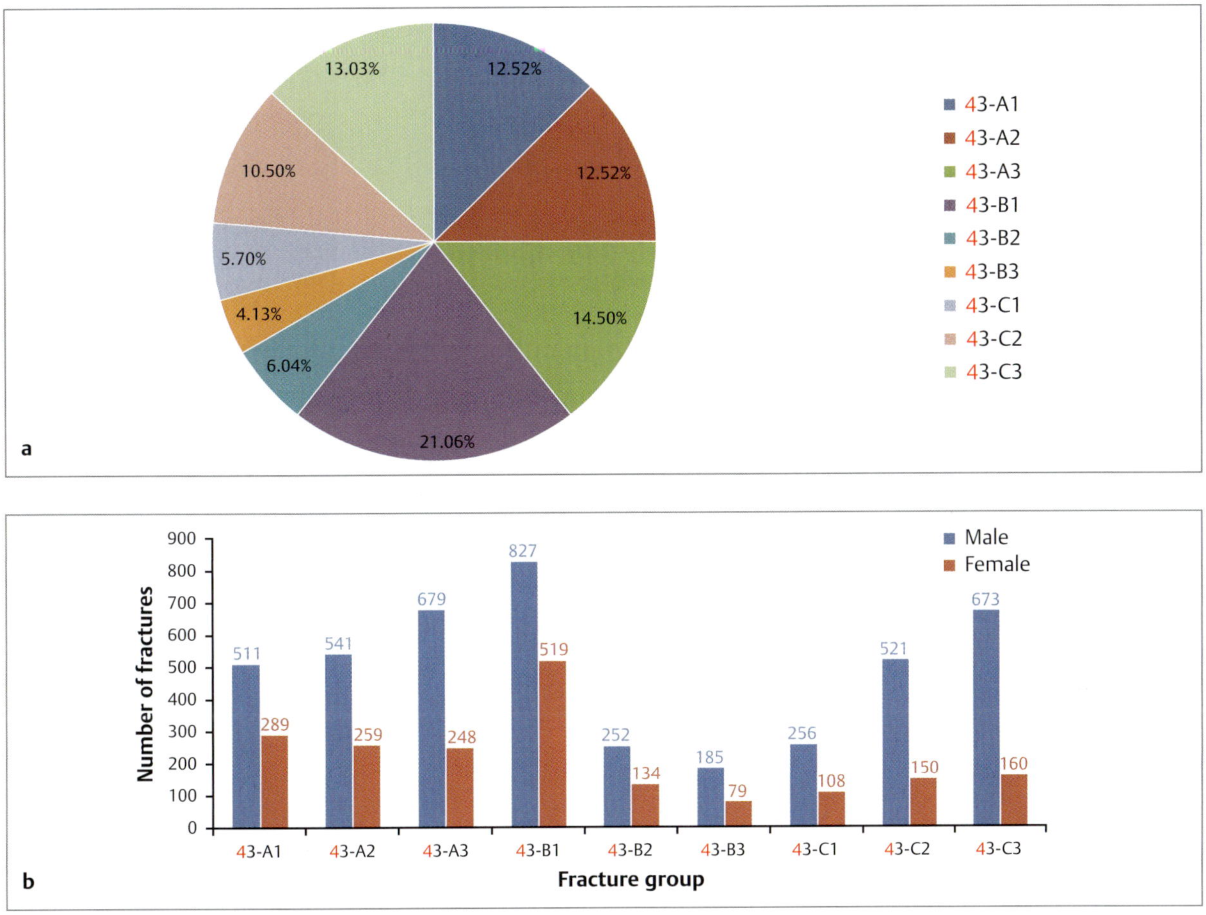

Fig. 5.17 **(a)** Fracture group distribution of 6,391 fractures of segment 43.
(b) Sex and fracture group distribution of 6,391 fractures of segment 43.

43-A Tibia/fibula, extra-articular fractures

43-A1
Simple
800 fractures
M: 511 (63.88%)
F: 289 (36.13%)
0.21% of total adult fractures
1.32% of adult tibia/fibula
12.52% of segment 43
31.66% of type 43-A

43-A1.1

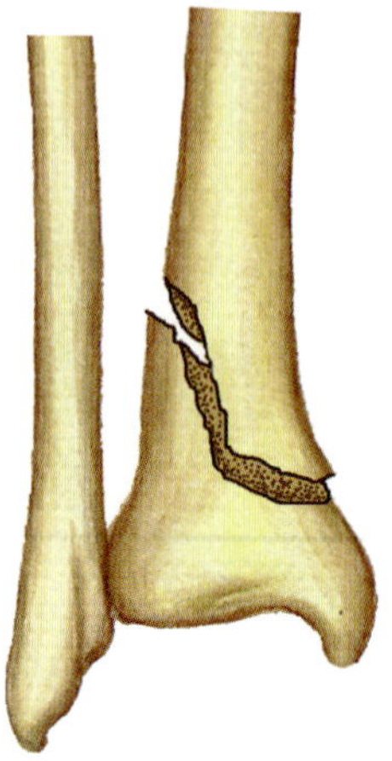

Spiral

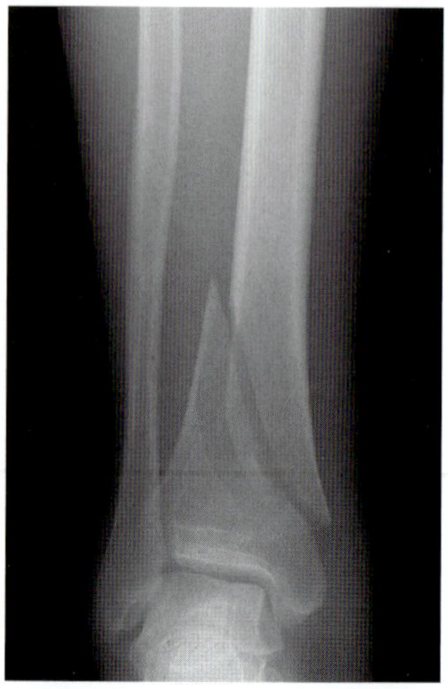

43-A1.2

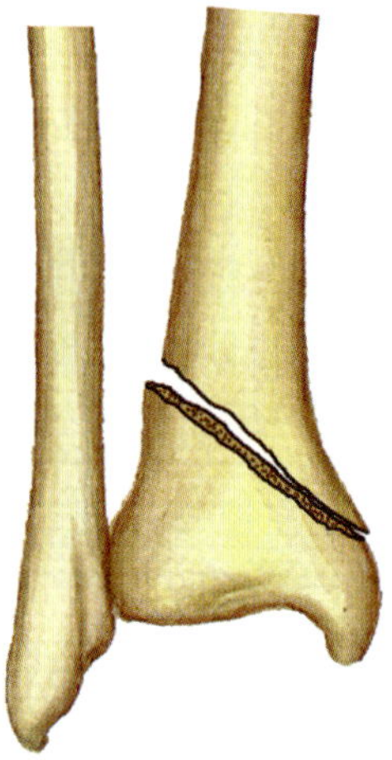

Oblique

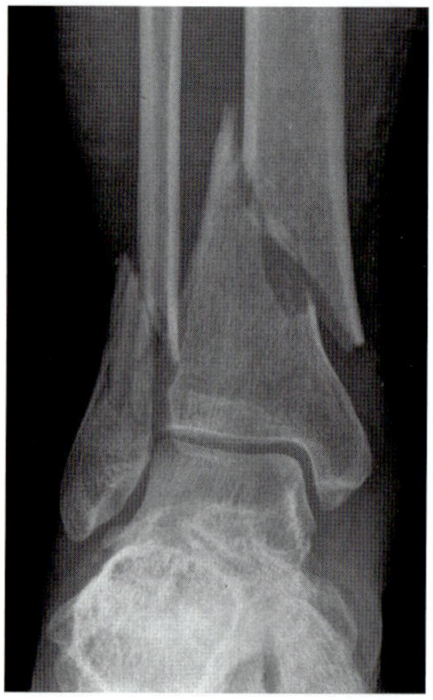

43-A1.3

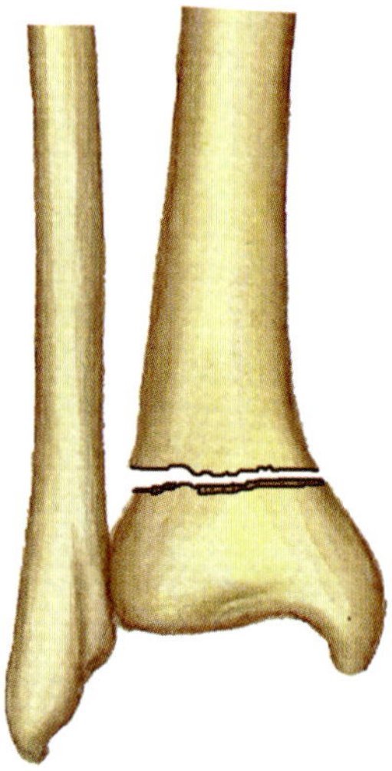

Transverse

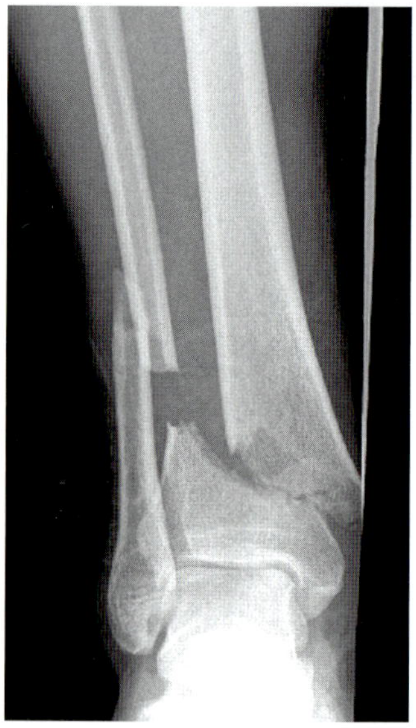

43-A Tibia/fibula, extra-articular fractures

43-A2
Wedge
800 fractures
M: 541 (67.63%)
F: 259 (32.37%)
0.21% of total adult fractures
1.32% of adult tibia/fibula
12.52% of segment 43
31.66% of type 43-A

43-A2.1

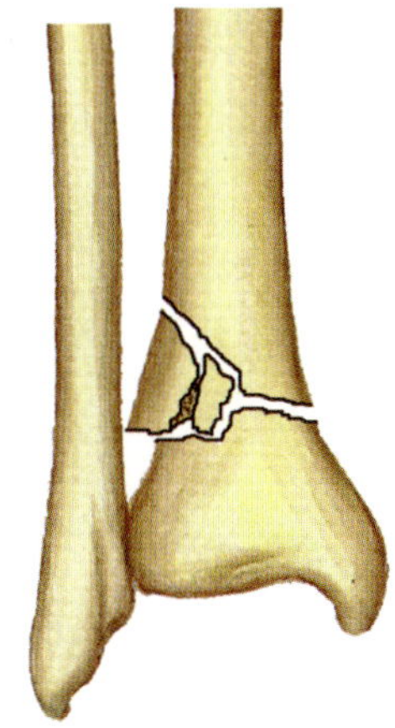

Posterolateral wedge

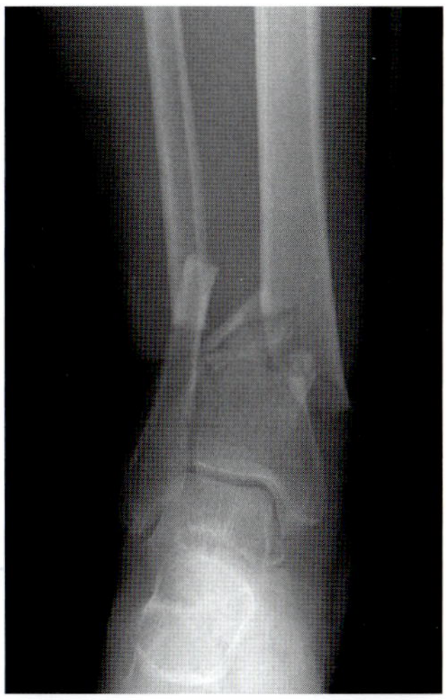

43-A2.2

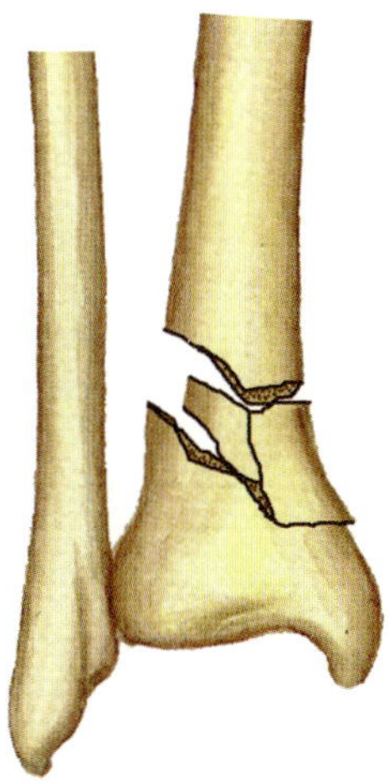

Anteromedial wedge

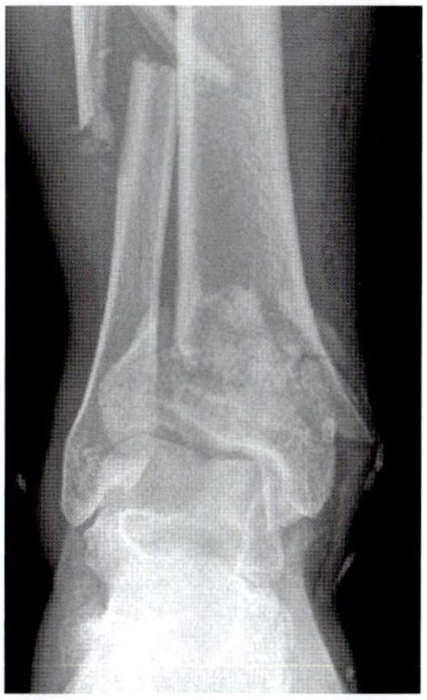

43-A2.3

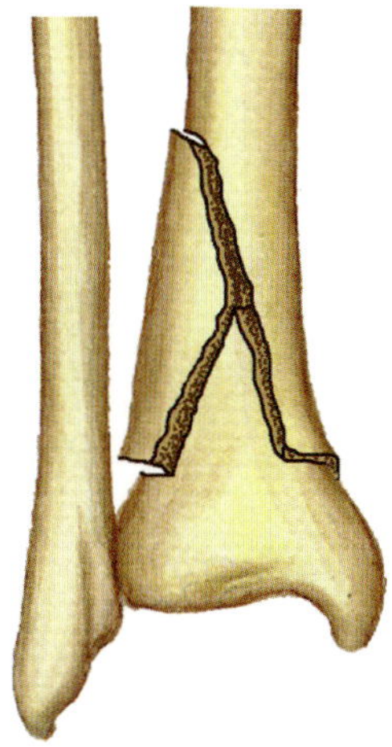

Fracture line extending into the diaphysis

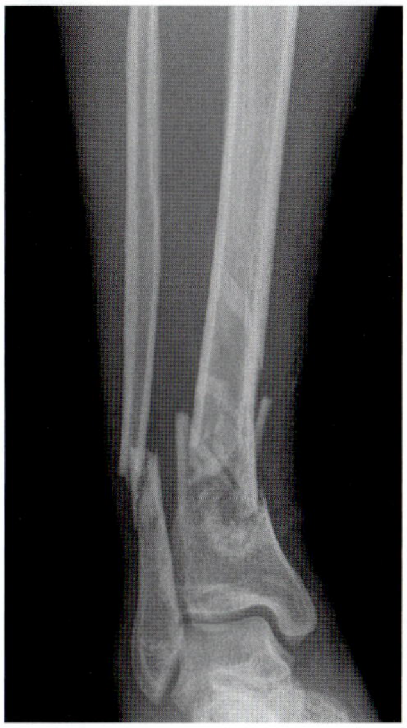

43-A Tibia/fibula, extra-articular fractures

43-A3
Complex
927 fractures
M: 679 (73.25%)
F: 248 (26.75%)
0.25% of total adult fractures
1.53% of adult tibia/fibula
14.50% of segment 43
36.68% of type 43-A

43-A3.1

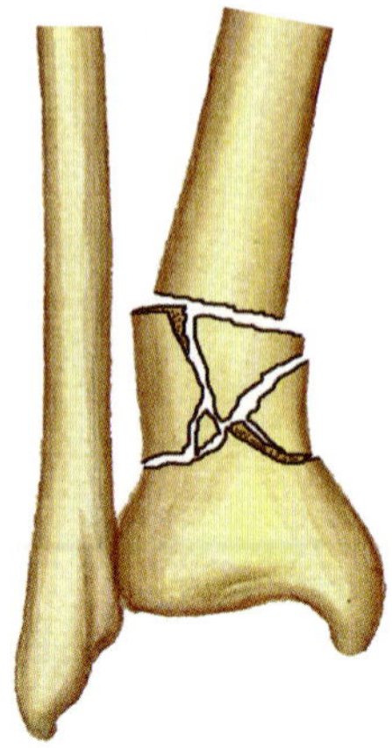

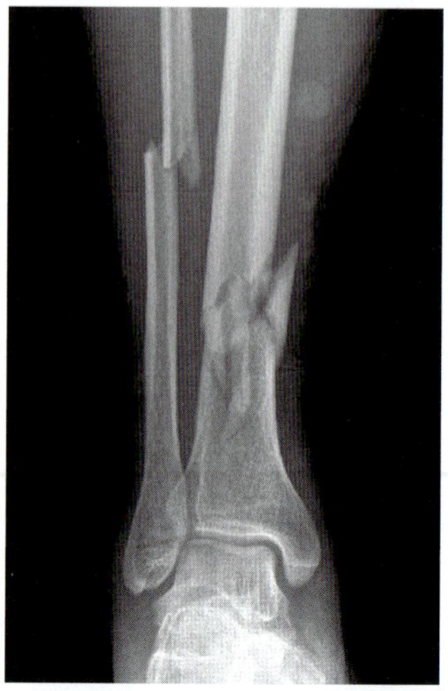

With three intermediate fragments

43-A3.2

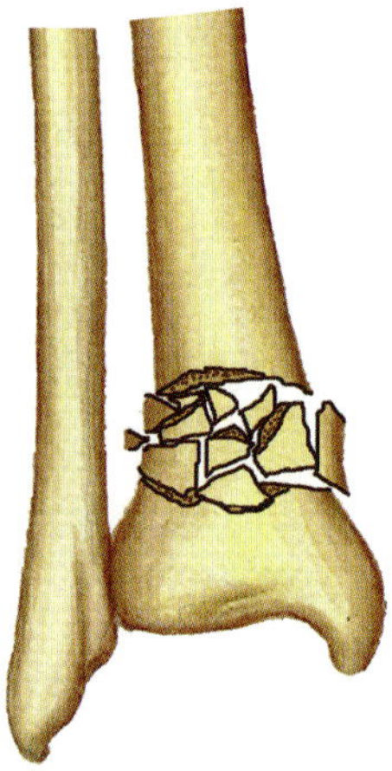

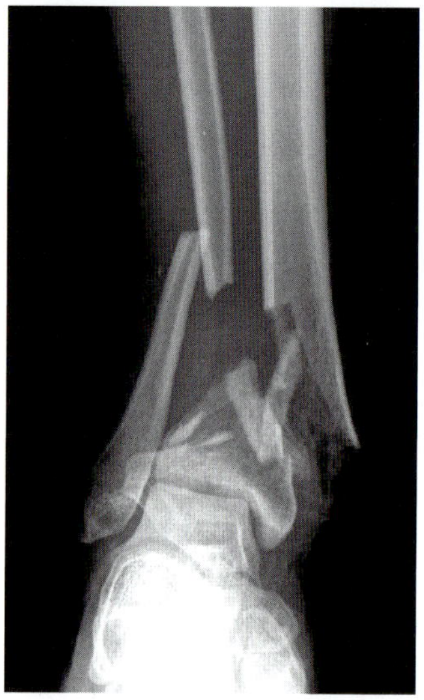

With more than three intermediate fragments

43-A3.3

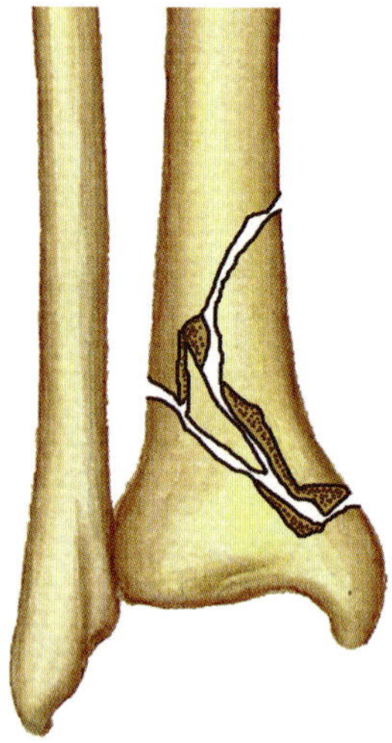

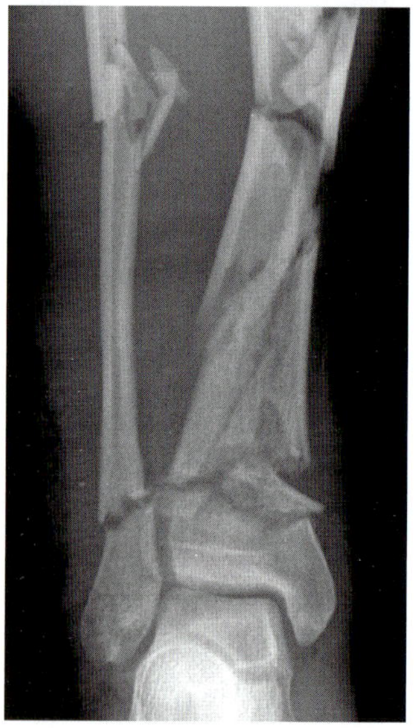

Fracture line extending into the diaphysis

43-B Tibia/fibula, partial articular fractures

43-B1
Pure split
1,346 fractures
M: 827 (61.44%)
F: 519 (38.56%)
0.36% of total adult fractures
2.22% of adult tibia/fibula
21.06% of segment 43
67.43% of type 43-B

43-B1.1

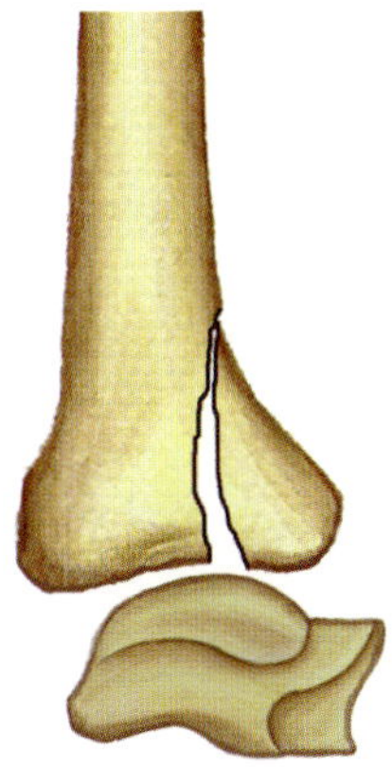

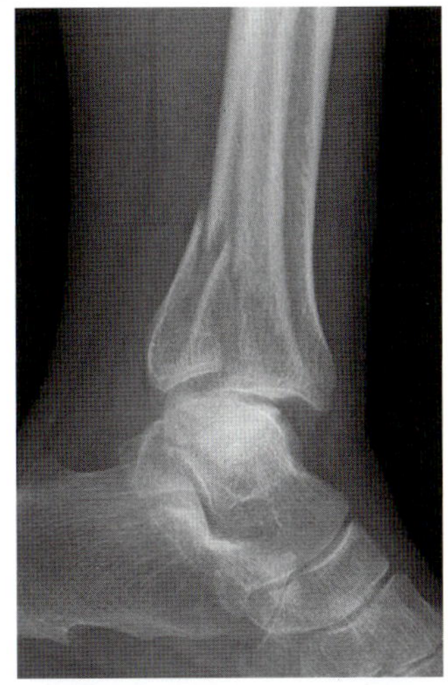

Frontal

43-B1.2

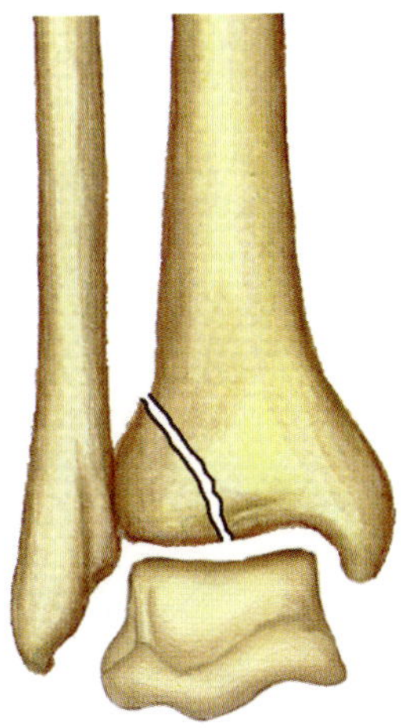

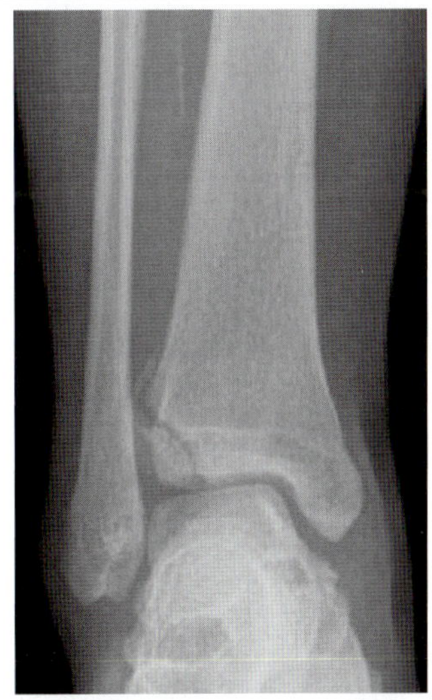

Sagittal

43-B1.3

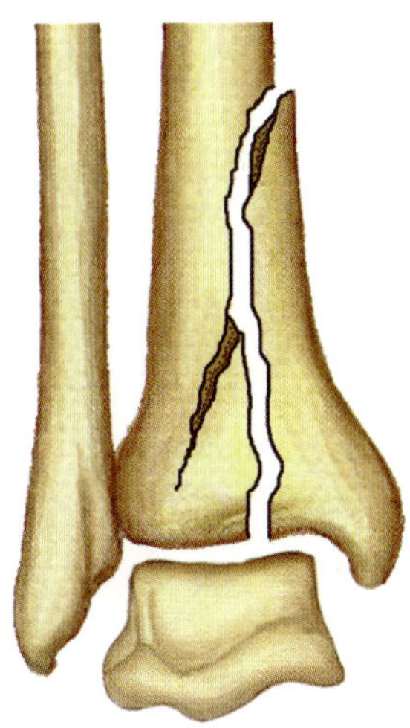

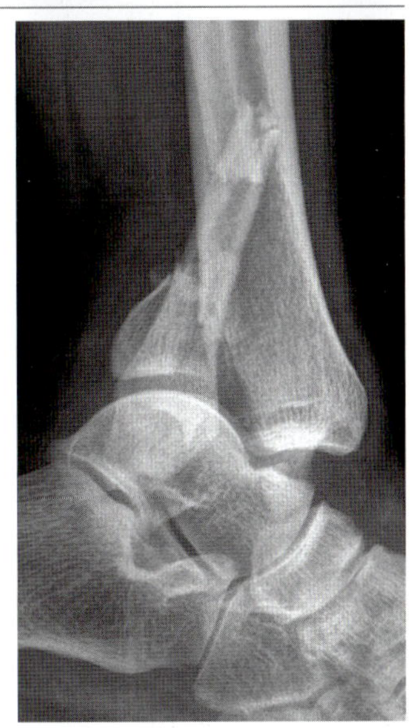

Metaphyseal multifragmentary

5

43-B Tibia/fibula, partial articular fractures

43-B2
Split depression
386 fractures
M: 252 (65.28%)
F: 134 (34.72%)
0.10% of total adult fractures
0.64% of adult tibia/fibula
6.04% of segment 43
19.34% of type 43-B

43-B2.1

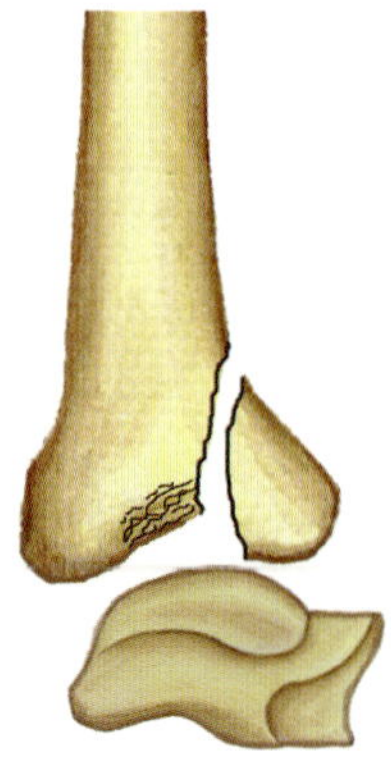

Frontal

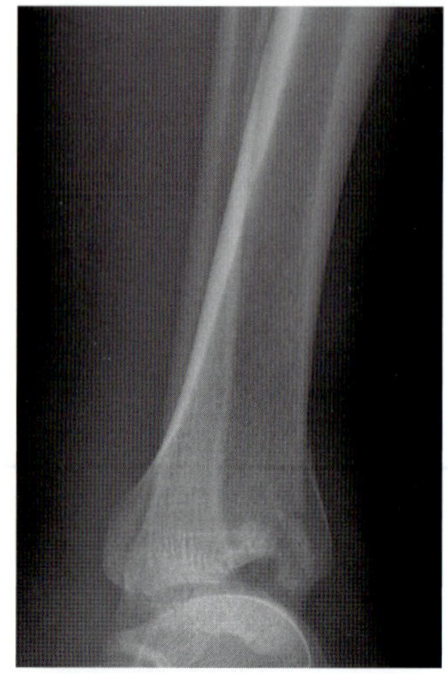

43-B2.2

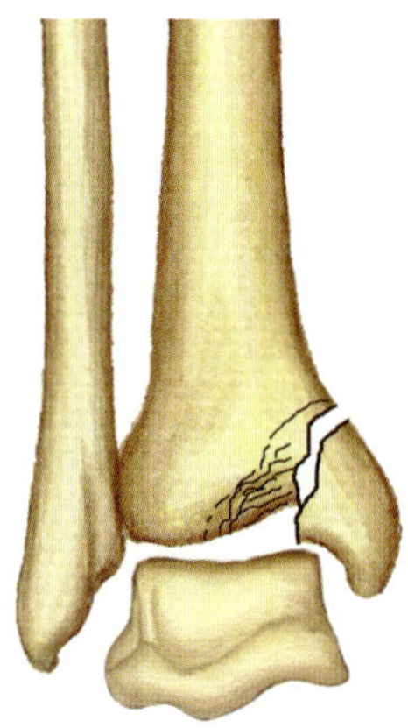

Sagittal

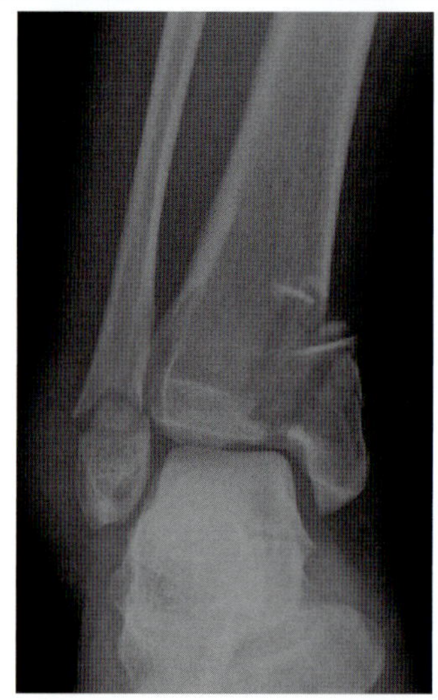

43-B2.3

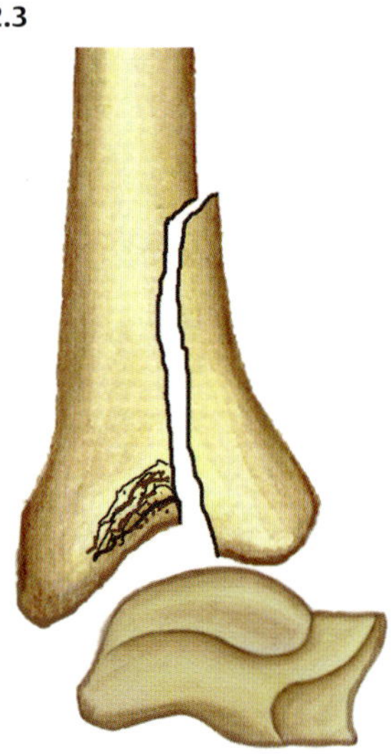

With central fragment

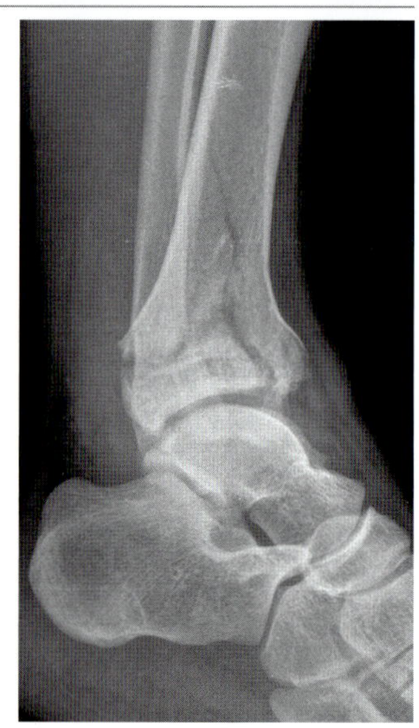

43-B Tibia/fibula, partial articular fractures

43-B3
Multifragmentary depression
264 fractures
M: 185 (70.08%)
F: 79 (29.92%)
0.07% of total adult fractures
0.44% of adult tibia/fibula
4.13% of segment 43
13.23% of type 43-B

43-B3.1

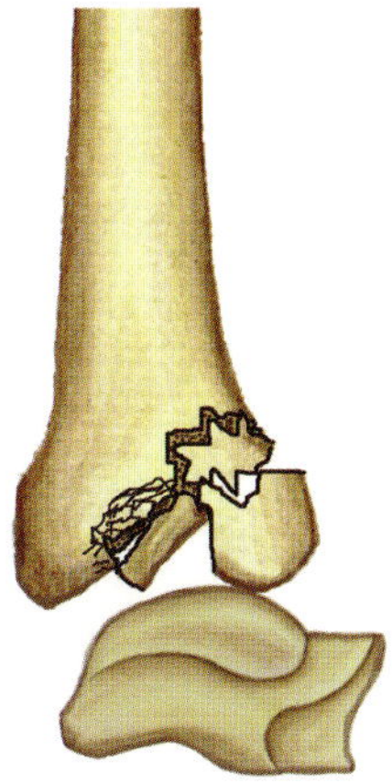

Frontal

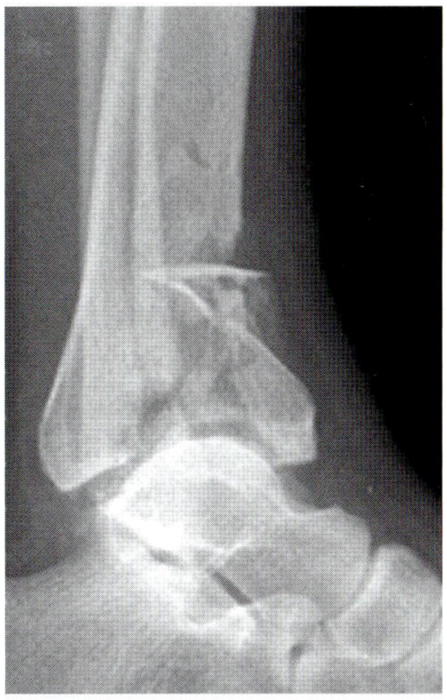

43-B3.2

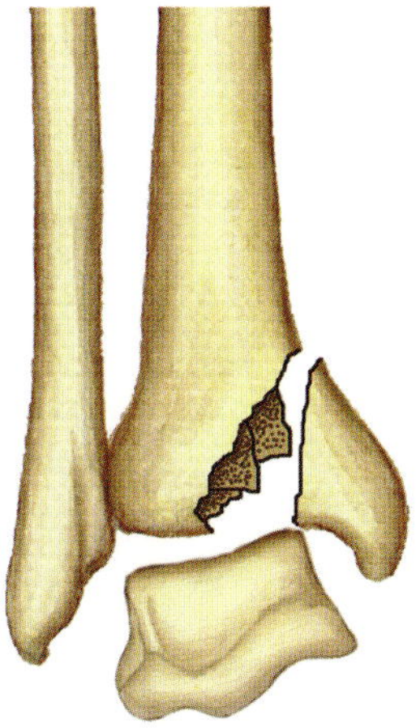

Sagittal

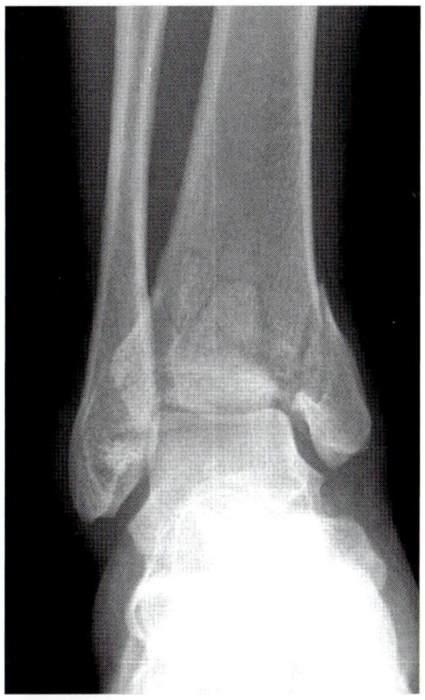

43-B3.3

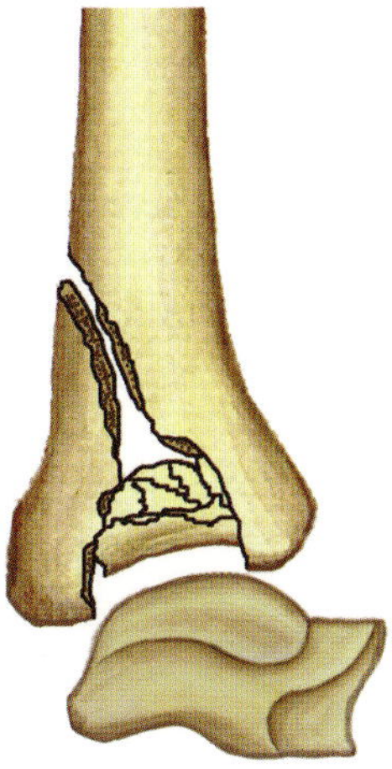

Metaphyseal multifragmentary

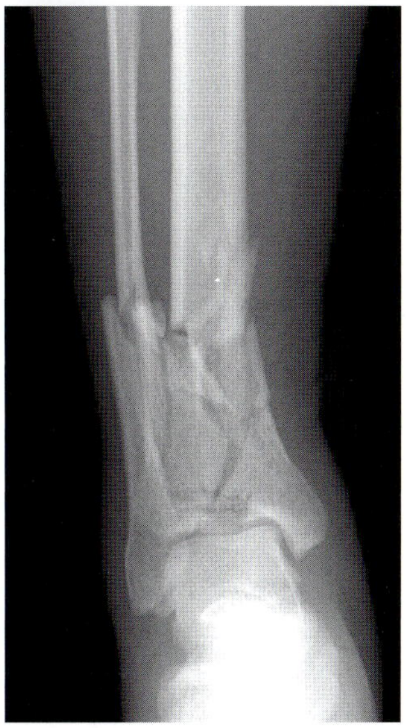

43-C Tibia/fibula, complete articular fractures

43-C1
Articular simple, metaphyseal simple
364 fractures
M: 256 (70.33%)
F: 108 (29.67%)
0.10% of total adult fractures
0.60% of adult tibia/fibula
5.70% of segment 43
19.49% of type 43-C

43-C1.1

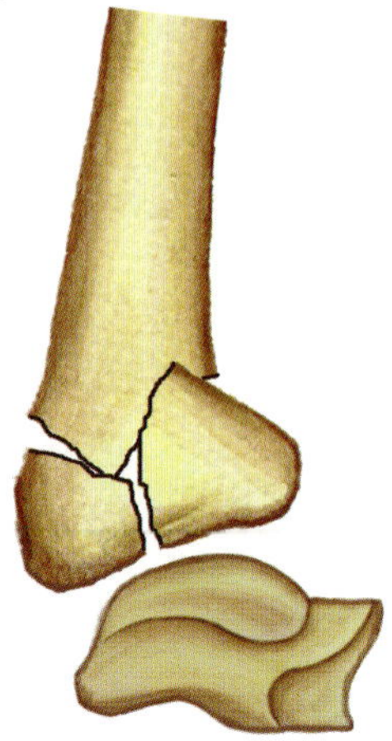

Without depression

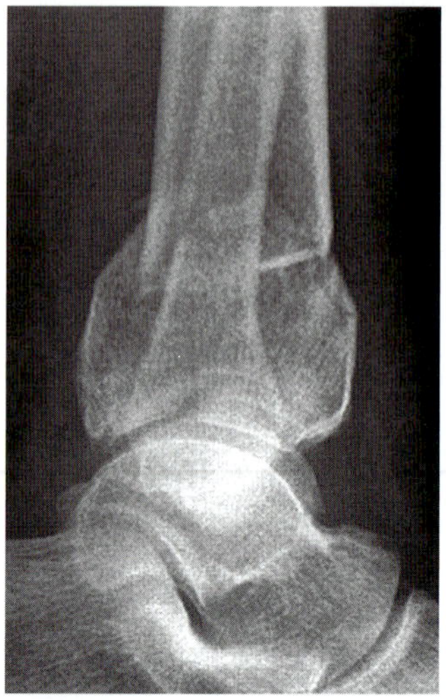

43-C1.2

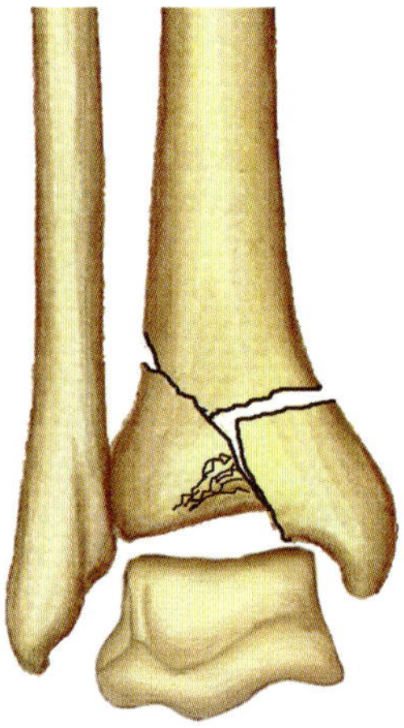

With depression

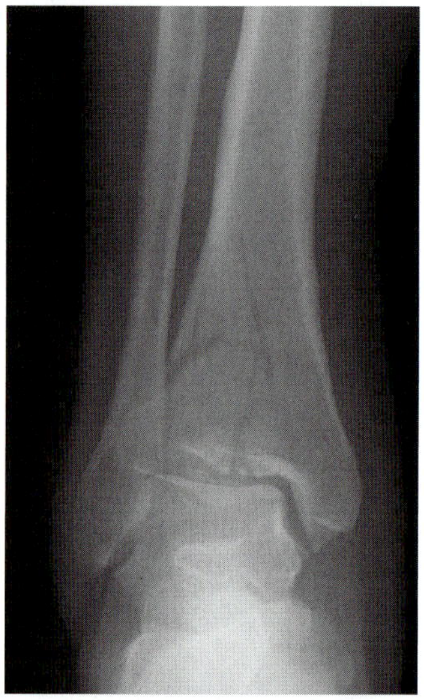

43-C1.3

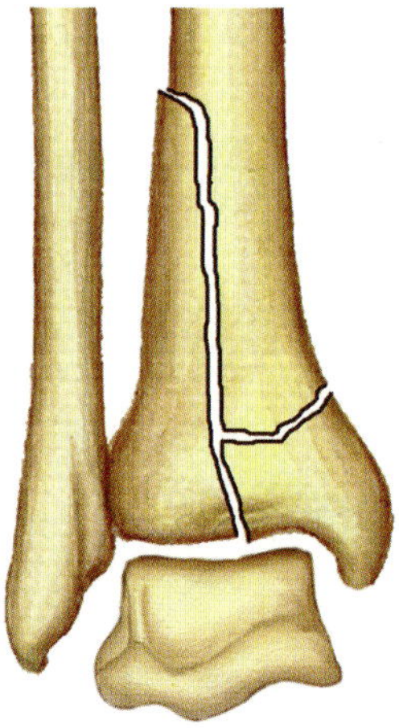

Fracture line extending into the diaphysis

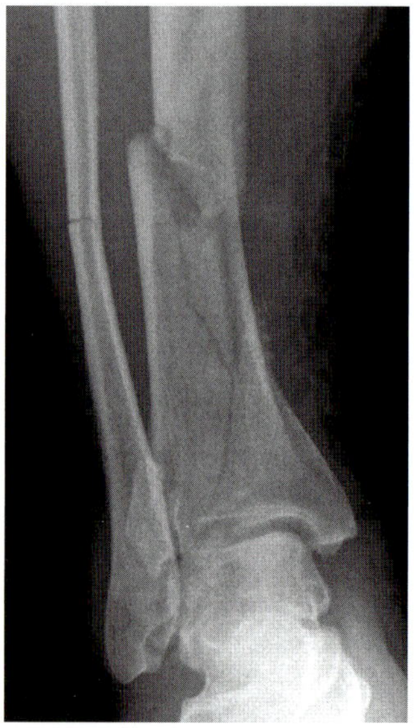

43-C Tibia/fibula, complete articular fractures

43-C2
Articular simple, metaphyseal multifragmentary
671 fractures
M: 521 (77.65%)
F: 150 (22.35%)
0.18% of total adult fractures
1.11% of adult tibia/fibula
10.50% of segment 43
35.92% of type 43-C

43-C2.1

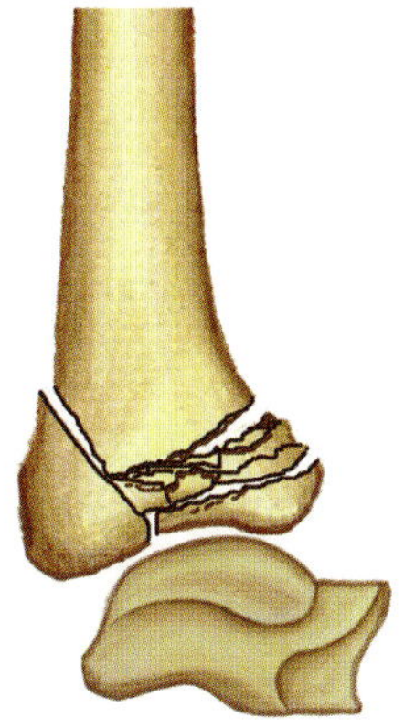

With asymmetric impaction

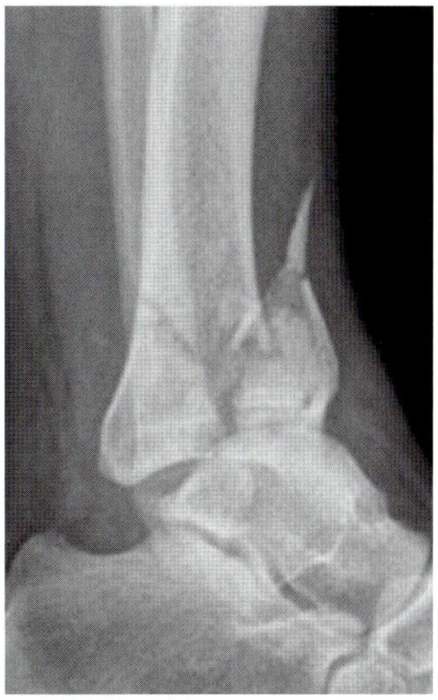

43-C2.2

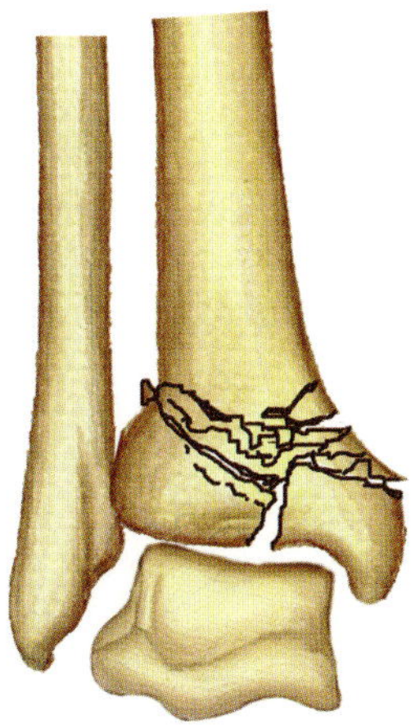

Without asymmetric impaction

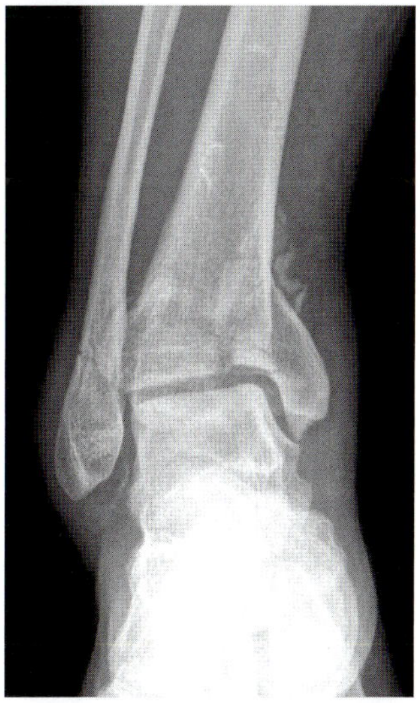

43-C2.3

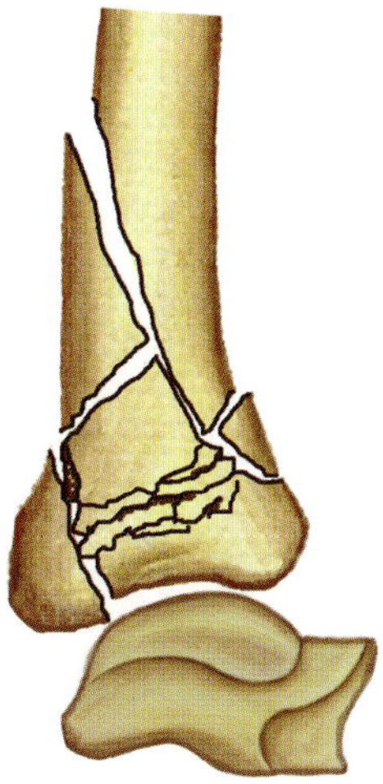

Fracture line extending into the diaphysis

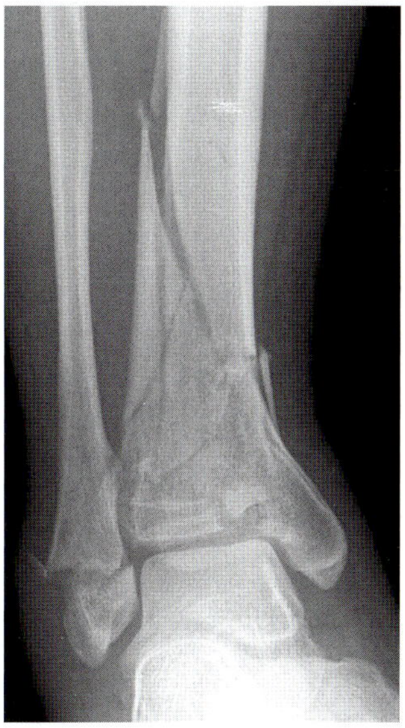

43-C Tibia/fibula, complete articular fractures

43-C3
Metaphyseal multifragmentary
833 Fractures
M: 673 (80.79%)
F: 160 (19.21%)
0.22% of total adult fractures
1.37% of adult tibia/fibula
13.03% of segment 43
44.59% of type 43-C

43-C3.1

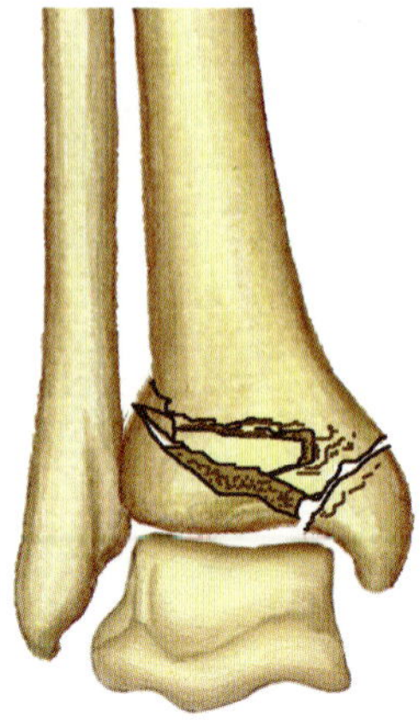

Epiphyseal

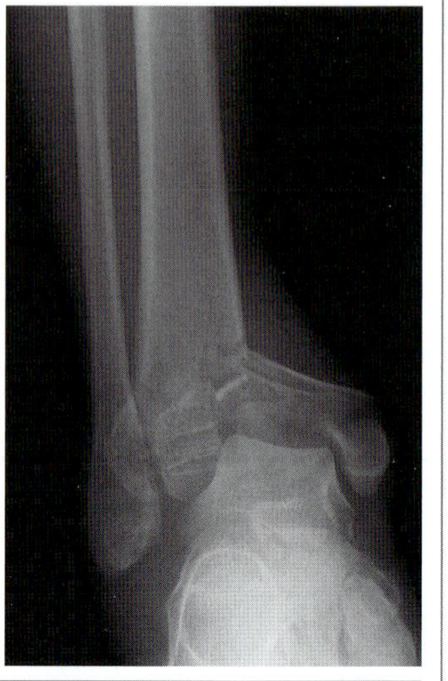

43-C3.2

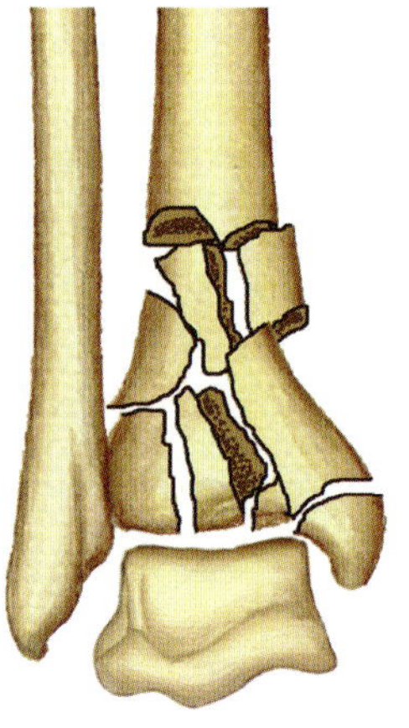

Epiphyseal + metaphyseal

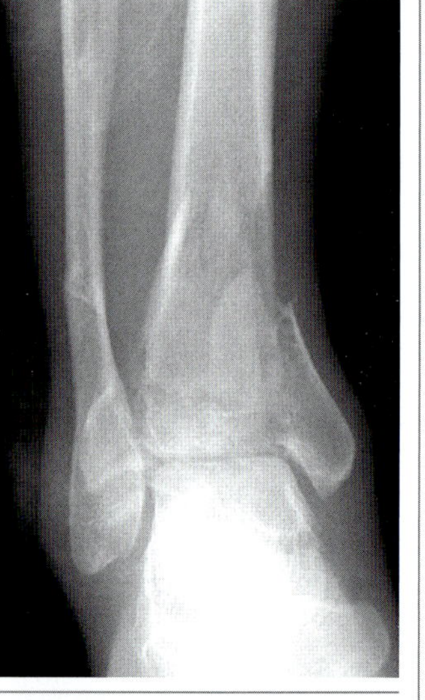

43-C3.3

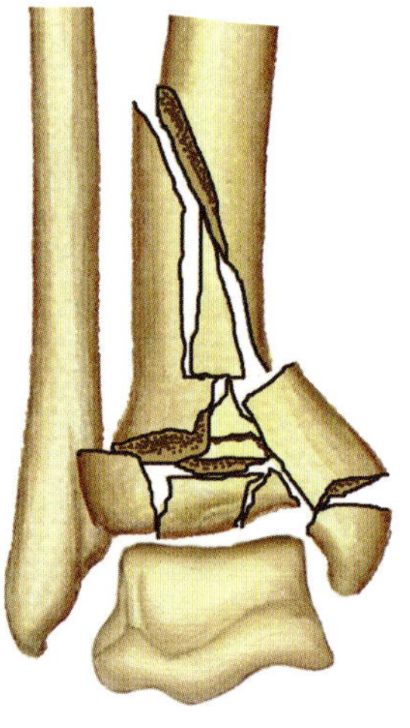

Epiphyseal, metaphyseal, and diaphyseal

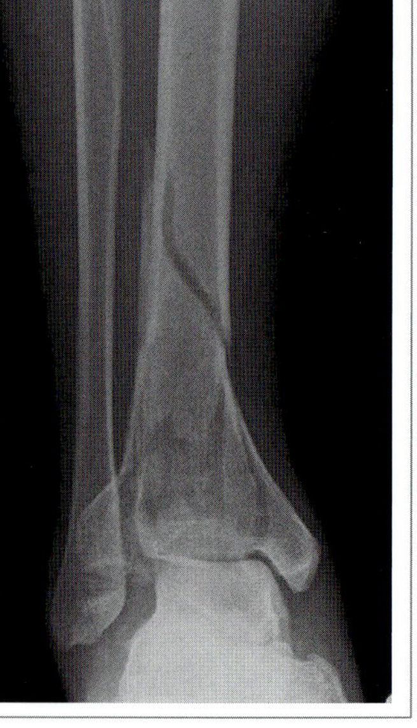

Injury Mechanism

Mechanisms of injury for tibia/fibula fractures can be divided into two categories: low-energy injuries such as ground level falls and athletic injuries involving twisting motions (accompanied by rotational force) can produce spiral fractures; and high-energy injuries that occur due to falls from a significant height and motor vehicle injuries. In either case, the resulting axial load forces transmitted through the talus to the distal tibia can cause depression of the articular surface and/or a split fracture of the distal tibia.

Diagnosis

Distal tibial fractures present with localized pain and swelling during the early stages of symptoms. The swelling may spread down to the ankle joint at a later time. Swelling, tenderness, and ecchymosis over the area of the Achilles tendon often suggest fracture of the posterior malleolus. The anteromedial surface of the tibia is subcutaneous, and the state of the skin and subcutaneous tissue is of enormous importance in influencing the wound-healing process. A careful assessment of skin, soft tissue, and neurovascular status should be performed early.

Radiographic examination should include standard AP, lateral, and mortise views (taken with the foot/ankle at 15 degrees of internal rotation) of the ankle joint. If necessary, additional X-ray films can be taken when the foot/ankle is held in external rotation at 45 degrees to visualize the anteromedial and posterolateral surface of the tibia. CT can further help to evaluate the degree of articular comminution and extent of articular depression.

Treatment

Several factors influence the treatment of distal tibial fractures, including age, general medical condition, severity of soft tissue injury, and fracture pattern. Closed fractures with minimal displacement or stable reduction can be managed successfully by nonsurgical treatment. Surgical intervention is indicated when fractures are unstable. Operative fixation methods include: screws, plating, a locking compression plate, and circular ring external fixation. The principle of open reduction and internal fixation is: (1) restoration of the length of the fibula; (2) reconstruction of the articular surface of the distal tibia; (3) bone grafting to ensure adequate bone tissue for the metaphyseal defect; and (4) plating of the medial surface of the tibia. A closed fracture with poor soft tissue status should be treated with talus traction first, and one should proceed to surgical intervention when the soft tissue status improves.

Malleolar Injury (Segment 44)

Anatomical Features

The lateral malleolus is the distal expansion of the fibula, whereas the medial malleolus is that of the tibia. Together they form a mortise—a rectangular recess into which the talus fits. The medial malleolus is a broader prominence, situated at a higher level and somewhat farther forward than the lateral malleolus. The tibia and fibula are connected to each other by the attachment of the interosseous ligament. Stability of the ankle mortise relies on the configuration of the osseous structures, the ligament, and the joint capsule. The interosseous membrane of the leg extends between the interosseous crests of the tibia and fibula. It also separates the muscles on the front from those on the back of the leg, and gives attachments to several muscles. The oblique fibers, for the most part, run downward and lateralward; a few fibers, however, pass in the opposite direction. They are continuous below with the interosseous ligament of the tibiofibular syndesmosis. The distal tibiofibular syndesmosis is between the convex medial surface of the distal end of the fibula and the rough concave fibular notch of the tibia. It is composed of the anterior and posterior tibiofibular ligaments, the interosseous membrane with its corresponding ligament, and the transverse tibiofibular ligament. The anterior tibiofibular ligament is a flat, triangular band of fibers, which extends obliquely downward and lateralward between the adjacent margins of the tibia and fibula, on the front aspect of the syndesmosis. The posterior tibiofibular ligament rests on the posterior surface of the syndesmosis. The transverse tibiofibular ligament lies deep to the posterior tibiofibular ligament. Because there are variations in the slope of the lateral malleolar surface of the talus, dorsiflexion of the foot, combined with slight external rotation of the fibula, can result in a small separation of the tibia and fibula. Normally the medial open space (between the talus and medial malleolus) should be less than 3 mm, and when it is greater than 3 mm, a lateral shift of the talus is present.

The ligaments of the ankle joint are grouped into two categories: the lateral collateral ligaments and the medial collateral ligaments. The lateral collateral ligaments include the anterior talofibular ligament, calcaneofibular ligament, and posterior talofibular ligament. The posterior talofibular ligament is the strongest fibrous ligament among the three. The medial collateral ligaments, so-called deltoid ligaments, are composed of superficial and deep components. The superficial components run from the medial malleolus to the navicular bone, the edge of the calcaneus, and the sustentaculum tali. The deep layers merge into the joint capsule.

AO Classification of Malleolar Injury

Based on AO classification, the malleolus is coded as the number 44 (**Plate 5.12**). Malleolar injury can be divided into three types defined by the level of the lateral malleolar lesion, in relation to the ligamentous complex of the syndesmosis: 44-A, infrasyndesmotic malleolar lesion; 44-B, trans-syndesmotic fibular fracture; and 44-C, suprasyndesmotic lesion (**Plate 5.13**).

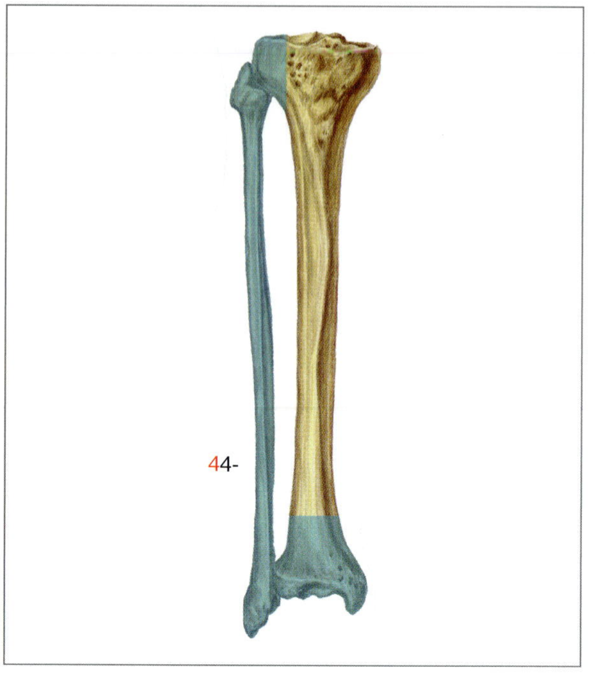

Plate 5.12

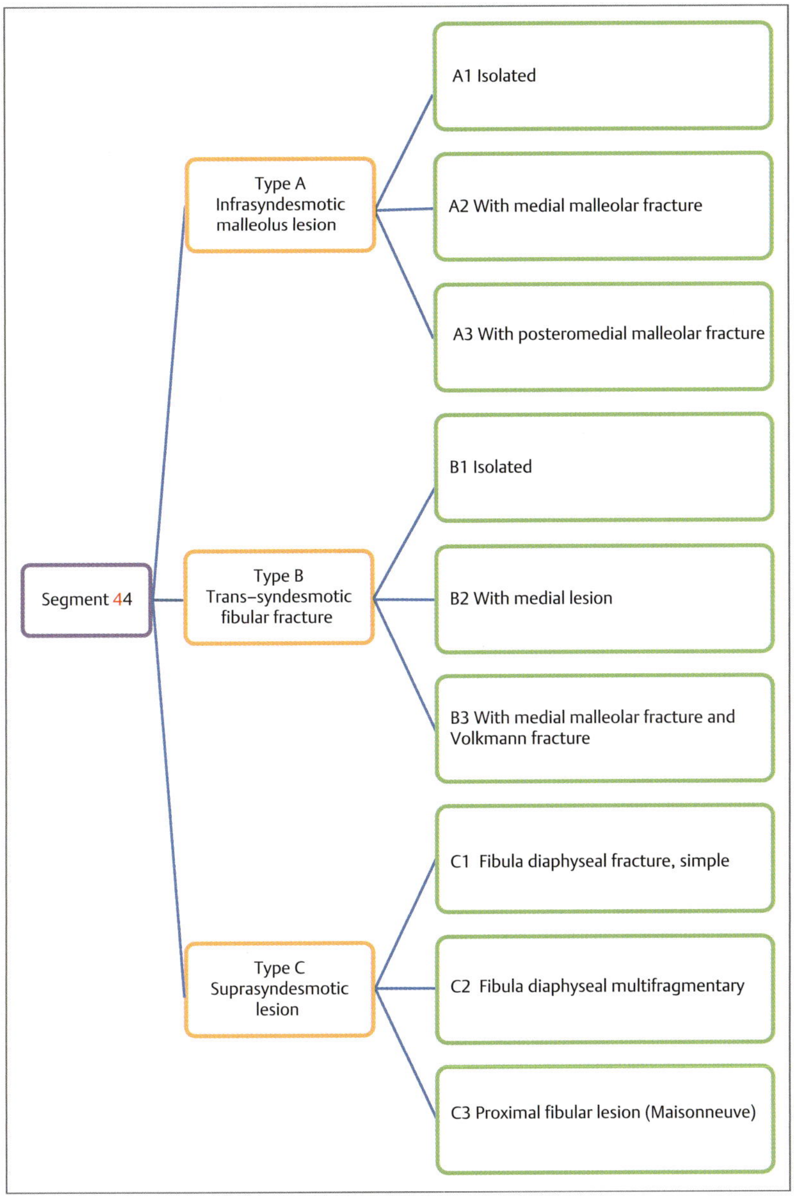
Segment 44
Type A
Infrasyndesmotic
malleolus lesion
A1 Isolated
A2 With medial malleolar fracture
A3 With posteromedial malleolar fracture
Type B
Trans–syndesmotic
fibular fracture
B1 Isolated
B2 With medial lesion
B3 With medial malleolar fracture and
Volkmann fracture
Type C
Suprasyndesmotic
lesion
C1 Fibula diaphyseal fracture, simple
C2 Fibula diaphyseal multifragmentary
C3 Proximal fibular lesion (Maisonneuve)

Plate 5.13

Clinical Epidemiologic Features of Malleolar Injury (Segment 44)

A total of 28,279 malleolar injuries were treated in 83 hospitals in China over a 2-year period from 2010 to 2011. All cases were reviewed and statistically studied; the fractures accounted for 46.65% of all tibia/fibula fractures in adults. Their epidemiologic features are as follows:

- More males than females
- The highest risk age group is 21–25 years. The most affected male age group is 21–25 years, while females aged 56–60 years have the highest risk.
- The most common fracture type among segment 44 fractures is type 44-A—the same fracture type for both males and females.
- The most common fracture group among segment 44 fractures is group 44-A1—group 44-A2 in males and group 44-A1 in females.

Fractures of Segment 44 by Sex

Table 5.18 Sex distribution of 28,279 fractures of segment 44

Sex	Number of fractures	Percentage (%)
Male	16,860	59.62
Female	11,419	40.38
Total	28,279	100.00

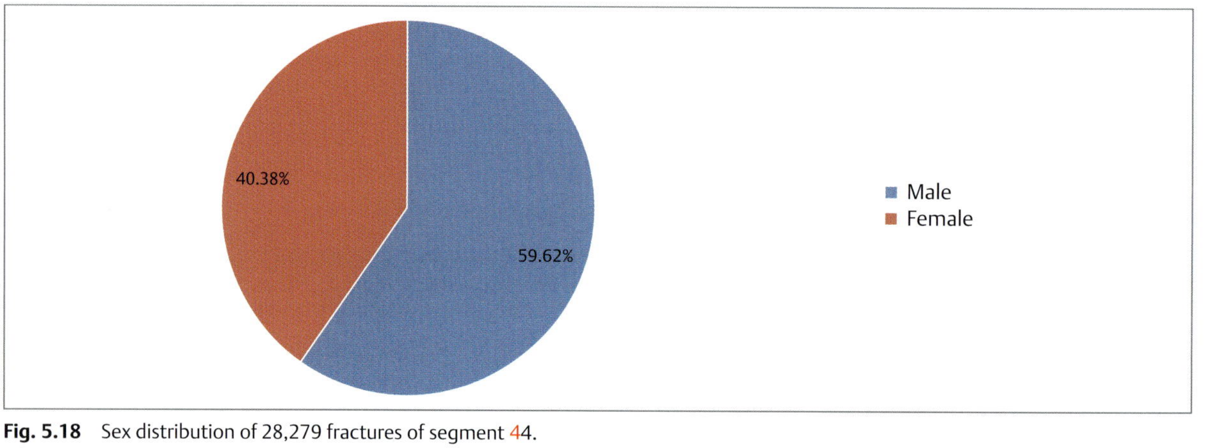

Fig. 5.18 Sex distribution of 28,279 fractures of segment 44.

Fractures of Segment 44 by Age Group

Table 5.19 Sex and age distribution of 28,279 fractures of segment 44

Age group (years)	Male	Female	Number of fractures	Percentage (%)
16–20	1,748	649	2,397	8.48
21–25	2,171	858	3,029	10.71
26–30	1,814	763	2,577	9.11
31–35	1,686	740	2,426	8.58
36–40	1,974	1,049	3,023	10.69
41–45	1,826	1,094	2,920	10.33
46–50	1,620	1,249	2,869	10.15
51–55	1,221	1,278	2,499	8.84
56–60	1,109	1,404	2,513	8.89
61–65	664	835	1,499	5.30
66–70	408	580	988	3.49
71–75	277	461	738	2.61
76–80	192	313	505	1.79
81–85	116	103	219	0.77
≥86	34	43	77	0.27
Total	16,860	11,419	28,279	100.00

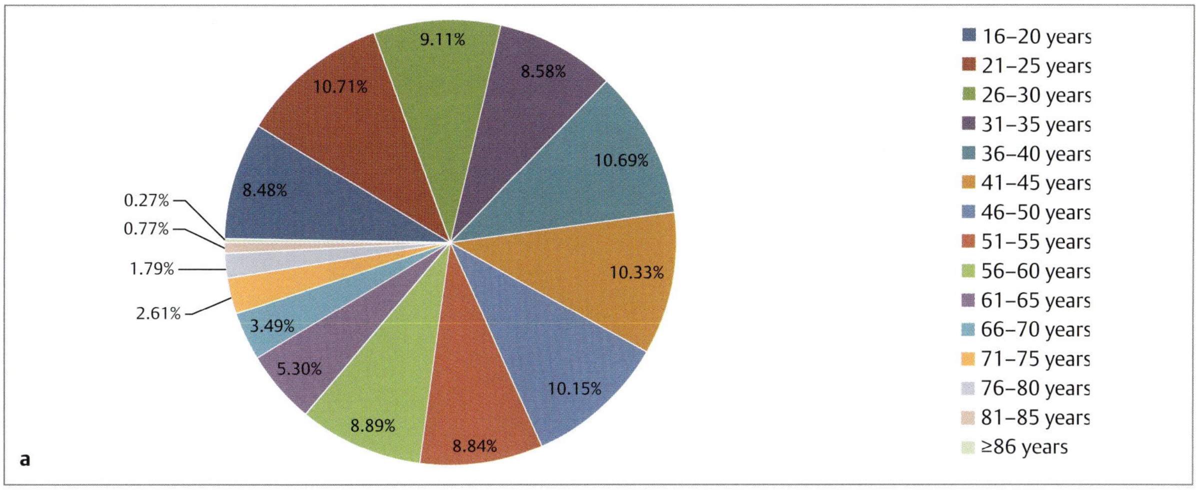

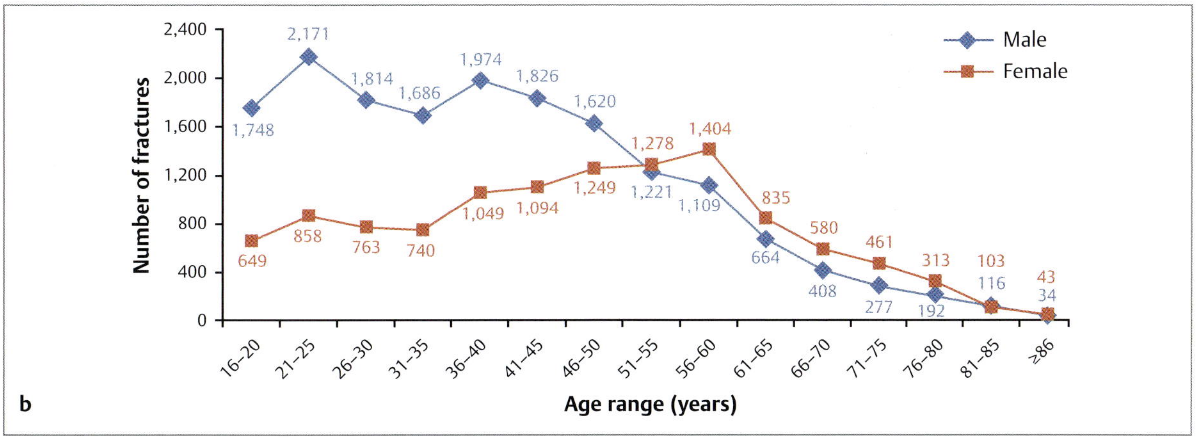

Fig. 5.19 **(a)** Age distribution of 28,279 fractures of segment 44.
(b) Age and sex distribution of 28,279 fractures of segment 44.

Fractures of Segment 44 by Fracture Type

Table 5.20 Sex and fracture type distribution of fractures of segment 44

Fracture type	Male	Female	Number of fractures	Percentage (%)
44-A	6,431	4,821	11,252	39.79
44-B	6,046	5,084	11,130	39.36
44-C	4,383	1,514	5,897	20.85
Total	16,860	11,419	28,279	100.00

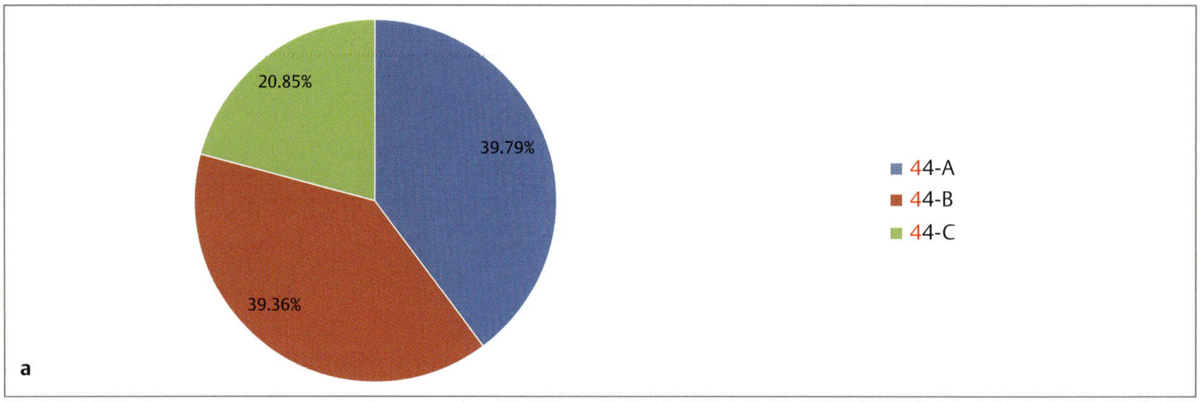

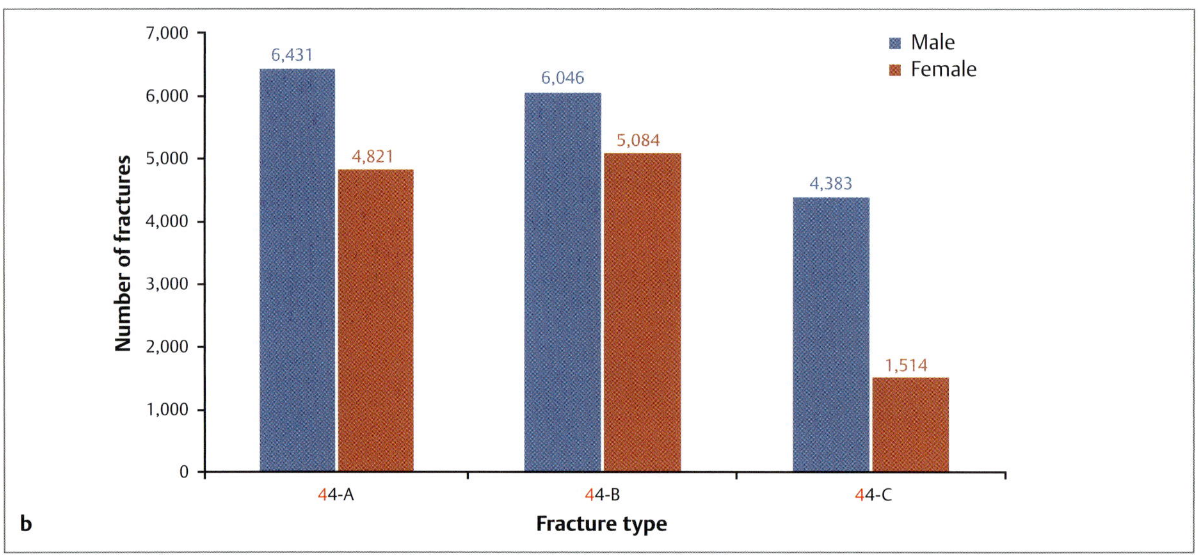

Fig. 5.20 **(a)** Fracture type distribution of 28,279 fractures of segment 44.
(b) Sex and fracture type distribution of 28,279 fractures of segment 44.

Table 5.21 Sex and fracture group distribution of 28,279 fractures of segment 44

Fracture group	Male	Female	Number of fractures	Percentage of segment 44 fractures (%)	Percentage of adult tibia/fibula fractures (%)
44-A1	3,898	3,652	7,550	26.70	12.46
44-A2	2,289	1,054	3,343	11.82	5.52
44-A3	244	115	359	1.27	0.59
44-B1	3,063	2,494	5,557	19.65	9.17
44-B2	2,072	1,709	3,781	13.37	6.24
44-B3	911	881	1,792	6.34	2.96
44-C1	2,299	806	3,105	10.98	5.12
44-C2	1,408	430	1,838	6.50	3.03
44-C3	676	278	954	3.37	1.57
Total	16,860	11,419	28,279	100.00	46.65

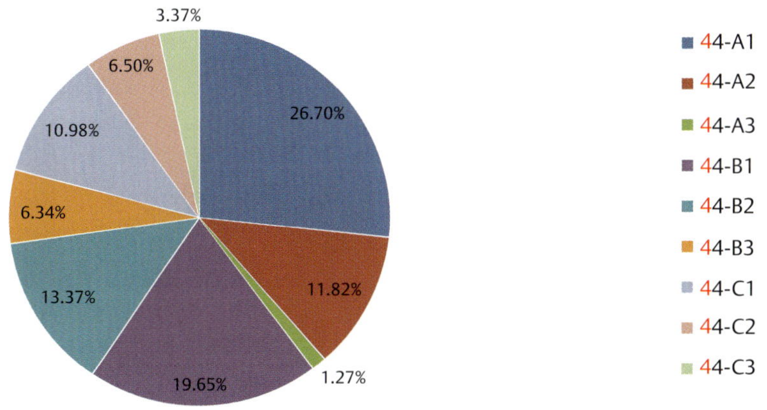

a

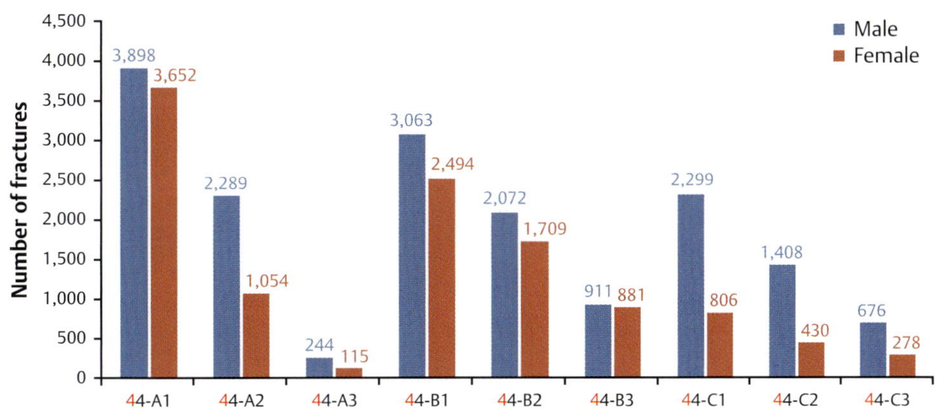

b

Fig. 5.21 **(a)** Fracture group distribution of 28,279 fractures of segment 44.
(b) Sex and fracture group distribution of 28,279 fractures of segment 44.

44-A Tibia/fibula malleolar segment, infrasyndesmotic lesion

44-A1
Isolated
7,550 fractures
M: 3,898 (51.63%)
F: 3,652 (48.37%)
2.02% of total adult fractures
12.46% of adult tibia/fibula
26.70% of segment 44
67.10% of type 44-A

44-A1.1

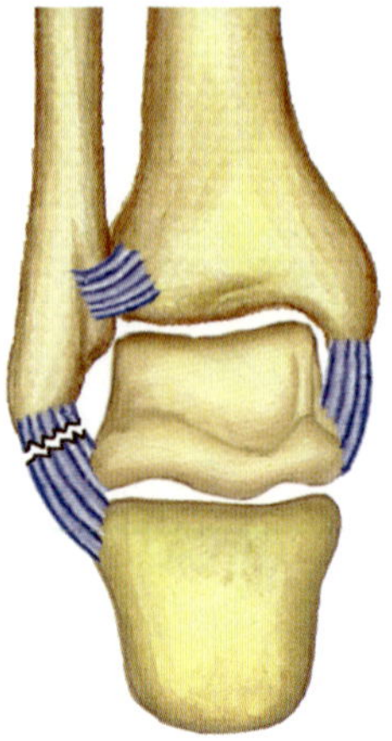

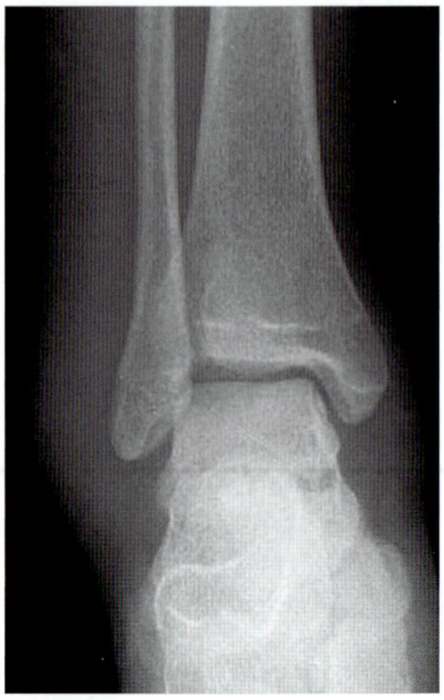

Rupture of the lateral collateral ligament

44-A1.2

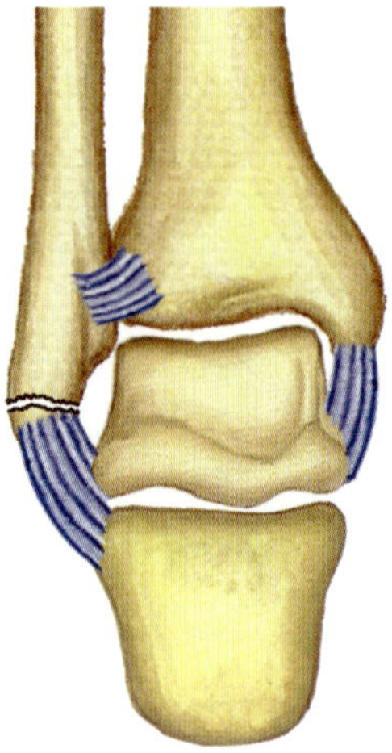

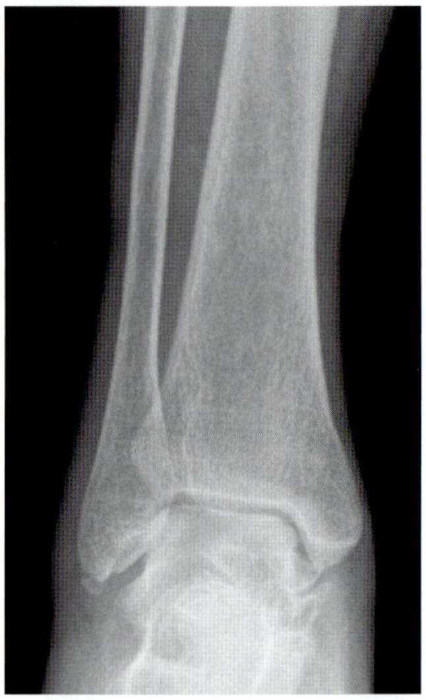

Avulsion of the tip of the lateral malleolus

44-A1.3

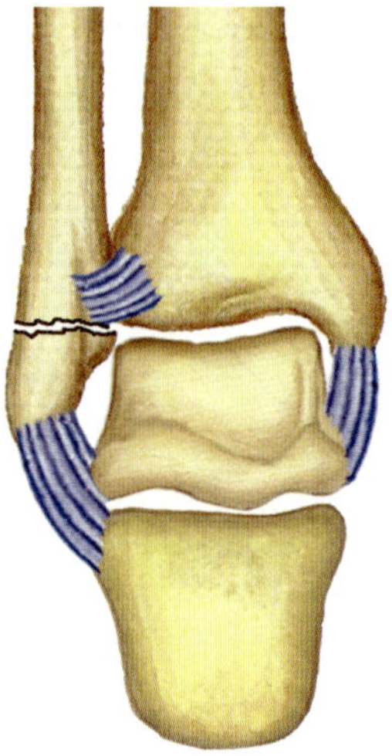

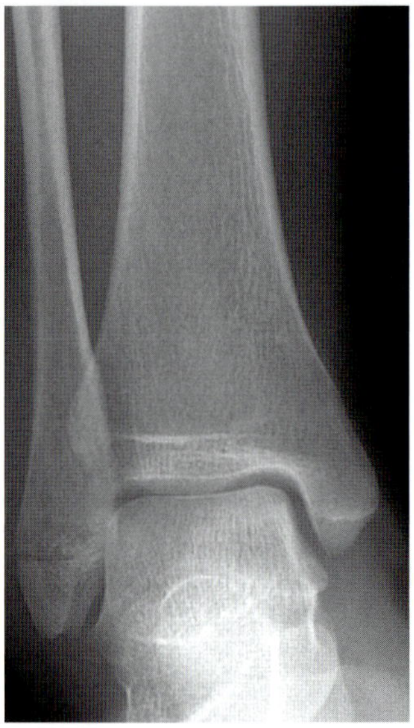

Transverse fracture, lateral malleolus

44-A Tibia/fibula malleolar segment, infrasyndesmotic lesion

44-A2
With fracture of the medial malleolus
3,343 fractures
M: 2,289 (68.47%)
F: 1,054 (31.53%)
0.89% of total adult fractures
5.52% of adult tibia/fibula
11.82% of segment 44
29.71% of type 44-A

44-A2.1

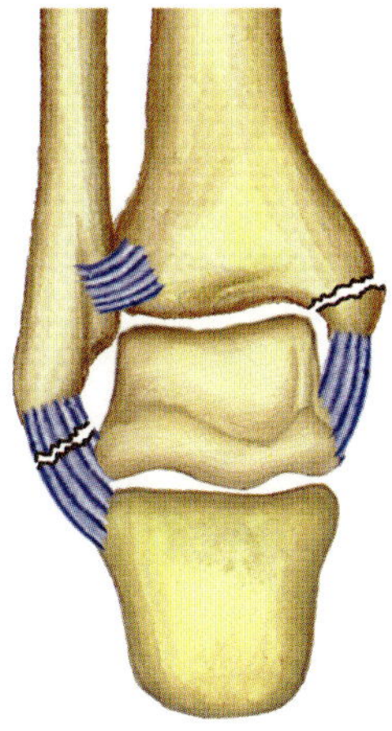

Rupture of the lateral collateral ligament

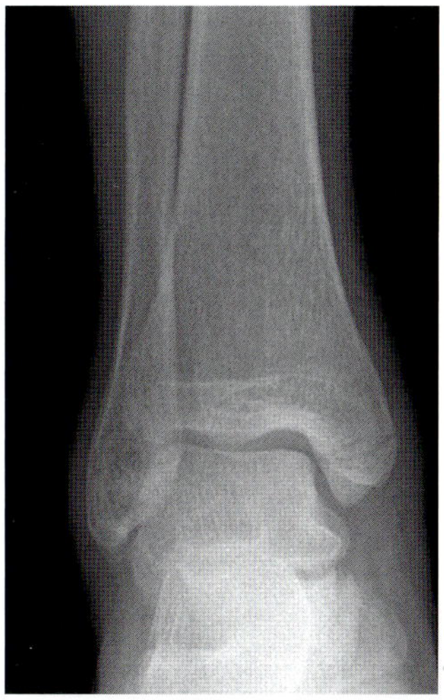

44-A2.2

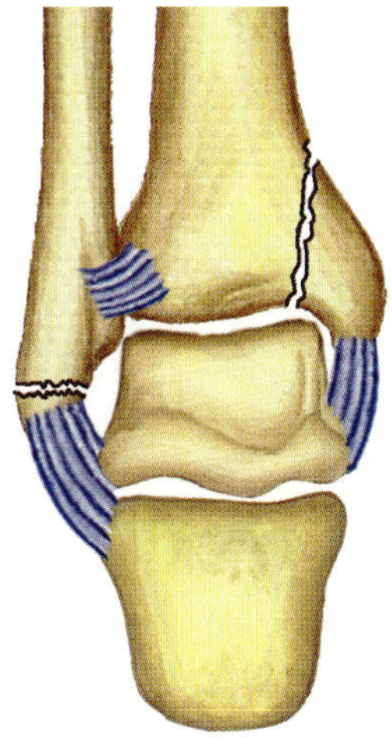

Avulsion of the tip of the lateral malleolus

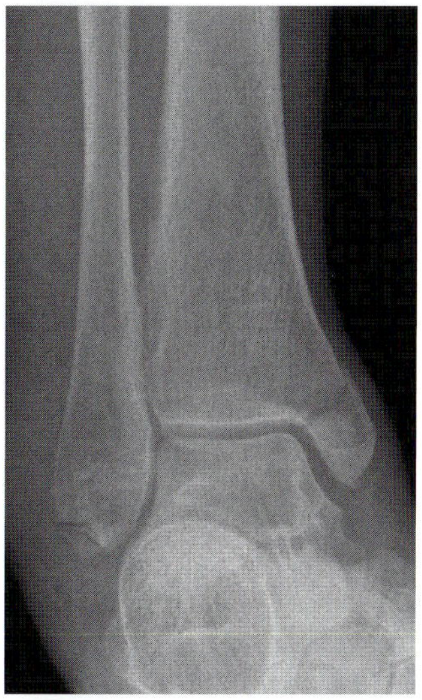

44-A2.3

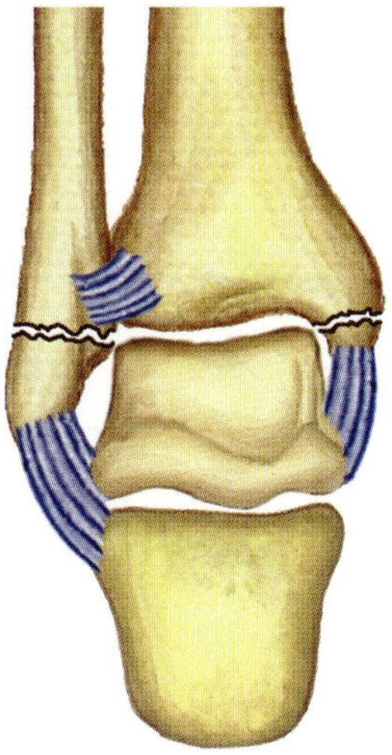

Transverse fracture, lateral malleolus

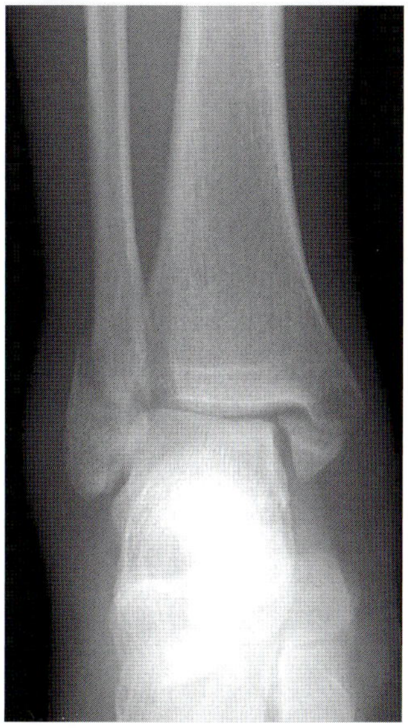

44-A Tibia/fibula malleolar segment, infrasyndesmotic lesion

44-A3
With posteromedial fracture
359 fractures
M: 244 (67.97%)
F: 115 (32.03%)
0.10% of total adult fractures
0.59% of adult tibia/fibula
1.27% of segment 44
3.19% of type 44-A

44-A3.1

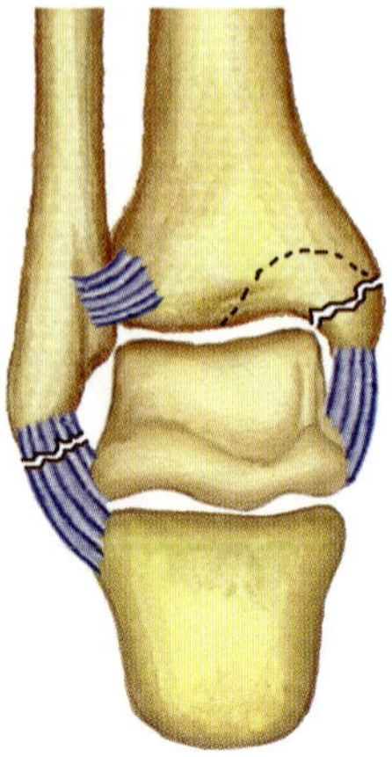

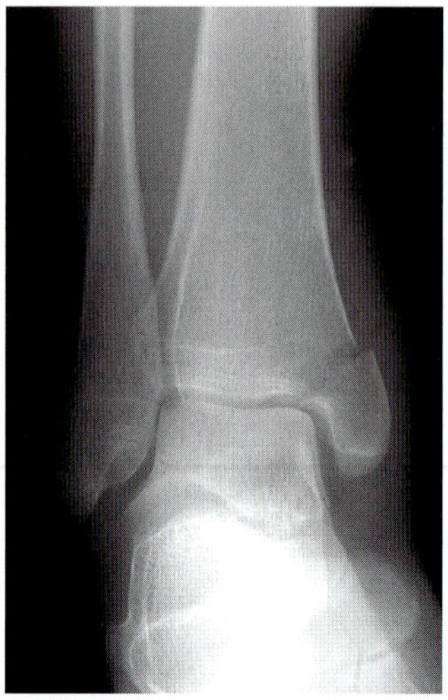

Rupture of the lateral collateral ligament

44-A3.2

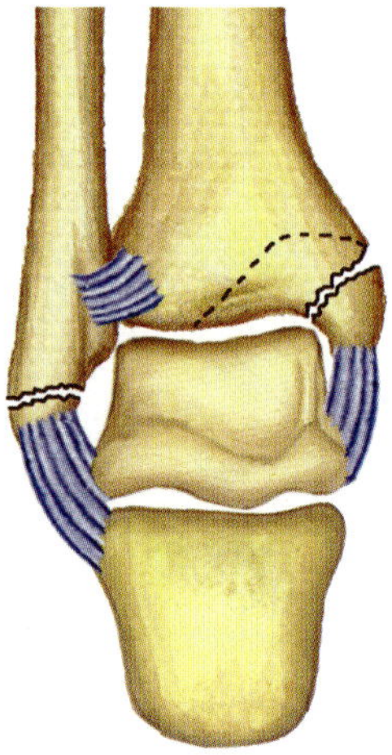

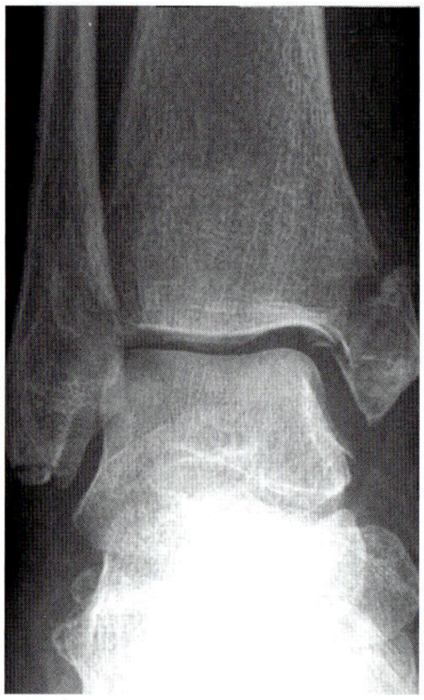

Avulsion of the tip of the lateral malleolus

44-A3.3

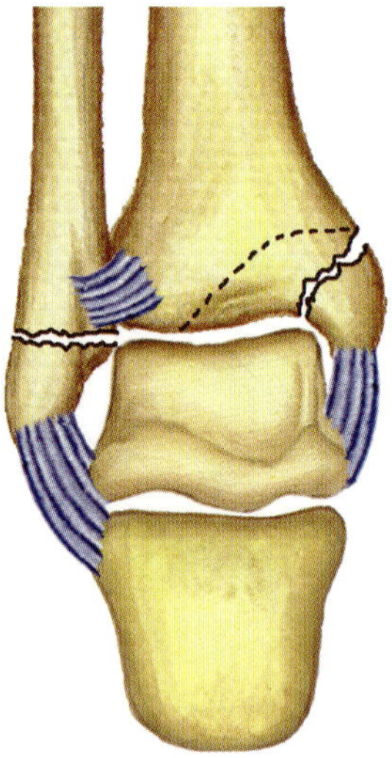

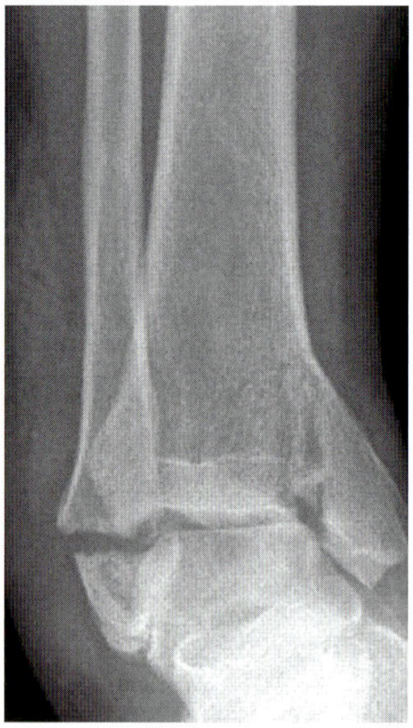

Transverse fracture, lateral malleolus

44-B Tibia/fibula malleolar segment, trans-syndesmotic fibular fractures

44-B1
Isolated
5,557 fractures
M: 3,063 (55.12%)
F: 2,494 (44.88%)
1.48% of total adult fractures
9.17% of adult tibia/fibula
19.65% of segment 44
49.93% of type 44-B

44-B1.1

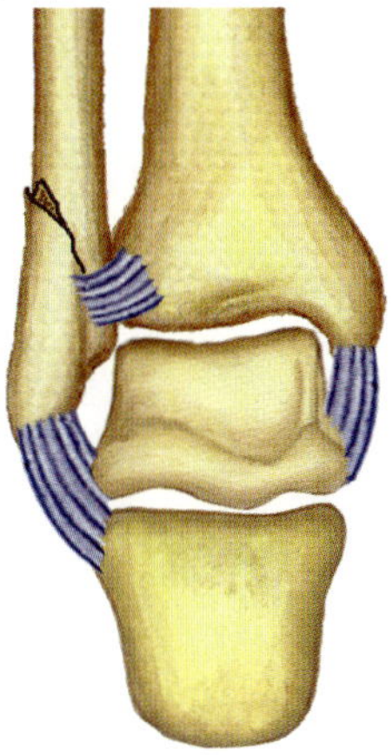

Fibular simple

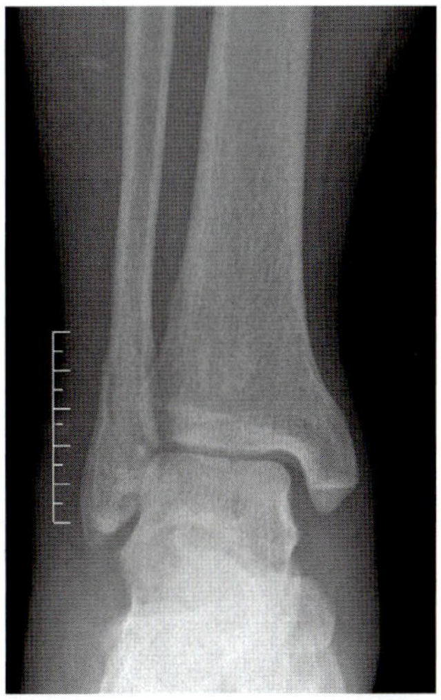

44-B1.2

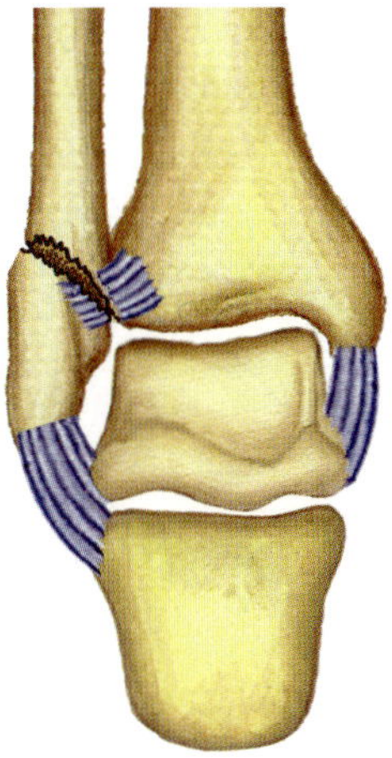

Fibular simple, with rupture of the anterior syndesmosis

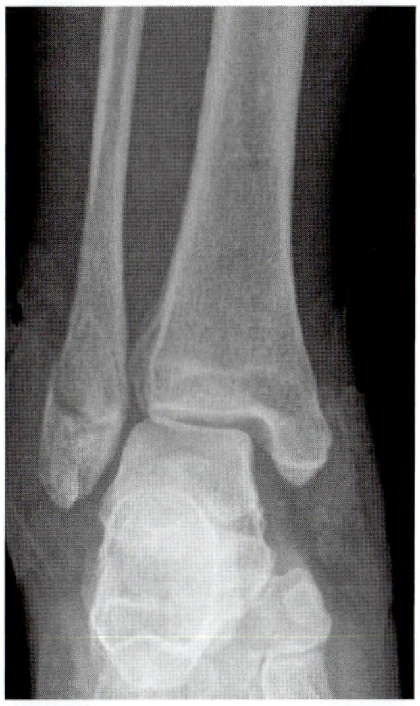

44-B1.3

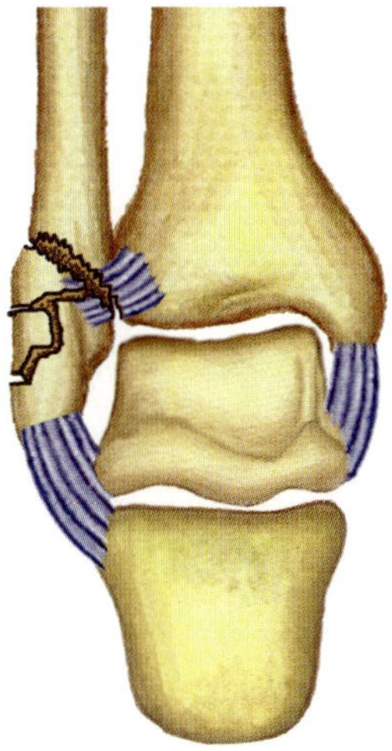

Fibular multifragmentary

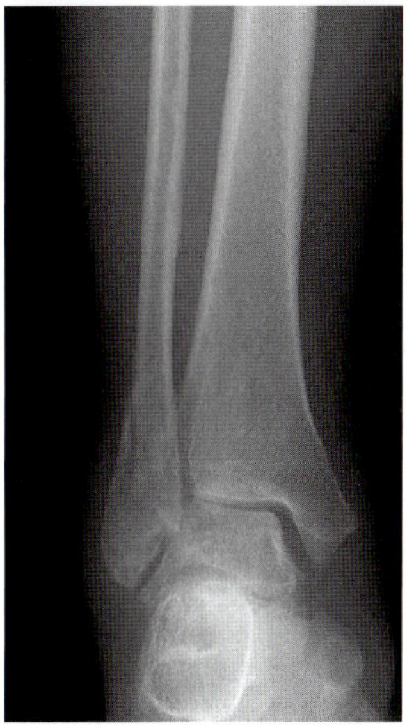

5

44-A Tibia/fibula malleolar segment, infrasyndesmotic lesion

44-B2
With medial lesion
3,781 fractures
M: 2,072 (54.80%)
F: 1,709 (45.20%)
1.01% of total adult fractures
6.24% of adult tibia/fibula
13.37% of segment 44
33.97% of type 44-B

44-B2.1

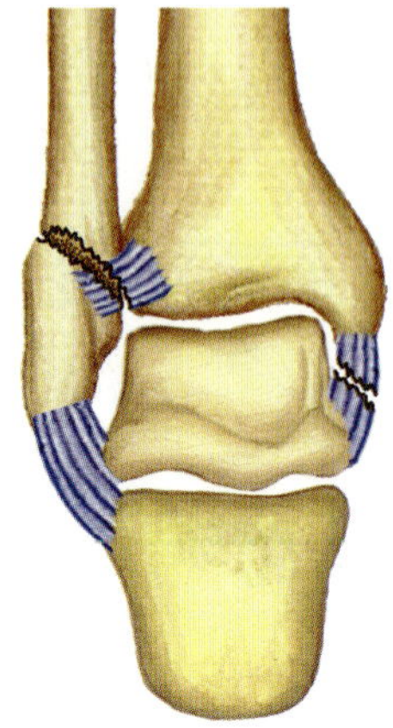

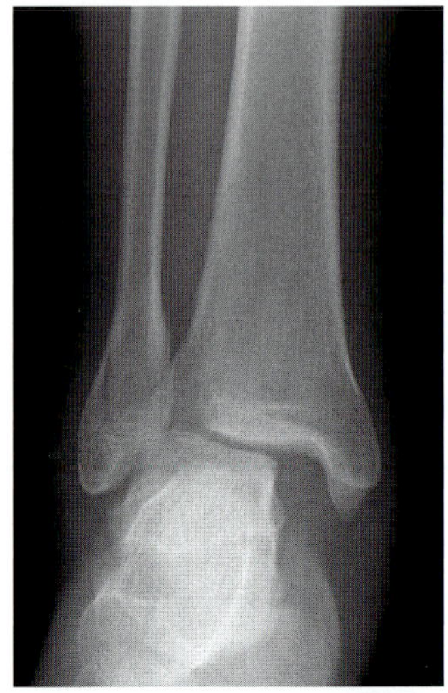

Fibular simple, with rupture of anterior syndesmosis + medial collateral ligament

44-B2.2

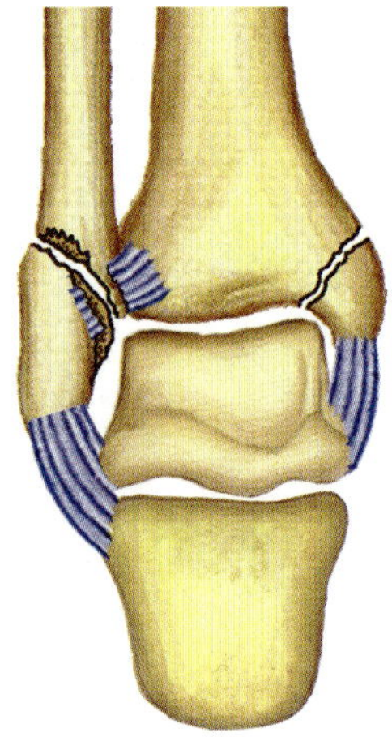

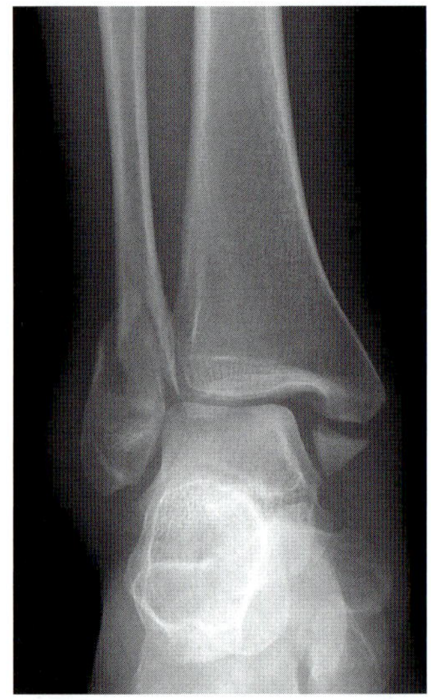

Fibular simple, with rupture of anterior syndesmosis + fracture of medial malleolus

44-B2.3

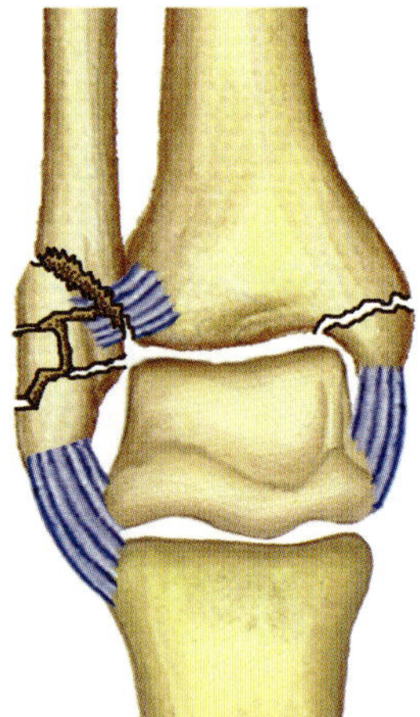

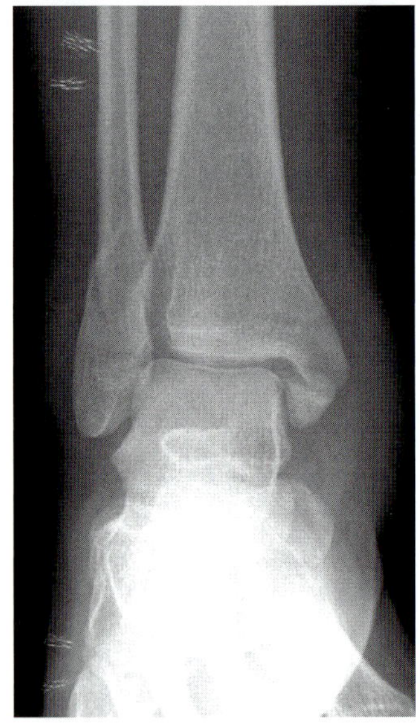

Fibular multifragmentary, with medial lesion

44-B Tibia/fibula malleolar segment, trans-syndesmotic fibular fractures

44-B3
With medial lesion and a Volkmann fracture
1,792 fractures
M: 911 (50.84%)
F: 881 (49.16%)
0.48% of total adult fractures
2.96% of adult tibia/fibula
6.34% of segment 44
16.10% of type 44-B

44-B3.1

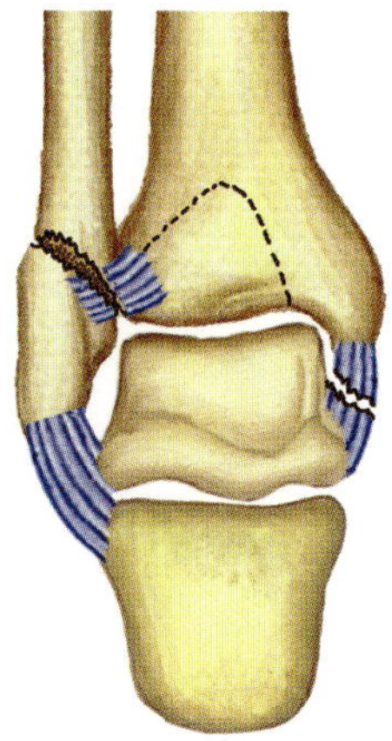

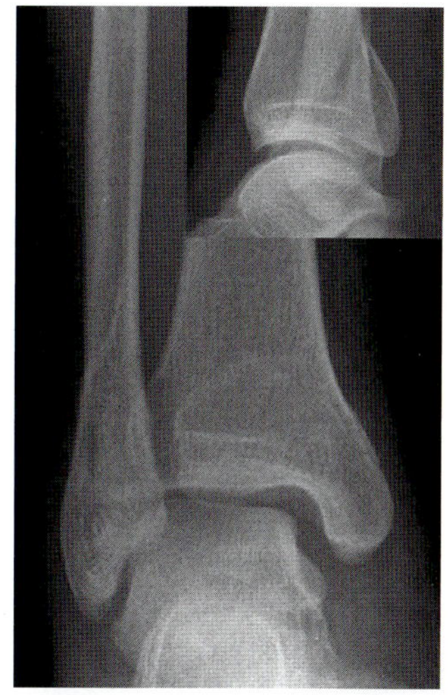

Fibular simple, with rupture of medial collateral ligament + a Volkmann fracture

44-B3.2

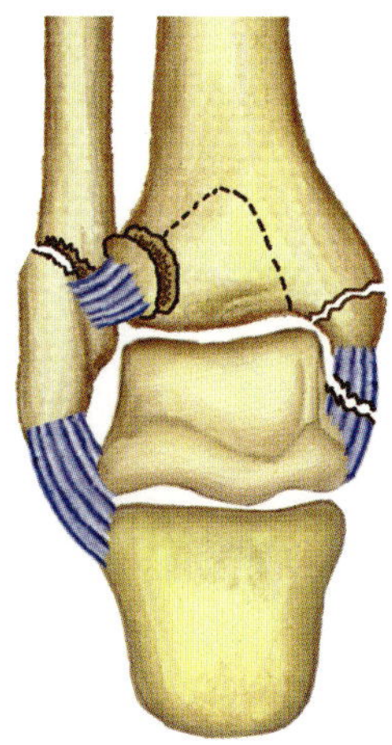

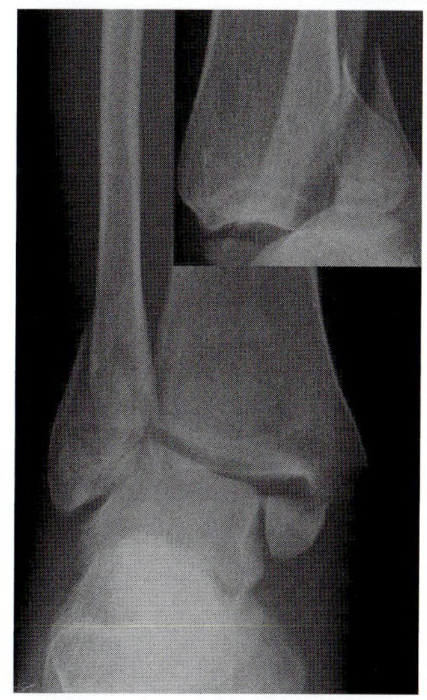

Fibular simple, with fracture of medial malleolus + a Volkmann fracture

44-B3.3

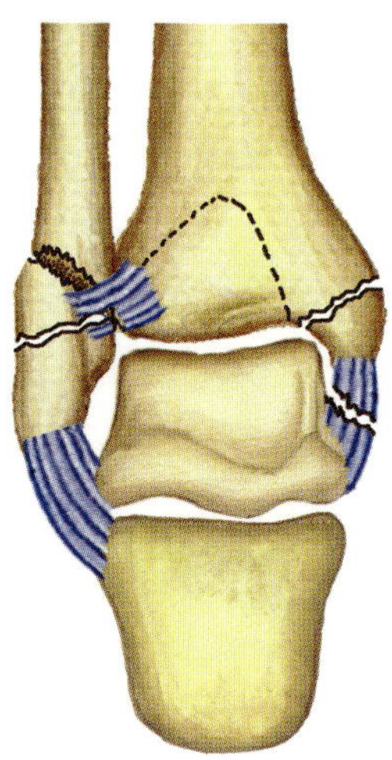

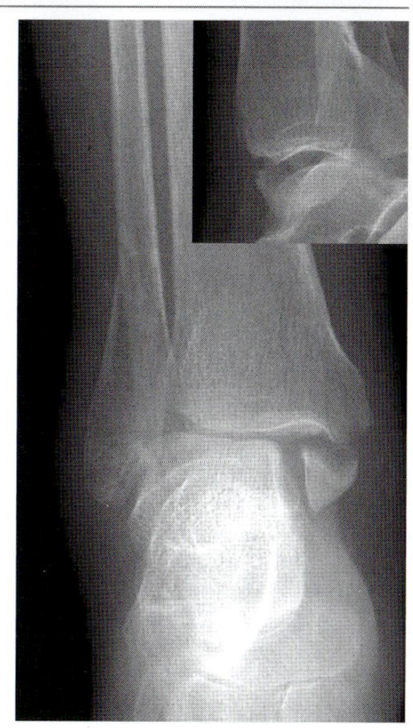

Fibular multifragmentary, with fracture of medial malleolus + a Volkmann fracture

44-C Tibia/fibula malleolar segment, suprasyndesmotic lesion

44-C1
Fibular diaphyseal simple
3,105 fractures
M: 2,299 (74.04%)
F: 806 (25.96%)
0.83% of total adult fractures
5.12% of adult tibia/fibula
10.98% of segment 44
52.65% of type 44-C

44-C1.1

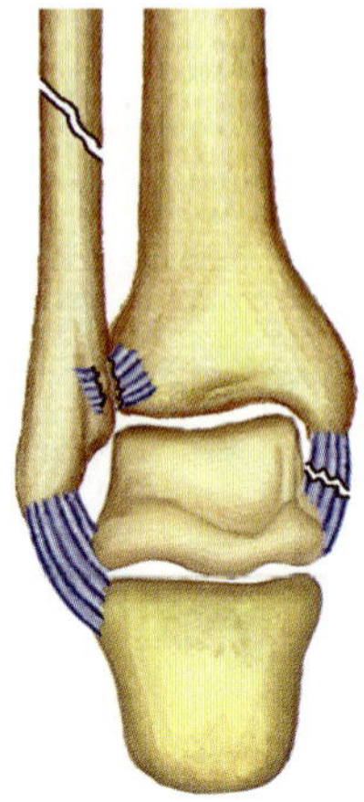

With rupture of medial collateral ligament

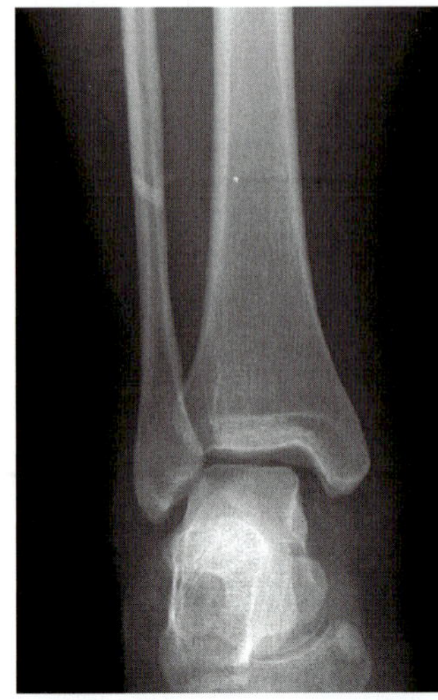

44-C1.2

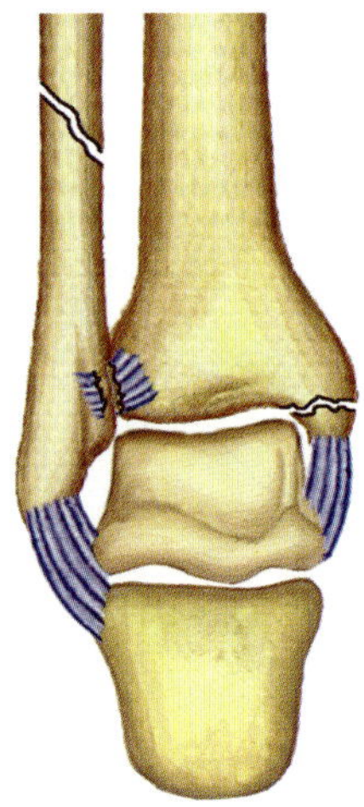

With fracture of medial malleolus

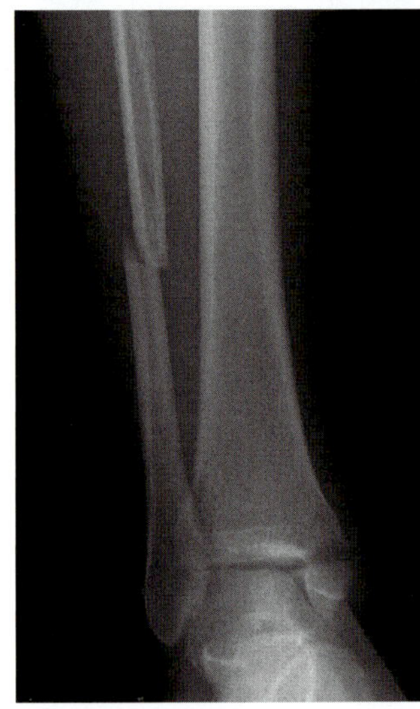

44-C1.3

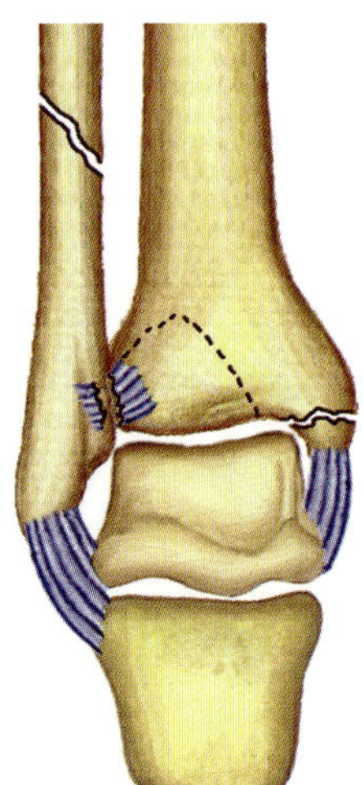

With fracture of medial malleolus
+ a Volkmann fracture

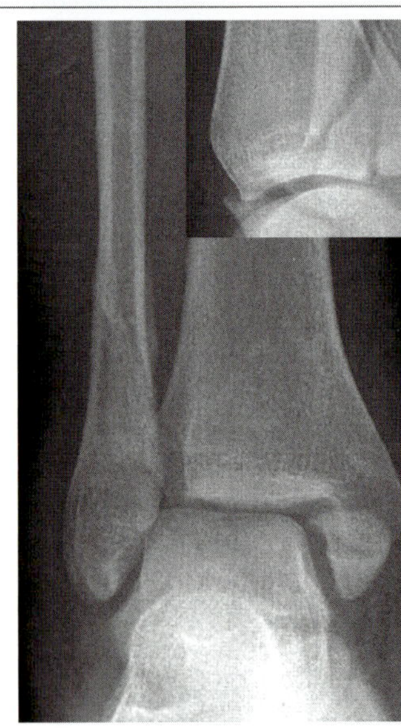

44-C Tibia/fibula malleolar segment, suprasyndesmotic lesion

44-C2
Fibular diaphyseal multifragmentary
1,838 fractures
M: 1,408 (76.61%)
F: 430 (23.39%)
0.49% of total adult fractures
3.03% of adult tibia/fibula
6.50% of segment 44
31.17% of type 44-C

44-C2.1

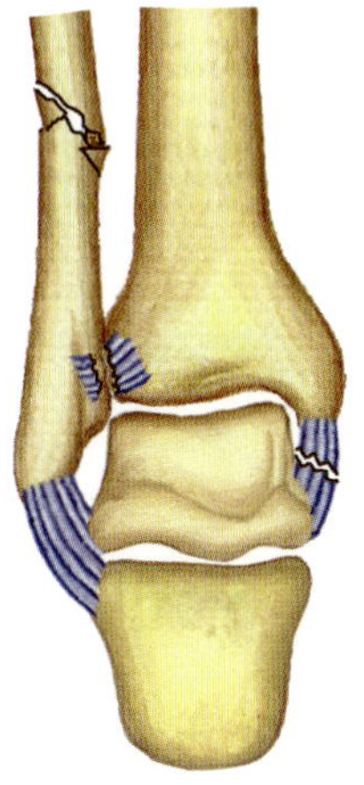

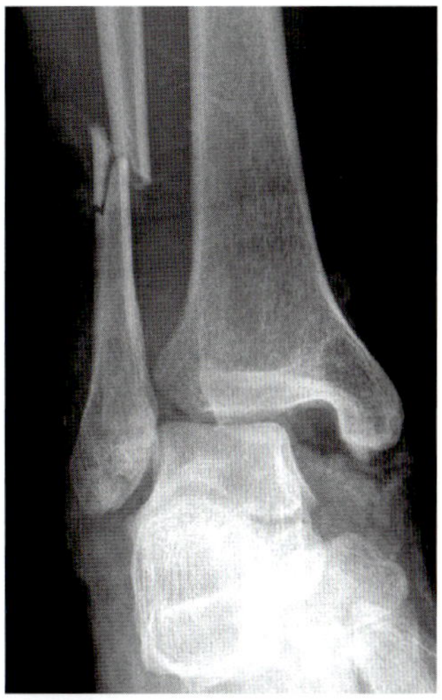

With rupture of medial collateral ligament

44-C2.2

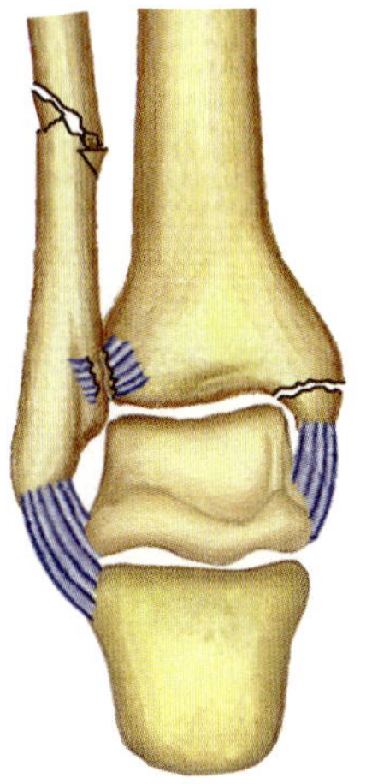

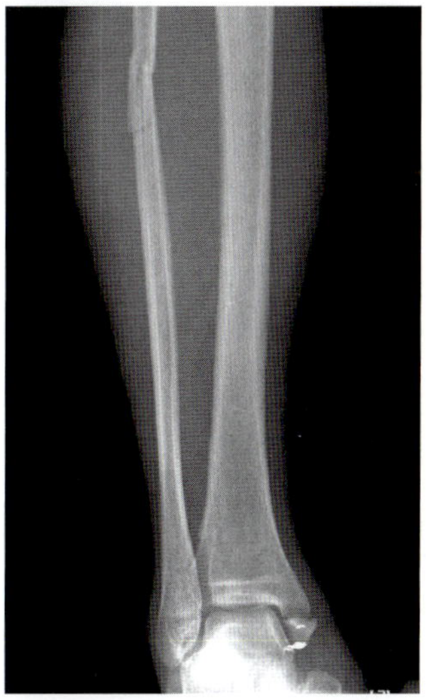

With fracture of medial malleolus

44-C2.3

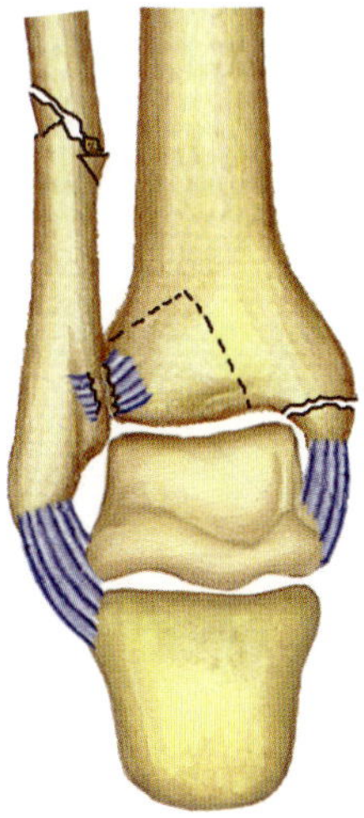

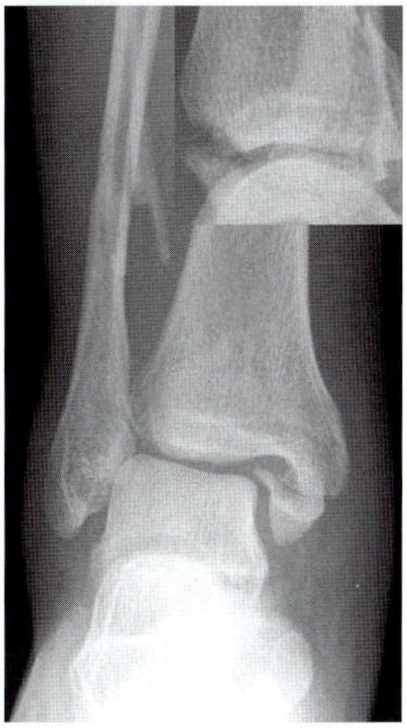

With fracture of medial malleolus
+ a Volkmann fracture

44-C Tibia/fibula malleolar segment, suprasyndesmotic lesion

44-C3
Proximal fibular fracture (Maisonneuve)
954 fractures
M: 676 (70.86%)
F: 278 (29.14%)
0.25% of total adult fractures
1.57% of adult tibia/fibula
3.37% of segment 44
16.18% of type 44-C

44-C3.1

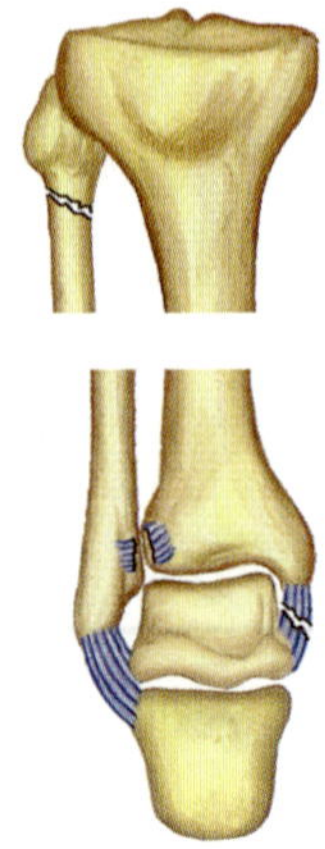

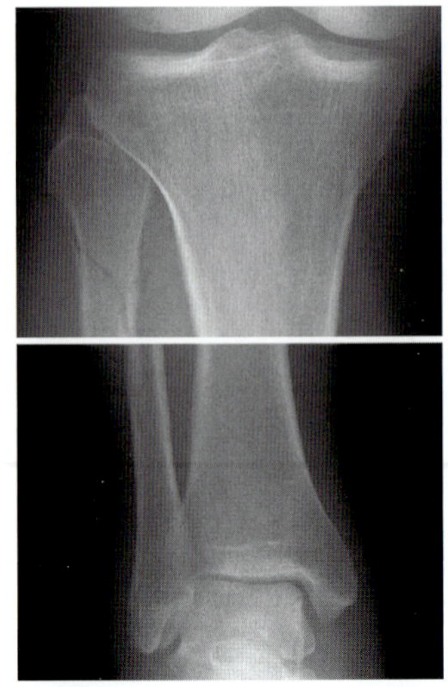

Without shortening,
without Volkmann fracture

44-C3.2

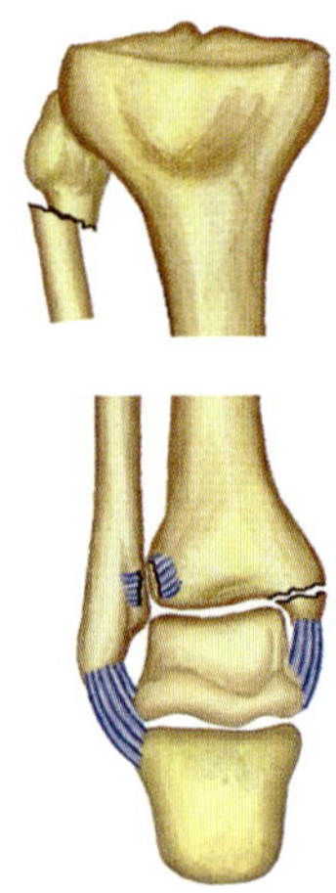

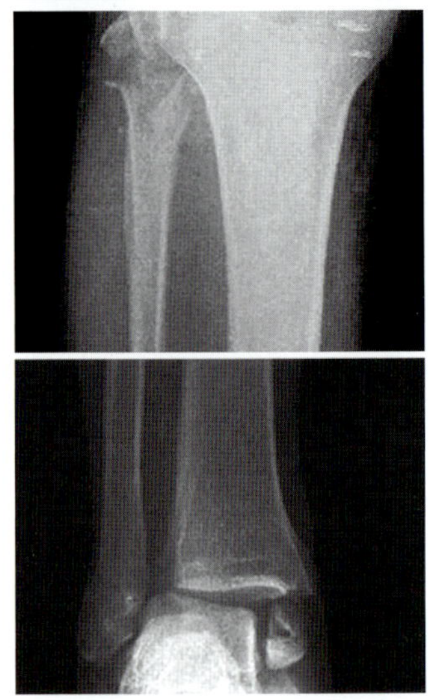

With shortening,
without Volkmann fracture

44-C3.3

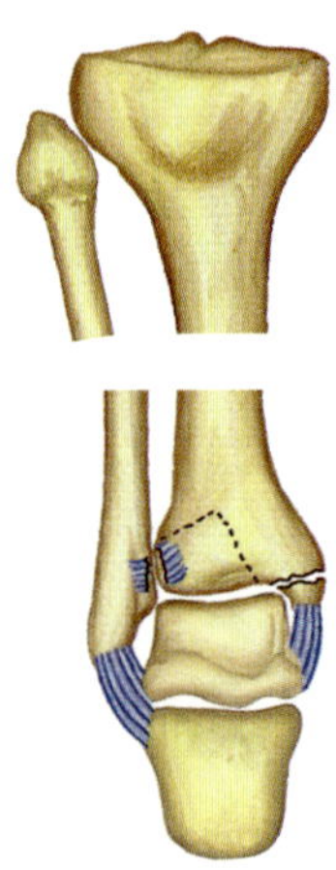

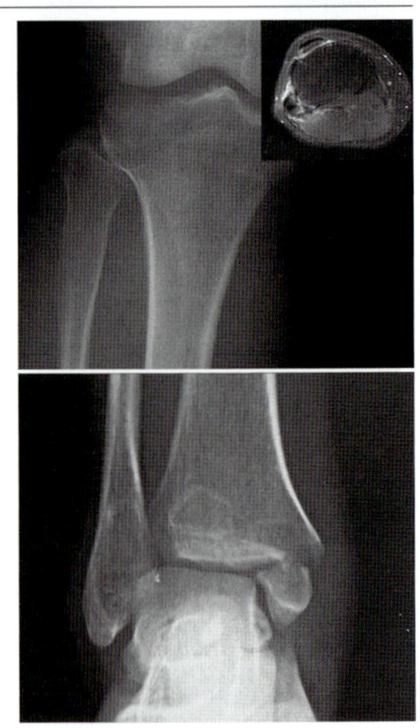

With dislocation of proximal fibula,
+ fracture of medial malleolus
+ a Volkmann fracture

Injury Mechanism

Ankle fractures are usually caused by an indirect mechanism, such as eversion, inversion, dorsiflexion, or plantar flexion. Injury to the ankle occurs when the foot is fixed on the ground in supination or pronation and an exorotation or adduction force is applied. The fracture type varies depending on the magnitude and direction of the force, and the position of the ankle at the time of injury.

Diagnosis

Ankle fractures usually present with swelling, pain, and deformity if the ankle joint is dislocated. With a partial or limited range of motion, patients experience the pain that becomes worse with activity. According to individual injury mechanisms, a careful evaluation of relevant ligament and osseous structures should be performed. Special attention should be paid to the ankle's range of motion, specifically for eversion/inversion and dorsiflexion/plantar flexion. If ligamentous injury is suspected, a comparison with the unaffected limb is helpful. Physicians should be aware of the possible association of fractures or dislocations of the proximal fibula, and the need to avoid a hasty underdiagnosis.

Radiographic evaluation of ankle injuries should include standard AP, lateral, and mortise views (taken with a 15-degree internal rotation of the foot). An additional oblique view can be obtained if necessary. A special X-ray, called a "stress test" can be performed after the acute stage has passed; it is very useful in determining the status of the ligamentous injury and the stability of the mortise joint. CT scan can be considered to further assess complex fractures or if plain films are inconclusive. MRI is indicated if ligamentous injury is suspected. Physicians should be aware of the possible associated fracture displacement of the diaphyseal or proximal fibula, for which an X-ray can be taken over the entire length of the tibia/fibula. An additional AP view of the proximal tibia/fibula can be helpful for diagnosis if a view of the entire length of the tibia/fibula cannot be obtained.

Treatment

The main principles of treatment in malleolar injury are anatomical reduction of the malleolus and restoration of the ankle joint mortise. Malleolus fractures can be divided into stable and unstable fractures.

Stable fractures are those where the lateral malleolus has an isolated fracture and the talus lies within the center of the ankle mortise without dislocation. Unstable fractures are fractures that do not fit into the "stable" category. Stable fractures of the ankle can usually be managed by nonsurgical treatment, such as a U-shaped or tubular casting. Minimally invasive plating or screw fixation can also be applied to facilitate early mobilization. Unstable fractures of the ankle should be treated by surgical intervention. Plating or screw fixation can be applied for rigid fixation and ligament repair, based on the fracture patterns and severity of the ligamentous injury.

Commonly Used Classification for Fracture of the Tibia and Fibula

Tibial Plateau Fractures

Overview

The Schatzker classification system is the most commonly used classification for tibial plateau fractures, and is based on the location and extent of the fracture and associated depression of the bone.

- *Type I*: split fracture of the lateral tibial plateau without articular depression.
- *Type II*: split fracture of the lateral tibial plateau with articular depression.
- *Type III*: isolated depression of the lateral plateau.
- *Type IV*: fracture of the medial plateau with associated intercondylar eminence avulsion.
- *Type V*: split bicondylar fracture.
- *Type VI*: split bicondylar fracture with diaphyseal, metaphyseal dissociation.

Patients who have tibial plateau fractures may experience swelling, pain, partial or limited active or passive range of motion, and varus or valgus deformity in severe cases. Fractures resulting from high-energy trauma are often associated with tension blisters, compartment syndrome, ligament rupture, and neurovascular injury. Radiographic evaluation should include standard AP and lateral views of the knee joint. Complex fractures resulting from high-energy injuries can be viewed with application of knee traction to better visualize the pattern and location of the fracture fragments; 40-degree internal and external oblique views can clearly show lateral and medial plateaus. An AP projection with an inclination of 15 degrees backward may be helpful in assessing the depression of the tibial plateau. Three-dimensional CT reconstruction and MRI can be used to further characterize fractures of the tibial plateau and assess the degree of articular comminution, as well as the extent of the depression. MRI is excellent for illustrating injuries of the anterior/posterior cruciate ligament, collateral ligament, and meniscus.

Most tibial plateau fractures are unstable fractures and require surgical intervention that strictly follows the principles of anatomical reduction, adequate bone grafting, and rigid fixation. Early non-weight-bearing mobilization exercises should be initiated to avoid joint stiffness and adhesion. Limited weight-bearing exercises, based on the stage of the fracture healing process can be conducted under the supervision of an experienced therapist.

Tibial plateau fractures

Type I
Split fracture of the lateral tibial plateau, without articular depression
881 fractures
M: 607 (68.90%)
F: 274 (31.10%)
14.15% of adult tibial plateau
1.45% of adult tibia/fibula
0.24% of total adult fractures

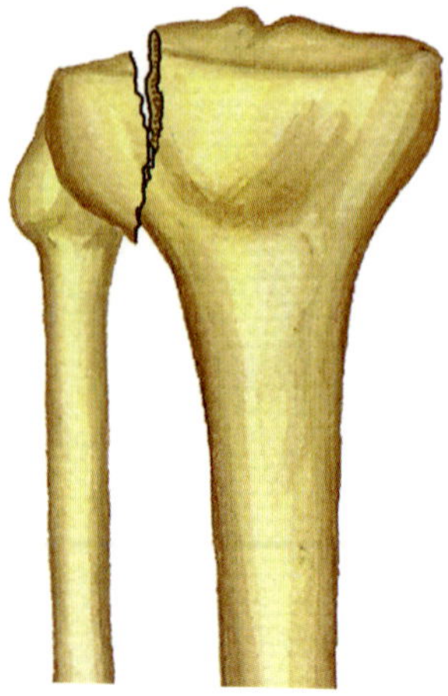

Type I

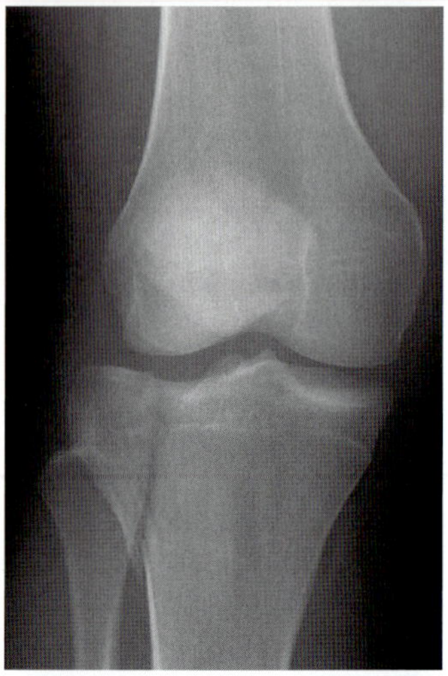

Type II
Split fracture of the lateral tibial plateau, with articular depression
909 fractures
M: 570 (62.71%)
F: 339 (37.29%)
14.6% of adult tibial plateau
1.50% of adult tibia/fibula
0.24% of total adult fractures

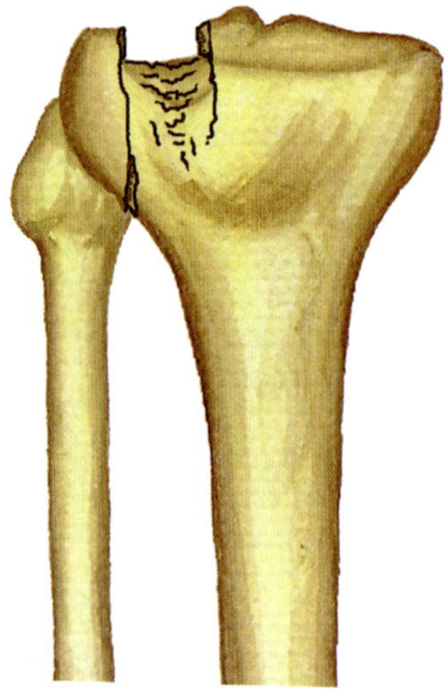

Type II

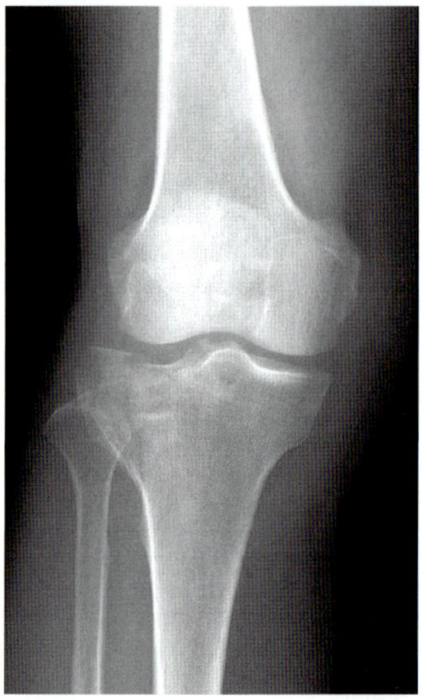

Type III
Isolated depression of the lateral plateau
960 fractures
M: 497 (51.77%)
F: 463 (48.23%)
15.42% of adult tibial plateau
1.58% of adult tibia/fibula
0.26% of total adult fractures

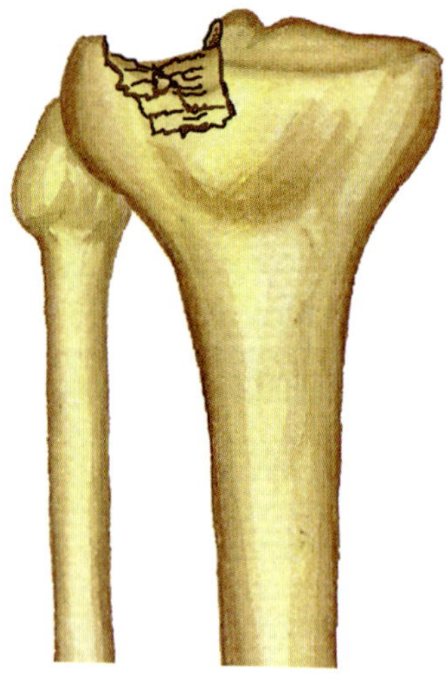

Type III

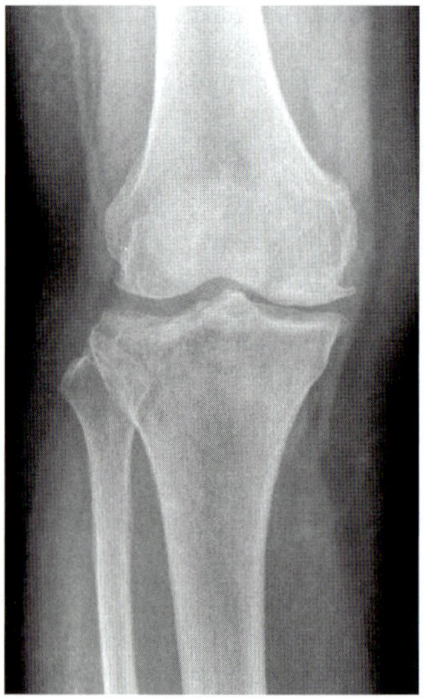

Type IV
Fracture of the medial plateau, with associated intercondylar eminence avulsion
1,278 fractures
M: 870 (68.08%)
F: 408 (31.92%)
20.52% of adult tibial plateau
2.11% of adult tibia/fibula
0.34% of total adult fractures

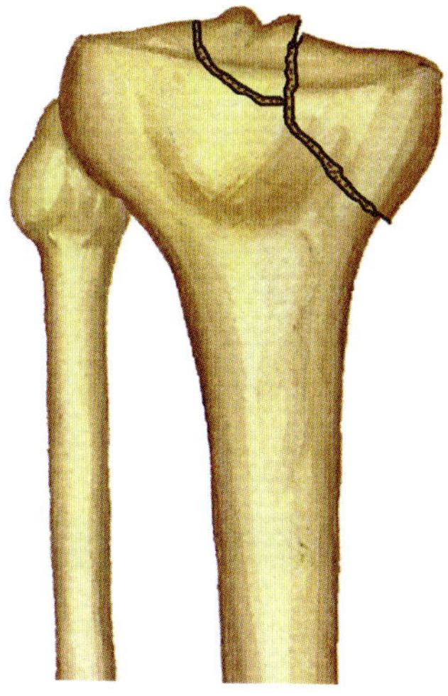

Type IV

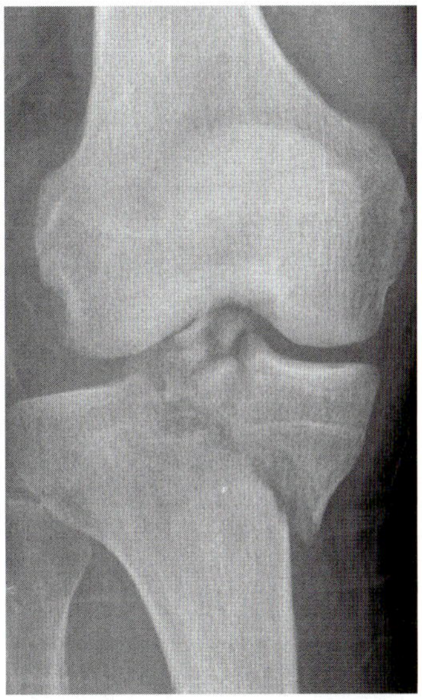

Type V
Split bicondylar fracture
511 fractures
M: 377 (73.78%)
F: 134 (26.22%)
8.21% of adult tibial plateau
0.84% of adult tibia/fibula
0.14% of total adult fractures

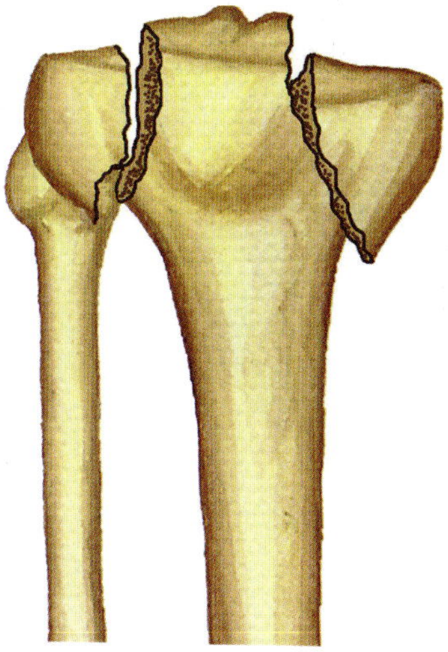

Type V

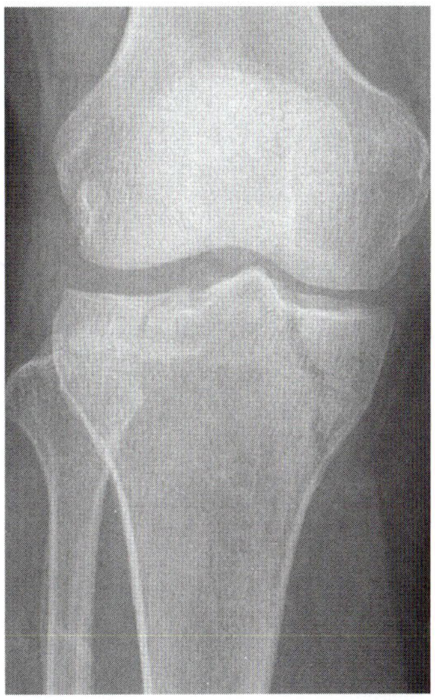

Type VI
Split bicondylar fracture, with diaphyseal, metaphyseal dissociation
1,688 fractures
M: 1,354 (80.21%)
F: 334 (19.79%)
27.11% of adult tibial plateau
2.78% of adult tibia/fibula
0.45% of total adult fractures

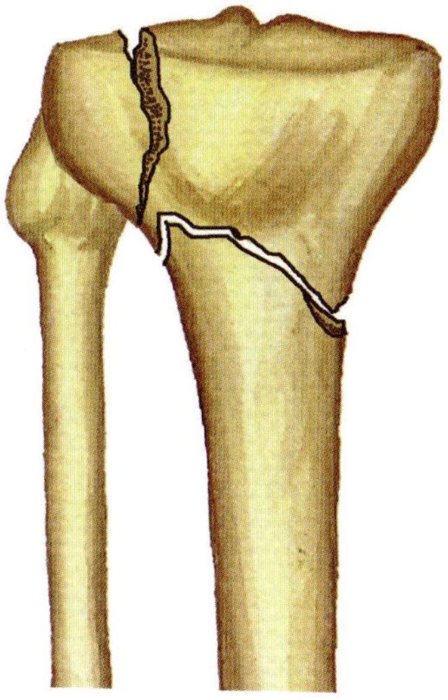

Type VI

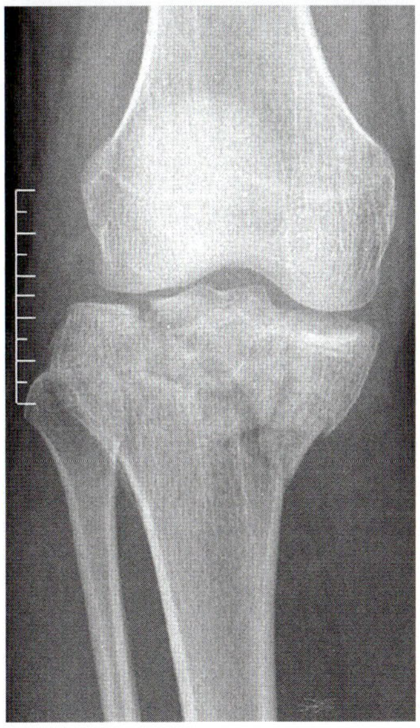

Clinical Epidemiologic Features of Tibial Plateau Fractures

A total of 6,227 tibial plateau fractures were treated in 83 hospitals in China over a 2-year period from 2010 to 2011. All cases were reviewed and statistically studied, the fractures accounted for 10.27% of all tibia/fibula fractures in adults and 1.66% of all types of fractures in adults. Their epidemiologic features are as follows:

- More males than females
- The highest risk age group is ages 41–45 years; the most affected male age group is 41–45 years, while females aged 56–60 years have the highest risk.
- The most common fracture type according to Schatzker classification is type VI; type VI for males, while type III is most common for females.

Tibial Plateau Fractures by Sex

Table 5.22 Sex distribution of 6,227 tibial plateau fractures

Sex	Number of fractures	Percentage (%)
Male	4,275	68.65
Female	1,952	31.35
Total	6,227	100.00

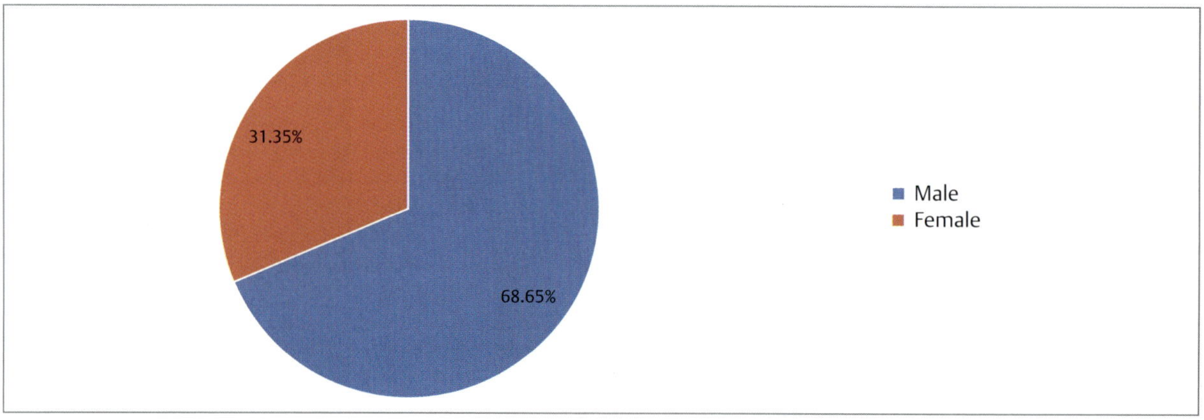

Fig. 5.22 Sex distribution of 6,227 tibial plateau fractures.

Tibial Plateau Fractures by Age Group

Table 5.23 Sex and age distribution of 6,227 tibial plateau fractures

Age group (years)	Male	Female	Number of fractures	Percentage (%)
16–20	169	55	224	3.60
21–25	266	67	333	5.35
26–30	296	86	382	6.13
31–35	423	125	548	8.80
36–40	624	171	795	12.77
41–45	694	206	900	14.45
46–50	607	232	839	13.47
51–55	459	247	706	11.34
56–60	338	276	614	9.86
61–65	185	181	366	5.88
66–70	90	117	207	3.32
71–75	65	67	132	2.12
76–80	36	75	111	1.78
81–85	19	30	49	0.79
≥86	4	17	21	0.34
Total	4,275	1,952	6,227	100.00

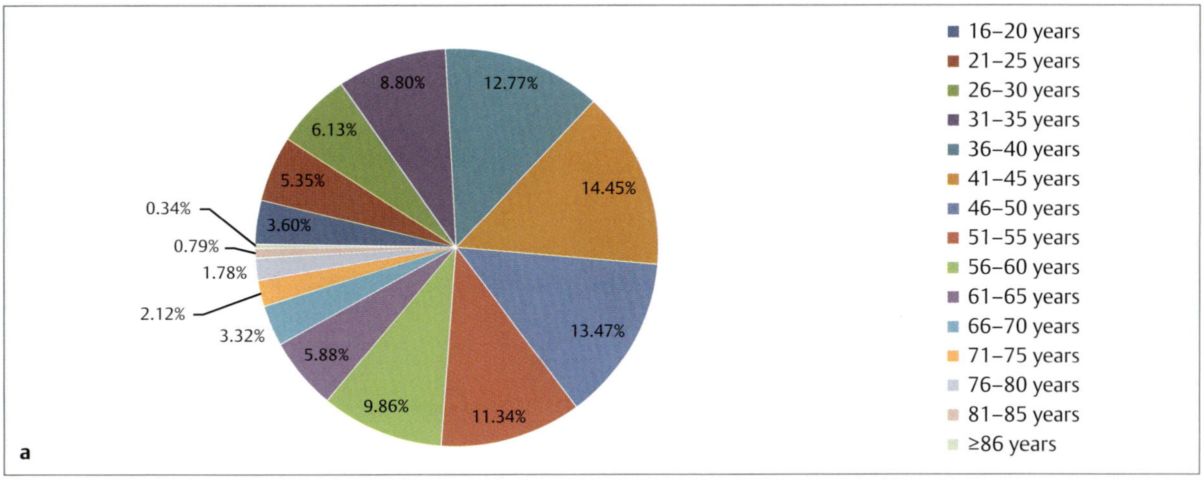

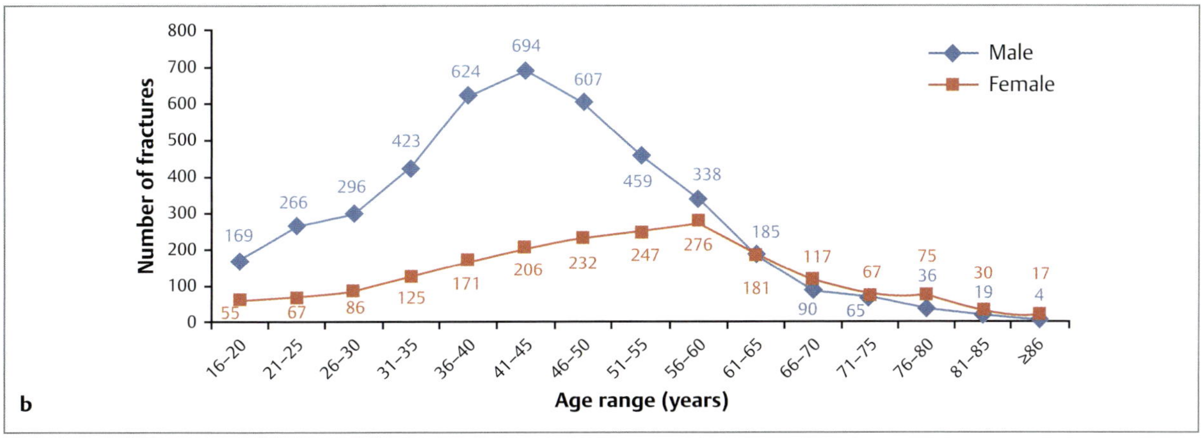

Fig. 5.23 **(a)** Age distribution of 6,227 tibial plateau fractures.
(b) Age and sex distribution of 6,227 tibial plateau fractures.

Tibial Plateau Fractures by Fracture Type Based on Schatzker Classification

Table 5.24 Sex and fracture type distribution of 6,227 tibial plateau fractures by Schatzker classification

Fracture type (Schatzker)	Male	Female	Number of fractures	Percentage (%)
I	607	274	881	14.15
II	570	339	909	14.60
III	497	463	960	15.42
IV	870	408	1,278	20.52
V	377	134	511	8.21
VI	1,354	334	1,688	27.11
Total	4,275	1,952	6,227	100.00

5

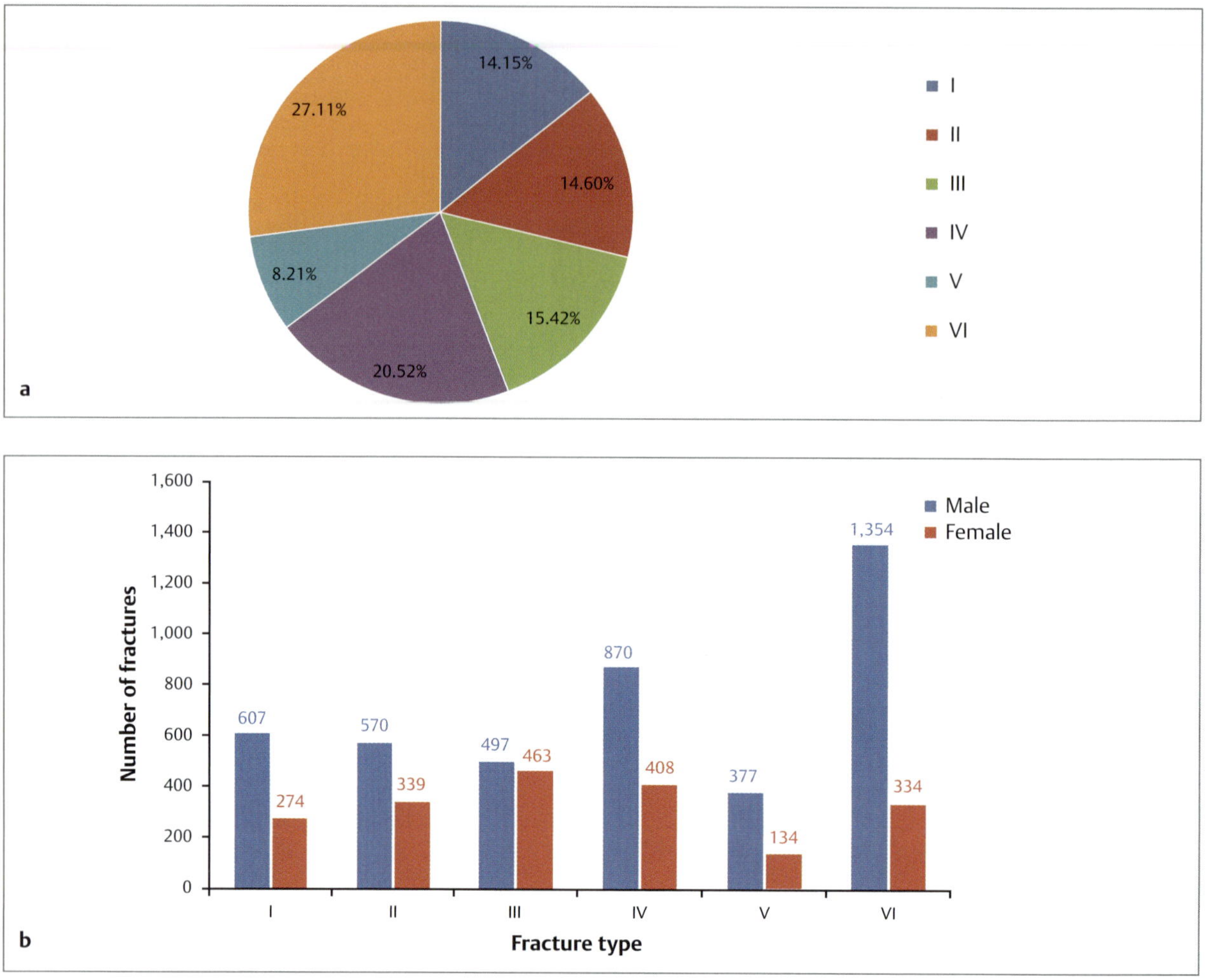

Fig. 5.24 **(a)** Fracture type distribution of 6,227 tibial plateau fractures by Schatzker classification. **(b)** Sex and fracture type distribution of 6,227 tibial plateau fractures by Schatzker classification.

Pilon Fractures

Overview

The Pilon fracture is a comminuted fracture of the distal tibia. Destot first described this type of compression injury in 1911, while Ruedi and Allgower divided it into three types:

- Type I: articular split fracture without significant displacement; it can be managed with conservative treatment.
- Type II: articular fracture displacement with articular incongruity but minimal comminution.
- Type III: severe articular comminution and articular impaction fracture.

Radiographic evaluations should include AP, lateral, and mortise views of the ankle joint, with the foot in 15 degrees of internal rotation. Additional views with the foot/ankle held in external rotation at 45 degrees can be obtained, if indicated, to visualize the anteromedial and posterolateral surface of the tibia. CT can be of great help in evaluating the degree of articular comminution and extent of articular depression. Stable Pilon fractures with minimal displacement are generally managed nonsurgically, while unstable Pilon fractures usually require surgical intervention. Operative approaches include: screw fixation, plating, use of a locking compression plate, circular ring external fixation, etc. Open reduction and internal fixation can be performed utilizing the following principles:

- Restoration of the fibular length
- Reconstruction of the articular surface of the distal tibia
- Restoration of the mortise structure
- Plating of the medial surface of the tibia.
- Adequate bone grafting to cover the metaphyseal defect

Closed fractures with poor soft tissue status should be treated first with talar traction, then one should proceed to surgical intervention after the soft tissue status has improved.

Pilon fractures by Ruedi and Allgower classification

Type I
Articular split fracture without significant displacement
1,532 fractures
M: 896 (58.49%)
F: 636 (41.51%)
39.65% of adult Pilon
2.53% of adult tibia/fibula
0.41% of total adult fractures

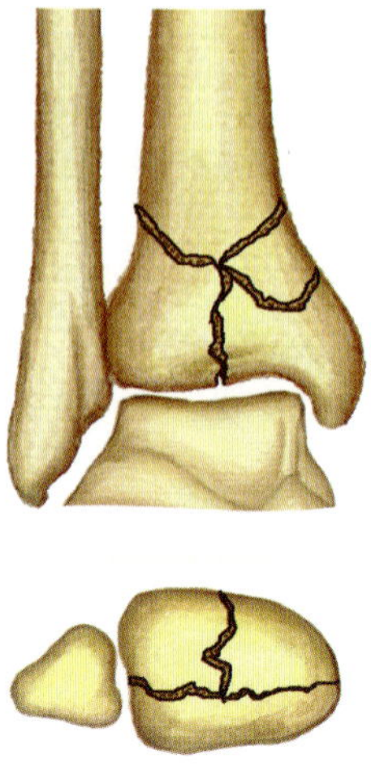

Type I

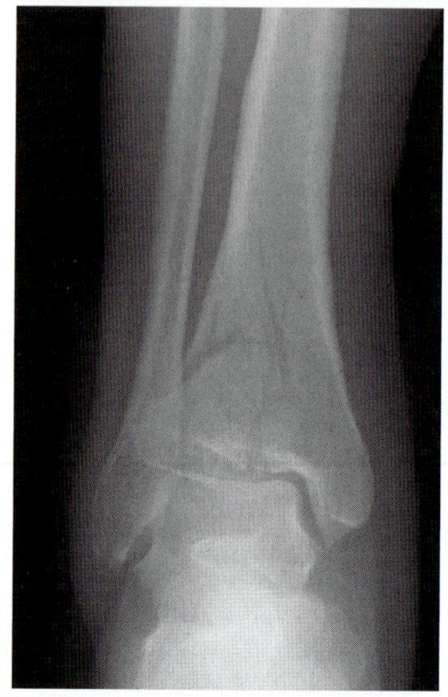

Type II
Articular fracture displacement with articular incongruity but minimal comminution
1,238 fractures
M: 924 (74.64%)
F: 314 (25.36%)
32.04% of adult Pilon
2.04% of adult tibia/fibula
0.33% of total adult fractures

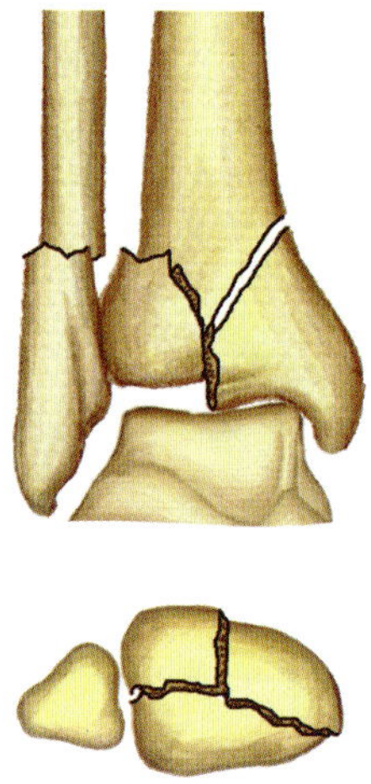

Type II

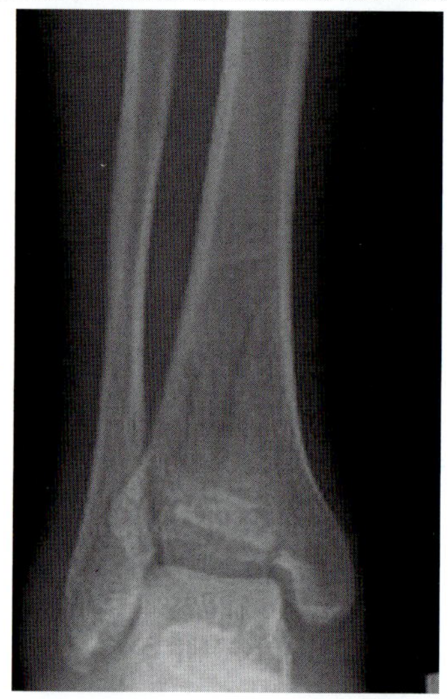

Type III
Severe articular comminution and articular impaction fracture
1,094 fractures
M: 894 (81.72%)
F: 200 (18.28%)
28.31% of adult Pilon
1.80% of adult tibia/fibula
0.29% of total adult fractures

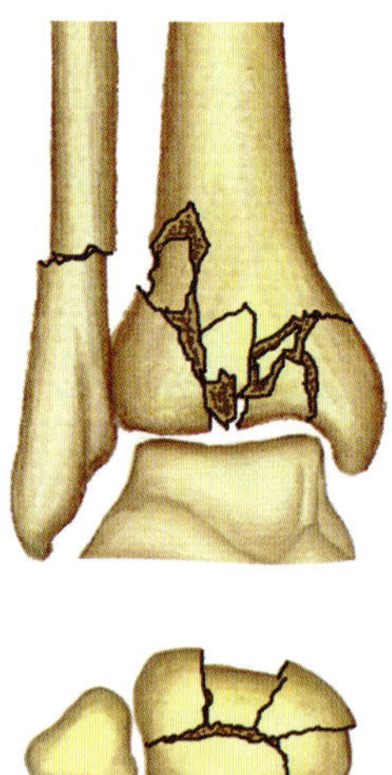

Type III

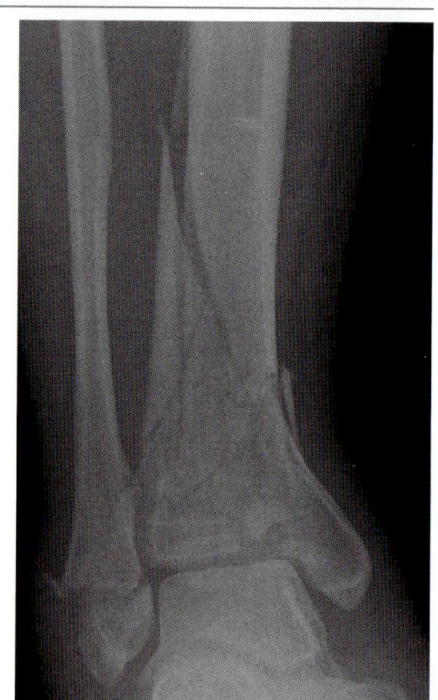

Epidemiologic Features of Pilon Fractures

A total of 3,864 Pilon fractures were treated in 83 hospitals in China over a 2-year period from 2010 to 2011. All cases were reviewed and statistically studied, the fractures accounted for 6.37% of all tibia/fibula fractures in adult, and 1.03% of all type of fractures in adults. Their epidemiologic features are as follows:

- More males than females
- The highest risk age group is 41–45 years; the most affected male age group is 41–45 years, while females aged 41–45 and 46–50 years have the highest risk.
- The most common fracture type according to Ruedi and Allgower classification is type I; type II for males, while type I is most common for females.

Pilon Fractures by Sex

Table 5.25 Sex distribution of 3,864 Pilon fractures

Sex	Number of fractures	Percentage (%)
Male	2,714	70.24
Female	1,150	29.76
Total	3,864	100.00

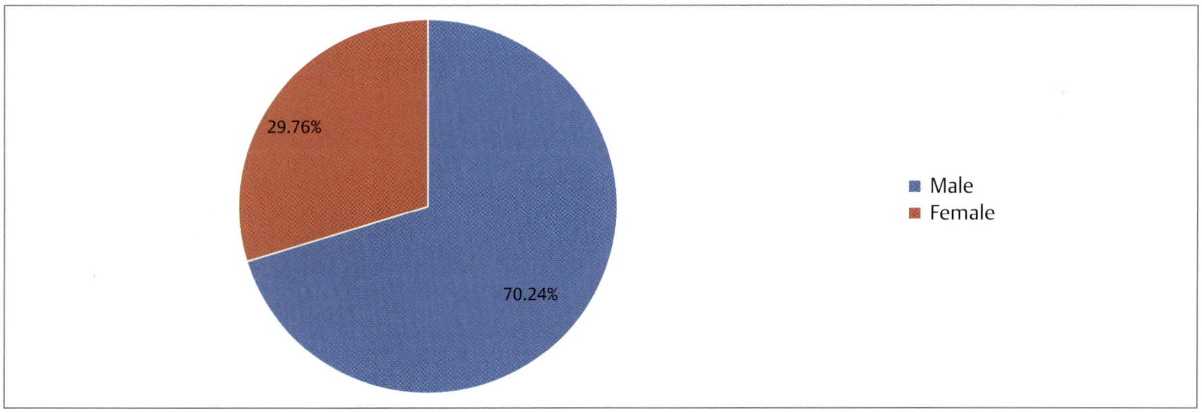

Fig. 5.25 Sex distribution of 3,864 Pilon fractures.

5

Pilon Fractures by Age Group

Table 5.26 Age and sex distribution of 3,864 Pilon fractures

Age group (years)	Male	Female	Number of fractures	Percentage (%)
16–20	146	29	175	4.53
21–25	201	72	273	7.07
26–30	275	86	361	9.34
31–35	346	76	422	10.92
36–40	407	127	534	13.82
41–45	460	136	596	15.42
46–50	297	136	433	11.21
51–55	213	135	348	9.01
56–60	156	128	284	7.35
61–65	107	61	168	4.35
66–70	42	61	103	2.67
71–75	30	33	63	1.63
76–80	15	28	43	1.11
81–85	15	23	38	0.98
≥86	4	19	23	0.60
Total	2,714	1,150	3,864	100.00

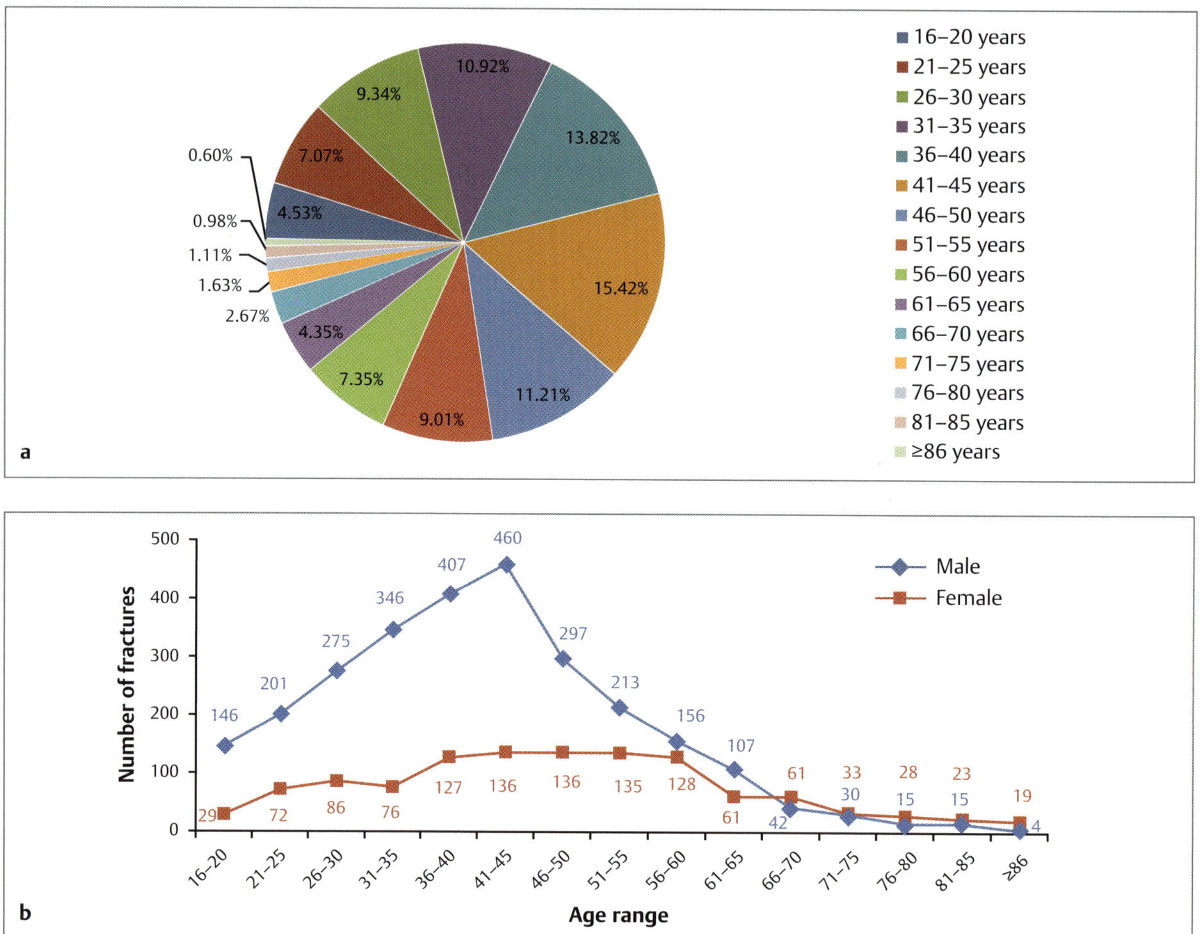

Fig. 5.26 **(a)** Age distribution of 3,864 Pilon fractures.
(b) Age and sex distribution of 3,864 Pilon fractures.

Fracture Type Distribution of Pilon Fractures by Ruedi and Allgower Classification

Table 5.27 Sex and fracture type distribution of 3,864 Pilon fractures by Ruedi and Allgower classification

Fracture type (Ruedi and Allgower)	Male	Female	Number of fractures	Percentage (%)
I	896	636	1,532	39.65
II	924	314	1,238	32.04
III	894	200	1,094	28.31
Total	2,714	1,150	3,864	100.00

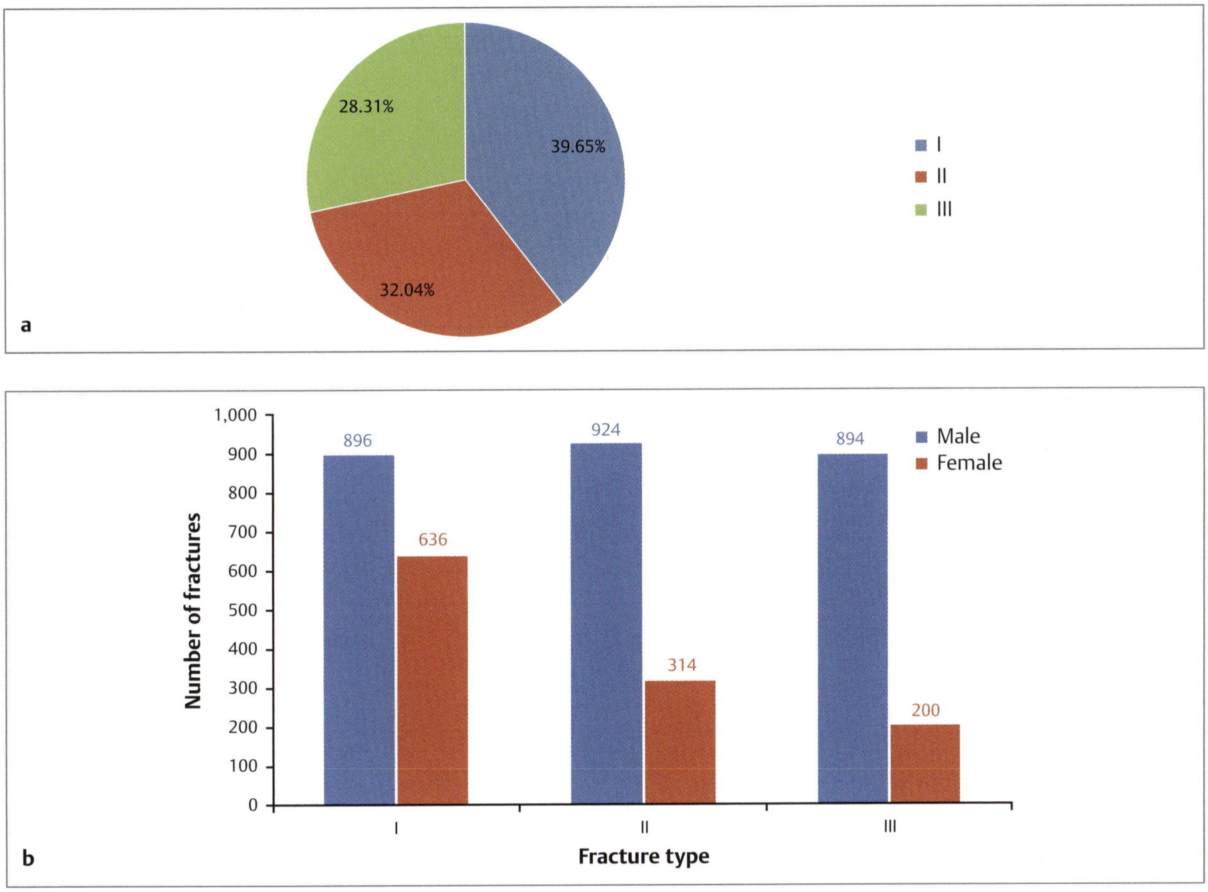

Fig. 5.27 **(a)** Fracture type distribution of 3,864 Pilon fractures by Ruedi and Allgower classification.
(b) Sex and fracture type distribution of 3,864 Pilon fractures by Ruedi and Allgower classification.

6 Fractures of the Spine

Overview

Anatomical Features

The spinal column consists of individual bony vertebrae and intervertebral disks that connect each vertebra in the front of the spine. A healthy spine provides strength, is flexible, and allows movement in several planes. Body movement and weight-bearing changes can produce an alteration in the geometry of the spine. The vertebral column is made of 26 separate vertebrae, and can be divided into five sections: cervical, thoracic, lumbar, sacral, and coccygeal. Because the sacrum and coccyx are fused with five sacral vertebrae and four coccygeal vertebrae, respectively, some believe the vertebral column is actually made up of 33 vertebral bones.

Each vertebra is composed of a body anteriorly and a neural arch posteriorly. The arch has two supporting pedicles and two arched laminae; it encloses an opening, the vertebral foramen, which helps to form the vertebral canal in which the spinal cord is housed. Seven processes arise from the vertebral arch: the central spinous process, two transverse processes, two superior facets, and two inferior facets. Three-quarters of the length of the vertebral column is from the vertebral bodies and one quarter is from the thickness of the intervertebral disks.

Two important concepts have emerged during the study of the spine's anatomical features. They are the two-column concept and three-column concept. In 1968, Kelly and Whitesides proposed a two-column concept that aided the assessment of angular deformation (**Plate 6.1**). The two columns, specifically the anterior and posterior columns, are defined as involving the vertebral bodies and neural arches,

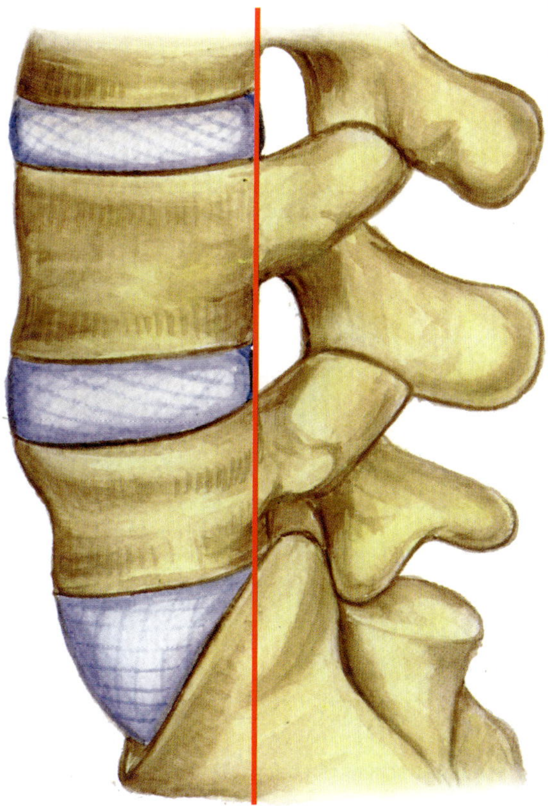

Delineation illustration of two-column spine concept

Plate 6.1

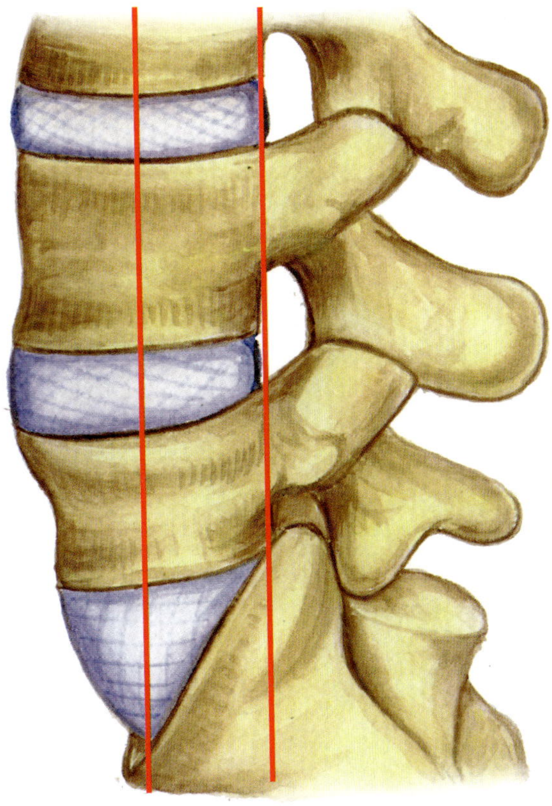

Delineation illustration of three-column spine concept

Plate 6.2

respectively, and are delineated by the posterior longitudinal ligament. The anterior column is composed of the anterior longitudinal ligament, posterior longitudinal ligament, and the vertebral body. The posterior column, otherwise known as the hollow column, is composed of the vertebral canal and the posterior ligamentous complex. Kelly and Whitesides highlighted the importance of the posterior ligamentous complex in the assessment of spine stability. However, the two-column concept is limited in assessing posterior nerve root injury in spine fractures, and has been gradually replaced by the three-column concept.

The three-column concept was introduced by Denis in 1983, and is able to reach better agreement with clinical observations regarding spine stability than the two-column concept (**Plate 6.2**). It divides the spine into three columns: the anterior, middle, and posterior columns. Using this scheme, the anterior column is composed of the anterior half of the vertebral body, the intervertebral disk, and the anterior longitudinal ligament; the middle column includes the posterior part of vertebral body and the disk, and the posterior longitudinal ligament; and the posterior column includes the pedicles, the facet joints, and the supraspinous ligaments. In 1984, McAfee proposed that the demarcation lies between the anterior and middle columns at the junction of the anterior two-thirds and posterior one-third of the vertebral body, instead of the midpoint of the vertebral body as proposed by Denis. With McAfee's scheme, fractures involving the middle column are unstable fractures. This concept is able to provide a better and more accurate assessment of spinal stability and neurologic injury.

AO Classification and Coding System for Spine Fractures

Based on AO classification, the spinal column is coded as the number 5. Cervical, thoracic, lumbar, and sacral fractures are assigned as numbers 51, 52, 53, and 54, respectively. Pelvic fractures always involve sacrococcygeal fractures; therefore, we put sacral and coccygeal fractures into the pelvic section during our statistical analysis.

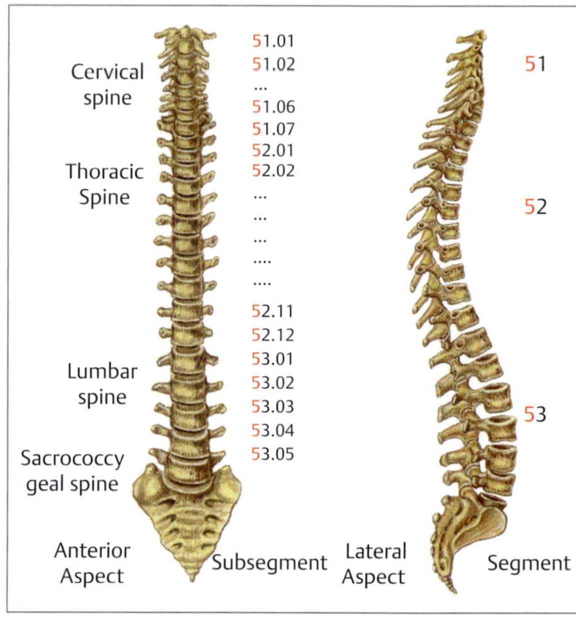

Plate 6.3

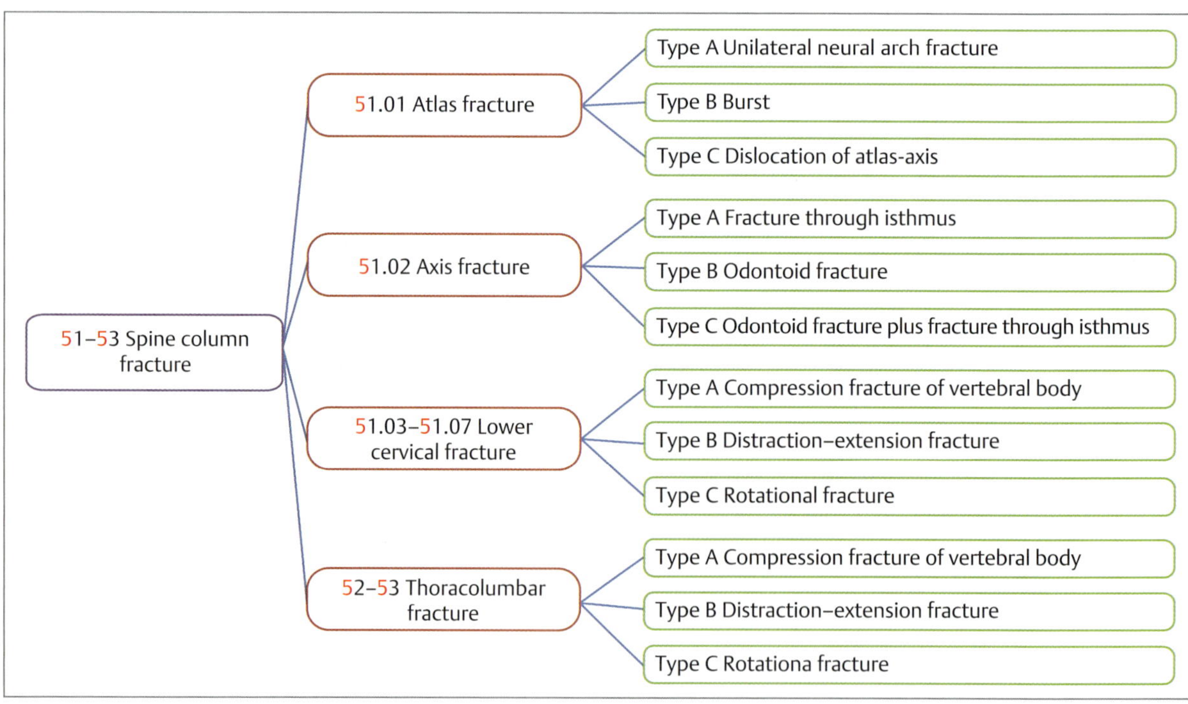

Plate 6.4

Because the atlas (51.01) and axis (51.02) have different anatomical features and unique functions from other cervical vertebrae, they require different methods of assessment regarding the stability and neurologic injury resulting from fractures. As such, AO classification describes vertebral column fractures into four sections: atlas, axis, lower cervical, and thoracolumbar fractures. The atlas and axis constitute the upper cervical spine.

For AO classification of spine fractures, the number 5 is assigned for the spine; 51 for cervical spine, 51.01–51.07 for vertebrae C1–C7, respectively (**Plate 6.3**); 52 for thoracic spine, 52.01–52.12 for vertebrae T1–T12, respectively; and 53 for lumbar spine, 53.01–53.05 for L1–L5, respectively (**Plate 6.4**).

Clinical Epidemiologic Features of Fractures of the Spinal Column

A total of 49,679 patients with 55,097 spinal column fractures were treated in 83 hospitals in China over a 2-year period from 2010 to 2011. All cases were reviewed and statistically studied, accounting for 11.97% of all patients with fractures and 12.76% of all types of fractures, respectively. Among these 49,679 patients, there were 517 children and 49,162 adults.

Epidemiologic features of fractures of the spinal column are as follows:

- More males than females
- The high-risk age group is 56–60 years. The most affected male age group is 41–45 years, while females aged 56–60 years have the highest risk.
- Thoracolumbar fractures occur more frequently than cervical or sacrococcygeal fractures.

Spinal Column Fractures by Sex

Table 6.1 Sex distribution of 49,679 patients with spinal column fractures

Sex	Number of patients	Percentage (%)
Male	25,280	50.89
Female	24,399	49.11
Total	49,679	100.00

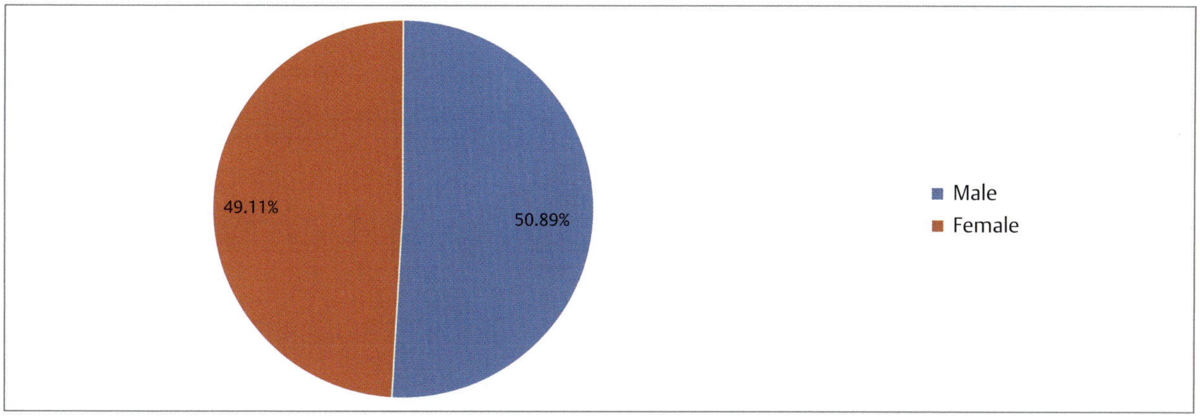

Fig. 6.1 Sex distribution of 49,679 patients with spinal column fractures.

6

Spinal Column Fractures by Age Group

Table 6.2 Age and sex distribution of 49,679 patients with spinal column fractures

Age group (years)	Male	Female	Number of patients	Percentage (%)
0–5	58	38	96	0.19
6–10	75	62	137	0.28
11–15	172	112	284	0.57
16–20	750	307	1,057	2.13
21–25	1,337	440	1,777	3.58
26–30	1,483	557	2,040	4.11
31–35	1,622	664	2,286	4.60
36–40	2,468	1,045	3,513	7.07
41–45	2,847	1,323	4,170	8.39
46–50	2,723	1,649	4,372	8.80
51–55	2,356	2,010	4,366	8.79
56–60	2,530	3,099	5,629	11.33
61–65	1,757	2,883	4,640	9.34
66–70	1,399	2,867	4,266	8.59
71–75	1,392	2,995	4,387	8.83
76–80	1,176	2,493	3,669	7.39
81–85	727	1,286	2,013	4.05
≥86	408	569	977	1.97
Total	25,280	24,399	49,679	100.00

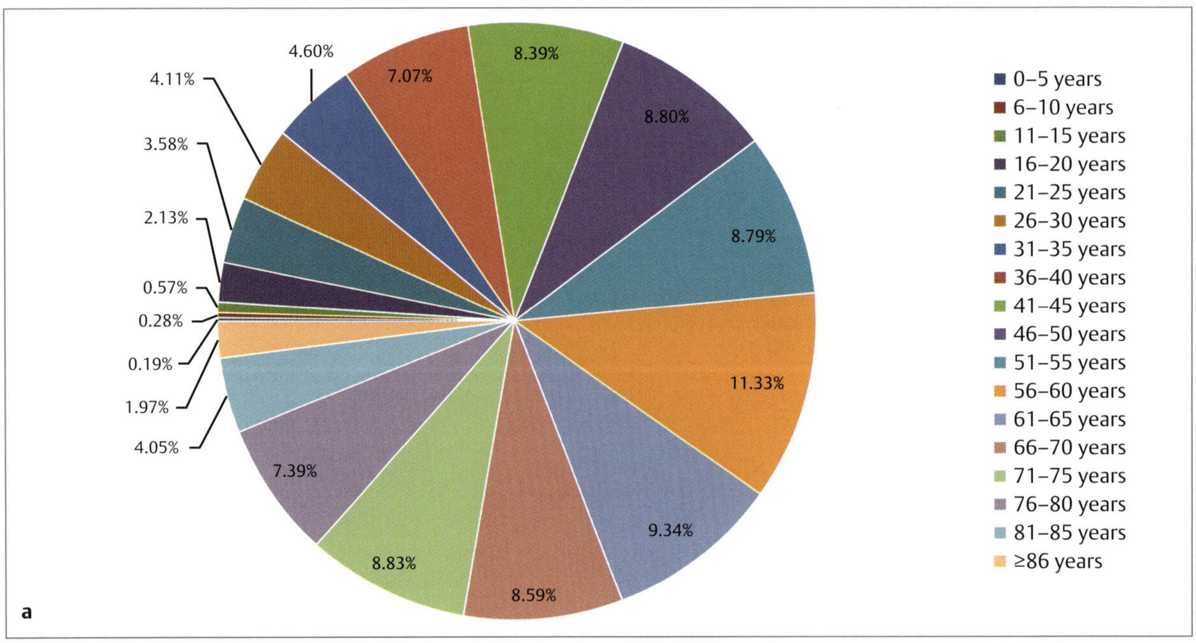

Fig. 6.2 **(a)** Age distribution of 49,679 patients with spinal column fractures.

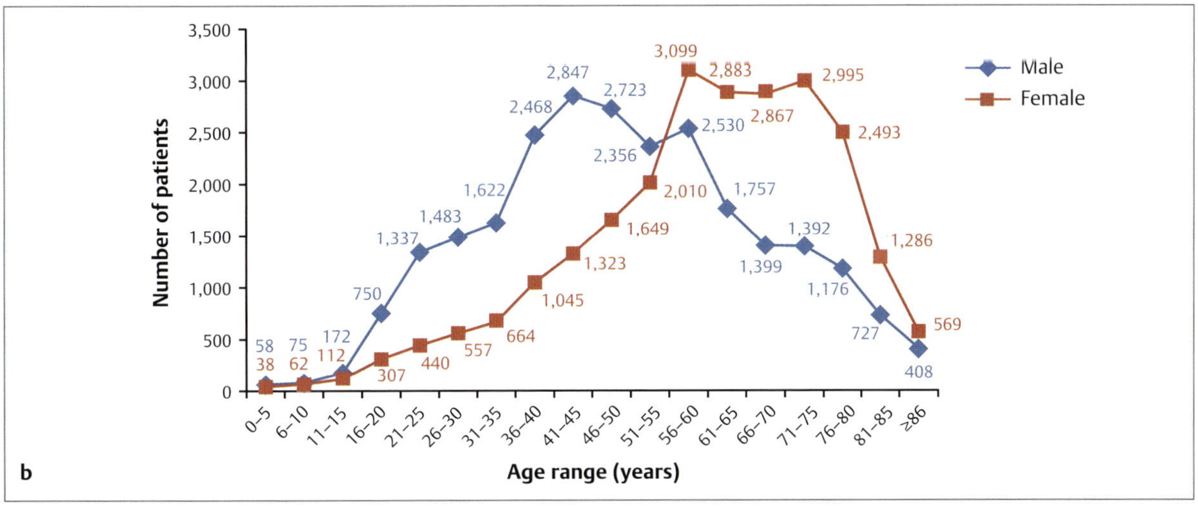

b

Fig. 6.2 (*continued*) **(b)** Age and sex distribution of 49,679 patients with spinal column fractures.

Spinal Column Fractures by Segment

Table 6.3 Sex and fracture subsegment distribution of 55,097 spinal column fractures

Subsegment	Male	Female	Number of fractures	Percentage (%)
51.01	189	118	307	0.56
51.02	694	417	1,111	2.02
51.03	200	74	274	0.50
51.04	314	114	428	0.78
51.05	619	223	842	1.53
51.06	433	191	624	1.13
51.07	128	44	172	0.31
52.01	593	748	1,341	2.43
52.02	112	201	313	0.57
52.03	62	63	125	0.23
52.04	92	99	191	0.35
52.05	107	111	218	0.40
52.06	164	198	362	0.66
52.07	233	280	513	0.93
52.08	243	316	559	1.01
52.09	232	289	521	0.95
52.10	282	388	670	1.22
52.11	1,337	1,660	2,997	5.44
52.12	4,657	5,535	10,192	18.50
53.01	9,399	8,970	18,369	33.34
53.02	3,918	3,547	7,465	13.55
53.03	1,863	1,788	3,651	6.63
53.04	1,320	1,259	2,579	4.68
53.05	603	670	1,273	2.31
Total	27,794	27,303	55,097	100.00

NB: This table has no corresponding figure.

Cervical Fractures (Segment 51)

Anatomical Features

The first two vertebral bodies in the cervical spine are called the atlas and the axis. They are very special with respect to their unique anatomical features and functions; therefore, assessment of injuries to the atlas and axis are very different from those to other vertebrae. The AO classification has special descriptions for fractures of the atlas and axis (**Plate 6.5**).

The atlas, a ring-shaped bone, is remarkable for having no body. It consists of anterior and posterior arches, and two lateral masses, from which two transverse processes project laterally and downward. Its superior articular facets articulate with the occipital condyles of the skull, and it forms the atlantoaxial joint with the dens of the axis. The two transverse processes of the atlas serve as an attachment site for muscles and ligaments, which assist in rotating the head. The foramen transversarium pierces the transverse processes of the atlas, and gives passage to the vertebral artery and vein. The anterior and posterior arches are thin, especially at their junction with the lateral mass, which is particularly susceptible to injury and, if damaged, may lead to fracture and dislocation.

The dens of the axis was originally part of the atlas, but became separated from the atlas during development; therefore, malformations commonly occur, such as absence of the dens of axis, hypoplasia or agenesis of the dens, occipital–atlas fusion, and atlas–axis fusion. These malformations may result in poor stability of the craniocervical region and compression of the spinal cord. The root of the dens is very thin, making it especially prone to injury. The resultant fracture and dislocation of the root would lead to a high risk of paraplegia or even death (**Plate 6.5**).

There are important ligaments between the atlas and axis, connecting two or more bones, chondrites, or other soft tissues. The atlantoaxial ligament complex provides stability to the atlantoaxial joint though it has great range of motion, and prevents hyperflexion or hyperextension of the joint (**Plate 6.6**). The upper cervical ligament is important in stabilizing the upper cervical spine and preventing neurologic injury. Loss of stability of the ligament can result in subluxation of C1–C2, and lead to lethal neurologic injuries.

Each vertebra in the lower cervical spine (C3–C7) consists of a vertebral body, a vertebral arch, which is formed by a pair of pedicles, and a pair of laminae (**Plate 6.7**). Each vertebra also has seven processes: four articular, two transverse, and one spinous. By comparison, cervical vertebrae are smaller than thoracolumbar vertebrae. The lateral aspect of each vertebral body has a superior projection (uncinate process) that forms Luschka's joints (uncovertebral joints) with a projection downward from the inferior surface of the vertebral body above. The transverse process is short and broad, with a wide groove for the existing spinal nerve on its upper surface. It gives attachment to a number of muscles. The bony protuberances at the end of the transverse processes are called the anterior and posterior tubercles, accordingly. The articular facets are inclined approximately 45 degrees from the horizontal plane. A characteristic feature of vertebrae C2 to C6 is a projection known as the bifid spinous process, whereas C7 has a prominent nonbifid spinous process that can be felt at the base of the neck.

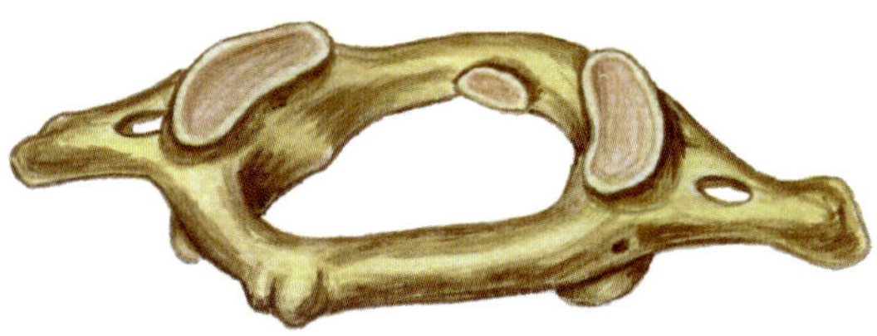

Oblique posterior–superior view of atlas

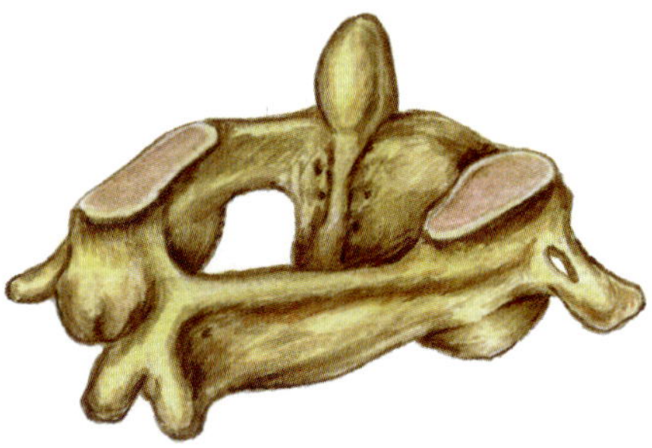

Oblique posterior–superior view of axis

Plate 6.5

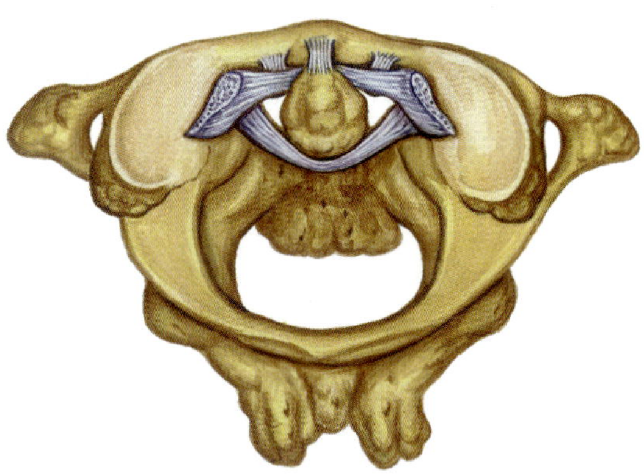

Superior view of atlantoaxial ligaments

Plate 6.6

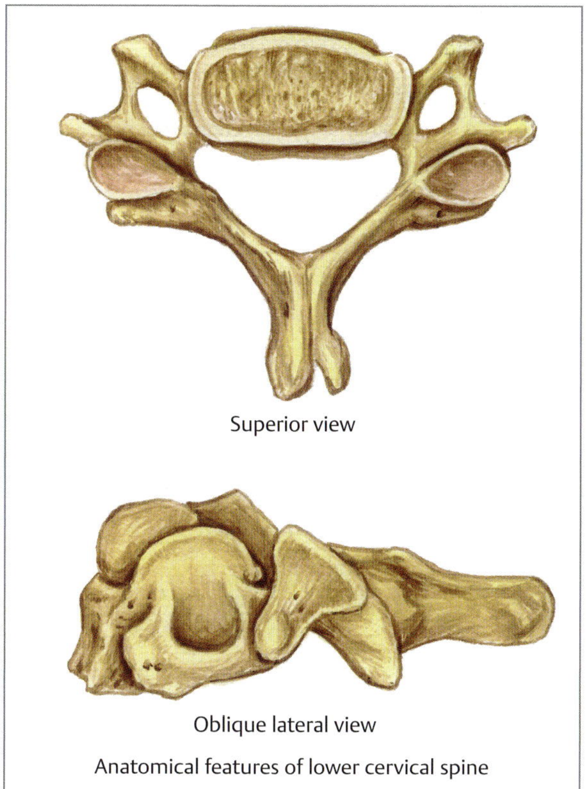

Plate 6.7

AO Classification of Cervical Spine Fractures

Based on AO classification, 51.01 (atlas) fractures can be divided into three types: A, unilateral neural arch fractures; B, burst fractures; and C, dislocation of the atlas–axis. 51.02 (axis) fractures can also be grouped into three types: A, fractures through the isthmus, including neural arch (ring) fractures or Hangman fractures; B, dens fractures; and C, fractures through the isthmus plus a dens fracture. AO classification for segments 51.03 to 51.07 (lower cervical spine) has three categories: A, compression fractures of the vertebral body; B, distraction injuries of the anterior and posterior elements; and C, rotational injuries with translation affecting the anterior and posterior elements (**Plate 6.8**).

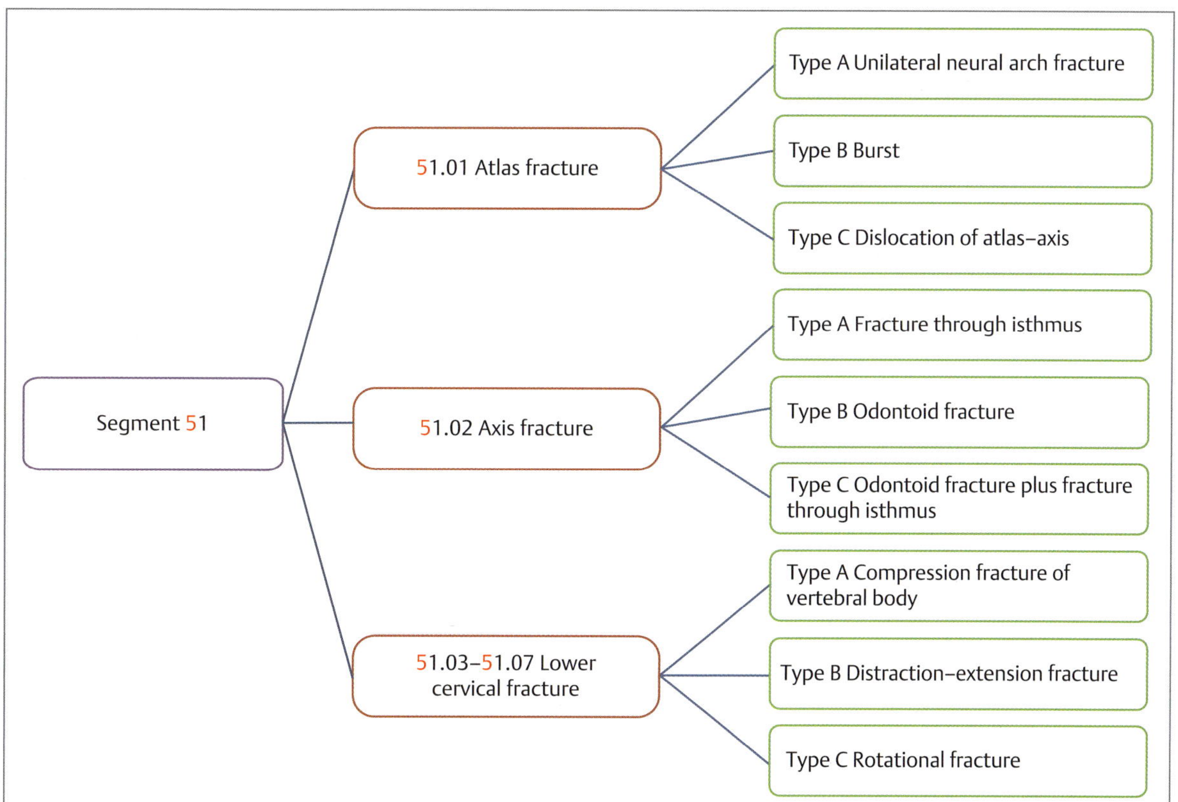

Plate 6.8

6

Clinical Epidemiologic Features of Fractures of the Upper Cervical Spine (Segment 51.01–51.02)

A total of 1,341 adult fractures of the upper cervical column were treated in 83 hospitals in China over a 2-year period from 2010 to 2011. All were reviewed and statistically studied, accounting for 2.46% of all spinal column fractures in adults. Their epidemiologic features are as follows:

- More males than females
- The highest risk age group is 41–50 years.
- The most common type of fracture among segment 51.01 (atlas) fractures is type A.
- The most common type of fracture among segment 51.02 (axis) fractures is type B.

Fractures of Segment 51.01–51.02 by Sex

Table 6.4 Sex distribution of 1,341 upper cervical spine fractures in adults

Sex	Number of fractures	Percentage (%)
Male	831	61.97
Female	510	38.03
Total	1,341	100.00

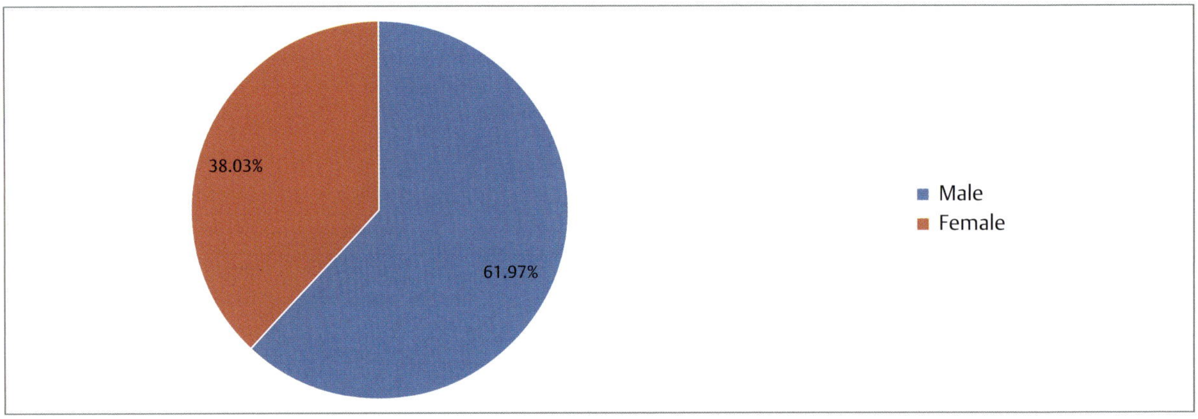

Fig. 6.4 Sex distribution of 1,341 upper cervical spine fractures in adults.

Fractures of Segment 51.01–51.02 by Age Group

Table 6.5 Age and sex distribution of 1,341 upper cervical spine fractures in adults

Age group (years)	Male	Female	Number of fractures	Percentage (%)
16–20	34	16	50	3.73
21–25	59	19	78	5.82
26–30	63	47	110	8.20
31–35	57	41	98	7.31
36–40	100	50	150	11.19
41–45	123	62	185	13.80
46–50	95	72	167	12.45
51–55	90	37	127	9.47
56–60	73	41	114	8.50
61–65	45	48	93	6.94
66–70	36	26	62	4.62
71–75	26	24	50	3.73
76–80	16	20	36	2.68
81–85	9	6	15	1.12
≥86	5	1	6	0.45
Total	831	510	1,341	100.00

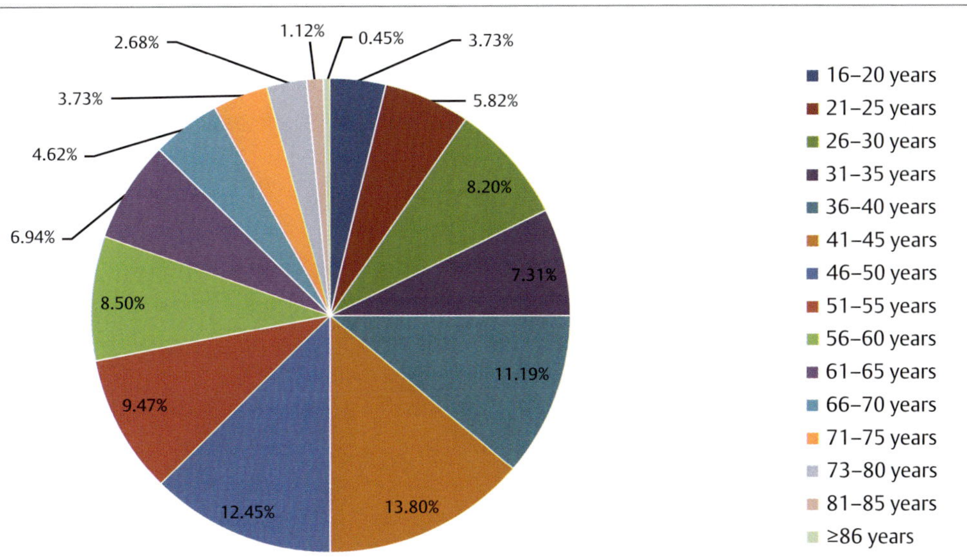

a

Fig. 6.5 **(a)** Age distribution of 1,341 upper cervical spine fractures in adults. (*Continued*)

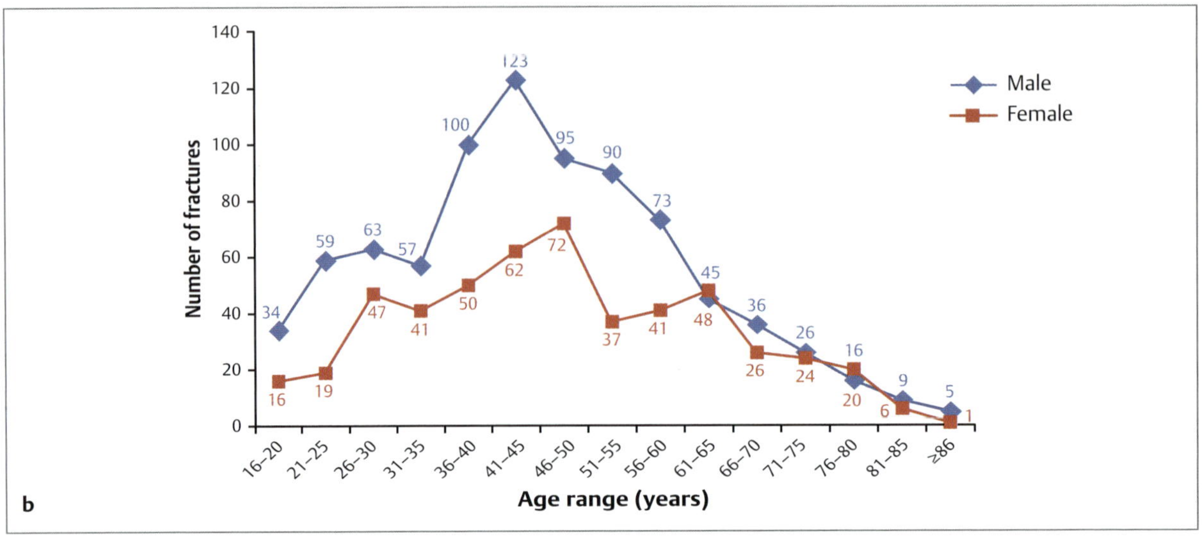

Fig. 6.5 (*continued*) **(b)** Age and sex distribution of 1,341 upper cervical spine fractures in adults.

Fractures of Segment 51.01–51.02 by Fracture Type

Segment 51.01 (Atlas) Fractures by Fracture Type

Table 6.6 Sex and fracture type distribution of 280 fractures of segment 51.01 in adults

Fracture type	Male	Female	Number of fractures	Percentage of 51.01 fractures (%)	Percentage of spine fractures (%)
51.01-A	87	53	140	50.00	0.26
51.01-B	28	20	48	17.14	0.09
51.01-C	57	35	92	32.86	0.17
Total	172	108	280	100.00	0.51

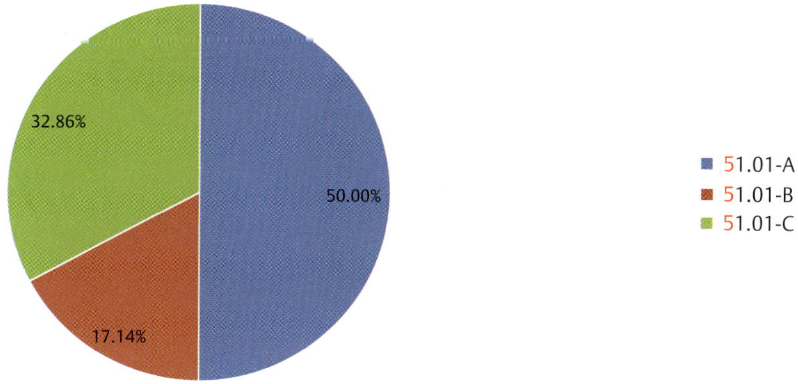

a

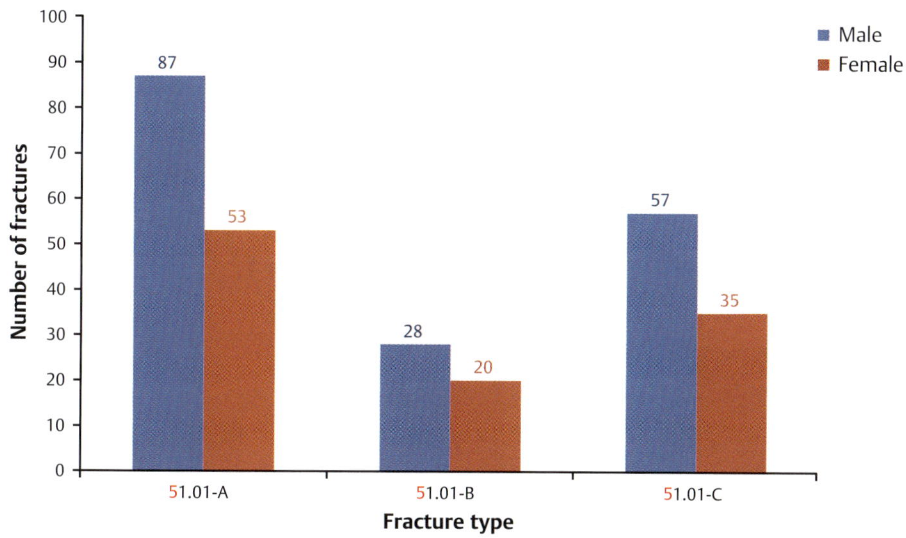

b

Fig. 6.6 **(a)** Fracture type distribution of 280 fractures of segment 51.01 in adults.
(b) Sex and fracture type distribution of 280 fractures of segment 51.01 in adults.

Segment 51.02 (Axis) Fractures by Fracture Type

Table 6.7 Sex and fracture type distribution of 1,061 fractures of segment 51.02 in adults

Fracture type	Male	Female	Number of fractures	Percentage of 51.02 fractures (%)	Percentage of spine fractures (%)
51.02-A	137	63	200	18.85	0.37
51.02-B	466	300	766	72.20	1.40
51.02-C	56	39	95	8.95	0.17
Total	659	402	1,061	100.00	1.95

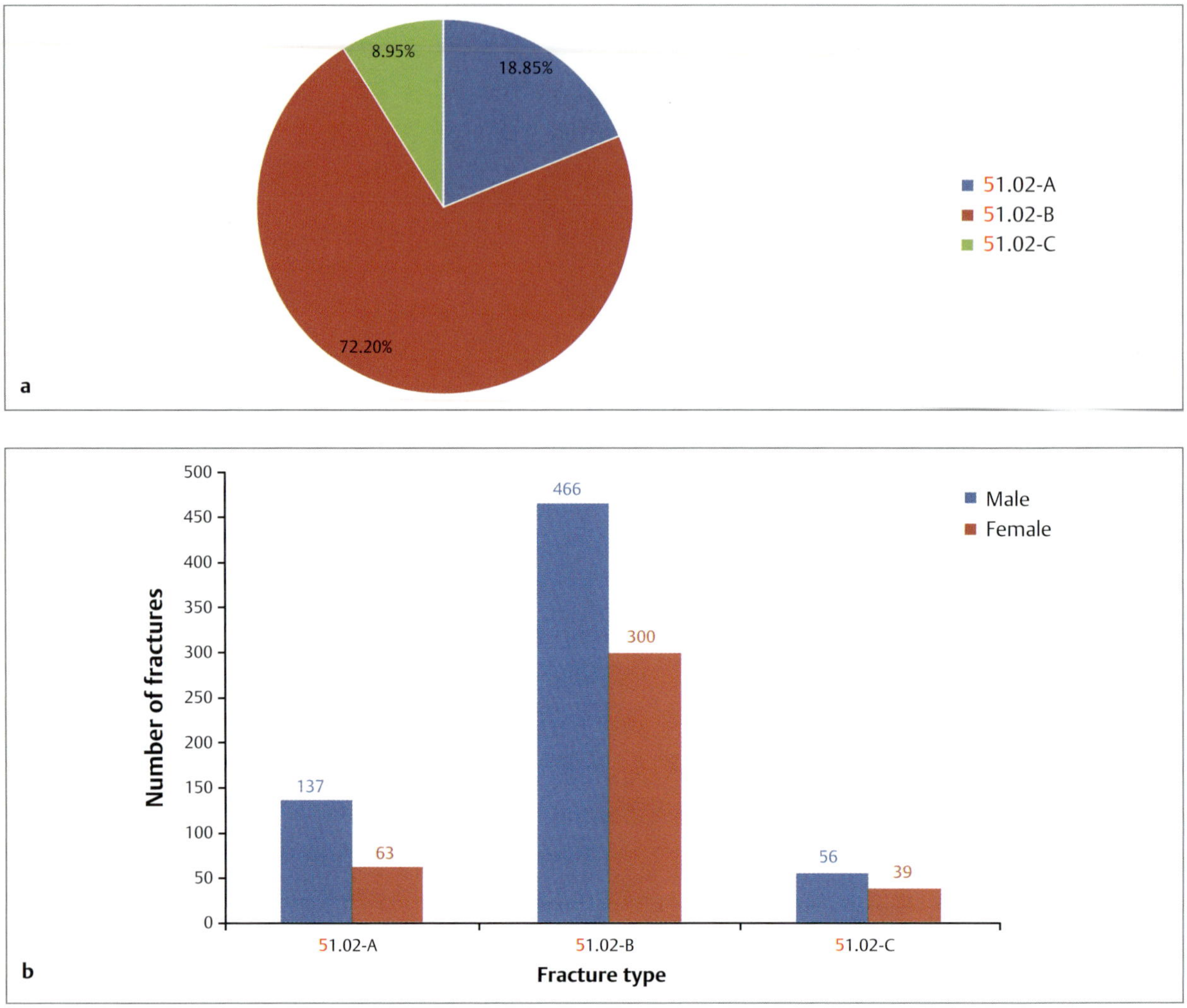

Fig. 6.7 (a) Fracture type distribution of 1,061 fractures of segment 51.02 in adults. **(b)** Sex and fracture type distribution of 1,061 fractures of segment 51.02 in adults.

Segment 51.01 (atlas) fractures

51.01-A
Unilateral neural arch fracture
140 fractures
M: 87 (62.14%)
F: 53 (37.86%)
0.04% of total adult fractures
0.26% of adult spinal column
3.86% of adult cervical column

51.01-A

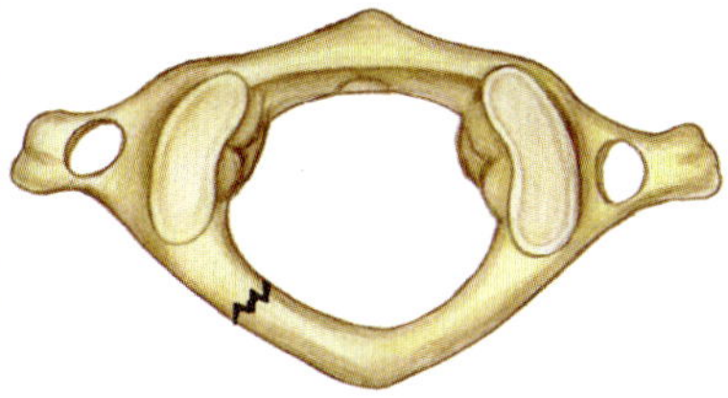

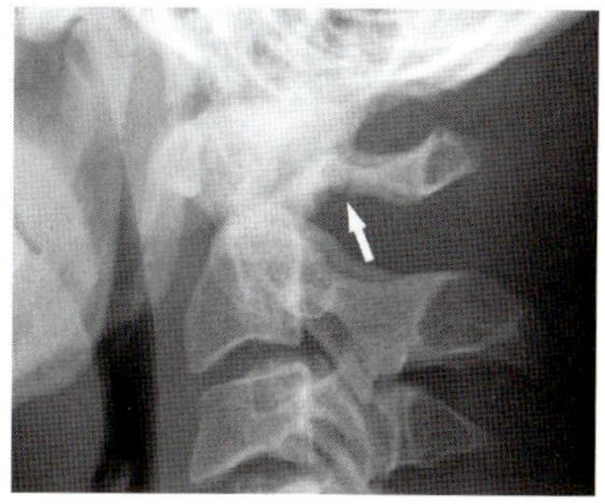

Unilateral neural arch fracture

51.01-B
Burst fracture
48 fractures
M: 28 (58.33%)
F: 20 (41.67%)
0.01% of total adult fractures
0.09% of adult spinal column
1.32% of adult cervical column

51.01-B

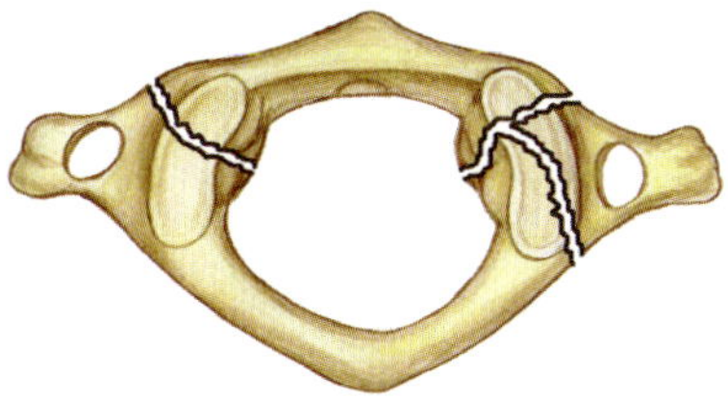

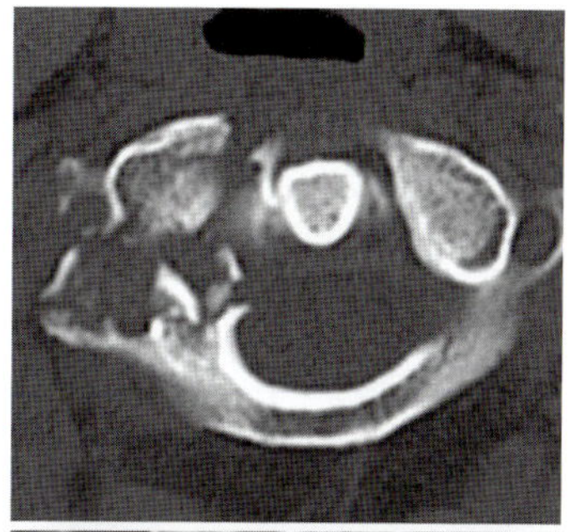

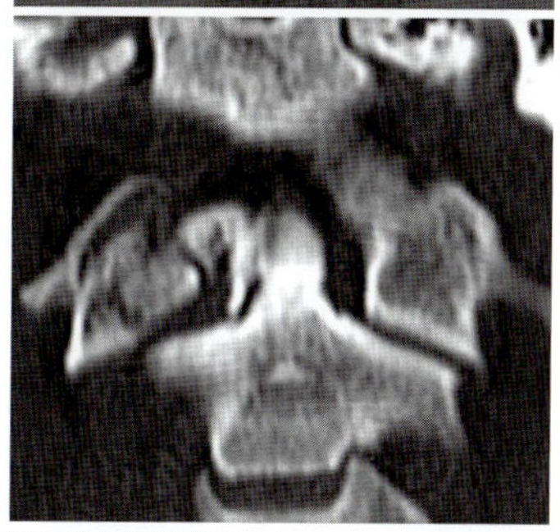

Burst fracture

51.01-C
Dislocation of atlas–axis
92 fractures
M: 57 (61.96%)
F: 35 (38.04%)
0.02% of total adult fractures
0.17% of adult spinal column
2.54% of adult cervical column

51.01-C

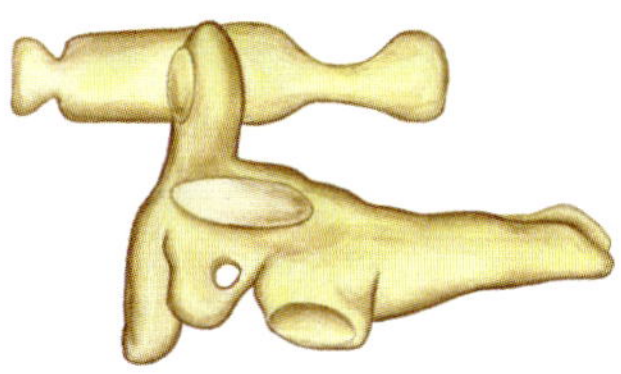

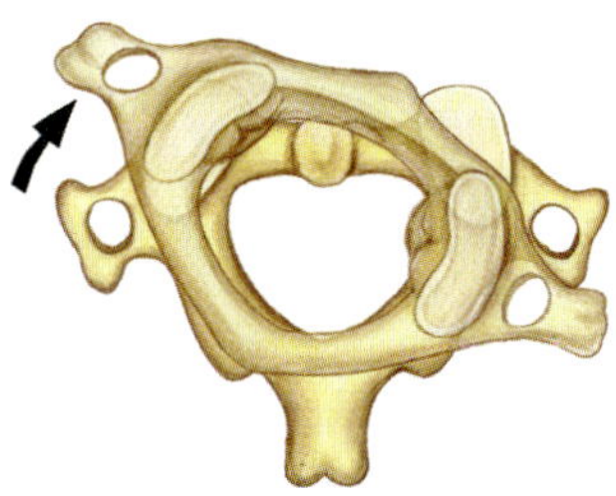

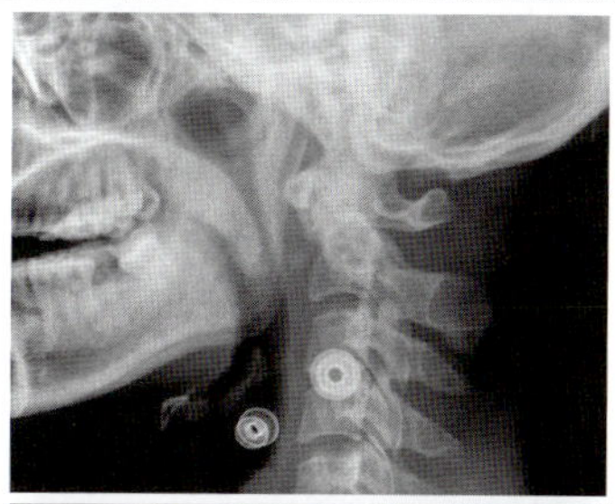

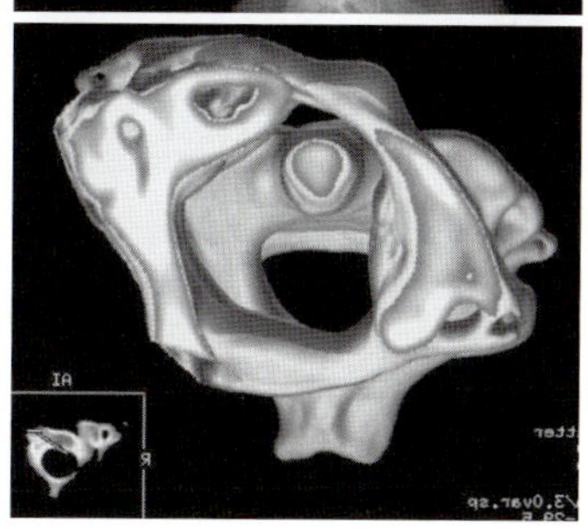

Dislocation of the atlas–axis

Segment 51.02 (axis) fracture

51.02-A
Fractures through isthmus
200 fractures
M: 137 (68.50%)
F: 63 (31.50%)
0.05% of total adult fractures
0.37% of adult spinal column
5.52% of adult cervical column

51.02-A

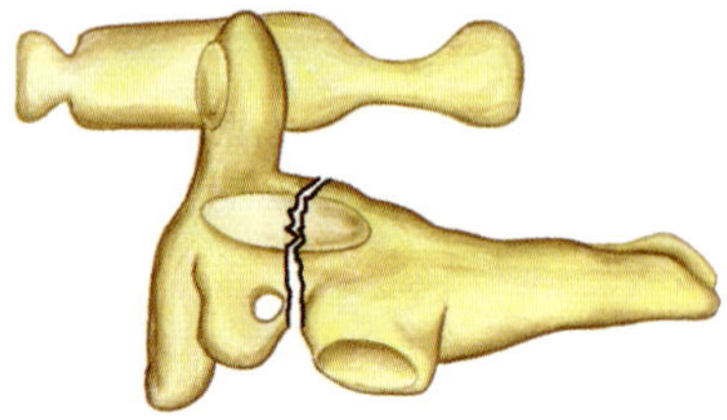

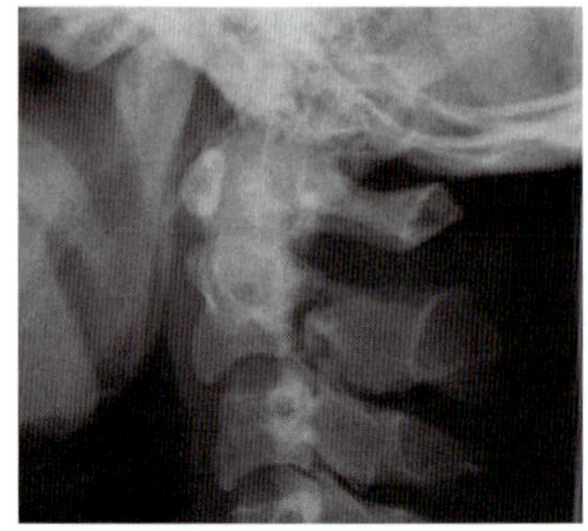

Fractures through isthmus

51.02-B
Odontoid fracture
766 fractures
M: 466 (60.84%)
F: 300 (39.16%)
0.20% of total adult fractures
1.40% of adult spinal column
21.14% of adult cervical column

51.02-B

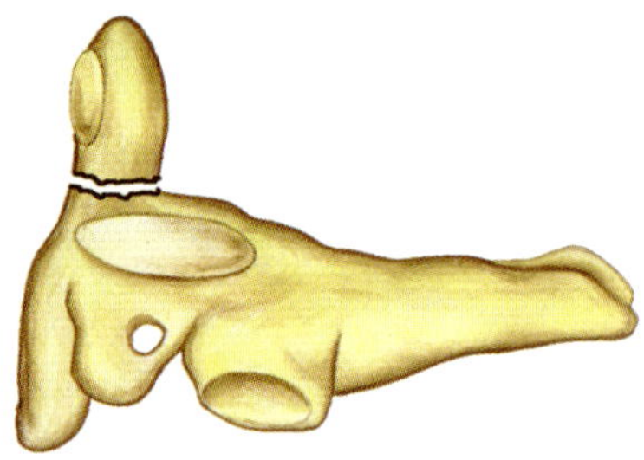

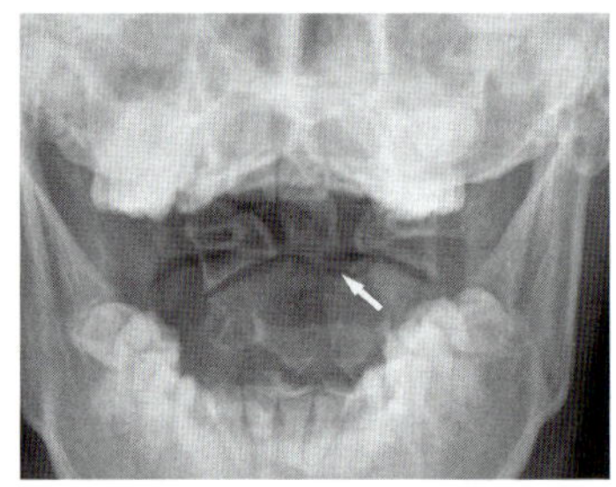

Odontoid fracture

51.02-C
Odontoid fracture plus fractures through isthmus
95 fractures
M: 56 (58.95%)
F: 39 (41.05%)
0.03% of total adult fractures
0.17% of adult spinal column
2.62% of adult cervical column

51.02-C

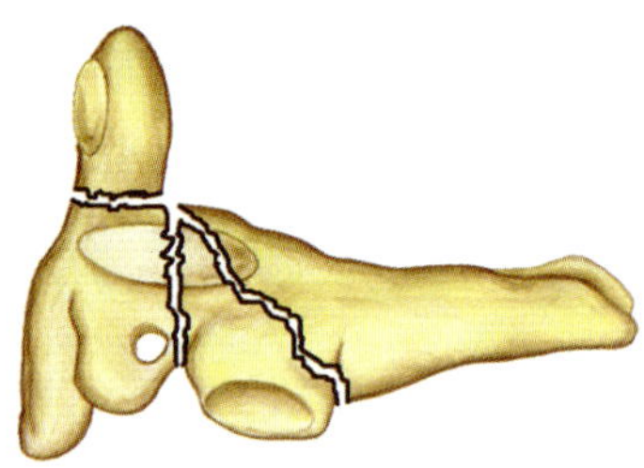

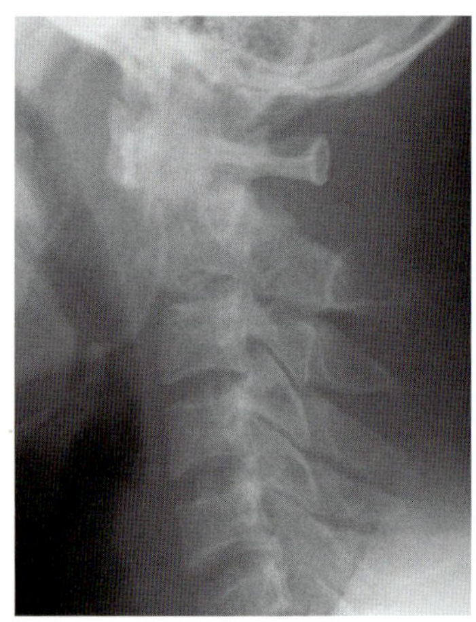

Odontoid fracture plus fractures through isthmus

Clinical Epidemiologic Features of Fractures of the Lower Cervical Spine (Segments 51.03–51.07)

A total of 2,282 adult fractures of the lower cervical column were treated in 83 hospitals in China over a 2-year period from 2010 to 2011. All were reviewed and statistically studied, accounting for 4.18% of all spinal column fractures in adults, and 0.61% of all types of fractures in adults. Their epidemiologic features are as follows:

- More males than females
- The highest risk age group is 46–50 years. The most affected male age group is 41–45 years, while females aged 51–55 years have the highest risk.
- The most common type of fracture among lower cervical spine fractures is type A—the same for both males and females.

Fractures of Segments 51.03–51.07 by Sex

Table 6.8 Sex distribution of 2,282 fractures of segments 51.03–51.07 in adults

Sex	Number of fractures	Percentage (%)
Male	1,657	72.61
Female	625	27.39
Total	2,282	100.00

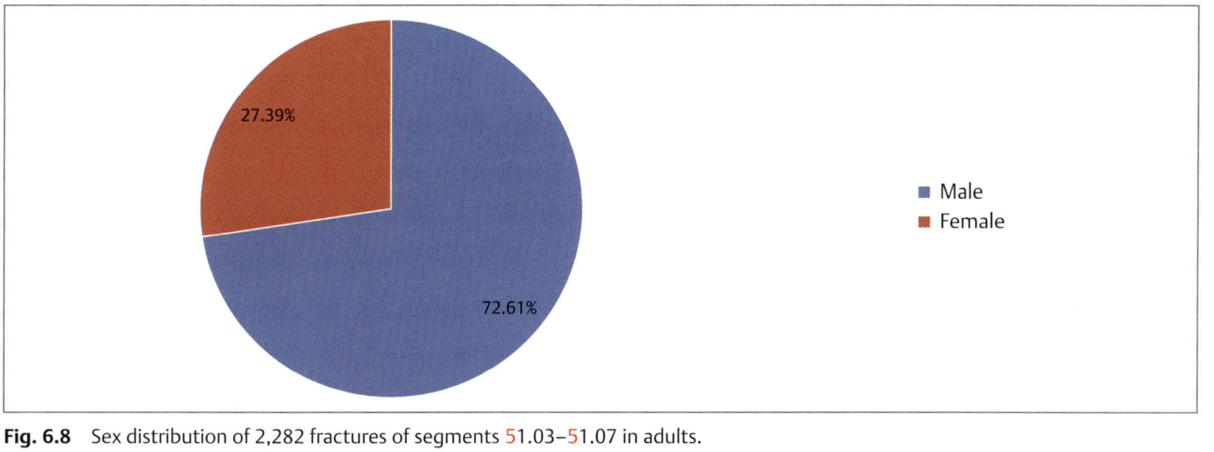

Fig. 6.8 Sex distribution of 2,282 fractures of segments 51.03–51.07 in adults.

Fractures of Segments 51.03–51.07 by Age Group

Table 6.9 Age and sex distribution of 2,282 fractures of segments 51.03–51.07 in adults

Age group (years)	Male	Female	Number of fractures	Percentage of 51.01–51.07 fractures (%)	Percentage of spine fractures (%)
16–20	46	11	57	2.50	0.10
21–25	107	26	133	5.83	0.24
26–30	137	30	167	7.32	0.31
31–35	123	35	158	6.92	0.29
36–40	193	56	249	10.91	0.46
41–45	199	76	275	12.05	0.50
46–50	197	81	278	12.18	0.51
51–55	173	87	260	11.39	0.48
56–60	183	66	249	10.91	0.46
61–65	113	62	175	7.67	0.32
66–70	70	41	111	4.86	0.20
71–75	60	26	86	3.77	0.16
76–80	37	17	54	2.37	0.10
81–85	14	7	21	0.92	0.04
≥86	5	4	9	0.39	0.02
Total	1,657	625	2,282	100.00	4.18

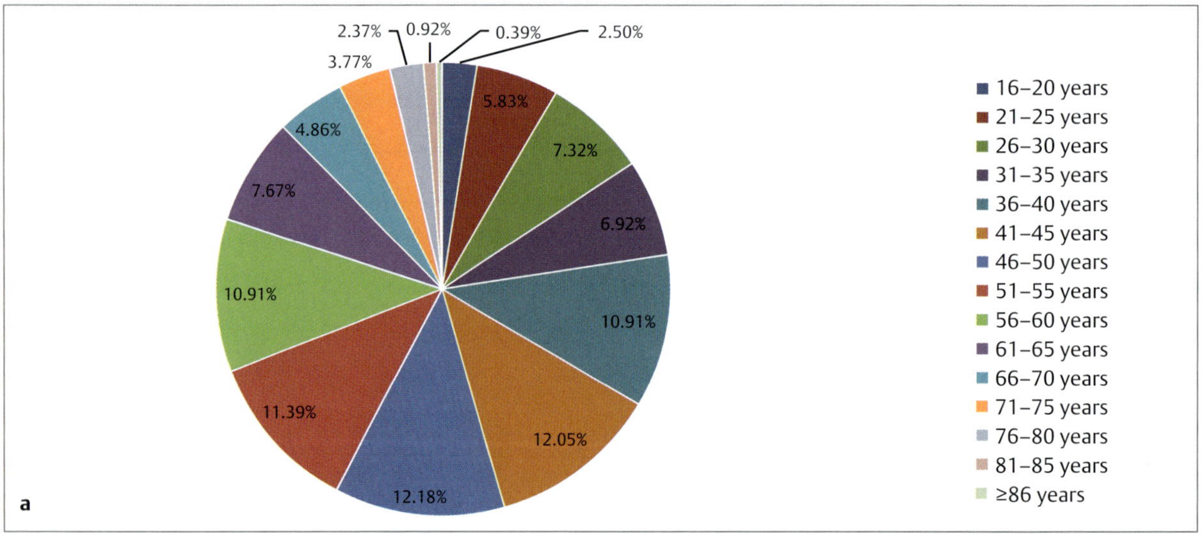

Fig. 6.9 **(a)** Age distribution of 2,282 fractures of segments 51.03–51.07 in adults.

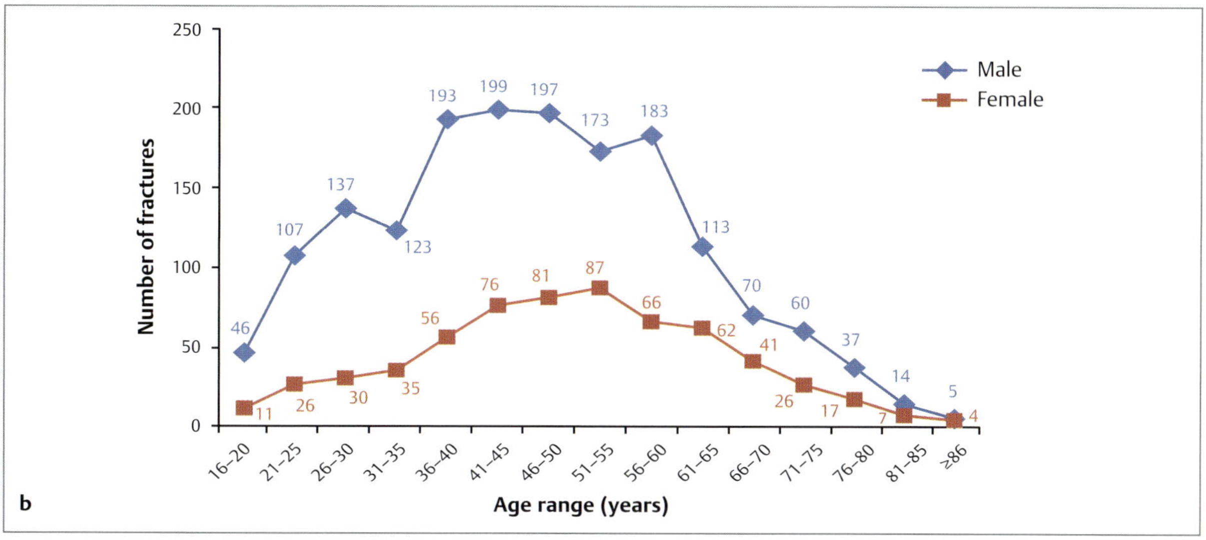

Fig. 6.9 (*continued*) **(b)** Age and sex distribution of 2,282 fractures of segments 51.03–51.07 in adults.

Fractures of Segments 51.03–51.07 by Fracture Type

Table 6.10 Sex and fracture type distribution of 2,282 fractures of segments 51.03–51.07 in adults

Fracture type	Male	Female	Number of fractures	Percentage (%)
51.03–51.07 A	996	439	1,435	62.88
51.03–51.07 B	537	152	689	30.19
51.03–51.07 C	124	34	158	6.92
Total	1,657	625	2,282	100.00

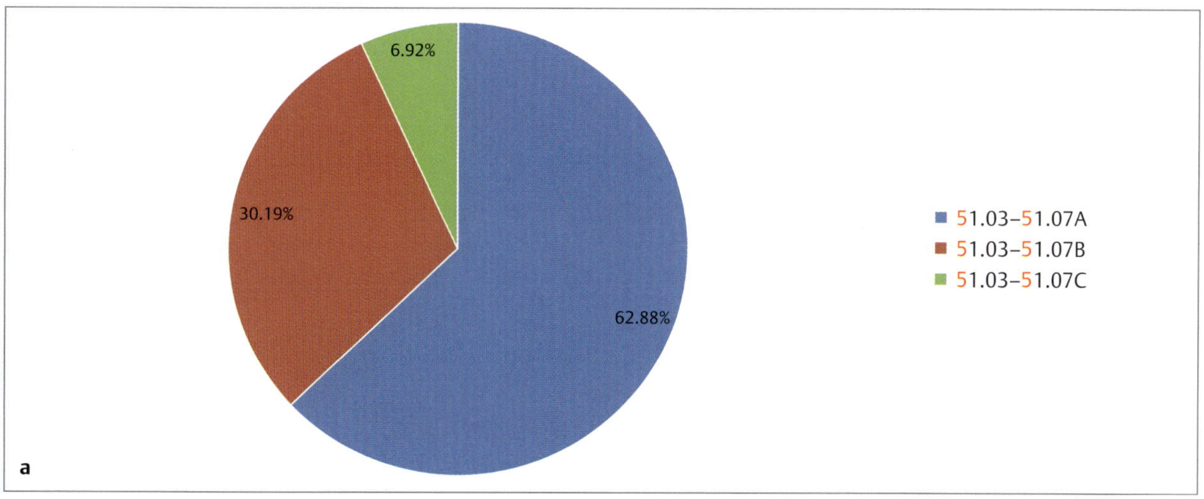

Fig. 6.10 **(a)** Fracture type distribution of 2,282 fractures of segments 51.03–51.07 in adults. (*Continued*)

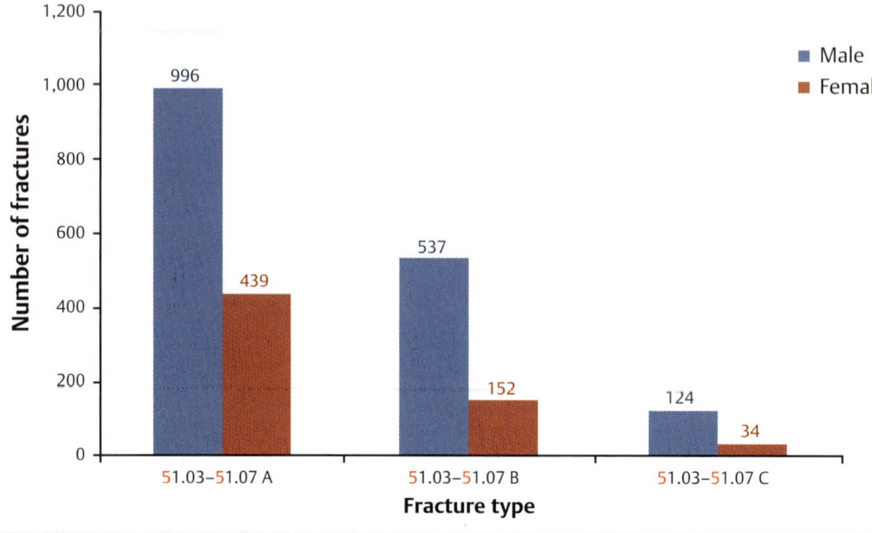

b

Fig. 6.10 (*continued*) **(b)** Sex and fracture type distribution of 2,282 fractures of segments 51.03–51.07 in adults.

51.03–51.07 Lower cervical spine fracture		
51.03–51.07- A **Compression fracture of vertebral body** 1,435 fractures M: 996 (69.41%) F: 439 (30.59%) 0. 38% of total adult fractures 2.63% of adult spine 39.61% of adult cervical	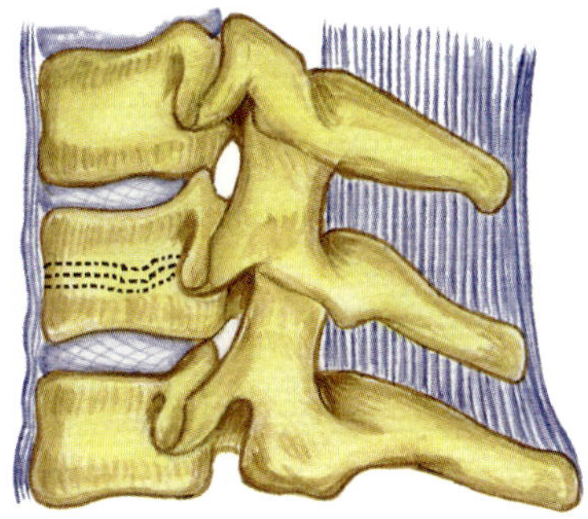 Compression fracture of vertebral body	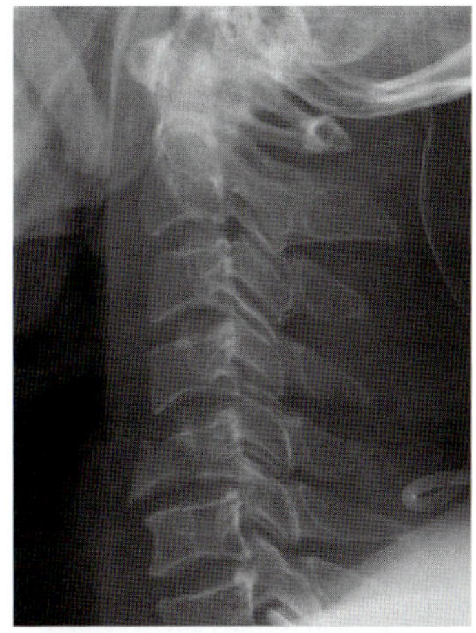
51.03–51.07- B **Distraction injuries of the anterior and posterior elements** 689 fractures M: 537 (77.94%) F: 152 (22.06%) 0.18% of total adult fractures 1.26% of adult spine 19.02% of adult cervical	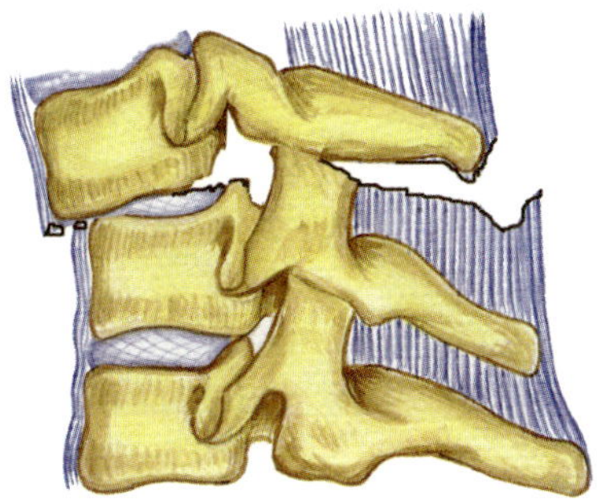 Distraction injuries of the anterior and posterior elements	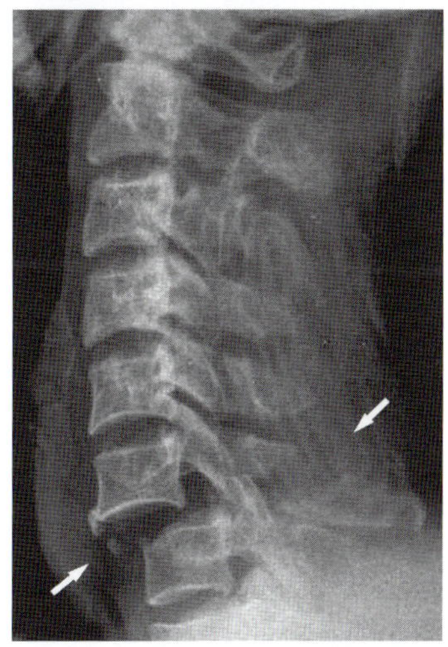
51.03–51.07- C **Rotation injuries with translation affecting the anterior and posterior elements** 158 fractures M: 124 (78.48%) F: 34 (21.52%) 0.04% of total adult fractures 0.29% of adult spine 4.36% of adult cervical	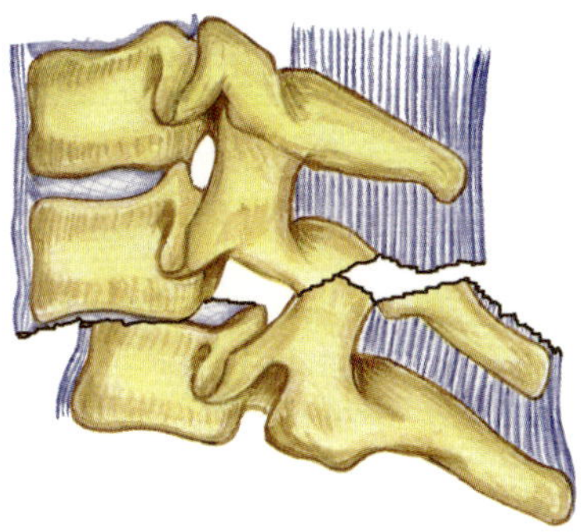 Rotation injuries with translation affecting the anterior and posterior elements	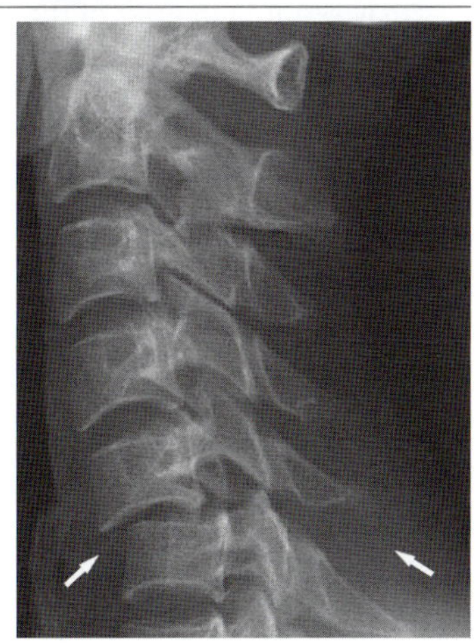

6

Injury Mechanism

The most common mechanism for cervical column fracture involves either direct or indirect force.

- *Direct force:* Less common; seen in traffic accidents, natural disasters (earthquake, tornado, etc.), or gunshot wounds, and are often associated with soft tissue damage, which should be noted.
- *Indirect force:* Relatively common; extreme forces can be transmitted to the vertebrae through the head, feet, or buttocks (e.g., when a heavy object is placed on top of the head, or when an individual falls from a significant height and lands on the feet or buttocks), and may involve fracture–dislocation of cervical bodies. Indirect forces can be grouped into five categories, according to the direction of the force applied on the vertebrae.
  - Vertical (axial) compressive forces: An example of this mechanism is when a compressive downward force is transmitted to a lower level in the cervical spine, the body of the vertebra can shatter outward, or be compressed, along with a possible fracture or disruption of the neural arch.
  - Flexion compressive forces: This mechanism can be described as the force produced when a person falls from a height and lands on the ground with their spine in flexion, due to an innate protective reflex. The resulting force, along with vertical axial compression, causes wedge compression of the cervical body. In severe cases, facet dislocation may occur.
  - Extension compressive forces: This can be explained as the force produced when a person strains to look up by bending the head back, as in athletic activities (e.g., gymnastics, diving, etc.). The effects of forceful posterior bending may result in injuries of the anterior longitudinal ligament, lamina, and facet joint.
  - Lateral compressive forces: This force is produced when a person falls from a height and lands on the ground unevenly, with the entire body leaning toward one side. The resulting force may cause unilateral compression of the cervical body, and facet injury.
  - Rotary compressive forces: This mechanism usually accompanies the injuries previously mentioned, and is relatively common. This force is produced when a person falls from a height and lands on the ground with their body in rotation.

Diagnosis

With a regular anteroposterior view (AP) of the C-spine alone it may be difficult to diagnose upper cervical fractures, which can be easily missed on X-ray images of the C-spine. A standard three-view C-spine trauma series, used for radiological screening of C-spine injuries, consists of AP, lateral, and open mouth odontoid views. An axial CT scan can be obtained for any questionable injury that cannot be visualized on plain radiographs. Based on individual injury mechanisms and clinical manifestations, if a patient presents with a suboccipital extradural hematoma radiographically, one should suspect the possibility of upper cervical fractures.

Plain radiographic evaluation is useful in detecting ligamentous injury. The normal distance between the anterior arch of the atlas and the odontoid process is 3–5 mm. A distance greater than 5 mm may indicate rupture of the transverse atlantal ligament and instability of the atlantoaxial joint. Radiographs may reveal an anterior shift of C1 on C2. The commonly used radiographic evaluations for stability of the atlantoaxial joint include: (1) AP open mouth view with 15-degree bending of the neck to the right and left; (2) lateral view of C-spine; and (3) cervical spine radiographs with the patient actively positioning their neck in extreme flexion and extension positions. If the cervical spine radiographs are inconclusive, CT scan, three-dimensional reformatting CT or MRI can be used to delineate bony details of the cervical spine, demonstrate fractures, and the extent of the bone injury.

On an AP open mouth radiograph, the medial aspect of the C1 lateral masses should be equidistant to the odontoid. The normal distance between the C1 lateral masses is ≤ 7 mm. A distance greater than 7 mm indicates a ruptured transverse ligament. If an atlantoaxial rotatory subluxation is suspected but not present on the open mouth view, the spinous process of C2 being out of alignment with the other cervical spinous process may likely indicate rotation of the atlas.

The vertebral body of C6 or C7 cannot be seen in some cases, for example, when the shoulders obscure this area in the lateral view. If this is the case, then traction on the upper extremities should be used to lower the shoulders. An improved visualization of the lower cervical spine can then be obtained. If the radiographs are still inconclusive, CT or MRI may be indicated for further investigation.

Treatment

The goal of treatment for upper cervical spine fractures is decompressing the injured spinal cord and nerve root, and providing stability to the spine. The fracture–dislocation of the cervical spine combined with a spinal cord injury requires open reduction, decompression, internal fixation, and interbody fusion with bone grafting. Generally speaking, ligamentous injury alone is usually treated nonsurgically, but with poor prognosis. However, some ligament injuries, such as an isolated unilateral alar ligament injury or a transverse ligament injury, should proceed with surgical intervention if conservative methods fail.

Nonsurgical treatments include: a semirigid collar, casting, skeletal traction, and Halo external fixation. The duration of the fixation is usually 2–4 months, depending on the reduction outcome with proper radiographic evidence.

Surgical treatment is indicated if conservative measures fail. The available internal fixation techniques include: odontoid screw fixation, C2–C3 anterior decompression of vertebral bodies and fusion, Gallie fusion, Brooks and Jenkins fusion for atlantoaxial arthrodesis, C1–C2 fusion with screw fixation, occipital cervical fusion, etc.

Usually, patients who sustain cervical spine injuries do not require further surgical intervention after treatment with nonsurgical methods (e.g., skeletal traction) if he or she has good spine stability and is without symptoms and signs of spinal cord or nerve root compression. The average healing time is 6–12 weeks with conservative treatment. If the clinical outcome is not satisfactory after the traction or external fixation is removed, surgical treatment should then be considered.

The primary indications for surgical intervention in cervical spine fracture include: fracture-dislocation of the cervical spine (malalignment of the spine), with neurologic deficits (evidence of spinal cord and nerve root compression); progressive neurologic deterioration (suggestive of persistent compression from bony or disk fragments); and an unstable fracture in the lower cervical spine. Neurologic deficits due to spinal cord or nerve root compression usually require surgical intervention for decompression. Patients with multiple injuries should have emergency surgery involving open reduction and internal fixation as soon as the patient's medical condition allows. For paralyzed patients, elective surgery is usually a better option than emergent surgery. An anterior or posterior approach can be applied depending on the fracture pattern. Available surgical methods include: anterior or posterior cervical decompression and fusion, posterior wiring fixation (including Bohlman's method, facet wiring, facet and spinous process wiring technique), lateral mass screw fixation, pedicle screw fixation, etc.

Further Classification of Cervical Spine Fractures

Anderson Classification of Odontoid Fractures

Anderson classified fractures of the odontoid process into three types:

- *Type I*: oblique avulsion fracture of the tip of the dens.
- *Type II*: fracture through the base of the odontoid process. Blood supply is often compromised in this type and associated with a high rate of nonunion fractures.
- *Type III*: fracture extends into the vertebral body of C2.

Most dens fractures can be identified on plain radiographs, except a type II fracture, which is easily missed on radiographs because the convex shape of the superior facet obscures this region. CT scanning with thick cuts can also miss a type II injury. Therefore, thin-section CT with sagittal reformation may be necessary to identify this type of odontoid fracture.

Hangman's Fracture

The Hangman's fracture consists of bilateral pedicle or pars fractures involving the vertebral body of C2. Associated with this fracture is anterior subluxation or dislocation of the C2 vertebral body. The mechanism of the injury is forcible hypertension of the head, which would occur during judicial hanging, thus this type of fracture was given the term Hangman's fracture. With this type of injury, spondylolisthesis of the axis is usually seen on a lateral view of the cervical spine, therefore the Hangman's fracture is also called traumatic spondylolisthesis of the axis.

Levine-Edwards Classification of Hangman's Fracture

- *Type I*: minimally displaced with no angulation; translation < 3 mm; stable.
- *Type II*: significant angulation at C2–C3; translation ≥ 3 mm; unstable; C2–C3 disk disrupted. Subclassified into flexion, extension, and listhetic types.
- *Type IIA*: avulsion of entire C2–C3 intervertebral disk in flexion, anterior longitudinal ligament intact. Severe angulation. No translation; unstable due to flexion-distraction injury.
- *Type III*: unilateral or bilateral anterior facet dislocation of C2 on C3, due to extension injury; severe angulation; unstable.

Allen-Ferguson Classification of Lower Cervical Spine Fractures

Allen described lower cervical injuries as six types of fractures: compressive flexion, vertical compression, distractive flexion, compressive extension, distractive extension, and lateral flexion. They are further classified into several subtypes according to their stage of progressive injury.

6

Anderson classification of odontoid fractures

Type I **Oblique avulsion fracture of tip of dens** 132 fractures M: 73 (55.30%) F: 59 (44.70%) 0.04% of total adult fractures 0.24% of adult spine 15.33% of adult odontoid	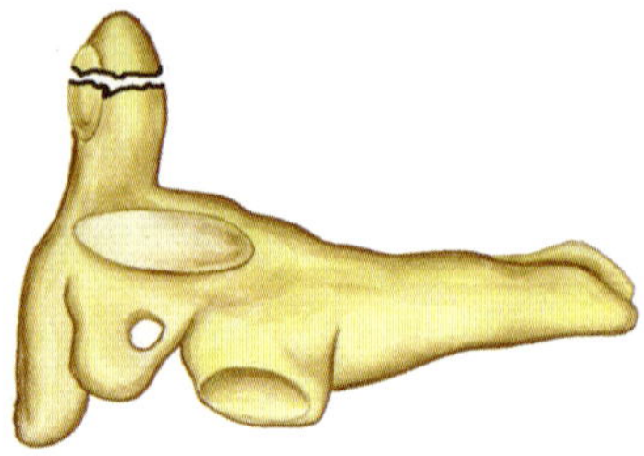 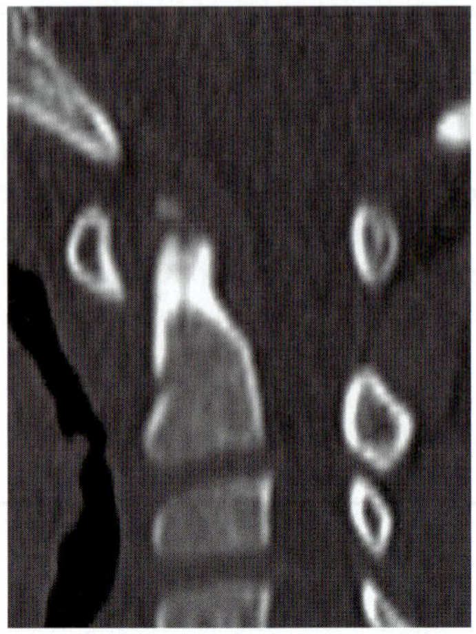 **Type I**
Type II **Fracture through the base of the odontoid process** 488 fractures M: 300 (61.48%) F: 188 (38.52%) 0.13% of total adult fractures 0.89% of adult spine 56.68% of adult odontoid	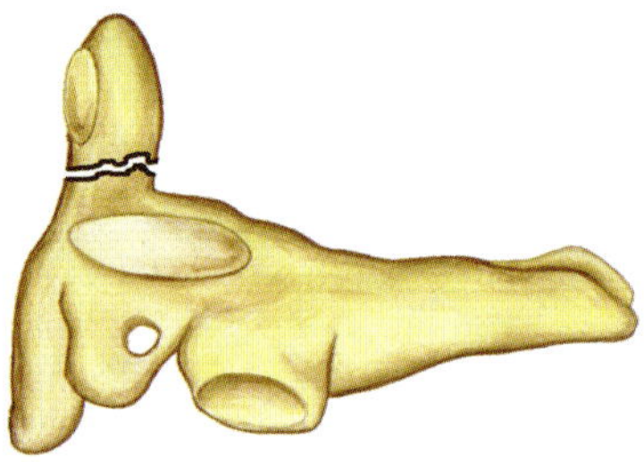 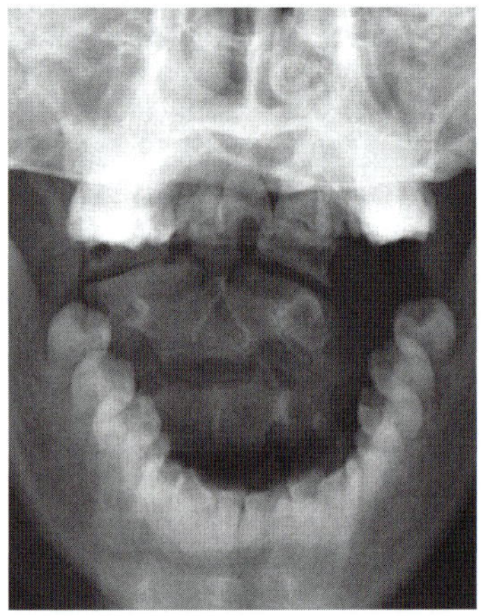 **Type II**
Type III **Fracture extends into the vertebral body of C2** 241 fractures M: 149 (61.83%) F: 92 (38.17%) 0.06% of total adult fractures 0.44% of adult spine 27.99% of adult odontoid	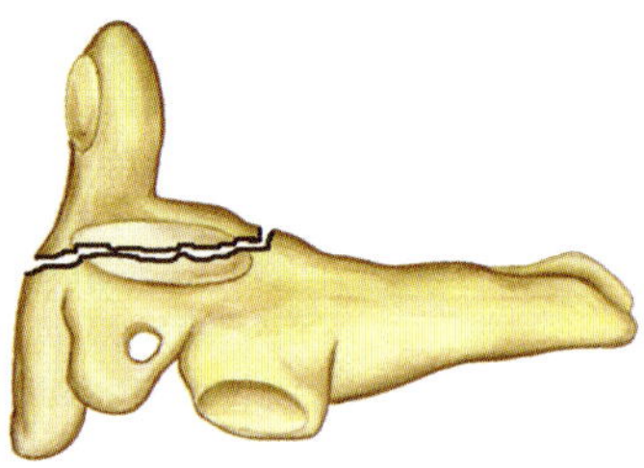 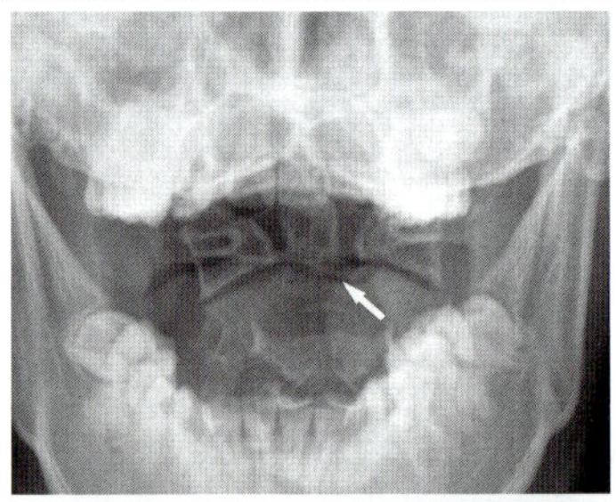 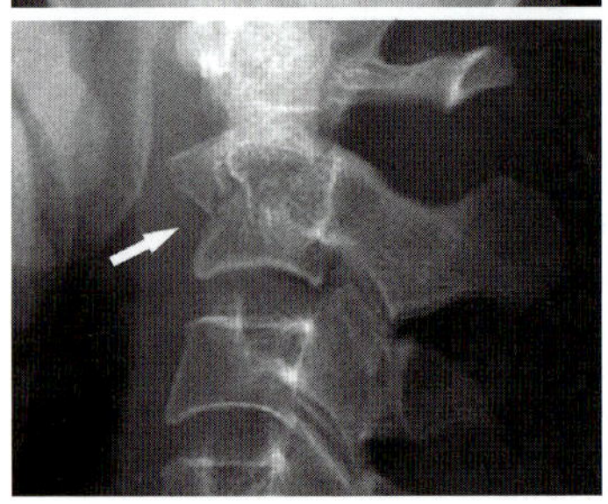 **Type III**

Levine-Edwards classification of Hangman's fracture

Type I
Minimally displaced with no angulation; translation < 3 mm; stable
207 fracture
M: 147 (71.01%)
F: 60 (28.99%)
0.06% of total adult fractures
0.38% of adult spine
70.17% of adult hangman's fracture

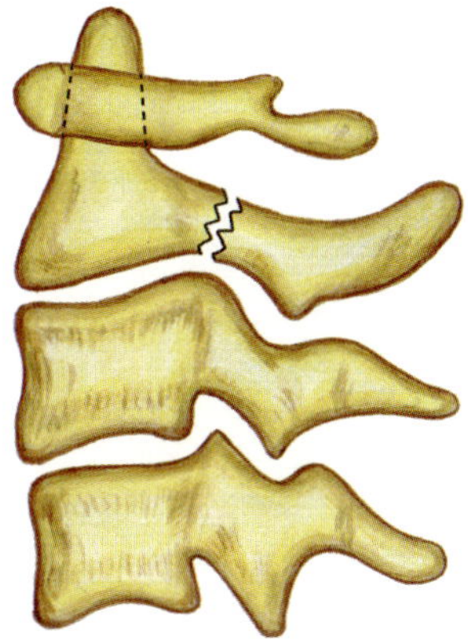

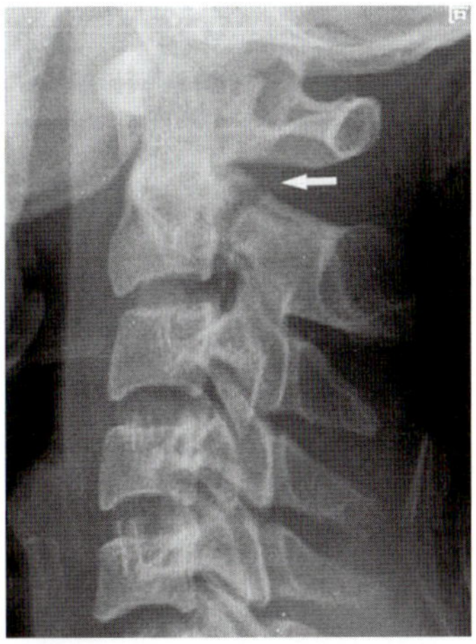

Type II
Significant angulation at C2–C3; translation ≥ 3 mm; unstable; C2–C3 disk disrupted; subclassified into flexion, extension, and listhetic types
44 fractures
M: 29 (65.91%)
F: 15 (34.09%)
0.01% of total adult fractures
0.08% of adult spine
14.92% of adult hangman's fracture

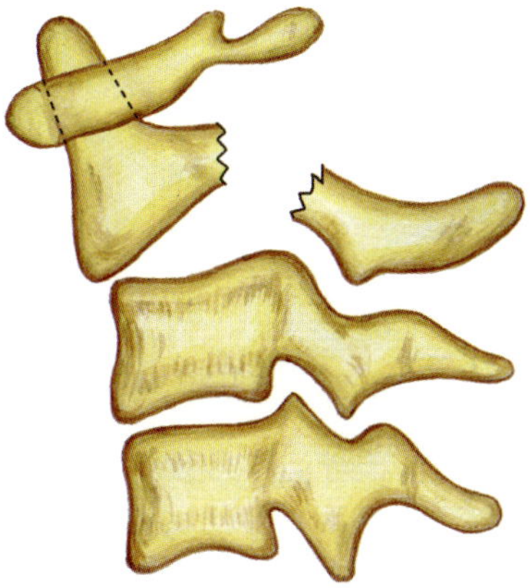

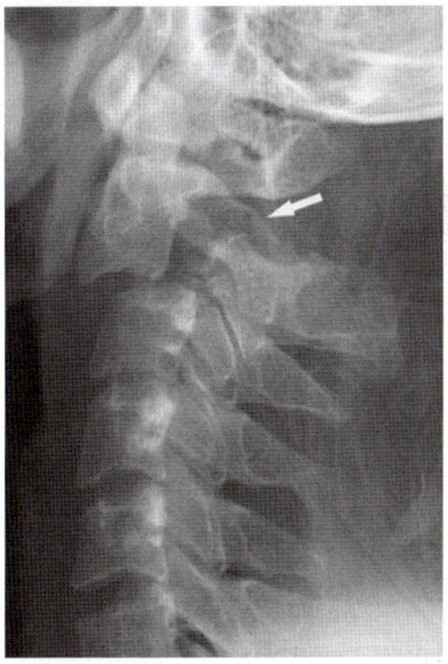

Type IIA
Avulsion of entire C2–C3 intervertebral disk in flexion, anterior longitudinal ligament intact; severe angulation; no translation; unstable due to flexion-distraction injury
9 fractures
M: 6 (66.67%)
F: 3 (33.33%)
0.002% of total adult fractures
0.02% of adult spine
3.05% of adult hangman's fracture

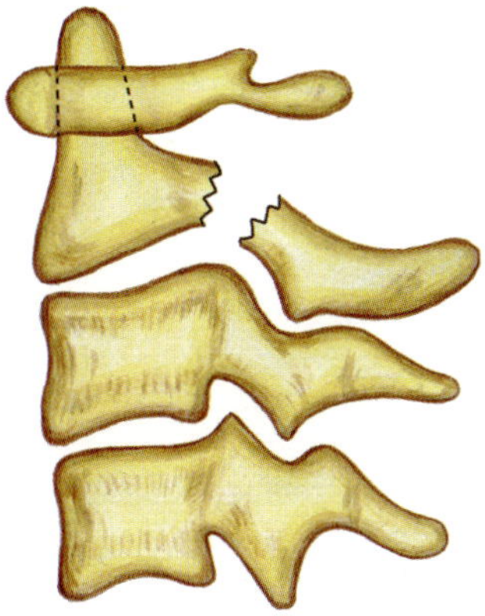

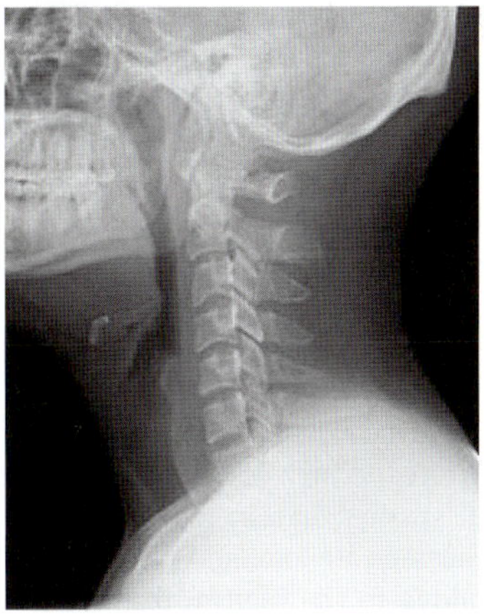

6

Levine-Edwards classification of Hangman's fracture	
Type III **Unilateral or bilateral anterior facet dislocation of C2 on C3, due to extension injury, severe angulation, unstable** 35 fractures M: 28 (80%) F: 7 (20%) 0.01% of total adult fractures 0.06% of adult spine 11.86% of adult hangman's fracture	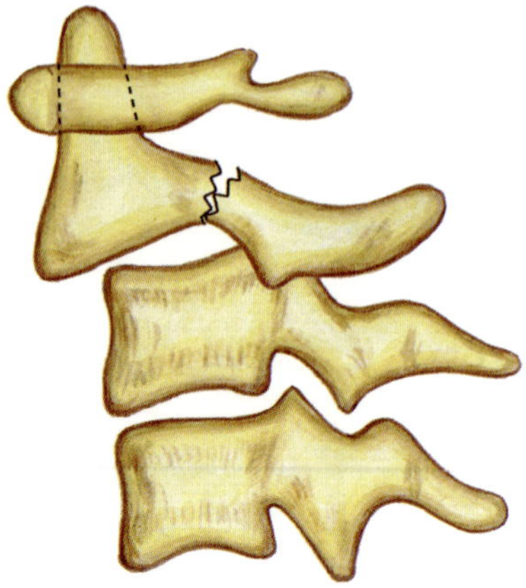 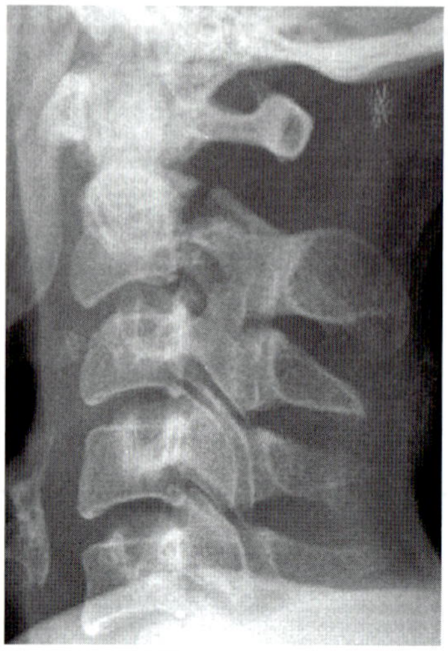

Thoracolumbar Fractures (Segments 52 and 53)

Anatomical Features

The thoracic spine is made up of 12 vertebrae. Each thoracic vertebra increases slightly in size from the neck down and each connects to an individual rib via a costovertebral joint on either side of spine. The costovertebral joint has two components that articulate with the vertebral column: the head of the ribs and the costotransverse joint. The head of each rib articulates with the superior facet of the same vertebral body and the inferior facet of the superior vertebra. The spinal canal is round in shape and relatively small. The pedicle bone is short but thin. The thoracic facet joints are oriented in a nearly coronal plane, which facilitates greater rotational movement, and are less likely to be displaced. The spinous processes are thin but long, and directed obliquely downward. These processes overlap from the fifth to the eighth vertebra. The transverse processes are thick and strong, directed obliquely backward and lateralward.

The lumbar vertebral body is large and wider from side to side than from front to back. The vertebral foramen within the arch is larger than in the thoracic vertebrae, but smaller than in the cervical vertebrae. The transverse processes are long and slender. The lumbar facet joints are oblique in the sagittal plane, and the superior facets are oriented medially with respect to the inferior facets of the superior vertebrae. The spinous processes are thick and broad, and project backward. There are wide intervals between each lumbar spinous process, which is helpful in the event of a lumbar puncture (**Plate 6.9**).

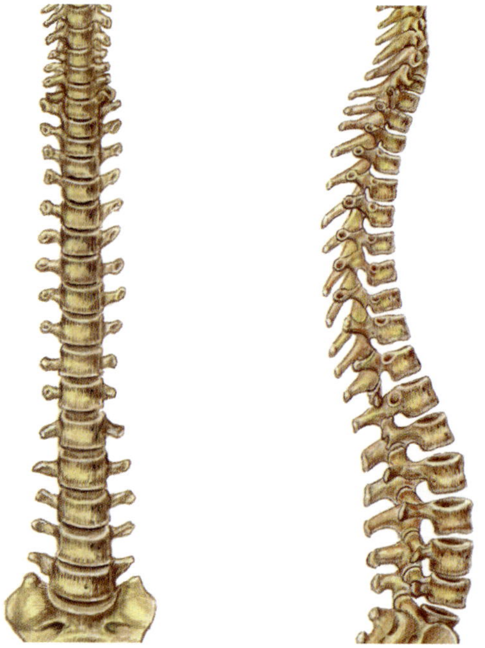

Anatomical illustration of thoracolumbar spine

Plate 6.9

AO Classification of Thoracolumbar Spine Fractures

Based on AO classification, the thoracic spine and lumbar spine are assigned the numbers 52 and 53, respectively. Thoracolumbar spine fractures are classified into three types: A, compression; B, flexion-distraction; and C, rotation (**Plate 6.10**).

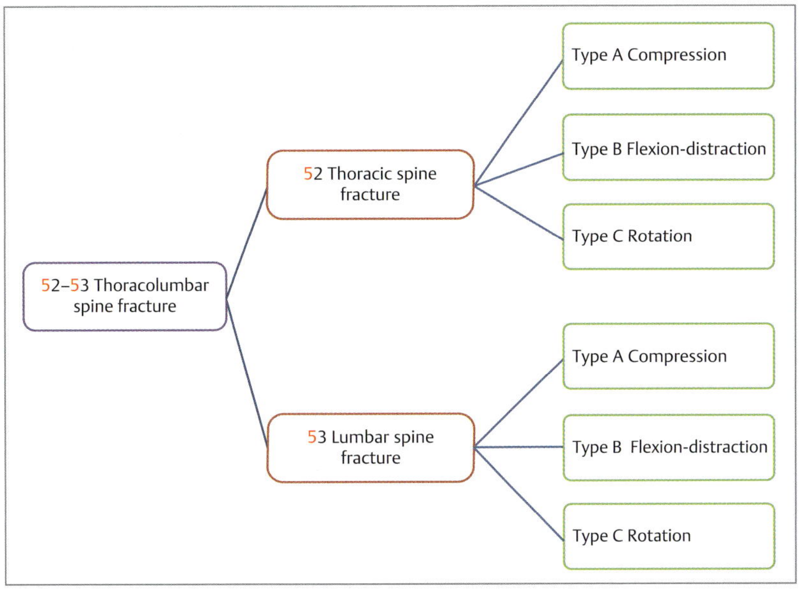

Plate 6.10

Clinical Epidemiologic Features of Fractures of the Thoracolumbar Spine (Segments 52 and 53)

A total of 50,910 adult thoracolumbar spine fractures were treated in 83 hospitals in China over a 2-year period from 2010 to 2011. All cases were reviewed and statistically studied; the fractures accounted for 93.36% of all adult spinal fractures. Their epidemiologic features are as follows:

- More females than males
- The highest risk age group is 56–60 years. The most affected male age group is 41–45 years, while females aged 71–75 have the highest risk.
- The most common type of fracture among thoracolumbar spine fractures is type A—the same for both males and females.
- The most common fracture group is group A1—the same for both males and females.

Fractures of Segment 52 and 53 by Sex

Table 6.11 Sex distribution of 50,910 fractures of segments 52 and 53 in adults

Sex	Number of fractures	Percentage (%)
Male	24,978	49.06
Female	25,932	50.94
Total	50,910	100.00

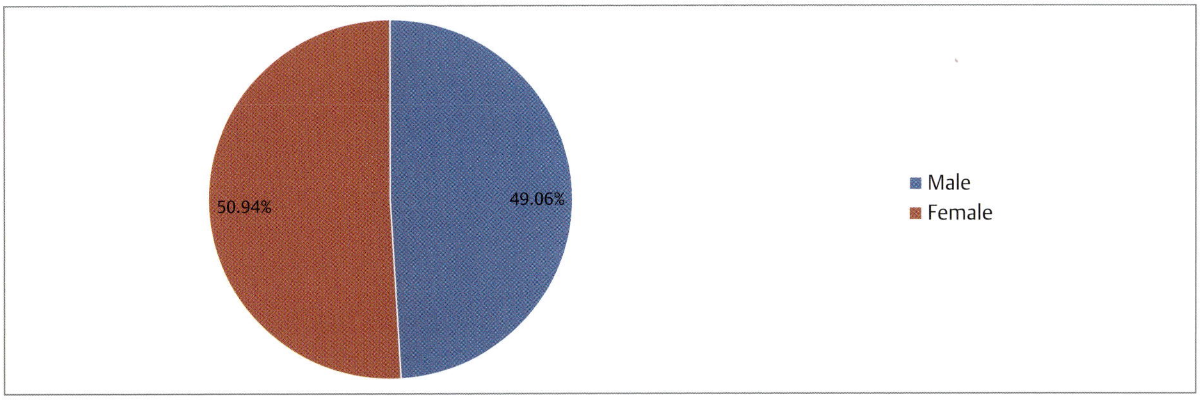

Fig. 6.11 Sex distribution of 50,910 fractures of segments 52 and 53 in adults.

6

Fractures of Segments 52 and 53 by Age Group

Table 6.12 Age and sex distribution of 50,910 fractures of segments 52 and 53 in adults

Age group (years)	Male	Female	Number of fractures	Percentage (%)
16–20	749	321	1,070	2.10
21–25	1,312	433	1,745	3.43
26–30	1,413	510	1,923	3.78
31–35	1,539	616	2,155	4.23
36–40	2,378	1,004	3,382	6.64
41–45	2,769	1,261	4,030	7.92
46–50	2,705	1,612	4,317	8.48
51–55	2,316	2,027	4,343	8.53
56–60	2,583	3,306	5,889	11.57
61–65	1,796	3,143	4,939	9.70
66–70	1,440	3,153	4,593	9.02
71–75	1,471	3,429	4,900	9.62
76–80	1,273	2,913	4,186	8.22
81–85	786	1,518	2,304	4.53
≥86	448	686	1,134	2.23
Total	24,978	25,932	50,910	100.00

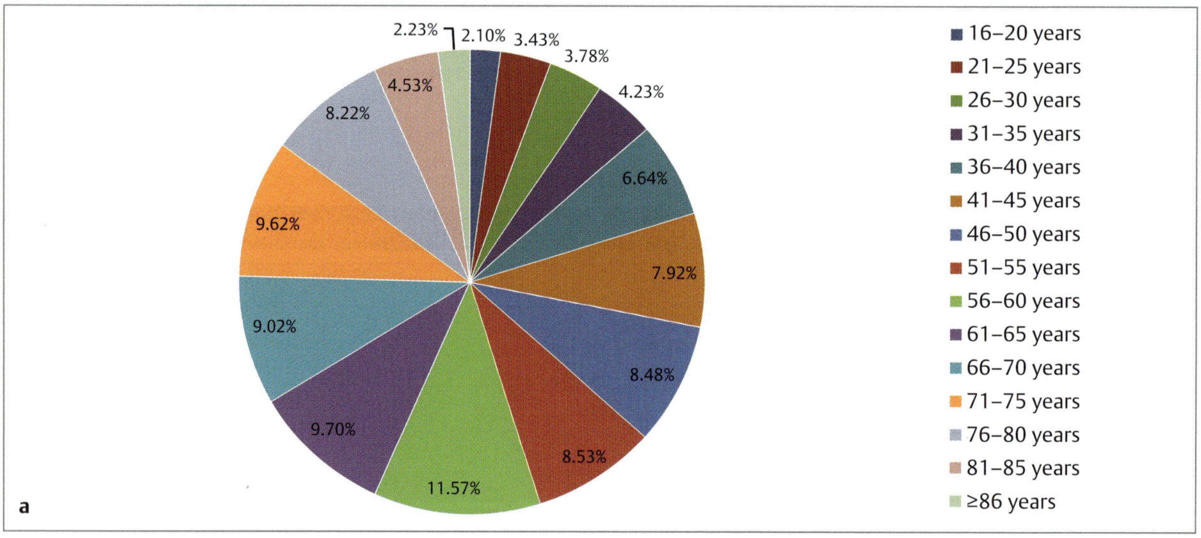

Fig. 6.12 **(a)** Age distribution of 50,910 fractures of segments 52 and 53 in adults.

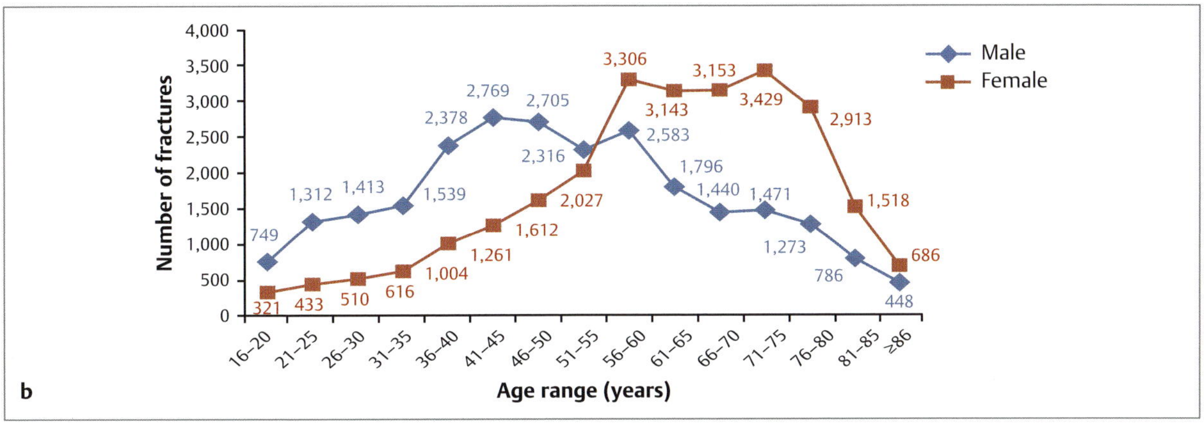

Fig. 6.12 (*continued*) **(b)** Age and sex distribution of 50,910 fractures of segments 52 and 53 in adults.

Fractures of Segments 52 and 53 by Fracture Type Based on AO Classification

Table 6.13 Sex and fracture type distribution of 50,910 fractures of segments 52 and 53 in adults

Fracture type	Male	Female	Number of fractures	Percentage (%)
52–53 A	22,668	23,883	46,551	91.44
52–53 B	1,663	1,651	3,314	6.51
52–53 C	647	398	1,045	2.05
Total	24,978	25,932	50,910	100.00

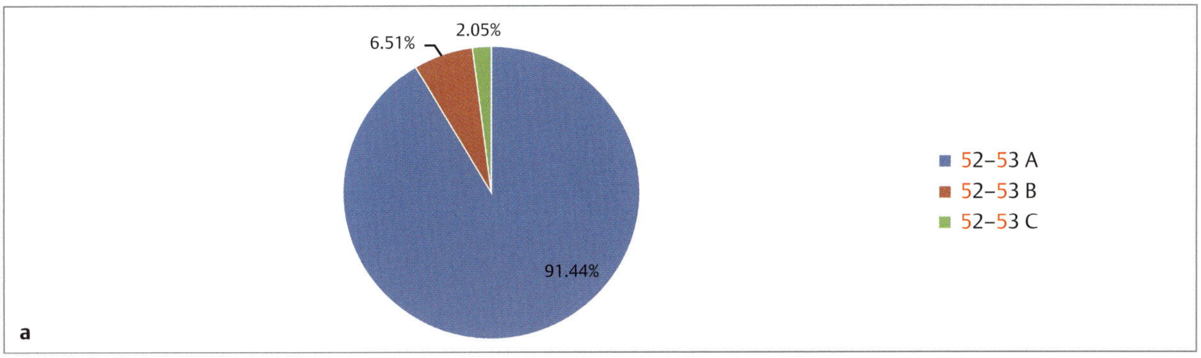

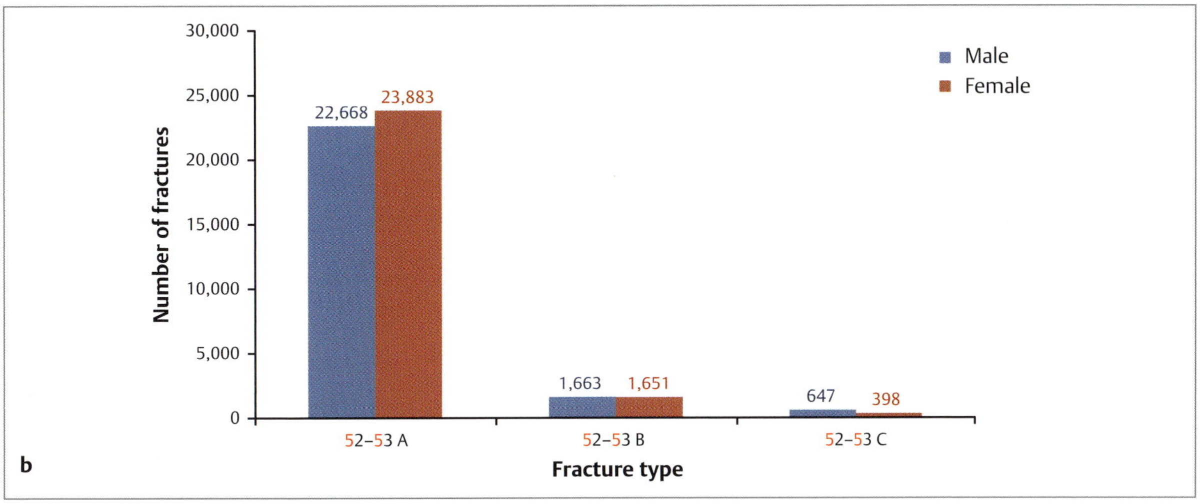

Fig. 6.13 **(a)** Fracture type distribution of 50,910 fractures of segments 52 and 53 in adults.
(b) Sex and fracture type distribution of 50,910 fractures of segments 52 and 53 in adults.

6

Fractures of Segments 52 and 53 by Fracture Group Based on AO Classification

Table 6.14 Sex and fracture group distribution of 50,910 fractures of segments 52 and 53 in adults

Fracture group	Male	Female	Number of fractures	Percentage (%)
A1	16,984	17,100	34,084	66.95
A2	1,988	1,776	3,764	7.39
A3	3,696	5,007	8,703	17.09
B1	900	996	1,896	3.72
B2	560	415	975	1.92
B3	203	240	443	0.87
C1	348	261	609	1.20
C2	222	102	324	0.64
C3	77	35	112	0.22
Total	24,978	25,932	50,910	100.00

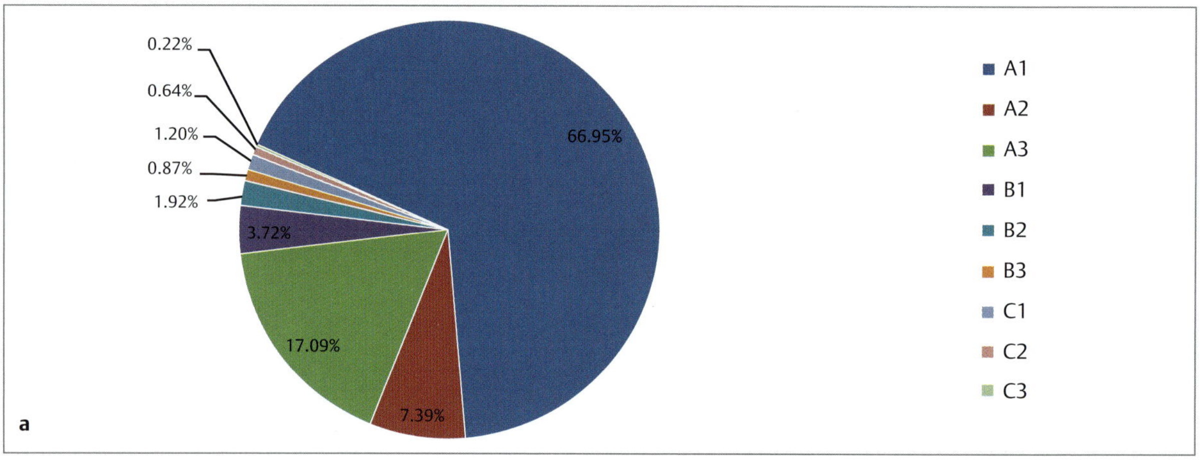

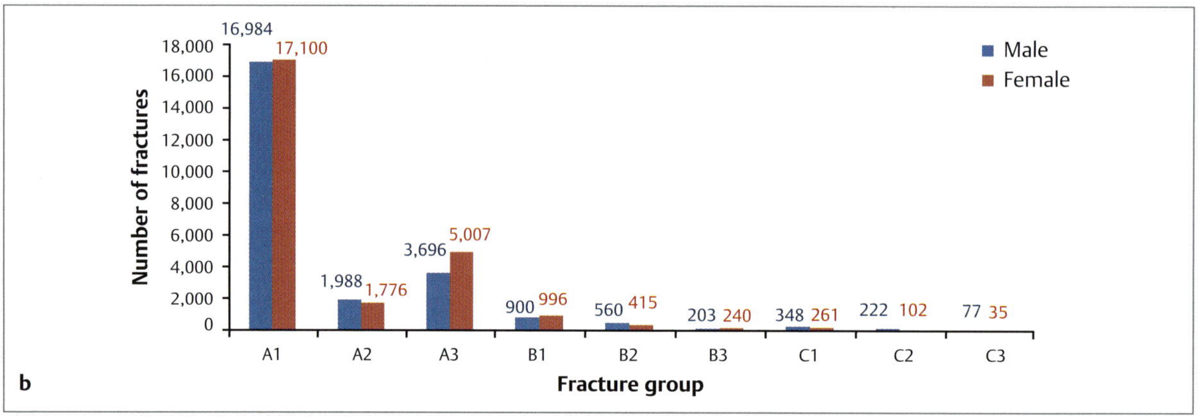

Fig. 6.14 **(a)** Fracture type distribution of 50,910 fractures of segments 52 and 53 in adults.
(b) Sex and fracture type distribution of 50,910 fractures of segments 52 and 53 in adults.

52–53-A Thoracolumbar spine, vertebral body compression

52–53-A1
Impaction fracture
34,084 fractures
M: 16,984 (49.83%)
F: 17,100 (50.17%)
9.1% of total adult fractures
62.5% of adult spine
66.95% of adult thoracolumbar spine

52–53-A1

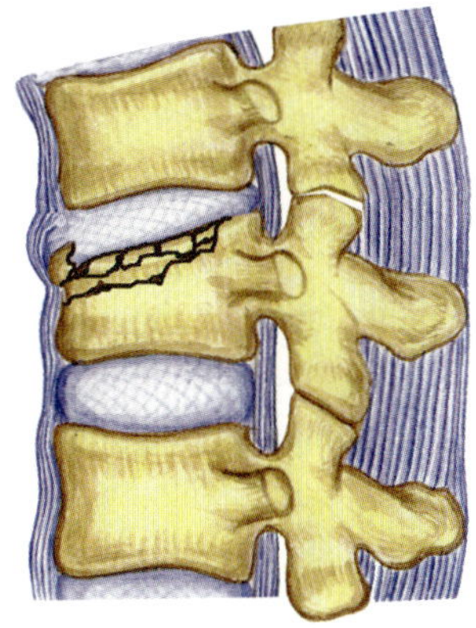

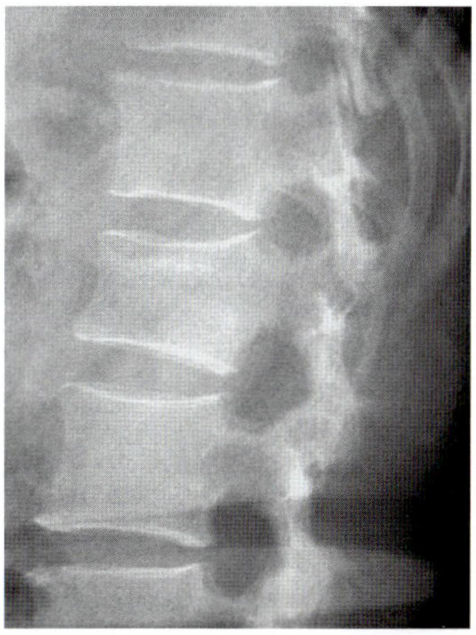

52–53-A2
Split fracture
3,764 fractures
M: 1,988 (52.82%)
F: 1,776 (47.18%)
1.01% of total adult fractures
6.9% of adult spine
7.39% of adult thoracolumbar spine

52–53-A2

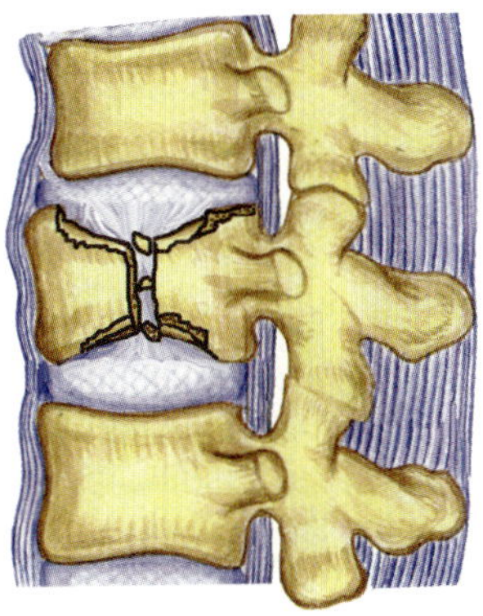

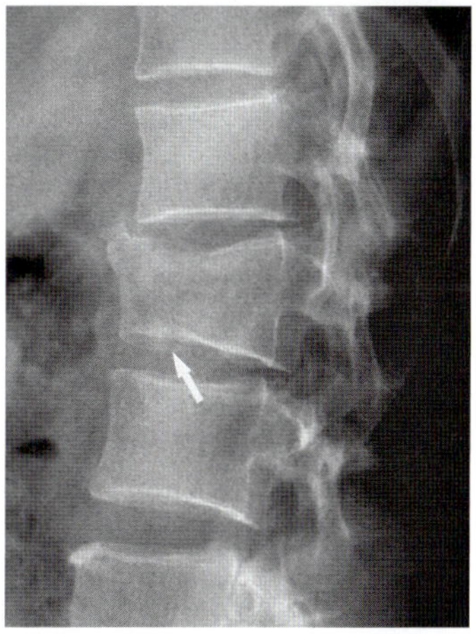

52–53-A3
Burst fracture
8,703 fractures
M: 3,696 (42.47%)
F: 5,007 (57.53%)
2.32% of total adult fractures
15.97% of adult spine
17.09% of adult thoracolumbar spine

52–53-A3

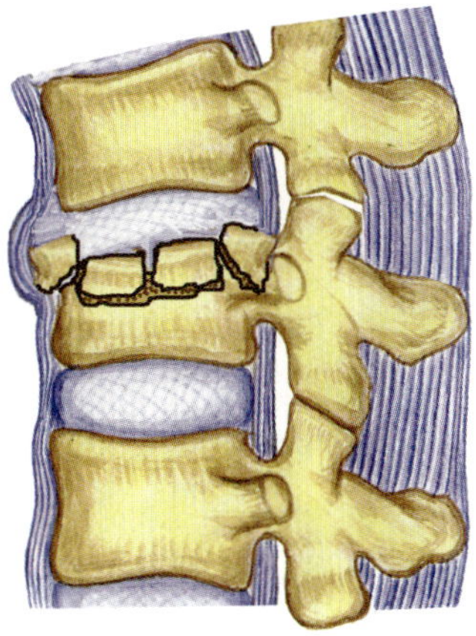

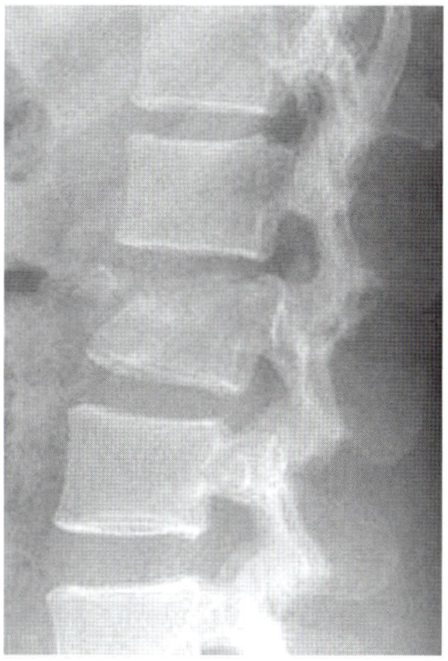

52–53-B Thoracolumbar spine, anterior and posterior injuries with flexion-distraction

52–53-B1
Posterior disruption predominantly ligamentous
1,896 fractures
M: 900 (47.47%)
F: 996 (52.53%)
0.51% of total adult fractures
3.48% of adult spine
3.72% of adult thoracolumbar spine

52–53-B1

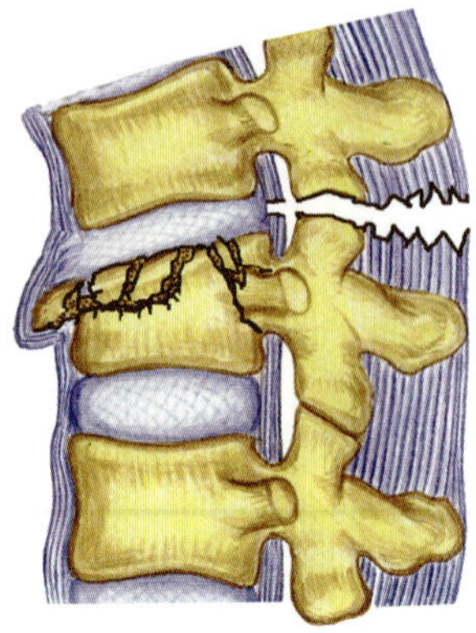

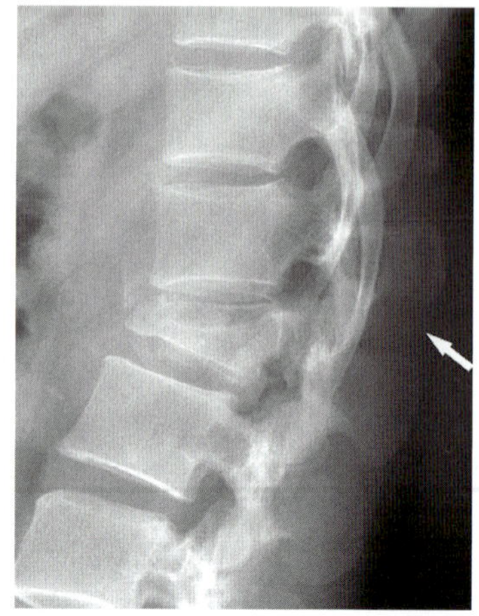

52–53-B2
Posterior disruption predominantly bony
975 fractures
M: 560 (57.44%)
F: 415 (42.56%)
0.26% of total adult fractures
1.79% of adult spine
1.92% of adult thoracolumbar spine

52–53-B2

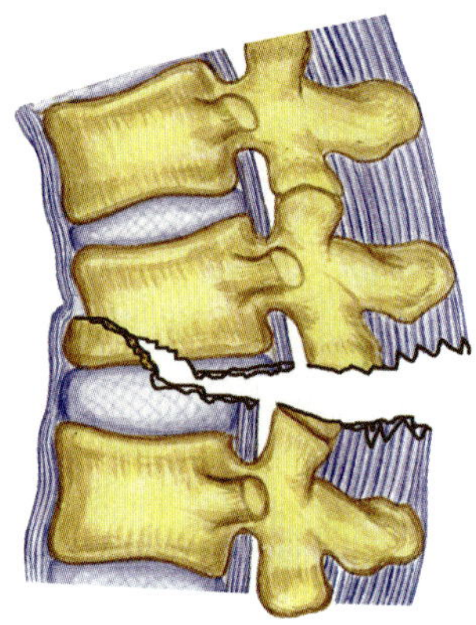

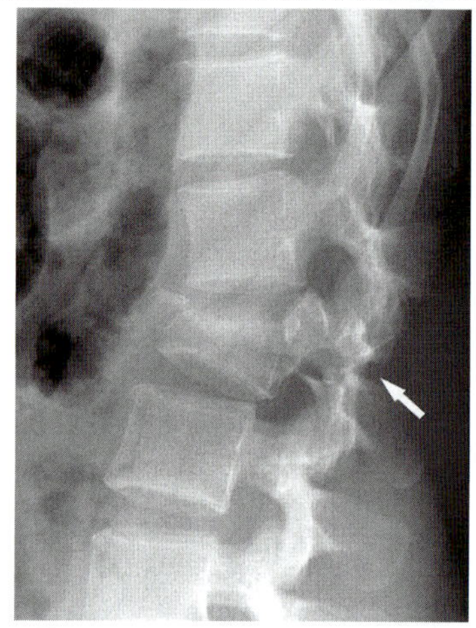

52–53-B3
Anterior disruption through disk
443 fractures
M: 203 (45.82%)
F: 240 (54.18%)
0.12% of total adult fractures
0.81% of adult spine
0.87% of adult thoracolumbar spine

52–53-B3

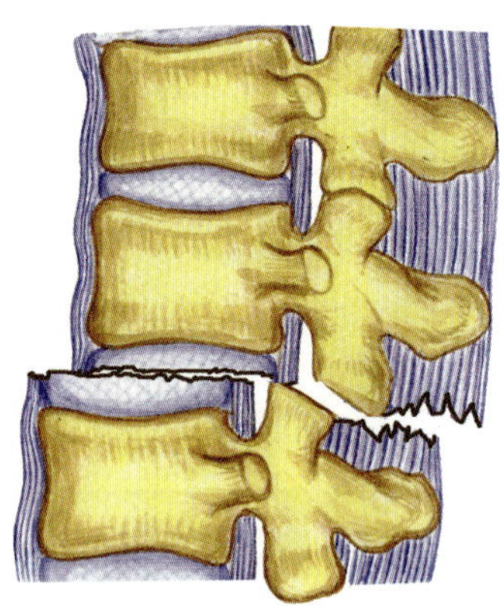

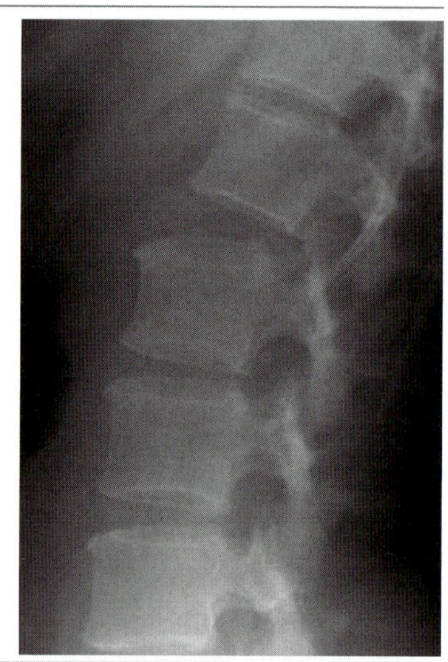

52–53-C Thoracolumbar spine, anterior and posterior element injury with rotation

52–53-C1
Type A injury with rotation
609 fractures
M: 348 (57.14%)
F: 261 (42.86%)
0.16% of total adult fractures
1.12% of adult spine
1.2% of adult thoracolumbar spine

52–53-C1

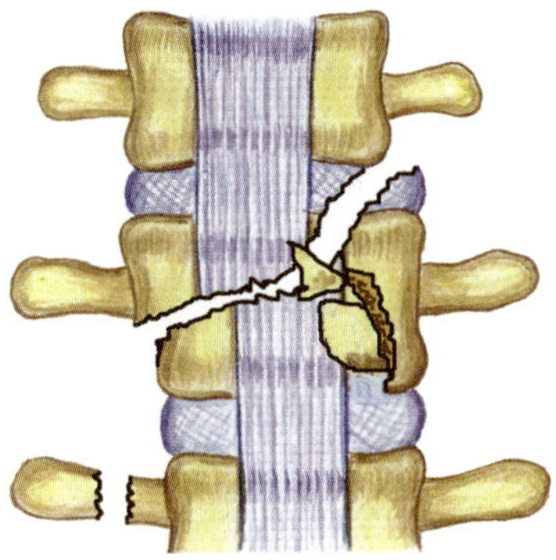

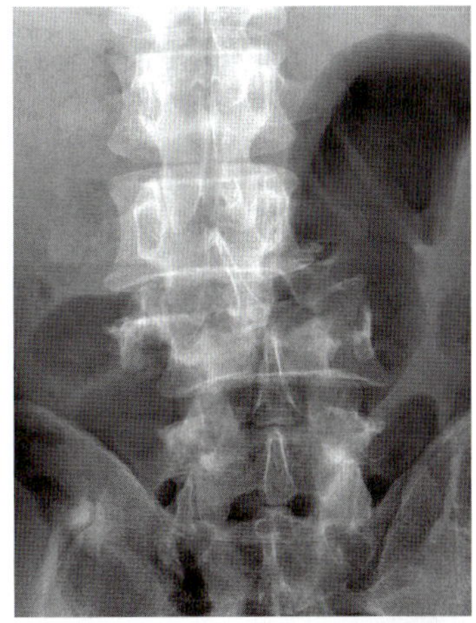

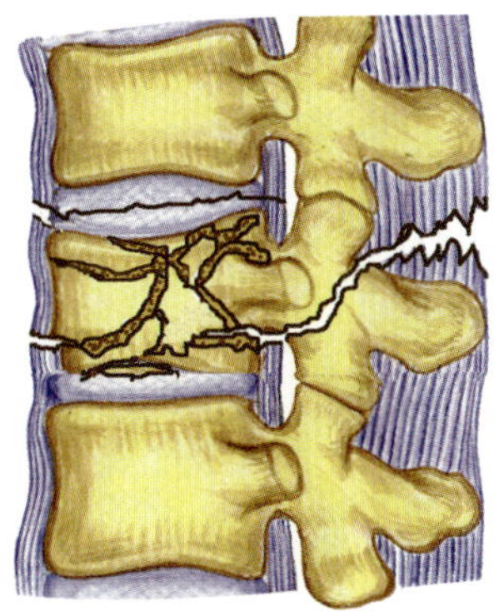

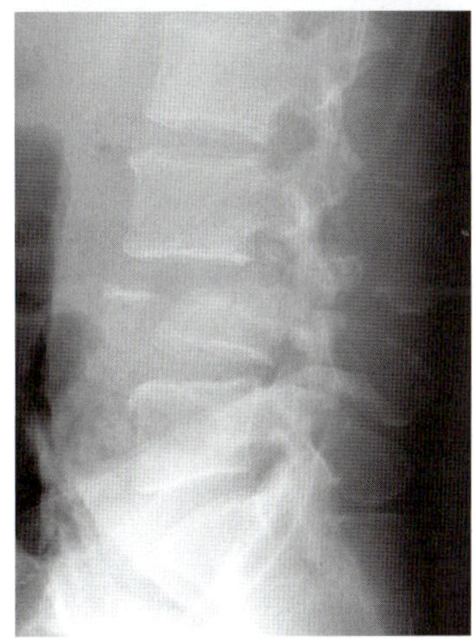

52–53-C Thoracolumbar spine, anterior and posterior element injury with rotation

52–53-C2
Type B injury with rotation
324 fractures
M: 222 (68.52%)
F: 102 (31.48%)
0.09% of total adult fractures
0.59% of adult spine
0.64% of adult thoracolumbar spine

52–53-C2

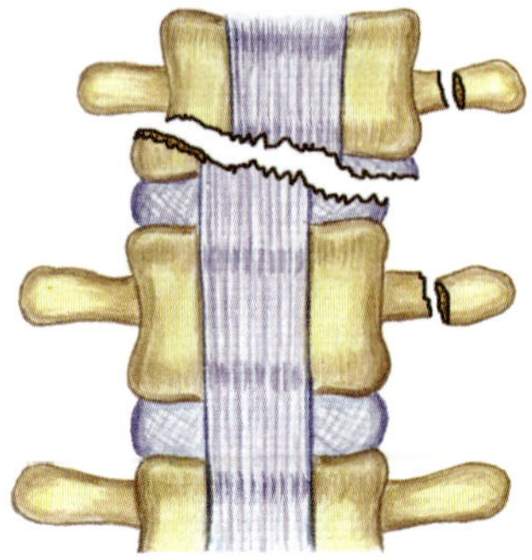

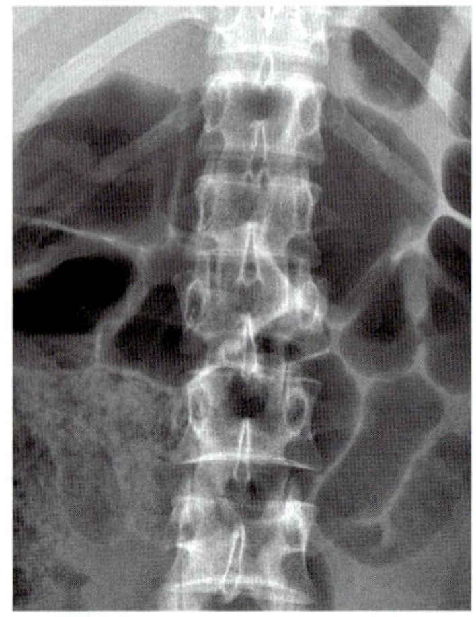

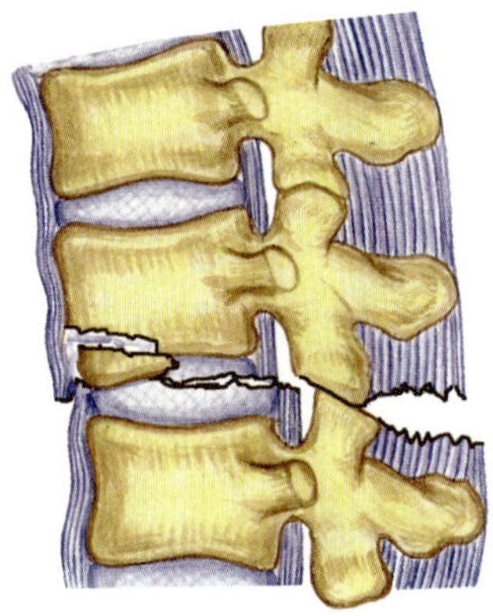

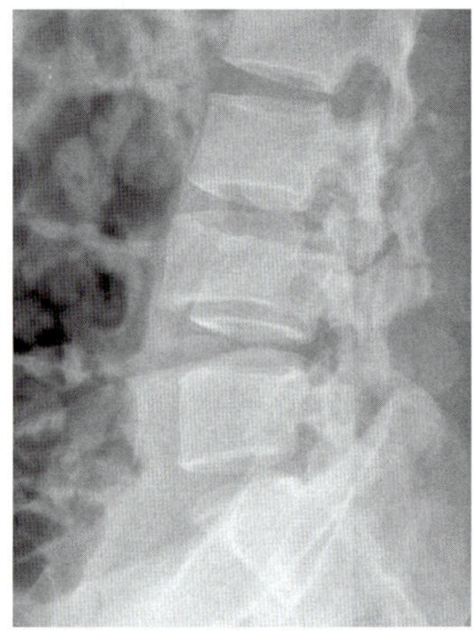

52–53-C3
Rotational shear injury
112 fractures
M: 77 (68.75%)
F: 35 (31.25%)
0.03% of total adult fractures
0.21% of adult spine
0.22% of adult thoracolumbar spine

52–53-C3

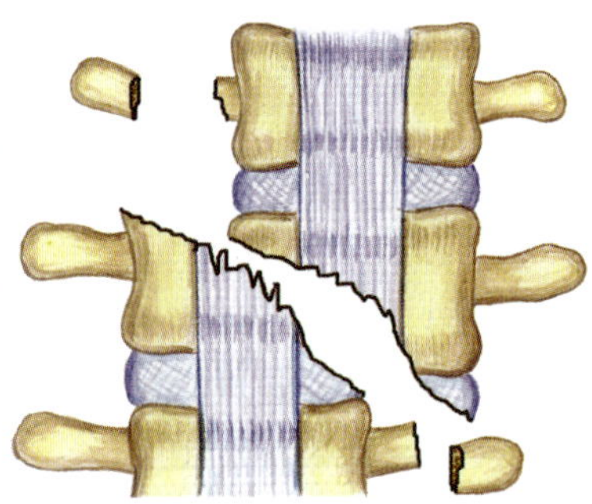

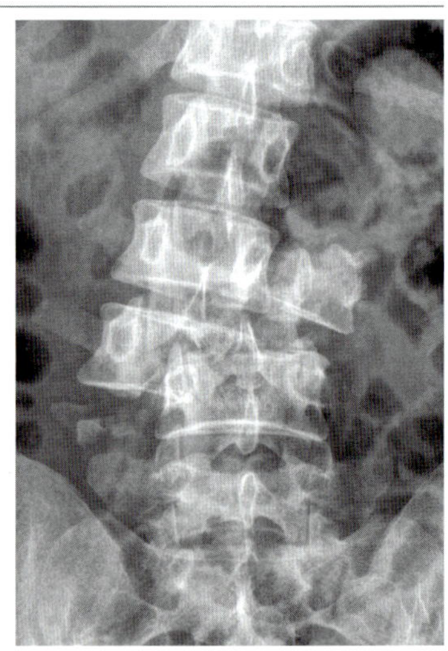

Injury Mechanism

Fractures of the thoracolumbar spine involve a number of injury mechanisms including: (1) axial compression, which usually results in a burst fracture; (2) flexion injury, often results in a compression fracture, with compression of the anterior column and distraction of the posterior column; (3) lateral compression, results in a lateral compression fracture, but the posterior ligament remains intact; (4) flexion rotation, always associated with varying degrees of spinal cord injury, also results in the disruption of posterior ligaments and capsule joints, and an oblique rupture of the vertebral body and disk; (5) flexion-distraction, results in axial rotation of the anterior column, and tension failures in both the anterior and posterior column—since it most commonly occurs in lap belt-restrained passengers, it is also called a seat belt type injury; (6) shear injury, results in failure of all three columns, most commonly in posteroanterior directions, radiographs show all three types of fractures and dislocations, which can be anterior, posterior, or lateral; and (7) distractive extension, results in compression of the posterior column, while the anterior column is pulled by the effect of extension-distraction.

Diagnosis

The diagnosis for thoracolumbar spine fractures is dependent on the clinical presentation, imaging studies, and the assessment of spine stability. Typical clinical presentations include pain, deformity and impaired function. AP and lateral radiographs of the thoracolumbar spine usually can detect the fracture and help in making the diagnosis. Conventional and computed axial tomography can be very important in assessing posterior element integrity and spinal canal encroachment. CT scans are very sensitive in detecting subtle fractures of posterior elements, especially a lamina fracture. MRI is useful in detecting the extent of damage to the spinal cord. MRI is most useful in patients when traumatic disk herniation, epidural hematoma, or spinal cord injury is suspected. Based on the three-column concept, posttraumatic spine stability is primarily dependent on the integrity of the middle column. The middle column remains intact in simple wedge compression injuries, which are thus stable fractures, whereas the anterior and middle column fail in burst fractures, making them unstable fractures.

Treatment

The principle treatments of thoracolumbar spine fracture are shown in **Plate 6.11**.

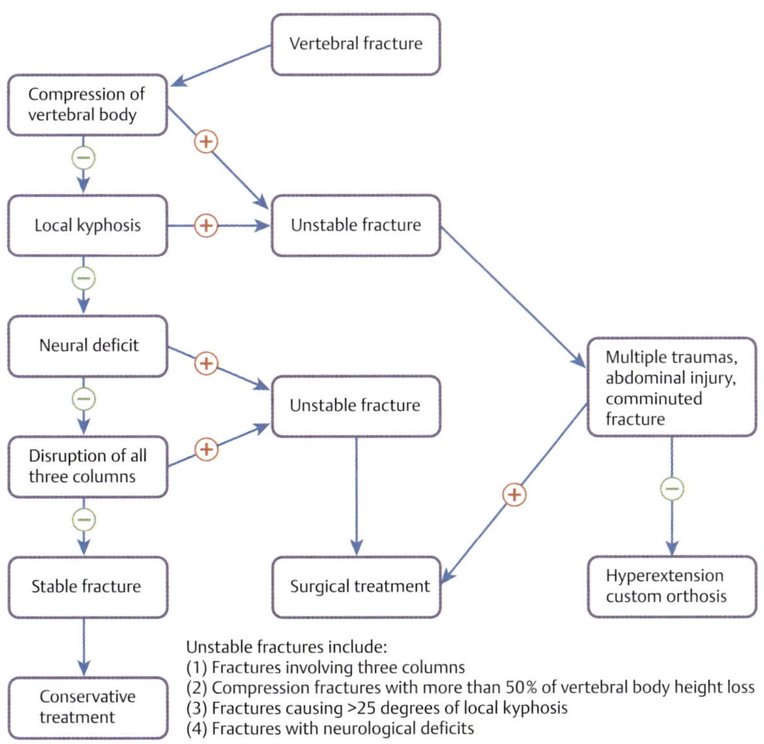

Unstable fractures include:
(1) Fractures involving three columns
(2) Compression fractures with more than 50% of vertebral body height loss
(3) Fractures causing >25 degrees of local kyphosis
(4) Fractures with neurological deficits

Plate 6.11

6

The management of thoracolumbar spine injury consists of conservative and surgical treatment. The indications for conservative treatment include: (1) stable fracture, with less than 50% of vertebral body height loss; (2) fracture of posterior elements without any signs of cord or multiple root compromise, and the canal encroachment is less than 50% of the cross-sectional area of the canal; or (3) burst fracture with an intact posterior column. In contrast, the following cases are more likely to require surgical intervention: (1) unstable fracture, even without evidence of neurologic injury; (2) burst fracture, where a fragment of more than 50% of the canal's cross-sectional area encroaches upon the canal; (3) burst fracture, complicated by neurologic signs; (4) fracture-dislocation or loss of joint congruity; (5) posterior decompression fails and requires a second surgery; (6) compression of the spinal cord, resulting from laminar fracture subsidence; and (7) presentation of delayed neurologic syndrome resulting from compression of the anterior cord by an old fracture, or progression of kyphosis.

Surgical procedures should be performed when patients become medically stable. The operative methods include: (1) posterior fracture reduction and fusion, and pedicle screw fixation; (2) anterior vertebrectomy, graft fusion, and internal fixation; and (3) combined AP decompression and graft fusion.

Further Classification of Thoracolumbar Spinal Fractures

Denis Classification

Denis classification of spinal injuries is one of the most commonly used classifications in clinical practice. It separates spinal injuries into 4 types and 10 subtypes, as illustrated by **Table 6.15**.

Of 50,910 thoracolumbar spine fractures, only 49,487 are able to be classified based on the Denis classification. Certain compound fracture types cannot be grouped into any category in the Denis system. Details are shown in the illustration below.

Table 6.15 Denis classification of thoracolumbar spinal fractures

Fracture Type	Subtype	Injury Force	Column involved	Stability
Compression fracture	–	Axial load	Anterior column	Stable
Burst fracture	A: Fracture of both endplates	Axial load	Anterior and middle columns	Unstable
	B: Fracture of superior endplate	Axial load, extension, flexion	Anterior and middle columns	May be unstable
	C: Fracture of inferior endplate	Axial load, extension, flexion	Anterior and middle columns	May be unstable
	D: Burst rotation fracture	Axial load, rotation	All three columns	Unstable
	E: Burst lateral flexion fracture	Lateral compressive load	All three columns	May be unstable
Chance fracture	–	Flexion-distraction	Middle and posterior columns	Unstable
Fracture dislocation	Flexion-rotation	Hyperextension and flexion, rotation	All three columns	Unstable
	Shear injury	Hyperextension and dislocation	All three columns	Unstable
	Flexion-distraction	Hyperflexion and distraction	All three columns	Unstable

Denis classification of thoracolumbar spine fractures

Type I **Axial compression** 36,904 fractures M: 18,401 (49.86%) F: 18,503 (50.14%) 9.86% of total adult fractures 67.67% of adult spine 72.49% of adult thoracolumbar spine	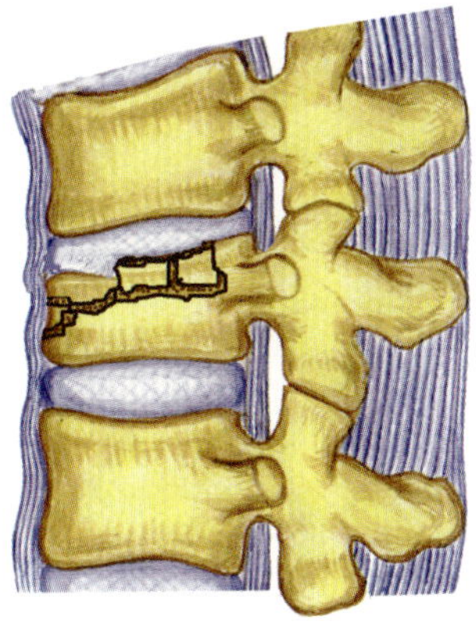 Axial compression	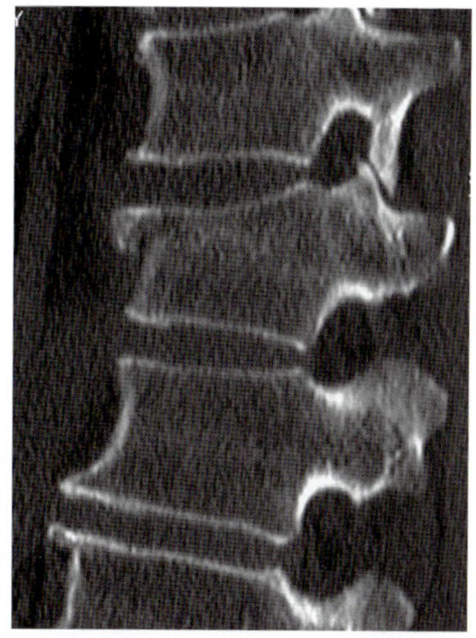
Type II **Burst fracture** 9,281 fractures M: 4,082 (43.98%) F: 5,199 (56.02%) 2.48% of total adult fractures 17.02% of adult spine 18.23% of adult thoracolumbar spine	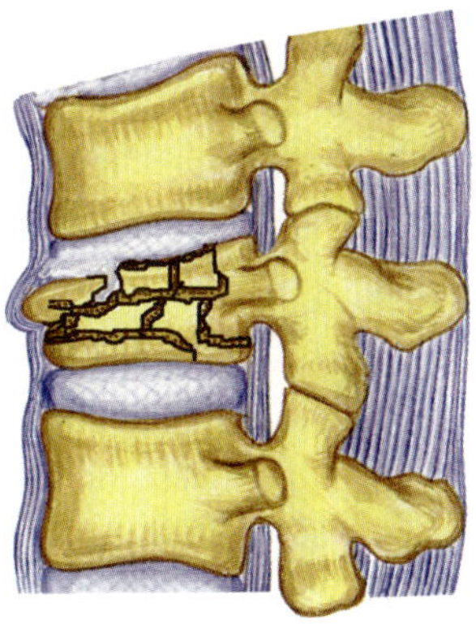 Burst fracture	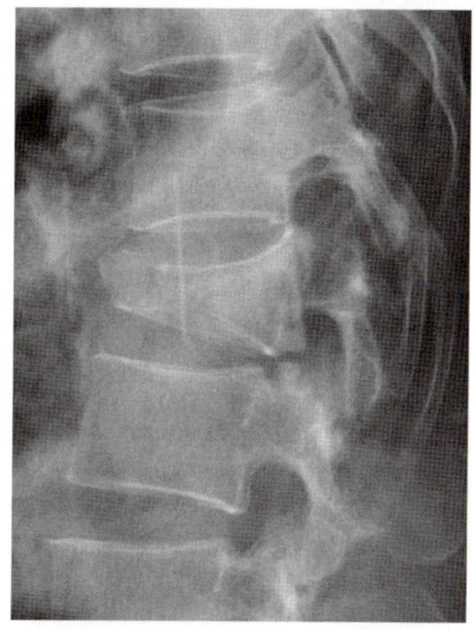
Type III **Chance fracture** 2,158 fractures M: 1,100 (50.97%) F: 1,058 (49.03%) 0.58% of total adult fractures 3.96% of adult spine 4.24% of adult thoracolumbar spine	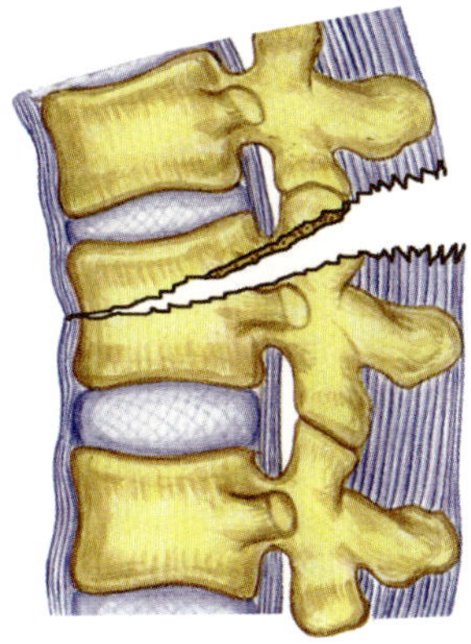 Chance fracture	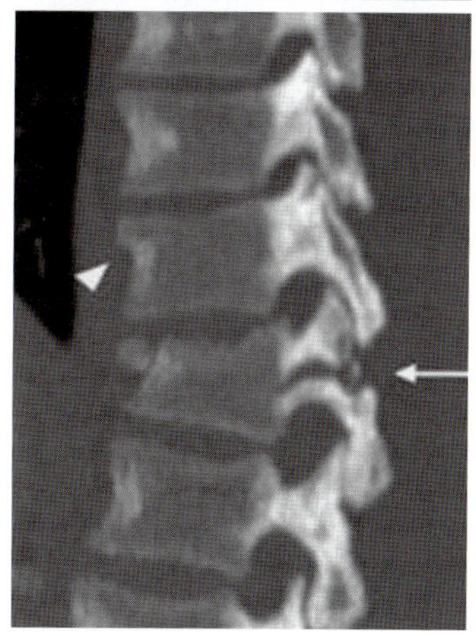

Denis classification of thoracolumbar spine fractures

Type IV
Fracture-dislocation
1,144 fractures
M: 693 (60.58%)
F: 451 (39.42%)
0.31% of total adult fractures
2.1% of adult spine
2.25% of adult thoracolumbar spine

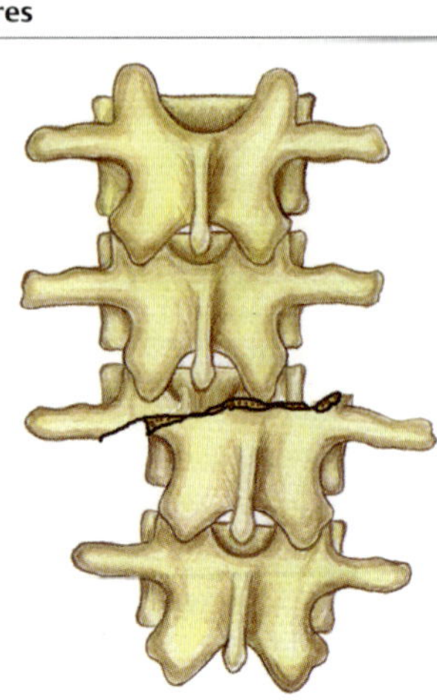

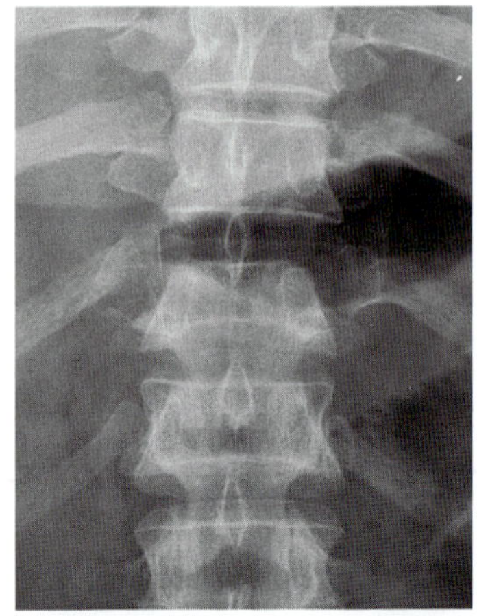

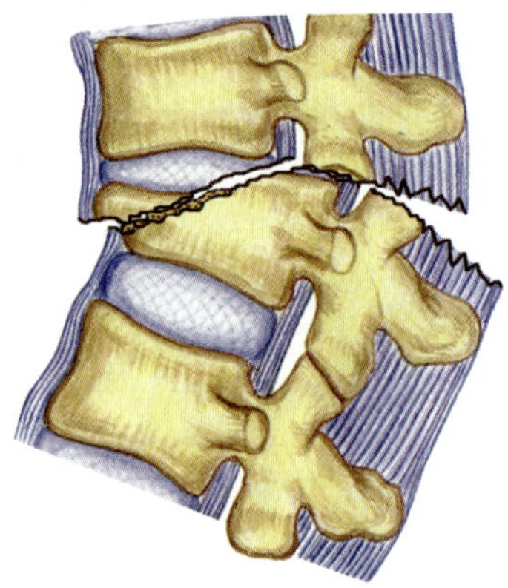

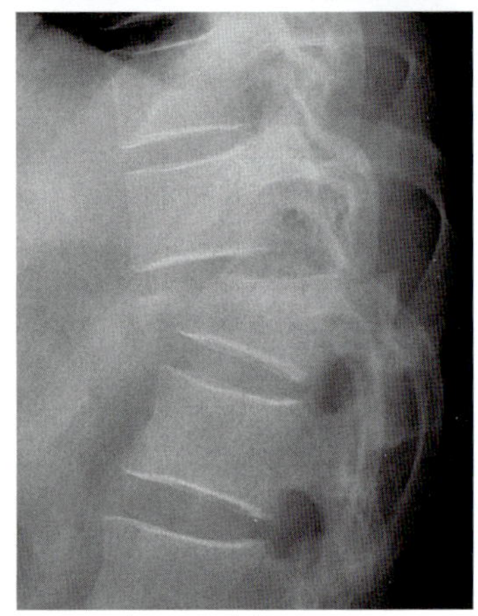

Fracture dislocation (lateral)

7 Fractures of the Pelvic Ring and Acetabulum

Overview

Anatomical Features

The pelvis is composed of four bones: the two hip bones laterally and in front, and the sacrum and coccyx behind (**Plate 7.1**). The hip bone is a large, flattened, irregularly shaped bone that forms the sides and anterior wall of the pelvic cavity together with its counterparts on the opposite side. It consists of three parts—the ilium, ischium, and pubis—which are fused into one bony structure in adults. The hip bone is narrowed in the middle and expanded above and below, with a large oval-shaped hole, the obturator foramen, on its inferior aspect. The acetabulum, a large cup-shaped articular cavity, is situated near the middle of the bone's outer surface. The external surface of the upper part of the hip bone is smooth and gives attachment to the gluteal muscles. The ilium is divided into two parts: the body and the ala. The ischium, the lower and back part of the hip bone, consists of three portions: a body and two rami. The pubis, which forms the anterior part of the hip bone, is divided into a body, and a superior and an inferior ramus. The pubic ramus is a very thin bone, making it an easy target for fractures. The sacrum is a triangular bone at the base of the spine and consists of five vertebrae that usually are completely fused into a single bone in adults. The sacral canal in the middle runs throughout the greater part of the bone; its walls are perforated by the anterior and posterior sacral foramina through which the sacral nerves pass. The coccyx, or tailbone, comprised of four fused vertebrae, articulates superiorly with the sacrum and extends downward as an individual piece (**Plates 7.2** and **7.3**).

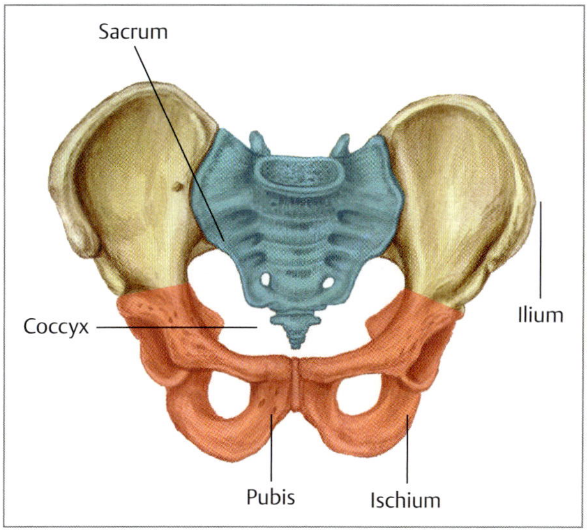

Plate 7.1

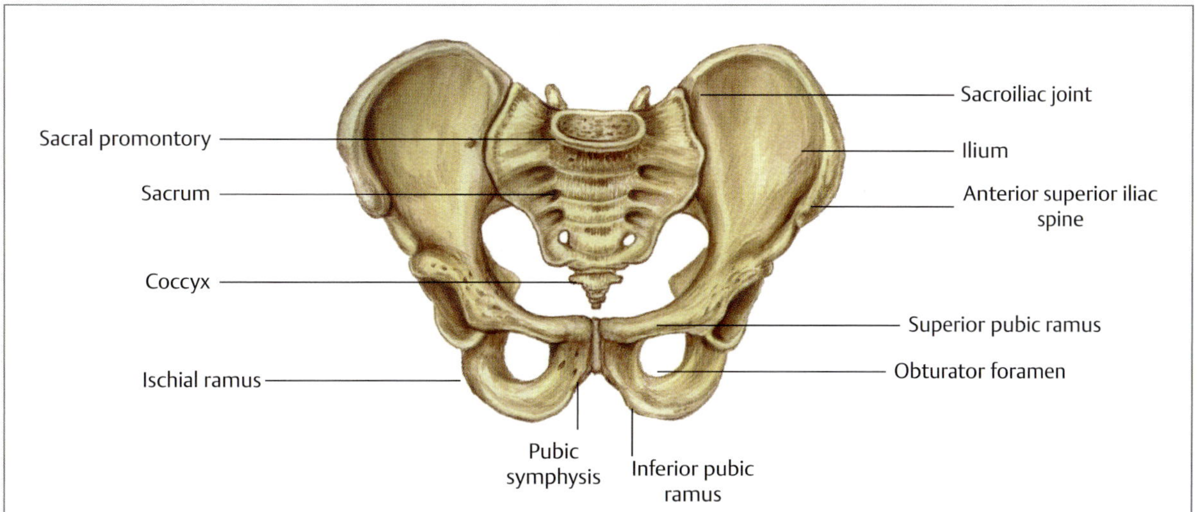

Anterior view of pelvis

Plate 7.2

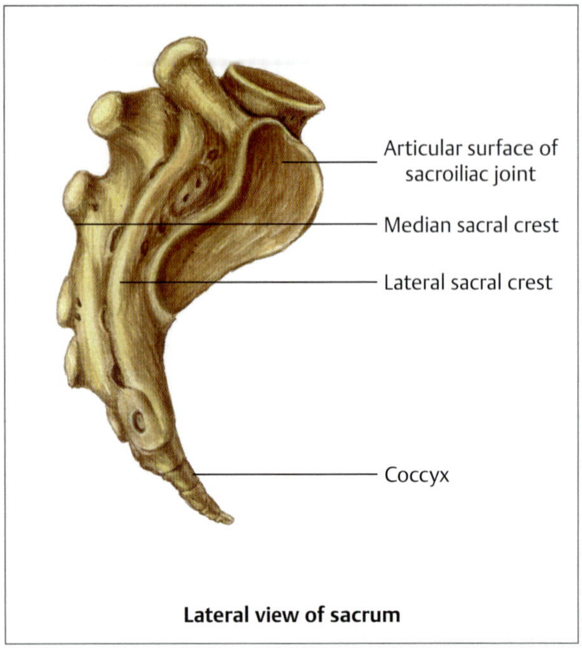

Plate 7.3

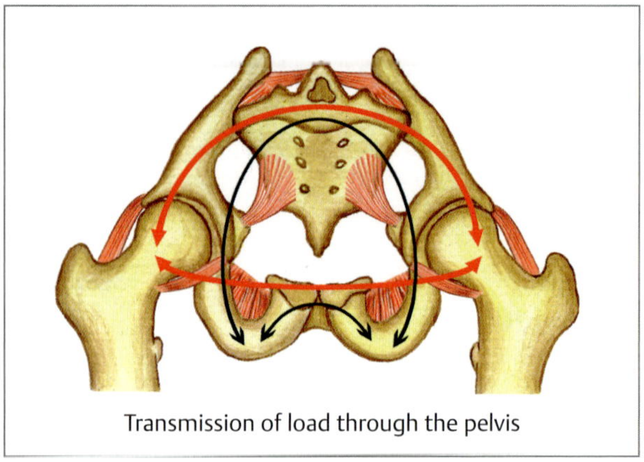

Plate 7.4

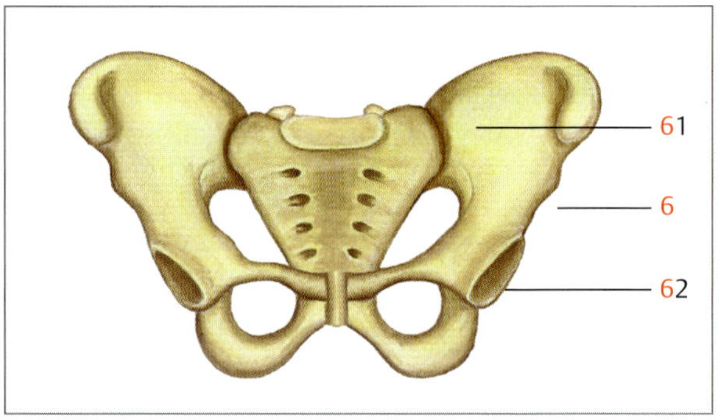

Plate 7.5

Based on fracture pattern, pelvic fractures can be divided into pelvic ring fractures and acetabular fractures. The pelvic ring is divided into an anterior and posterior ring by the acetabulum. The acetabulum is divided into the anterior column, the posterior column, and more.

In the erect posture, the pelvis is inclined forward so that the anterior superior iliac spines and the front of the top of the symphysis pubis are in the same coronal plane. When an individual is standing, their weight is transmitted from the upper body and trunk, through the spine, the sacrum, sacroiliac joint, and acetabulum, and continues down to the lower extremities. When an individual is in the sitting position, their weight is transmitted down the spine, the sacrum, and sacroiliac joint to the ischium (**Plate 7.4**).

AO Classification and Coding System for Fractures of the Pelvic Ring and Acetabulum

According to the AO fracture classification principle, the pelvis is considered one unit, with the location code of 6. The following section is divided into discussions of the pelvic ring and acetabulum. The numbers 61 and 62 are used to represent the pelvic ring and acetabulum, respectively (**Plates 7.5** and **7.6**).

Clinical Epidemiologic Features of Fractures of the Pelvic Ring and Acetabulum

A total of 14,420 patients with 14,555 fractures of the pelvic ring and/or acetabulum were treated in 83 hospitals in China over a 2-year period from 2010 to 2011. All cases were reviewed and statistically studied, comprising 3.48% of all patients with fractures and 3.37% of all types of fractures. Of a total 14,420 patients, there were 685 children with 687 fractures, accounting for 1.25% of pediatric patients with fractures, and 1.20% of all types of fractures in children. The rest of the 13,735 adult patients had 13,868 fractures, represent 3.81% of adult patients with fractures, and 3.70% of all types of fractures in adults.

Epidemiologic features of fractures of the pelvic ring and acetabulum are the following:

- More males than females
- The high risk age groups are 36–40 years and 41–45 years, while the high risk age group for males is 41–45 years, 36–40 years, and 41–45 years for females.
- Pelvic ring fractures occur more frequently than acetabular fractures.

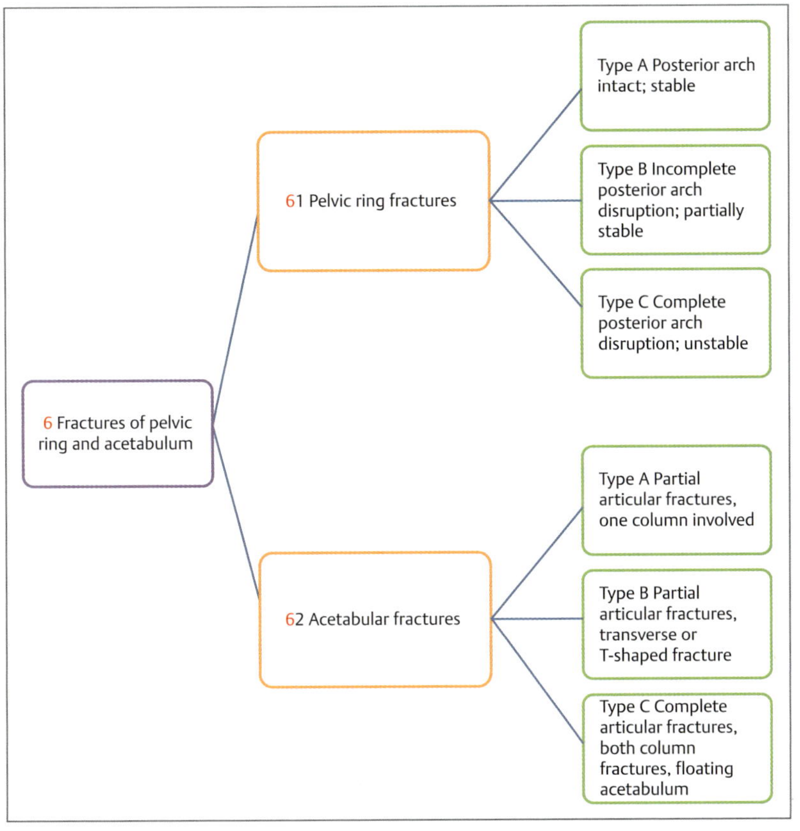

Plate 7.6

Fractures of the Pelvic Ring and Acetabulum by Sex

Table 7.1 Sex distribution of 14,420 patients with fractures of the pelvic ring and acetabulum

Sex	Number of patients	Percentage (%)
Male	7,892	54.73
Female	6,528	45.27
Total	14,420	100.00

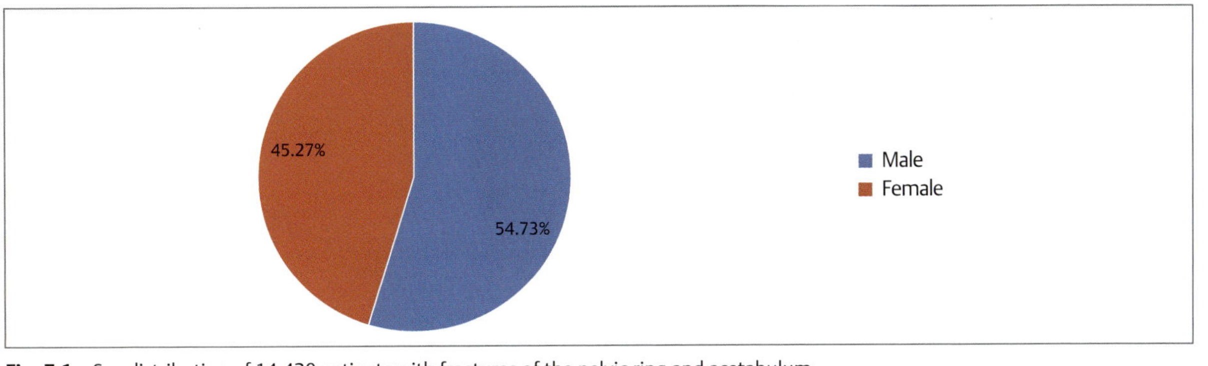

Fig. 7.1 Sex distribution of 14,420 patients with fractures of the pelvic ring and acetabulum.

Fractures of the Pelvic Ring and Acetabulum by Age Group

Table 7.2 Age and sex distribution of 14,420 patients with fractures of the pelvic ring and acetabulum

Age group (years)	Male	Female	Number of patients	Percentage (%)
0–5	60	86	146	1.01
6–10	98	109	207	1.44
11–15	201	131	332	2.30
16–20	407	237	644	4.47
21–25	720	549	1,269	8.80
26–30	728	569	1,297	8.99
31–35	723	518	1,241	8.61
36–40	941	738	1,679	11.64
41–45	983	738	1,721	11.93
46–50	857	581	1,438	9.97
51–55	648	491	1,139	7.90
56–60	565	438	1,003	6.96
61–65	292	302	594	4.12
66–70	236	268	504	3.50
71–75	174	269	443	3.07
76–80	134	234	368	2.55
81–85	82	169	251	1.74
≥86	43	101	144	1.00
Total	7,892	6,528	14,420	100.00

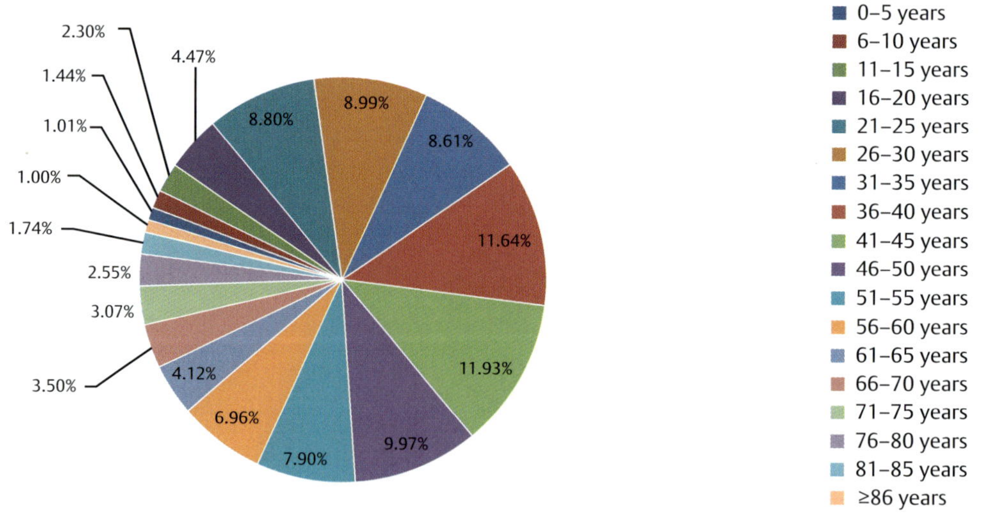

a

Fig. 7.2 **(a)** Age distribution of 14,420 patients with fractures of the pelvic ring and acetabulum.

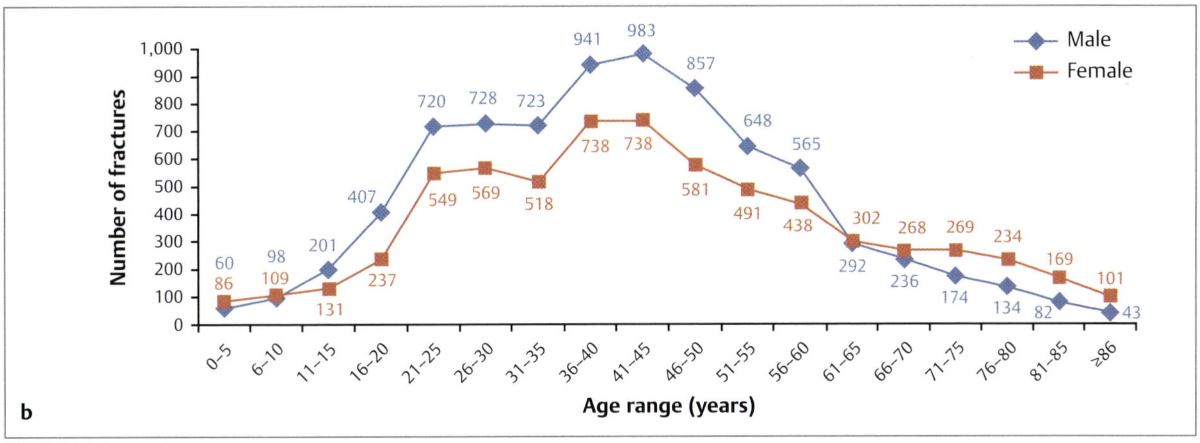

Fig. 7.2 (*continued*) **(b)** Age and sex distribution of 14,420 patients with fractures of the pelvic ring and acetabulum.

Fractures of the Pelvic Ring and Acetabulum by Fracture Location Based on the AO Classification

Fractures of the Pelvic Ring and Acetabulum in Adults by Fracture Segment Based on the AO Classification

Table 7.3 Segment distribution of 13,868 fractures of the pelvic ring and acetabulum in adults

Segment	Number of fractures	Percentage (%)
61	10,694	77.11
62	3,174	22.89
Total	13,868	100.00

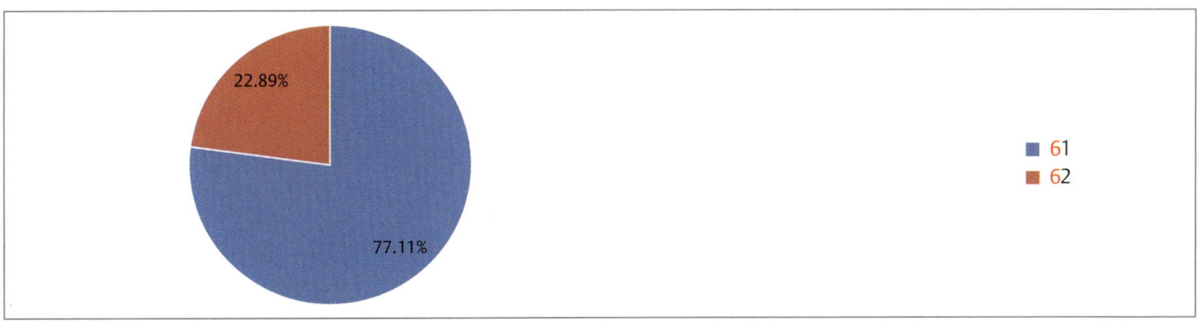

Fig. 7.3 Segment distribution of 13,868 fractures of the pelvic ring and acetabulum in adults.

Fractures of the Pelvic Ring and Acetabulum in Children by Fracture Location

Table 7.4 Fracture location distribution of 687 fractures of the pelvic ring and acetabulum in children

Fracture location	Number of fractures	Percentage (%)
Pelvic ring	568	82.68
Acetabulum	119	17.32
Total	687	100.00

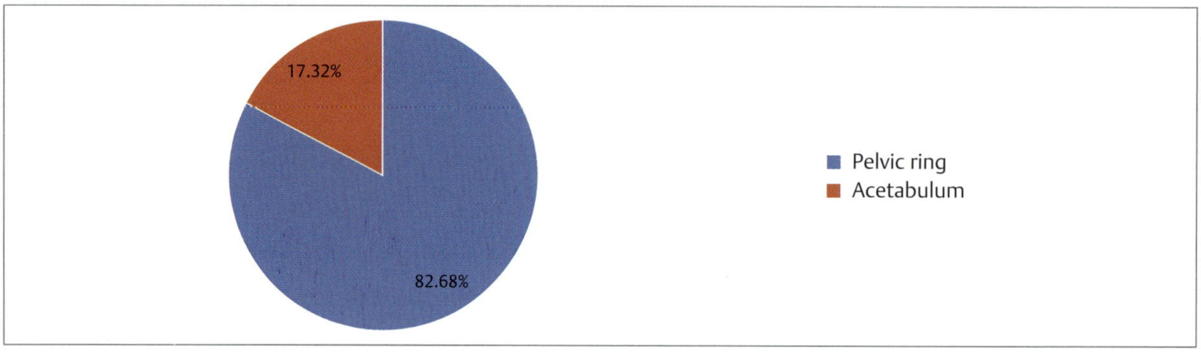

Fig. 7.4 Fracture location distribution of 687 fractures of the pelvic ring and acetabulum in children.

Fractures of the Pelvic Ring and Acetabulum in Children by Sex

Table 7.5 Sex distribution of 568 pediatric patients with pelvic ring fractures

Sex	Number of patients	Percentage (%)
Male	296	52.11
Female	272	47.89
Total	568	100.00

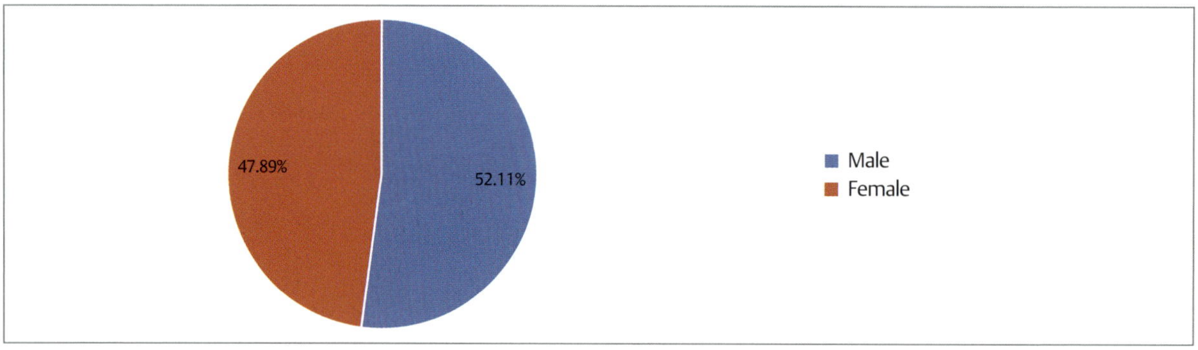

Fig. 7.5 Sex distribution of 568 pediatric patients with pelvic ring fractures.

Table 7.6 Sex distribution of 119 pediatric patients with acetabulum fractures (2 children had pelvic ring fracture and acetabulum fracture at the same time)

Sex	Number of patients	Percentage (%)
Male	63	52.94
Female	56	47.06
Total	119	100.00

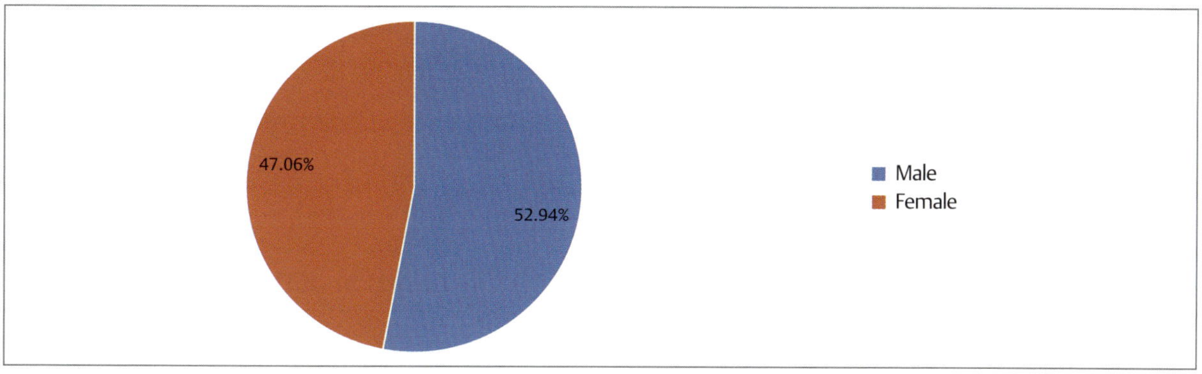

Fig. 7.6 Sex distribution of 119 pediatric patients with acetabulum fractures.

7

Pelvic Ring Fractures (Segment 61)

Anatomical Features

The pelvic ring is made up of paired innominate, pubic, ischial, and sacral bones. It is joined posteriorly by the sacroiliac joints and ligaments, and anteriorly by the pubic symphysis. The ischial bones, pubic rami, and pubic symphysis comprise the anterior ring. The sacroiliac joint is formed between the two auricular, or ear-shaped, articular surfaces of the ilium and sacrum, and connects to the posterior pelvic ring. The upper part of the sacroiliac articulation is formed by ligaments connecting the sacrum and ilium, while the lower part is separated by a space containing synovial fluid, thus comprising a synovial joint. The sacroiliac joint, together with the posterior sacroiliac, sacrotuberous, and sacrospinous ligaments, as well as muscles and fascia of the pelvic floor, form the sacroiliac complex—a very important structure that maintains the stability of the pelvis. The sacrotuberous and sacrospinous ligaments enclose the greater and lesser sciatic notch, which forms the greater sciatic foramen and the lesser sciatic foramen respectively, through which muscles, vessels, and nerves pass (**Plate 7.7**).

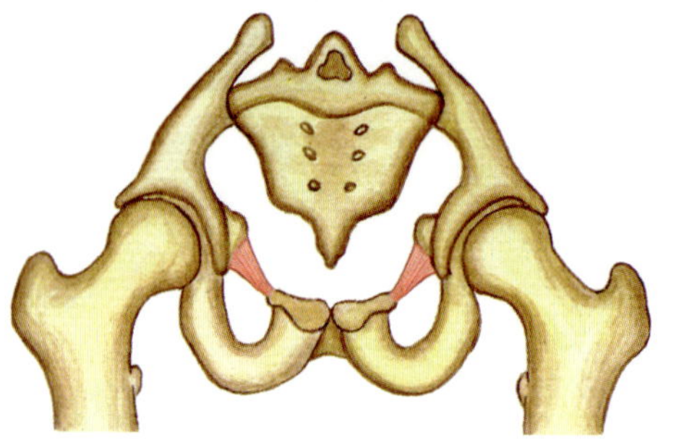

Plate 7.8

AO Classification of Pelvic Ring Fractures

Based on AO classification, the location code for the pelvic ring is the number 61. According to the mechanism of injury, fracture location, and the stability of the pelvis, segment 61 fractures can be further divided into: 61-A, posterior arch intact, stable; 61-B, incomplete posterior arch disruption, partially stable; and 61-C, complete posterior arch disruption, unstable (**Plates 7.8** and **7.9**).

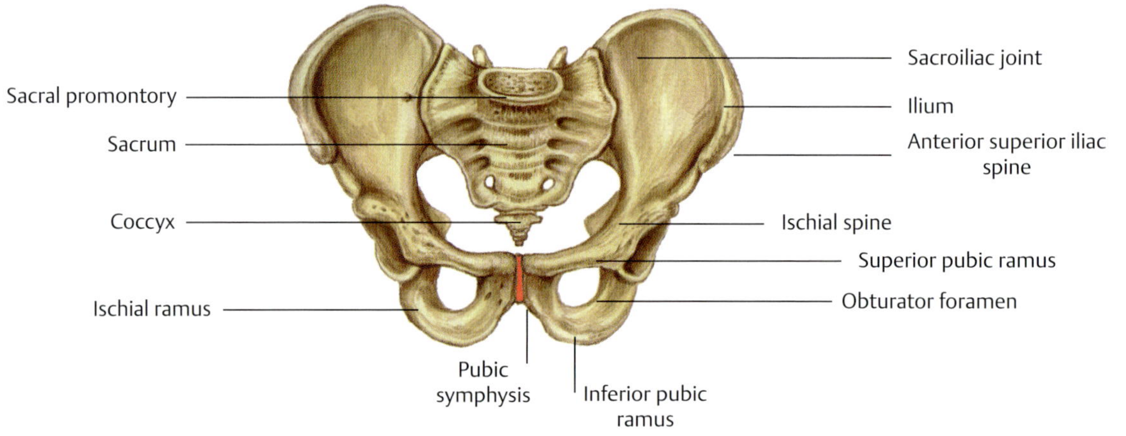

Anterior view of pelvis

Plate 7.7

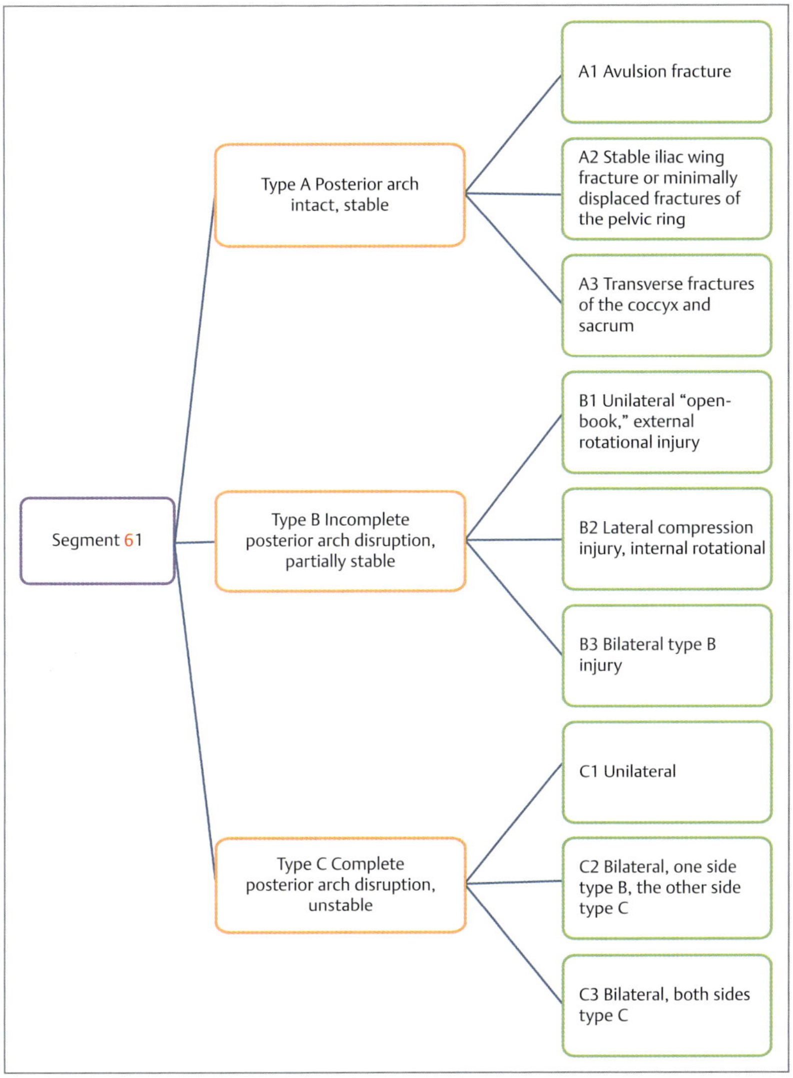

Plate 7.9

Clinical Epidemiologic Features of Pelvic Ring Fractures (Segment 61)

A total of 10,672 adult patients with 10,694 pelvic ring fractures were treated in 83 hospitals in China over a 2-year period from 2010 to 2011. All cases were reviewed and statistically studied, comprising 2.96% of all adult patients with fractures and 2.86% of all types of fractures.

Epidemiologic features of pelvic ring fractures are the following:

- Slightly more females than males
- The high risk age group is between ages 36 and 40, and ages 41 and 45; although the group 41–45 years is the high risk group for males, age group 36–40 is so for females.
- The most common fracture type of segment 61 fractures is type A—the same fracture type for both males and females.
- The most common fracture group of segment 61 fractures is group A2, the same group for males, and the most common fracture group for females is group A3.

Fractures of Segment 61 by Sex

Table 7.7 Sex distribution of 10,694 fractures of segment 61

Sex	Number of fractures	Percentage (%)
Male	5,343	49.96
Female	5,351	50.04
Total	10,694	100.00

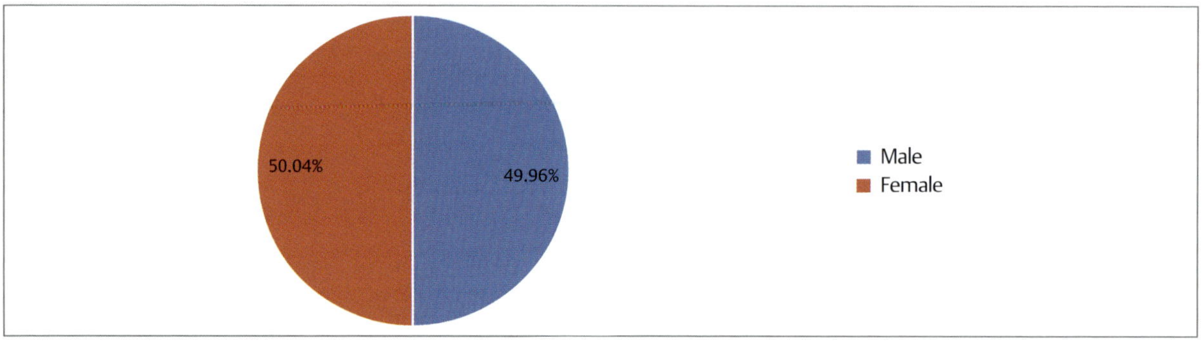

Fig. 7.7 Sex distribution of 10,694 fractures of segment 61.

Fractures of Segment 61 by Age Group

Table 7.8 Age and sex distribution of 10,694 fractures of segment 61

Age group (years)	Male	Female	Number of fractures	Percentage (%)
16–20	320	209	529	4.95
21–25	538	479	1,017	9.51
26–30	551	521	1,072	10.02
31–35	488	478	966	9.03
36–40	654	652	1,306	12.21
41–45	700	630	1,330	12.44
46–50	604	480	1,084	10.14
51–55	426	396	822	7.69
56–60	383	361	744	6.96
61–65	196	246	442	4.13
66–70	160	227	387	3.62
71–75	127	236	363	3.39
76–80	101	196	297	2.78
81–85	58	151	209	1.95
≥86	37	89	126	1.18
Total	5,343	5,351	10,694	100.00

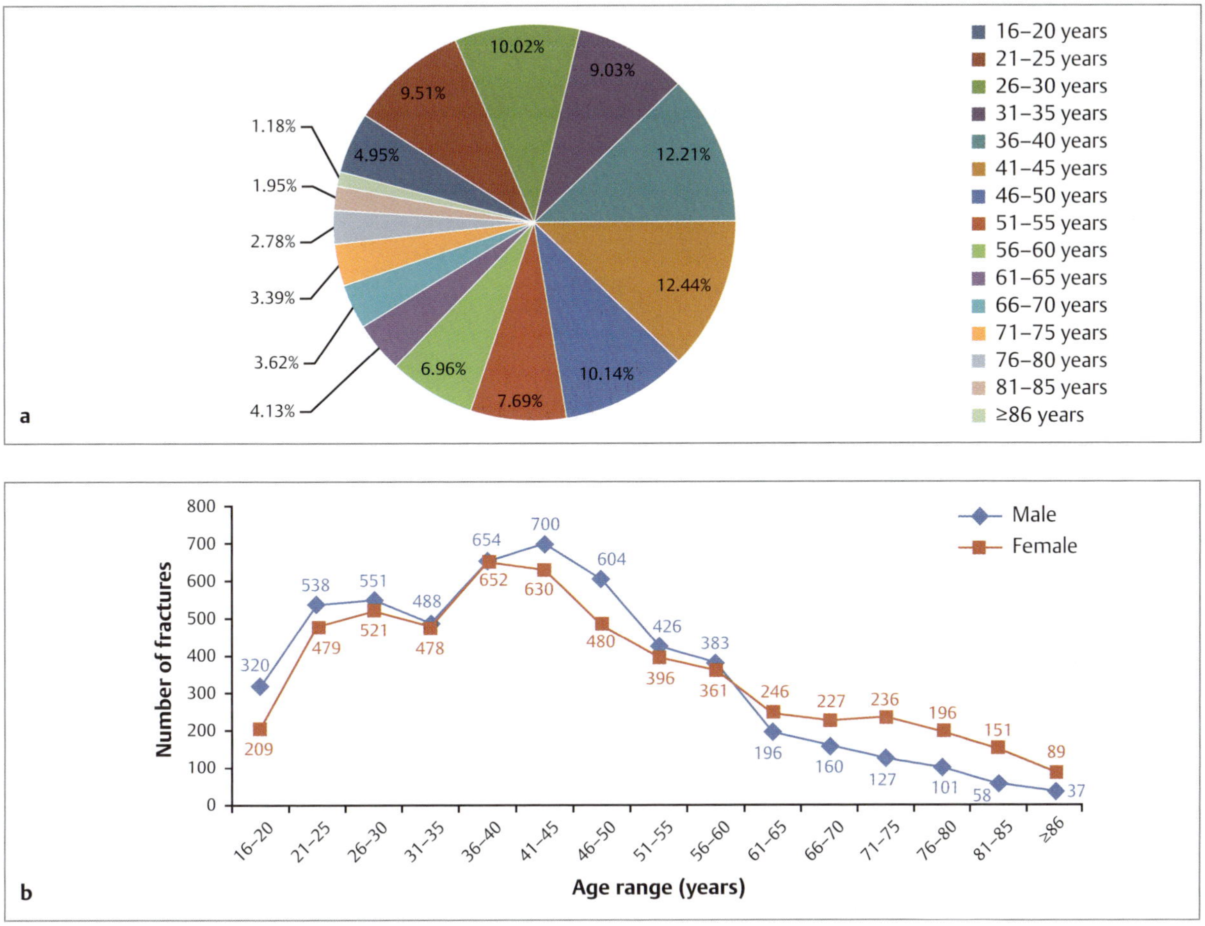

Fig. 7.8 **(a)** Age distribution of 10,694 fractures of segment 61.
(b) Age and sex distribution of 10,694 fractures of segment 61.

Fractures of Segment 61 by Fracture Type

Table 7.9 Sex and fracture type distribution of 10,694 fractures of segment 61

Fracture type	Male	Female	Number of fractures	Percentage (%)
61-A	4,240	4,680	8,920	83.41
61-B	768	503	1,271	11.89
61-C	335	168	503	4.70
Total	5,343	5,351	10,694	100.00

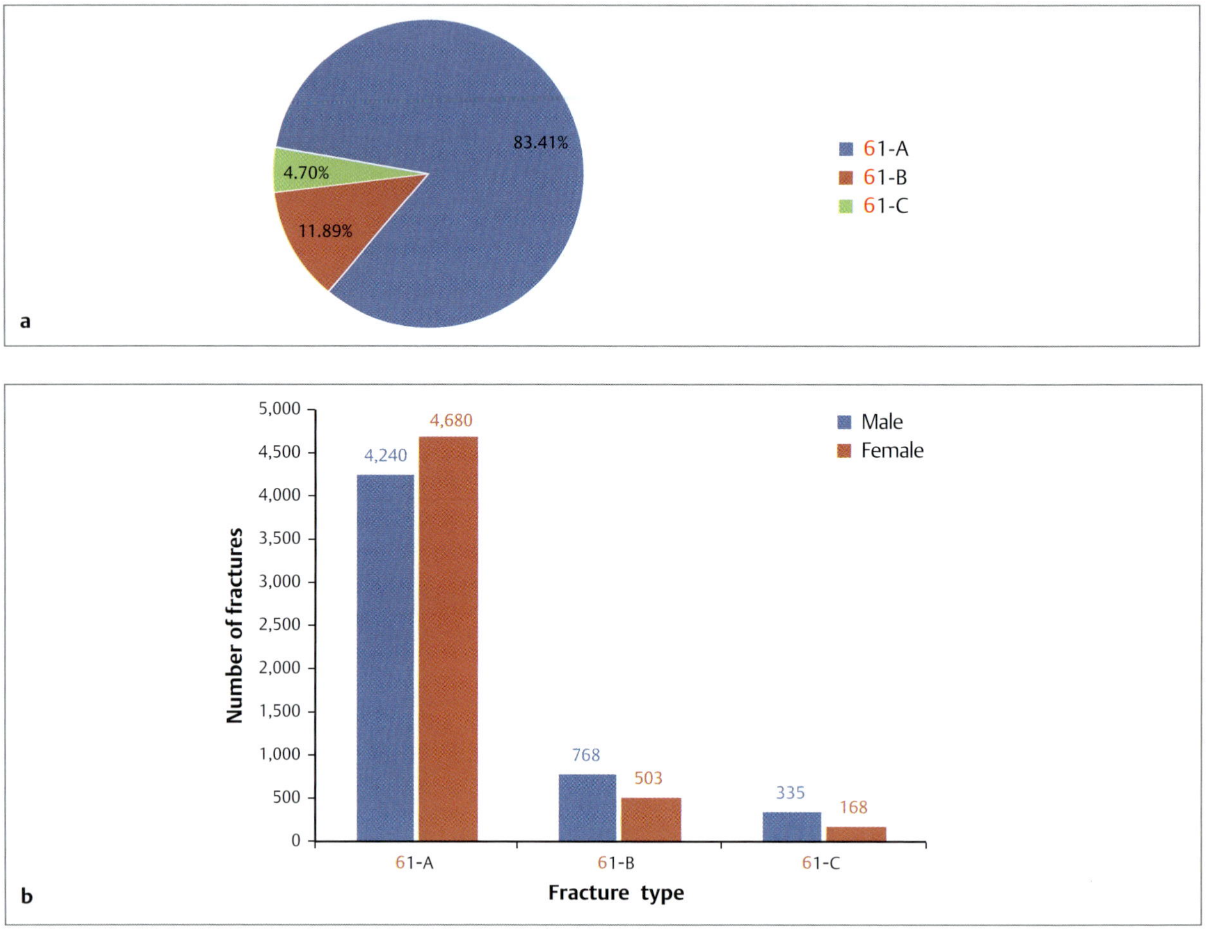

Fig. 7.9 **(a)** Fracture type distributions of 10,694 fractures of segment 61.
(b) Sex and fracture type distribution of 10,694 fractures of segment 61.

Table 7.10 Sex and fracture group distribution of 10,694 fractures of segment 61

Fracture group	Male	Female	Number of fractures	Percentage of segment 61 fractures (%)	Percentage of fractures of pelvic ring and acetabulum in adults (%)
61-A1	342	170	512	4.79	3.69
61-A2	2,862	2,129	4,991	46.67	35.99
61-A3	1,036	2,381	3,417	31.95	24.64
61-B1	449	324	773	7.23	5.57
61-B2	276	143	419	3.92	3.02
61-B3	43	36	79	0.74	0.57
61-C1	238	126	364	3.40	2.62
61-C2	66	26	92	0.86	0.66
61-C3	31	16	47	0.44	0.34
Total	5,343	5,351	10,694	100.00	77.11

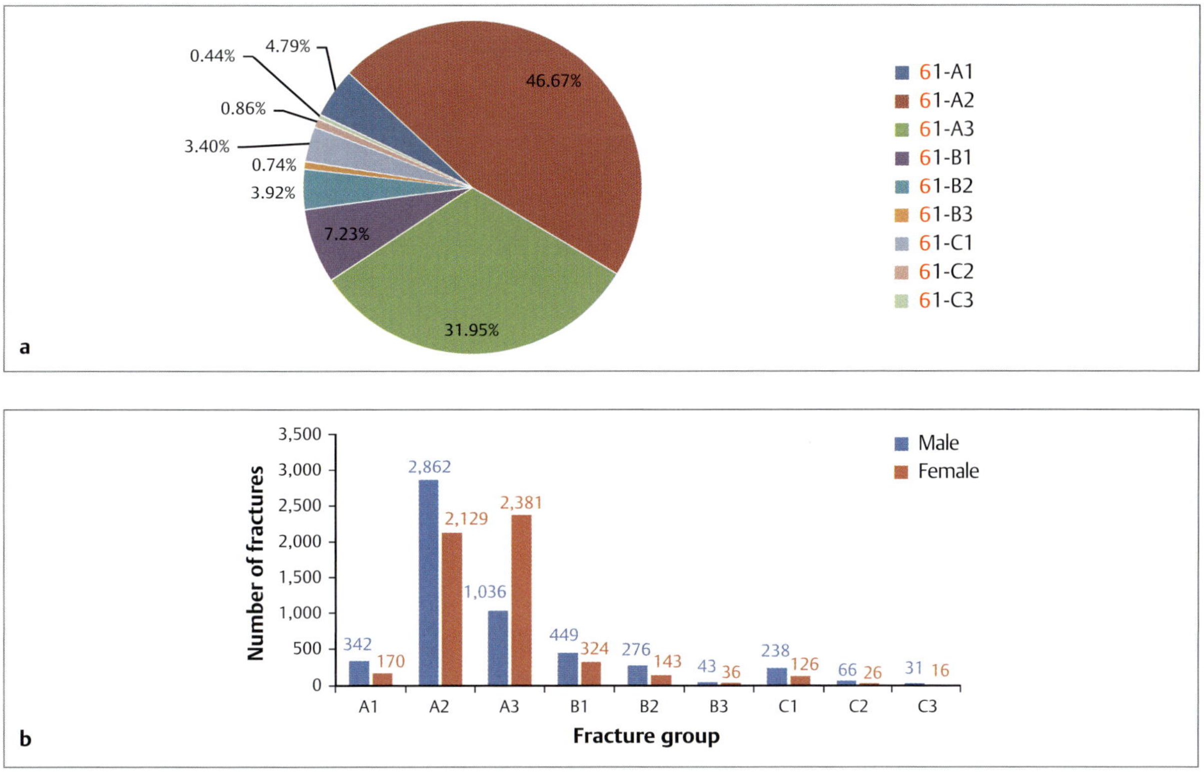

Fig. 7.10 **(a)** Fracture group distribution of 10,694 fractures of segment 61.
(b) Sex and fracture group distribution of 10,694 fractures of segment 61.

61-A Pelvic ring posterior arch intact, stable fractures

61-A1
Avulsion fracture
512 fractures
M: 342 (66.8%)
F: 170 (33.2%)
0.14% of total adult fractures
3.69% of adult pelvic ring and acetabulum
4.79% of segment 61
5.74% of type 61-A

61-A1.1

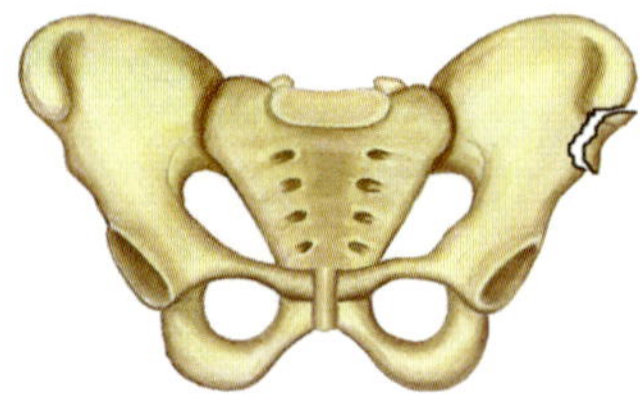

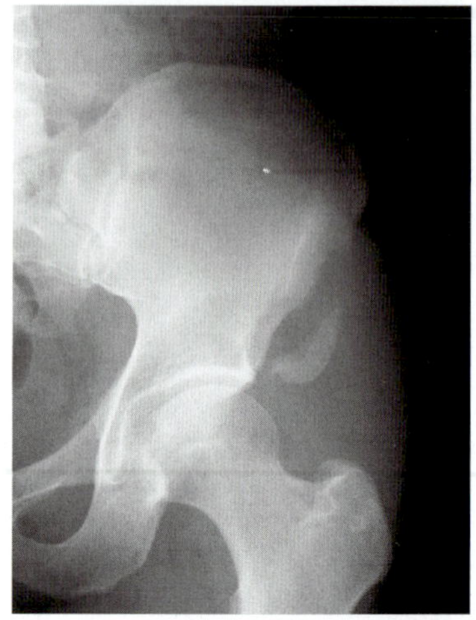

Fracture involving anterior superior iliac spine, anterior inferior iliac spine, or pubic spine

61-A1.2

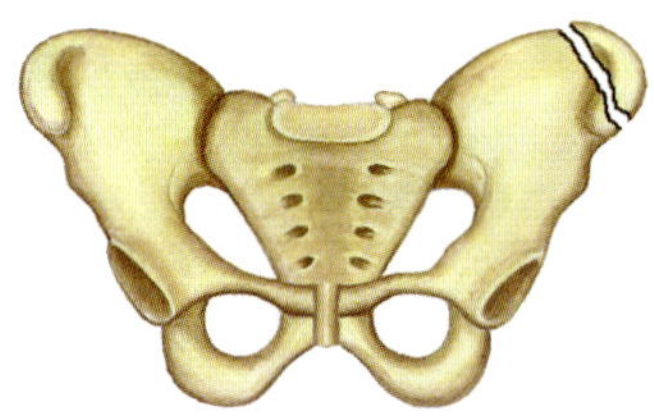

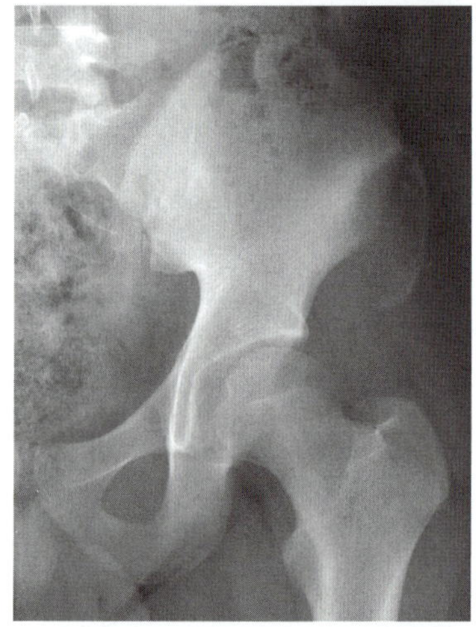

Iliac crest

61-A1.3

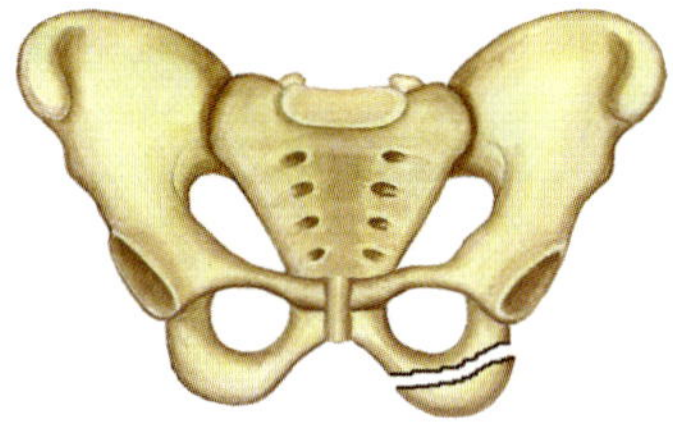

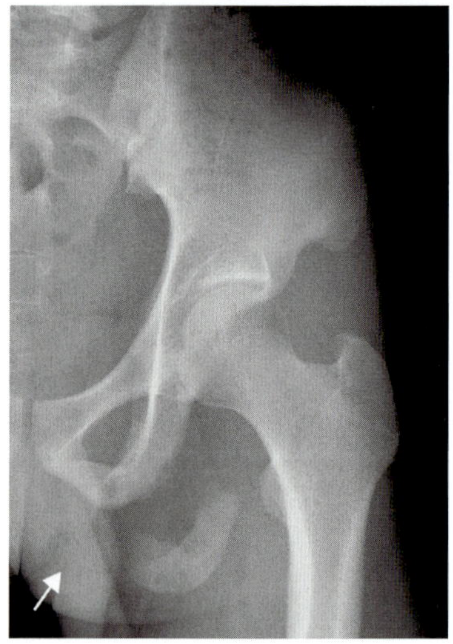

Ischial tuberosity

61-A Pelvic ring posterior arch intact, stable fractures

61-A2

Stable iliac wing fracture or minimally displaced fractures of the pelvic ring (result of a direct blow to the ilium)

4,991 fractures
M: 2,862 (57.34%)
F: 2,129 (42.66%)
1.33% of total adult fractures
35.99% of adult pelvic ring and acetabulum
46.67% of segment 61
55.95% of type 61-A

61-A2.1

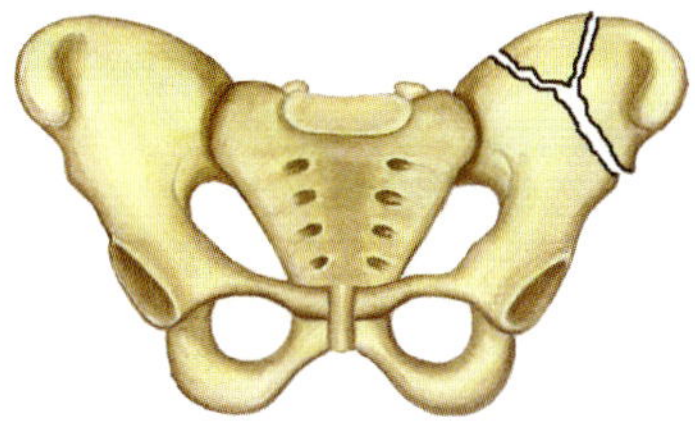

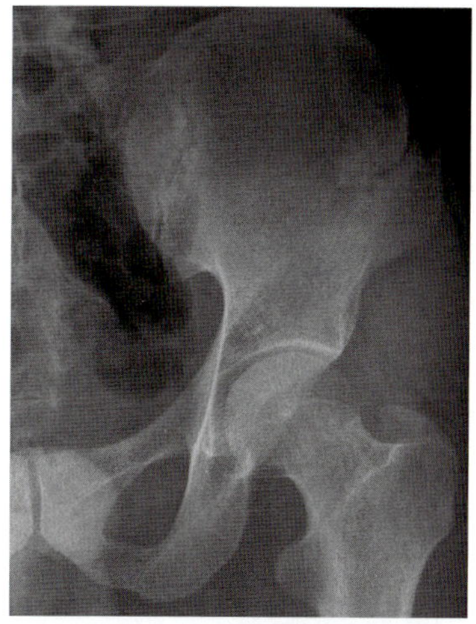

Iliac wing fracture, with one or more fragments

61-A2.2

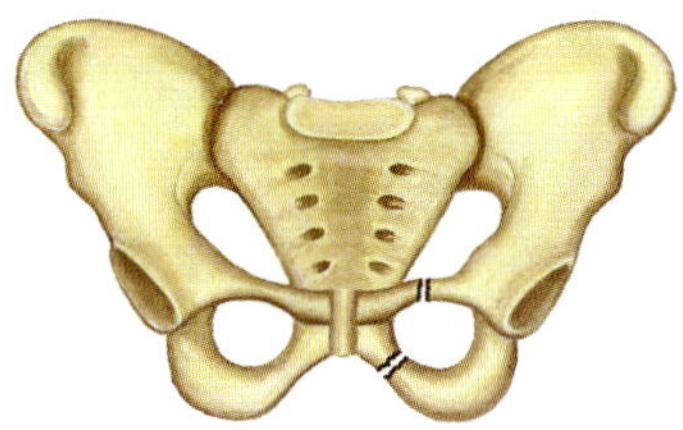

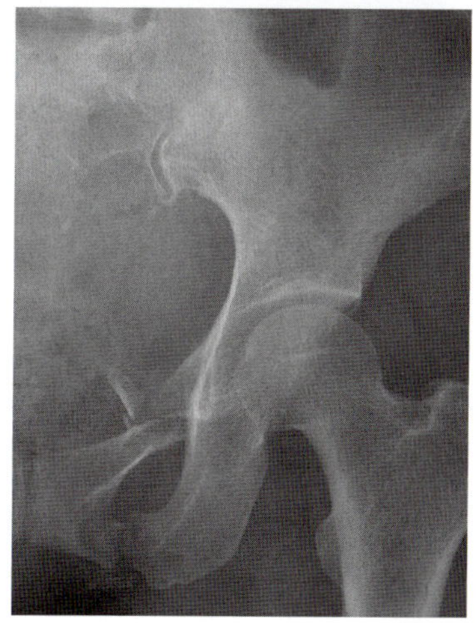

Unilateral pubic rami fracture

61-A2.3

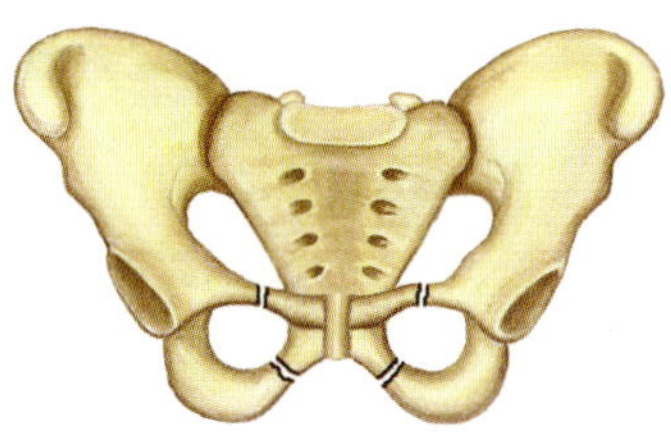

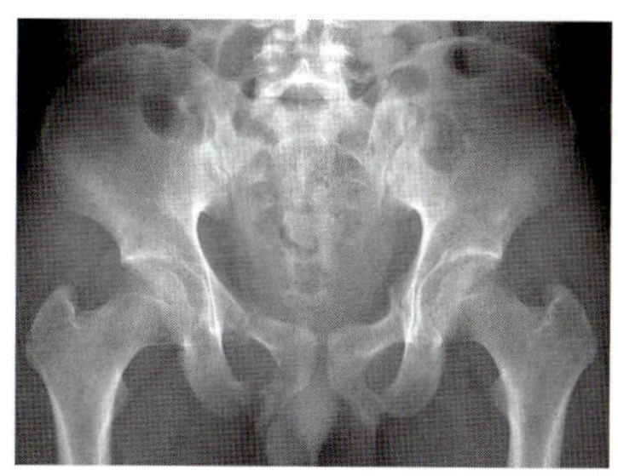

Bilateral pubic rami fracture

61-A Pelvic ring posterior arch intact, stable fractures

61-A3
Transverse fractures of the coccyx and sacrum
3,417 fractures
M: 1,036 (30.32%)
F: 2,381 (69.68%)
0.91% of total adult fractures
24.64% of adult pelvic ring and acetabulum
31.95% of segment 61
38.31% of type 61-A

61-A3.1

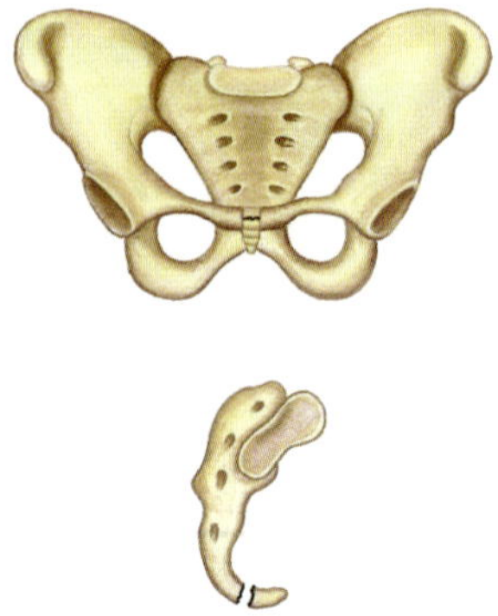

Sacrococcygeal dislocation

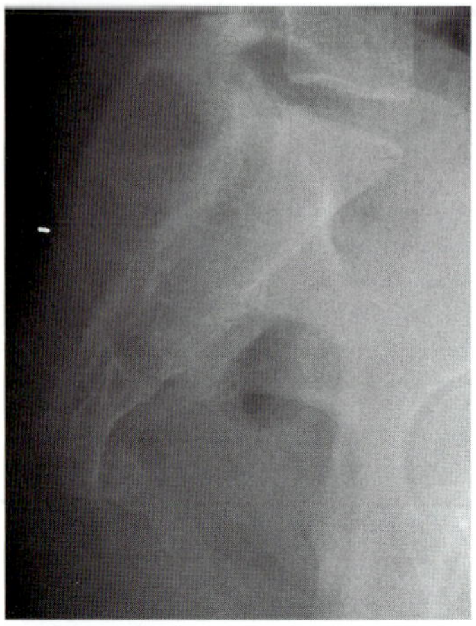

61-A3.2

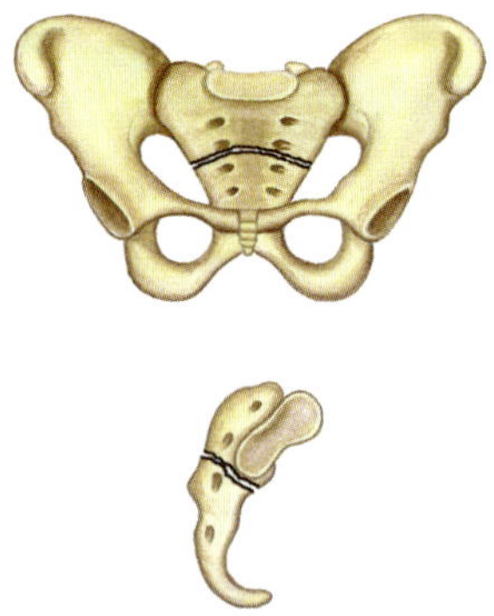

Nondisplaced sacral fracture

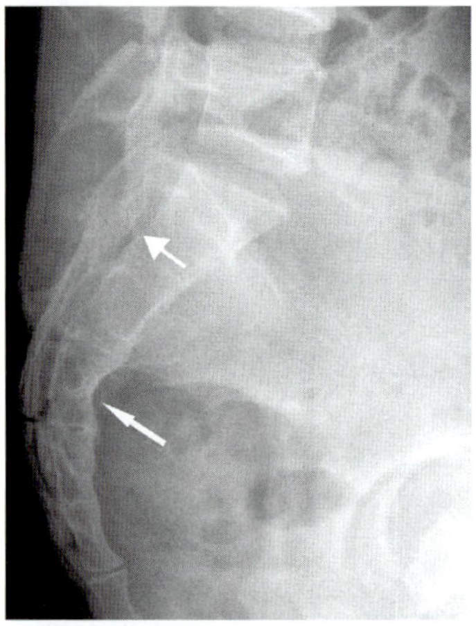

61-A3.3

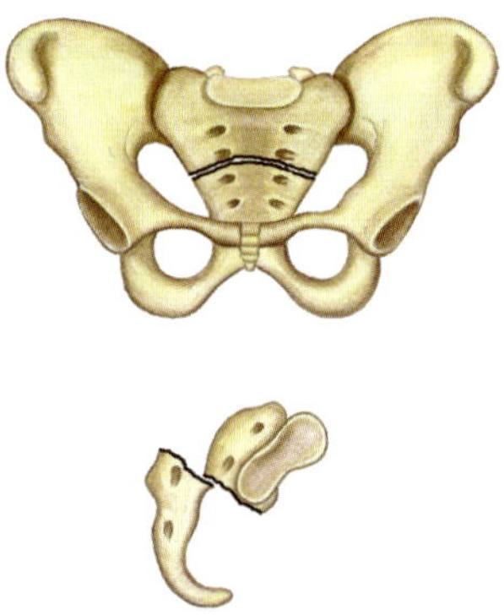

Displaced sacral fracture

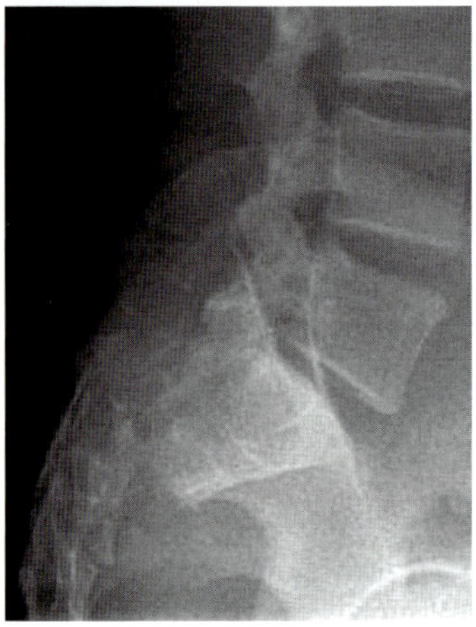

61-B Pelvic ring incomplete posterior arch disruption, partial stable fractures

61-B1
Unilateral open book injury (external rotational instability)
773 fractures
M: 449 (58.09%)
F: 324 (41.91%)
0.21% of total adult fractures
5.57% of adult pelvic ring and acetabulum
7.23% of segment 61
60.82% of type 61-B

*A injury includes: ipsilateral pubic or pubic rami fracture; contralateral pubic or pubic rami fracture; bilateral pubic or pubic rami fracture; isolated symphysis pubis separation ≥ 2.5 cm; isolated symphysis pubis separation < 2.5 cm; isolated symphysis separation, or locked; symphysis separation + ipsilateral pubic or ramus fracture; symphysis separation + contralateral pubic or ramus fracture; symphysis separation + bilateral pubic or rami fracture; without anterior lesion

61-B1.1

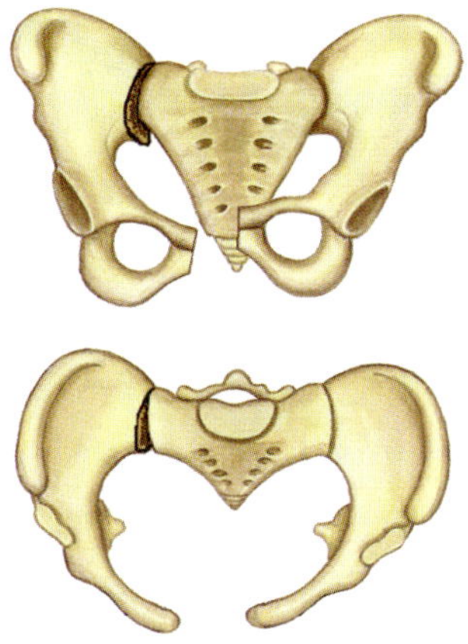

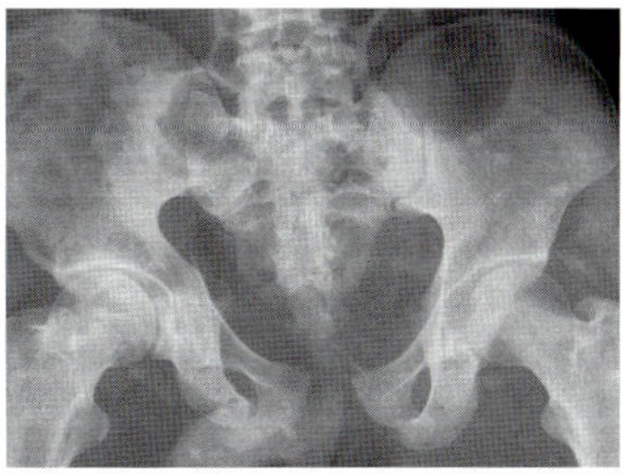

Anterior sacroiliac joint disruption + A injury*

61-B1.2

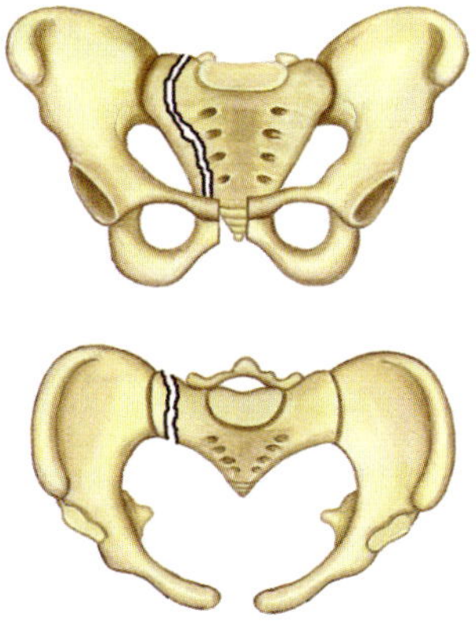

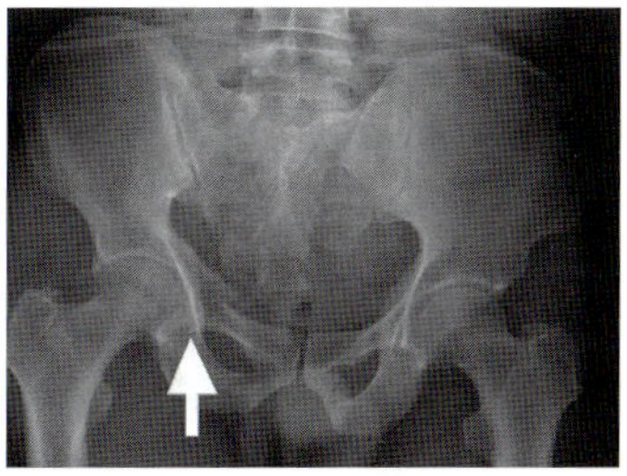

Sacral fracture + A injury*

61-B Pelvic ring incomplete posterior arch disruption, partial stable fractures

61-B2
Lateral compression injury (internal rotational instability)
419 fractures
M: 276 (65.87%)
F: 143 (34.13%)
0.11% of total adult fractures
3.02% of adult pelvic ring and acetabulum
3.92% of segment 61
32.97 % of type 61-B

*A injury includes: ipsilateral pubic or pubic rami fracture; contralateral pubic or pubic rami fracture; bilateral pubic or pubic rami fracture; isolated symphysis pubis separation ≥ 2.5 cm; isolated symphysis pubis separation < 2.5 cm; isolated symphysis separation, or locked; symphysis separation + ipsilateral pubic or ramus fracture; symphysis separation + contralateral pubic or ramus fracture; symphysis separation + bilateral pubic or rami fracture; without anterior lesion

61-B2.1

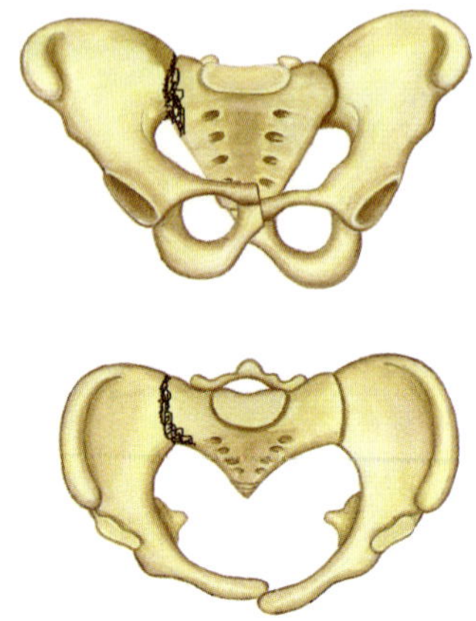

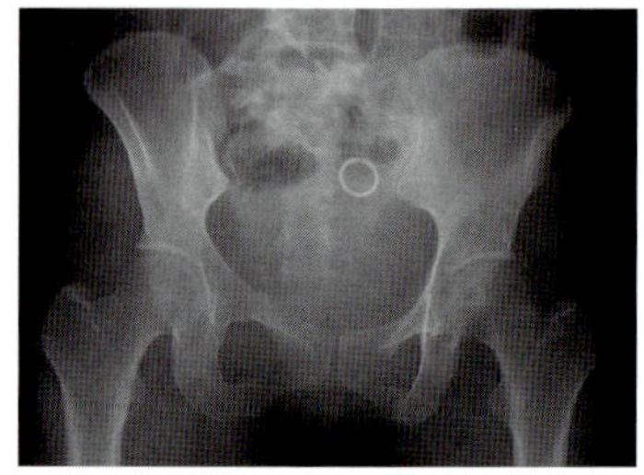

Ipsilateral, anterior sacral buckle fracture + A injury*

61-B2.2

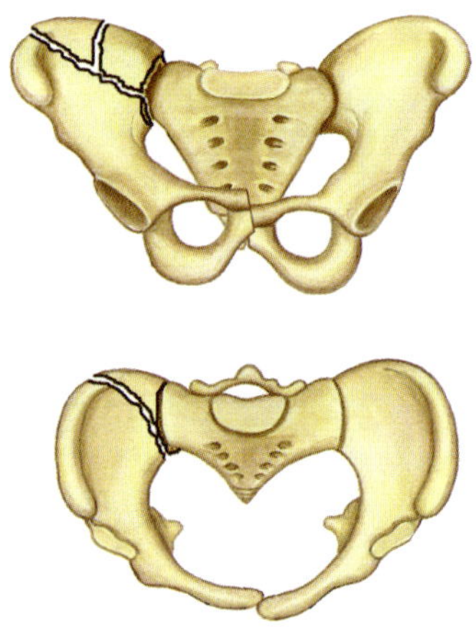

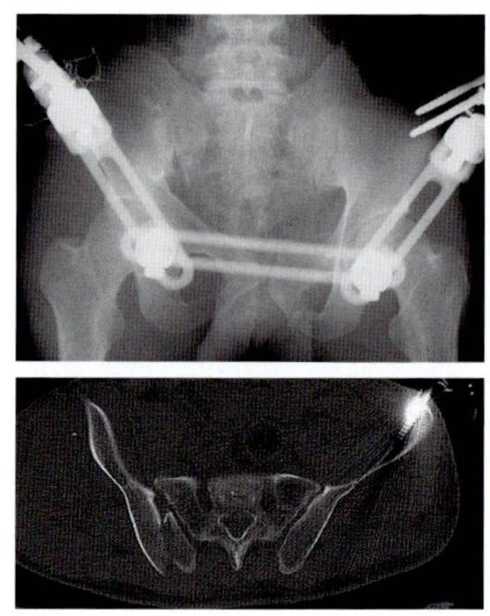

Contralateral, partial sacroiliac joint fracture/subluxation (bucket handle) + A injury*

61-B2.3

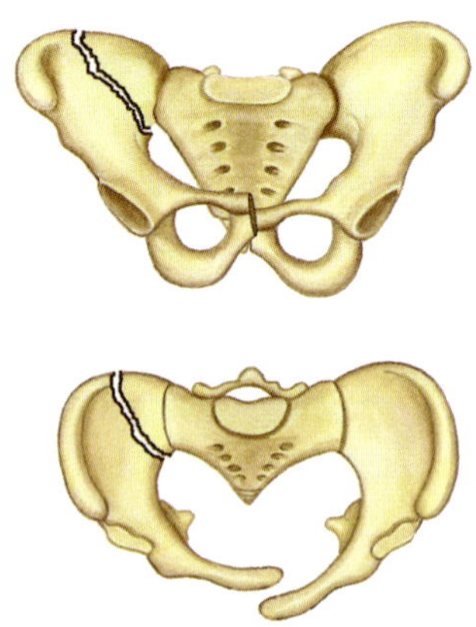

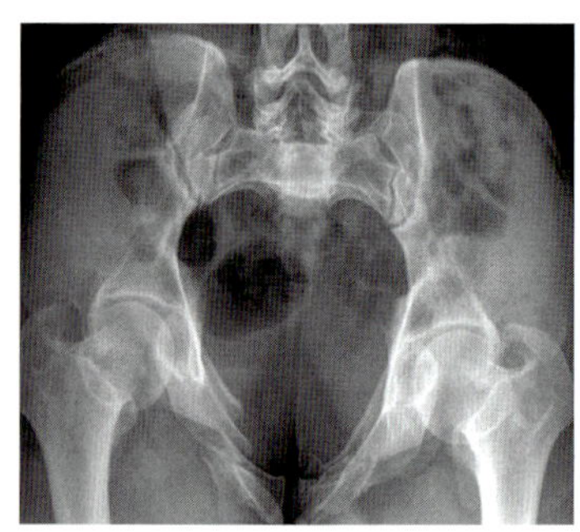

Incomplete posterior iliac fracture + A injury*

61-B Pelvic ring incomplete posterior arch disruption, partial stable fractures

61-B3
Bilateral type B injury
79 fractures
M: 43 (54.43%)
F: 36 (45.57%)
0.02% of total adult fractures
0.57% of adult pelvic ring and acetabulum
0.74% of segment 61
6.22% of type 61-B

61-B3.1

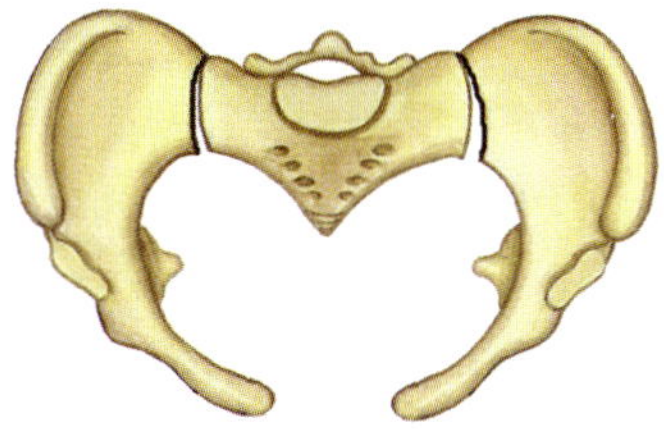

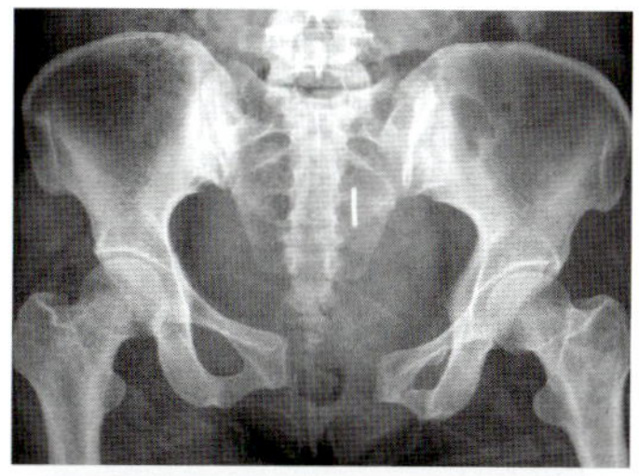

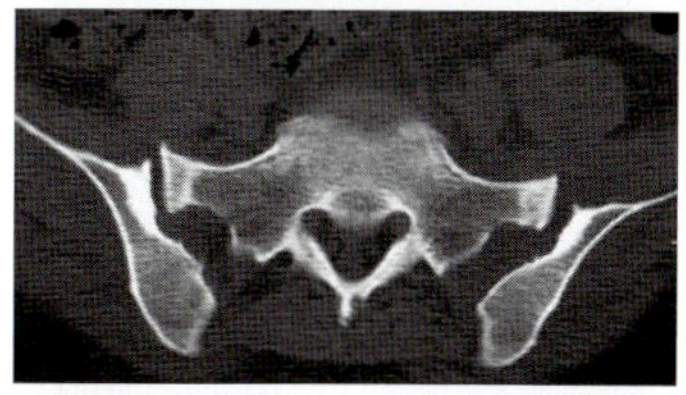

Bilateral type B1 injury

61-B3.2

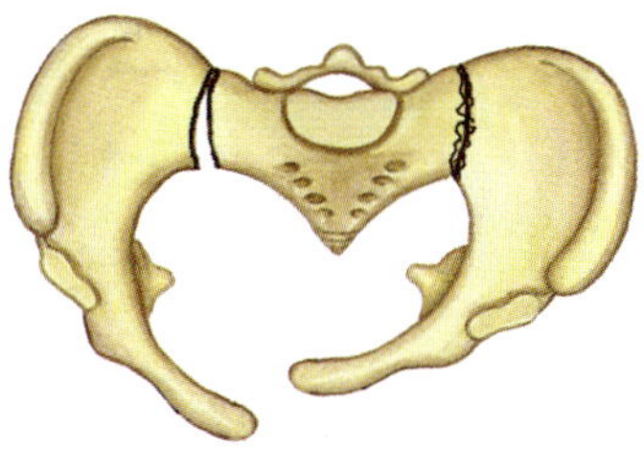

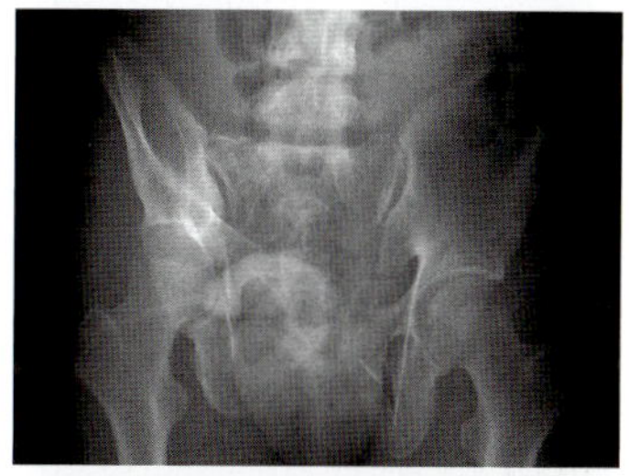

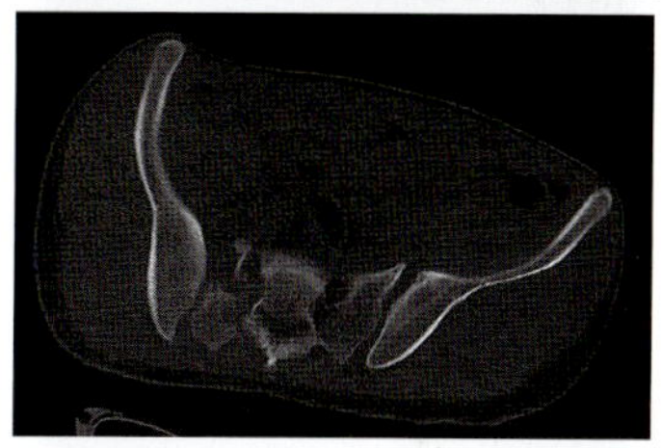

One side type B1 injury, the other side type B2 injury

61-B3.3

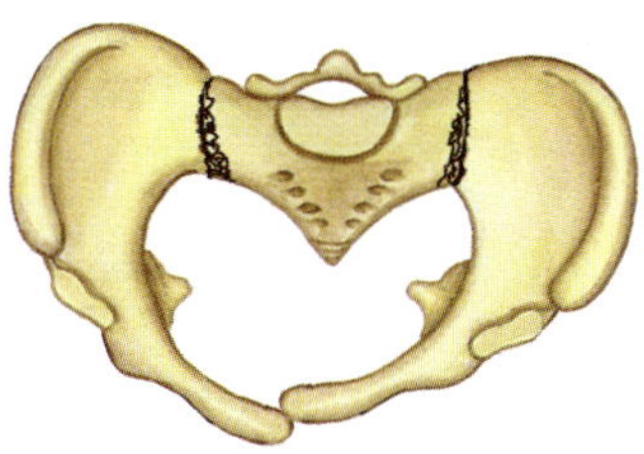

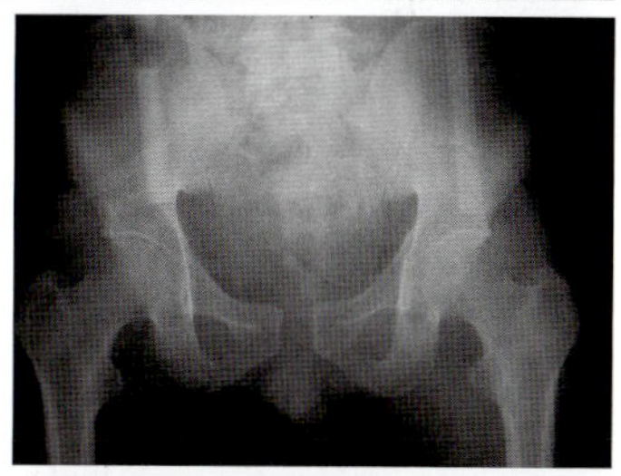

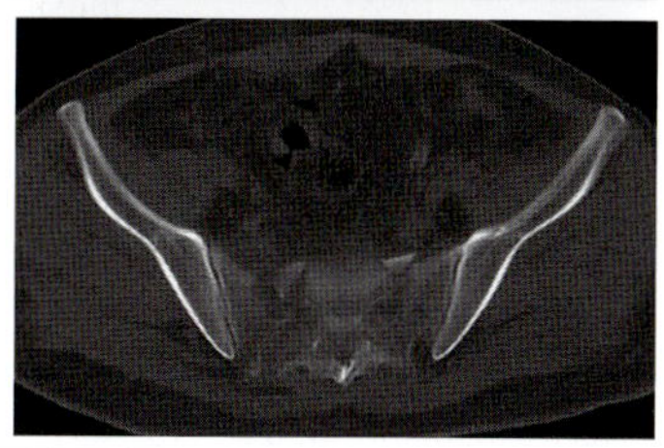

Bilateral type B2 injury

61-C Pelvic ring complete posterior arch disruption, unstable fractures

61-C1
Unilateral
364 fractures
M: 238 (65.38%)
F: 126 (34.62%)
0.1% of total adult fractures
2.62% of adult pelvic ring and acetabulum
3.4% of segment 61
72.37% of type 61-C

61-C1.1

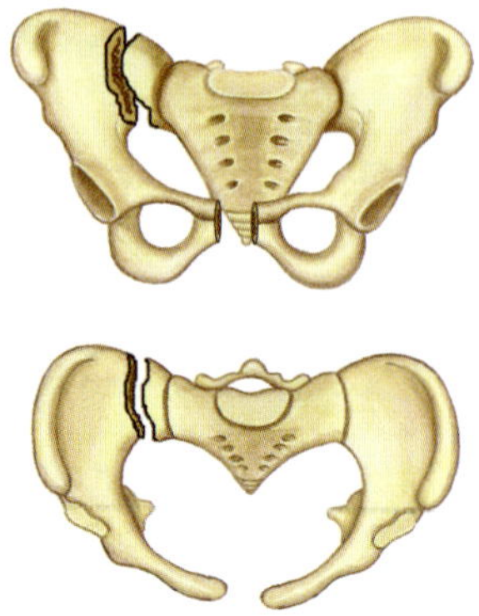

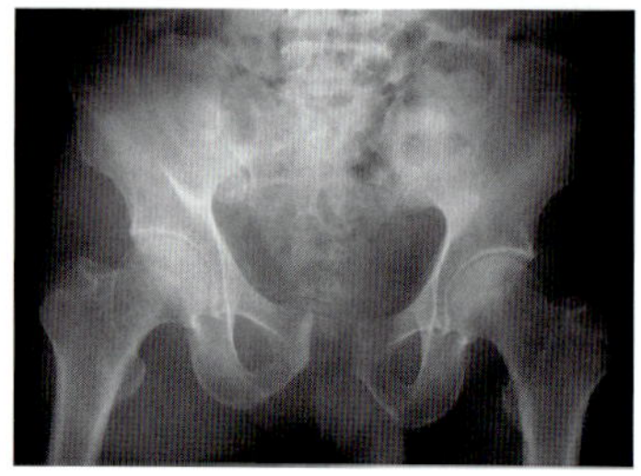

Fracture of ilium + A injury*

61-C1.2

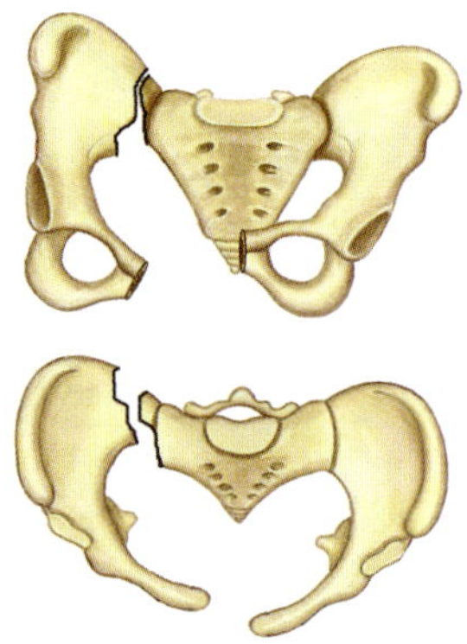

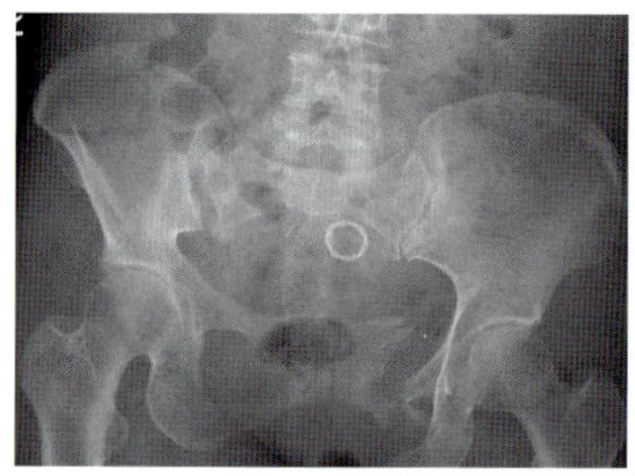

Sacroiliac dislocation or fracture dislocation + A injury*

61-C1.3

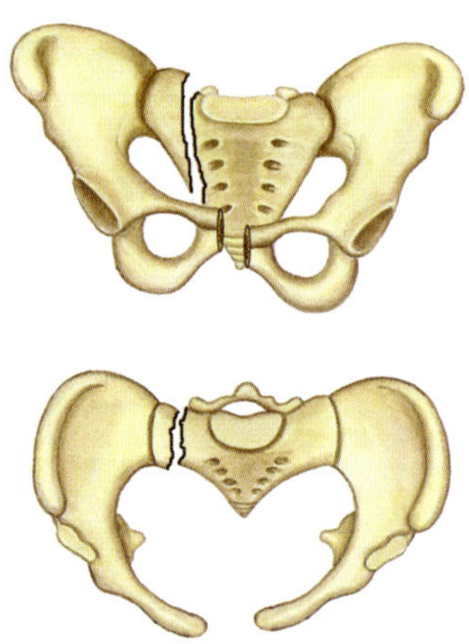

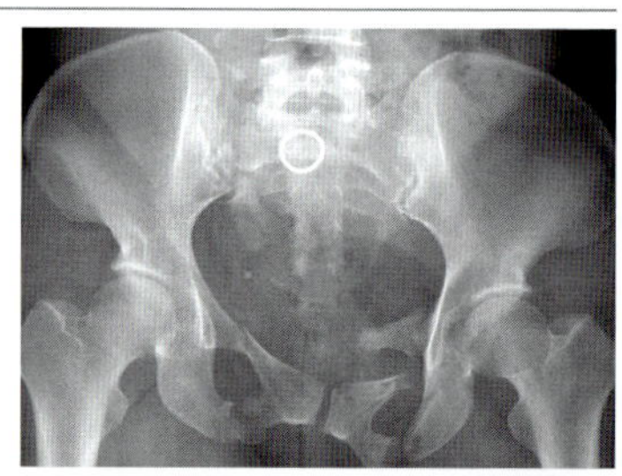

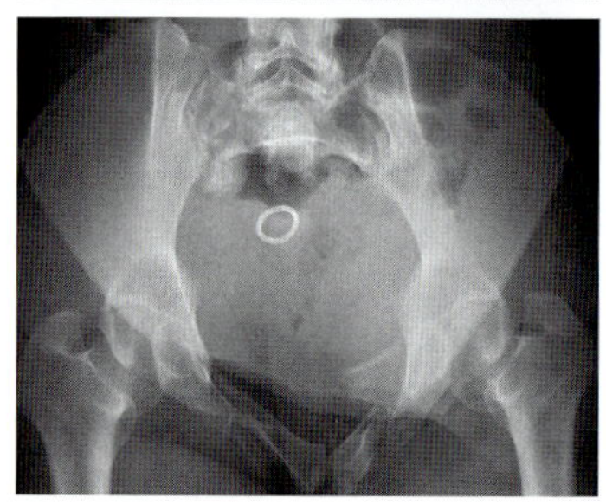

Fracture of sacrum (lateral, medial, or through the sacral foramina) + A injury*

*A injury includes: ipsilateral pubic or pubic rami fracture; contralateral pubic or pubic rami fracture; bilateral pubic or pubic rami fracture; isolated symphysis pubis separation ≥ 2.5 cm; isolated symphysis pubis separation < 2.5 cm; isolated symphysis separation, or locked; symphysis separation + ipsilateral pubic or ramus fracture; symphysis separation + contralateral pubic or ramus fracture; symphysis separation + bilateral pubic or rami fracture; without anterior lesion

61-C Pelvic ring complete posterior arch disruption, unstable fractures

61-C2
Bilateral, one side type B, the other side type C
92 fractures
M: 66 (71.74%)
F: 26 (28.26%)
0.02% of total adult fractures
0.66% of adult pelvic ring and acetabulum
0.86% of segment 61
18.29% of type 61-C

*A injury includes: ipsilateral pubic or pubic rami fracture; contralateral pubic or pubic rami fracture; bilateral pubic or pubic rami fracture; isolated symphysis pubis separation ≥ 2.5 cm; isolated symphysis pubis separation < 2.5 cm; isolated symphysis separation, or locked; symphysis separation + ipsilateral pubic or ramus fracture; symphysis separation + contralateral pubic or ramus fracture; symphysis separation + bilateral pubic or rami fracture; without anterior lesion

61-C2.1

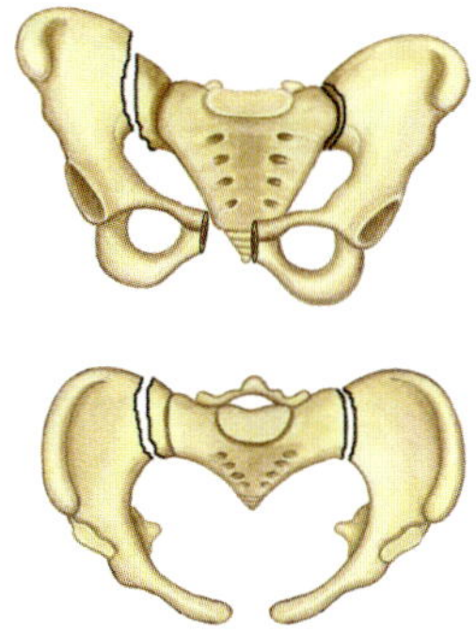
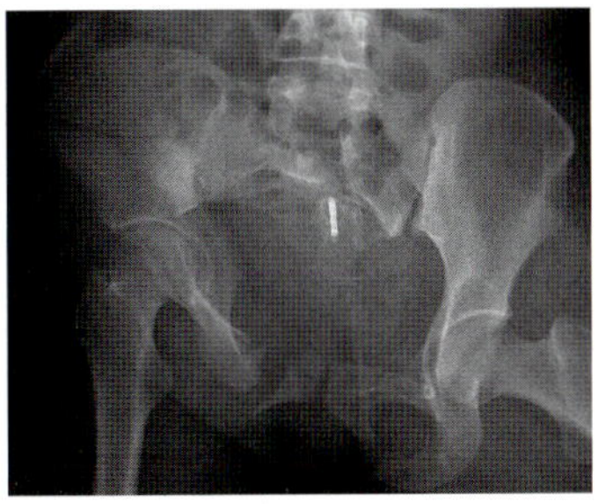

Ipsilateral C1 lesion through the ilium, contralateral B1 or B2 injury + A injury*

61-C2.2

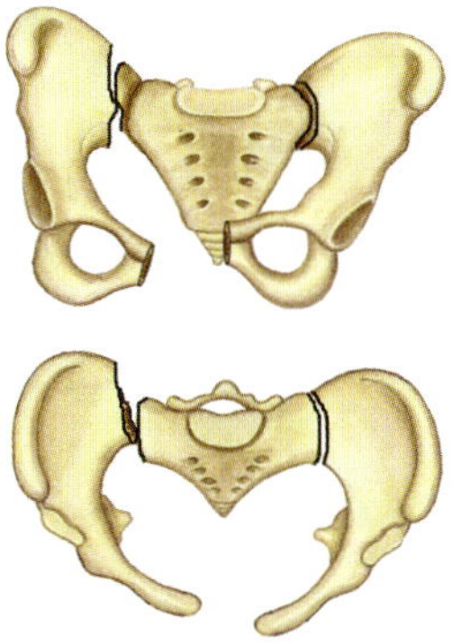
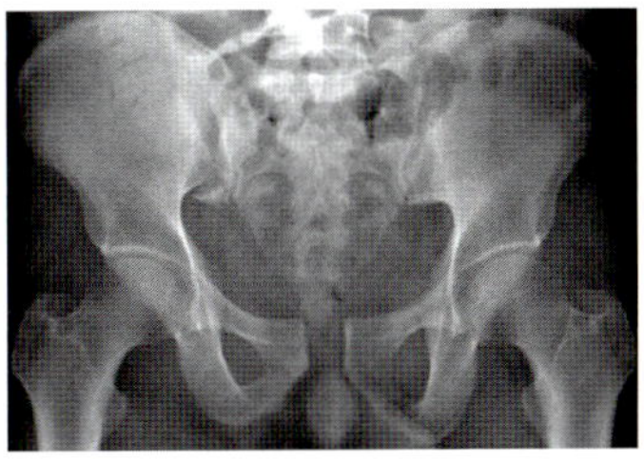

Ipsilateral C1 lesion through the sacroiliac joint (transiliac fracture dislocation, pure dislocation, transsacral fracture dislocation), contralateral B1 or B2 injury + A injury*

61-C2.3

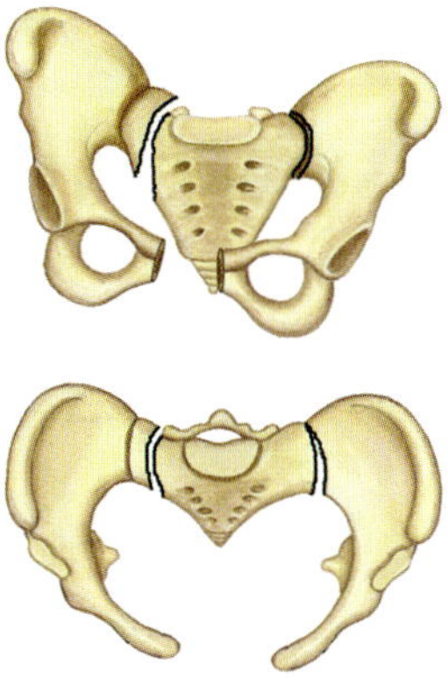
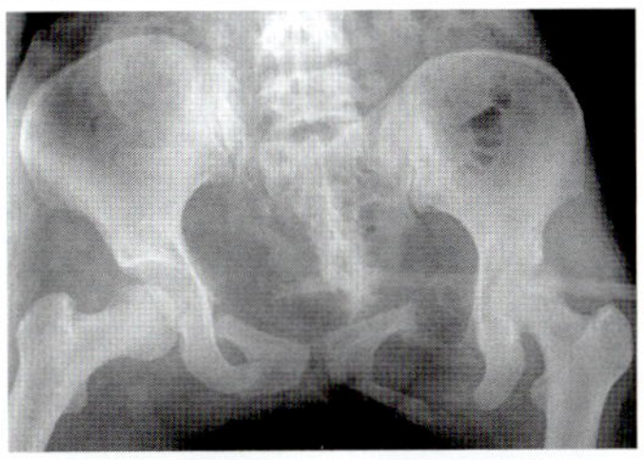
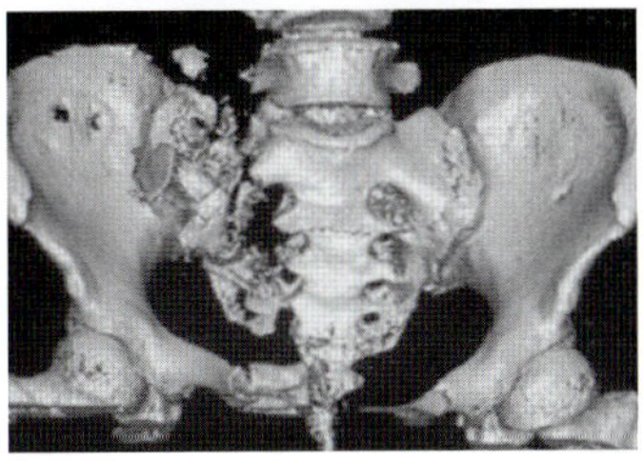

Ipsilateral C1 lesion through the sacrum (lateral, medial, or through the sacral foramina) contralateral B1 or B2 injury + A injury*

61-C Pelvic ring complete posterior arch disruption, unstable fracture

61-C3
Bilateral, both type C
47 fractures
M: 31 (65.96%)
F: 16 (34.04%)
0.01% of total adult fractures
0.34% of adult pelvic ring and acetabulum
0.44% of segment 61
9.34% of type 61-C

61-C3.1

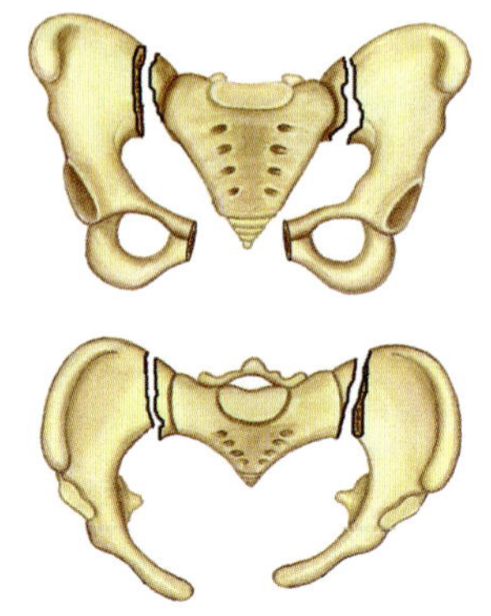

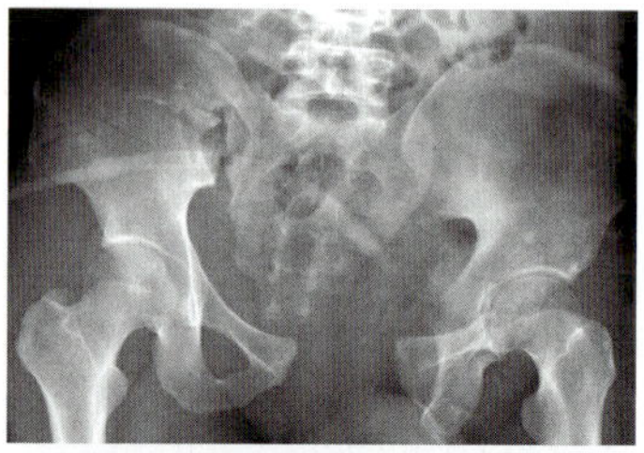

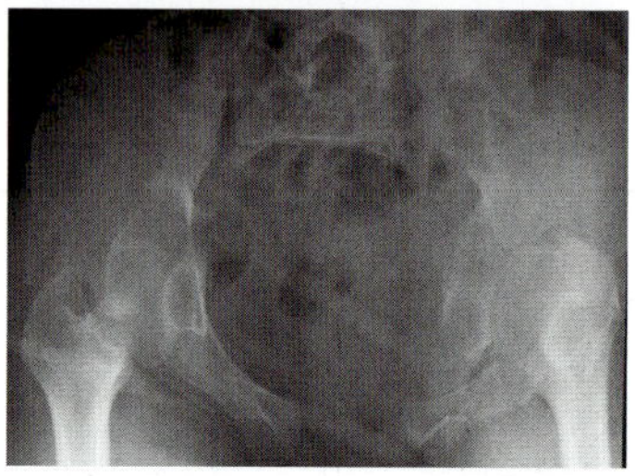

Extrasacral on both sides (ilium, transiliac SI joint fracture/dislocation, transsacral SI joint fracture/dislocation, SI joint dislocation)

61-C3.2

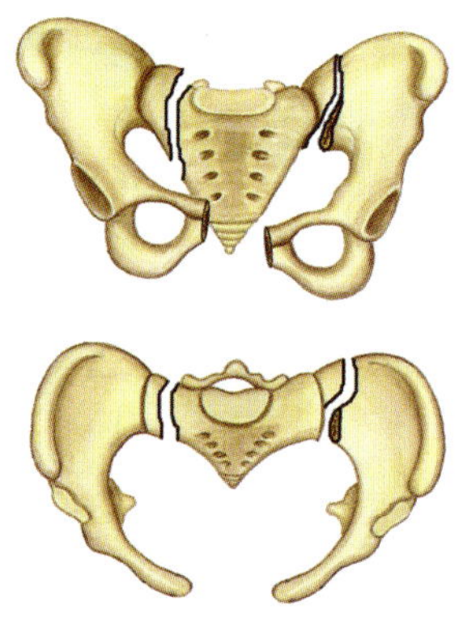

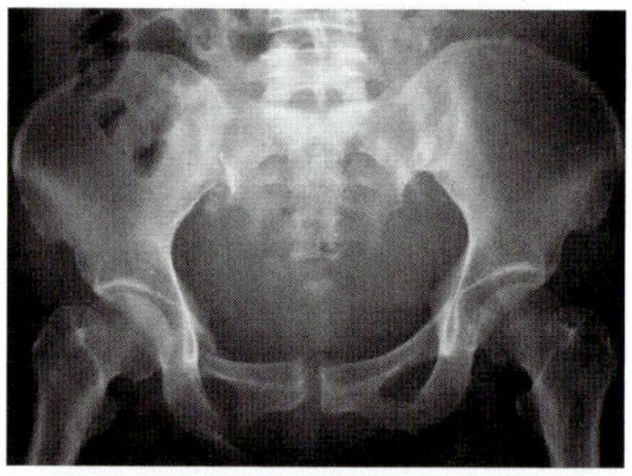

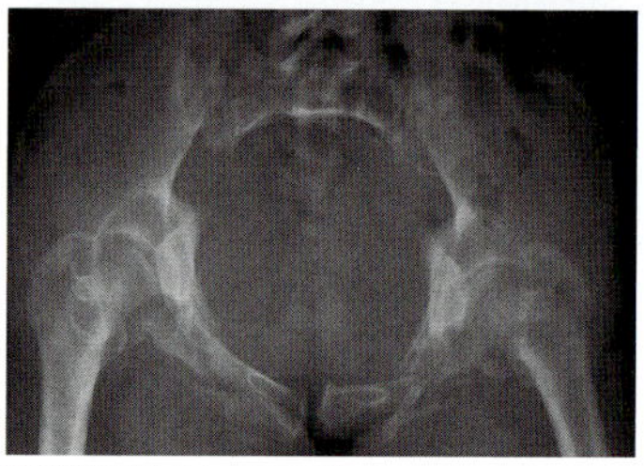

One side C1 lesion through the sacrum (lateral, medial or through the sacral foramina), the other side extra sacral lesion + A injury*

61-C3.3

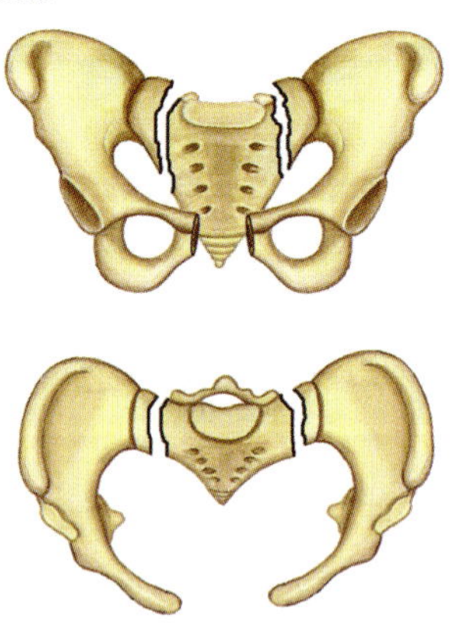

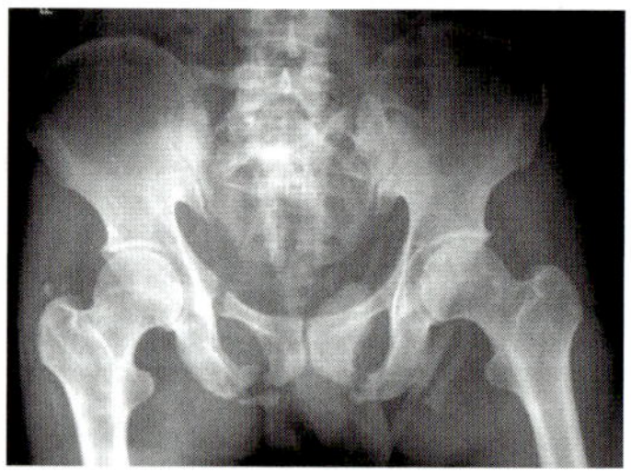

Sacral lesion on both sides (lateral, medial, or through the sacral foramina)0 + A injury*

*A injury includes: ipsilateral pubic or pubic rami fracture; contralateral pubic or pubic rami fracture; bilateral pubic or pubic rami fracture; isolated symphysis pubis separation ≥ 2.5 cm; isolated symphysis pubis separation < 2.5 cm; isolated symphysis separation, or locked; symphysis separation + ipsilateral pubic or ramus fracture; symphysis separation + contralateral pubic or ramus fracture; symphysis separation + bilateral pubic or rami fracture; without anterior lesion

Injury Mechanism

Pelvic ring fractures involve direct or indirect mechanisms. The direct mechanism includes a direct blow, motor vehicle crash, crush injury, fall, etc. Based on the direction of the force, the injury mechanisms can be classified into the following types: anteroposterior (AP) compression, lateral compression, and vertical shear. Different forces can result in different types of pelvic ring fractures. Indirect forces usually result in avulsion fractures from the traction of muscles or tendons.

The force of anteroposterior compression usually produces an "open-book"-type injury, that is, a symphysis disruption, by acting on the posterior superior spine and symphysis pubis, or by forced external rotation through the hip joints unilaterally or bilaterally. If more force is applied, the anterior ligaments of the sacroiliac joint and the sacrospinous ligament may also be injured, and the posterior dislocation of the sacroiliac joint, which is the traditional dislocation of the sacroiliac joint, may occur. In rare conditions, enormous anteroposterior force can lead to anterior dislocation of the sacroiliac joint, in which the ilium dislocates anterior to the sacrum and often combines with symphyseal diastasis and fractures of pubic rami and ilia. Different locations upon which the AP compression is applied may lead to different types of open-book injuries.

The force of lateral compression can be transmitted by a direct blow to the iliac crest, often causing an internal rotation of the hemipelvis, or the so called "bucket-handle" fracture. Lateral compression may also cause an ipsilateral injury through the femoral head, occasionally causing contralateral injury. The injuries caused by internal rotation account for the majority of pelvic fractures.

Shearing forces in the vertical plane can cause marked displacement of bony structures of the pelvic ring, and gross disruption of soft tissue structures.

Complex forces, resulting from a combination of these injury patterns, often cause associated acetabular fractures. The most common combined mechanism is lateral compression and vertical shearing. The combined injury of the acetabulum and posterior pelvic ring can be described by three patterns: acetabular fractures, associated with ipsilateral, contralateral, or bilateral posterior pelvic ring injuries.

Diagnosis

Pelvic ring injuries are generally high-energy fractures and frequently associated with multiple injuries. Evaluation of the patient should begin with an initial assessment to form a general impression of the degree or severity of the injury, such as to assess hemodynamic status, and the presence of other severe associated injuries. Physical examination should note the morphology of the pelvis and hip joint, as well as the function of the lower extremities. A careful examination of the painful area should be performed. The pelvic compression and separation test, Gaenslen's maneuver, and the Yeoman test can be used to assess an injury and point to appropriate imaging studies.

The radiographic evaluation includes the anteroposterior (AP), inlet, outlet, and Judet views of the pelvis. An AP pelvis is usually sufficient to uncover most pelvic injuries. Abnormalities depicted on the AP view can direct the need for the next set of radiographs, which usually include inlet and outlet views of the pelvis in pelvic ring fractures, and Judet (oblique) radiographs of the pelvis in acetabular fractures. Inlet radiographs of the pelvis allow the evaluation of pelvic brim integrity, AP displacement of the hemipelvis, internal/external rotation of the hemipelvis, and sacral impaction. Outlet views of the pelvis allow for confirmation of vertical displacement of the hemipelvis. Judet views of the pelvis illustrate the anterior and posterior columns of the acetabulum, free of superimposition. Computed tomography (CT) or magnetic resonance imaging (MRI) should be performed when plain diagnostic radiographs are inconclusive, with regard to pelvic fractures, or the presence of concomitant visceral or neurovascular injuries are suspected.

Treatment

Patients with hemodynamic instability require emergency rehydration, and temporary stabilization of pelvic fractures, such as by pelvic ring pocket and external fixation, to decrease hemorrhage. Interventional radiology therapy can be applied if necessary. For instance, patients who sustain type B or C injuries often have concomitant severe bony and soft tissue injuries, for example, massive internal bleeding is commonly associated with complete sacroiliac joint disruption. To prevent recurrence of hemorrhage in such patients, temporary fracture stabilization should be performed.

For hemodynamically stable patients, surgical intervention should be performed 5–7 days after the injury. Either an external fixation device or open reduction fixation is used for isolated anterior arch fractures. The treatment of choice for unstable pelvic fractures is anatomical reduction and rigid internal fixation. In addition, minimally invasive methods, such as percutaneous iliosacral screw fixation for fracture dislocations of the sacroiliac joint, are increasingly applied in the clinical setting. The sacral pedicle axial view projection is an optimal radiographic technique for percutaneous placement of iliosacral screws in clinical practice. AO classification of pelvis fractures provides a guide in selecting appropriate surgical plans: type A2 and B1 injuries, in which symphysis separation is less than 2.5 cm, can be managed nonsurgically; however, if symphysis disruption is greater than 2.5 cm, either an external fixation device or plate fixation can be applied; type B2 injuries, being relatively mild, only require reduction and maintenance in proper position; type B3 injuries with shortening of the limb > 1.5 cm should be considered for internal fixation. Operative reduction and internal fixation should be performed if the fracture fragments protrude into the perineal region. Type C fractures should be treated with an anterior external fixation device combined with skeletal traction (8–12 weeks), or operative reduction and internal fixation. In addition to iliosacral screw fixation, posterior pelvic disruptions can be treated with the use of posterior tension band plate and the minimally invasive adjustable plate (MIAP). The MIAP conforms to the irregular shape of the posterior pelvic ring and can be used without prebending. This plate also has a role in reducing compressed or separated fractures/dislocations. Favorable clinical and radiological outcomes can be achieved in treating posterior pelvic disruptions with MIAP.

Acetabular Fractures (Segment 62)

Anatomical Features

The acetabulum is a hemispherical horseshoe-shaped articular cavity, with a diameter of 3.5 cm, that articulates with the head of the femur. It is formed at the confluence of the ilium, ischium, and pubis, and is situated near the middle of the outer surface of the hip bone, between the anterior superior iliac spine and ischial tuberosity (**Plate 7.10**). The hip joint is enclosed in a strong fibrous capsule and surrounding musculature, which provide a good amount of stability. At the lower brim of the acetabulum is the acetabular notch. The external surface of the acetabulum is partly articular, partly nonarticular; the articular segment forms a curved, crescent moon–shaped surface, the lunate surface; the nonarticular portion contributes to a circular depression, the acetabular fossa, situated at the bottom of the acetabulum, inside which the Haversian gland is located and enhances the depth of the hip joint.

The acetabulum is divided into an anterior and posterior column, and dome (**Plates 7.11** and **7.12**). The anterior column (iliopectineal) begins at the iliac wing and extends down the anterior portion of the acetabulum, through the superior pubic ramus to the symphysis pubis. It is composed of the iliac crest, the iliac spines, the anterior wall, anterior half of the acetabulum, and the superior pubic ramus, and can be divided into three major parts: the iliac, acetabular, and pubic portions. The posterior column (ilioischial line) begins at the sciatic notch and extends down the posterior acetabulum into the ischium. It is composed of dense bone superior to the sciatic notch, posterior wall, and posterior half of the acetabulum and the ischium. The dome, or roof of the acetabulum, formed by the iliac bone, is the weight-bearing surface, making up 40% of the acetabulum.

AO Classification of Acetabular Fractures

Based on the AO fracture classification, the location code for the acetabulum is the number 62. According to fracture patterns, acetabular fractures can be divided into three types: A, partial articular fracture, involving one column; B, partial articular fracture, transverse; and C, complete articular fracture, involving both columns (**Plate 7.13**).

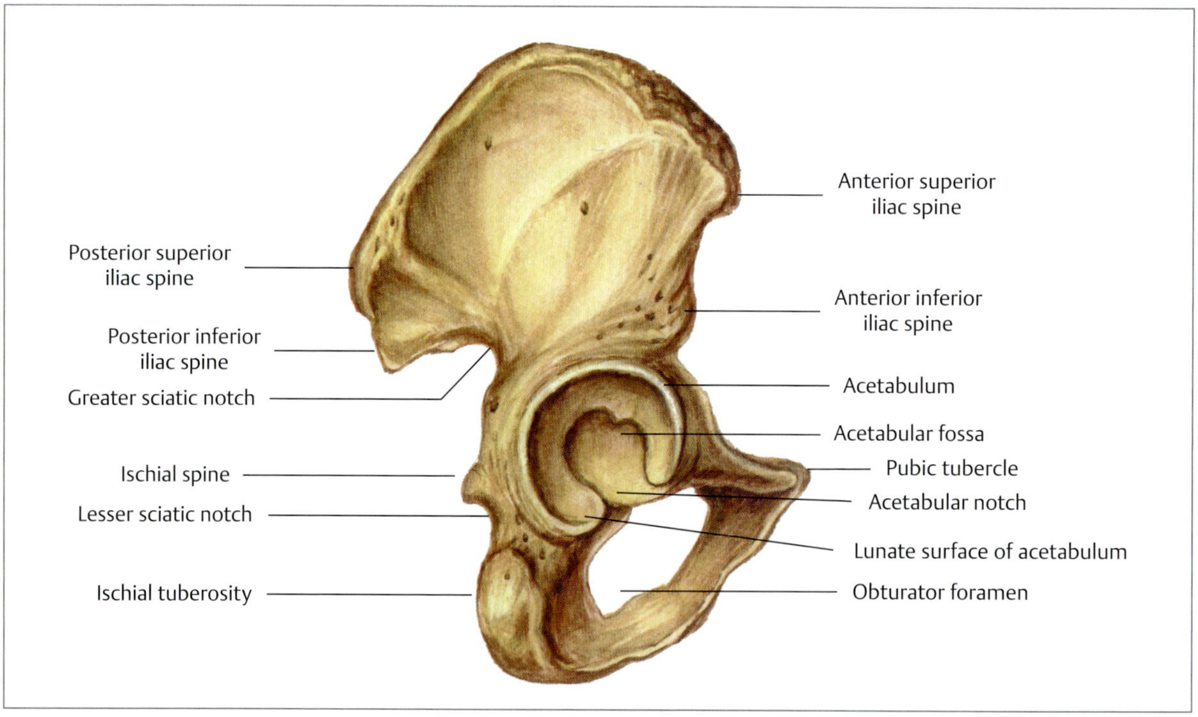

Plate 7.10

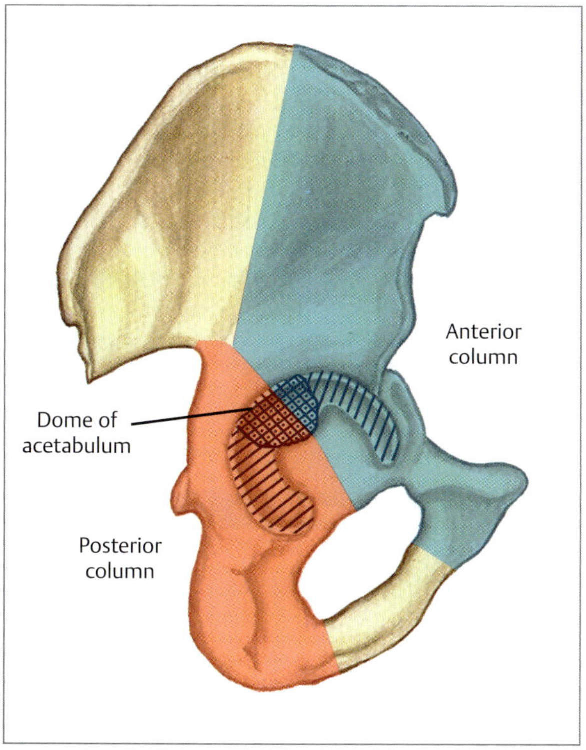

Plate 7.11

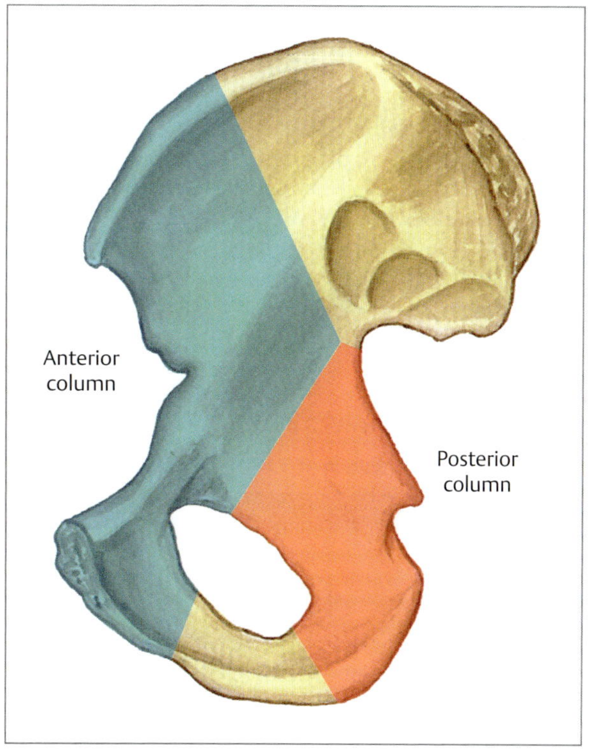

Plate 7.12

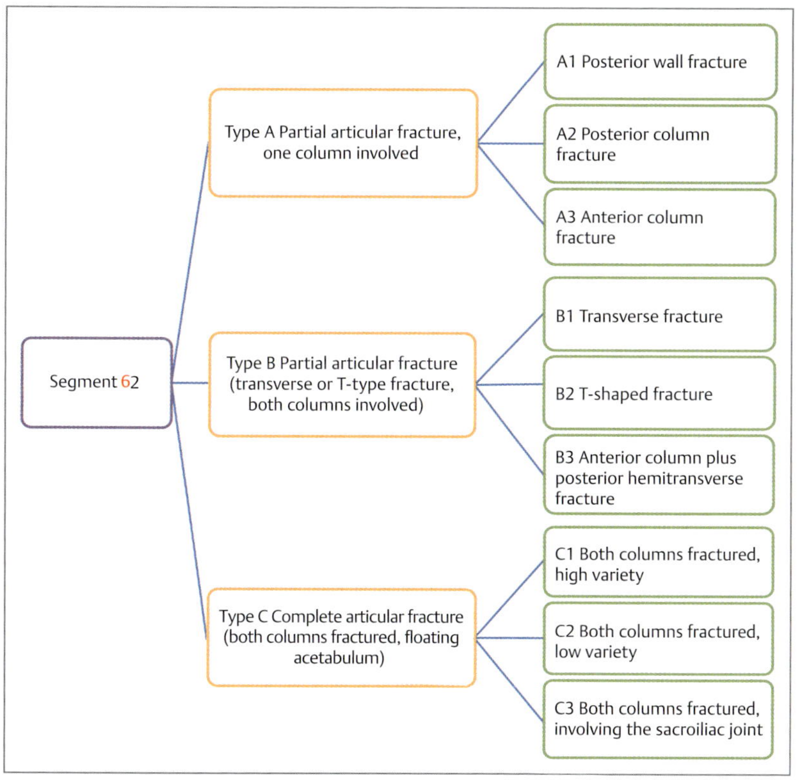

Plate 7.13

Clinical Epidemiologic Features of Acetabular Fractures (Segment 62)

A total of 3,131 adult patients with 3,174 pelvic ring fractures, including 43 patients with bilateral acetabular fracture, were treated in 83 hospitals in China over a 2-year period from 2010 to 2011. All cases were reviewed and statistically studied. Acetabular fractures comprise 22.89% of adult fractures of the pelvic ring and acetabulum.

Epidemiologic features of pelvic ring fractures are the following:

- More males than females
- The high risk age group is 41–45, while age group 36–40 is the high risk group for males, ages 41–45 is the high risk group for females.
- The most common fracture type of segment 62 fractures is type 62-A—the same fracture type for both males and females.
- The most common fracture group of segment 62 fractures is group 62-A1—the same group for males, while the most common fracture group for females is 62-A2.

Fractures of Segment 62 by Sex

Table 7.11 Sex distribution of 3,174 fractures of segment 62

Sex	Number of fractures	Percentage (%)
Male	2,286	72.02
Female	888	27.98
Total	3,174	100.00

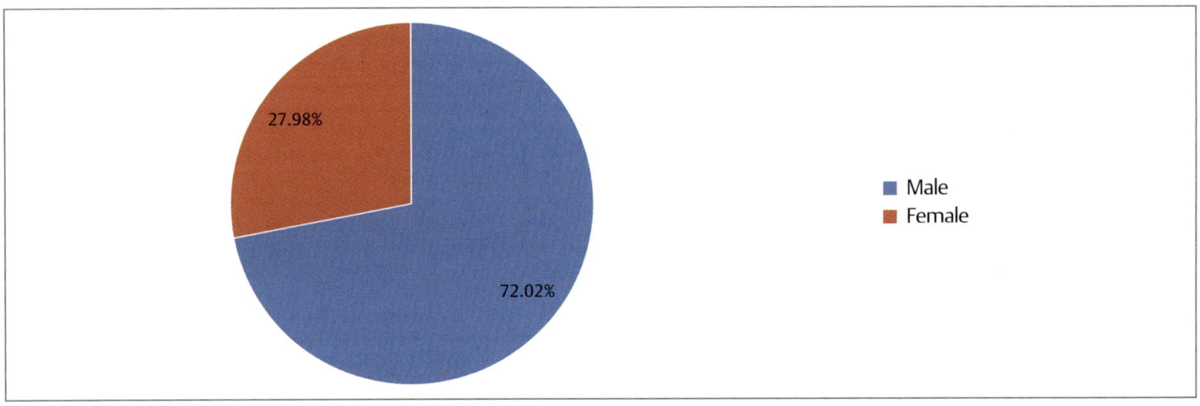

Fig. 7.11 Sex distribution of 3,174 fractures of segment 62.

Fractures of Segment 62 by Fracture Side

Table 7.12 Fracture side distribution of 3,131 patients with fractures of segment 62

Fracture side	Number of patients	Percentage (%)
Left	1,713	54.71
Right	1,375	43.92
Both	43	1.37
Total	3,131	100.00

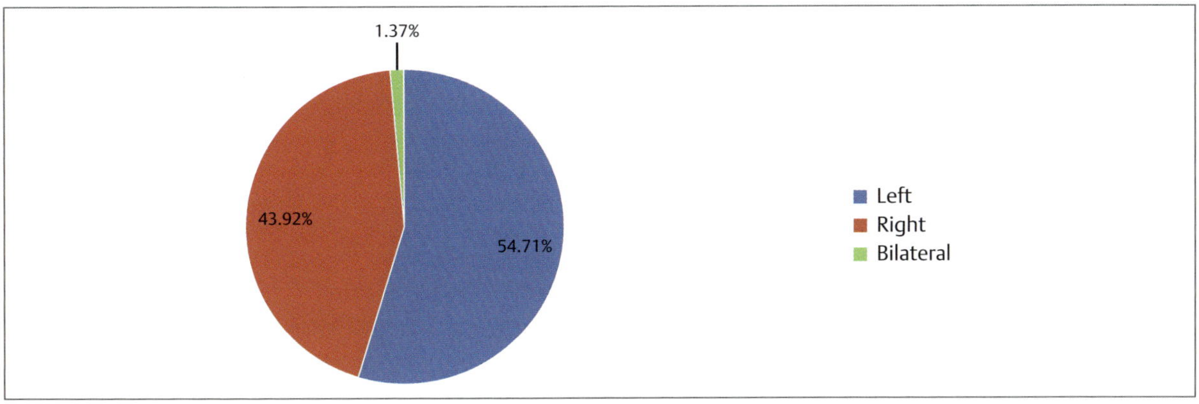

Fig. 7.12 Fracture side distribution of 3,131 patients with fractures of segment 62.

Fractures of Segment 62 by Age Group

Table 7.13 Age and sex distribution of 3,131 fractures of segment 62

Age group (years)	Male	Female	Total number of fractures	Percentage (%)
16–20	89	28	117	3.74
21–25	187	72	259	8.27
26–30	187	50	237	7.57
31–35	239	44	283	9.04
36–40	296	91	387	12.36
41–45	289	118	407	13.00
46–50	262	103	365	11.66
51–55	227	95	322	10.28
56–60	188	78	266	8.50
61–65	98	58	156	4.98
66–70	77	41	118	3.77
71–75	49	33	82	2.62
76–80	33	38	71	2.27
81–85	24	19	43	1.37
≥86	6	12	18	0.57
Total	2,251	880	3,131	100.00

7

7

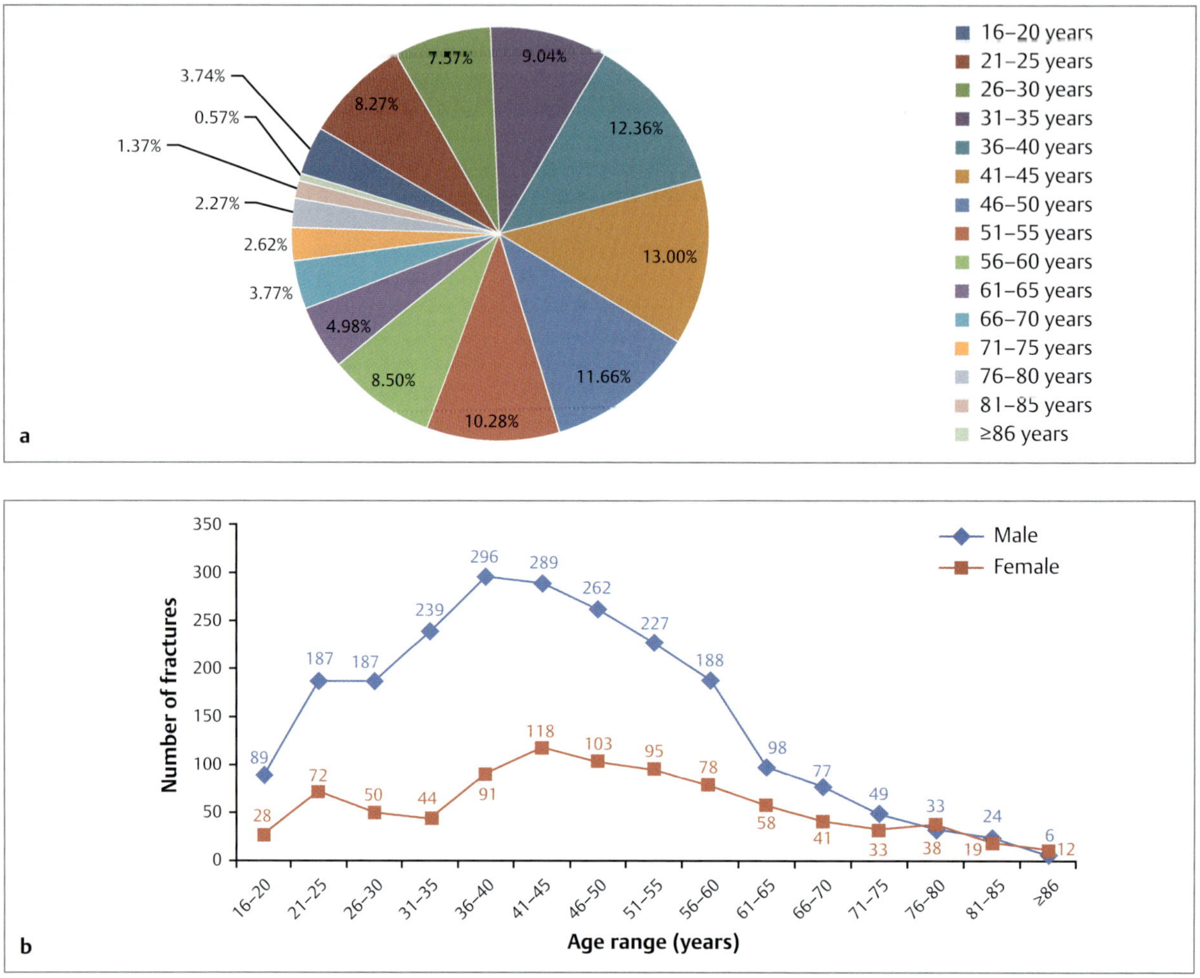

Fig. 7.13 **(a)** Age distribution of 3,131 fractures of segment 62.
(b) Age and sex distribution of 3,131 fractures of segment 62.

Fractures of Segment 62 by Fracture Type

Table 7.14 Sex and fracture type distribution of 3,174 fractures of segment 62

Fracture type	Male	Female	Number of fractures	Percentage (%)
62-A	1,237	516	1,753	55.23
62-B	784	286	1,070	33.71
62-C	265	86	351	11.06
Total	2,286	888	3,174	100.00

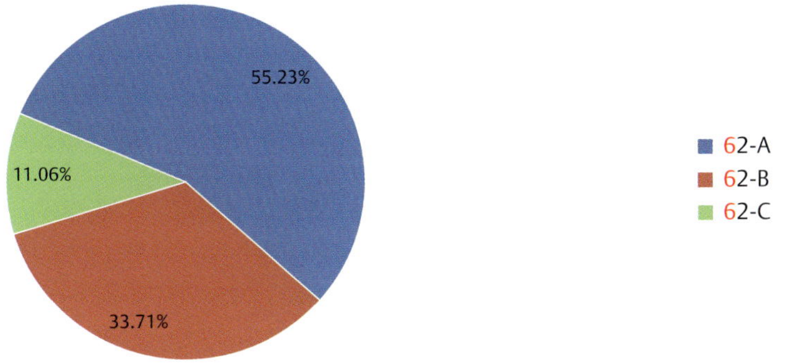

a

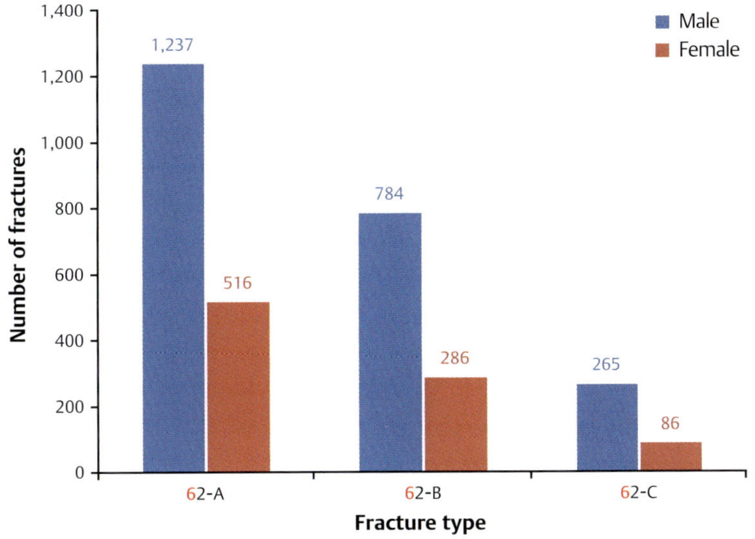

b

Fig. 7.14 **(a)** Fracture type distribution of 3,174 fractures of segment 62.
(b) Sex and fracture type distribution of 3,174 fractures of segment 62.

7

Table 7.15 Sex and fracture group distribution of 3,174 fractures of segment 62

Fracture group	Male	Female	Number of fractures	Percentage of segment 62 fractures (%)	Percentage of fractures of pelvic ring and acetabulum in adults (%)
62-A1	557	165	722	22.75	5.21
62-A2	396	217	613	19.31	4.42
62-A3	284	134	418	13.17	3.01
62-B1	466	175	641	20.20	4.62
62-B2	185	81	266	8.38	1.92
62-B3	133	30	163	5.14	1.18
62-C1	91	29	120	3.78	0.87
62-C2	127	28	155	4.88	1.12
62-C3	47	29	76	2.39	0.55
Total	2,286	888	3,174	100.00	22.89

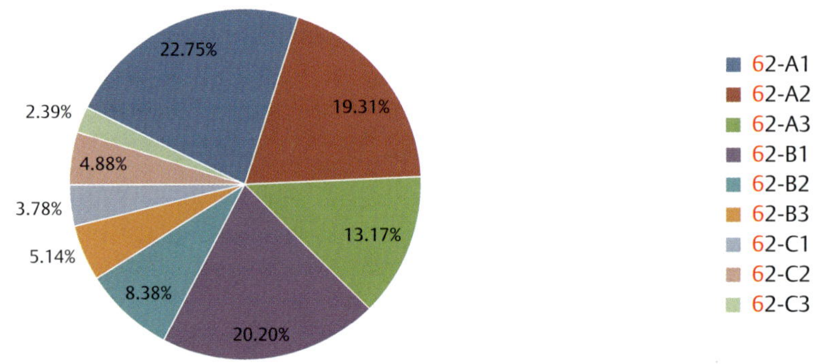

a

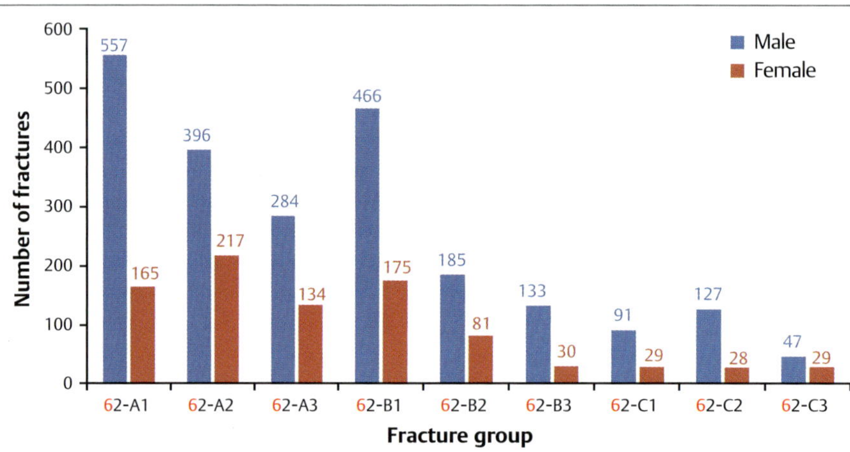

b

Fig. 7.15 **(a)** Fracture group distribution of 3,174 fractures of segment 62.
(b) Sex and fracture group distribution of 3,174 fractures of segment 62.

62-A Acetabular partial articular fracture, one column involved

62-A1
Posterior wall fracture
722 fractures
M: 557 (77.15%)
F: 165 (22.85%)
0.19% of total adult fractures
5.21% of adult pelvis and acetabulum
22.75% of segment 62
41.19% of type 62-A

62-A1.1

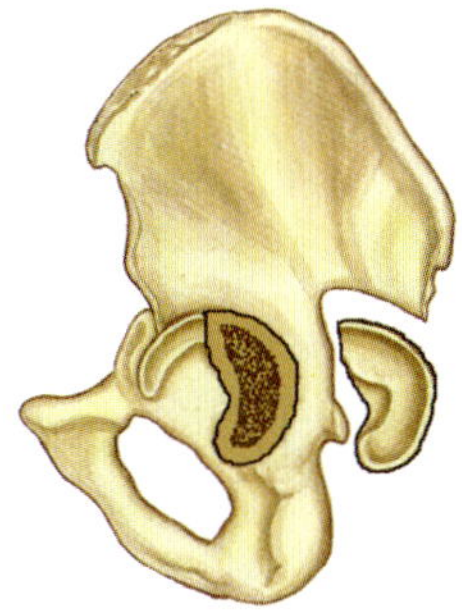

Pure fracture dislocation, one fragment in the posterior, posterosuperior, or posteroinferior

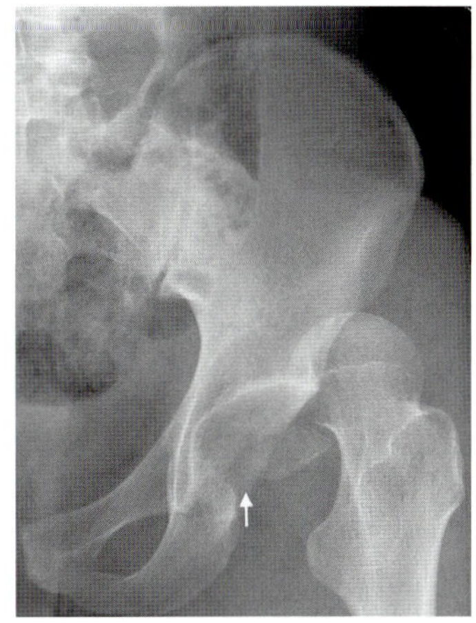

62-A1.2

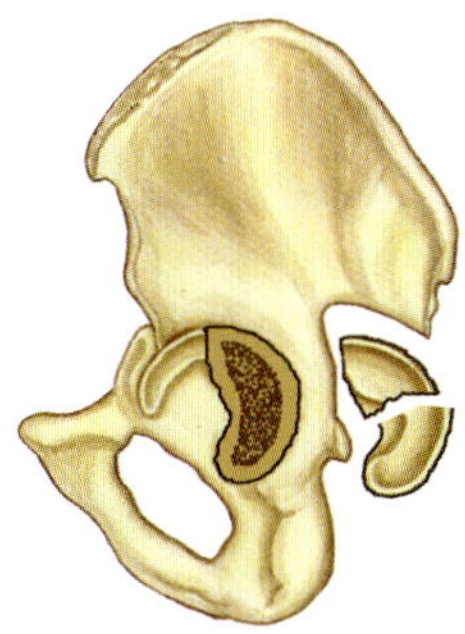

Pure fracture dislocation, multifragmentary in posterior, posterosuperior, or posteroinferior

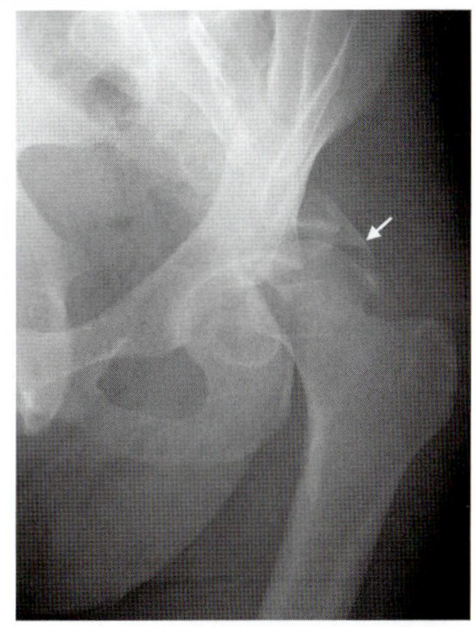

62-A1.3

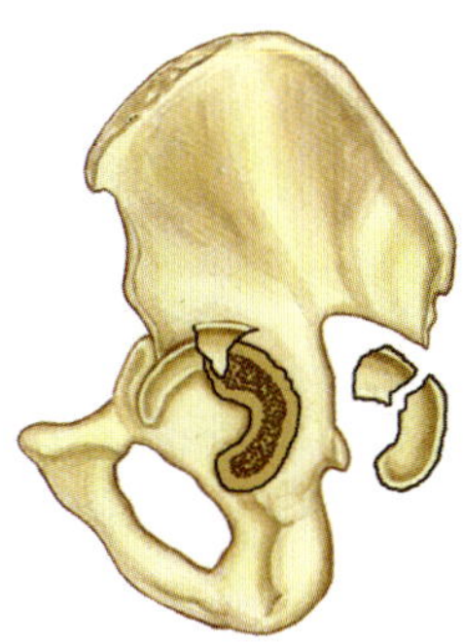

Fracture dislocation, with marginal impaction in posterior, posterosuperior, or posteroinferior

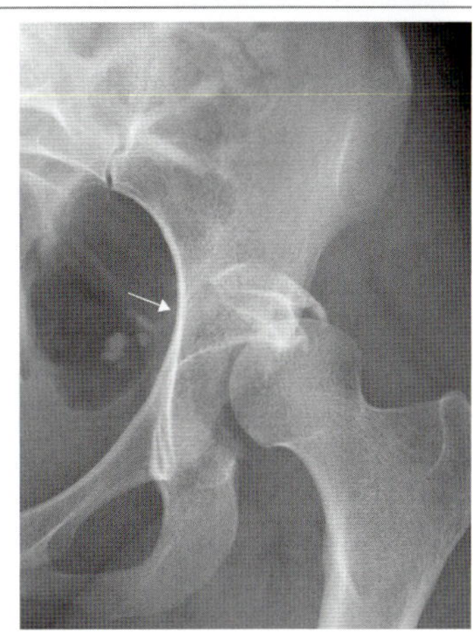

62-A Acetabular partial articular fracture, one column involved

62-A2
Posterior column fracture
613 fractures
M: 396 (64.6%)
F: 217 (35.4%)
0.16% of total adult fractures
4.42% of adult pelvis and acetabulum
19.31% of segment 62
34.97% of type 62-A

62-A2.1

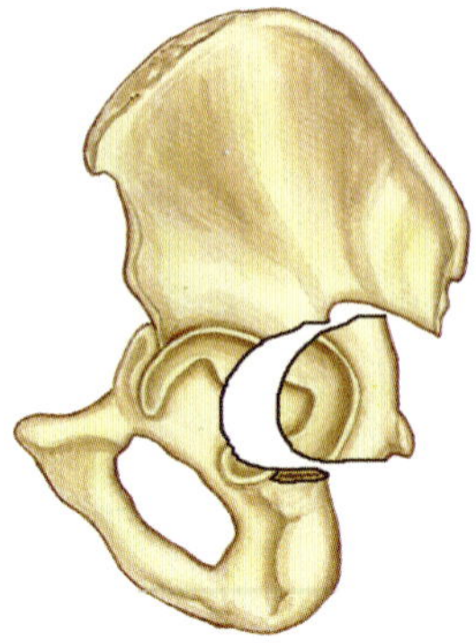

Through the ischium

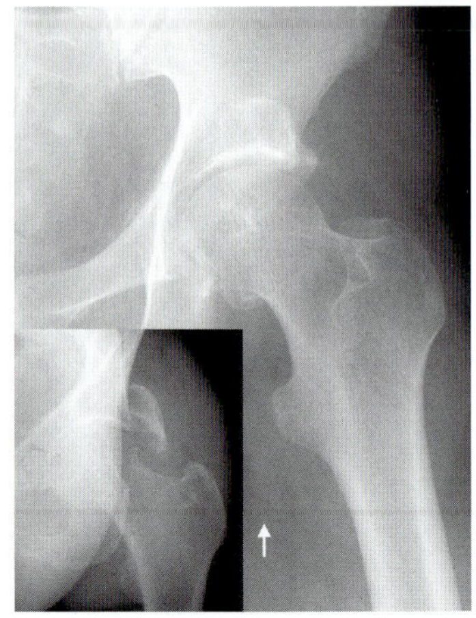

62-A2.2

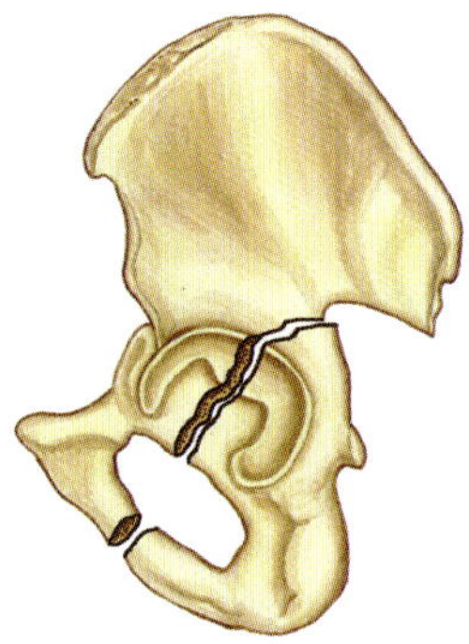

Through the obturator foramen (preserving tear drop or involving tear drop)

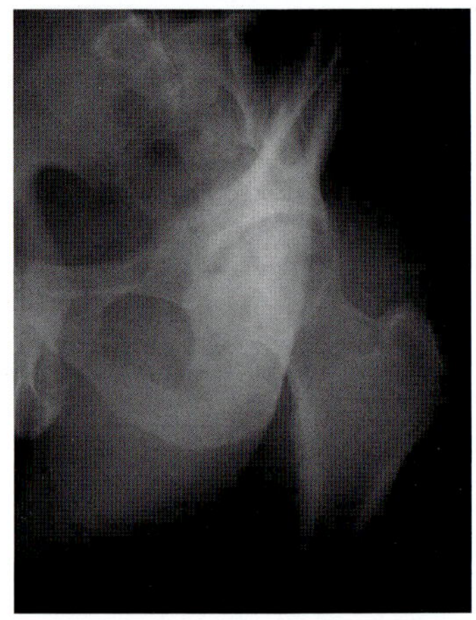

62-A2.3

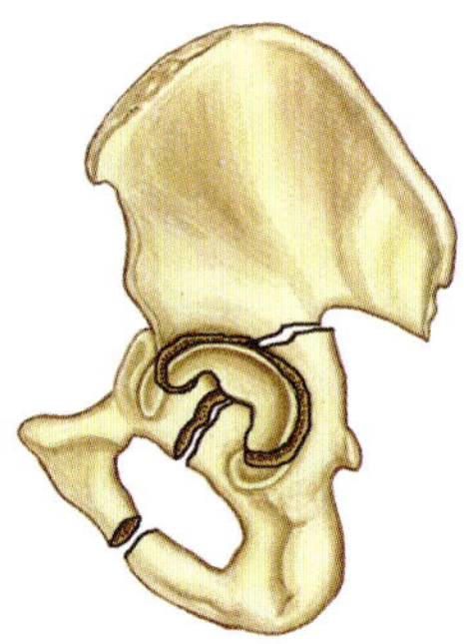

Associated with posterior wall fracture in posterior, posterosuperior or posteroinferior

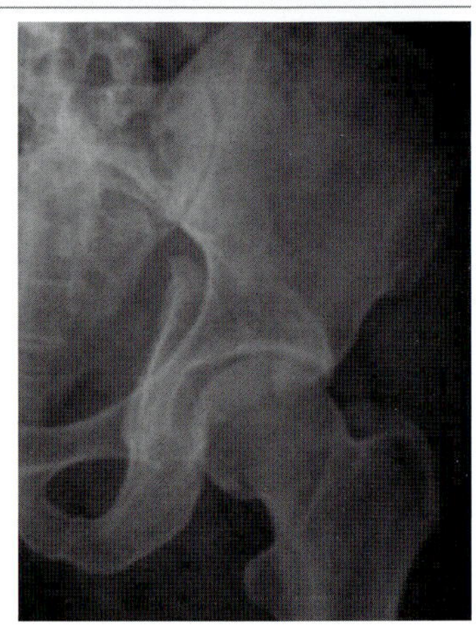

62-A Acetabular partial articular fracture, one column involved

62-A3
Anterior column fracture
418 fractures
M: 284 (67.94%)
F: 134 (32.06%)
0.11% of total adult fractures
3.01% of adult pelvis and acetabulum
13.17% of segment 62
23.84% of type 62-A

62-A3.1

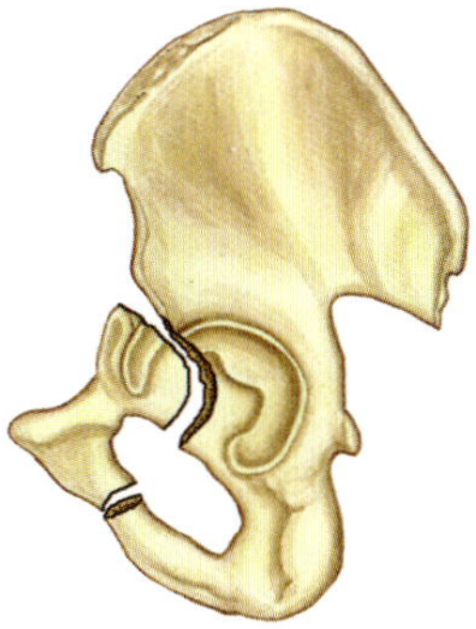

Anterior wall fracture, with one or more fragments

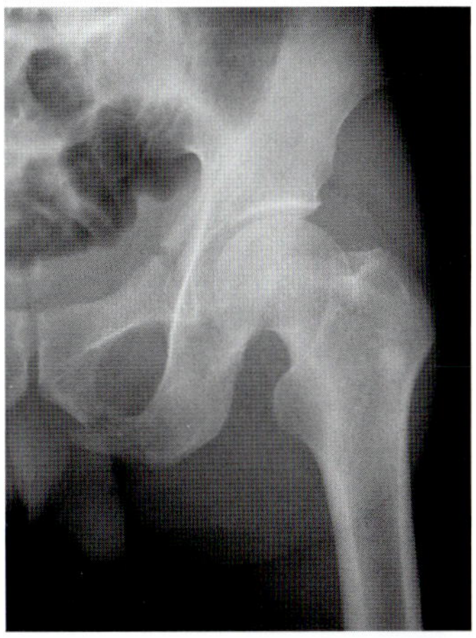

62-A3.2

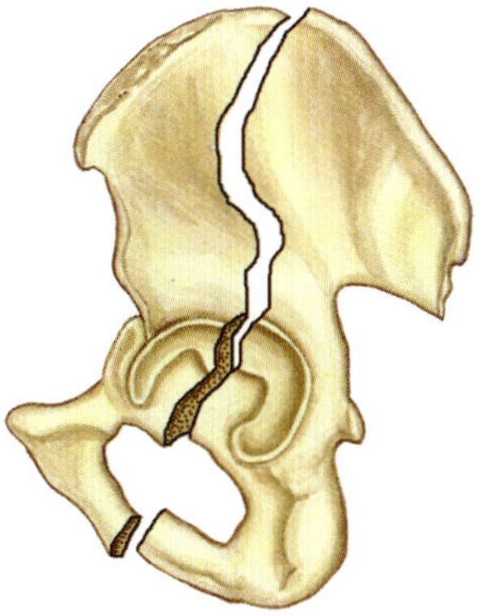

Anterior column fracture, high fracture to iliac crest, with one or more fragments

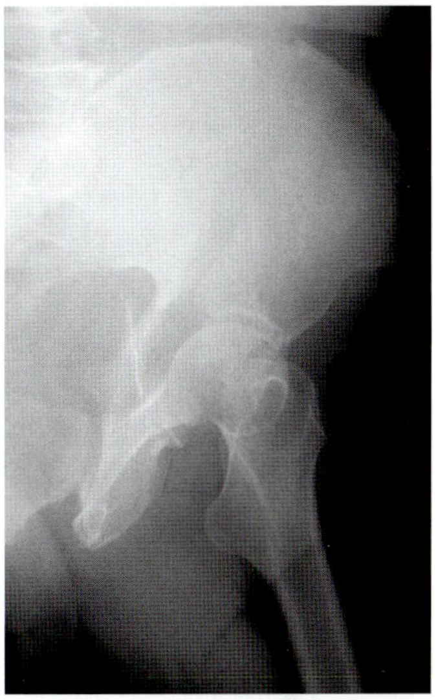

62-A3.3

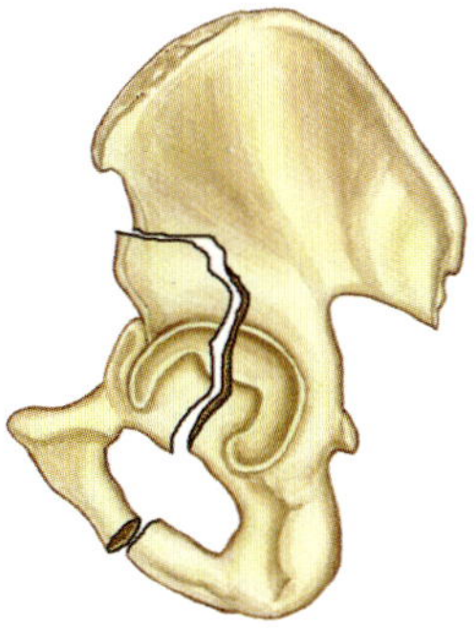

Anterior column fracture, low fracture to anterior border, with one or more fragments

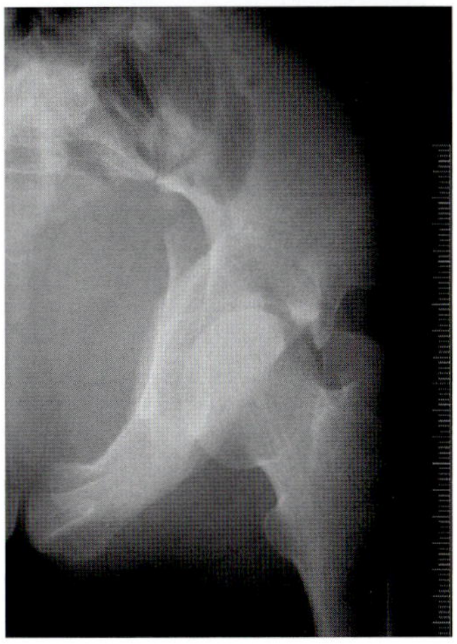

62-B Acetabular partial articular fracture, transverse

62-B1
Transverse
641 fractures
M: 466 (72.7%)
F: 175 (27.3%)
0.17% of total adult fractures
4.62% of adult pelvis and acetabulum
20.2% of segment 62
59.91% of type 62-B

62-B1.1

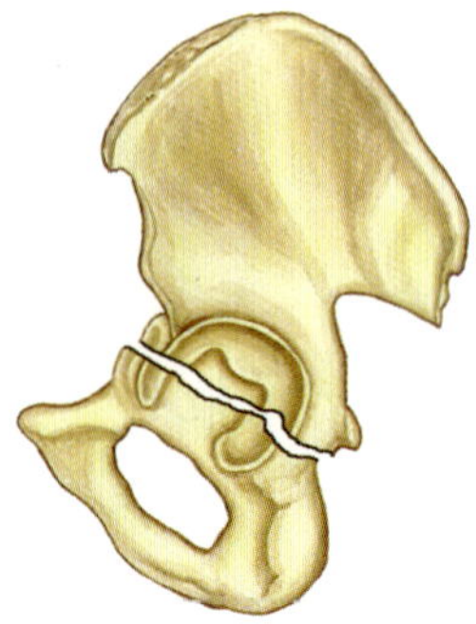

Infratectal

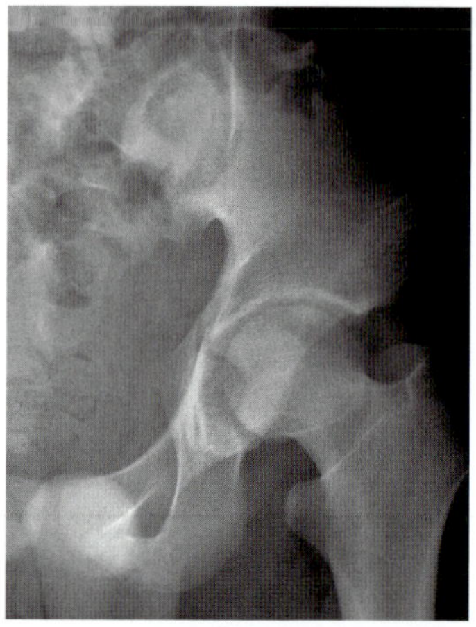

62-B1.2

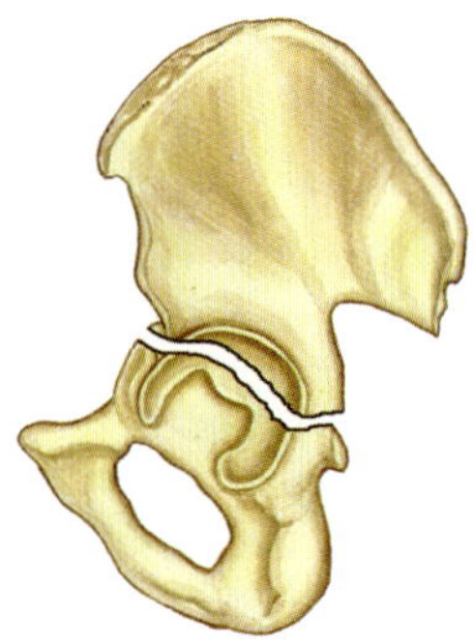

Juxtatectal

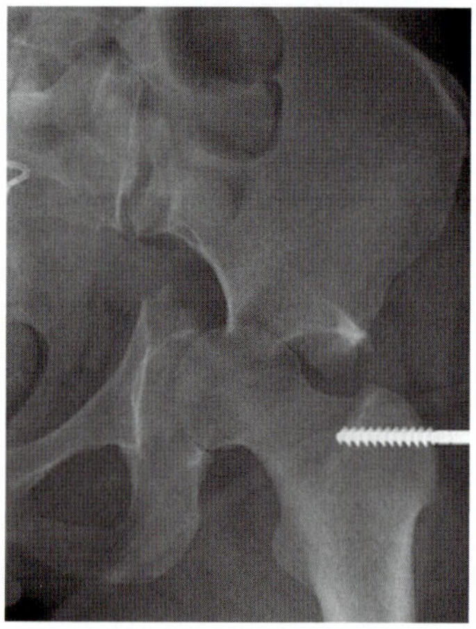

62-B1.3

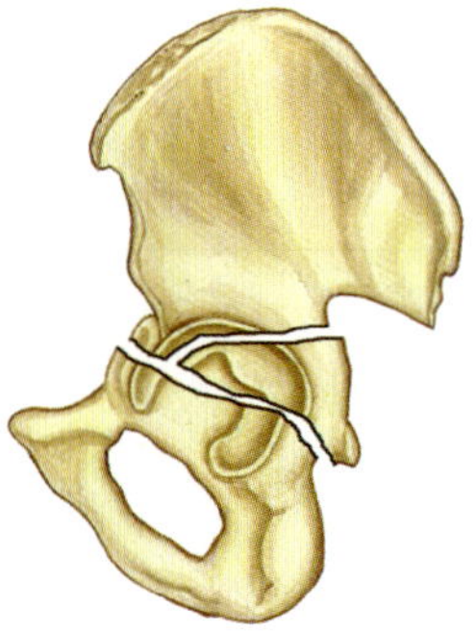

Transtectal

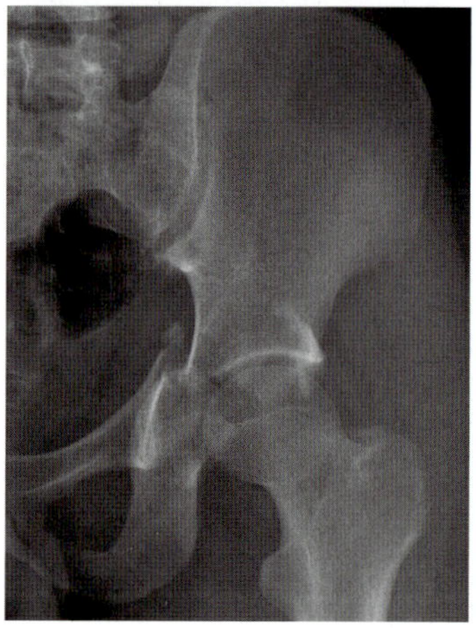

62-B Acetabular partial articular fracture, transverse

62-B2
T-shaped
266 fractures
M: 185 (69.55%)
F: 81 (30.45%)
0.07% of total adult fractures
1.92% of adult pelvis and acetabulum
8.38% of segment 62
24.86% of type 62-B

62-B2.1

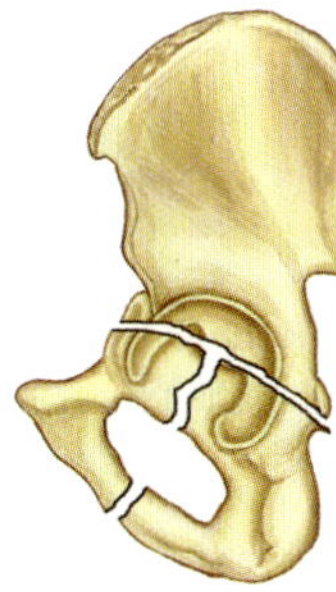

Infratectal fracture (stem posterior, stem through obturator foramen, stem anterior)

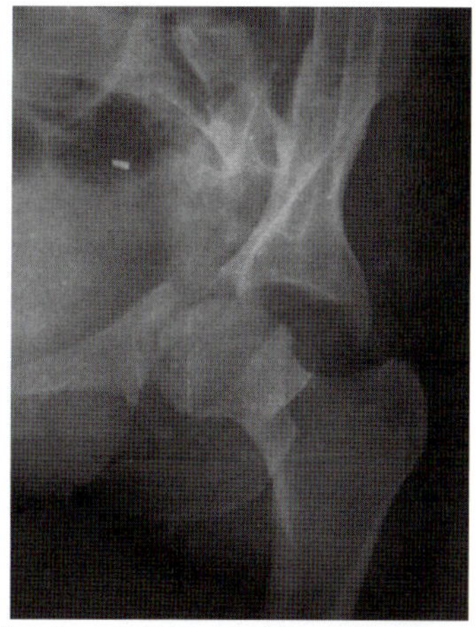

62-B2.2

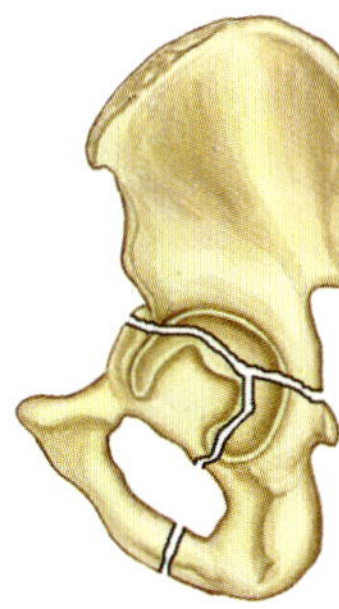

Juxtatectal fracture (stem posterior, stem through obturator foramen, stem anterior)

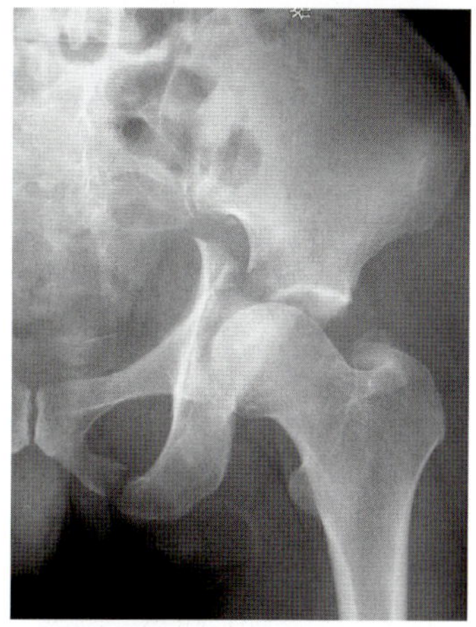

62-B2.3

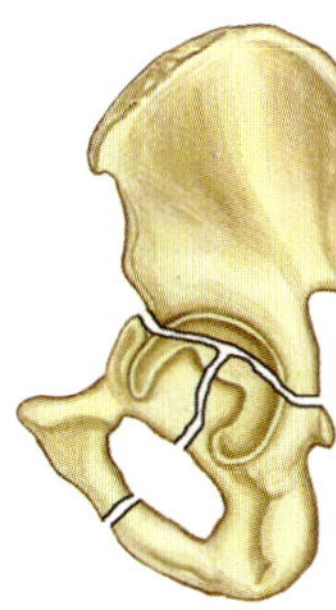

Transtectal fracture (stem posterior, stem through obturator foramen, stem anterior)

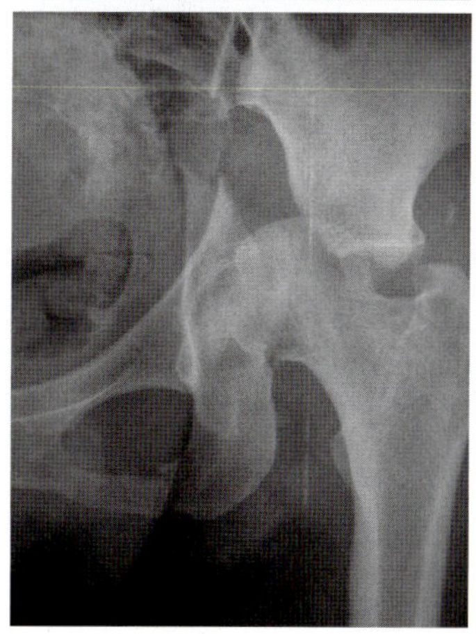

62-B Acetabular partial articular fracture, transverse

62-B3
Anterior column, posterior hemitransverse
163 fractures
M: 133 (81.6%)
F: 30 (18.4%)
0.04% of total adult fractures
1.18% of adult pelvis and acetabulum
5.14% of segment 62
15.23% of type 62-A

62-B3.1

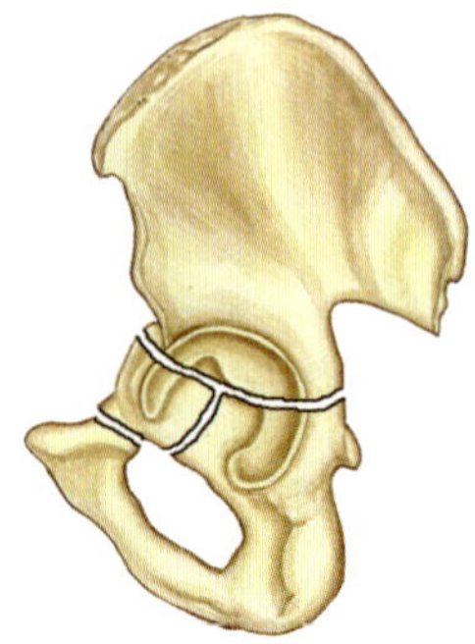

Anterior wall

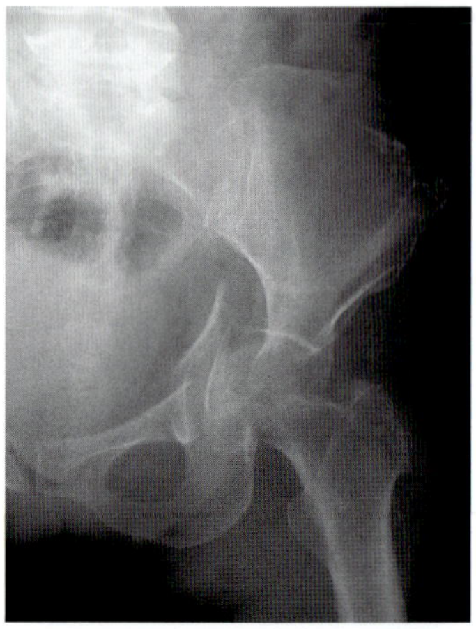

62-B3.2

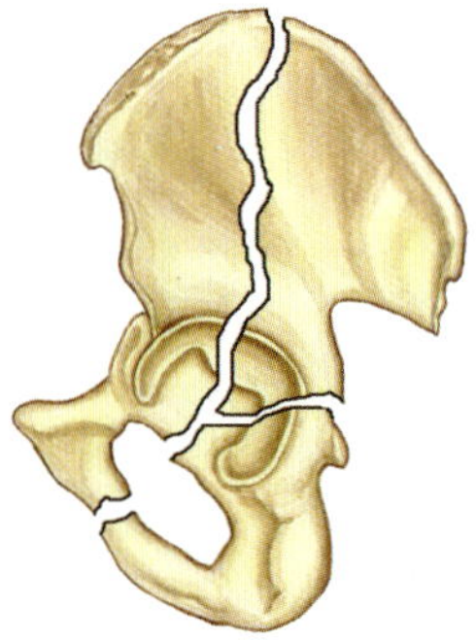

Anterior column high

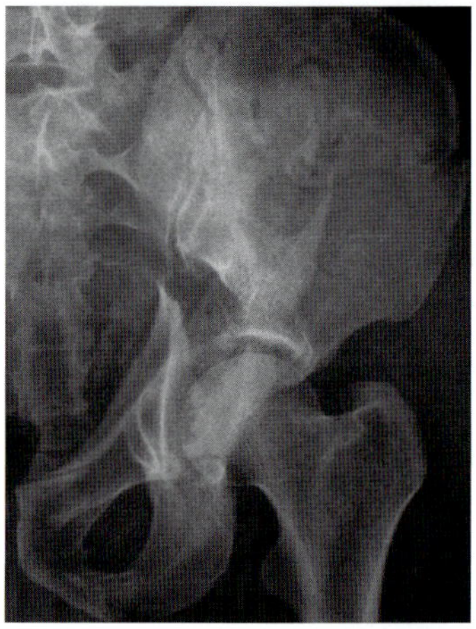

62-B3.3

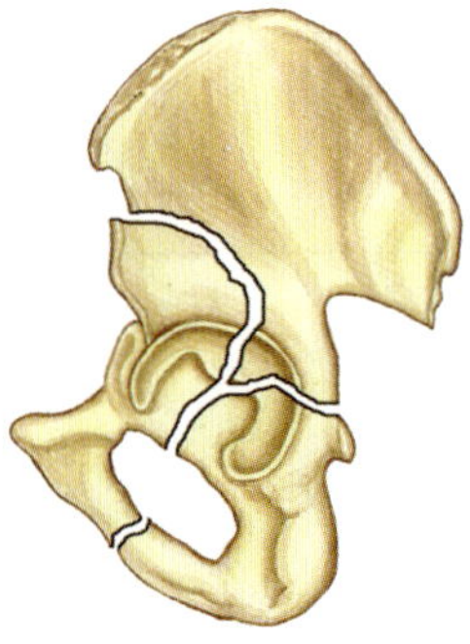

Anterior column low

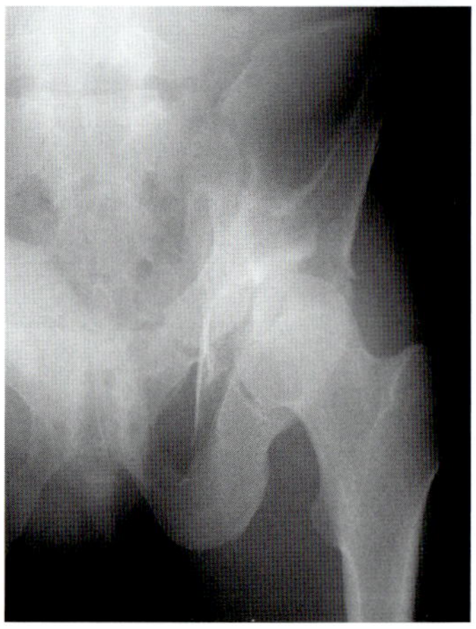

62-C Acetabular complete articular fracture, both columns (floating acetabulum)

62-C1
High
120 fractures
M: 91 (75.83%)
F: 29 (24.17%)
0.03% of total adult fractures
0.87% of adult pelvis and acetabulum
3.78% of segment 62
34.19% of type 62-C

62-C1.1

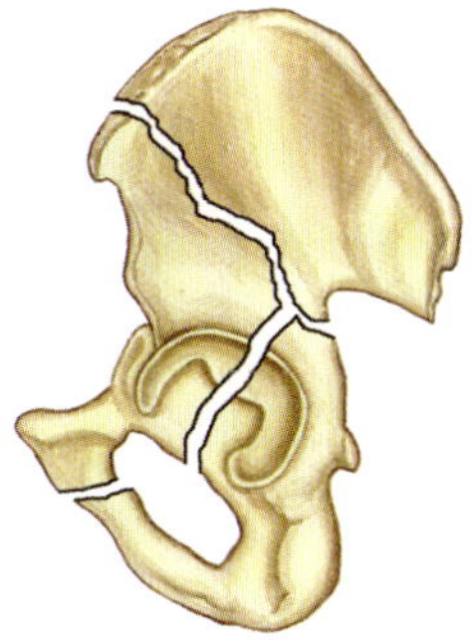

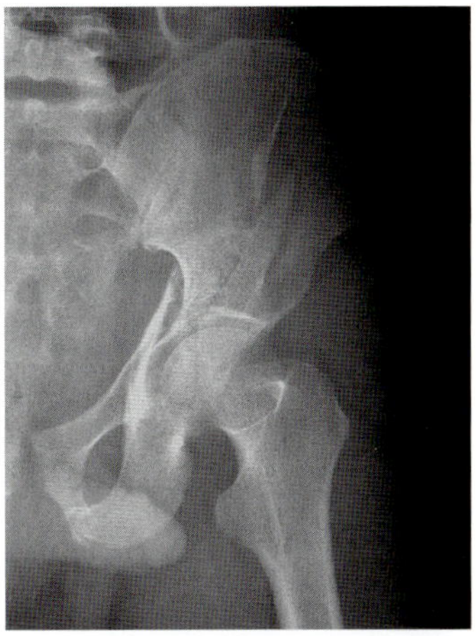

Both columns simple

62-C1.2

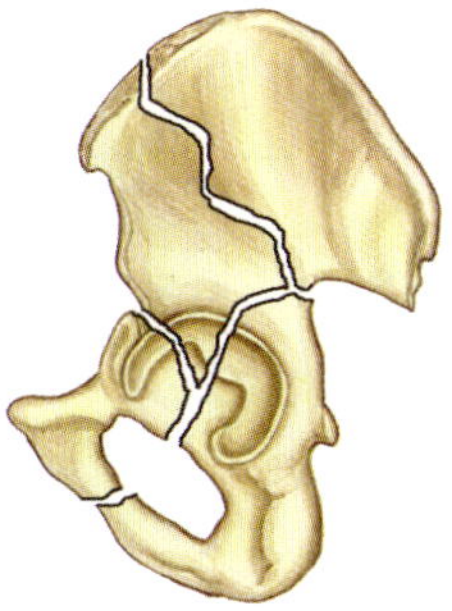

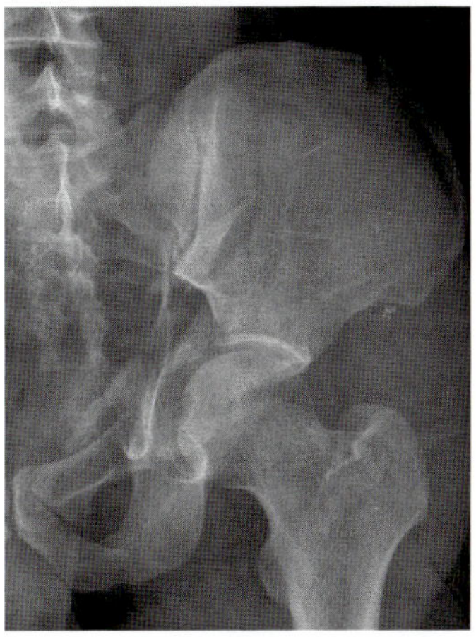

Posterior column simple, anterior column multifragmentary

62-C1.3

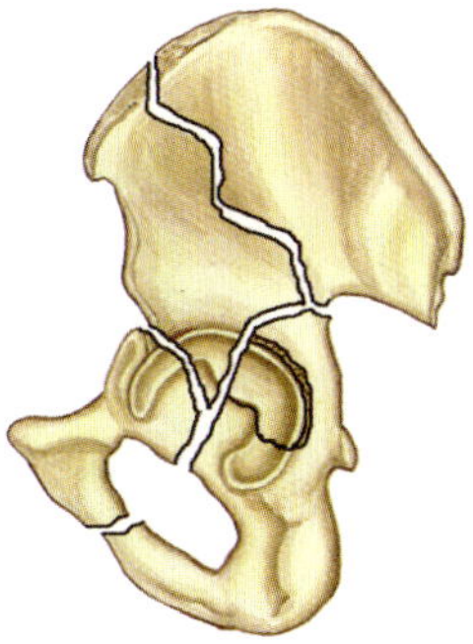

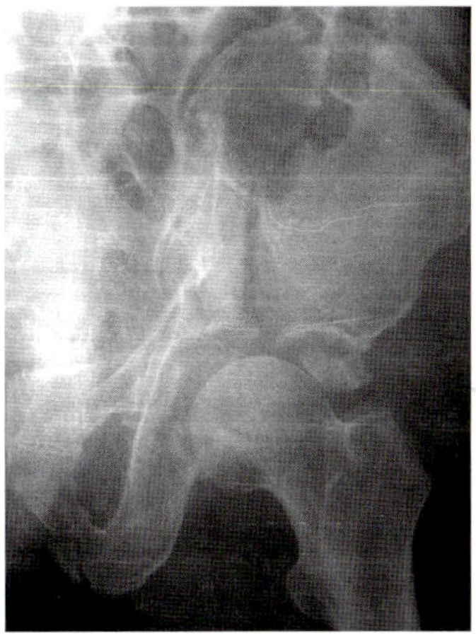

Posterior column and posterior wall

62-C Acetabular complete articular fracture, both columns (floating acetabulum)

62-C2
Low
155 fractures
M: 127 (81.94%)
F: 28 (18.06%)
0.04% of total adult fractures
1.12% of adult pelvis and acetabulum
4.88% of segment 62
44.16% of type 62-C

62-C2.1

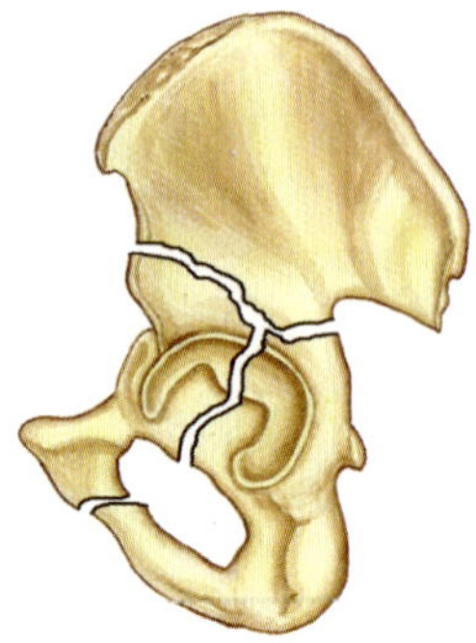

Both columns simple

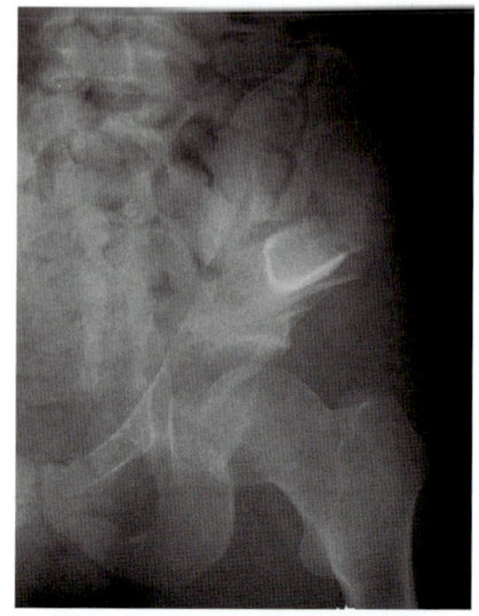

62-C2.2

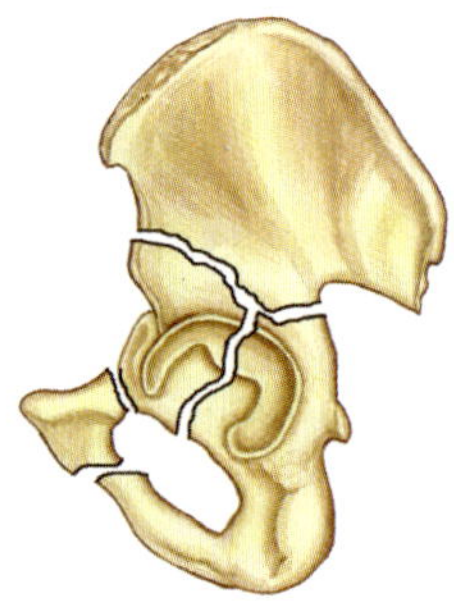

Posterior column simple, anterior column multifragmentary

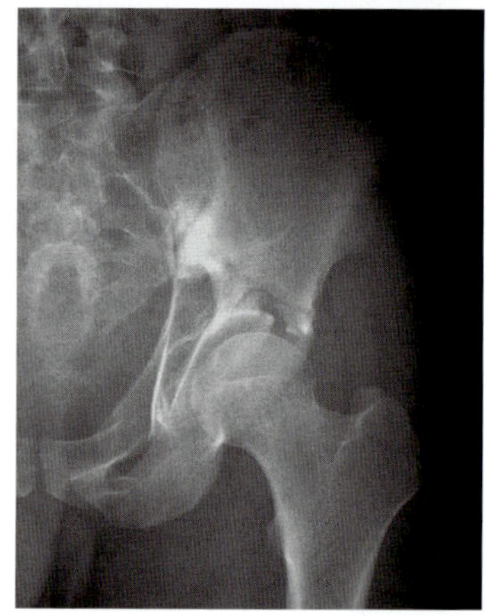

62-C2.3

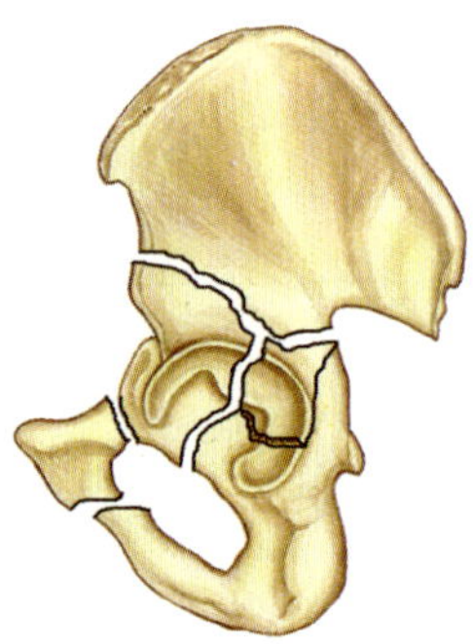

Posterior column and posterior wall

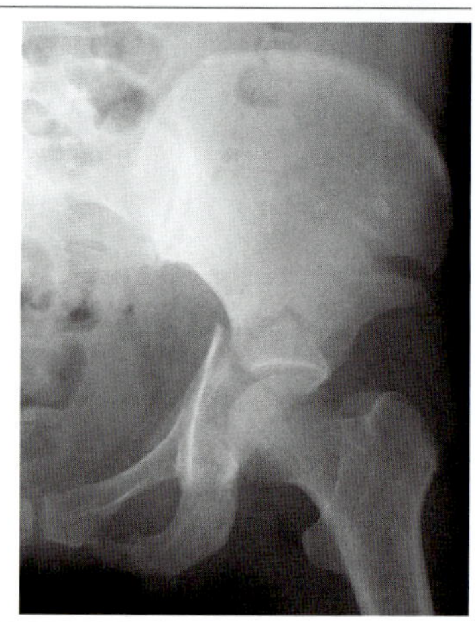

62-C Acetabular complete articular fracture, both columns (floating acetabulum)

62-C3
Involving sacroiliac joint
76 fractures
M: 47 (61.84%)
F: 29 (38.16%)
0.02% of total adult fractures
0.55% of adult pelvis and acetabulum
2.39% of segment 62
21.65% of type 62-C

62-C3.1

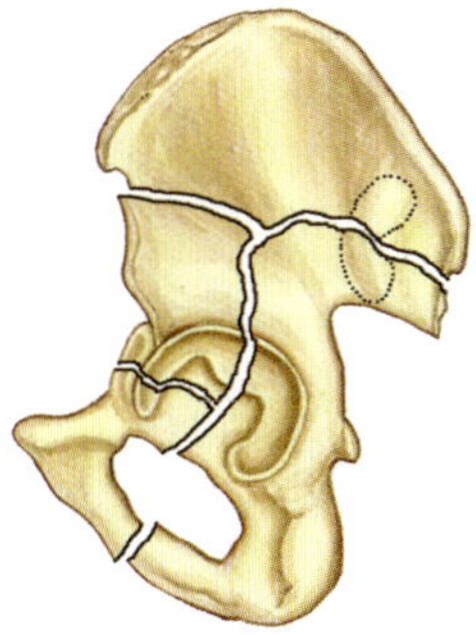

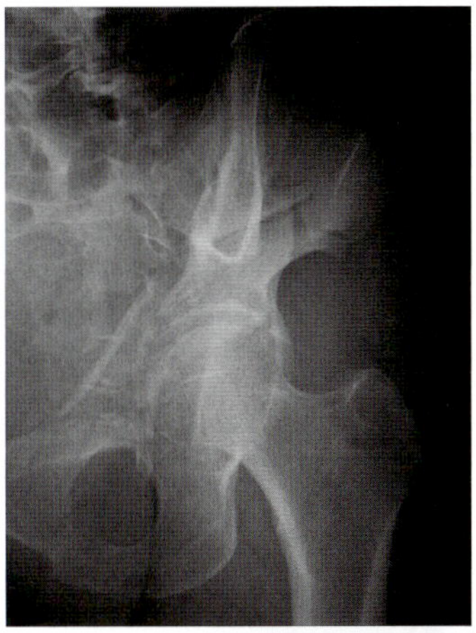

Anterior wall (anterior column high/low, simple; high/low multifragmentary)

62-C3.2

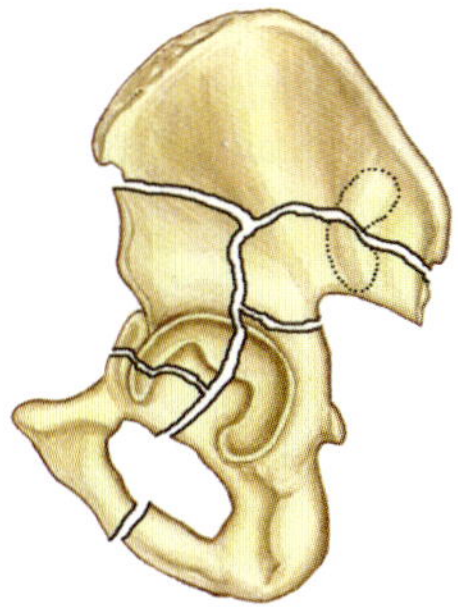

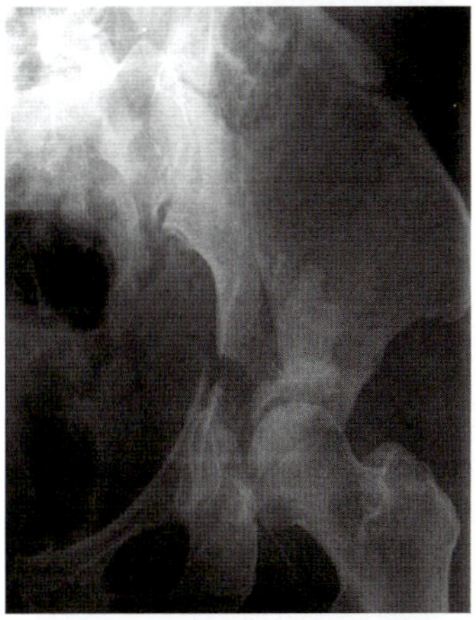

Posterior column multifragmentary, anterior column high

62-C3.3

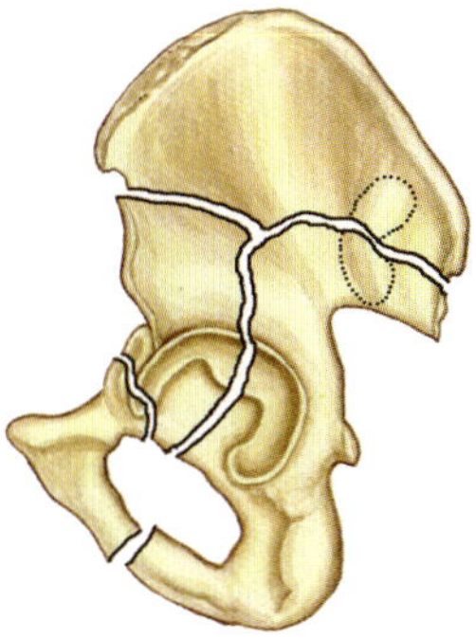

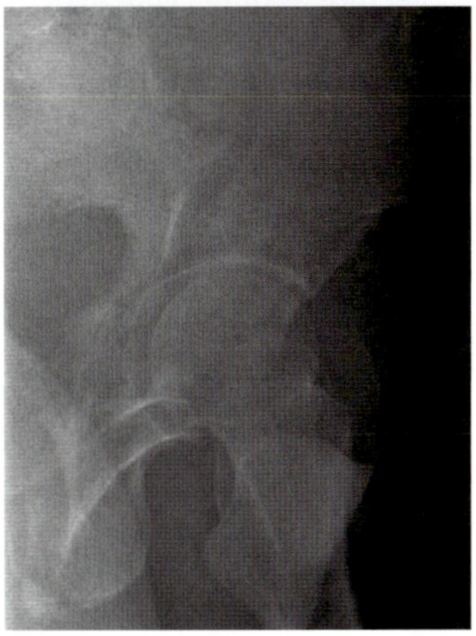

Posterior column and posterior wall

Injury Mechanism

Most acetabular fractures occur as a result of high-energy trauma such as motor vehicle accidents or falls from a height. Occasionally, this injury can also be caused by epileptic seizures. Most injuries occur when force is exerted on the femur (greater tuberosity, neck, or head), passes through the femoral head, and is transferred to the acetabulum; axial compression injuries along the femur can also lead to acetabular fractures. The position of the femoral head at the time of injury, as well as the direction and magnitude of the force determine the pattern of acetabular injury. Flexion and internal rotation of the hip predispose to posterior column injuries, while extension and external rotation of the hip predispose to anterior column injuries.

Diagnosis

Acetabular fractures typically present as groin and hip pain, exacerbated by passive hip motion. Range of motion is limited by pain, local tenderness to palpation is noted, and the heel percussion test is positive. Radiographic evaluation includes AP views of the pelvis that provide a general impression of the pelvic ring. Iliac oblique views illustrate the ilioischial line (posterior column) and anterior wall, while obturator oblique views illustrate the iliopectineal line (anterior column) of the pelvis and posterior wall. If the clinical presentation is highly suggestive of a fracture, and X-ray findings fail to demonstrate a subtle fracture, a CT scan of the pelvis, including three-dimensional reformatted images, may be required to assist in conceptualizing the fracture pattern, and thereby help in the planning of orthopaedic surgery. For hemodynamically unstable patients with acetabular fractures, angiography can greatly assist in making the diagnosis, and embolotherapy can be performed at the same time (**Plates 7.14, 7.15,** and **7.16**).

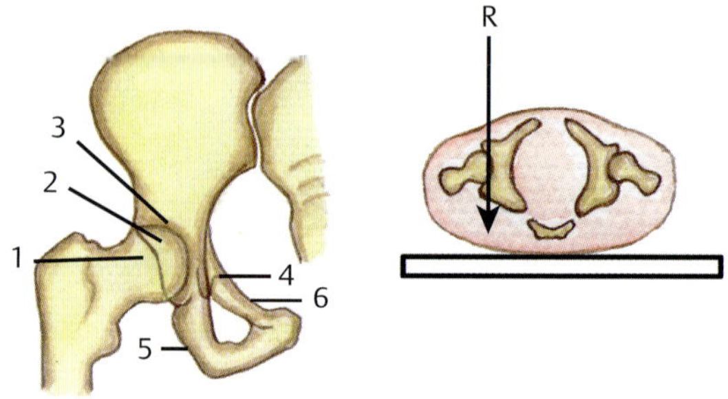

AP view showing (1) the posterior wall; (2) the anterior wall; (3) the dome of the acetabulum; (4) the tear drop; (5) the ilioischial line (posterior column); and (6) the iliopubic line (anterior column). R = radiation beam

Plate 7.14

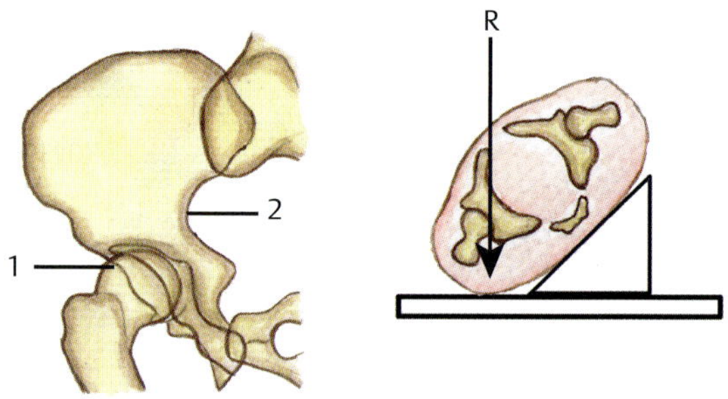

External (iliac) oblique view showing:
(1) the anterior wall; and (2) the posterior column.
R = radiation beam

Plate 7.15

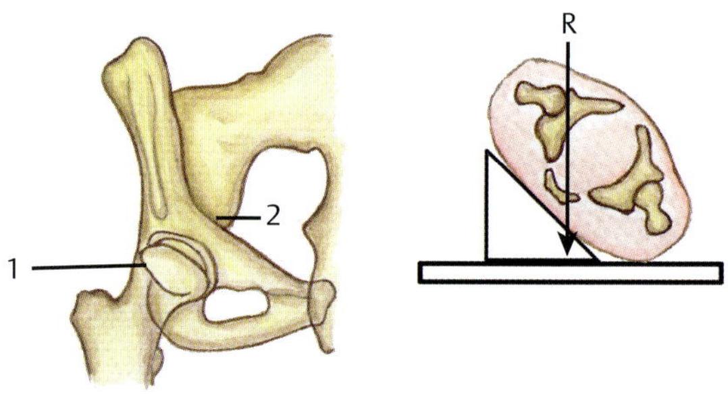

Internal (obturator) oblique view showing:
(1) the posterior wall; and (2) the anterior column.
R = radiation beam

Plate 7.16

Treatment

Indications for nonsurgical treatment:

- Fractures with no displacement or displacement ≤ 3 mm.
- Displaced fractures but the weight-bearing area of the acetabulum remains intact.
- Both columns with fracture displacement and secondary congruence.
- Pure posterior wall fractures including ≤ 40% of the acetabulum, with a stable stress test.

Surgical Treatment

The goal of surgical intervention for acetabular fractures is to reconstruct the articular surface, and to restore the congruity and stability of the hip joint. The surgical objective for severe comminuted acetabular fractures is to help ensure adequate bone stock for further arthroplasty. W-shaped acetabular angular plate can be used in the operation to fix the end of fracture, which can prevent the screw into the joint effectively and reduce complications.

Indications for open reduction and internal fixation

- Articular displacement of more than 3 mm.
- Incarcerated intra-articular fragments or impaction of the articular surface that lead to incongruity.
- Posterior displacement of the femoral head, associated with a posterior wall fracture, which leads to instability of the hip joint.
- Transverse fractures of the acetabulum associated with a posterior dislocation of the hip joint.
- Posterior wall fractures associated with sciatic nerve injuries.
- Associated with ipsilateral femoral neck fractures or diaphyseal femur fractures.

Timing of operation

Ideally, closed fractures should be treated with surgical treatment usually between the third and seventh day after the time of injury. Beyond 3 weeks, an anatomical reduction becomes progressively harder to obtain.

Reduction criteria

To achieve reconstruction of various acetabular components, concentric reduction of the femoral head under an adequate portion of the weight-bearing dome of the acetabulum, and anatomical reduction (displacement < 3 mm).

Other Classifications for Fractures of the Pelvic Ring and Acetabulum

Tile Classification of Pelvic Ring Fractures

Overview

Tile classification for pelvic ring fractures was established in 1986 by Tile and colleagues, based on the stability of a posterior lesion, its direction, and the nature of the force involved. This classification was modified and refined in 1988. The Tile classification has gained widespread recognition from AO/ASIF, OTA, and SICOT et al. AO classification of pelvic ring fractures has been developed and refined over years of practice, based on the Tile system. Tile classification of pelvic ring fractures is illustrated in the tables that follow (**Plate 7.17**).

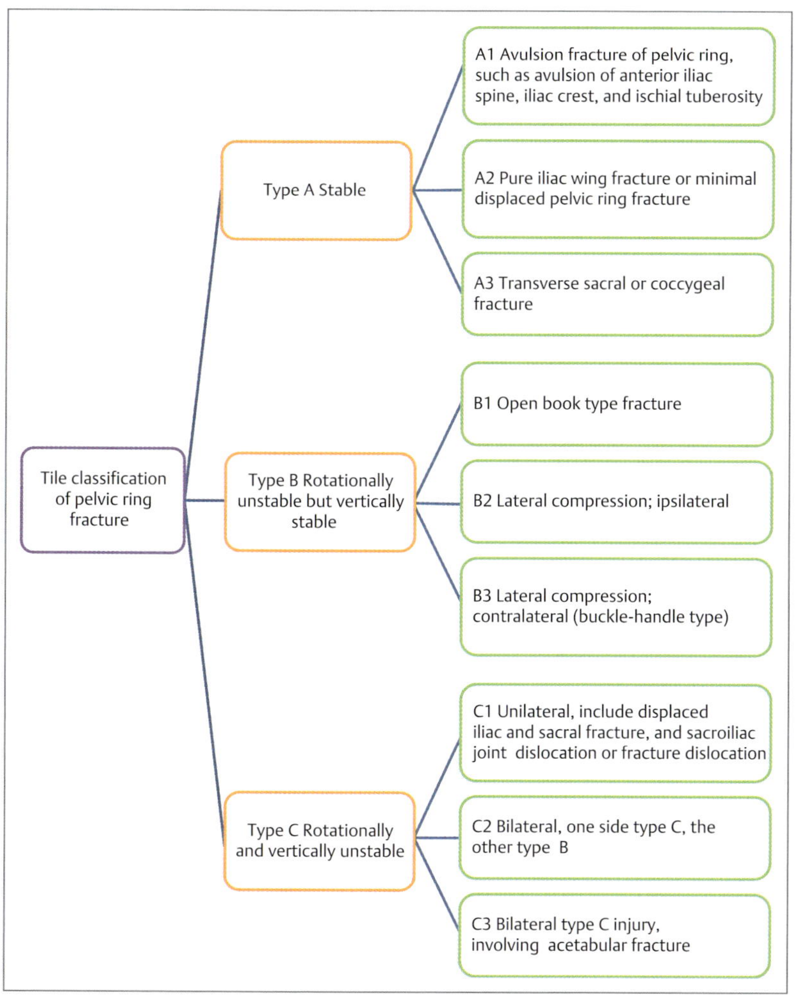

Plate 7.17

<table>
<tr><th colspan="3">Tile classification, type A</th></tr>
<tr><td rowspan="3">Tile type A
Stable</td><td>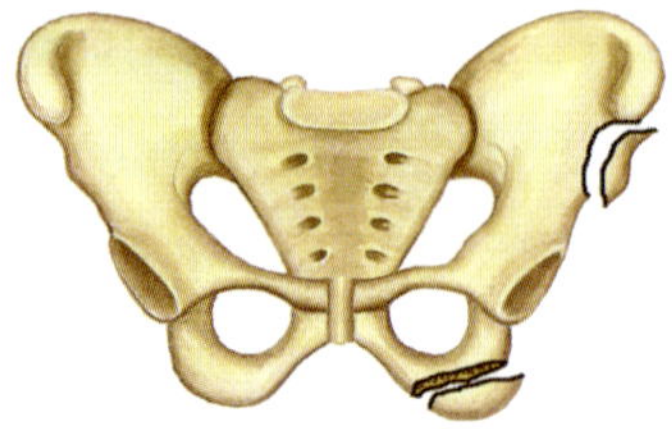
A1 Avulsion fracture, without disruption of the pelvic ring</td><td>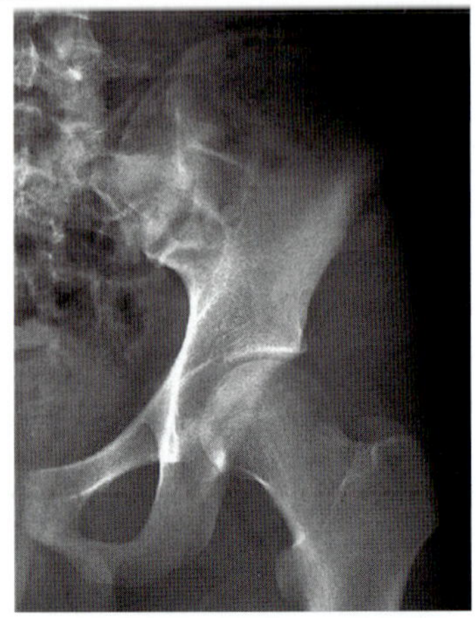</td></tr>
<tr><td>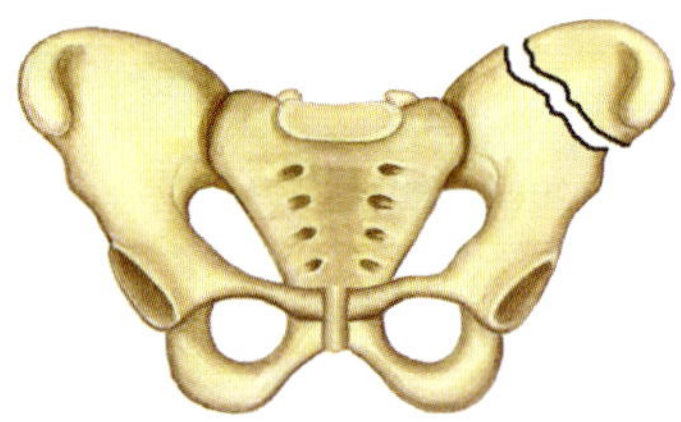
A2 Pure iliac wing fracture with minimal displacement</td><td>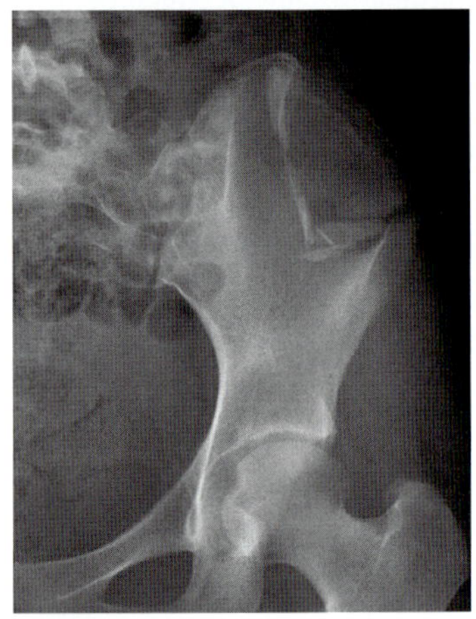</td></tr>
<tr><td>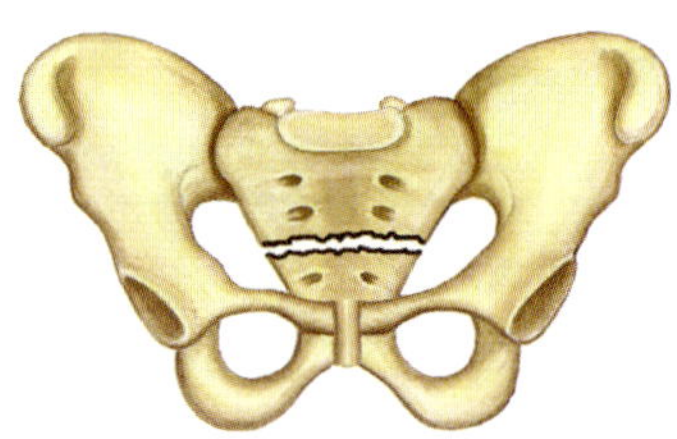
A3 Transverse sacral or coccygeal fracture</td><td>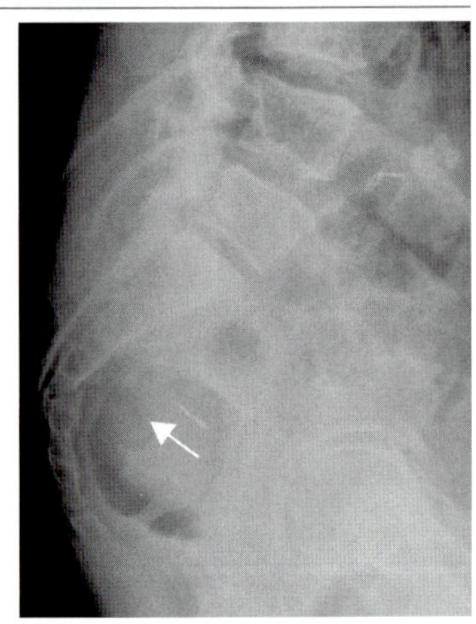</td></tr>
</table>

Tile classification, type B	
Type B **Rotationally unstable, vertically stable**	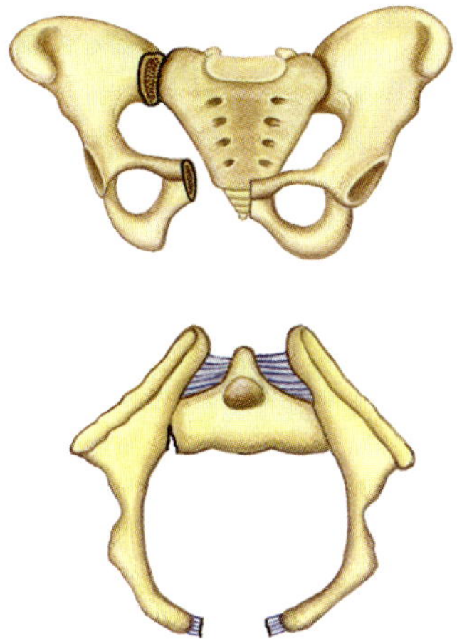 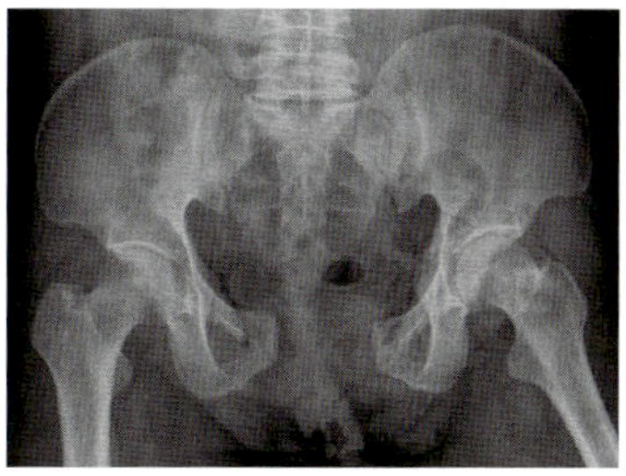 B1 "open-book"-type injury
	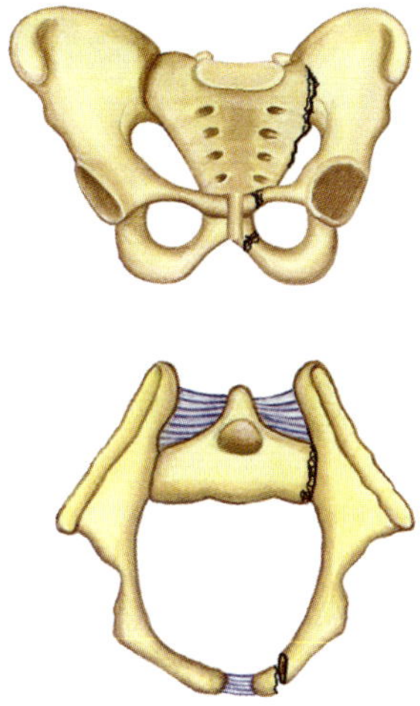 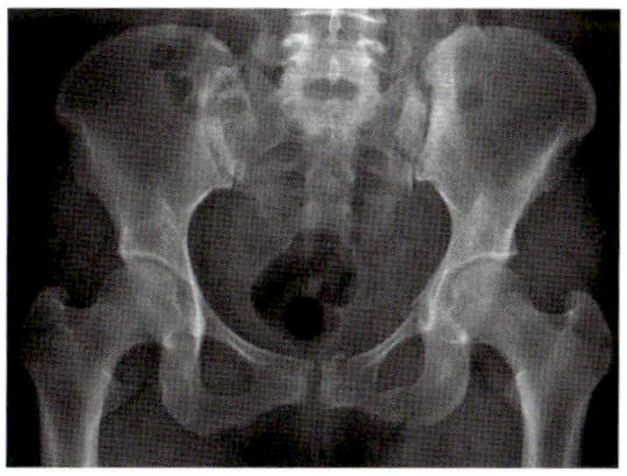 B2 Lateral compression, ipsilateral
	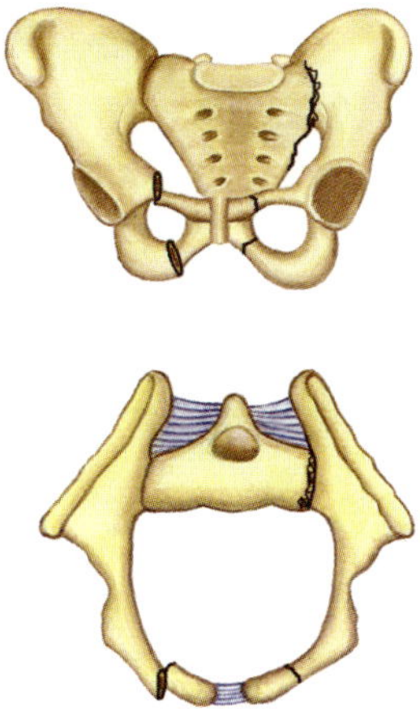 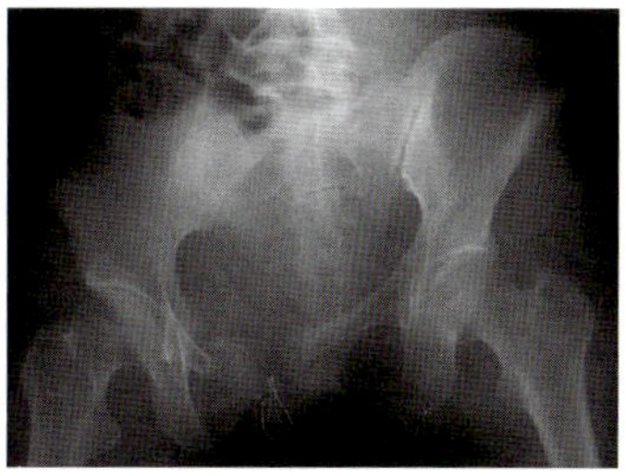 B3 Lateral compression, contralateral ("bucket handle"-type)

Tile classification, type C

Type C
Rotationally and vertically unstable

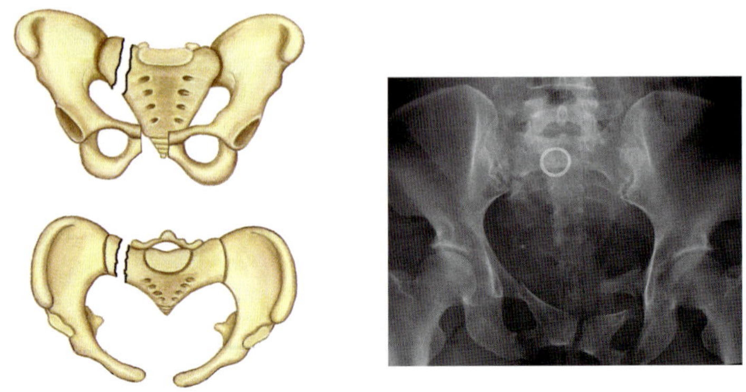

C1 Unilateral injury

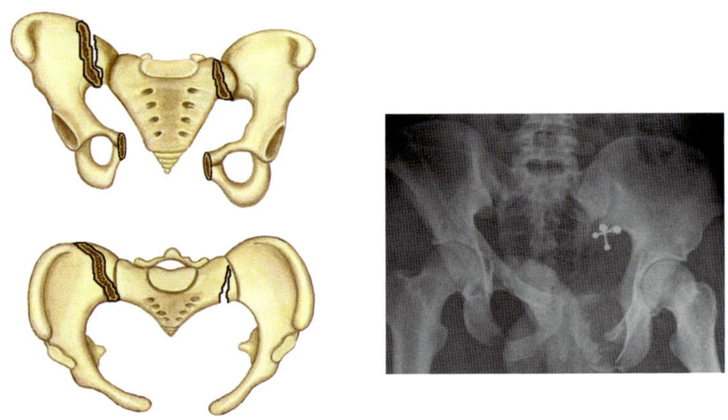

C2 Bilateral injury, ipsilateral vertically unstable, contralateral rotationally unstable

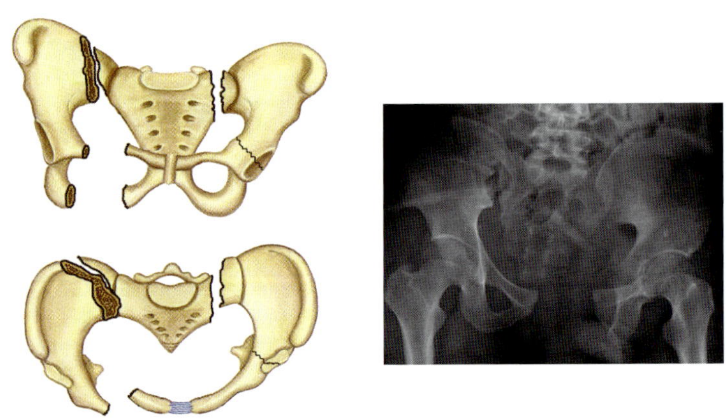

C3 Bilateral type C injury, involving an acetabular fracture

Young–Burgess Classification of Pelvic Ring Fractures

Overview

In 1990, based on the Tile concept of pelvic ring fractures, Young and Burgess developed and established their own classification to describe pelvic ring fractures that classify all pelvic ring fractures as one of four major groups: lateral compression (LC), anteroposterior compression (APC), vertical shear (VS), or combined mechanism injury (CM). Anteroposterior compression injuries are those in which the disruptive force is in the sagittal plane, as seen in blows to the front of the pelvis, commonly occurring in a motor vehicle accident. The resultant force tends to disrupt the anterior pelvis, either by fracturing the pubic rami, ischial rami, or by producing a diastasis of the pubic symphysis; as further force is applied, a typical "open-book"-type injury will occur. The force from a lateral compression injury is from the side and is associated with horizontal pubic rami fractures or interlocking of the pubic symphysis. With increasing lateral force, a typical lateral compression pelvic fracture will occur. This classification is based on the mechanism of injury and the direction of the injury force that allows for an accurate and timely application of the appropriate treatment, which, consequently, contributes to a more favorable outcome. According to the Young–Burgess classification, acetabular fractures (AF) are separate injuries. AF and LC injuries are commonly seen in car accidents while APC and AF frequently occur in motorcycle accidents. Crush trauma usually results from APC type injuries while falls from a height usually result from VS and LC type injuries. LC and APC injuries have a high rate of concomitant visceral injuries. APC injuries have a high incidence of brain, abdominal visceral, pelvic vascular injuries, and retroperitoneal hematomas, while concomitant arterial injuries are more frequently encountered during LC injury. LC and APC injuries have high mortality rates. Brain damage is commonly the cause of death in the LC injury, while acute respiratory distress syndrome (ARDS), sepsis, and shock are common causes of death for patients with APC injuries (**Plate 7.18**).

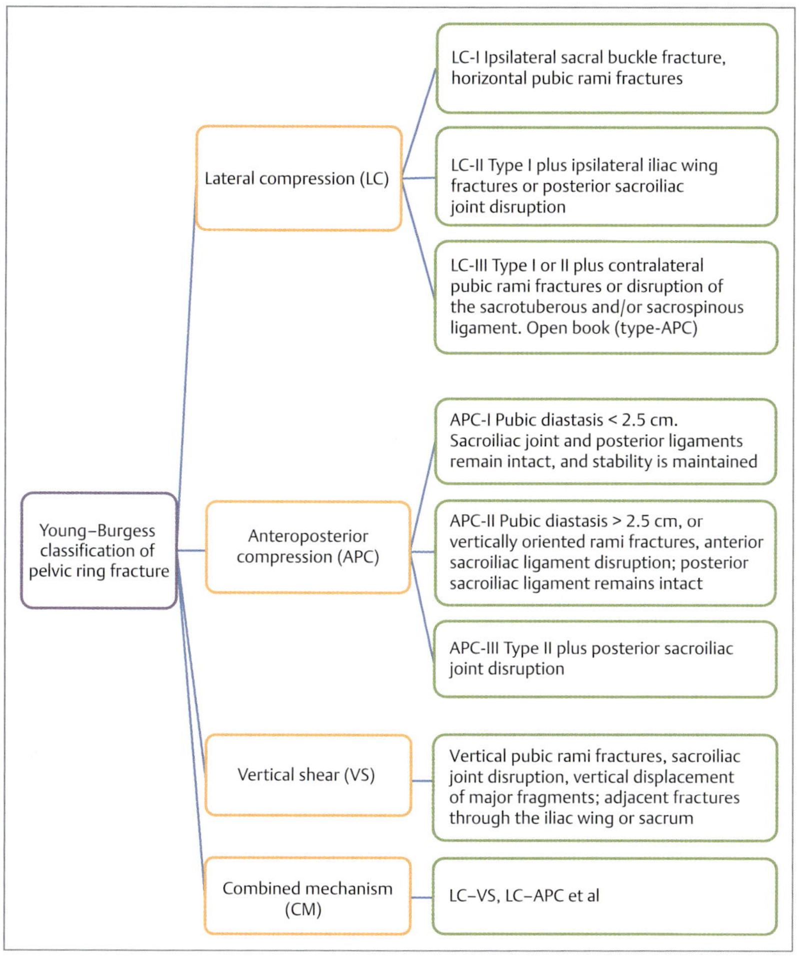

Plate 7.18

Management includes initial bed rest and early mobilization for LC injuries, open reduction and internal fixation for APC injuries. Hemodynamically stable patients with VS/APC injuries can be treated nonsurgically initially, with possible delayed open reduction and internal fixation. Emergency external fixation should be performed first for hemodynamically unstable patients. Surgical exploration should proceed if there is major visceral or vascular damage, and internal fixation can be performed simultaneously.

Epidemiologic Features of Pelvic Ring Fractures based on the Young–Burgess Classification

We retrospectively reviewed 1,956 pelvic ring fractures that fit into the description of the Young–Burgess classification system over a period of 2 years, from 2010 to 2011. These cases account for 17.37% of all pelvic ring fractures and 13.44% of all fractures of the pelvic ring and acetabulum, respectively.

Epidemiologic features of pelvic ring fractures based on the Young–Burgess classification are the following:
- More males than females
- The high risk age group is between ages 41 and 45, the same age group for both males and females.
- The most common fracture type of Young–Burgess fractures is type APC while the most common fracture group is group APC-II, the same type group for both males and females.

Pelvic Ring Fractures Based on the Young–Burgess Classification by Sex

Table 7.16 Sex distribution of 1,956 Young–Burgess fractures

Sex	Number of fractures	Percentage (%)
Male	1,205	61.61
Female	751	38.39
Total	1,956	100.00

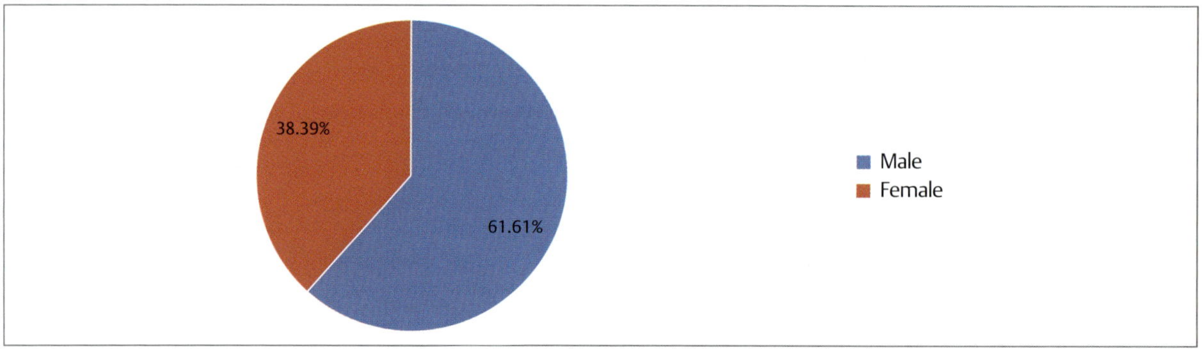

Fig. 7.16 Sex distribution of 1,956 Young–Burgess fractures.

Pelvic Ring Fractures Based on the Young–Burgess Classification by Age Group

Table 7.17 Age and sex distribution of 1,956 Young–Burgess fractures

Age group (years)	Male	Female	Number of fractures	Percentage (%)	Percentage of pelvic ring fractures (%)
0–5	11	7	18	0.92	0.16
6–10	18	19	37	1.89	0.33
11–15	40	24	64	3.27	0.57
16–20	81	40	121	6.19	1.07
21–25	117	90	207	10.58	1.84
26–30	118	66	184	9.41	1.63
31–35	94	54	148	7.57	1.31
36–40	133	87	220	11.25	1.95
41–45	159	100	259	13.24	2.30
46–50	133	61	194	9.92	1.72
51–55	114	44	158	8.08	1.40
56–60	80	45	125	6.39	1.11
61–65	28	16	44	2.25	0.39
66–70	33	27	60	3.07	0.53
71–75	22	26	48	2.45	0.43
76–80	15	20	35	1.79	0.31
81–85	7	11	18	0.92	0.16
≥86	2	14	16	0.82	0.14
Total	1,205	751	1,956	100.00	17.37

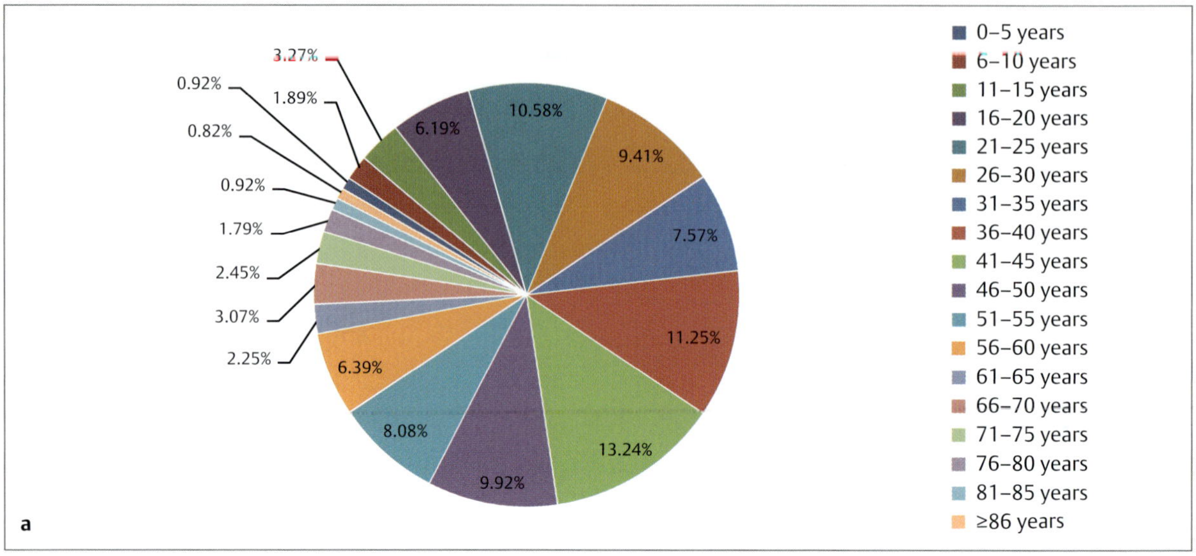

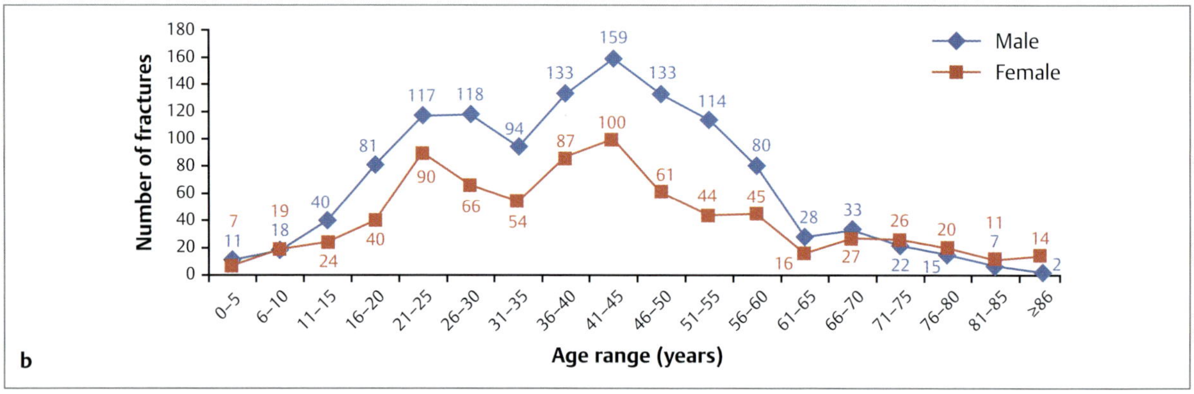

Fig. 7.17 **(a)** Age distribution of 1,956 Young–Burgess fractures.
(b) Age and sex distribution of 1,956 Young–Burgess fractures.

Pelvic Ring Fractures Based on the Young–Burgess Classification by Fracture Type

Table 7.18 Sex and fracture type distribution of 1,956 Young–Burgess fractures

Fracture type	Male	Female	Number of fractures	Percentage (%)	Percentage of pelvic ring fractures (%)
LC	342	188	530	27.10	4.71
APC	652	461	1,113	56.90	9.88
VS	112	58	170	8.69	1.51
CM	99	44	143	7.31	1.27
Total	1,205	751	1,956	100.00	17.37

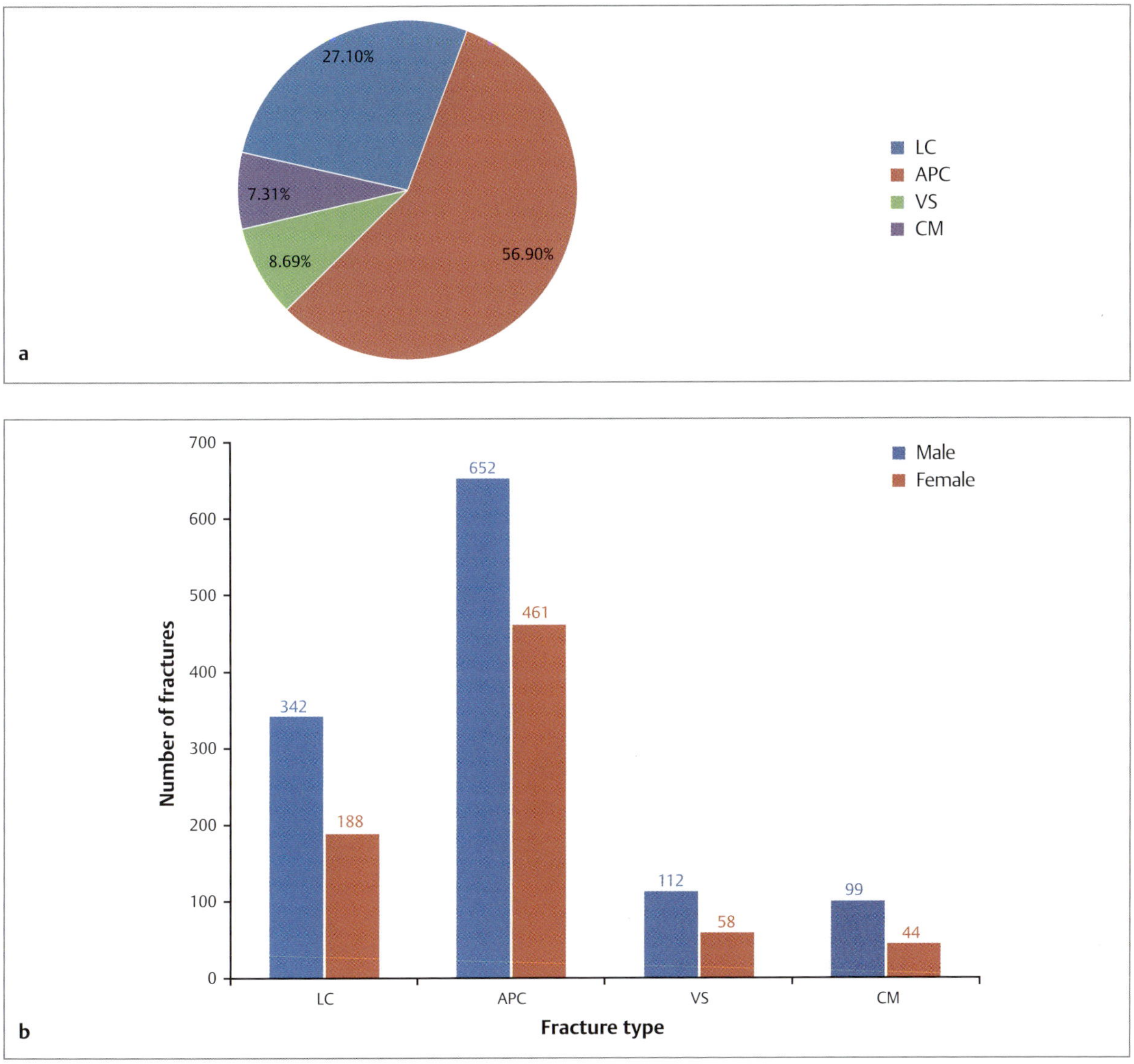

Fig. 7.18 **(a)** Fracture type distribution of 1,956 Young–Burgess fractures.
(b) Sex and fracture type distribution of 1,956 Young–Burgess fractures.

Table 7.19 Sex and fracture group distribution of 1,956 Young–Burgess fractures

Fracture group	Male	Female	Number of fractures	Percentage (%)	Percentage of pelvic ring fractures (%)
LC-I	238	142	380	19.43	3.37
LC-II	94	43	137	7.00	1.22
LC-III	10	3	13	0.66	0.12
APC-I	142	92	234	11.96	2.08
APC-II	375	298	673	34.41	5.98
APC-III	135	71	206	10.53	1.83
VS	112	58	170	8.69	1.51
CM	99	44	143	7.31	1.27
Total	1,205	751	1,956	100.00	17.37

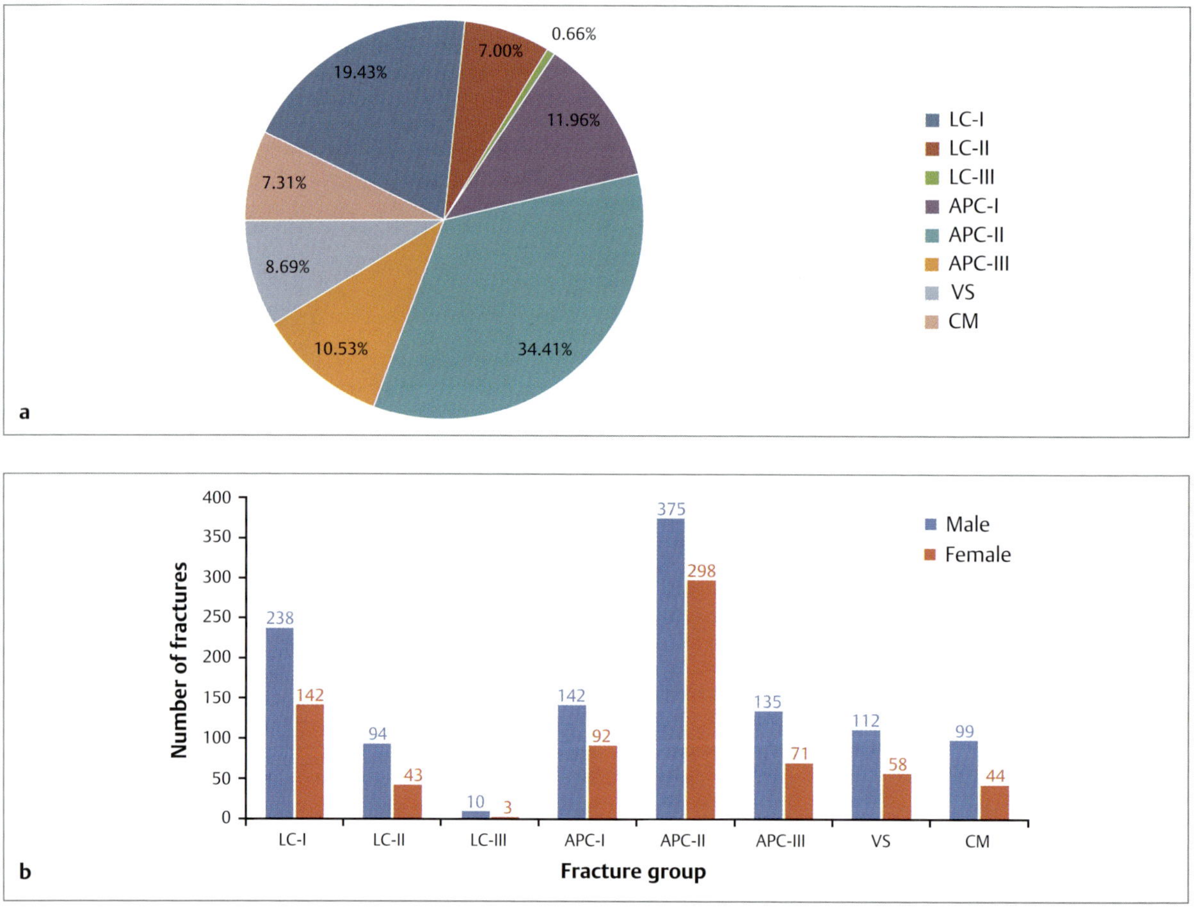

Fig. 7.19 **(a)** Fracture group distribution of 1,956 Young–Burgess fractures.
(b) Sex and fracture type distribution of 1,956 Young–Burgess fractures.

Lateral compression injury (LC)	
LC-I **Ipsilateral sacral buckle fracture, horizontal pubic rami fractures; stable** 380 fractures M: 238 (62.63%) F: 142 (37.37%) 19.43% of Young–Burgess	**LC-I** 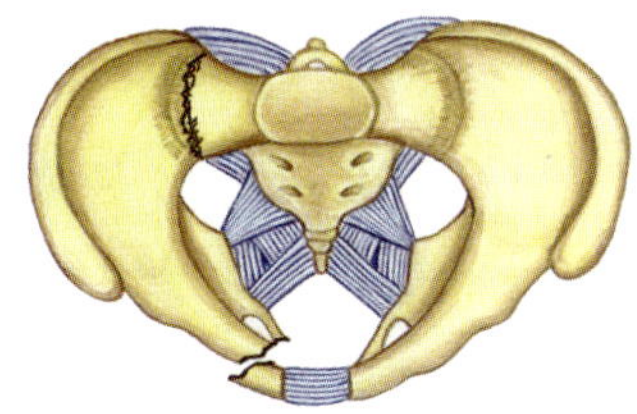 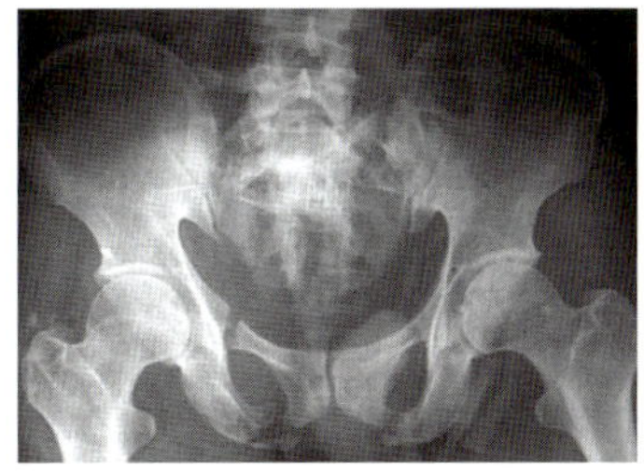 The injury force is directed posteriorly to the lateral aspect of the hemipelvis, resulting in an ipsilateral sacral buckle fracture and horizontal pubic rami fractures; stable
LC-II **LC-I plus ipsilateral iliac wing fractures or posterior SI joint disruption** 137 fractures M: 94 (68.61%) F: 43 (31.39%) 7% of Young–Burgess	**LC-II** 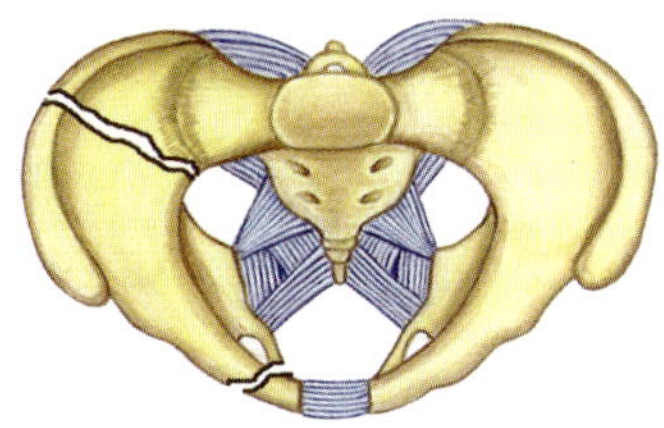 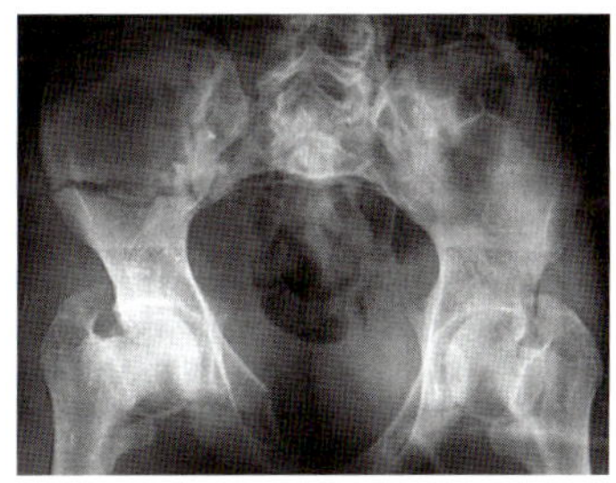 The injury force is anteriorly directed to the lateral part of the hemipelvis, resulting in ipsilateral sacral buckle fractures and horizontal pubic rami fractures, which are associated with fracture of the ipsilateral iliac wing or disruption of the ipsilateral posterior SI joint
LC-III **LC-I or II plus contralateral pubic rami fractures or disruption of the sacrotuberous and/or sacrospinous ligament; "open-book"-type (APC)** 13 fractures M: 10 (76.92%) F: 3 (23.08%) 0.66% of Young–Burgess	**LC-III** 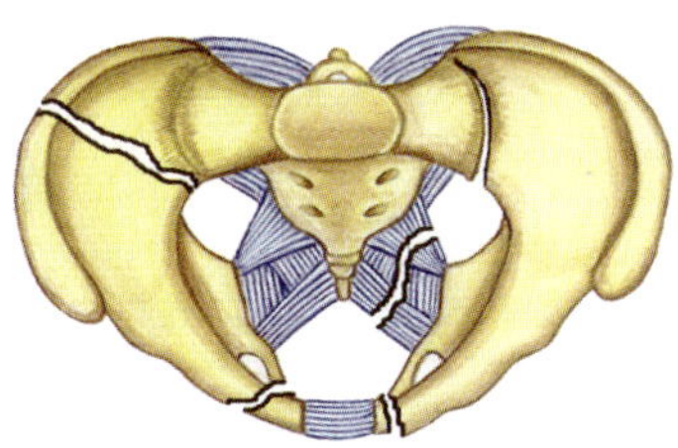 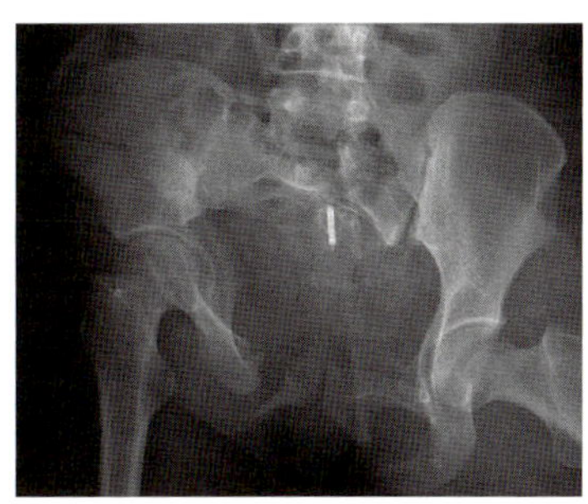 The force travels from the ipsilateral side to the contralateral side, resulting in an ipsilateral sacral buckle fracture or iliac fracture with contralateral external rotation. Contralateral vertical pubic rami fractures or disruption of the sacrotuberous and/or sacrospinous ligaments may occur.

Anteroposterior compression (APC)	
APC-I **Pubic diastasis < 2.5 cm, SI joint and posterior ligaments remain intact, and stability is maintained** 234 fractures M: 142 (60.68%) F: 92 (39.32%) 11.96% of Young–Burgess	**APC-I** 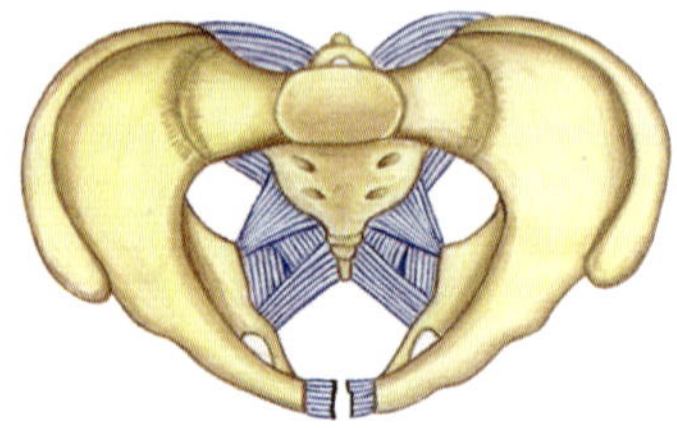 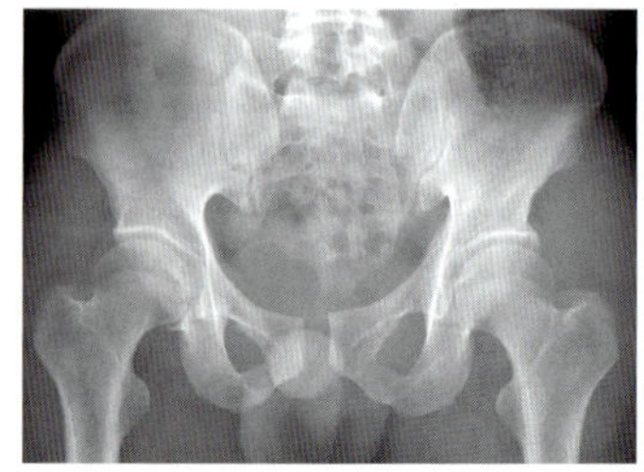 Pubic diastasis < 2.5 cm; with no or minimal disruption of the SI joint. Stable with no posterior disruption.
APC-II **Pubic diastasis > 2.5 cm, vertically oriented rami fractures, or anterior SI joint disruption. Posterior SI joint ligament remains intact** 673 fractures M: 375 (55.72%) F: 298 (44.28%) 34.41% of Young–Burgess	**APC-II** 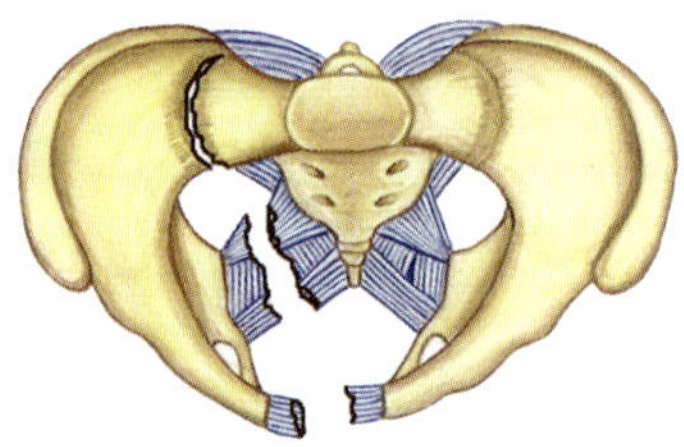 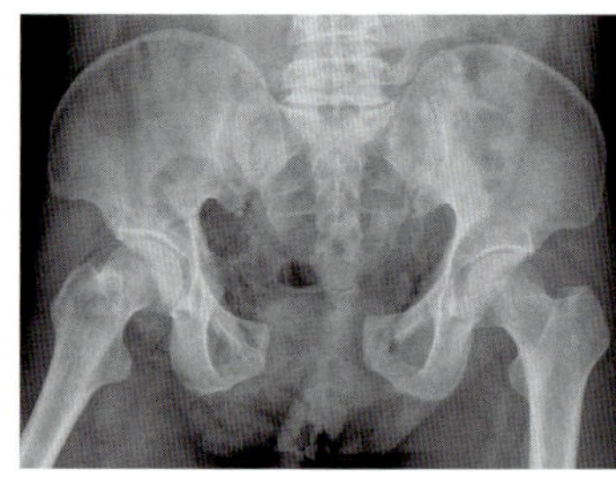 Pubic diastasis > 2.5 cm, or vertically oriented rami fractures; disrupted sacrospinous, sacrotuberous and anterior sacroiliac ligaments
APC-III **Type II plus posterior SI joint disruption** 206 fractures M: 135 (65.53%) F: 71 (34.47%) 10.53% of Young–Burgess	**APC-III** 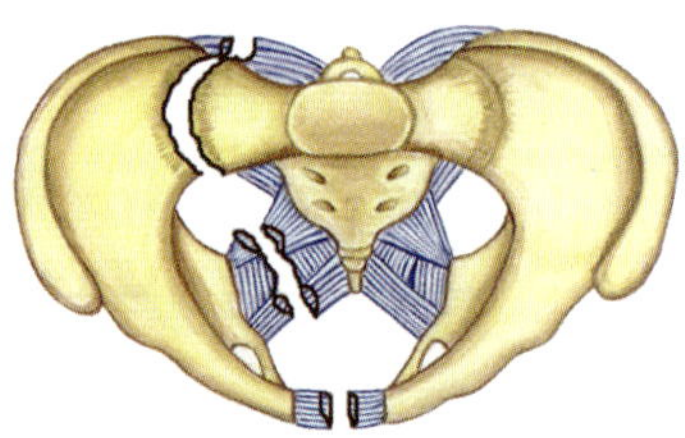 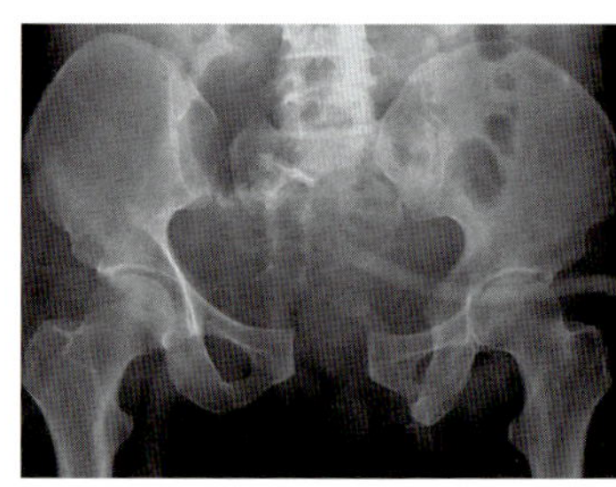 Pubic diastasis > 2.5 cm, or vertically oriented rami fractures; complete disruption of the anterior and posterior ligaments yields a rotationally and vertically unstable pelvis

Vertical shear (VS)

VS
Pubic diastasis, vertical pubic rami fractures, SI joint disruption, or vertical displacement of major fragments; adjacent fractures through the iliac wing or sacrum
170 fractures
M: 112 (65.88%)
F: 58 (34.12%)
8.69% of Young–Burgess

VS-I

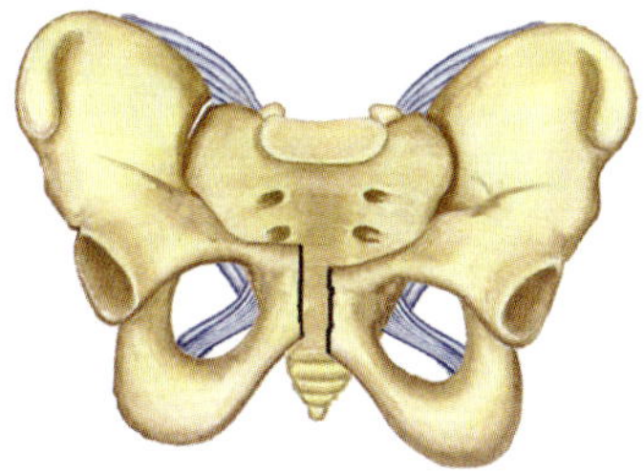

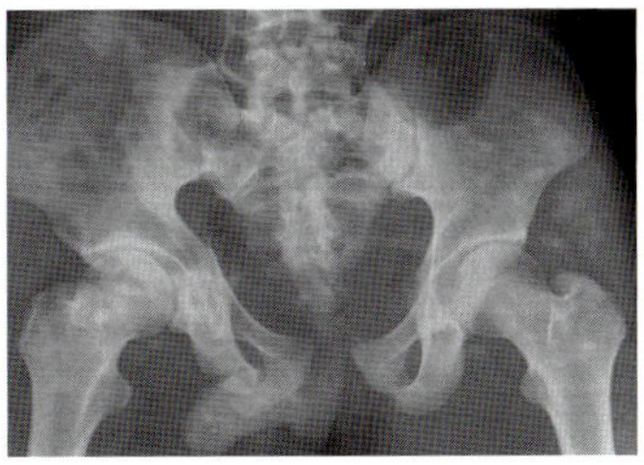

Pubic diastasis

VS-II

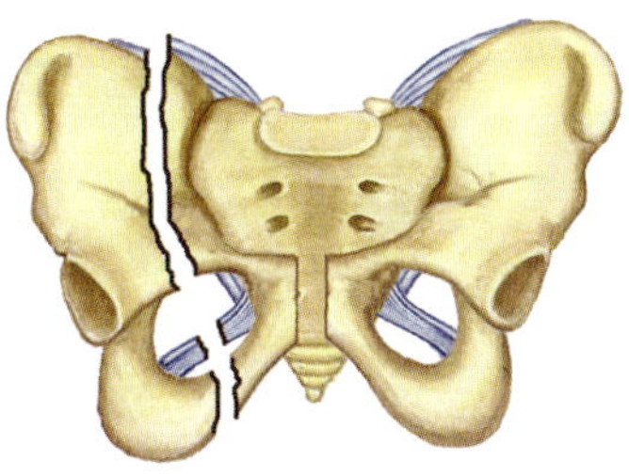

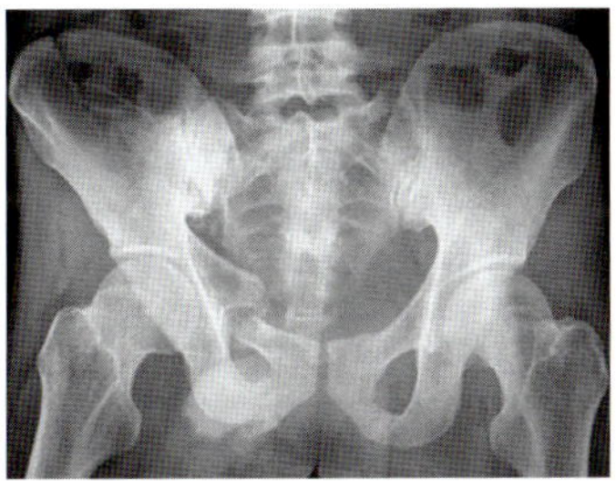

Vertical pubic rami fractures, vertical displacement, and an iliac fracture

VS-III

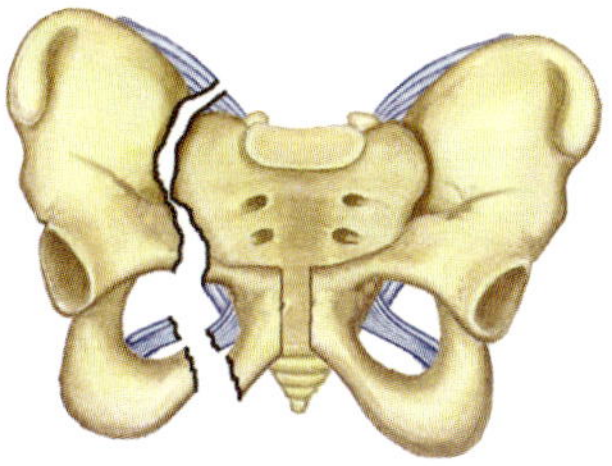

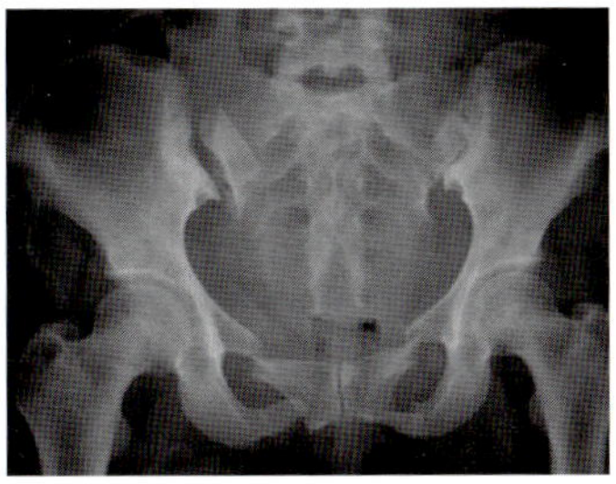

Vertical pubic rami fractures, vertical displacement, SI joint disruption, and a sacral fracture

<table>
<tr><th colspan="2">Combined mechanism (CM)</th></tr>
<tr><td rowspan="2">CM
Horizontal or vertical fracture of the anterior and/or posterior pelvic ring, involving more than one pattern of injury, with different combinations of injury types (LC-VS, LC-APC et al)
143 fractures
M: 99 (69.23%)
F: 44 (30.77%)
7.31% of Young–Burgess</td><td>CM-I
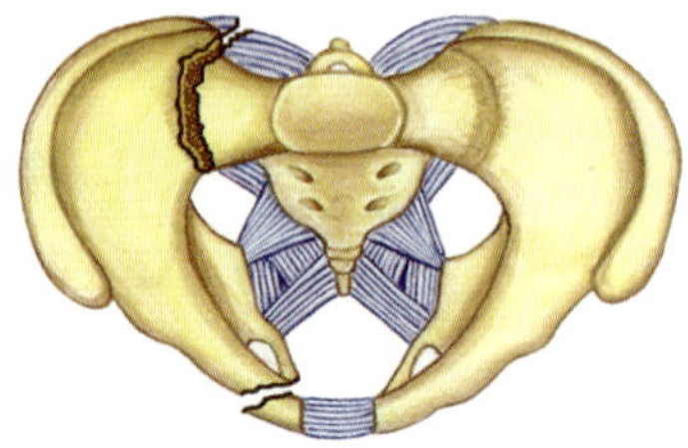 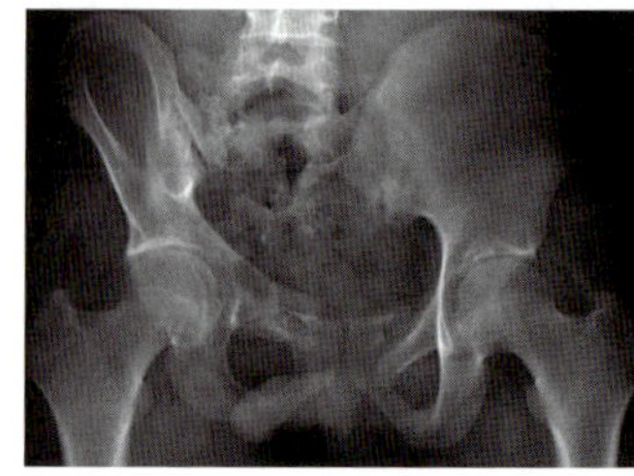
Anterolateral force</td></tr>
<tr><td>CM-II
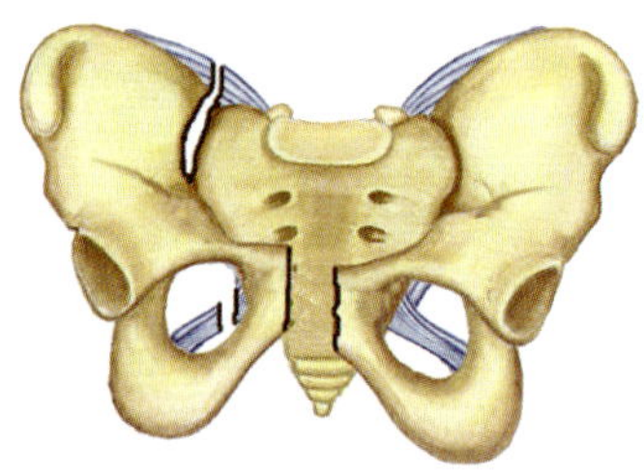 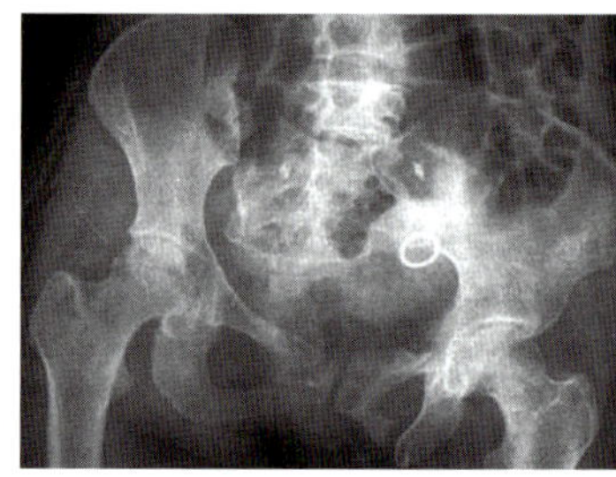
Anterovertical force</td></tr>
</table>

Letournel Classification of Pelvic Ring Fractures

Letournel devised a classification of pelvic ring fractures into anterior pelvic (ring) fractures and posterior pelvic (ring) fractures, according to the anatomical site of injury. Determination of injury site can help in assessing the severity of the injury and provide a guide in selecting the appropriate treatment (**Plate 7.19**).

- Anterior pelvic (ring) fracture
  - *Type I*: Isolated pubic diastasis
  - *Type II*: Vertical fracture of obturator foramen or adjacent pubic ramus
  - *Type III*: Acetabular fracture
- Posterior pelvic (ring) fracture
  - *Type I*: Iliac fracture without involvement of sacroiliac joint
  - *Type II*: Semilunar fracture and sacroiliac joint fracture dislocation, involving fracture of ilium or sacrum
  - *Type III*: Pure separation of sacroiliac joint
  - *Type IV*: Sacral fracture

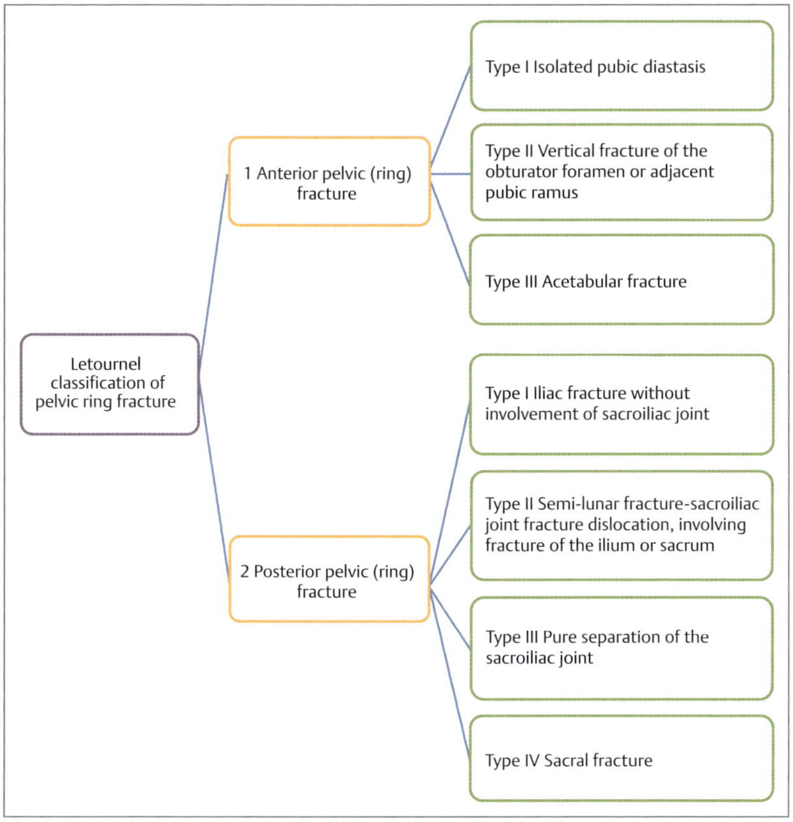

Plate 7.19

Special Type of Pelvic Ring Fracture

Bilateral Sacroiliac Dislocation with an Intact Anterior Pelvic Ring

This type of injury is rarely seen in practice; it usually occurs when both legs are in hyperflexion. This rare type of injury is characterized by bilateral SI dislocation while the anterior pelvic ring remains intact.

Disruption of the pelvic ring with associated avulsion fracture of acetabulum is not a rare type of injury, but it has a different prognosis from pure pelvic fractures, which are more dependent on the acetabular component than upon the pelvic ring disruption. CT imaging studies reveal that a considerable number of acetabular fractures are associated with sacroiliac disruption and/or pelvic ring fracture.

Letournel–Judet Classification of Acetabular Fractures

Overview

The classification method of Letournel and Judet is the most widely used classification of acetabular fractures in clinical practice and research. It classifies acetabular fractures into two basic types: simple fracture patterns and complex fracture patterns. Simple fracture patterns belong to a group of fractures in which only a wall or column is fractured, while complex patterns are combinations of the simple patterns (**Plate 7.20**).

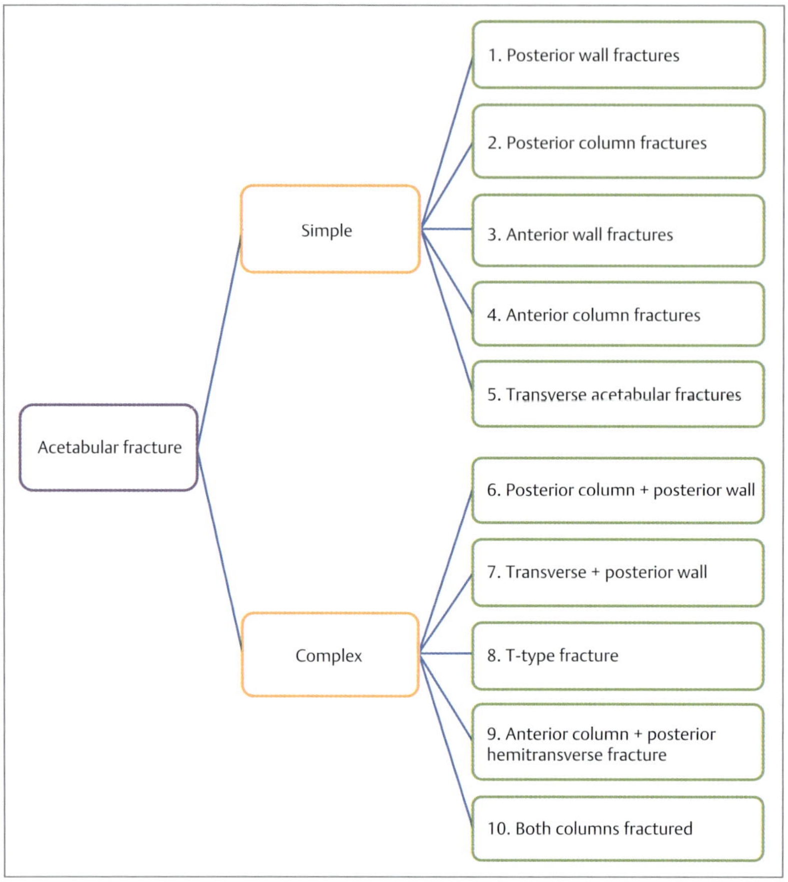

Plate 7.20

Epidemiologic Features of Acetabular Fractures Based on the Letournel –Judet Classification

We retrospectively reviewed 2,905 patients with 2,945 acetabular fractures that fit into the description of the Letournel–Judet classification system over a period of 2 years, from 2010 to 2011. These cases include 90 pediatric patients each with unilateral injuries and 2,815 adult patients with a total number of 2,855 acetabular fractures, and 40 patients sustained bilateral fractures.

Epidemiologic features of acetabular fractures based on the Letournel–Judet classification are the following:

- More males than females
- The most common fracture type of the Letournel type of acetabular fractures is Letournel-1, the same type for males, while the most common fracture type for females is Letournel-2.

Table 7.20 Sex and fracture group distribution of 2,945 acetabular fractures by the Letournel classification

Fracture group	Male	Female	Number of fractures	Percentage (%)	Percentage of fractures of pelvic ring and acetabulum (%)
Letournel-1	531	163	694	23.57	4.77
Letournel-2	325	203	528	17.93	3.63
Letournel-3	86	40	126	4.28	0.87
Letournel-4	194	91	285	9.68	1.96
Letournel-5	315	125	440	14.94	3.02
Letournel-6	79	9	88	2.99	0.60
Letournel-7	152	51	203	6.89	1.39
Letournel-8	110	47	157	5.33	1.08
Letournel-9	80	35	115	3.90	0.79
Letournel-10	242	67	309	10.49	2.12
Total	2,114	831	2,945	100.00	20.23

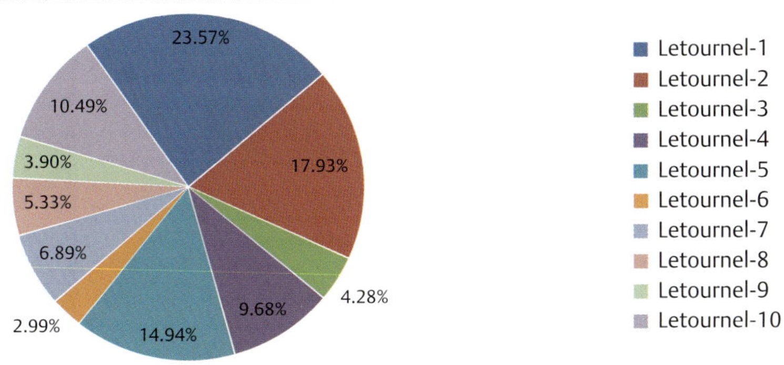

a

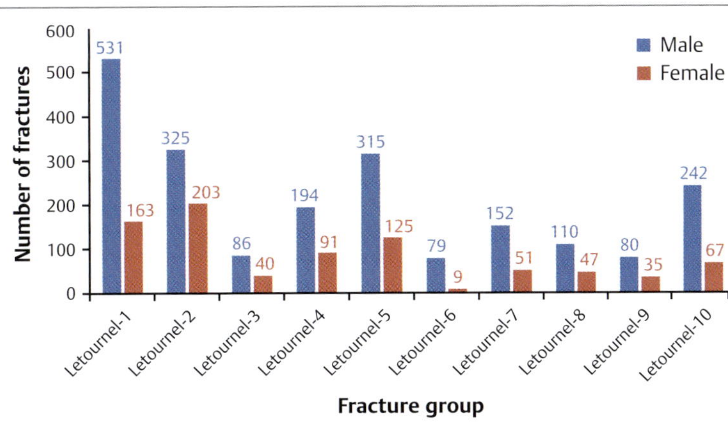

b

Fig. 7.20 **(a)** Fracture group distribution of 2,945 acetabular fractures by the Letournel classification.
(b) Sex and fracture group distribution of 2,945 acetabular fractures by the Letournel classification.

Letournel-1 **Posterior wall fractures** 694 fractures M: 531 (76.51%) F: 163 (23.49%) 23.57% acetabular	**Letournel-1** 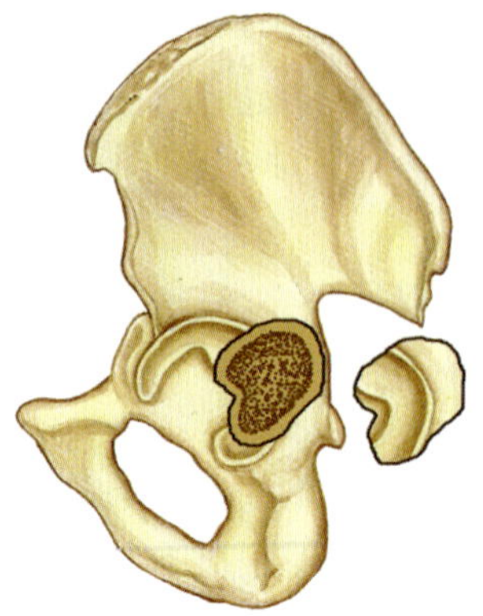	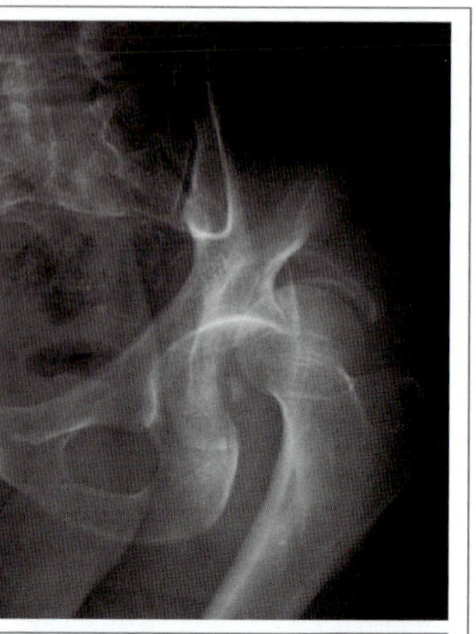
Letournel-2 **Posterior column fractures** 528 fractures M: 325 (61.55%) F: 203 (38.45%) 17.93% acetabular	**Letournel-2** 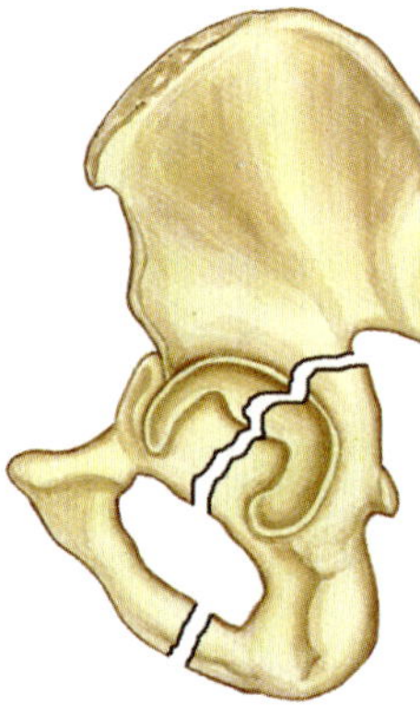	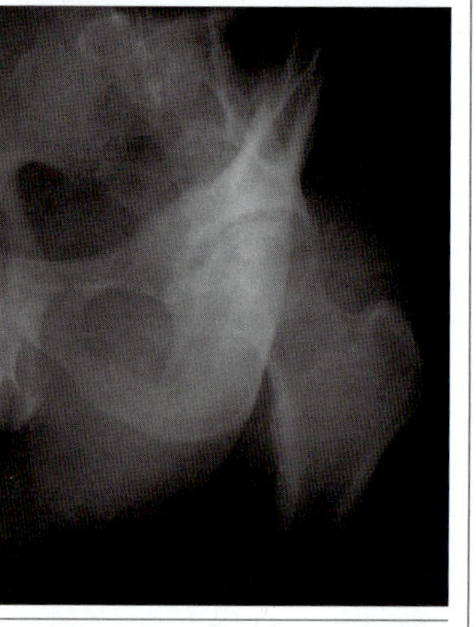
Letournel-3 **Anterior wall fractures** 126 fractures M: 86 (68.25%) F: 40 (31.75%) 4.28% acetabular	**Letournel-3** 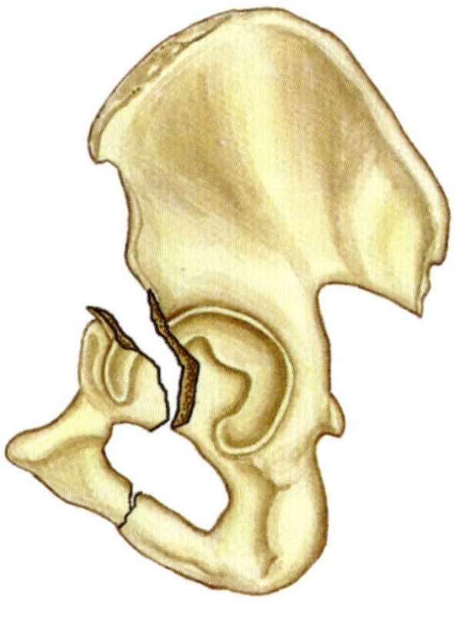	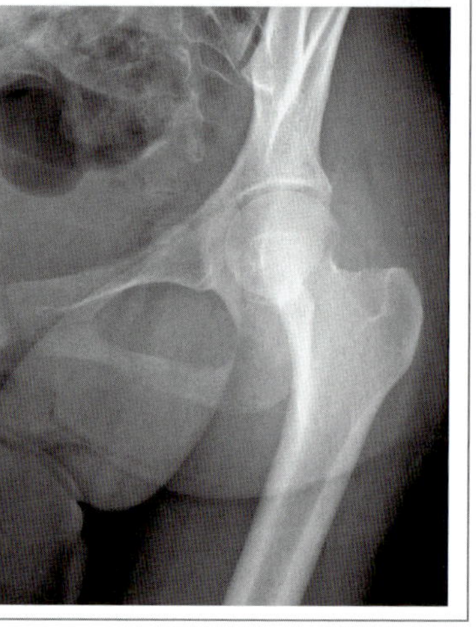

Letournel-4 **Anterior column fractures** 285 fractures M: 194 (68.07%) F: 91 (31.93%) 9.68% acetabular	**Letournel-4** 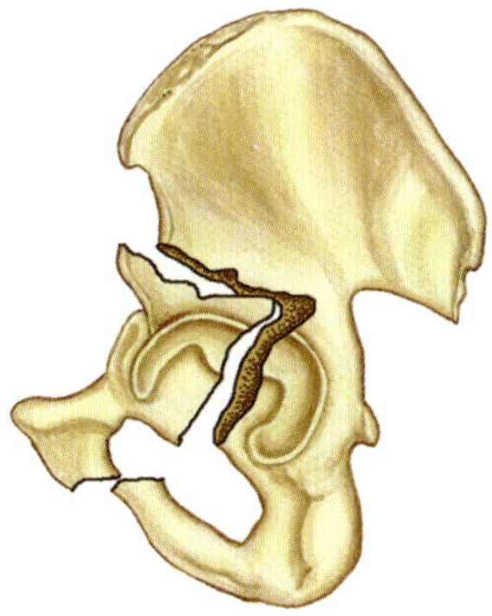 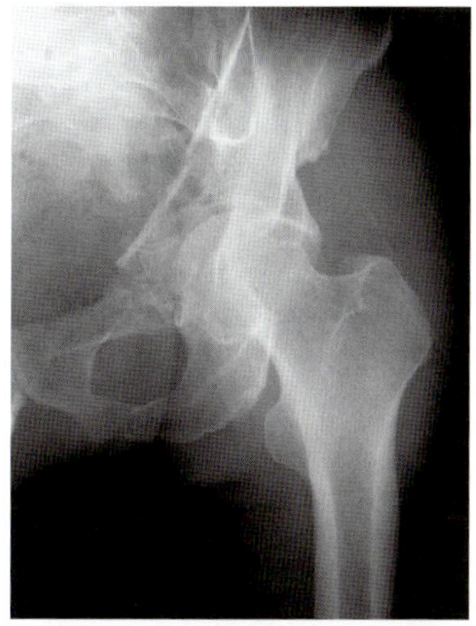
Letournel-5 **Transverse acetabular fractures** 440 fractures M: 315 (71.59%) F: 125 (28.41%) 14.94% acetabular	**Letournel-5** 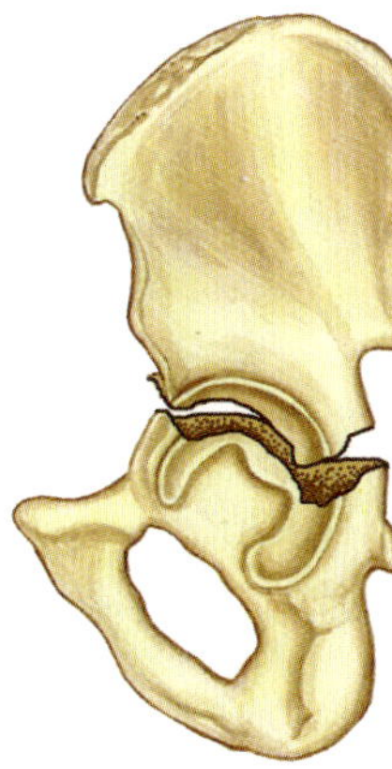 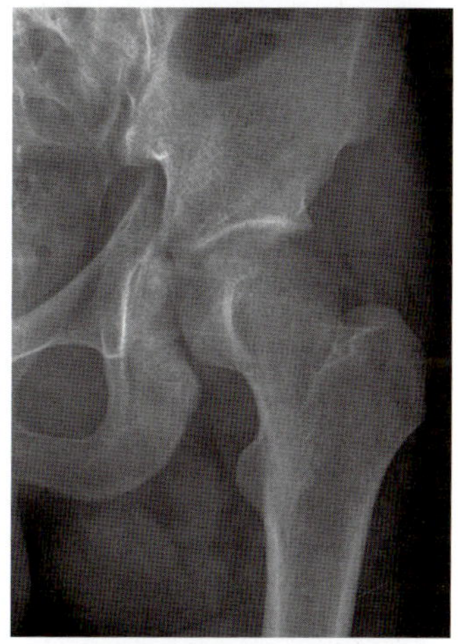
Letournel-6 **Posterior wall + posterior column** 88 fractures M: 79 (89.77%) F: 9 (10.23%) 2.99% acetabular	**Letournel-6** 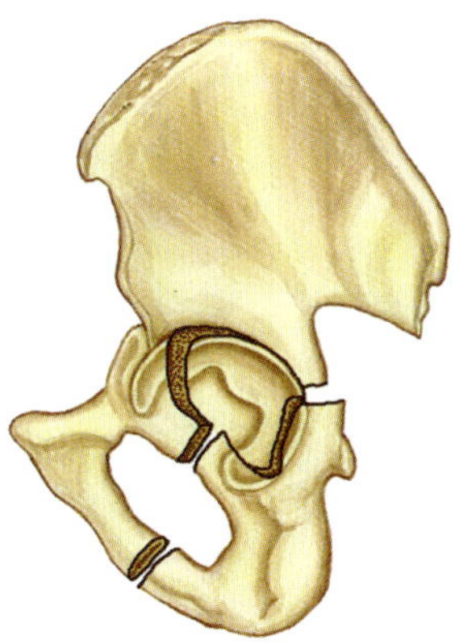 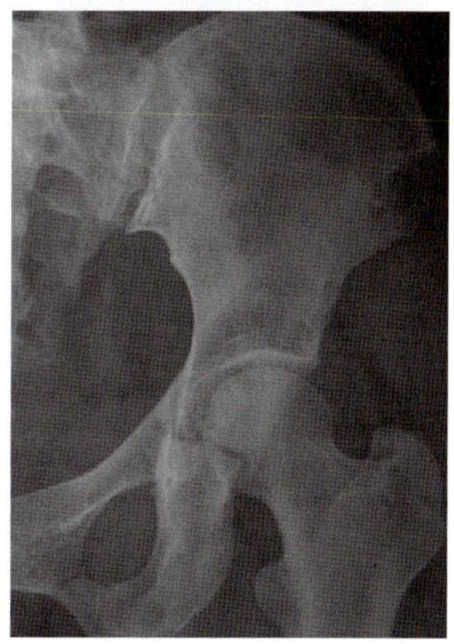

Letournel-7 **Transverse + posterior wall** 203 fractures M: 152 (74.88%) F: 51 (25.12%) 6.89% acetabular	**Letournel-7** 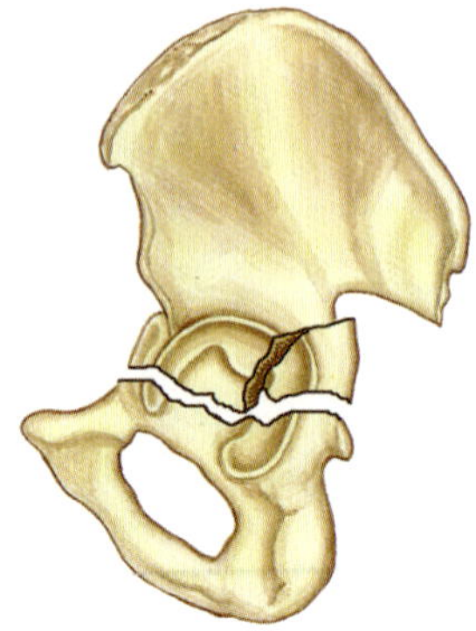	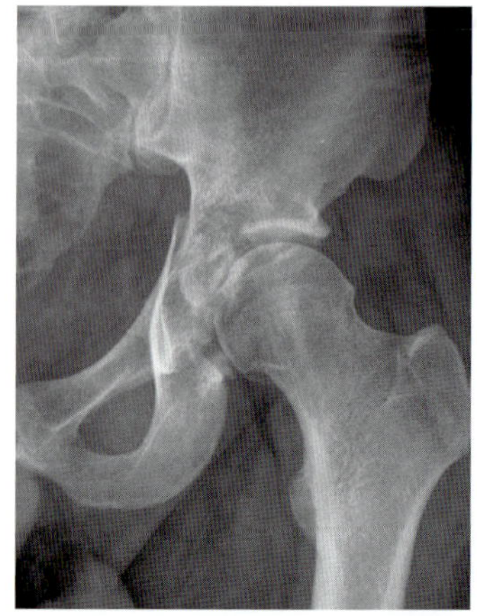
Letournel-8 **T-type fractures** 157 fractures M: 110 (70.06%) F: 47 (29.94%) 5.33% acetabular	**Letournel-8** 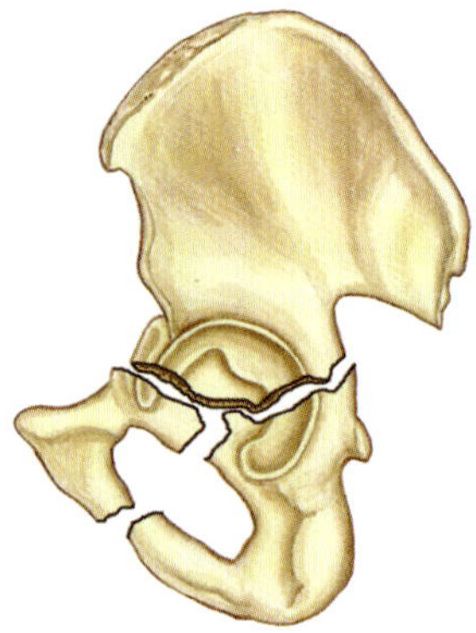	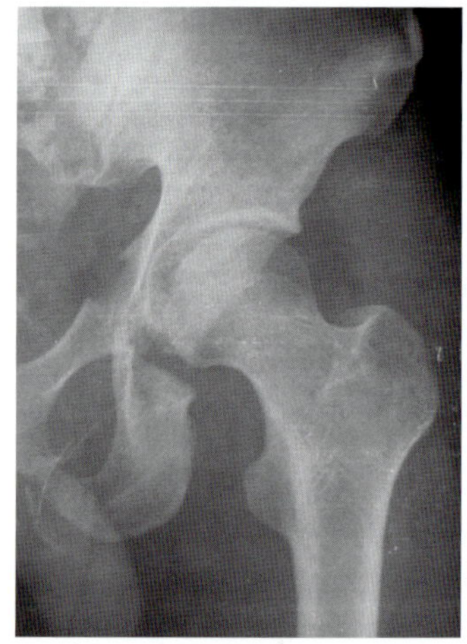
Letournel-9 **Anterior column + posterior hemitransverse fractures** 115 fractures M: 80 (69.57%) F: 35 (30.43%) 3.90% acetabular	**Letournel-9** 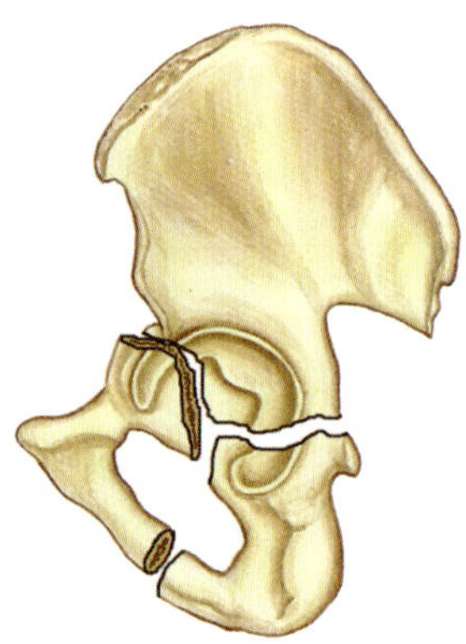	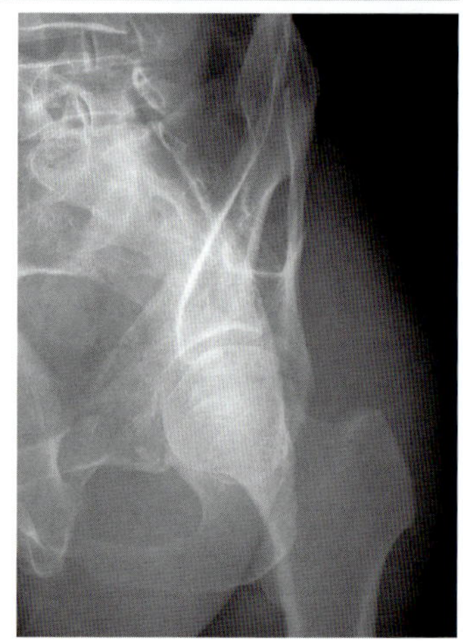

Letournel-10 **Both column fractured** 309 fractures M: 242 (78.32%) F: 67 (21.68%) 10.49% acetabular	**Letournel-10** 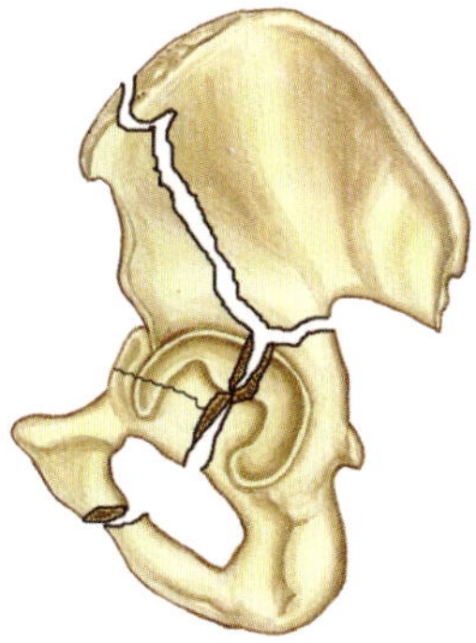 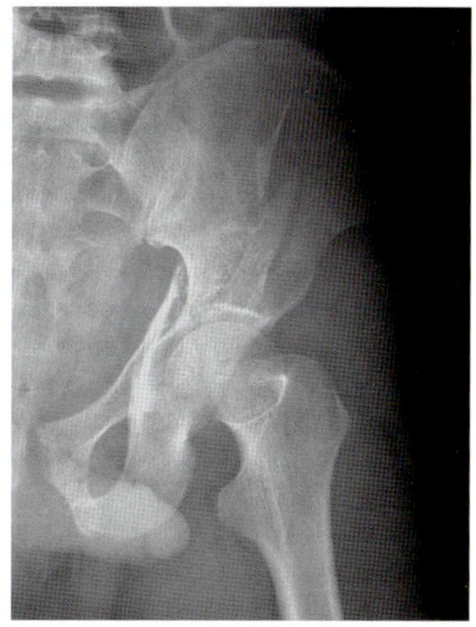

Tile Classification of Acetabular Fractures

- Nondisplaced acetabular fracture
- Displaced acetabular fracture. It is further divided into three types (**Plate 7.21**):
  - *Type I*: Fracture of the posterior part of the acetabulum with or without posterior dislocation
    - *Type IA*: Posterior column fracture
    - *Type IB*: Posterior wall fracture with associated posterior column or transverse fractures
  - *Type II:* Fracture of anterior part of the acetabulum with or without anterior dislocation
    - *Type IIA*: Anterior column fracture
    - *Type IIB*: Anterior wall fracture
    - *Type IIC*: With associated anterior or transverse fractures
  - *Type III:* Transverse fracture with or without central dislocation of the hip
    - *Type IIIA*: Pure transverse fracture
    - *Type IIIB*: T-type fractures
    - *Type IIIC*: With associated transverse or acetabular wall fractures
    - *Type IIID*: Bilateral column fractures

Plate 7.21

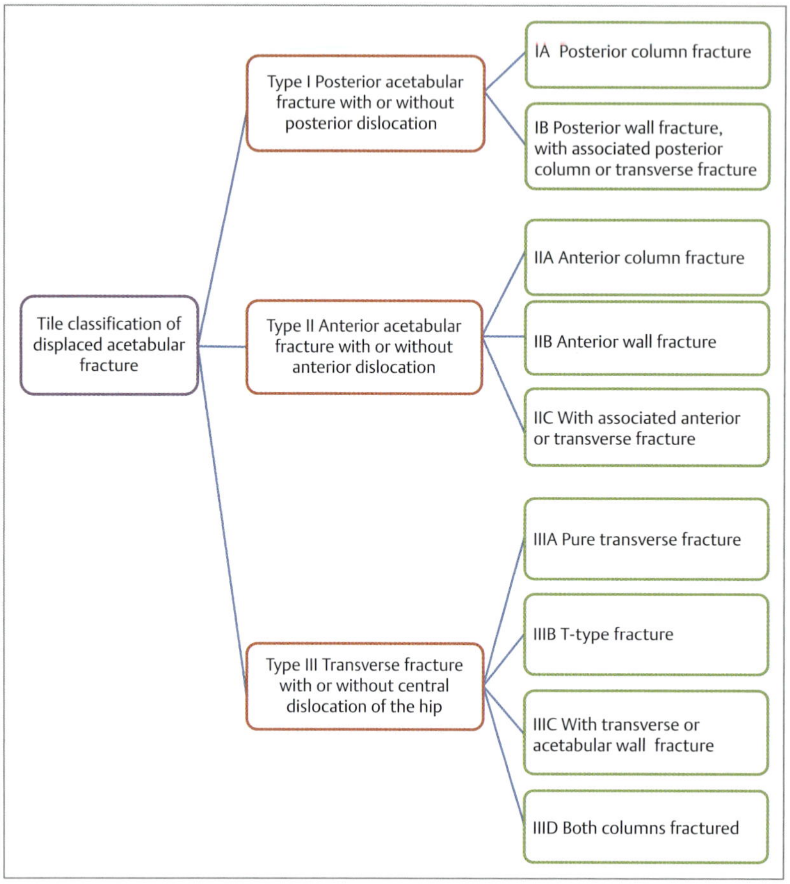
Tile classification of displaced acetabular fracture
Type I Posterior acetabular fracture with or without posterior dislocation
IA Posterior column fracture
IB Posterior wall fracture, with associated posterior column or transverse fracture
Type II Anterior acetabular fracture with or without anterior dislocation
IIA Anterior column fracture
IIB Anterior wall fracture
IIC With associated anterior or transverse fracture
Type III Transverse fracture with or without central dislocation of the hip
IIIA Pure transverse fracture
IIIB T-type fracture
IIIC With transverse or acetabular wall fracture
IIID Both columns fractured

7

8 Fractures of the Hand

Overview

Anatomical Features

The skeleton of the hand consists of 8 small carpal bones (wrist), 5 metacarpals (palm), 14 phalanges (fingers), and 2 sesamoid bones (**Plate 8.1**).

The carpus is made up of eight carpal bones, which are arranged into two rows: a proximal and distal row. The proximal row from lateral to medial contains the scaphoid, lunate, triquetral, and pisiform bones; all of these except the pisiform bone are part of the radiocarpal joint. The distal row contains, in the same order, the trapezium, trapezoid, capitate, and hamate bones, which are all involved in the formation of the carpometacarpal joints. The metacarpus consists of five cylindrical bones, each of which is made up of three parts: a body, base, and head. There are 14 phalanges on each hand: 3 for each finger and 2 for the thumb. Each finger has a proximal, middle, and distal phalange except the pollex, which only has proximal and distal phalanx.

OTA Classification and Coding System for Hand Fractures

Based on the Orthopaedic Trauma Association (OTA) classification for fractures, a hand fracture is coded as the number 7, and the numeric codes for fractures of each individual bone are as follows: 71, lunate; 72, scaphoid; 73, capitate; 74, hamate; 75, carpal bone on the ulnar side (triquetral and pisiform bones); 76, carpal bone on the radial side (trapezium and trapezoid bones); 77, metacarpal bones; 78, phalanx bones; and 79, multiple hand fractures (**Plate 8.2**).

Clinical Epidemiologic Features of Hand Fractures

A total of 62,555 patients with 63,730 hand fractures were treated in 83 hospitals in China over a 2-year period from 2010 to 2011. All cases were reviewed and statistically studied; the fractures accounted for 15.08% of all fractured patients and 14.76% of all types of fractures. Among these 62,555 patients, there were 4,847 children with 4,881 hand fractures, accounting for 8.87% of pediatric patients with fractures, and 8.50% of all types of fractures in children. The rest of the 57,708 adult patients had 58,849 fractures, representing 16.02% of adult patients with fractures, and 15.72% of all types of fractures in adults.

Epidemiologic features of hand fractures are as follows:

- More males than females
- More right-side than left-side injuries
- The high-risk age group is 21–25 years, the same age group for males whereas the high-risk age group for females is 36–40 years
- Phalanx fractures are the most common fractures of the hand.

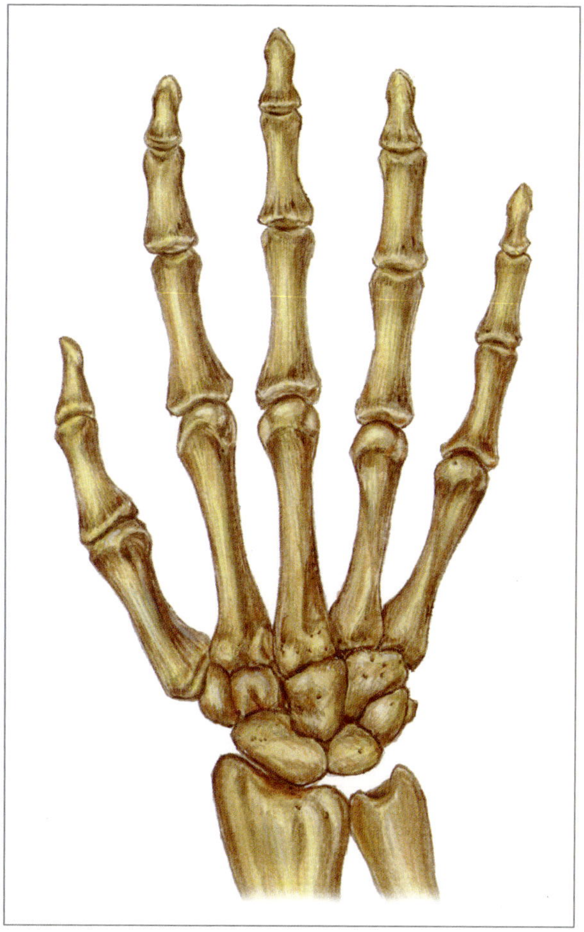

Plate 8.1

Plate 8.2

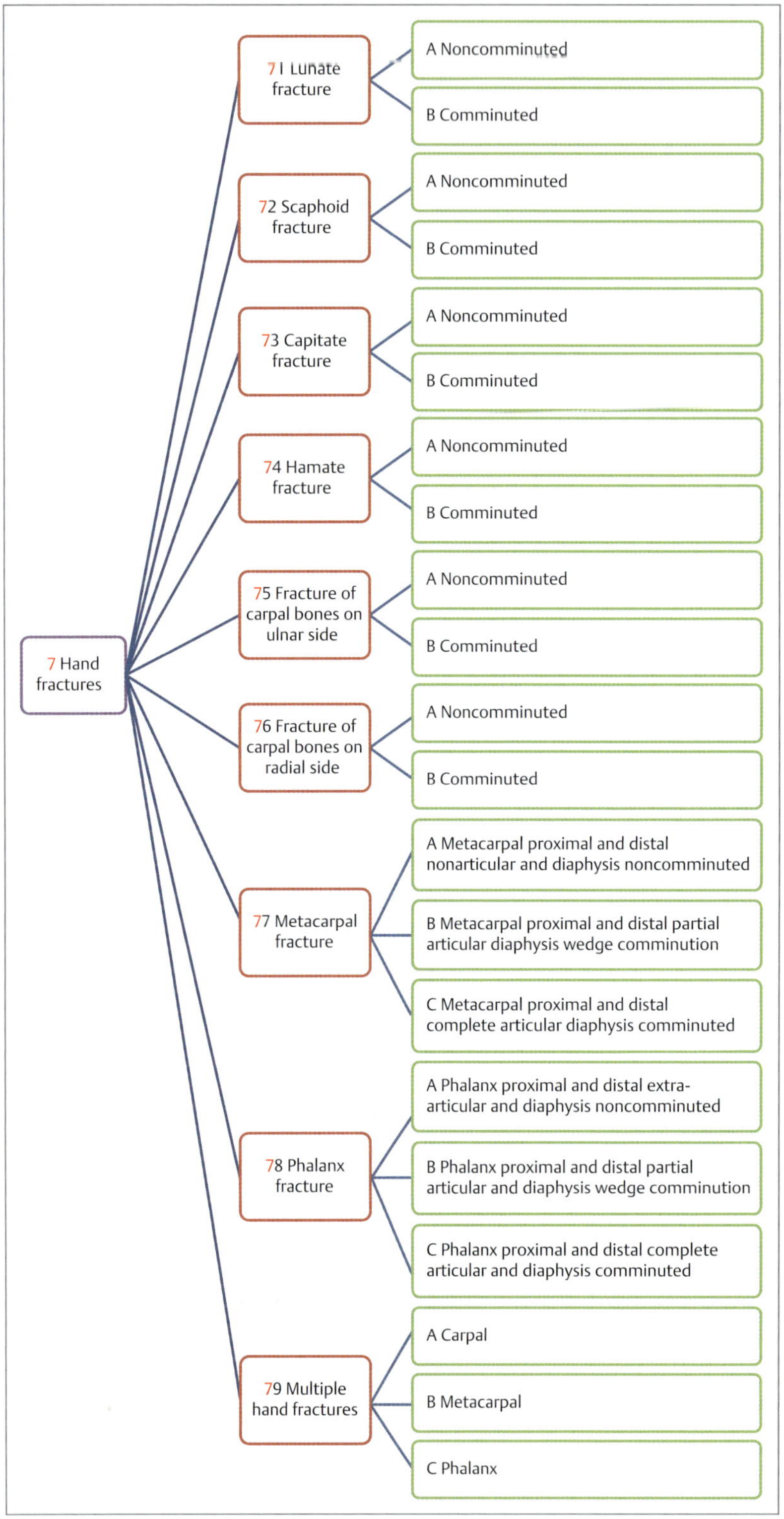
7 Hand fractures
71 Lunate fracture
A Noncomminuted
B Comminuted
72 Scaphoid fracture
A Noncomminuted
B Comminuted
73 Capitate fracture
A Noncomminuted
B Comminuted
74 Hamate fracture
A Noncomminuted
B Comminuted
75 Fracture of carpal bones on ulnar side
A Noncomminuted
B Comminuted
76 Fracture of carpal bones on radial side
A Noncomminuted
B Comminuted
77 Metacarpal fracture
A Metacarpal proximal and distal nonarticular and diaphysis noncomminuted
B Metacarpal proximal and distal partial articular diaphysis wedge comminution
C Metacarpal proximal and distal complete articular diaphysis comminuted
78 Phalanx fracture
A Phalanx proximal and distal extra-articular and diaphysis noncomminuted
B Phalanx proximal and distal partial articular and diaphysis wedge comminution
C Phalanx proximal and distal complete articular and diaphysis comminuted
79 Multiple hand fractures
A Carpal
B Metacarpal
C Phalanx

8

Hand Fractures by Sex

Table 8.1 Sex distribution of 62,555 patients with hand fractures

Sex	Number of patients	Percentage (%)
Male	48,799	78.01
Female	13,756	21.99
Total	62,555	100.00

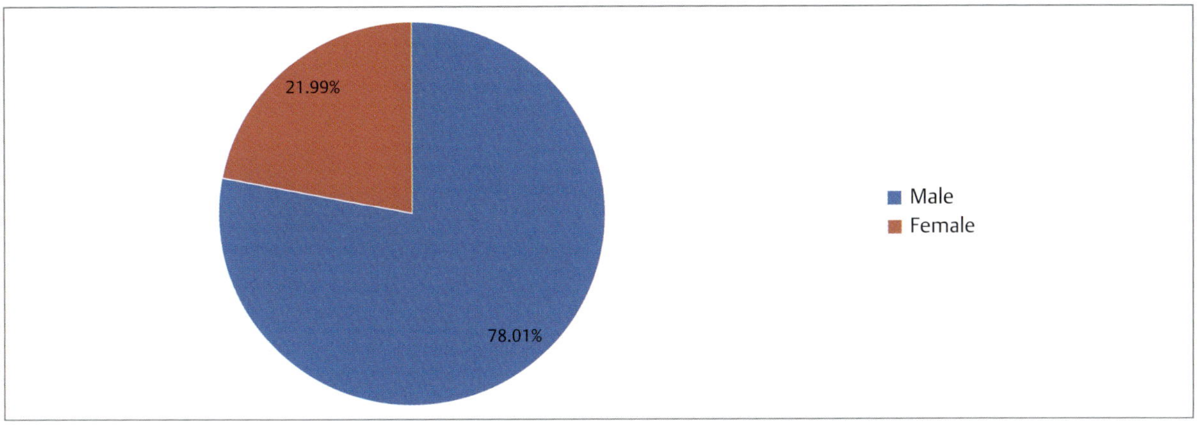

Fig. 8.1 Sex distribution of 62,555 patients with hand fractures.

Hand Fractures by Fracture Side

Table 8.2 Fracture side distribution of 62,555 patients with hand fractures

Fracture side	Number of patients	Percentage (%)
Left	30,291	48.42
Right	31,999	51.15
Bilateral	265	0.42
Total	62,555	100.00

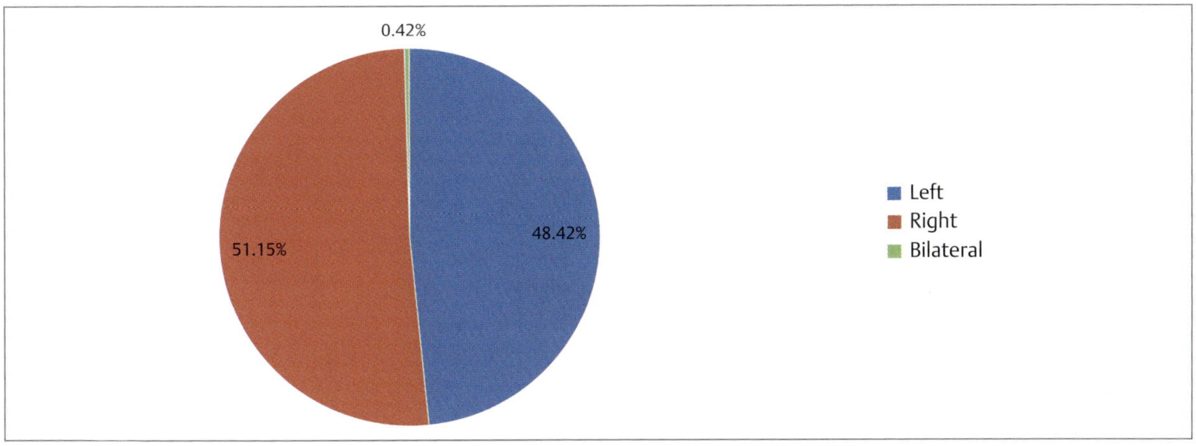

Fig. 8.2 Fracture side distribution of 62,555 patients with hand fractures.

8

Hand Fractures by Age Group

Table 8.3 Age and sex distribution of 62,555 patients with hand fractures

Age group (years)	Male	Female	Number of patients	Percentage (%)
0–5	1,031	510	1,541	2.46
6–10	943	435	1,378	2.20
11–15	1,591	337	1,928	3.08
16–20	5,327	868	6,195	9.90
21–25	7,499	1,147	8,646	13.82
26–30	5,972	1,218	7,190	11.49
31–35	4,995	1,314	6,309	10.09
36–40	5,697	1,840	7,537	12.05
41–45	5,172	1,811	6,983	11.16
46–50	4,006	1,383	5,389	8.61
51–55	2,633	893	3,526	5.64
56–60	2,052	794	2,846	4.55
61–65	926	455	1,381	2.21
66–70	371	298	669	1.07
71–75	292	192	484	0.77
76–80	170	161	331	0.53
81–85	75	64	139	0.22
≥86	47	36	83	0.13
Total	48,799	13,756	62,555	100.00

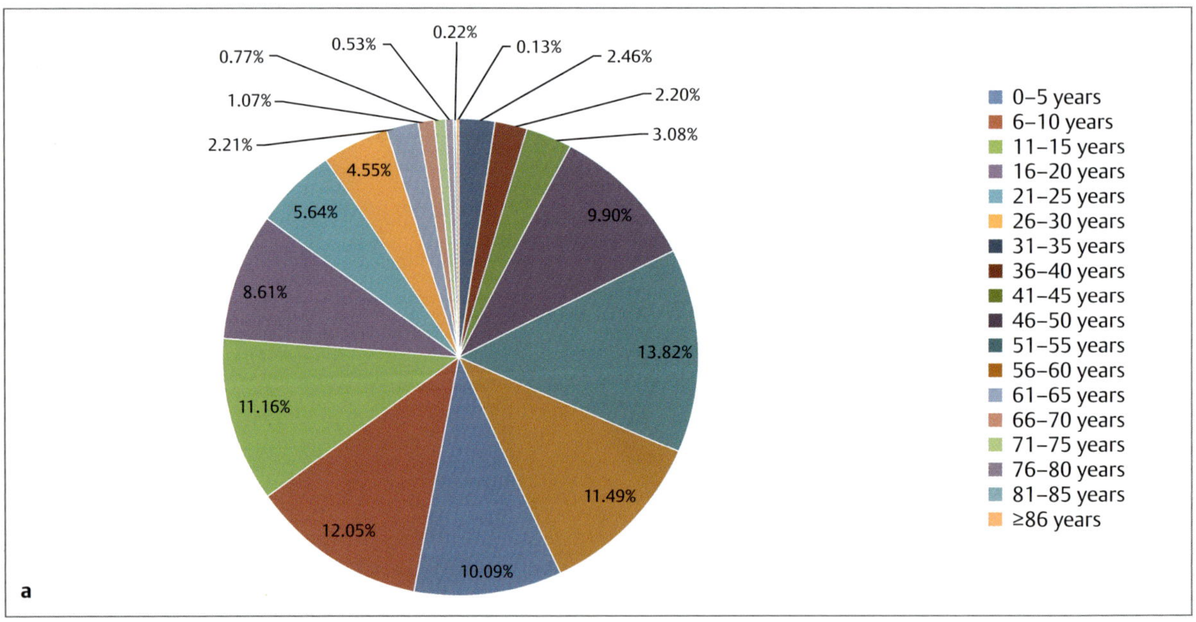

Fig. 8.3 **(a)** Age distribution of 62,555 patients with hand fractures.

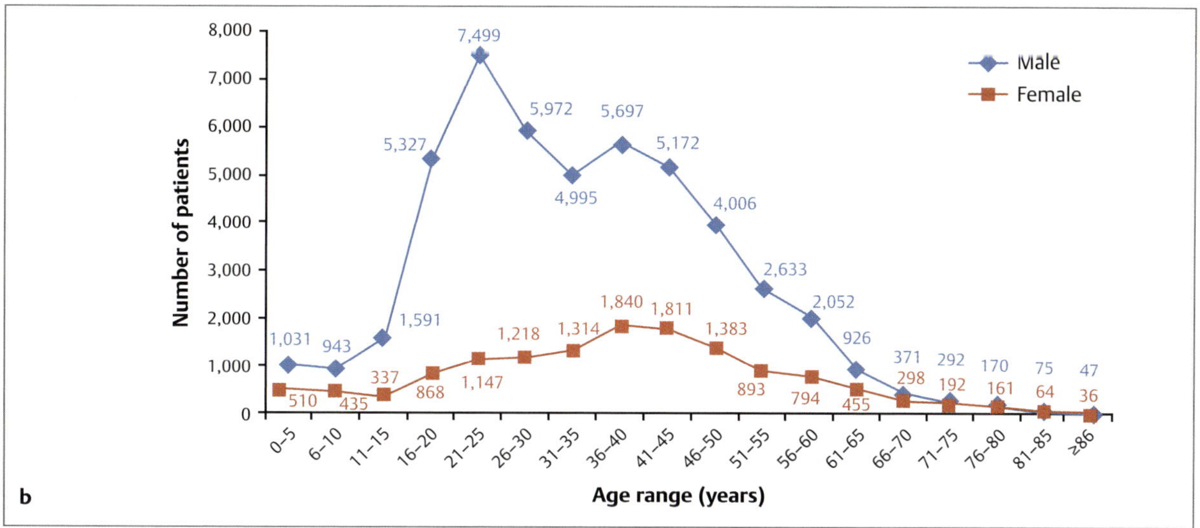

Fig. 8.3 (*continued*) **(b)** Age and sex distribution of 62,555 patients with hand fractures.

Hand Fractures by Fracture Location

Hand Fractures by Locations in Adults Based on OTA Classification

Table 8.4 Fracture location distribution of 58,849 hand fractures in adults

Fracture location	Number of fractures	Percentage (%)
71–76 (carpals)	3,064	5.21
77 (metacarpals)	10,145	17.24
78 (phalanx)	33,843	57.51
79 (multiple)	11,797	20.05
Total	58,849	100.00

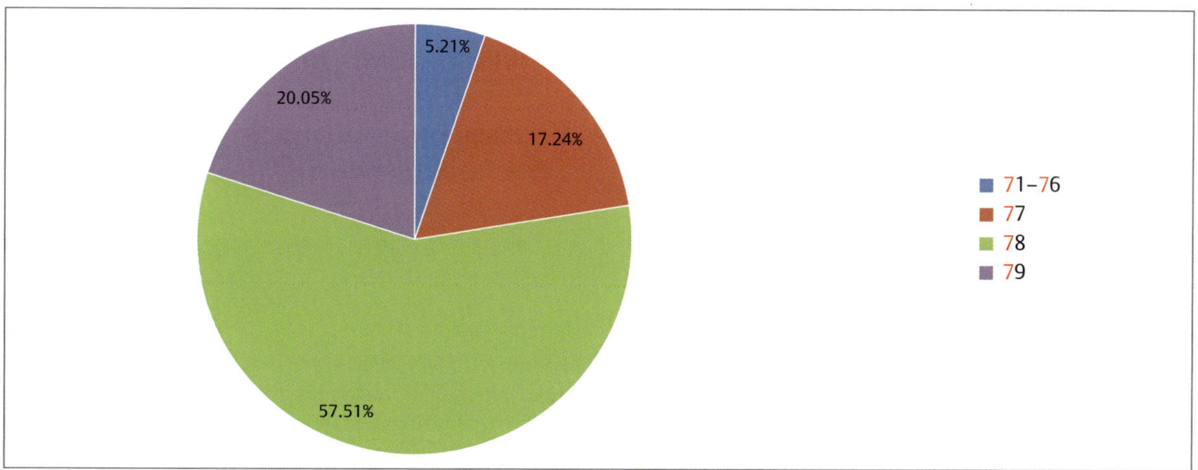

Fig. 8.4 Fracture location distribution of 58,849 hand fractures in adults.

Hand Fractures by Locations in Children

Table 8.5 Fracture location distribution of 4,881 hand fractures in children

Fracture location	Number of fractures	Percentage (%)
Carpals	95	1.95
Metacarpals	884	18.11
Phalanx	3,902	79.94
Total	4,881	100.00

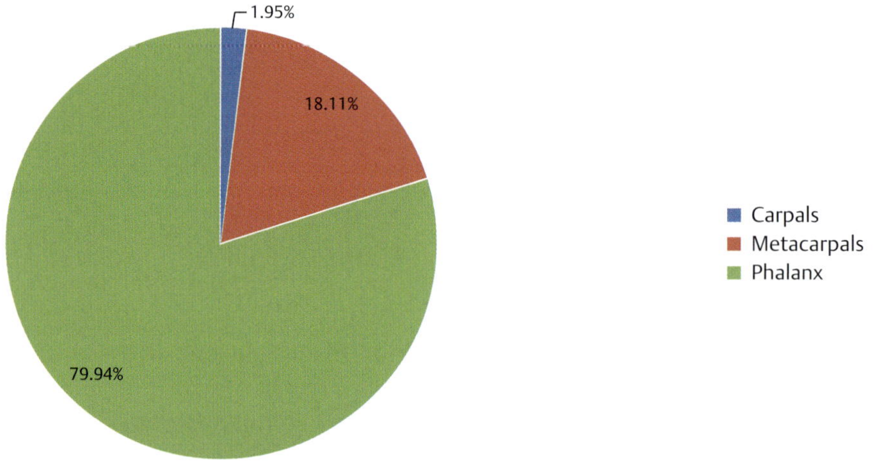

Fig. 8.5 Fracture location distribution of 4,881 hand fractures in children.

8

Carpal Fractures (Segments 71–76)

Anatomical Features

There are eight carpal bones, arranged in two rows. Those of the proximal row, from lateral to medial, are the scaphoid, lunate, triangular, and pisiform; those of the distal row, in the same order, are the trapezium, trapezoid, capitate, and hamate. From the proximal row, the superior articular surface of the scaphoid, lunate, and triangular are connected by ligaments, present a convex surface, and articulate with the inferior surface of the radius and articular disk, forming the radiocarpal joint; the distal row of carpal bones articulates with the proximal bases of the five metacarpal bones, forming the carpometacarpal joints. Carpals are short bones; each bone (except the pisiform) has six surfaces. The anterior and posterior surfaces, which make ligamentous attachment, are rough. The surfaces where the carpal bones make contact with contiguous bones are all articular, thus covered with articular cartilage, and are involved in the formation of the joint. The construction of these short bones provides complex but limited movement.

OTA Classification of Carpal Fractures

Carpal fractures are classified based on OTA classification as follows: 71, lunate; 72, scaphoid; 73, capitate; 74, hamate; 75, ulnar carpal bones; and 76, radial carpal bones (**Plate 8.3**).

Clinical Epidemiologic Features of Carpal Fractures (Segments 71–76)

A total of 3,057 patients with 3,064 carpal fractures were treated in 83 hospitals in China over a 2-year period from 2010 to 2011. All cases were reviewed and statistically studied; the fractures accounted for 5.30% of all adult patients with hand fractures and 5.21% of hand fractures in adults. Their epidemiologic features are as follows:

- More males than females
- The high-risk age group is 21–25 years—the same age group for males whereas the high-risk age group for females is 56–60 years.
- Scaphoid fractures (72) are the most common of carpal bone fractures (71–76).

Plate 8.3

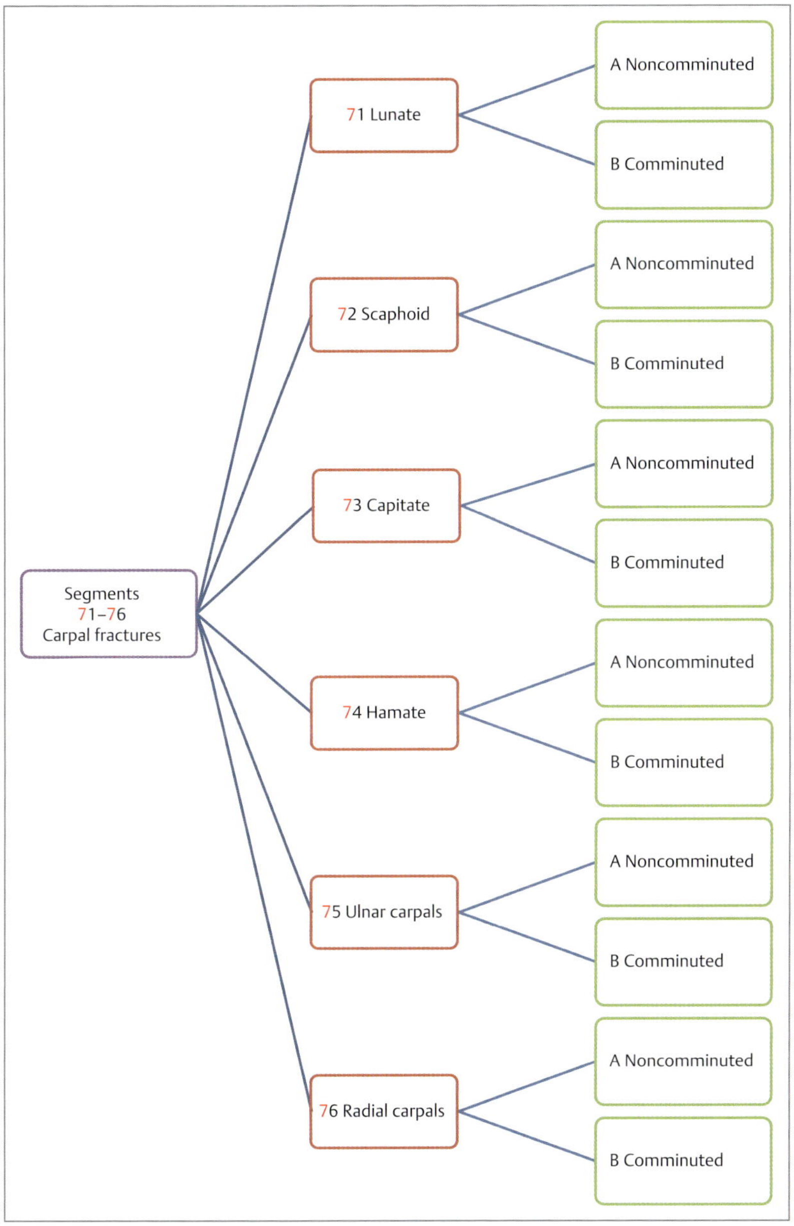
Segments
71–76
Carpal fractures
71 Lunate
72 Scaphoid
73 Capitate
74 Hamate
75 Ulnar carpals
76 Radial carpals
A Noncomminuted
B Comminuted
A Noncomminuted
B Comminuted
A Noncomminuted
B Comminuted
A Noncomminuted
B Comminuted
A Noncomminuted
B Comminuted
A Noncomminuted
B Comminuted

Carpal Fractures (Segments 71–76) by Sex

Table 8.6 Sex distribution of 3,057 patients with fractures of carpal bones (segments 71–76)

Sex	Number of patients	Percentage (%)
Male	2,284	74.71
Female	773	25.29
Total	3,057	100.00

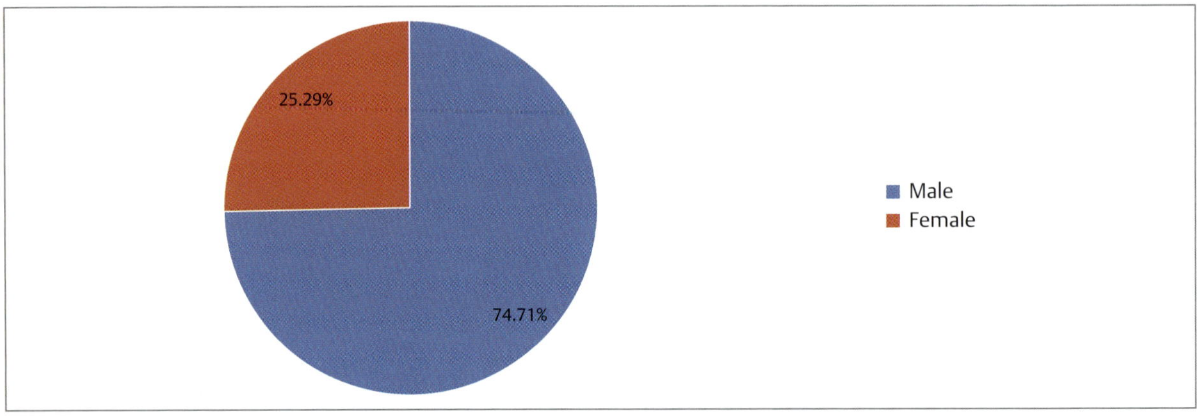

Fig. 8.6 Sex distribution of 3,057 patients with carpal fractures.

Carpal Fractures (Segments 71–76) by Age Group

Table 8.7 Age and sex distribution of 3,057 patients with fractures of the carpal bones (segments 71–76)

Age group (years)	Male	Female	Number of patients	Percentage (%)
16–20	291	47	338	11.06
21–25	405	62	467	15.28
26–30	360	49	409	13.38
31–35	243	57	300	9.81
36–40	252	82	334	10.93
41–45	201	77	278	9.09
46–50	168	86	254	8.31
51–55	112	83	195	6.38
56–60	80	100	180	5.89
61–65	58	45	103	3.37
66–70	23	38	61	2.00
71–75	41	25	66	2.16
76–80	28	16	44	1.44
81–85	18	4	22	0.72
≥86	4	2	6	0.20
Total	2,284	773	3,057	100.00

8

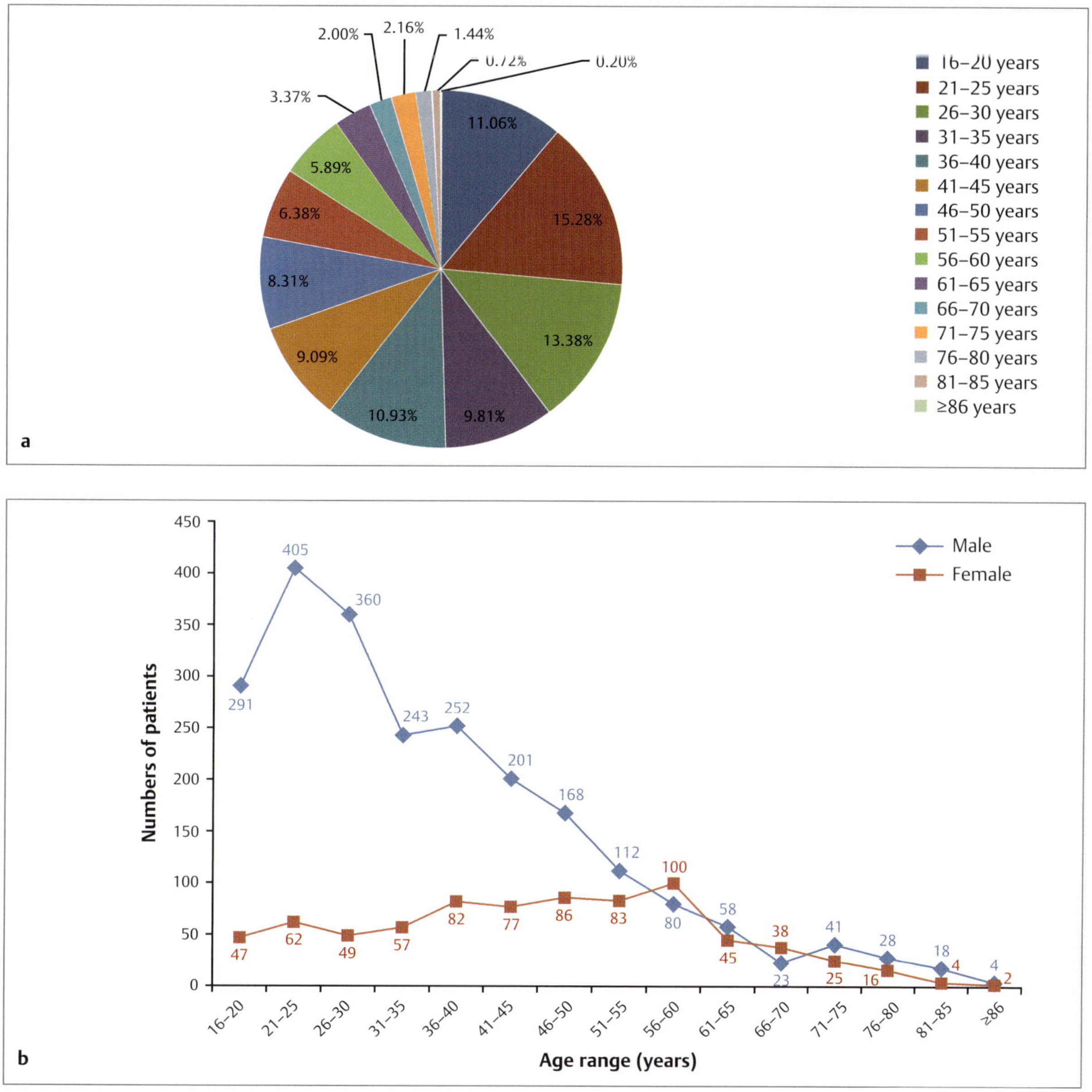

Fig. 8.7 **(a)** Age distribution of 3,057 patients with carpal fractures.
(b) Age and sex distribution of 3,057 patients with carpal fractures.

Carpal Fractures (Segments 71–76) by Fracture Type

Table 8.8 Sex and fracture type distribution of 3,064 fractures of carpal bones (segments 71–76)

Fracture type	Male	Female	Number of fractures	Percentage (%)
71 (lunate)	82	34	116	3.79
72 (scaphoid)	1,634	471	2,105	68.70
73 (capitate)	104	53	157	5.12
74 (hamate)	104	34	138	4.50
75 (ulnar carpal bones)	247	118	365	11.91
76 (radial carpal bones)	119	64	183	5.97
Total	2,290	774	3,064	100.00

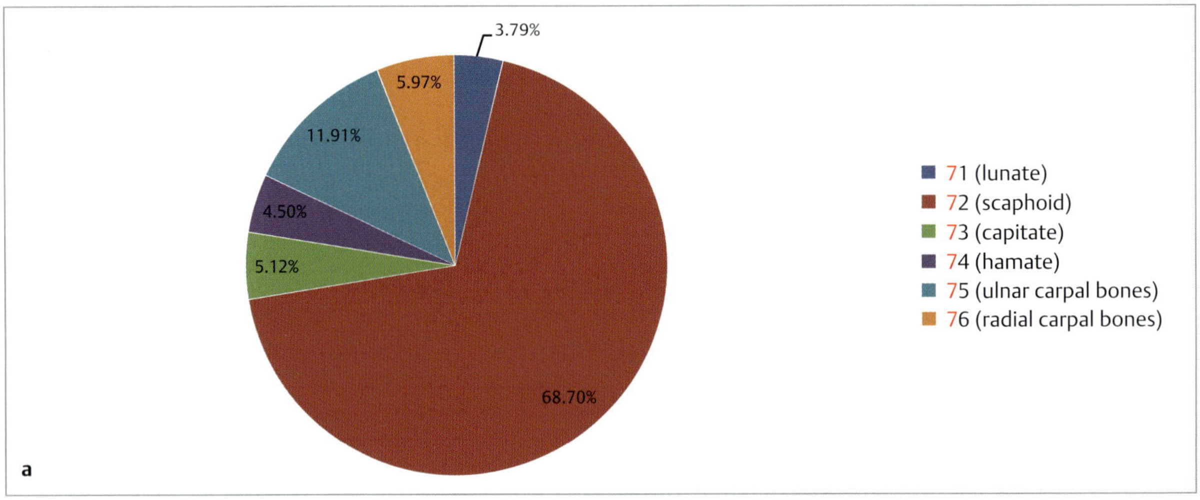

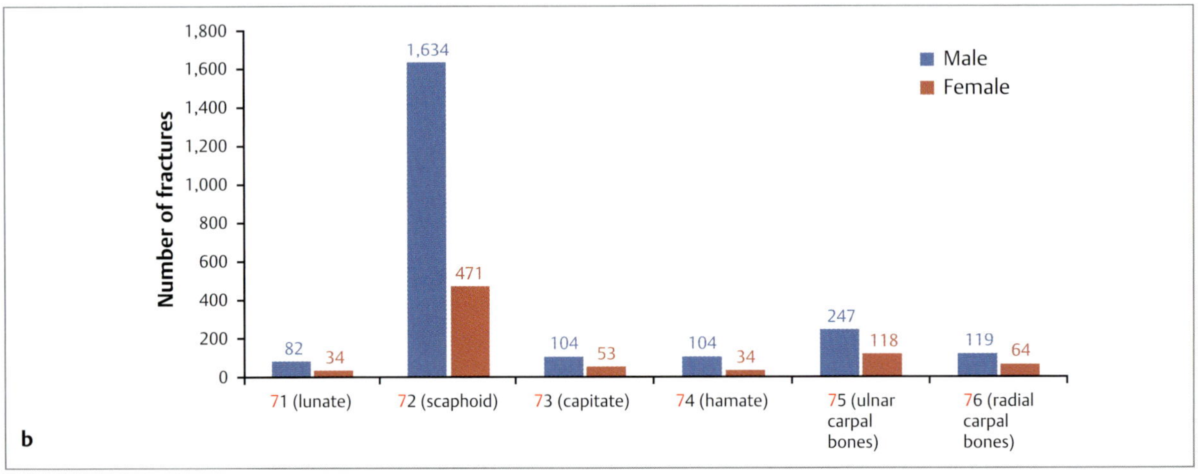

Fig. 8.8 **(a)** Fracture type distribution of 3,064 fractures of carpal bones (segments 71–76).
(b) Sex and fracture type distribution of 3,064 fractures of carpal bones (segments 71–76).

Table 8.9 Sex and fracture group distribution of 3,064 fractures of carpal bones (segments 71–76)

Fracture group	Male	Female	Number of fractures	Percentage of carpal bone fractures (segments 71–76) (%)	Percentage of fractures of the hand in adults (%)
71-A	69	28	97	3.17	0.16
71-B	13	6	19	0.62	0.03
72-A	1,419	419	1,838	59.99	3.12
72-B	215	52	267	8.71	0.45
73-A	76	36	112	3.66	0.19
73-B	28	17	45	1.47	0.08
74-A	93	30	123	4.01	0.21
74-B	11	4	15	0.49	0.03
75-A	213	99	312	10.18	0.53
75-B	34	19	53	1.73	0.09
76-A	94	51	145	4.73	0.25
76-B	25	13	38	1.24	0.06
Total	2,290	774	3,064	100.00	5.21

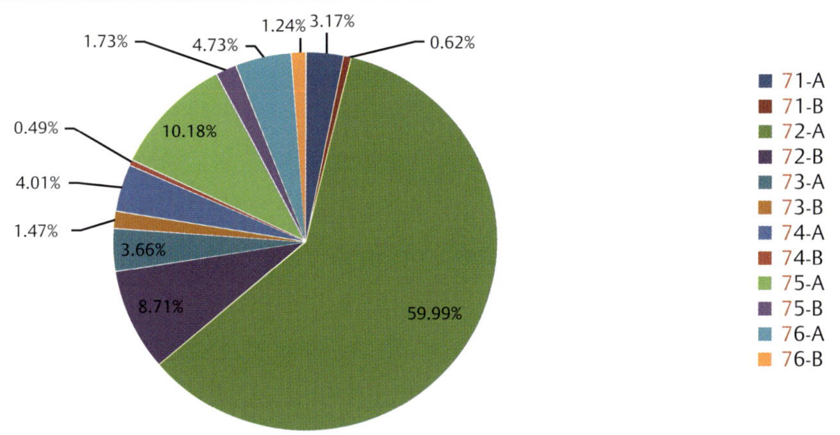

a

Fig. 8.9 **(a)** Fracture group distribution of 3,064 fractures of carpal bones (segments 71–76). (*Continued*)

8

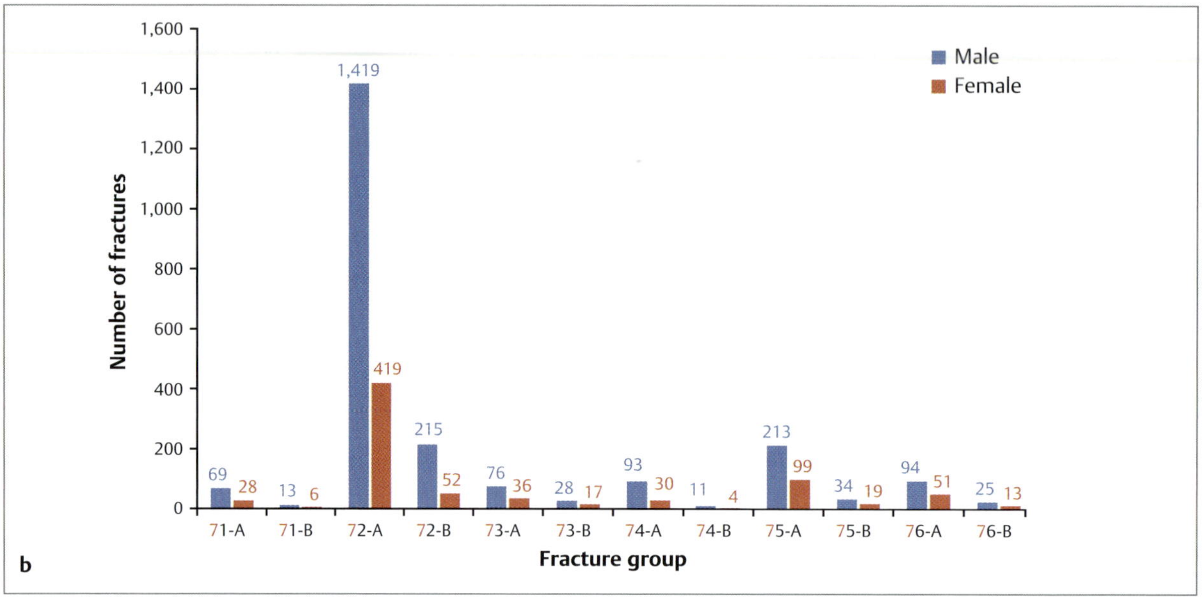

Fig. 8.9 (*continued*) **(b)** Sex and fracture group distribution of 3,064 fractures of carpal bones (segments 71–76).

8

71 Lunate fractures

71-A Noncomminuted 97 fractures M: 69 (71.13%) F: 28 (28.87%) 0.03% of total adult fractures 0.16% of adult hand fractures 3.17% of adult carpal fractures 83.62% of adult lunate fractures	**71-A** 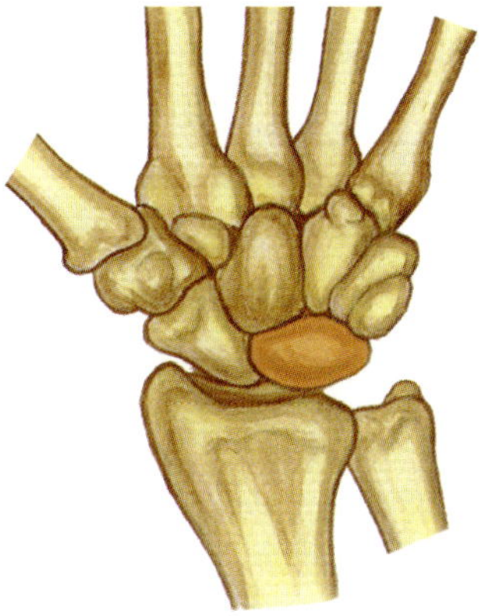 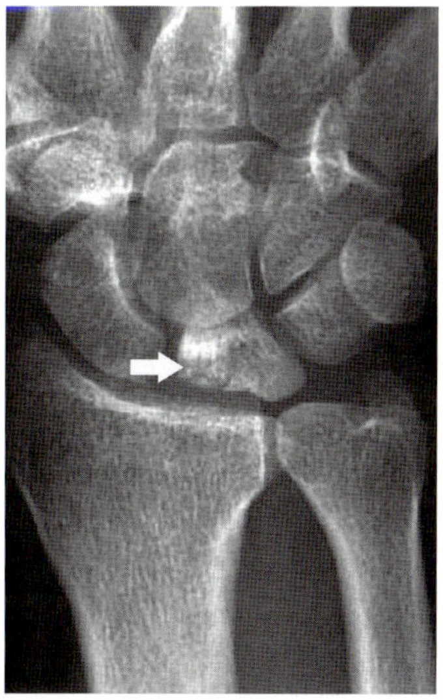 Anteroposterior view 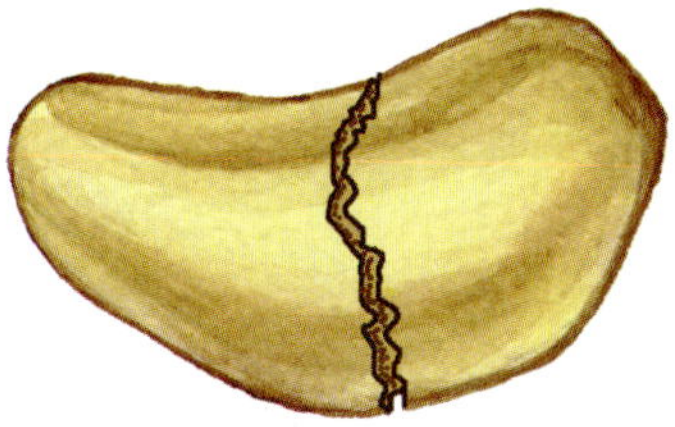 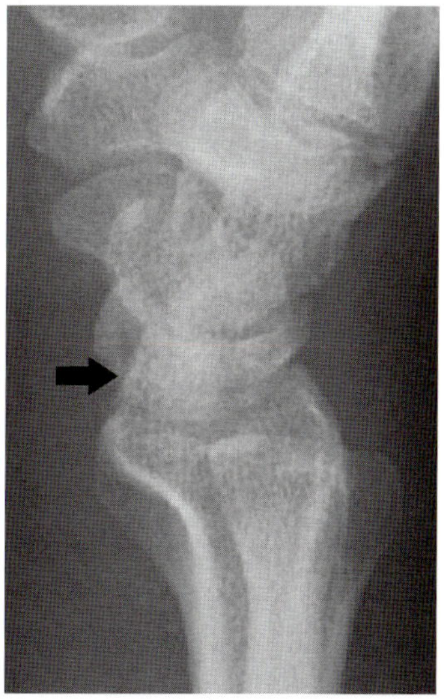 Lateral view
71-B Comminuted 19 fractures M: 13 (68.42%) F: 6 (31.58%) 0.01% of total adult fractures 0.03% of adult hand fractures 0.62% of adult carpal fractures 16.38% of adult lunate fractures	**71-B** 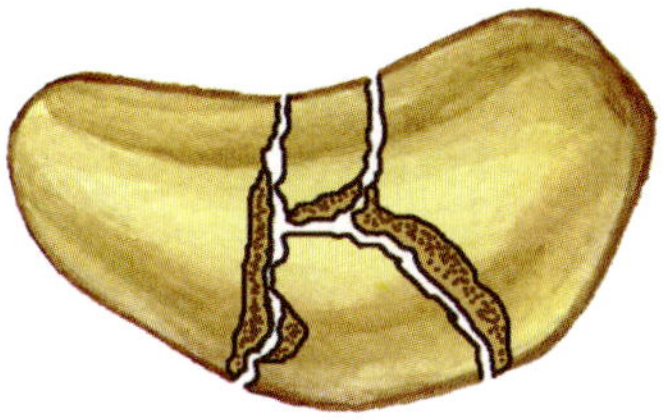 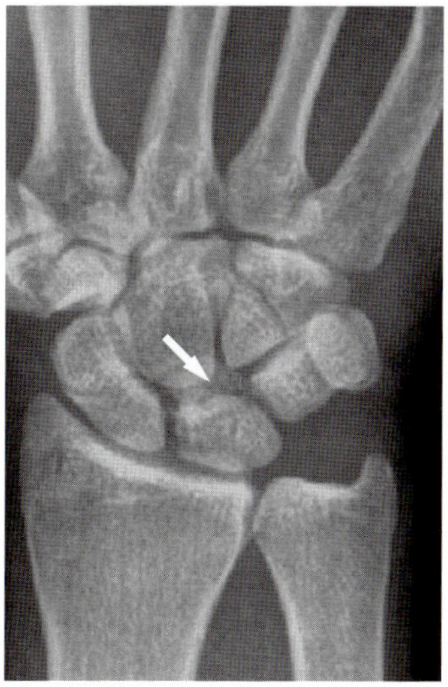

8

72 Scaphoid fractures

72-A Noncomminuted

1,838 fractures
M: 1,419 (77.20%)
F: 419 (22.80%)
0.49% of total adult fractures
3.12% of adult hand fractures
59.99% of adult carpal fractures
87.32% of adult scaphoid fractures

72-A1

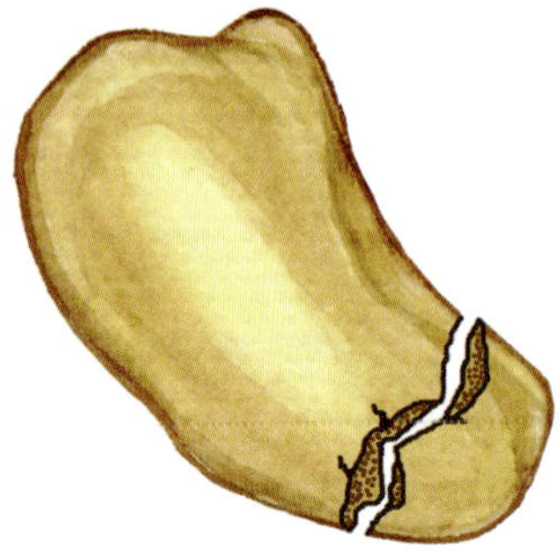

Proximal pole

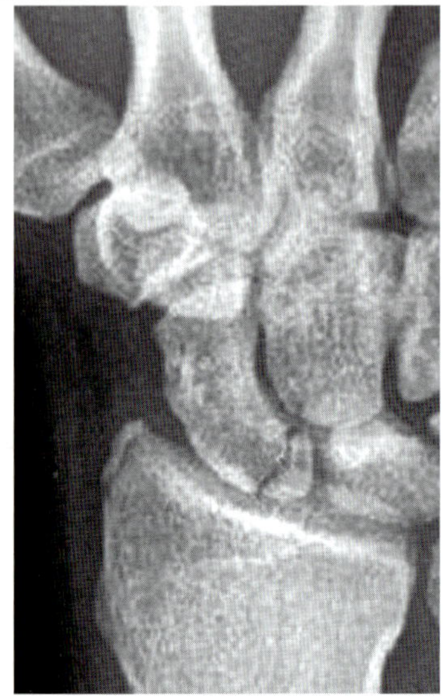

72-A2

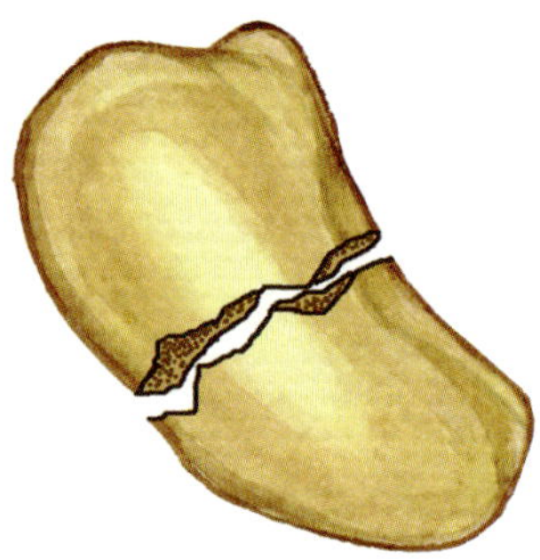

Waist

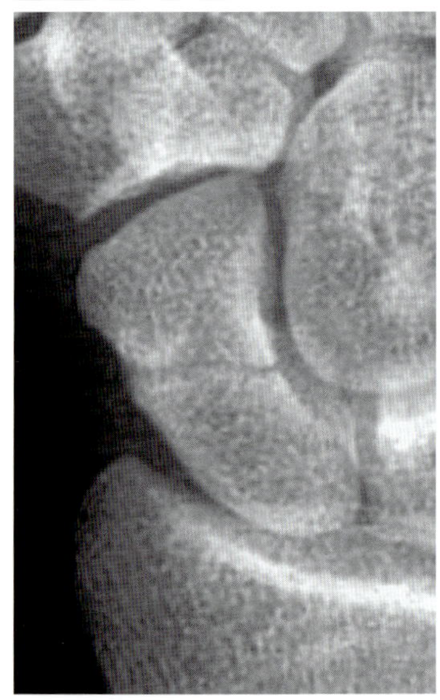

72-A3

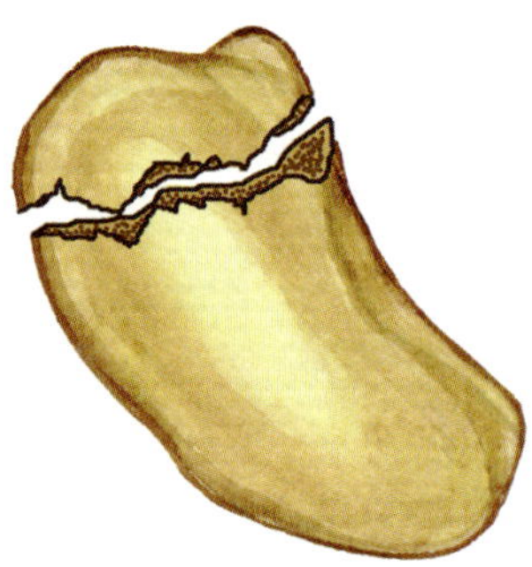

Distal pole

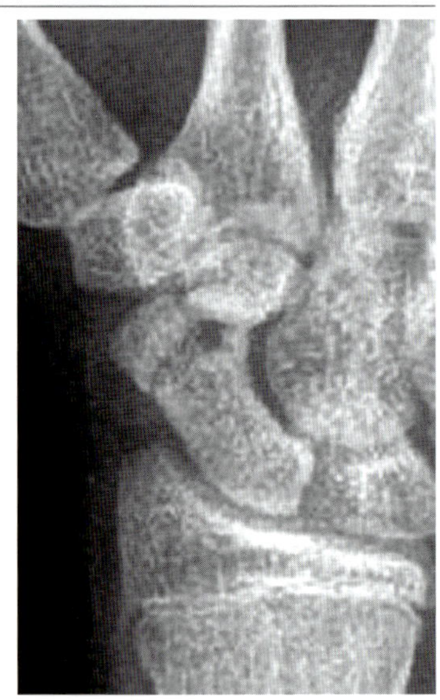

72 Scaphoid fractures

72-B Comminuted
267 fractures
M: 215 (80.52%)
F: 52 (19.48%)
0.07% of total adult fractures
0.45% of adult hand fractures
8.71% of adult carpal fractures
12.68% of adult scaphoid fractures

72-B1

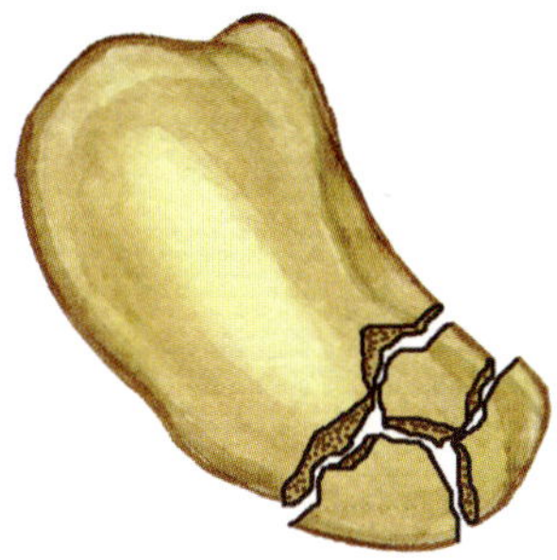

Proximal pole

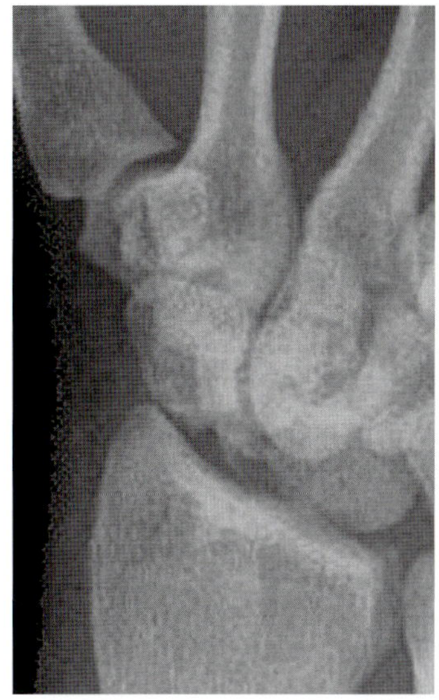

72-B2

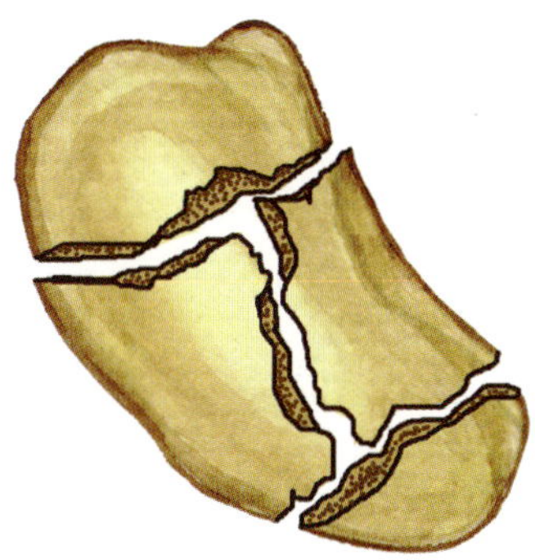

Waist

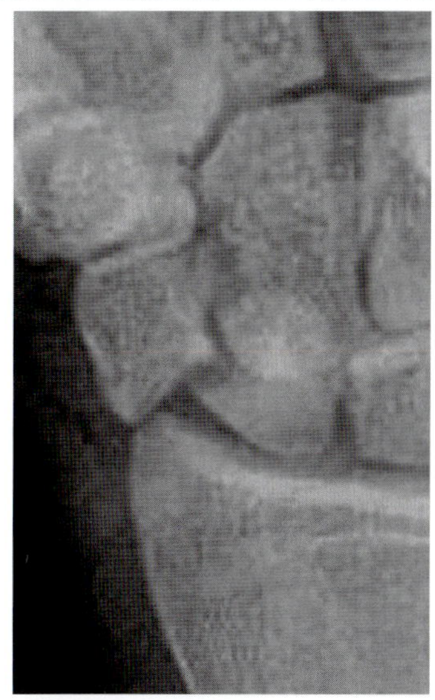

72-B3

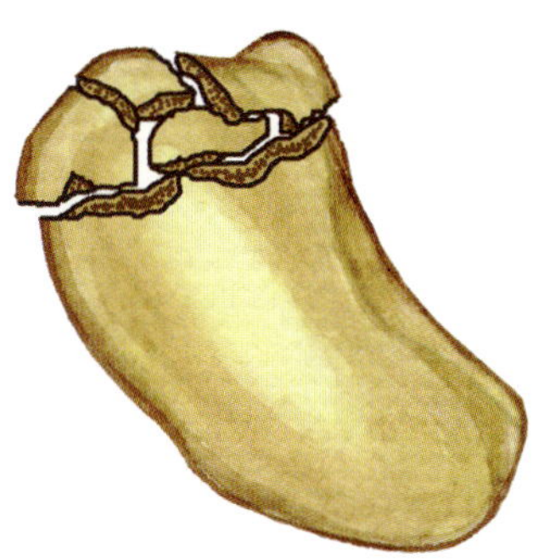

Distal pole

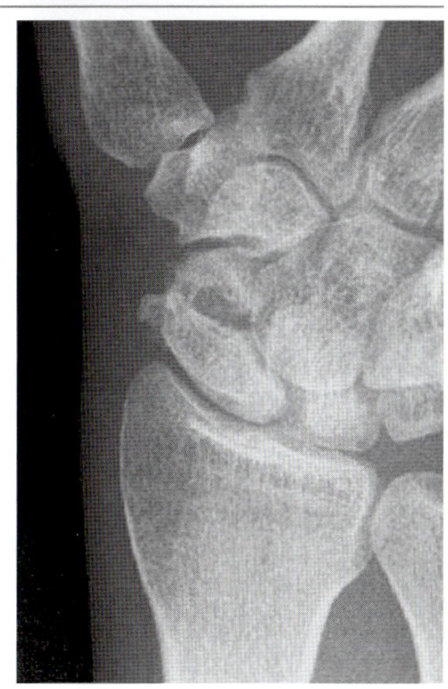

73 Capitate fractures

73-A Noncomminuted

112 fractures
M: 76 (67.86%)
F: 36 (32.14%)
0.03% of total adult fractures
0.19% of adult hand fractures
3.66% of adult carpal fractures
71.34% of adult capitate fractures

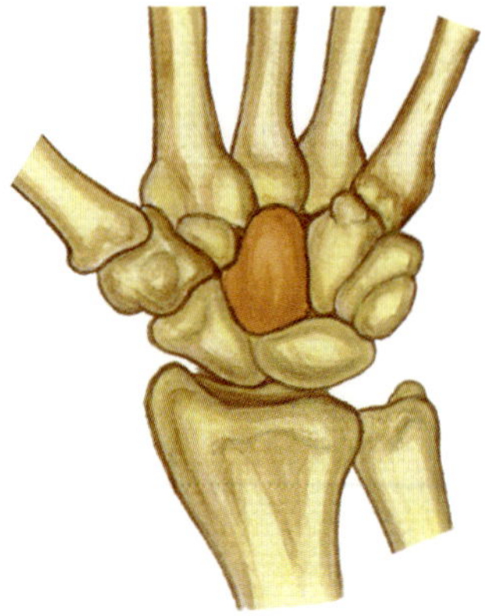

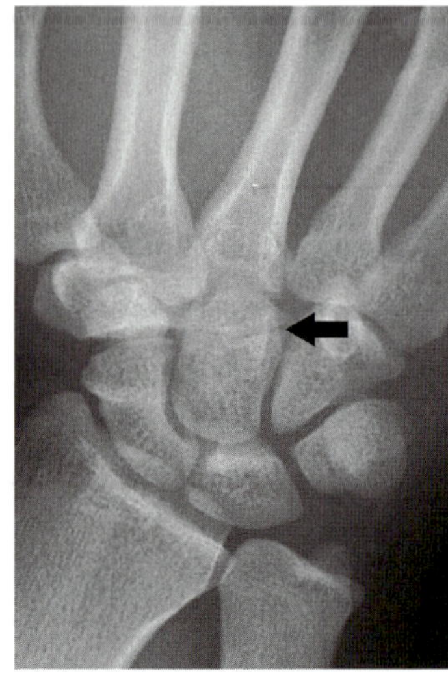

Anteroposterior view

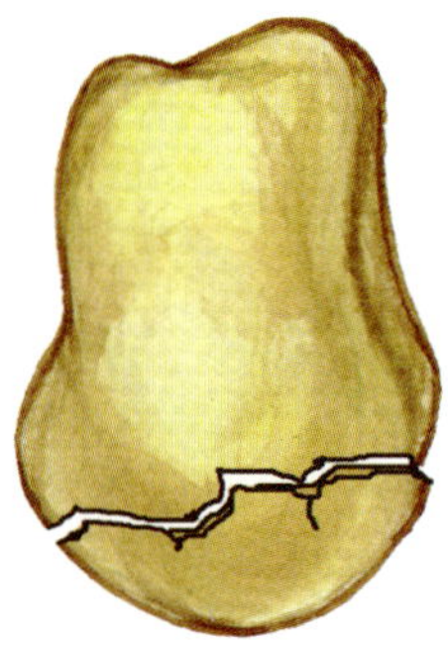

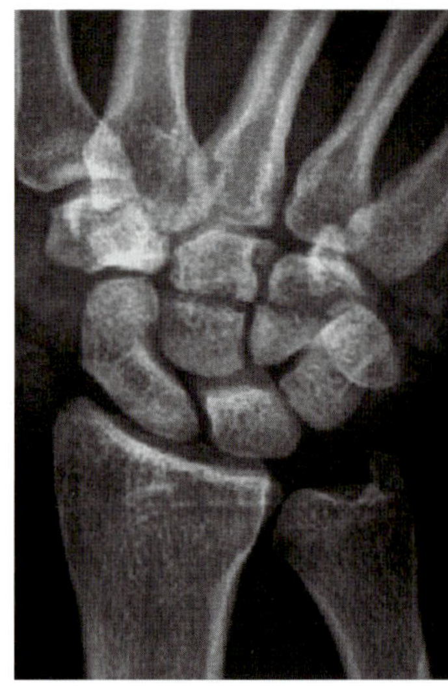

Lateral view

73-B Comminuted

45 fractures
M: 28 (62.22%)
F: 17 (37.78%)
0.01% of total adult fractures
0.08% of total hand fractures
1.47% of total carpal fractures
28.66% of total capitate fractures

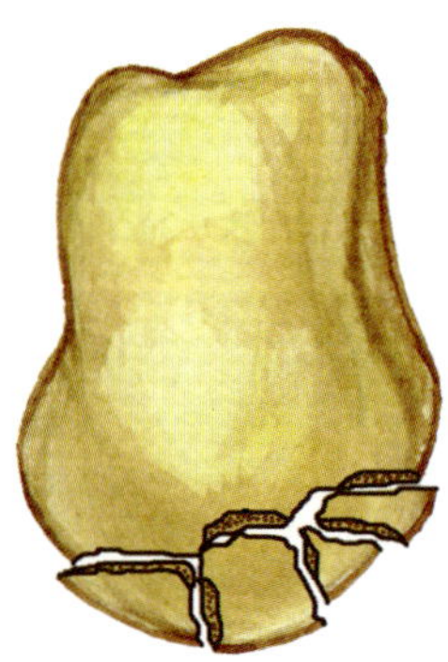

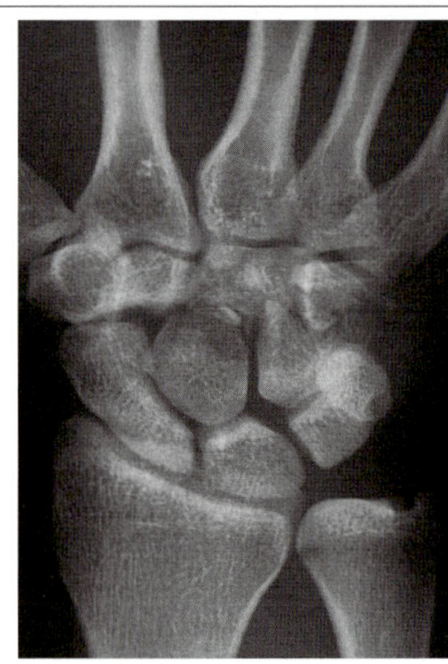

74 Hamate fractures

74-A Noncomminuted

123 fractures
M: 93 (75.61%)
F: 30 (24.39%)
0.03% of total adult fractures
0.21% of total hand fractures
4.01% of total carpal fractures
89.13% of total hamate fractures

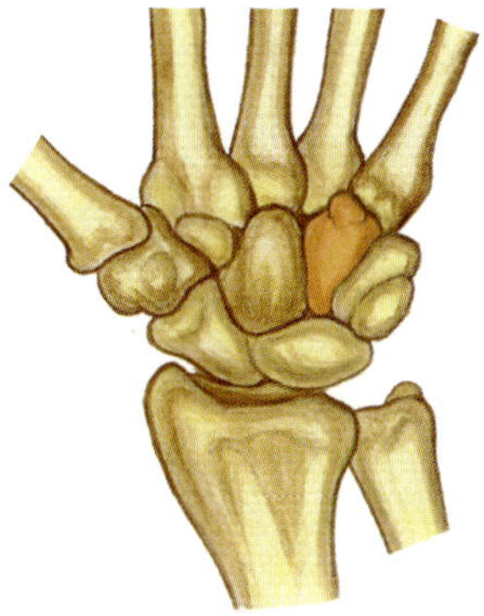

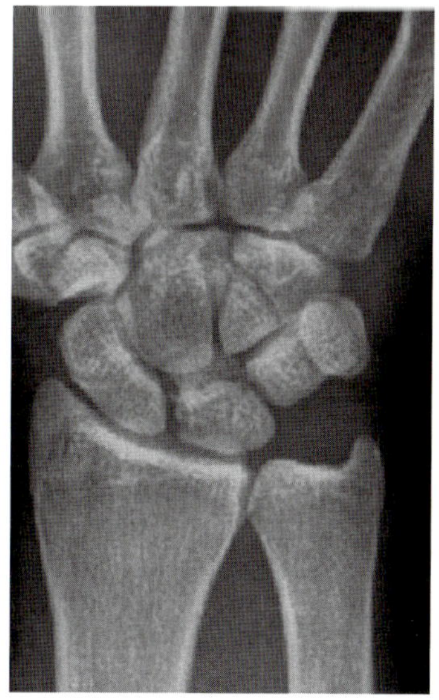

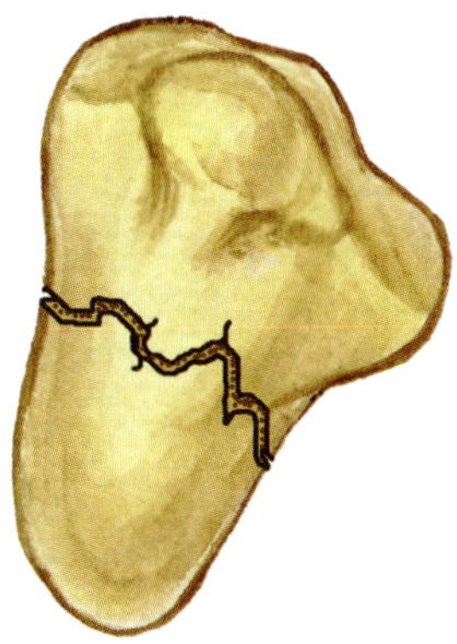

74-B Comminuted

15 fractures
M: 11 (73.33%)
F: 4 (26.67%)
0.004% of total adult fractures
0.03% of total hand fractures
0.49% of total carpal fractures
10.87% of total hamate fractures

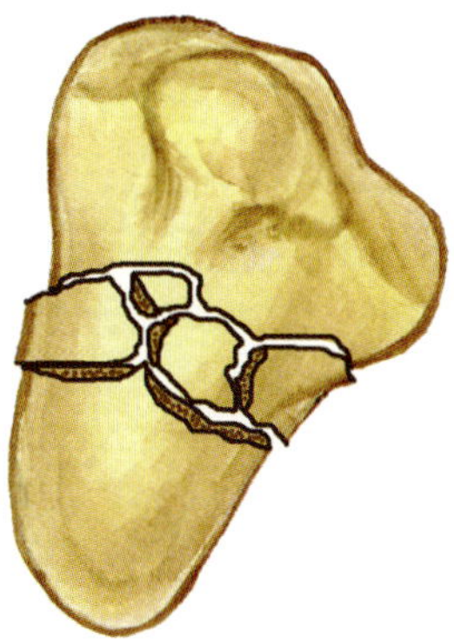

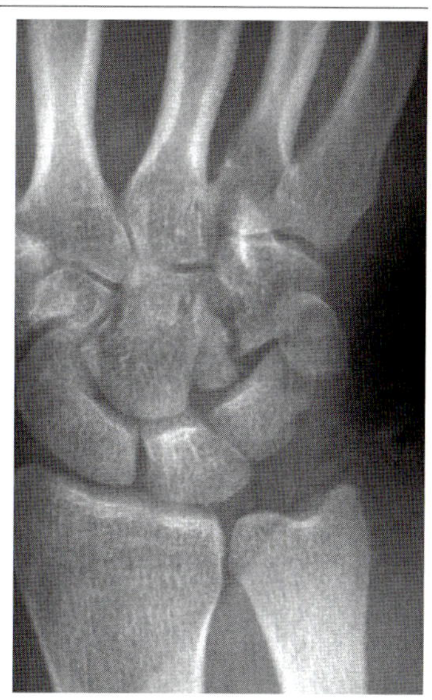

75 Ulnar carpal fractures (triquetrum, pisiform)

75-A Noncomminuted
312 fractures
M: 213 (68.27%)
F: 99 (31.73%)
0.08% of total adult fractures
0.53% of adult hand fractures
10.18% of adult carpal fractures
85.48% of adult ulnar carpal fractures

75-A1

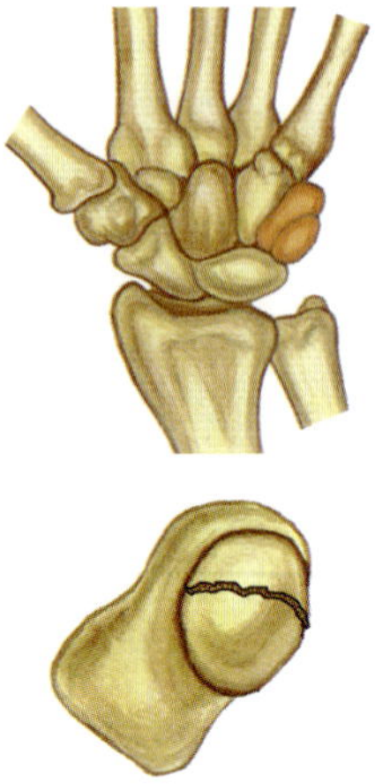

Pisiform

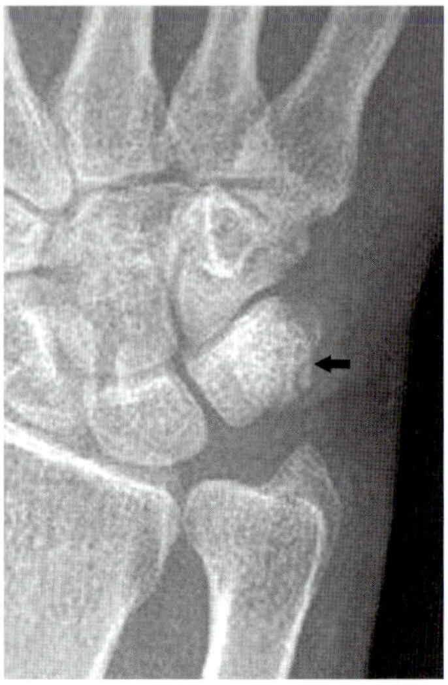

75-A2

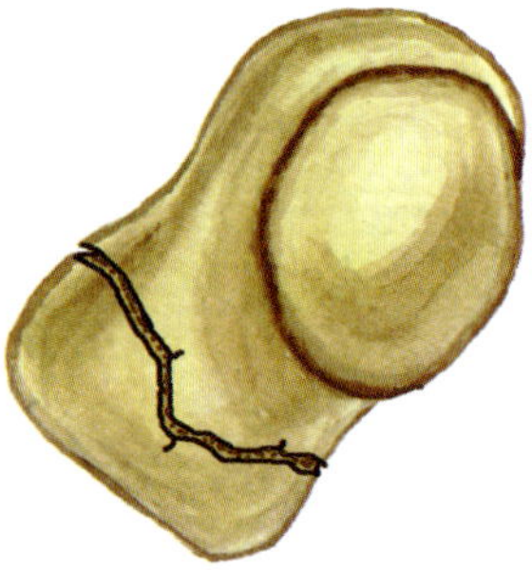

Triquetrum

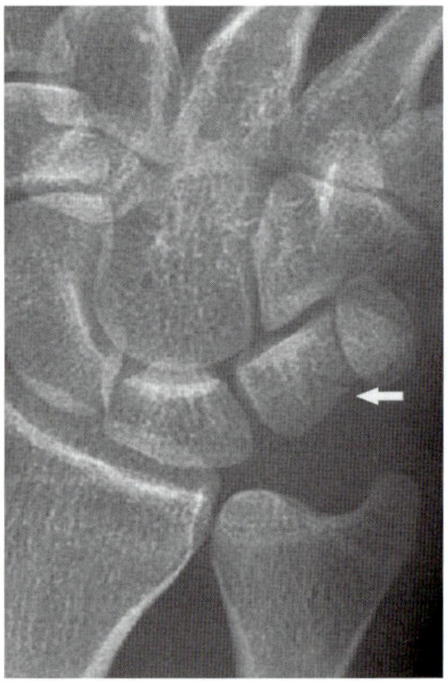

Anteroposterior view

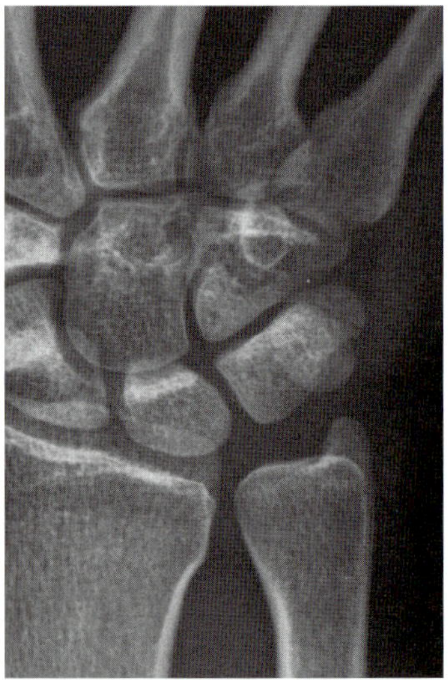

Lateral view

75-B Comminuted
53 fractures
M: 34 (64.15%)
F: 19 (35.85%)
0.01% of total adult fractures
0.09% of adult hand fractures
1.73% of adult carpal fractures
14.52% of adult ulnar carpal fractures

75-B1

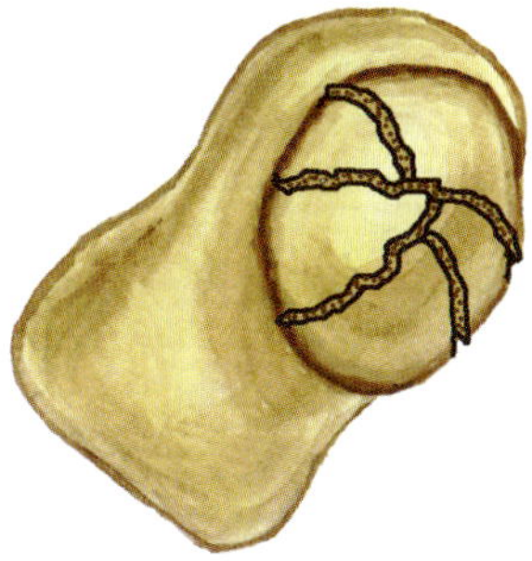

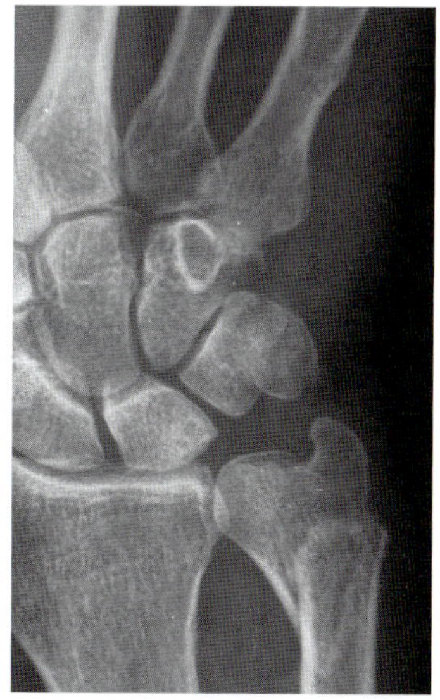

Pisiform

75-B2

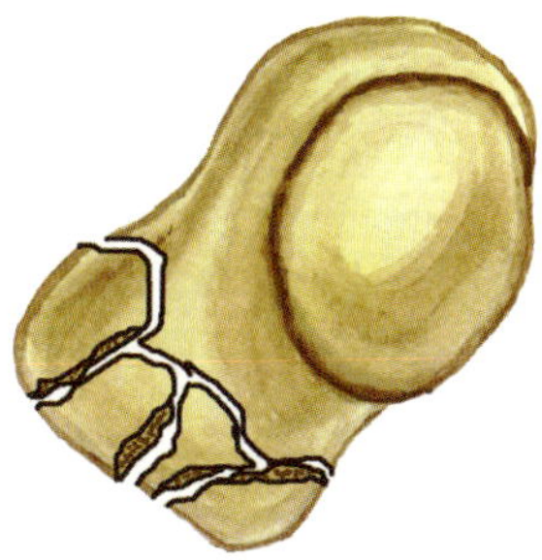

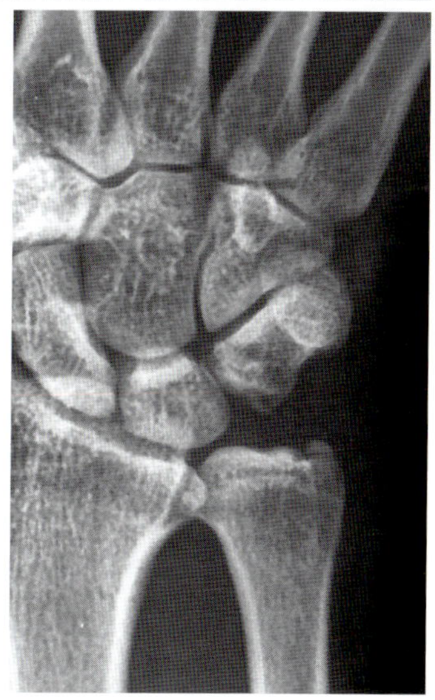

Triquetrum

76 Radial carpal fractures (trapezium, trapezoid)

76-A Noncomminuted

145 fractures
M: 94 (64.83%)
F: 51 (35.17%)
0.04% of total adult fractures
0.25% of adult hand fractures
4.73% of adult carpal fractures
79.23% of adult radial carpal fractures

76-A1

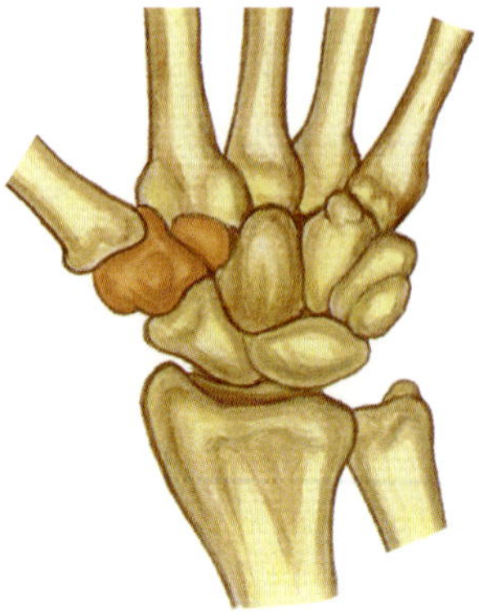

Trapezium

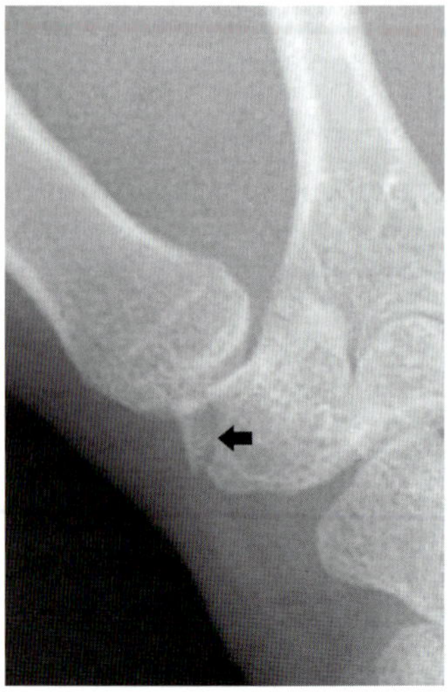

Anteroposterior view

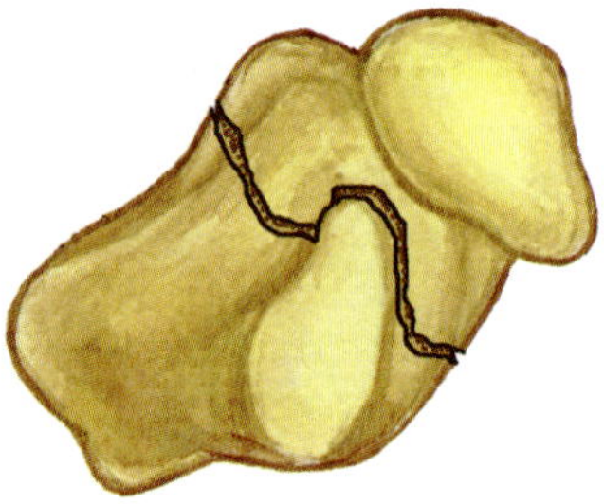

Trapezium

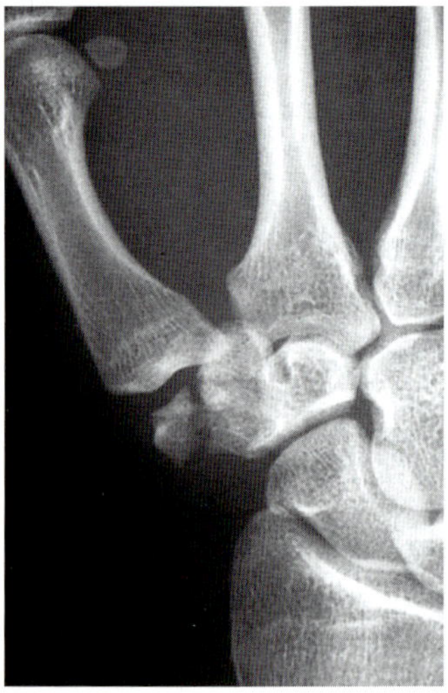

Lateral view

76-A2

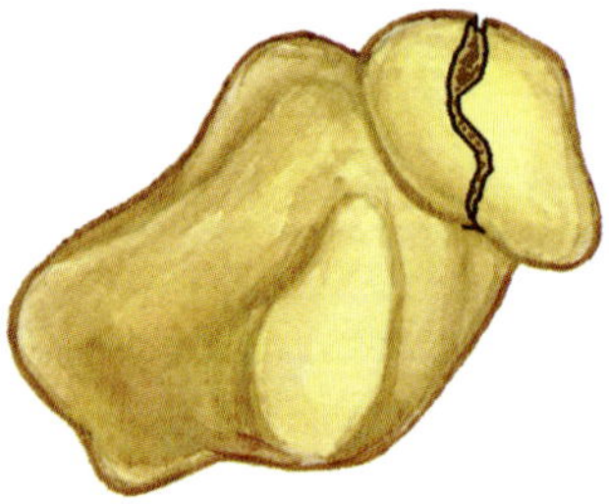

Trapezoid

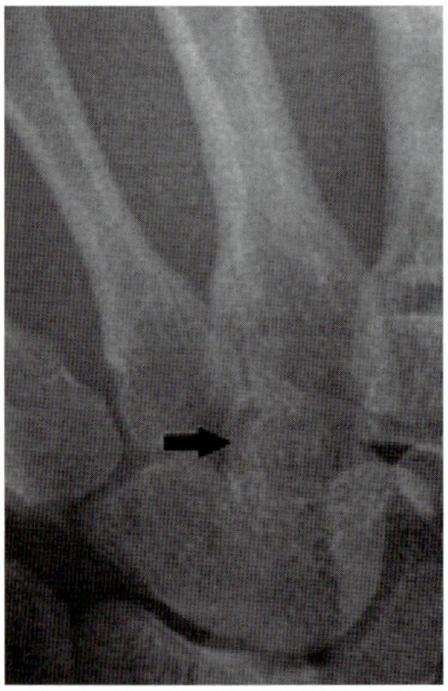

76-B Comminuted

38 fractures
M: 25 (65.79%)
F: 13 (34.21%)
0.01% of total adult fractures
0.06% of adult hand fractures
1.24% of adult carpal fractures
20.77% of adult radial carpal fractures

76-B1

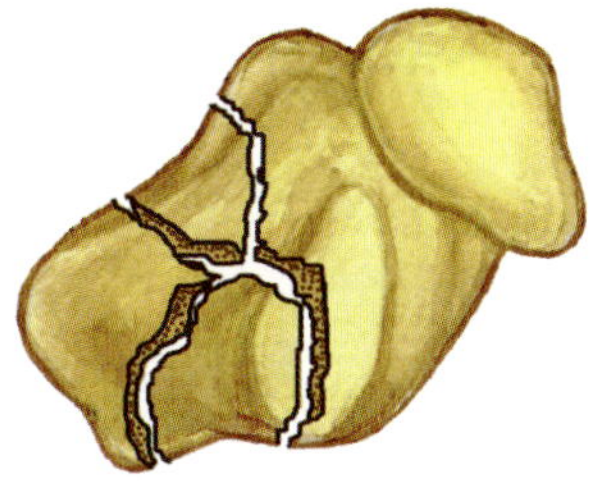

Trapezium

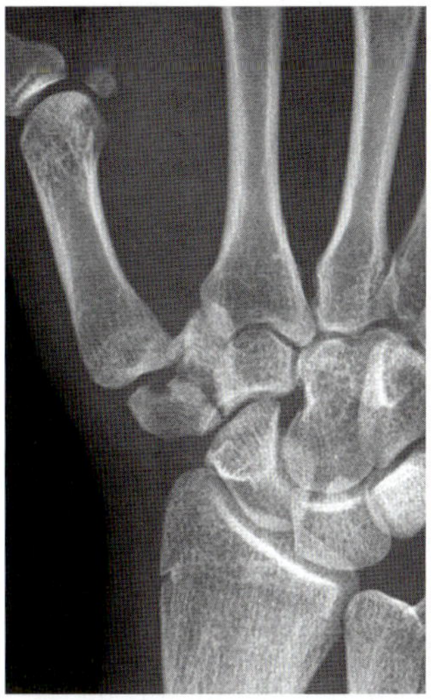

76-B2

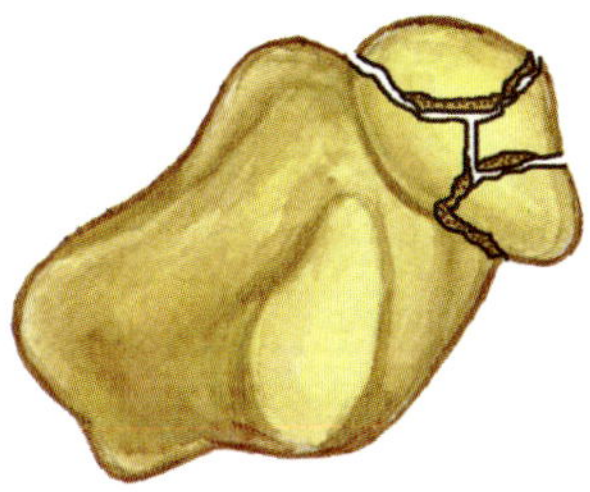

Trapezoid

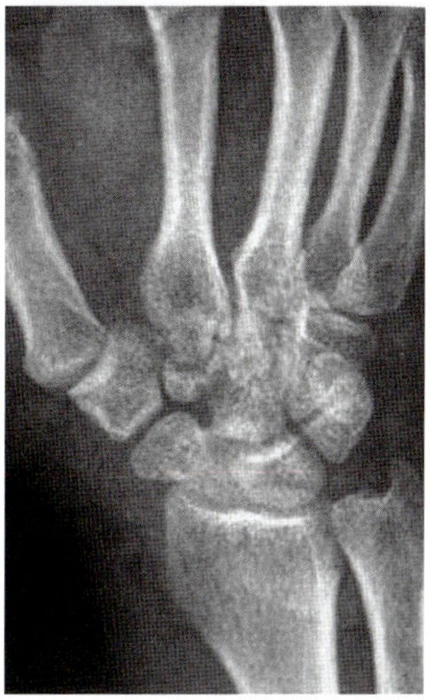

Injury Mechanism

Most carpal fractures are a result of axial loading on the outstretched palm and an extended wrist—for example, from a fall on an outstretched hand or motor vehicle collision. A direct blow to the dorsum of the hand, a crush injury, or cutting through the dorsum of the hand can also cause this type of injury.

Diagnosis

Most patients present with history of a fall on an outstretched hand, or a traumatic event like a motor vehicle accident. If palpation of each carpal bone and the intercarpal ligaments elicit pain and apparent local tenderness, one should strongly suspect the presence of fractures. Where carpal fracture is suspected, X-rays of anteroposterior (AP), lateral, and oblique views are needed. Bone scans and computed tomography (CT) scans are sometimes helpful if the plain X-ray is inconclusive for fracture.

Treatment

8

Most carpal fractures can be treated with nonsurgical intervention, except scaphoid fractures. The indications for nonsurgical treatment are as follows:

- Nondisplaced carpal fracture
- Stable wrist joint injury, with less than 2 mm fracture displacement
- Stable wrist joint injury, with less than 1 mm intra-articular fracture step-off
- Isolated ligamentous rupture, in elderly low-demand patients
- Hamate fracture with the hook intact
- Pisiform fracture

The treatment principle for scaphoid fractures is discussed in the next section.

Further Classification for Scaphoid Fractures

Anatomical Features and Coding System

The scaphoid bone is the largest bone of the wrist bone's proximal row. It is situated between the hand and forearm at the radial side of the carpus, and plays an important role in the formation of the radiocarpal joint. The scaphoid bone received its name from its resemblance to a boat, its long axis being from above, downward, lateralward, and forward. The dorsal surface has a rough groove, and a rounded projection called a tubercle, which is elevated at its lower and lateral part, and is directed forward; it gives attachment to the transverse carpal ligament and is sometimes the origin of a few fibers of the abductor pollicis brevis. The scaphoid has a central narrowing or waist, which is at high risk for fracture.

The proximal pole of the scaphoid is completely covered with cartilage, and receives a very limited vascular supply from a ligamentous structure (radioscapholunate ligament), in contrast to the distal two-thirds of the bone, which appears to have its own abundant blood supply. Therefore, any displaced fracture involving the proximal half of the scaphoid will severely jeopardize the vascularity of the proximal portion and may result in increased risk of avascular necrosis of that portion of the bone.

Based on AO classification, scaphoid fractures are classified into three subtypes: A, avulsion fracture of the tubercle; B, fracture of the waist; and C, multiple fragments or comminuted fractures.

Russe classified scaphoid fractures as horizontal oblique, transverse, or vertical oblique, based on the direction of the fracture line.

Clinical Epidemiologic Features of Scaphoid Fractures in Adults

A total of 2,101 adult patients with 2,105 scaphoid fractures were treated in 83 hospitals in China over a 2-year period from 2010 to 2011. All cases were reviewed and statistically studied, accounting for 68.73% of all adult patients with carpal fractures and 68.70% of carpal fractures in adults. Their epidemiologic features are as follows:

- The number of men greatly outweighs the number of women.
- The high-risk age group is 21–25 years—the same age group for men while there is no apparent high-risk age group for women.
- The waist of the scaphoid is the most frequent fracture site.

Scaphoid Fractures by Sex

Table 8.10 Sex distribution of 2,101 patients with scaphoid fractures

Sex	Number of patients	Percentage (%)
Male	1,630	77.58
Female	471	22.42
Total	2,101	100.00

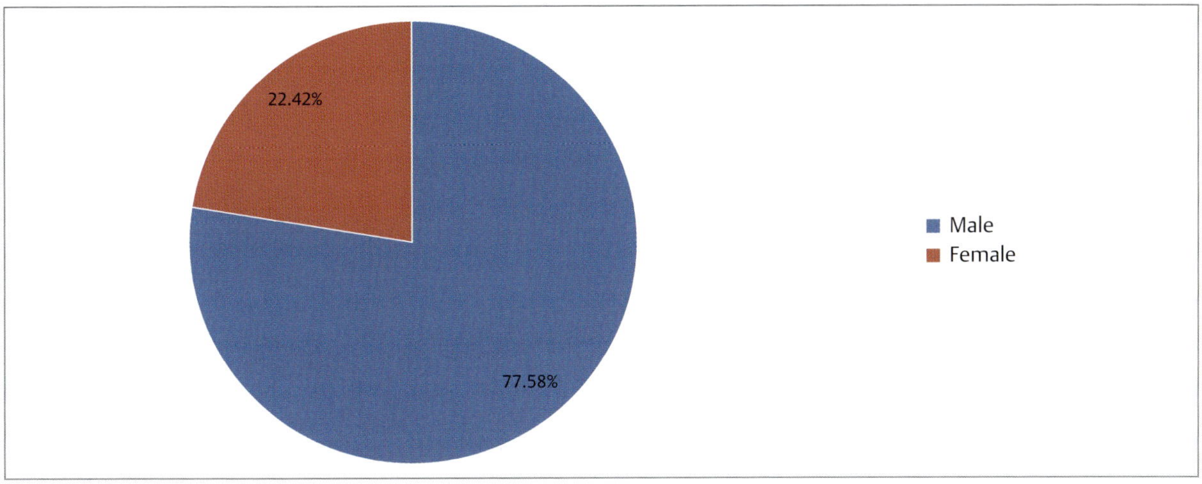

Fig. 8.10 Sex distribution of 2,101 patients with scaphoid fractures.

Scaphoid Fractures by Age Group

Table 8.11 Age and sex distribution of 2,101 patients with scaphoid fractures

Age group (years)	Male	Female	Number of fractures	Percentage (%)
16–20	214	37	251	11.95
21–25	322	44	366	17.42
26–30	276	31	307	14.61
31–35	177	34	211	10.04
36–40	180	50	230	10.95
41–45	141	47	188	8.95
46–50	102	61	163	7.76
51–55	68	44	112	5.33
56–60	54	60	114	5.43
61–65	38	26	64	3.05
66–70	14	14	28	1.33
71–75	22	11	33	1.57
76–80	13	10	23	1.09
81–85	8	1	9	0.43
≥86	1	1	2	0.10
Total	1,630	471	2,101	100.00

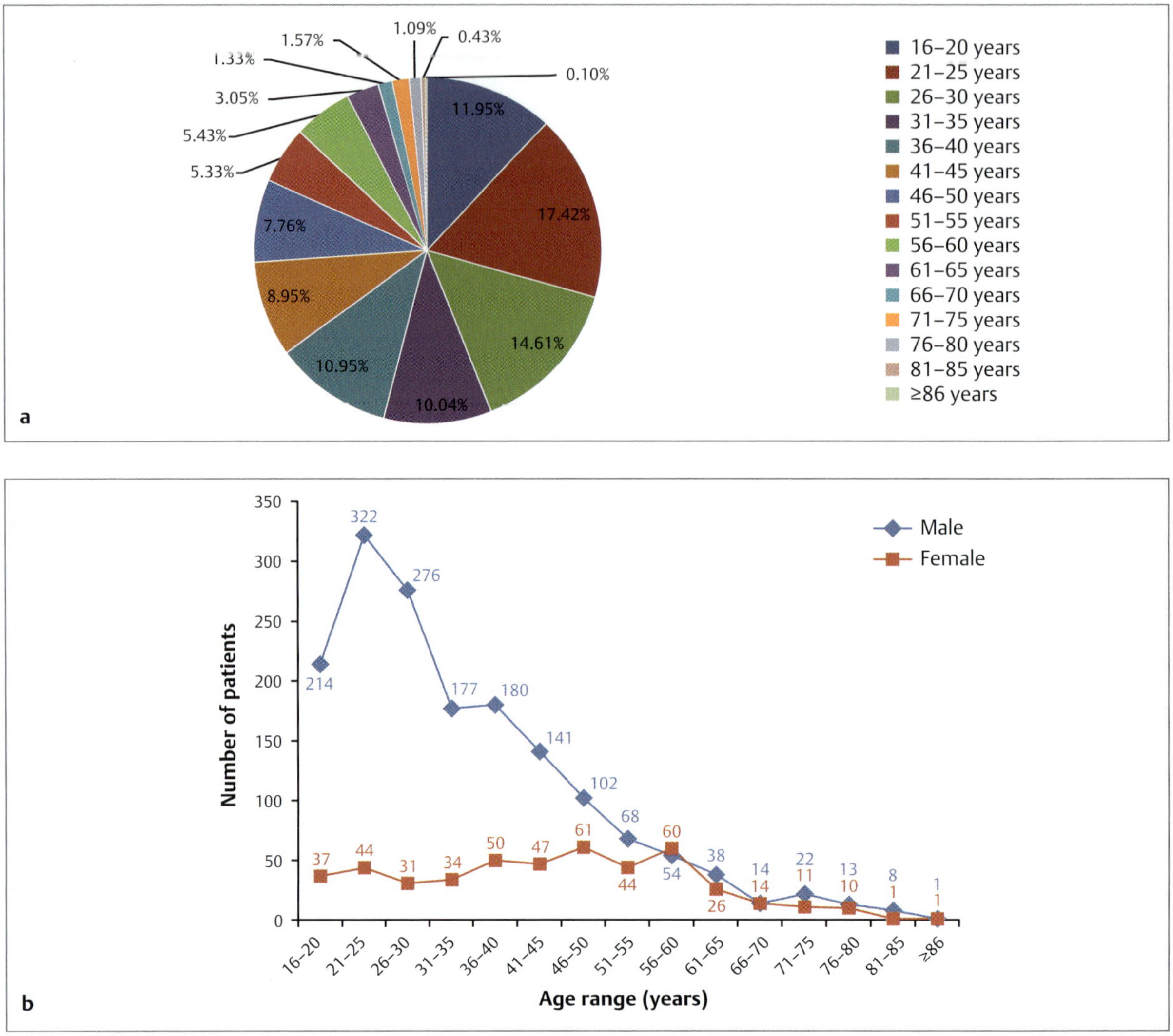

Fig. 8.11 **(a)** Age distribution of 2,101 patients with scaphoid fractures.
(b) Age and sex distribution of 2,101 patients with scaphoid fractures.

Scaphoid Fractures by Fracture Type Based on AO Classification

Table 8.12 Sex and fracture type distribution of 2,105 scaphoid fractures based on AO classification

Fracture type	Male	Female	Number of fractures	Percentage (%)	Percentage of carpal fractures (%)	Percentage of hand fractures (%)
A	233	79	312	14.82	10.18	0.53
B	1,272	365	1,637	77.77	53.43	2.78
C	129	27	156	7.41	5.09	0.27
Total	1,634	471	2,105	100.00	68.70	3.58

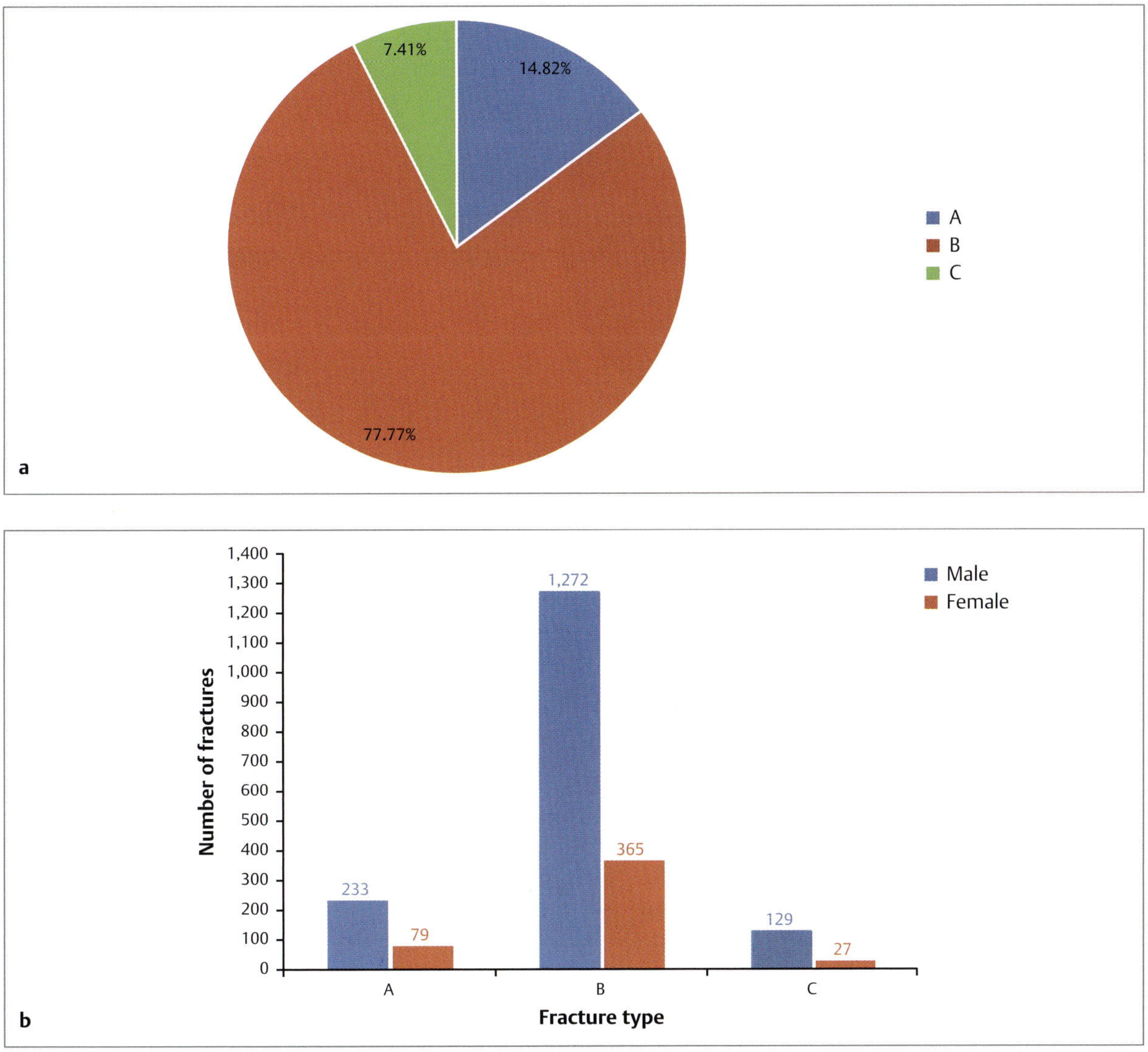

Fig. 8.12 **(a)** Fracture type distribution of 2,105 scaphoid fractures based on AO classification. **(b)** Sex and fracture type distribution of 2,105 scaphoid fractures based on AO classification.

Scaphoid Fractures by Fracture Type Based on Russe Classification

Table 8.13 Fracture pattern distribution of 2,105 scaphoid fractures by Russe classification

Fracture pattern	Male	Female	Number of fractures	Percentage (%)	Percentage of carpal fractures (%)	Percentage of hand fractures (%)
Horizontal	698	197	895	42.52	29.21	1.52
Transverse	865	257	1,122	53.30	36.62	1.91
Vertical	71	17	88	4.18	2.87	0.15
Total	1,634	471	2,105	100.00	68.70	3.58

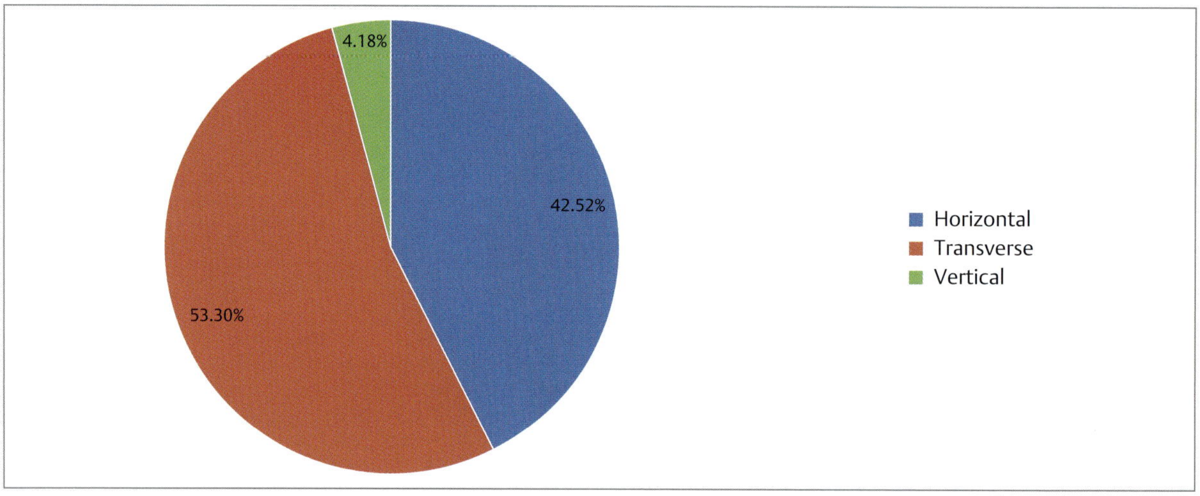

Fig. 8.13 Fracture pattern distribution of 2,105 scaphoid fractures by Russe classification.

<table>
<tr><th colspan="3">AO classification of scaphoid fractures</th></tr>
<tr><td>Type A
312 fractures
M: 233 (74.68%)
F: 79 (25.32%)
0.08% of total adult fractures
0.53% of adult hand fractures
10.18% of adult carpal fractures
14.82% of adult scaphoid fractures
Avulsion fracture of tubercle</td><td>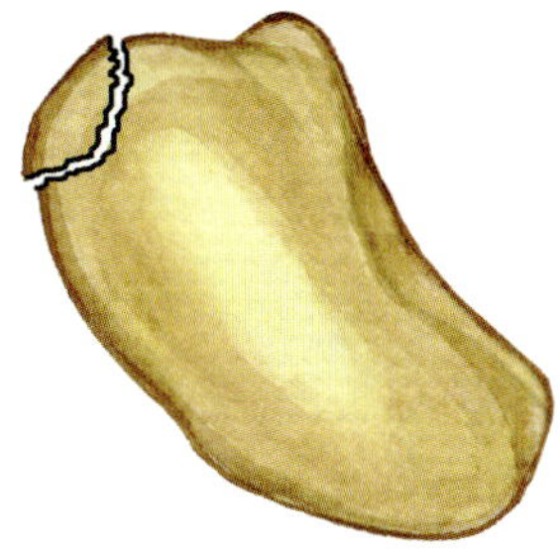
Avulsion fracture of tubercle</td><td>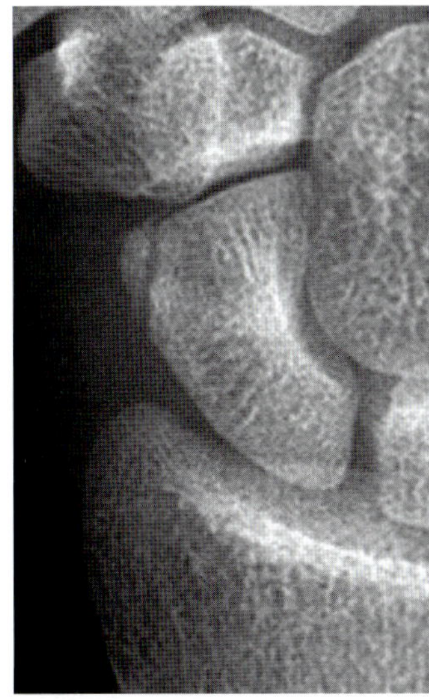</td></tr>
<tr><td>Type B
1,637 fractures
M: 1,272 (77.7%)
F: 365 (22.3%)
0.44% of total adult fractures
2.78% of adult hand fractures
53.43% of adult carpal fractures
77.77% of adult scaphoid fractures</td><td>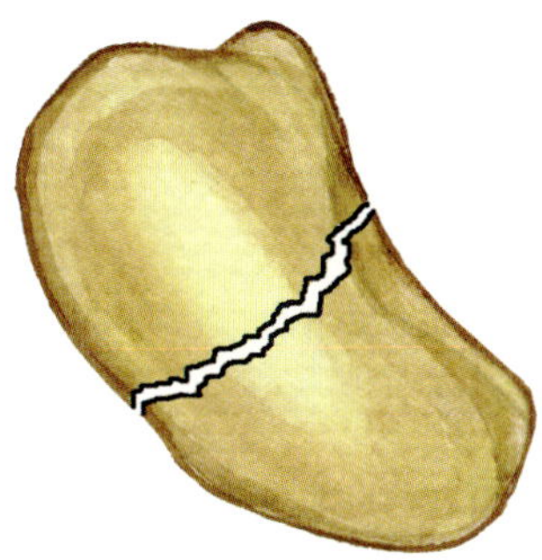
Waist fractures</td><td>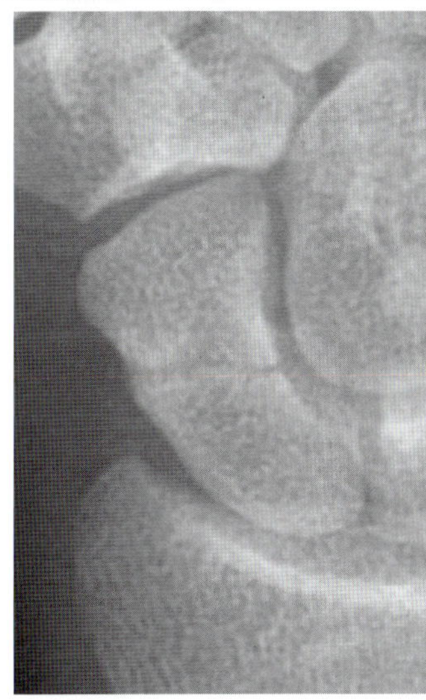</td></tr>
<tr><td>Type C
156 fractures
M: 129 (82.69%)
F: 27 (17.31%)
0.04% of total adult fractures
0.27% of adult hand fractures
5.09% of adult carpal fractures
7.41% of adult scaphoid fractures</td><td>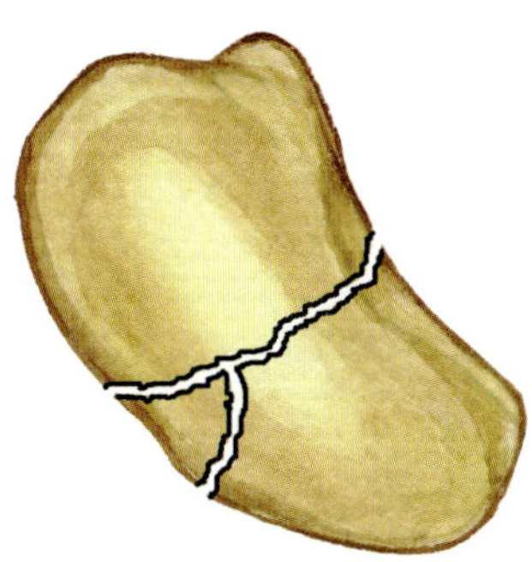
Multiple fragments or comminuted fractures</td><td>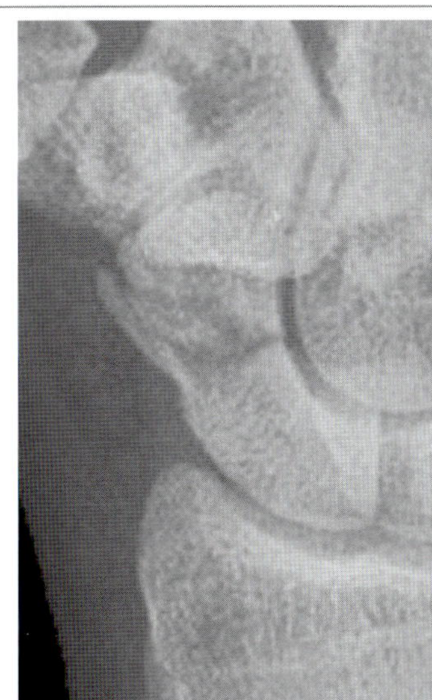</td></tr>
</table>

Russe classification of scaphoid fractures		
Horizontal 895 fractures M: 698 (77.99%) F: 197 (22.01%) 0.24% of total adult fractures 1.52% of adult hand fractures 29.21% of adult carpal fractures 42.52% of adult scaphoid fractures	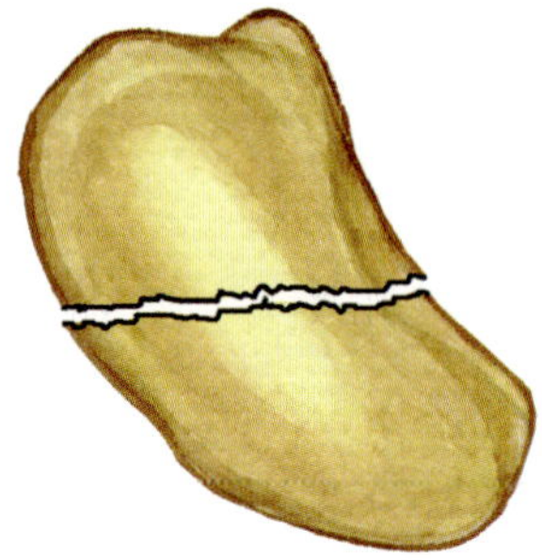	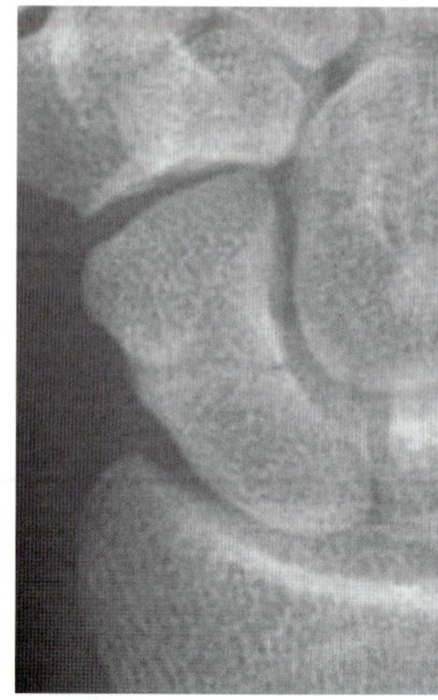
Transverse 1,122 fractures M: 865 (77.09%) F: 257 (22.91%) 0.30% of total adult fractures 1.91% of adult hand fractures 36.62% of adult carpal fractures 53.3% of adult scaphoid fractures	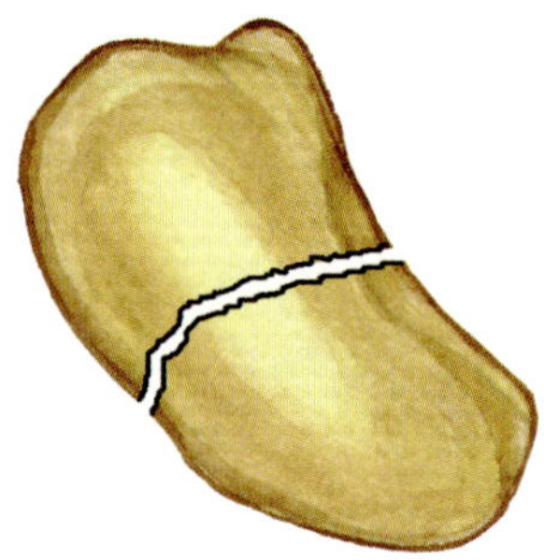	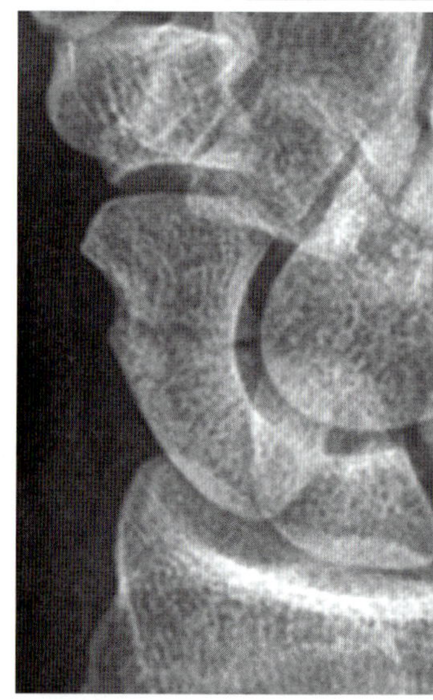
Vertical 88 fractures M: 71 (80.68%) F: 17 (19.32%) 0.02% of total adult fractures 0.15% of adult hand fractures 2.87% of adult carpal fractures 4.18% of adult scaphoid fractures	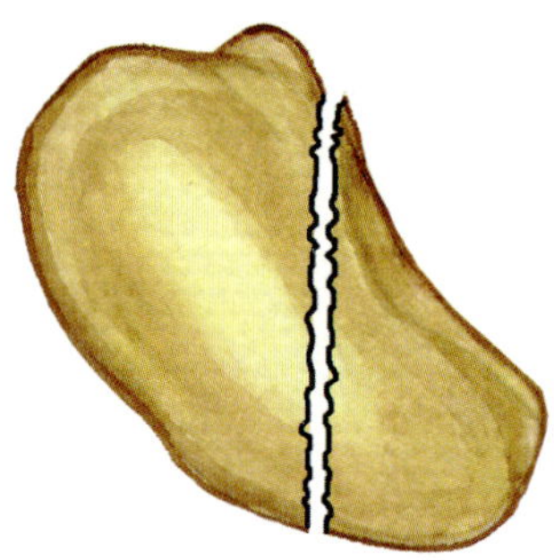	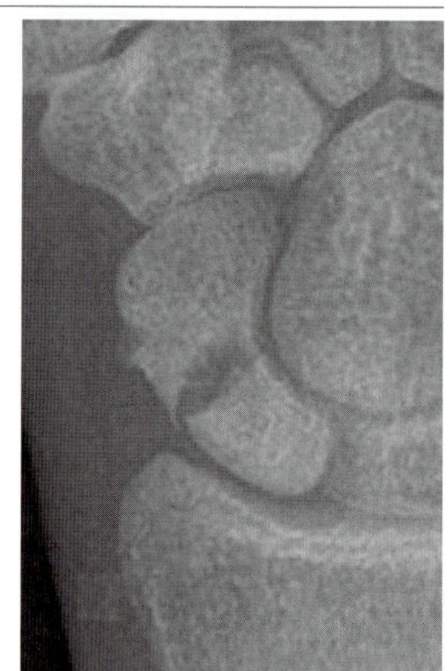

Injury Mechanism

The scaphoid usually fractures secondary to excessive compression, which produces changes in the scaphoid itself or its surrounding structures. Because of the anatomical features of the waist of the scaphoid, thin and across two rows of the carpal bones, it is an easy target for fracture when subject to compression-force injuries. The typical injury mechanism is a fall on the outstretched hand, with the wrist in extension and radial deviation.

Diagnosis

Patients usually present with history of a fall, with the wrist in dorsiflexion, or a traumatic event. Dorsal wrist pain is elicited when the wrist is dorsiflexed. Tenderness is usually present in the area under the styloid process of the radius, in the area of the volar scaphoid tubercle, or in the anatomical snuffbox. There may be discomfort or pain elicited from the scaphoid with percussion of the head of the second and third metacarpal bone. X-ray helps rule out a scaphoid fracture. Standard radiographs should include posteroanterior (PA), lateral, oblique, and ulnar-deviated "clenched fist" PA views. The fracture may not be visible on plain radiographs initially. If plain radiographs are inconclusive but a scaphoid fracture is still suspected, a CT scan can be performed or the radiographs should be repeated in 1–2 weeks; by then, the bone will have had a chance to undergo visible resorptive changes as a response to the fracture, making the fracture visible on X-ray.

Treatment

Stable scaphoid fractures or fractures that can be manually reduced can be managed nonsurgically. A thumb spica cast is used for 8–12 weeks. Failure of nonsurgical treatment or acutely displaced scaphoid fractures warrant open reduction and internal fixation, usually with a Kirschner wire (K-wire) or screws (cannulated or Herbert screws). To make sure the bones are healing, a long arm cast might be needed for 6–8 weeks after surgery, followed by a short-arm thumb spica cast for another 6–8 weeks.

Metacarpal Fractures (Segment 77)

Anatomical Features

Each metacarpus consists of three parts: a body, head, and base. The base articulates with the carpus, and with the adjoining metacarpal bones. The body is prismoid in form and curved, so as to be convex in the longitudinal direction posteriorly, and concave anteriorly. The medial and lateral surfaces are concave for the attachment of the interossei. There is a tubercle on either side of the head for attachment of the collateral ligaments of the metacarpophalangeal joint. The dorsal surface, which is broad and flat, supports the extensor tendons.

OTA Classification of Metacarpal Fractures

Based on OTA classification, metacarpal fractures are classified as the following: 77-A, metacarpal proximal and distal extra-articular and diaphysis noncomminuted; 77-B, metacarpal proximal and distal partial articular and diaphysis wedge comminuted; and 77-C, metacarpal proximal and distal complete articular and diaphysis comminuted (**Plate 8.4**).

Clinical Epidemiologic Features of Metacarpal Fractures in Adults (Segment 77)

A total of 10,124 adult patients with 10,145 metacarpal fractures were treated in 83 hospitals in China over a 2-year period from 2010 to 2011. All cases were reviewed and statistically studied, the fractures accounted for 17.54% of all adult patients with fractured hands and 17.24% of hand fractures in adults. Their epidemiologic features are as follows:

- More males than females
- The high-risk age group is 21–25 years—the same age group for males whereas the high-risk age groups for females are 36–40 years and 41–45 years
- The most commonly seen fracture type is type 77-A—the same for both males and females
- The most commonly seen fracture group is group 77-A2—the same for both males and females
- The number of fractures of the fifth metacarpal outweighs the number of any other metacarpal fracture.

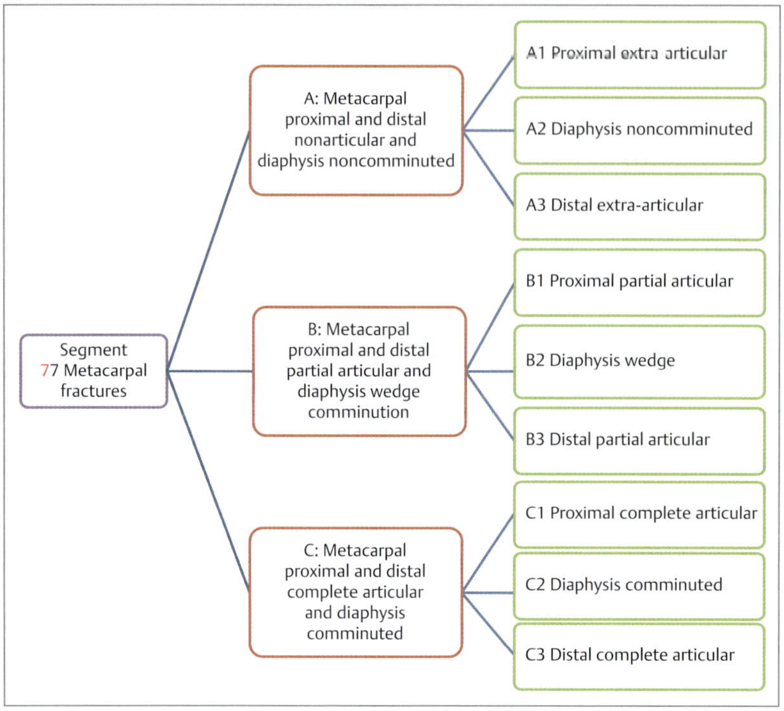

Plate 8.4

Metacarpal Fractures (Segment 77) by Sex

Table 8.14 Sex distribution of 10,124 patients with metacarpal bone (segment 77) fractures

Sex	Number of patients	Percentage (%)
Male	8,392	82.89
Female	1,732	17.11
Total	10,124	100.00

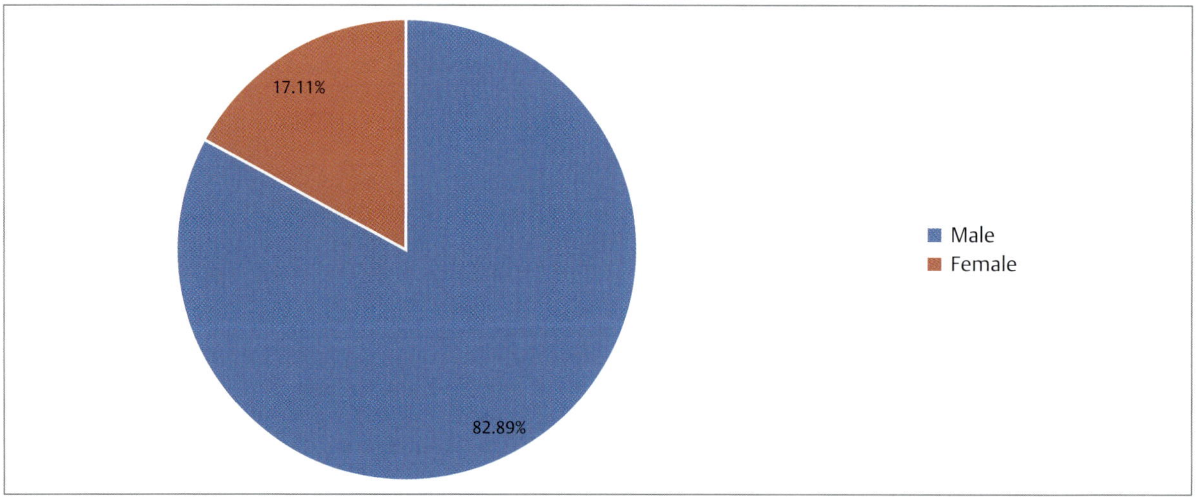

Fig. 8.14 Sex distribution of 10,124 patients with metacarpal bone (segment 77) fractures.

Metacarpal Fractures (Segment 77) by Age Group

Table 8.15 Age and sex distribution of 10,124 patients with fractures of metacarpal bones (segment 77)

Age group (years)	Male	Female	Number of patients	Percentage (%)
16–20	1,136	104	1,240	12.25
21–25	1,666	177	1,843	18.20
26–30	1,376	149	1,525	15.06
31–35	1,004	178	1,182	11.68
36–40	882	200	1,082	10.69
41–45	771	201	972	9.60
46–50	572	160	732	7.23
51–55	369	145	514	5.08
56–60	283	148	431	4.26
61–65	143	89	232	2.29
66–70	70	77	147	1.45
71–75	59	39	98	0.97
76–80	42	42	84	0.83
81–85	14	17	31	0.31
≥86	5	6	11	0.11
Total	8,392	1,732	10,124	100.00

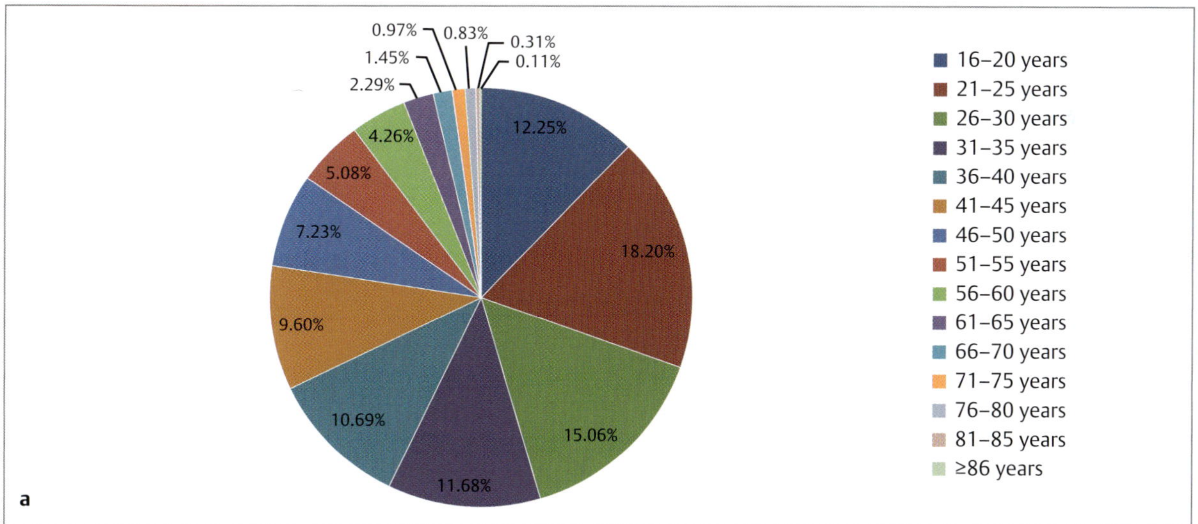

Fig. 8.15 **(a)** Age distribution of 10,124 patients with fractures of metacarpal bones (segment 77). (*Continued*)

8

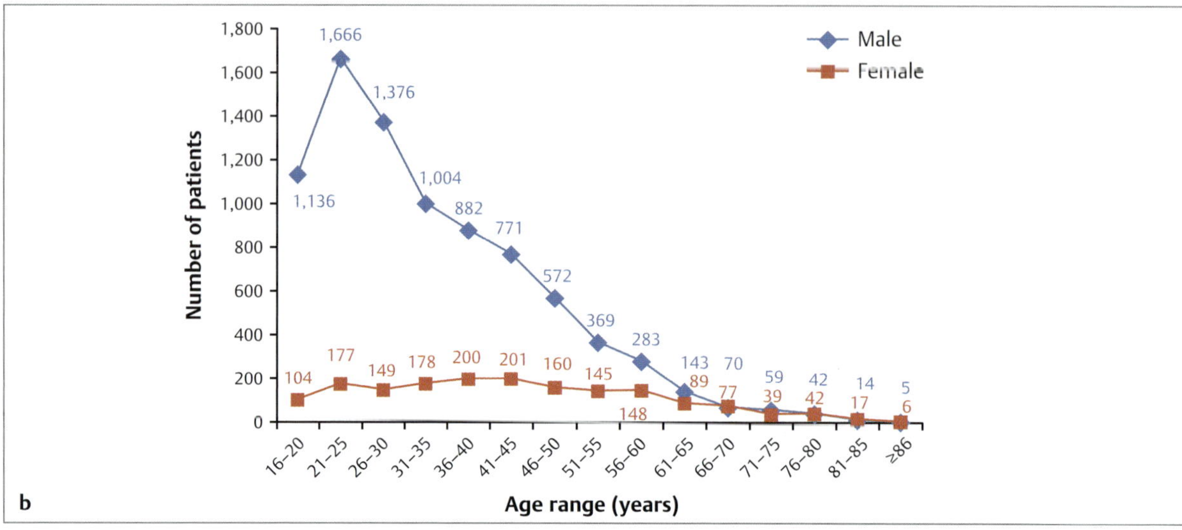

Fig. 8.15 (*continued*) **(b)** Age and sex distribution of 10,124 patients with fractures of metacarpal bones (segment 77).

Metacarpal Fractures (Segment 77) by Fracture Type

Table 8.16 Sex and fracture type distribution of 10,145 fractures of metacarpal bones (segment 77)

Fracture type	Male	Female	Number of fractures	Percentage (%)
77-A	5,975	1,190	7,165	70.63
77-B	1,687	412	2,099	20.69
77-C	749	132	881	8.68
Total	8,411	1,734	10,145	100.00

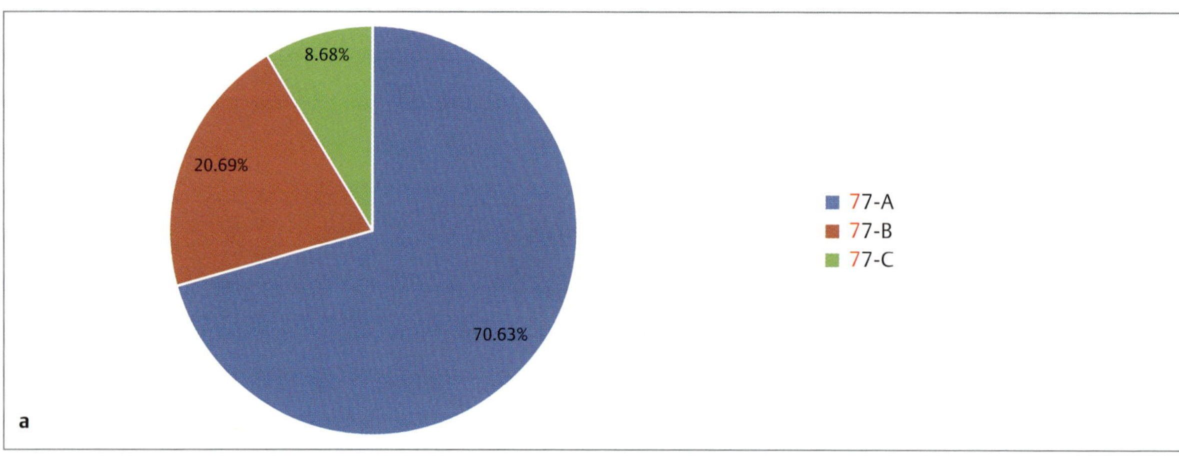

Fig. 8.16 **(a)** Fracture type distribution of 10,145 fractures of metacarpal bones (segment 77).

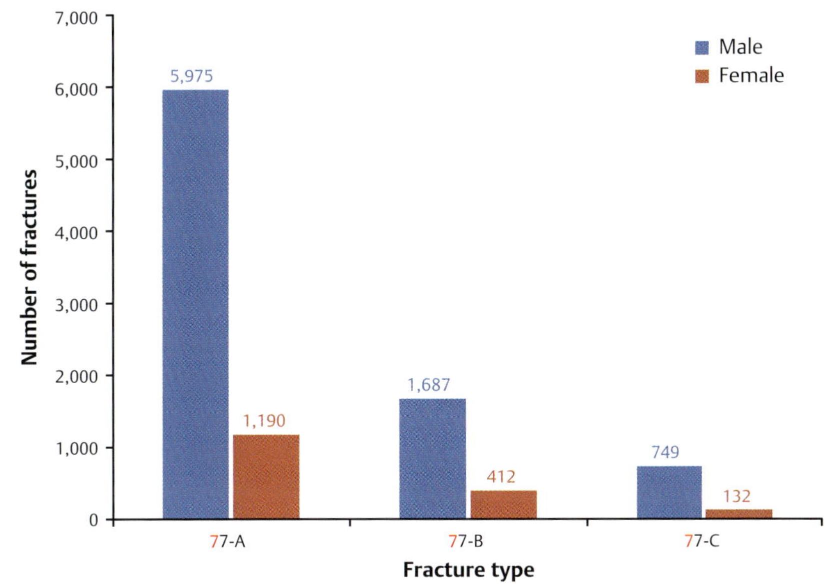

b

Fig. 8.16 (*continued*) **(b)** Sex and fracture type distribution of 10,145 fractures of metacarpal bones (segment 77).

Table 8.17 Sex and fracture group distribution of 10,145 fractures of metacarpal bones (segment 77)

Fracture group	Male	Female	Number of fractures	Percentage (%)
77-A1	1,488	318	1,806	17.80
77-A2	2,443	573	3,016	29.73
77-A3	2,044	299	2,343	23.10
77-B1	993	248	1,241	12.23
77-B2	446	105	551	5.43
77-B3	248	59	307	3.03
77-C1	406	53	459	4.52
77-C2	242	54	296	2.92
77-C3	101	25	126	1.24
Total	8,411	1,734	10,145	100.00

8

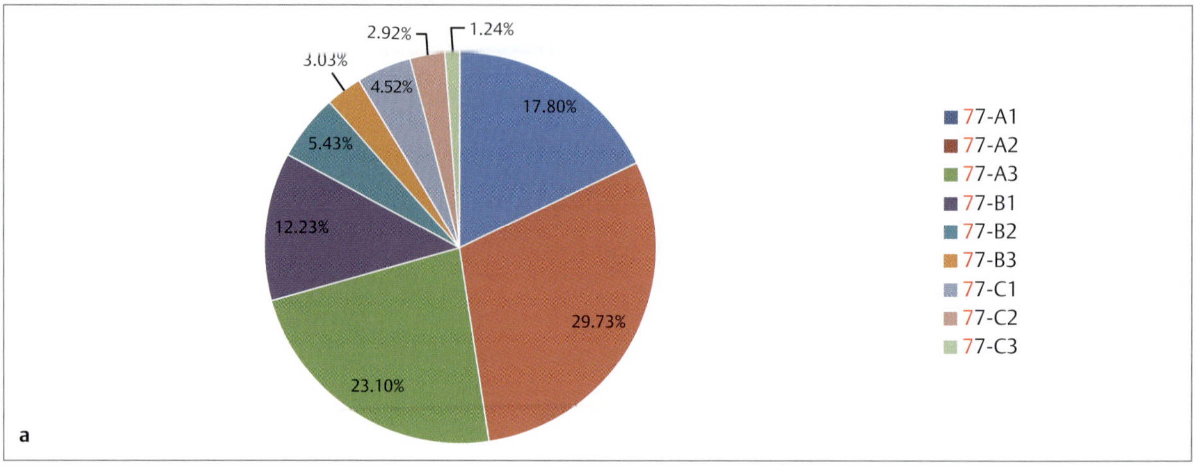

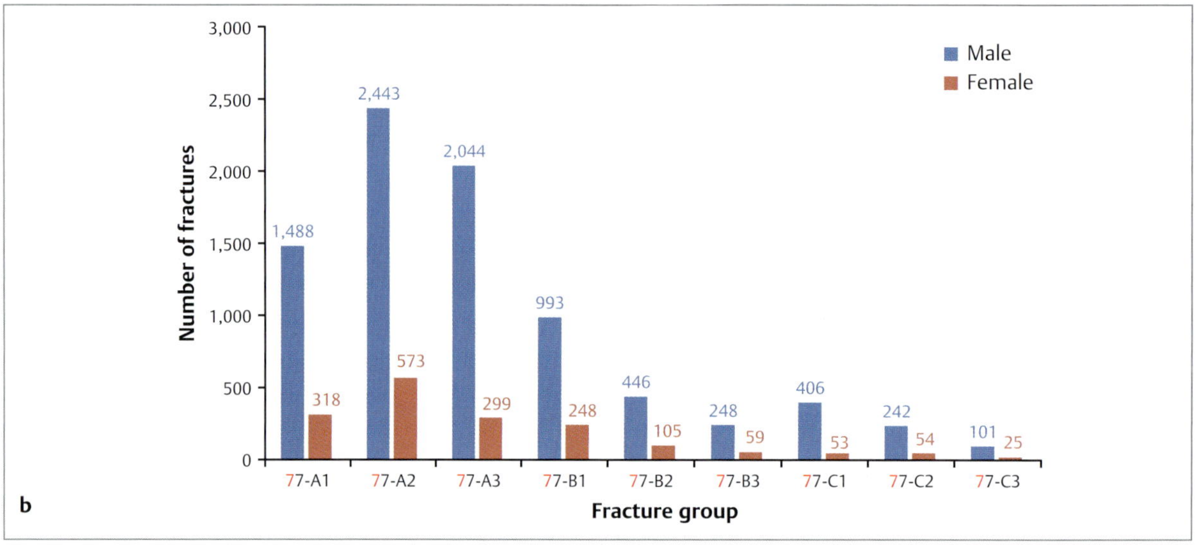

Fig. 8.17 **(a)** Fracture group distribution of 10,145 fractures of metacarpal bones (segment 77).
(b) Sex and fracture group distribution of 10,145 fractures of metacarpal bones (segment 77).

Metacarpal Fractures by Individual Metacarpal Bone

Table 8.18 Sex distribution of 10,145 metacarpal fractures by individual metacarpal bone

Number of metacarpal	Male	Female	Number of fractures	Percentage (%)
1st	1,453	322	1,775	17.50
2nd	907	190	1,097	10.81
3rd	727	200	927	9.14
4th	1,569	397	1,966	19.38
5th	3,755	625	4,380	43.17
Total	8,411	1,734	10,145	100.00

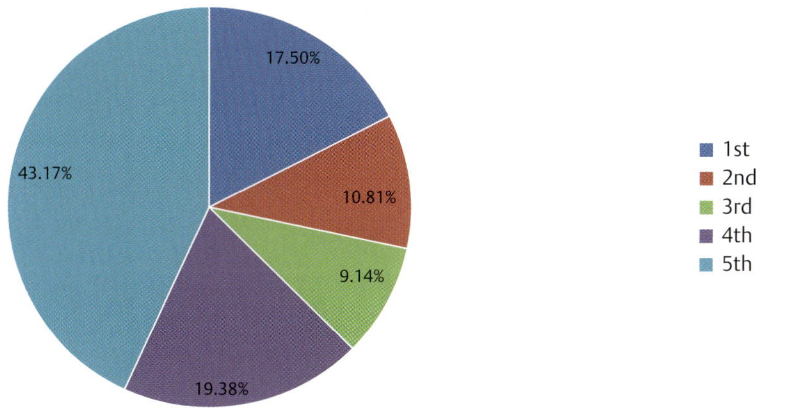

a

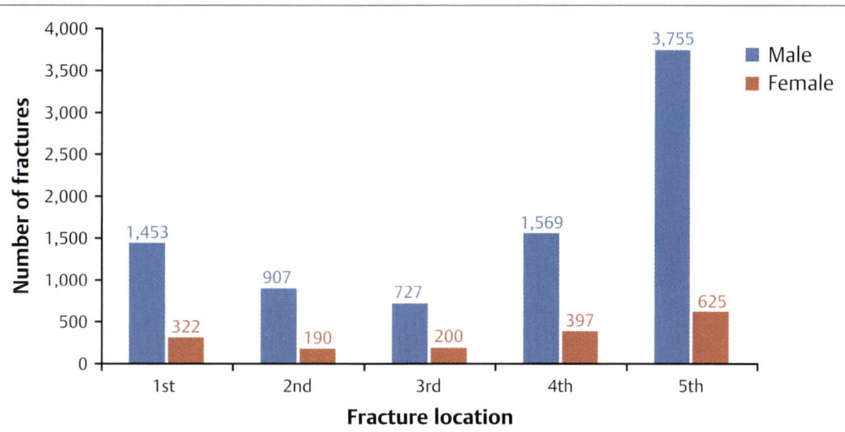

b

Fig. 8.18 **(a)** Distribution of 10,145 fractures of metacarpal bones by individual metacarpal bone.
(b) Sex distribution of 10,145 fractures of metacarpal bones by individual metacarpal bone.

77-A Metacarpal proximal and distal nonarticular and diaphysis noncomminuted

77-A1
Proximal extra-articular
1,806 fractures
M: 1,488 (82.39%)
F: 318 (17.61%)
0.48% of total adult fractures
3.07% of adult hand fractures
17.80% of adult metacarpal fractures
25.21% of type 77-A fractures

77-A1.1

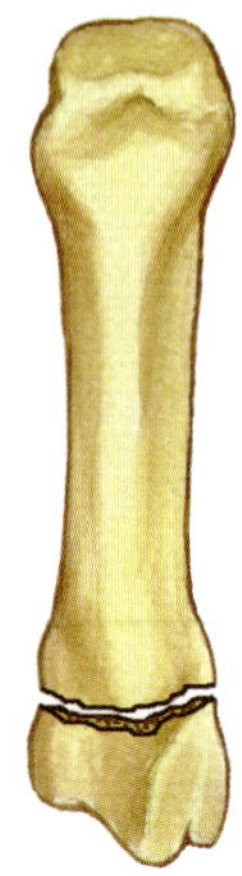

Simple

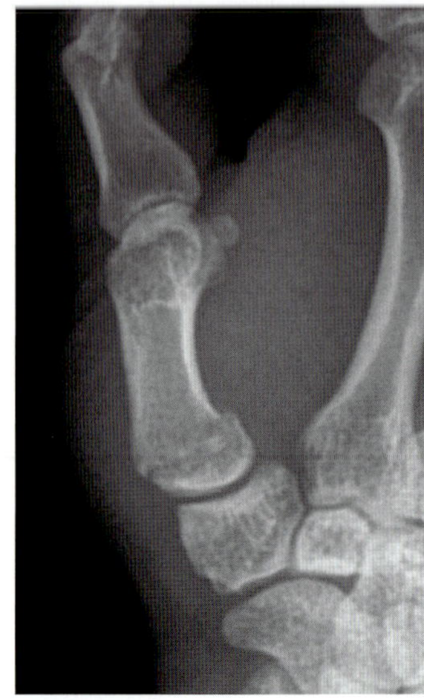

77-A1.2

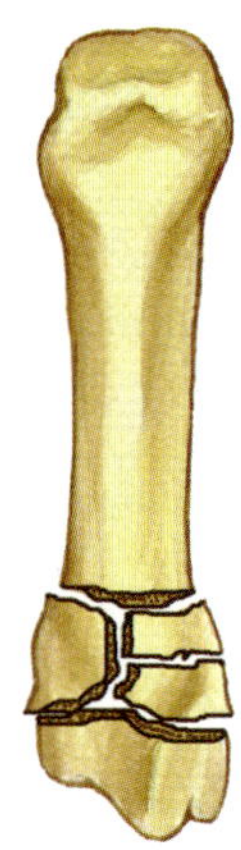

Wedge or comminuted

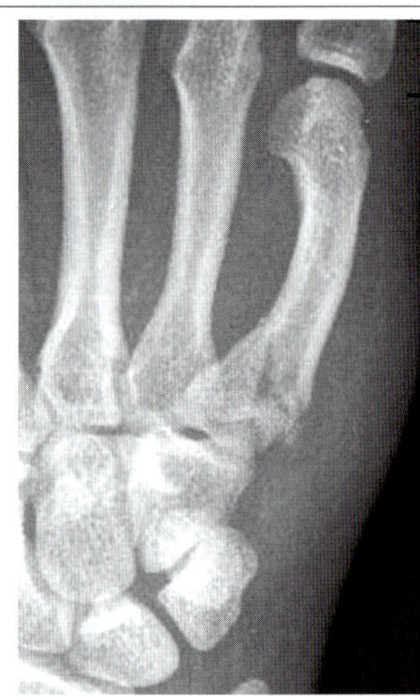

77-A Metacarpal proximal and distal nonarticular and diaphysis noncomminuted

77-A2
Diaphysis noncomminuted
3,016 fractures
M: 2,443 (81.00%)
F: 573 (19.00%)
0.81% of total adult fractures
5.12% of adult hand fractures
29.73% of adult metacarpal fractures
42.09% of type 77-A fractures

77-A2.1

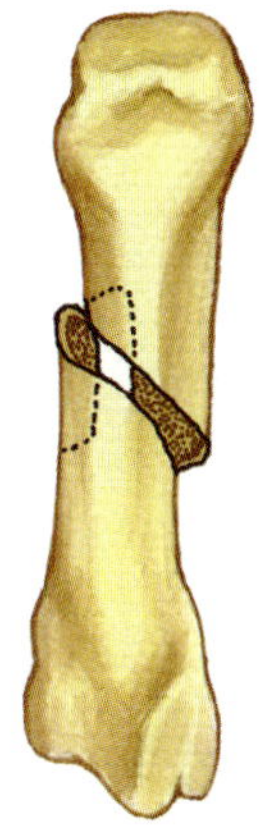

Spiral

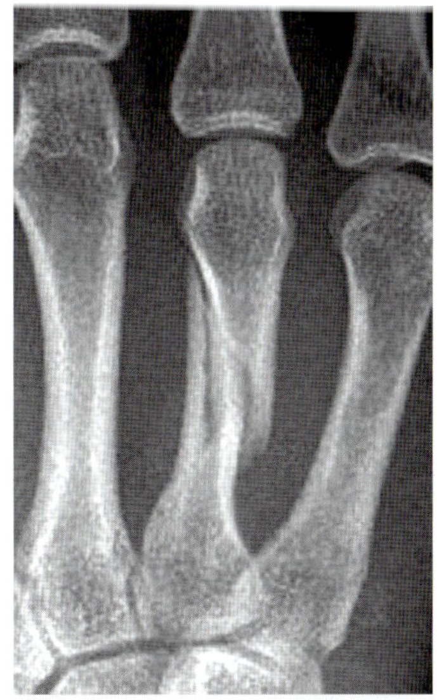

77-A2.2

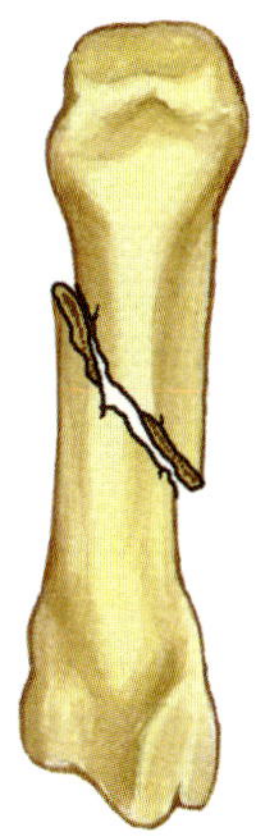

Oblique

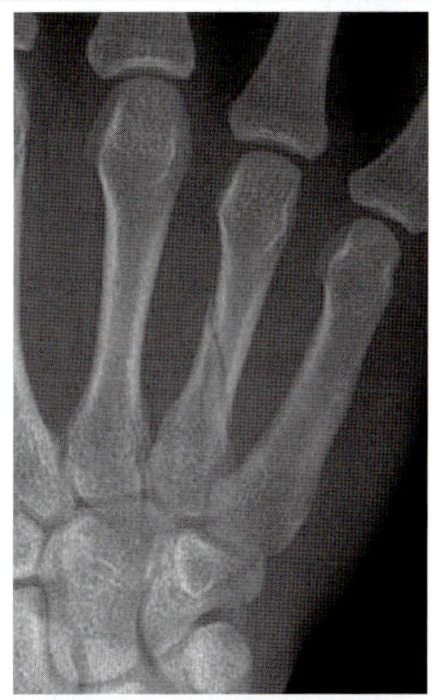

77-A2.3

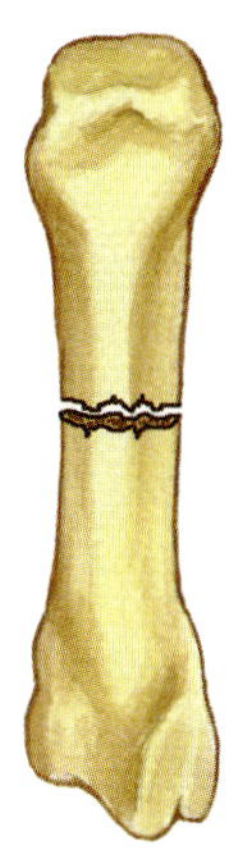

Transverse

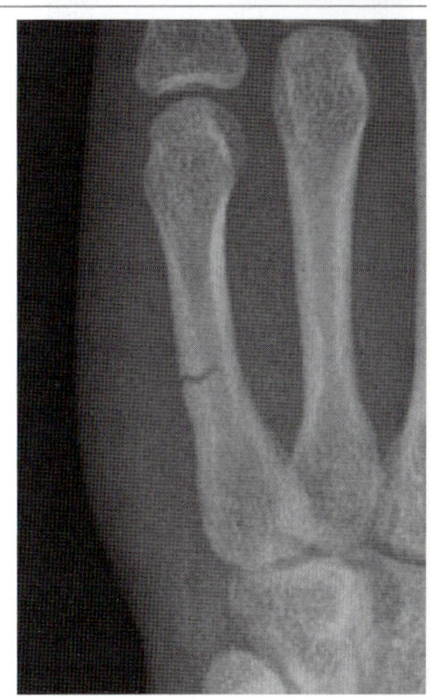

77-A Metacarpal proximal and distal nonarticular and diaphysis noncomminuted

77-A3
Distal extra-articular
2,343 fractures
M: 2,044 (87.24%)
F: 299 (12.76%)
0.63% of total adult fractures
3.98% of adult hand fractures
23.10% of adult metacarpal fractures
32.70% of type 77-A fractures

77-A3.1

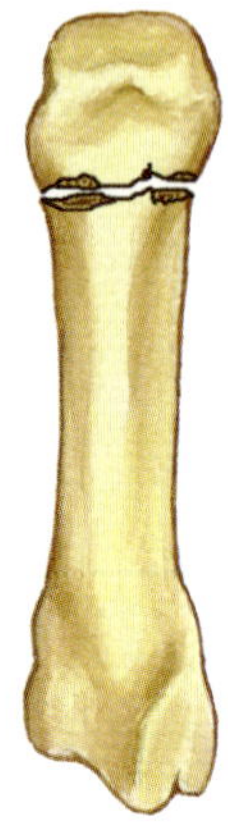

Simple

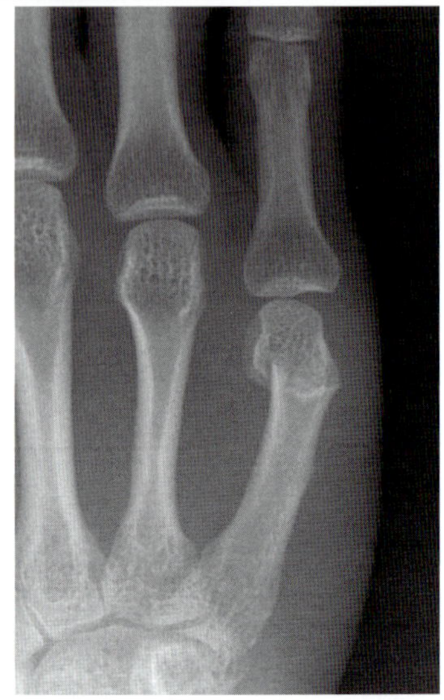

77-A3.2

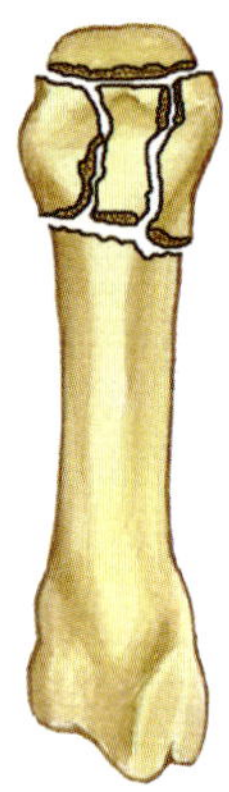

Comminuted

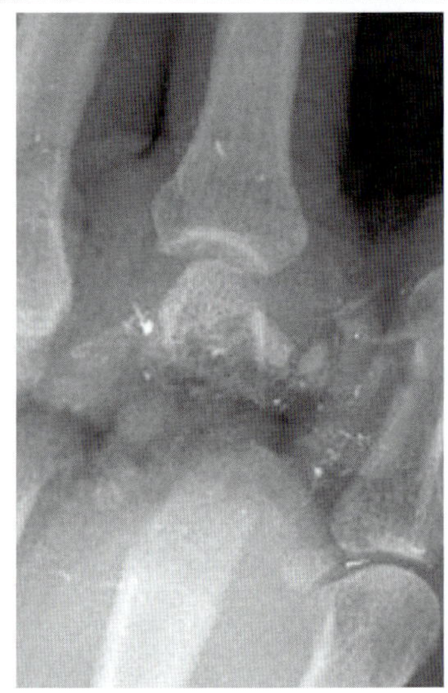

77-B Metacarpal proximal and distal partial articular and diaphysis wedge comminution

77-B1
Proximal partial articular

1,241 fractures
M: 993 (80.02%)
F: 248 (19.98%)
0.33% of total adult fractures
2.11% of adult hand fractures
12.23% of adult metacarpal fractures
59.12% of type 77-B fractures

77-B1.1

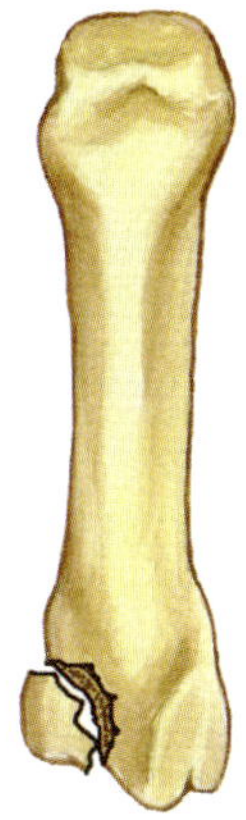

Avulsion or split

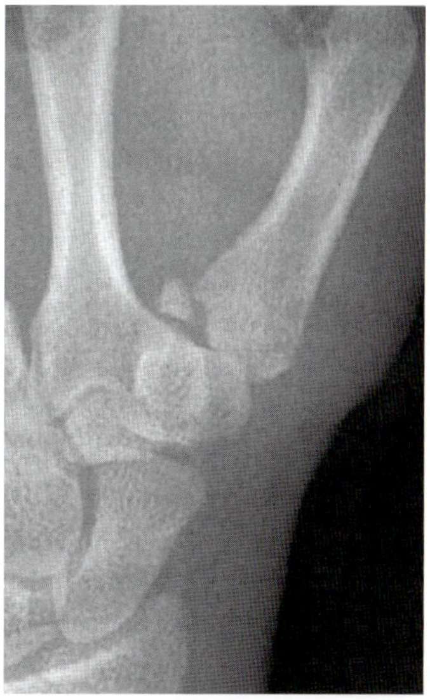

77-B1.2

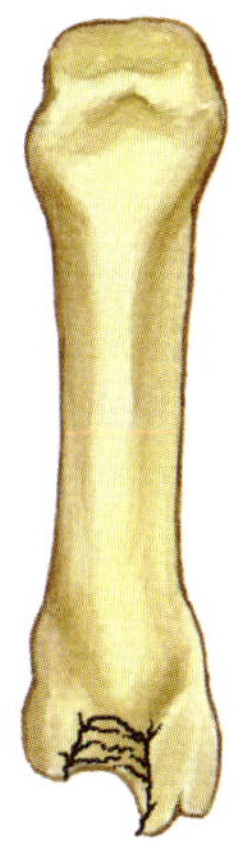

Depression

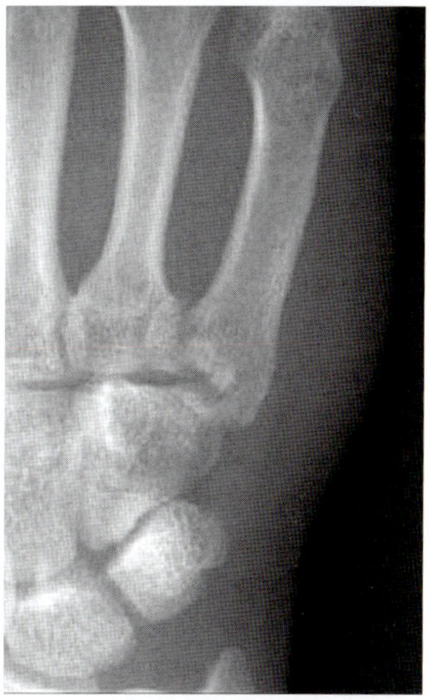

77-B1.3

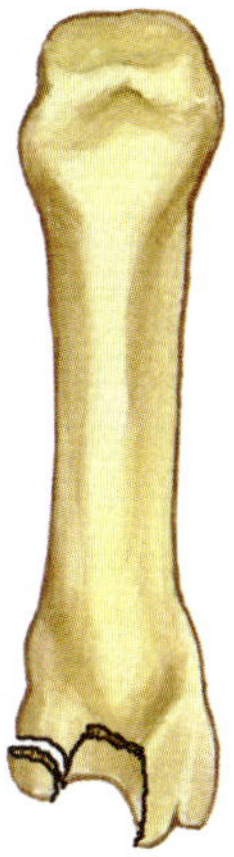

Split/depression

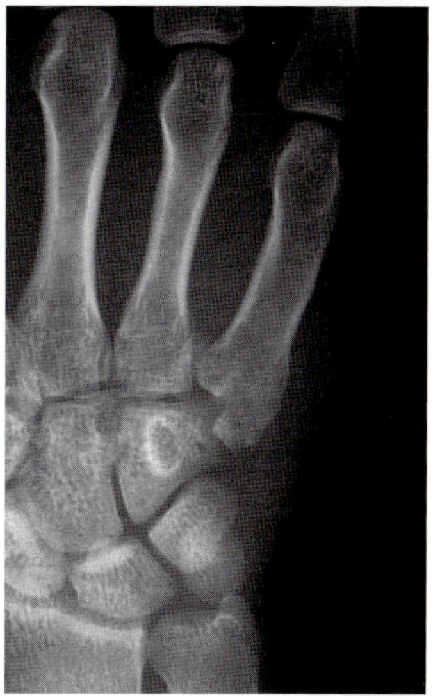

77-B Metacarpal proximal and distal partial articular and diaphysis wedge comminution

77-B2
Diaphysis wedge
551 fractures
M: 446 (80.94%)
F: 105 (19.06%)
0.15% of total adult fractures
0.94% of adult hand fractures
5.43% of adult metacarpal fractures
26.25% of type 77-B fractures

77-B2.1

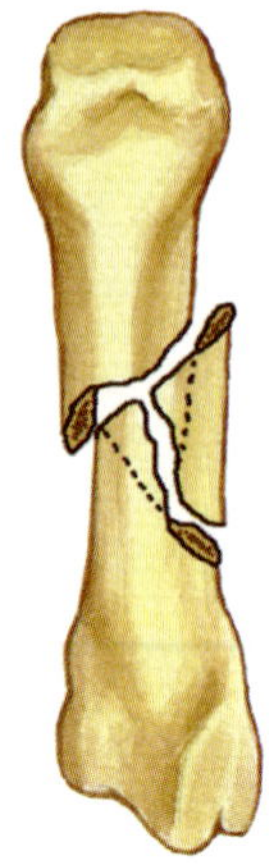

Spiral wedge

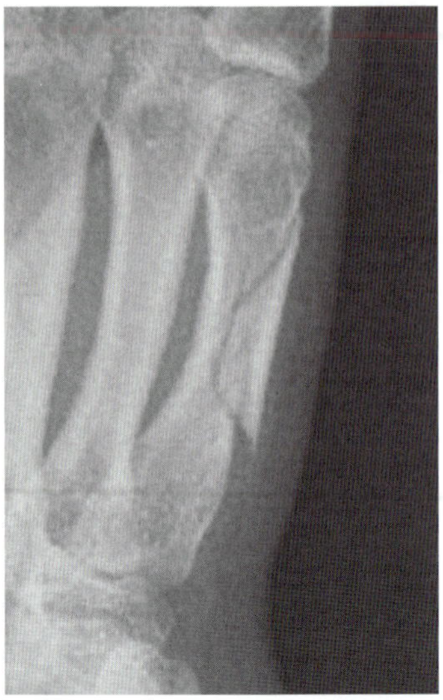

77-B2.2

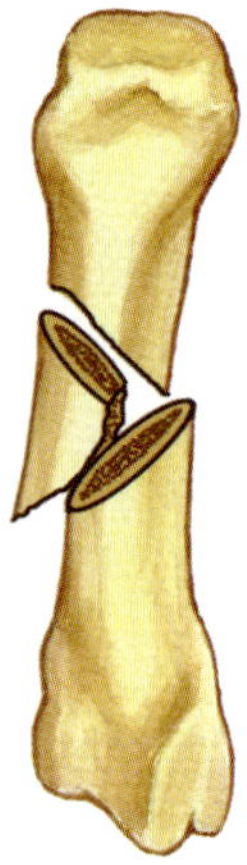

Bending wedge

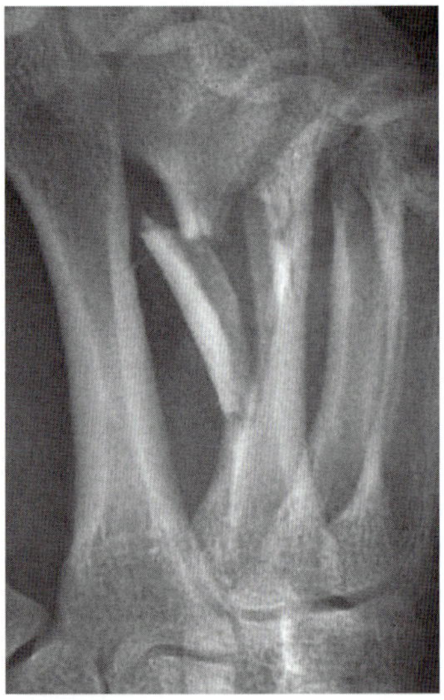

77-B2.3

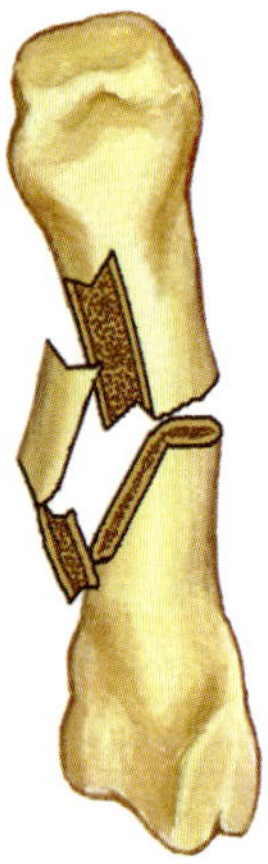

Comminuted

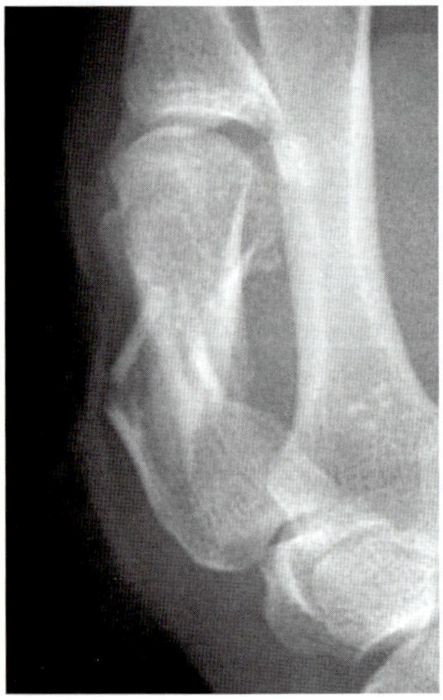

77-B Metacarpal proximal and distal partial articular and diaphysis wedge comminution

77-B3
Distal partial articular
307 fractures
M: 248 (80.78%)
F: 59 (19.22%)
0.08% of total adult fractures
0.52% of adult hand fractures
3.03% of adult metacarpal fractures
14.63% of type 77-B fractures

77-B3.1

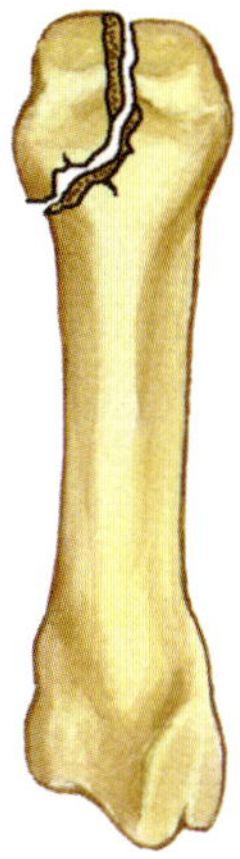

Avulsion or split

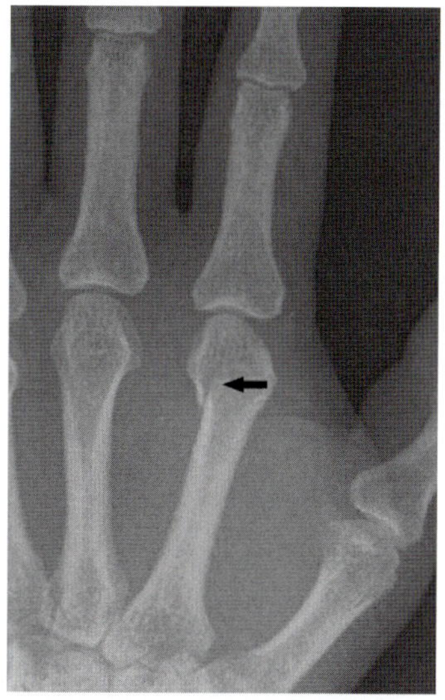

77-B3.2

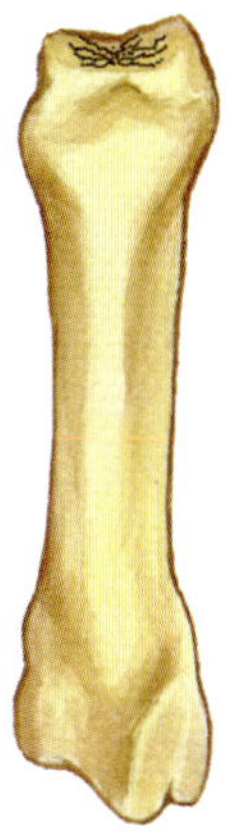

Depression

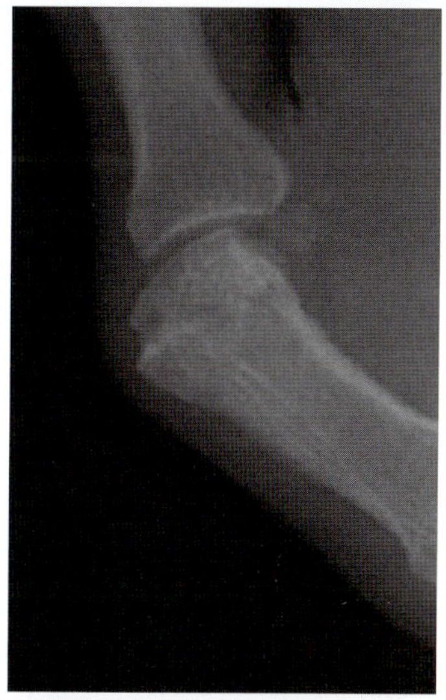

77-B3.3

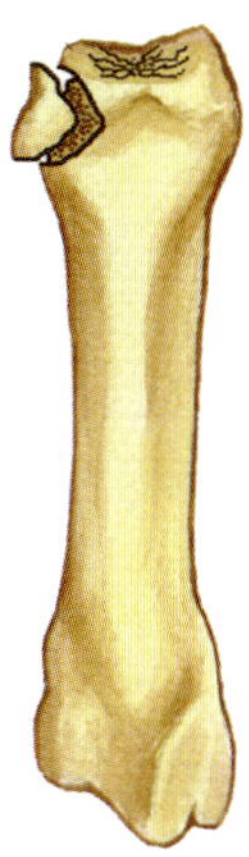

Split/depression

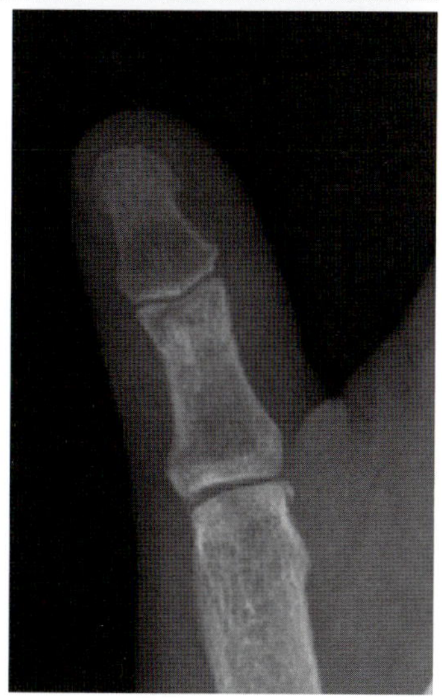

77-C Metacarpal proximal and distal complete articular and diaphysis comminuted

77-C1
Proximal complete articular
459 fractures
M: 406 (88.45%)
F: 53 (11.55%)
0.12% of total adult fractures
0.78% of adult hand fractures
4.52% of adult metacarpal fractures
52.10% of type 77-C fractures

77-C1.1

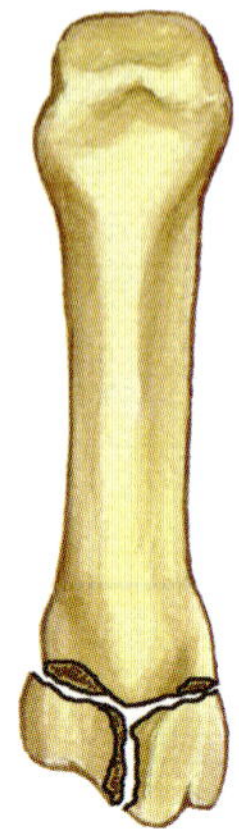

Noncomminuted
articular and metaphysis

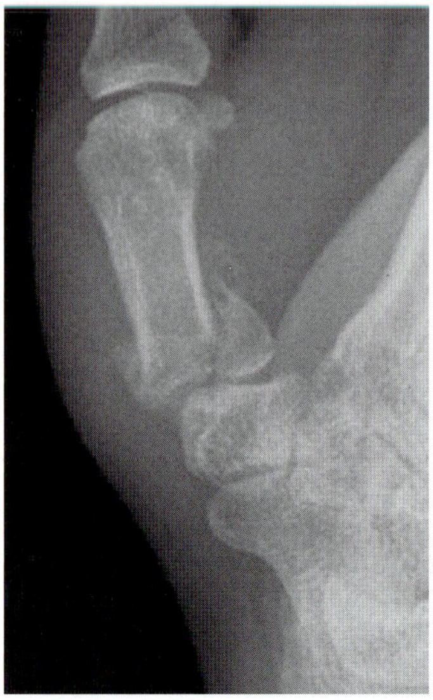

77-C1.2

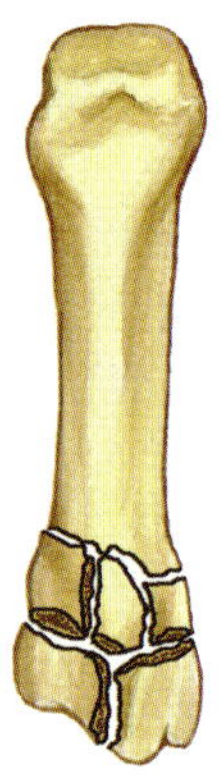

Noncomminuted
articular, comminuted metaphysis

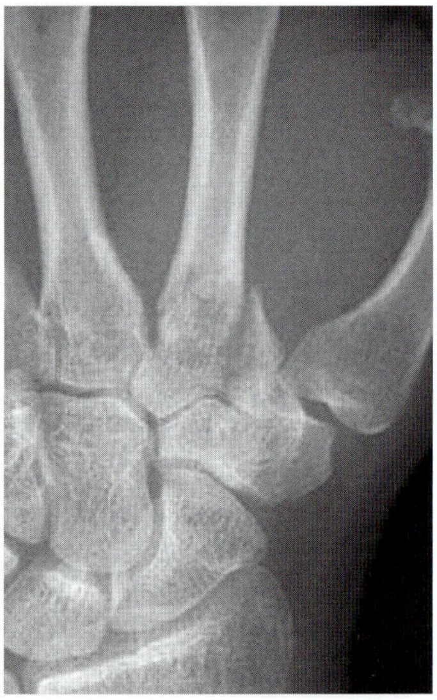

77-C1.3

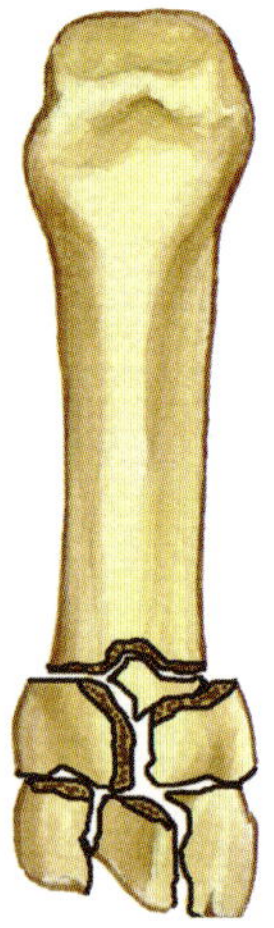

Comminuted articular

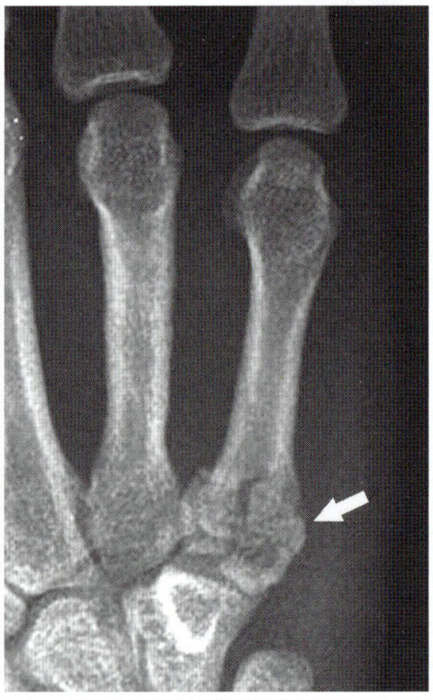

77-C Metacarpal proximal and distal complete articular and diaphysis comminuted

77-C2
Diaphysis comminuted
296 fractures
M: 242 (81.76%)
F: 54 (18.24%)
0.08% of total adult fractures
0.50% of adult hand fractures
2.92% of adult metacarpal fractures
33.60% of type 77-C fractures

77-C2.1

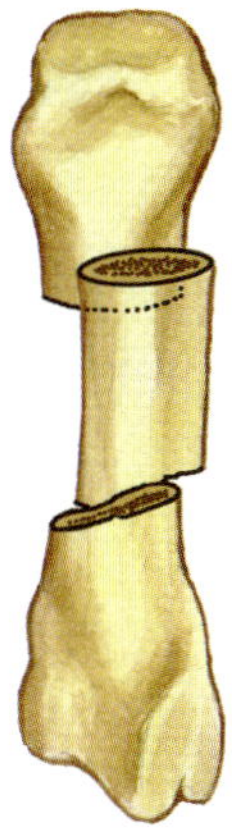

Segmental

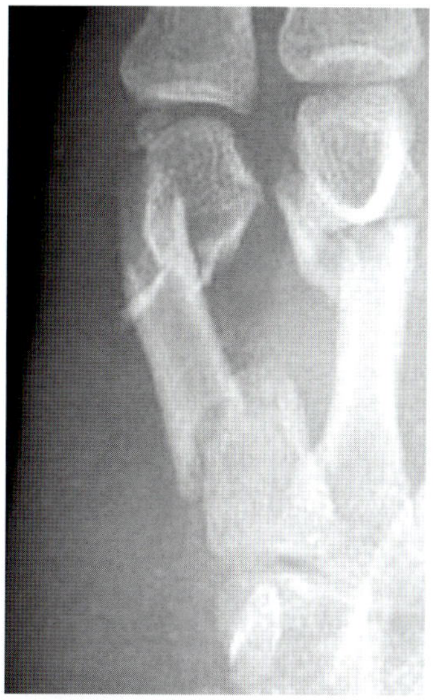

77-C2.2

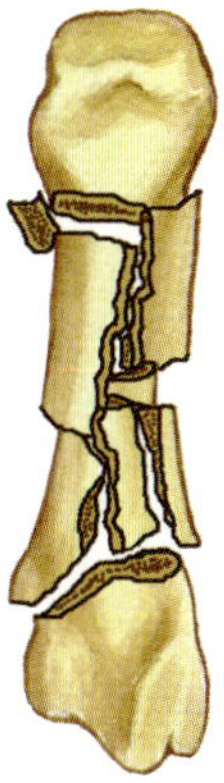

Complex comminuted

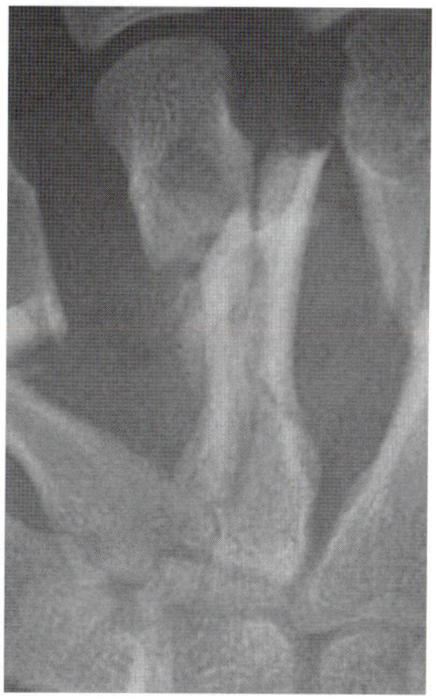

8

77-C Metacarpal proximal and distal complete articular and diaphysis comminuted

77-C3
Distal articular
126 fractures
M: 101 (80.16%)
F: 25 (19.84%)
0.03% of total adult fractures
0.21% of adult hand fractures
1.24% of adult metacarpal fractures
14.30% of type 77-C fractures

77-C3.1

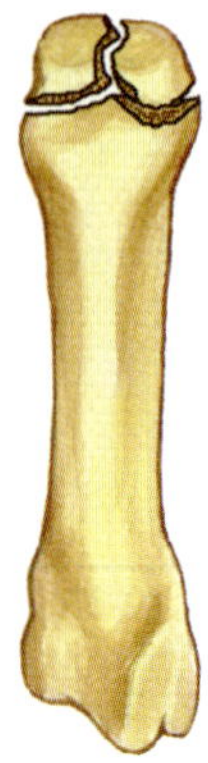

Simple articular/metaphysis

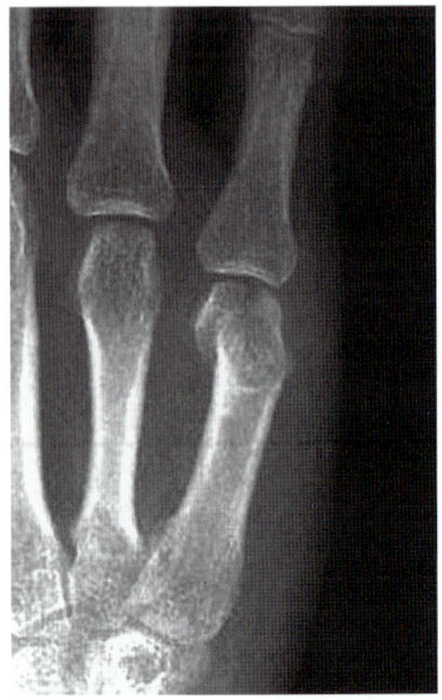

77-C3.2

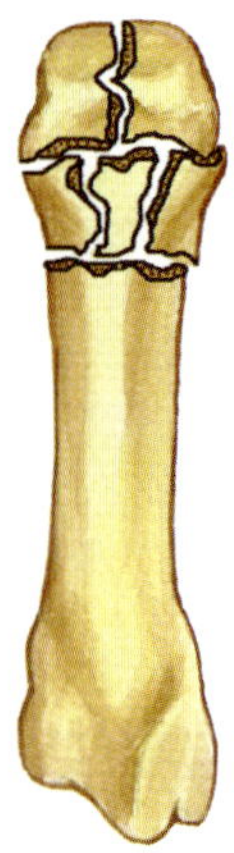

Simple articular/comminuted metaphysis

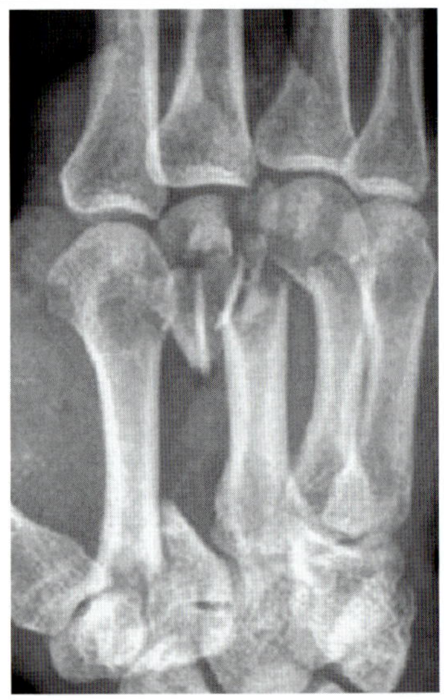

77-C3.3

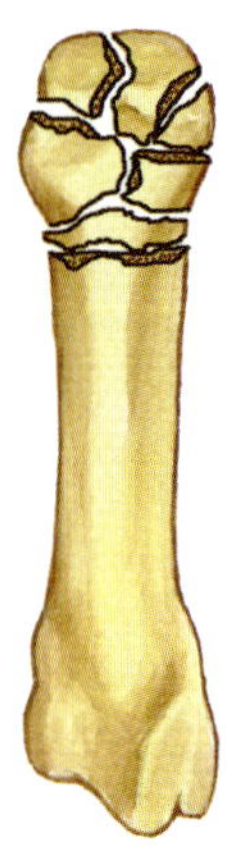

Comminuted articular

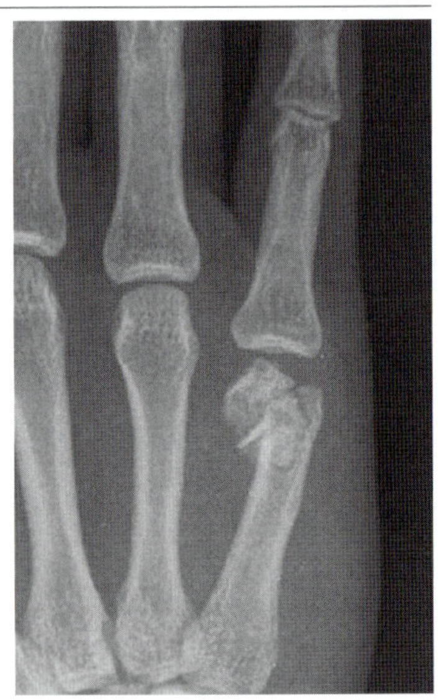

Injury Mechanism

Fractures of metacarpals generally occur with a straightforward history of trauma. Injury to the first metacarpal shaft occurs when an axial or torsional force is transmitted through a partially flexed thumb metacarpal. Because of the pull of the thenar muscles and the abductor pollicis longus, the proximal fragment may be angularly displaced dorsally and radially, with the thumb in adduction. Rotational deformity of the thumb may also be present. Fractures of the second to fifth metacarpals usually occur as a result of compression or torsional force injuries.

Diagnosis

Diagnosis is usually directed by trauma history and clinical examination. Pain, swelling, deformity, tenderness, and loss of motion are common with any fractures or dislocation. Standard radiographs including AP and lateral views of the hand should be performed to help define the nature of the fracture, and the degree of the displacement.

Treatment

Most metacarpal fractures can be managed nonoperatively, utilizing closed reduction and casting or splinting, with a good long-term clinical outcome. Indications for open reduction and internal fixation (plating or K-wire), or closed reduction and percutaneous wire fixation include the following: (1) displaced intra-articular fractures; (2) avulsion fractures associated with torn ligaments or tendons; (3) failure to achieve or maintain acceptable reduction using closed techniques; (4) multiple hand fractures; and (5) open fractures.

Further Classification of Base Fracture of the First Metacarpal Bone

Anatomical Features and Classification

The base of the first metacarpal bone presents a concavo-convex surface, which forms the carpometacarpal joint of the thumb, with its reciprocal articular surface formed by the greater multangular bone. The joint, having saddle-shaped surfaces, is capable of moving in all directions, which allows the thumb freedom of motion described as extension and flexion (parallel to the palm), abduction and adduction (at right angles to the palm), as well as some rotation. The joint is surrounded by a thick but loose joint capsule that is reinforced by several ligaments. The laxity of the joint capsule permits a great amount of movement by the thumb.

Fractures of the base of the first metacarpal are particularly common. Based on the X-ray appearance, fractures of the thumb metacarpal are classified into four patterns:

- *Type I* injury is a fracture-dislocation of the base of the thumb metacarpal, a so-called Bennett's fracture. This injury usually occurs as a result of axially directed forces or torsional forces transmitted through the partially flexed metacarpal shaft. A proximal metacarpal fragment maintains its ulnar aspect attachment to the trapezium via the volar ligament. The distal aspect of the metacarpal is usually subluxated radially and dorsally by the adductor pollicis. The proximal aspect of this fragment is pulled proximally by the abductor pollicis longus.
- *Type II* injuries are known as Rolando fractures, and can be thought of as a comminuted version of a Bennett fracture, in which the fragments may form a T or Y pattern at the base of the metacarpal.
- *Type III* fractures are extra-articular, either transverse or, less commonly, oblique.
- *Type IV* fractures are extra-articular pediatric injuries involving the proximal physis, and are not commonly associated with dislocation.

8

Clinical Epidemiologic Features of Fractures of the Base of the First Metacarpal Bone

A total of 1,243 patients with 1,244 fractures of the base of first metacarpal bone were treated in 83 hospitals in China over a 2-year period from 2010 to 2011. All cases were reviewed and statistically studied, and accounted for 1.99% of all patients with hand fractures and 1.95% of hand fractures.

Epidemiologic features of fractures of the base of the first metacarpal bone are as follows:

- More males than females
- The high-risk age group is 21–25 years—the same age group for males and the high-risk age group for females is 51–55 years
- Type III fractures are the most common type of fracture of the base of the first metacarpal bone.

Fractures of the Base of the First Metacarpal Bone by Sex

Table 8.19 Sex distribution of 1,243 patients with fractures of the base of the first metacarpal bone

Sex	Number of patients	Percentage (%)
Male	1,016	81.74
Female	227	18.26
Total	1,243	100.00

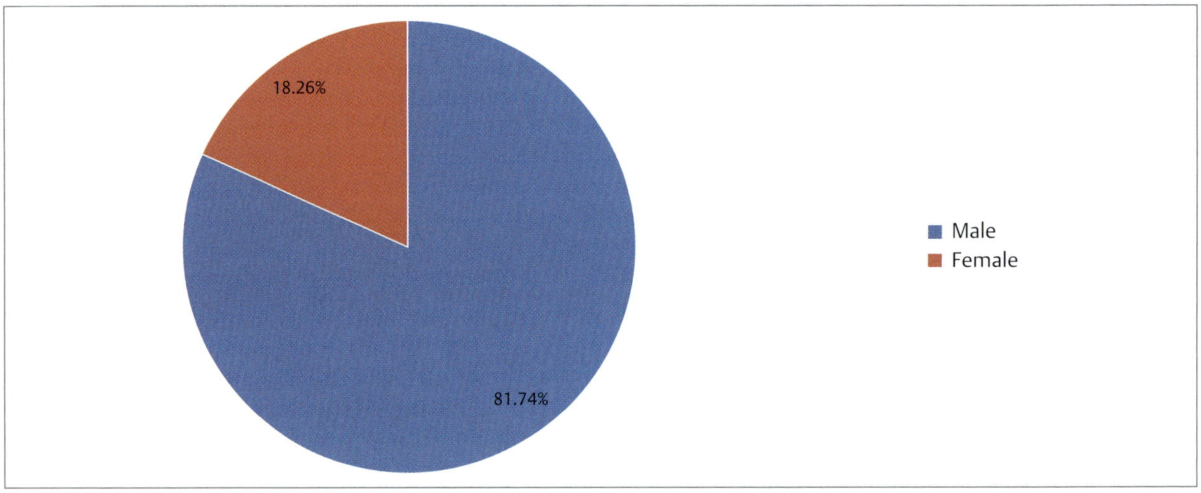

Fig. 8.19 Sex distribution of 1,243 patients with fractures of the base of the first metacarpal bone.

Fractures of the Base of the First Metacarpal Bone by Age Group

Table 8.20 Age and sex distribution of 1,243 patients with fractures of the base of the first metacarpal bone

Age group (years)	Male	Female	Number of patients	Percentage (%)
0–5	6	1	7	0.56
6–10	9	0	9	0.72
11–15	20	11	31	2.49
16–20	88	5	93	7.48
21–25	143	13	156	12.55
26–30	134	14	148	11.91
31–35	115	10	125	10.06
36–40	119	20	139	11.18
41–45	103	20	123	9.90
46–50	99	24	123	9.90
51–55	62	32	94	7.56
56–60	57	25	82	6.60
61–65	21	14	35	2.82
66–70	11	17	28	2.25
71–75	14	8	22	1.77
76–80	10	10	20	1.61
81–85	4	2	6	0.48
≥86	1	1	2	0.16
Total	1,016	227	1,243	100

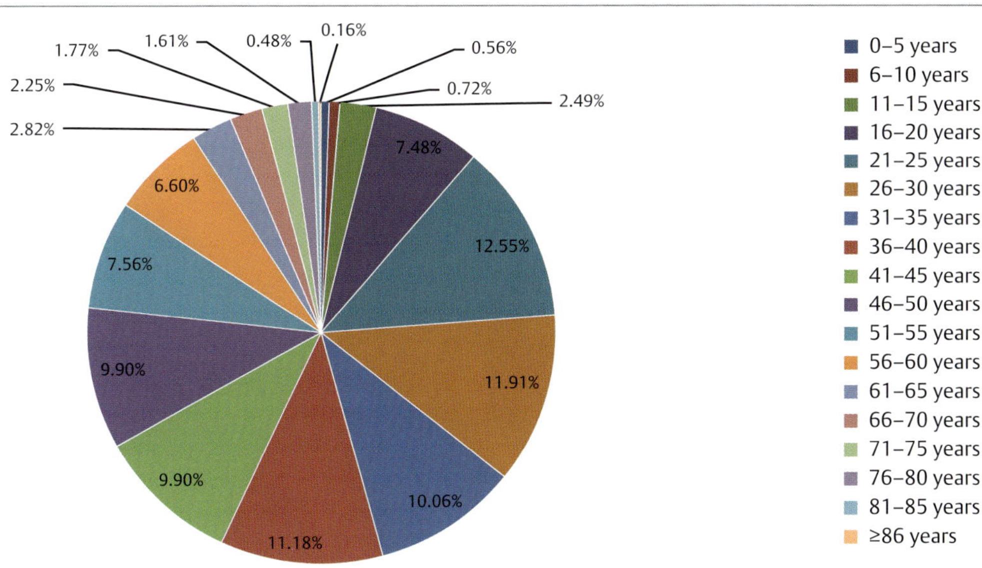

a

Fig. 8.20 **(a)** Age distribution of 1,243 patients with fractures of the base of the first metacarpal bone. (*Continued*)

8

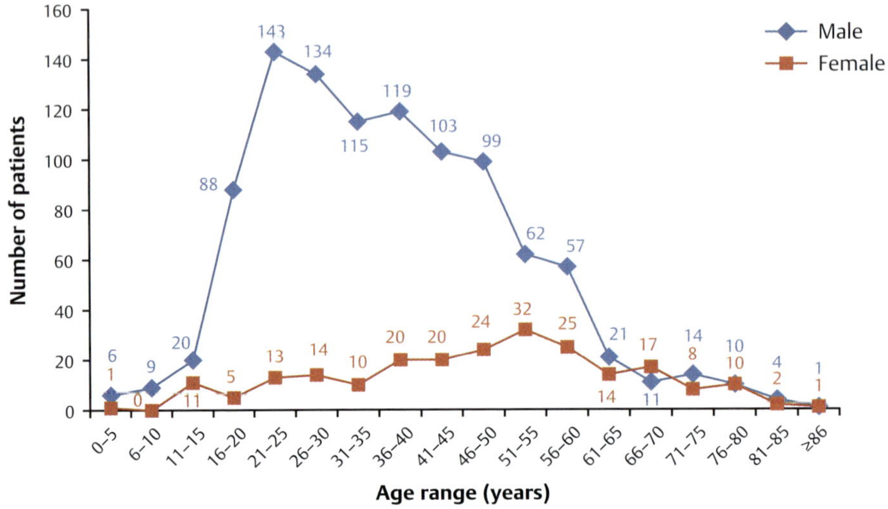

b

Fig. 8.20 (*continued*) **(b)** Age and sex distribution of 1,243 patients with fractures of the base of the first metacarpal bone.

Fractures of the Base of the First Metacarpal Bone by Fracture Type

Table 8.21 Fracture type distribution of 1,244 fractures of the base of the first metacarpal bone

Fracture type	Male	Female	Number of fractures	Percentage	Percentage of metacarpal fractures (%)	Percentage of hand fractures (%)
I	385	95	480	38.59	4.38	0.75
II	135	17	152	12.22	1.39	0.24
III	462	103	565	45.42	5.16	0.89
IV	35	12	47	3.78	0.43	0.07
Total	1,017	227	1,244	100.00	11.36	1.95

A total of 10,951 isolated metacarpal fractures in adults and children were treated.

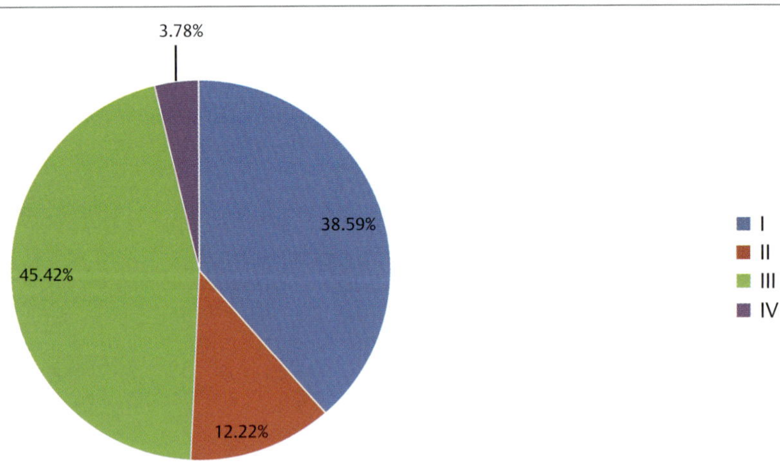

Fig. 8.21 Fracture type distribution of 1,244 fractures of the base of the first metacarpal bone.

Fractures of the base of the first metacarpal bone	
Type I 480 fractures M: 385 (80.21%) F: 95 (19.79%) 0.11% of total fractures 0.75% of hand fractures 4.38% of all metacarpal fractures 25.28% of the first metacarpal fractures 38.59% of the base of the first metacarpal fractures	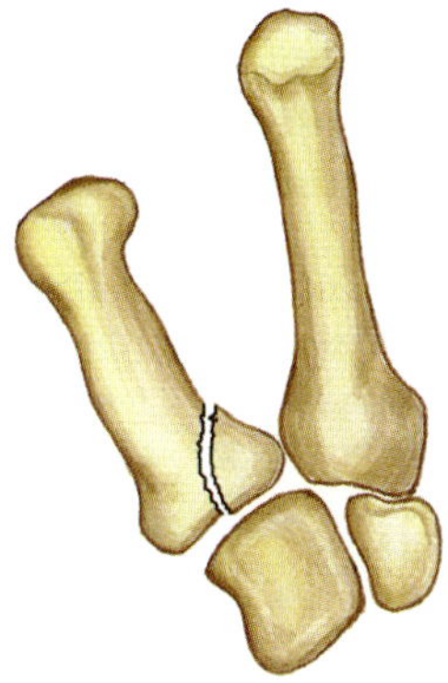 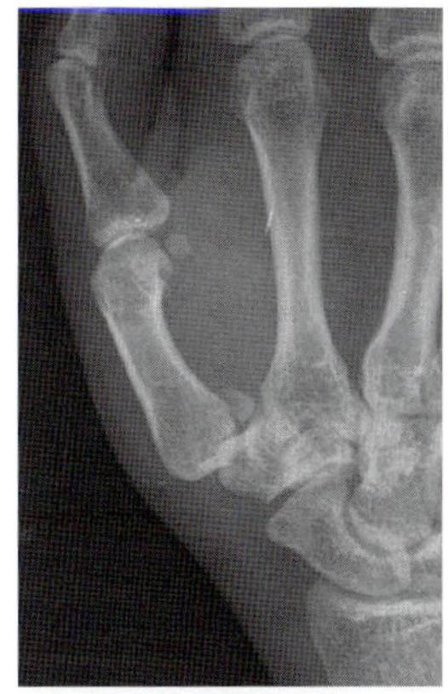
Type II 152 fractures M: 135 (88.82%) F: 17 (11.18%) 0.04% of total fractures 0.24% of hand fractures 1.39% of all metacarpal fractures 8.00% of the first metacarpal fractures 12.22% of the base of the first metacarpal fractures	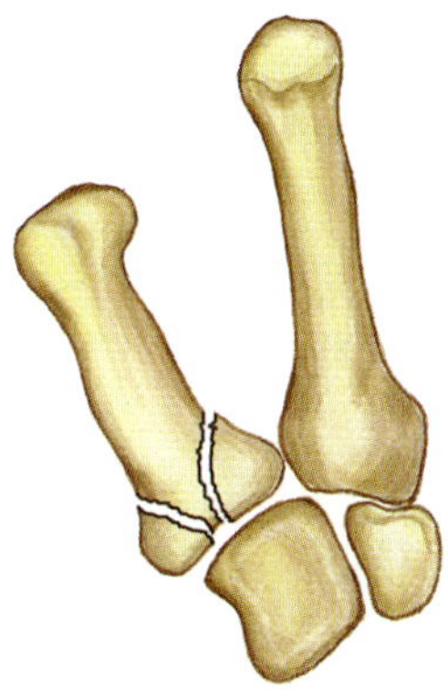 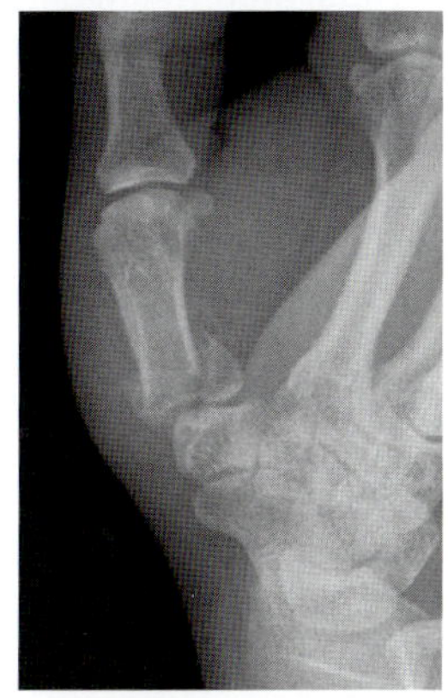
Type III 565 fractures M: 462 (81.77%) F: 103 (18.23%) 0.13% of total fractures 0.89% of hand fractures 5.16% of all metacarpal bones fractures 29.75% of the first metacarpal fractures 45.42% of the base of the first metacarpal fractures	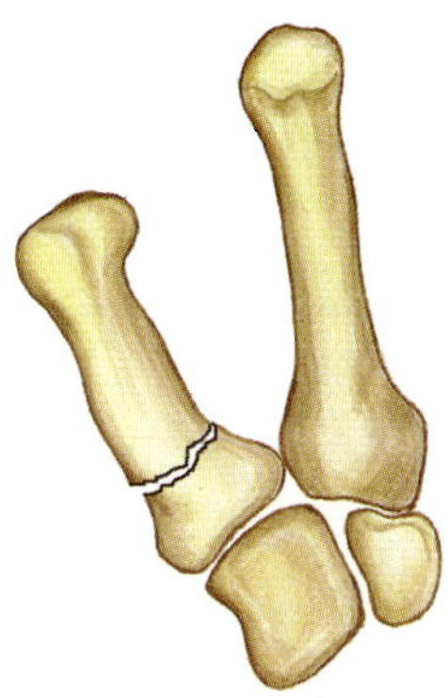 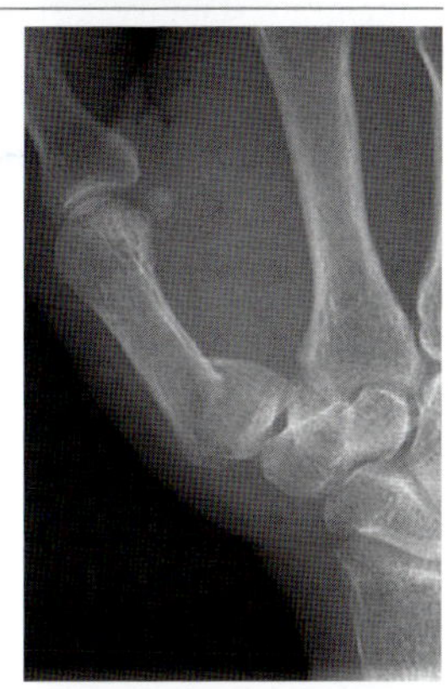
Type IV 47 fractures M: 35 (74.47%) F: 12 (25.53%) 0.01% of total fractures 0.07% of hand fractures 0.43% of all metacarpal bones fractures 2.47% of the first metacarpal fractures 3.78% of the base of the first metacarpal fractures	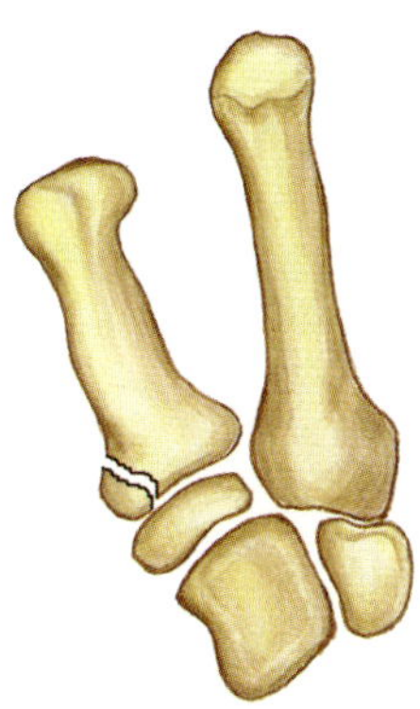 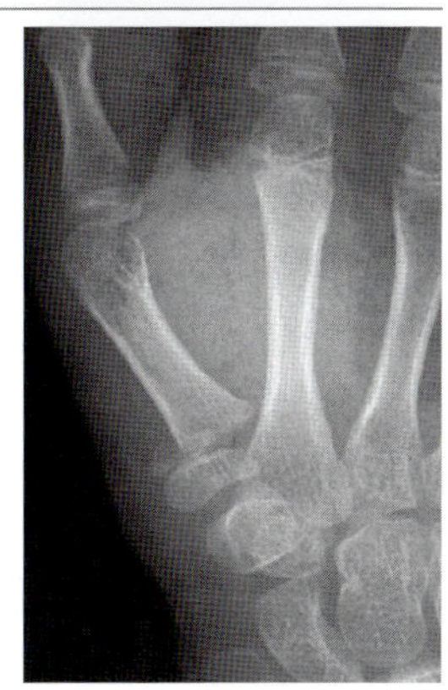

Injury Mechanism

This type of injury usually occurs from indirect force. The distal fragment is usually adducted and displaced volarly secondary to the pull of the flexor pollicis longus and adductor pollicis. The thumb carpometacarpal joint is a saddle-shaped joint. When the ulnar aspect of the thumb's metacarpal base is fractured, the small triangle-shaped fragment remains in its correct anatomical region and the main body of the first metacarpal is typically displaced radially and dorsally, due to the pull of the thumb extensors.

Diagnosis

Usually it is not difficult to make a diagnosis, with a straightforward trauma history and clinical examination. Swelling, pain, tenderness over the base of the thumb, loss of function (thumb opposition and abduction), and radial and dorsal angulation of the thumb base are common symptoms that indicate the presence of the fracture. There is no apparent impairment in the motion of the metacarpophalangeal joints and interphalangeal joints. The diagnosis should be confirmed by radiographs, and CT scan if indicated.

Treatment

Closed reduction can be initiated but it is usually difficult to maintain the reduction. If the reduction is adequate and can maintain stability, a short-arm cast is applied so as to exclude the web space for 4–6 weeks. Open reduction and internal fixation or percutaneous K-wire fixation should be attempted if the fracture does not reduce adequately, or it is too difficult to maintain the reduction. The fixator should be removed as soon as radiographic features show healing of the fractures. During rehabilitation, exercise with an active range of motion should be encouraged.

Phalanx Fractures (Segment 78)

Anatomical Features

There are 14 phalanges on each hand, three of each finger, and two of each thumb. The three types of phalanges are: the proximal phalanx, the middle phalanx (not present in the thumb), and the distal phalanx. The phalanges are all long tubular bones, each having a base, shaft, and head (also called the trochlea of the phalanx). The head of the distal phalanx is pointed, with a palmar tuberosity for attachment of the finger pulp. The shaft resides between the head and the base. On the base of each phalanx is a concave surface for articulations. The shaft is wider at the base and tapers toward the head in all phalanges. The palmar surface is slightly concave, while the dorsal surface is convex and flat on either side.

OTA Classification of Phalanx Fractures

The OTA classified phalanx fractures into three types as follows: 78-A, phalanx proximal and distal extra-articular and diaphysis noncomminuted; 78-B, phalanx proximal and distal partial articular and diaphysis wedge comminuted; and 78-C, phalanx proximal and distal complete articular and diaphysis comminuted (**Plate 8.5**).

8

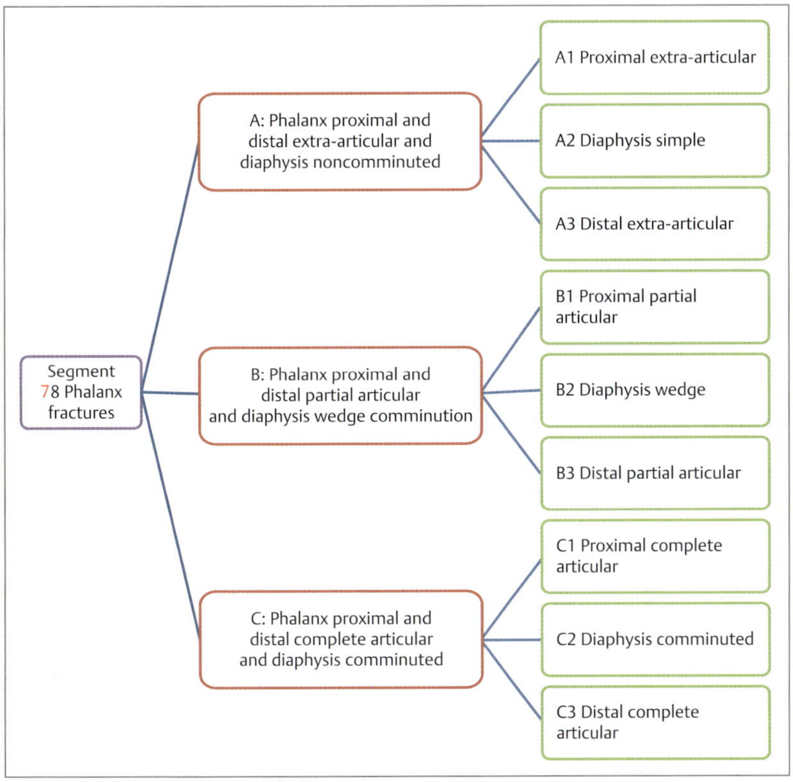

Plate 8.5

Clinical Epidemiologic Features of Phalanx Fractures (Segment 78)

A total of 33,737 adult patients with 33,843 phalanx fractures were treated in 83 hospitals in China over a 2-year period from 2010 to 2011. All cases were reviewed and statistically studied, accounting for 58.46% of all hand fractured adult patients and 57.51% of all hand fractures in adults. Their epidemiologic features are as follows:

- More males than females
- The high-risk age group is 21–25 years—the same age group for males while the high-risk age group for females is 36–40 years.
- The most common phalanx fracture is Type 78-A—the same fracture type for both males and females.
- The most common fracture group is group 78-A3—the same fracture group for both males and females.
- Fractures of the index phalanx are more common than those of other phalanges.

Phalanx Fractures by Sex

Table 8.22 Sex distribution of 33,737 patients with phalanx fractures (segment 78)

Sex	Number of patients	Percentage (%)
Male	26,112	77.40
Female	7,625	22.60
Total	33,737	100.00

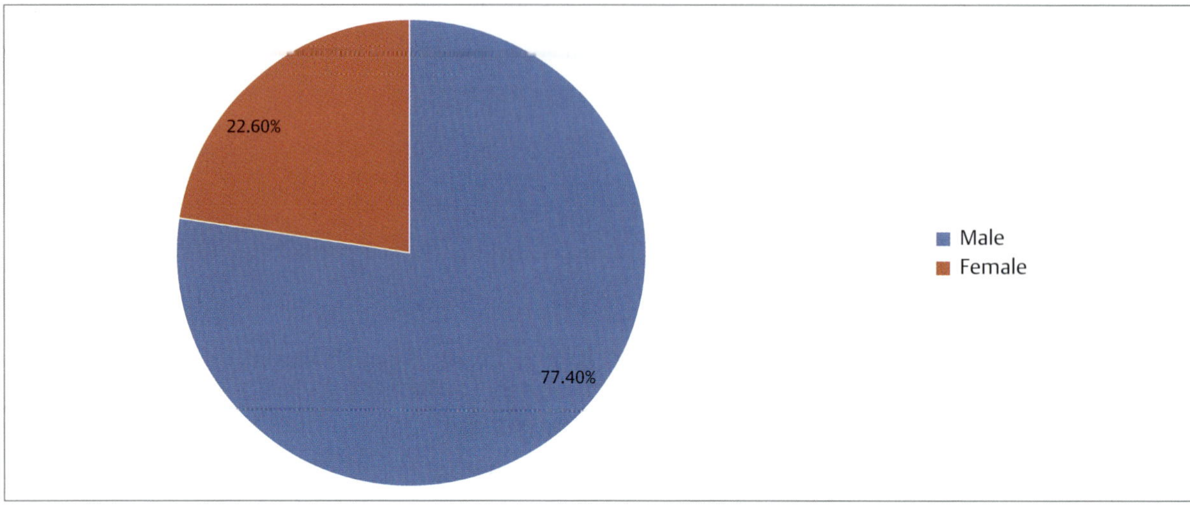

Fig. 8.22 Sex distribution of 33,737 patients with phalanx fractures (segment 78).

Phalanx Fractures by Age Group

Table 8.23 Age and sex distribution of 33,737 patients with phalanx fractures (78)

Age group (years)	Male	Female	Number of patients	Percentage (%)
16–20	2,953	540	3,493	10.35
21–25	4,127	710	4,837	14.34
26–30	3,176	806	3,982	11.80
31–35	2,827	813	3,640	10.79
36–40	3,498	1,178	4,676	13.86
41-45	3,160	1,115	4,275	12.67
46–50	2,465	861	3,326	9.86
51–55	1,630	513	2,143	6.35
56–60	1,241	440	1,681	4.98
61–65	548	257	805	2.39
66–70	202	148	350	1.04
71–75	134	100	234	0.69
76–80	79	82	161	0.48
81–85	35	38	73	0.22
≥86	37	24	61	0.18
Total	26,112	7,625	33,737	100.00

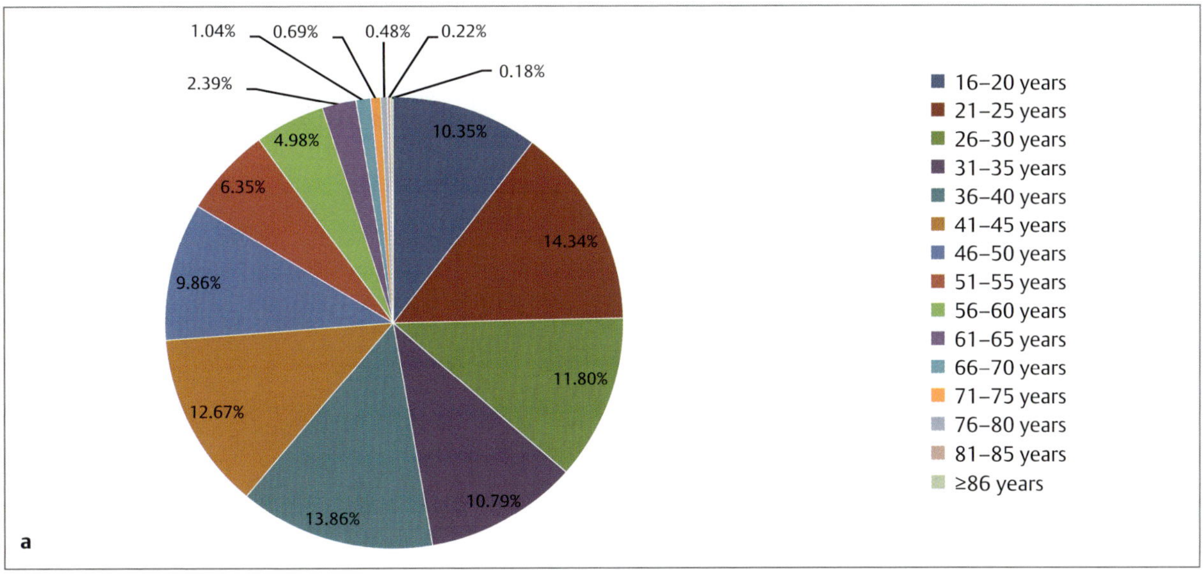

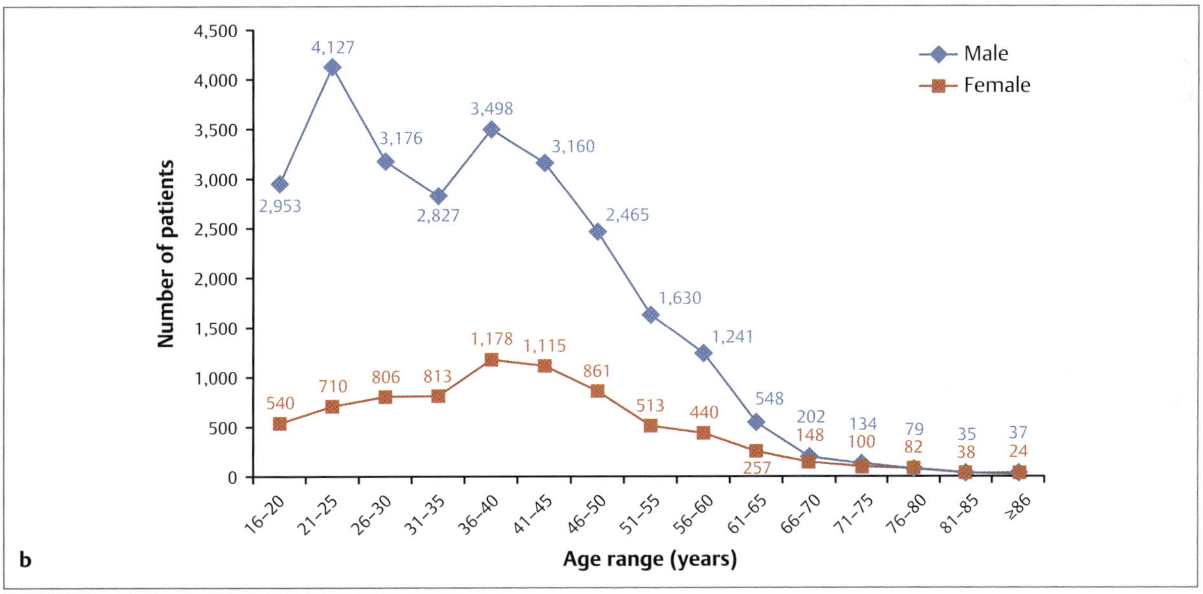

Fig. 8.23 **(a)** Age distribution of 33,737 patients with phalanx fractures (segment 78).
(b) Age and sex distribution of 33,737 patients with phalanx fractures (segment 78).

Phalanx Fractures by Fracture Type

Table 8.24 Sex and fracture type distribution of 33,843 fractures of the phalanx (segment 78)

Fracture type	Male	Female	Number of fractures	Percentage (%)
78-A	16,334	4,662	20,996	62.04
78-B	5,964	1,933	7,897	23.33
78-C	3,898	1,052	4,950	14.63
Total	26,196	7,647	33,843	100.00

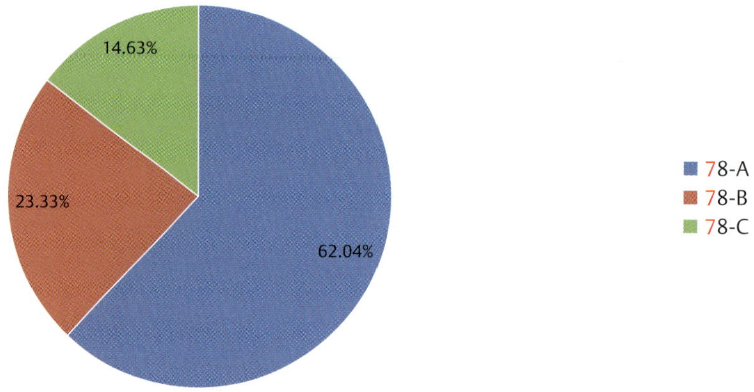

a

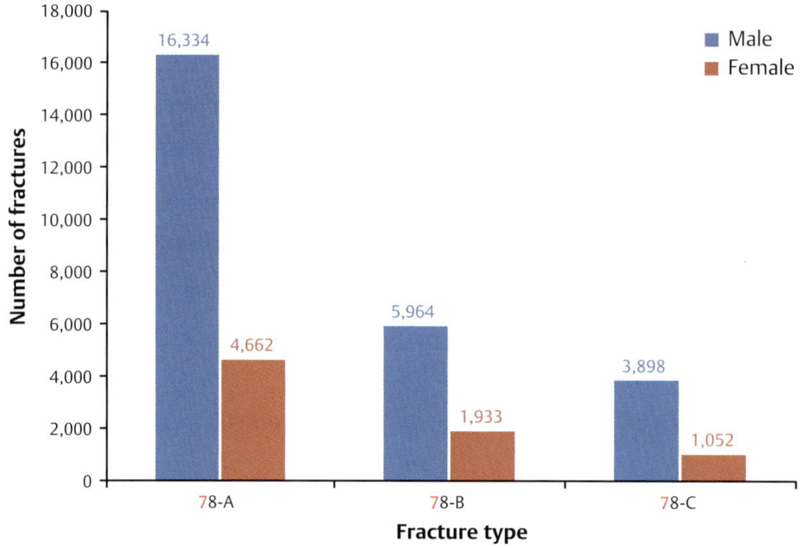

b

Fig. 8.24 **(a)** Fracture type distribution of 33,843 fractures of the phalanx (segment 78). **(b)** Sex and fracture type distribution of 33,843 fractures of the phalanx (78).

Table 8.25 Sex and fracture group distribution of 33,843 fractures of the phalanx (segment 78)

Fracture group	Male	Female	Number of fractures	Percentage (%)
78-A1	2,733	826	3,559	10.52
78-A2	4,567	1,250	5,817	17.19
78-A3	9,034	2,586	11,620	34.34
78-B1	2,797	1,103	3,900	11.52
78-B2	1,278	283	1,561	4.61
78-B3	1,889	547	2,436	7.20
78-C1	1,114	306	1,420	4.20
78-C2	1,899	523	2,422	7.16
78-C3	885	223	1,108	3.27
Total	26,196	7,647	33,843	100.00

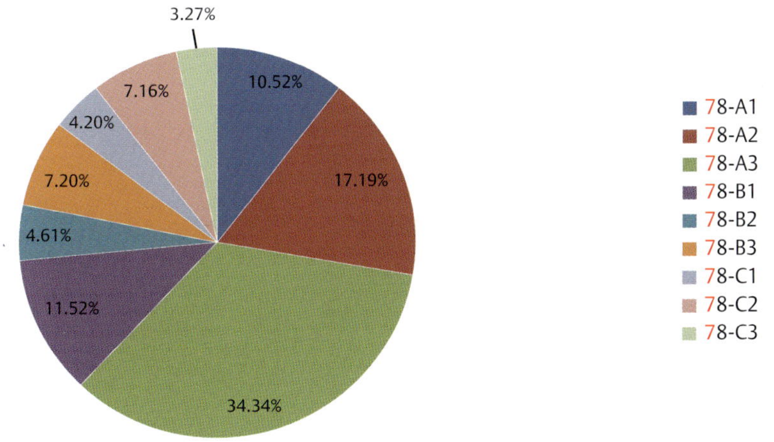

a

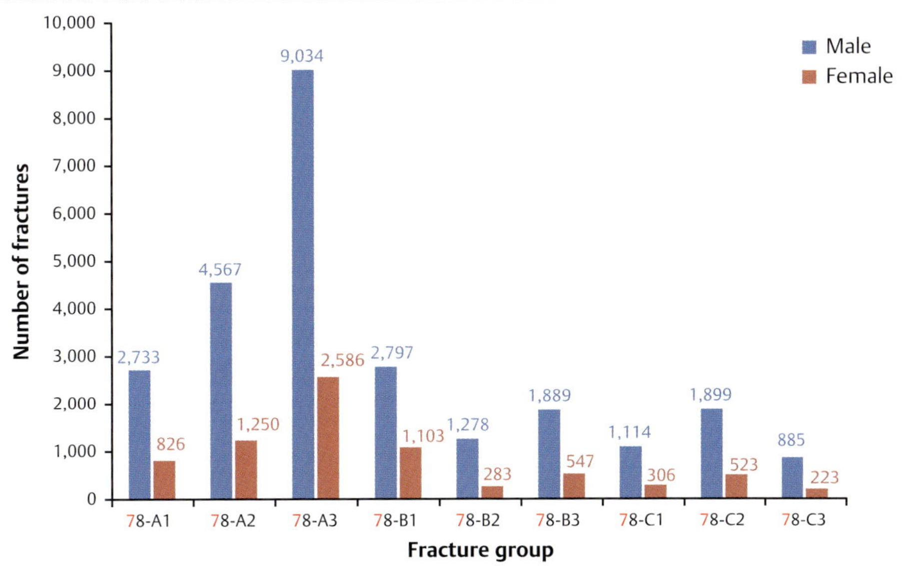

b

Fig. 8.25 **(a)** Fracture group distribution of 33,843 fractures of the phalanx (segment 78).
(b) Sex and fracture group distribution of 33,843 fractures of the phalanx (segment 78).

Phalanx Fractures by Individual Finger

Table 8.26 Sex distribution of 33,843 phalanx fractures by individual finger

Finger	Male	Female	Number of fractures	Percentage (%)	Percentage of hand fractures (%)
Thumb	5,203	1,330	6,533	19.30	11.10
Index	6,498	1,945	8,443	24.95	14.35
Middle	5,200	1,625	6,825	20.17	11.60
Ring	4,522	1,431	5,953	17.59	10.12
Little	4,773	1,316	6,089	17.99	10.35
Total	26,196	7,647	33,843	100.00	57.51

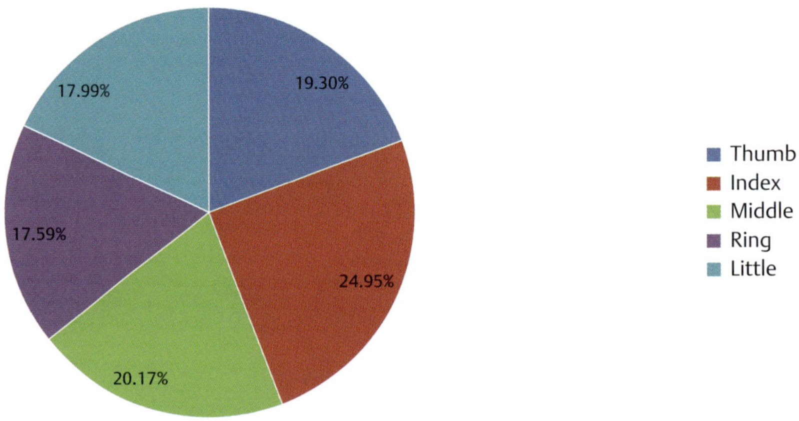

a

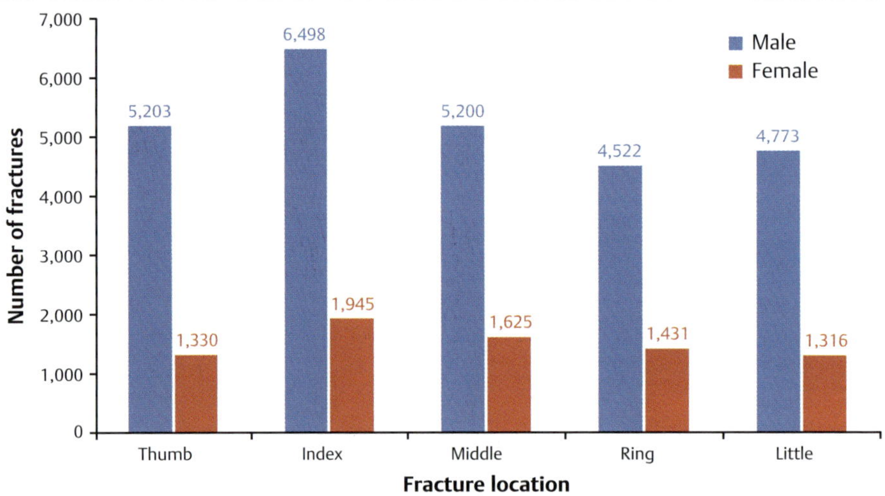

b

Fig. 8.26 **(a)** Distribution of 33,843 phalanx fractures by individual finger.
(b) Sex distribution of 33,843 phalanx fractures by individual finger.

78-A Phalanx proximal and distal extra-articular and diaphysis noncomminuted

78-A1
Proximal extra-articular
3,559 fractures
M: 2,733 (76.79%)
F: 826 (23.21%)
0.95% of total adult fractures
6.05% of adult hand fractures
10.52% of adult phalanx fractures
16.95% of type 78-A fractures

78-A1.1

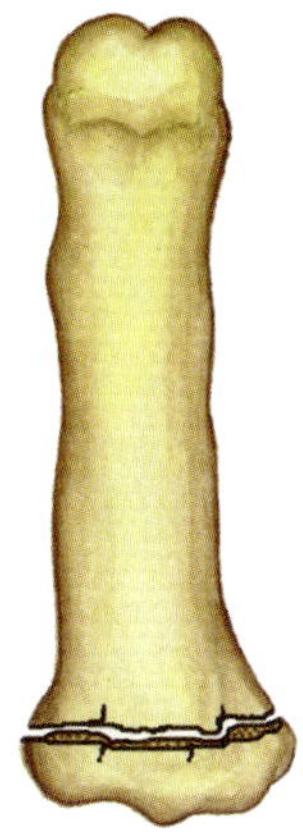

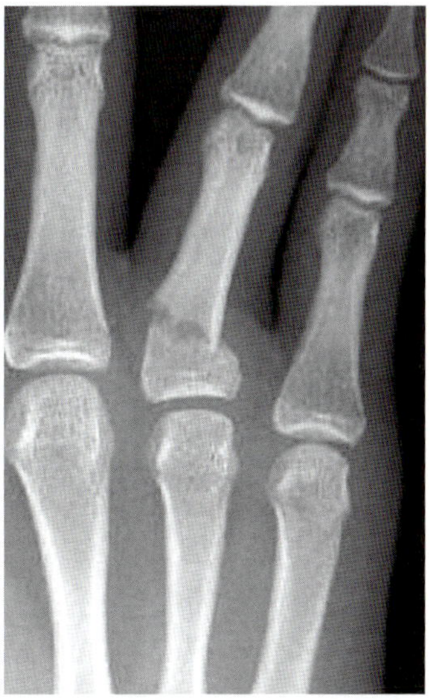

Extra-articular, simple

78-A1.2

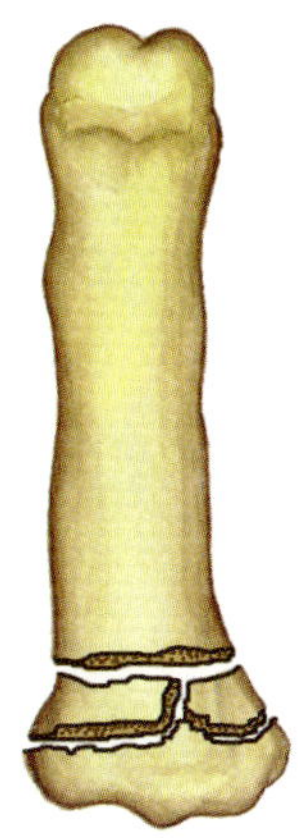

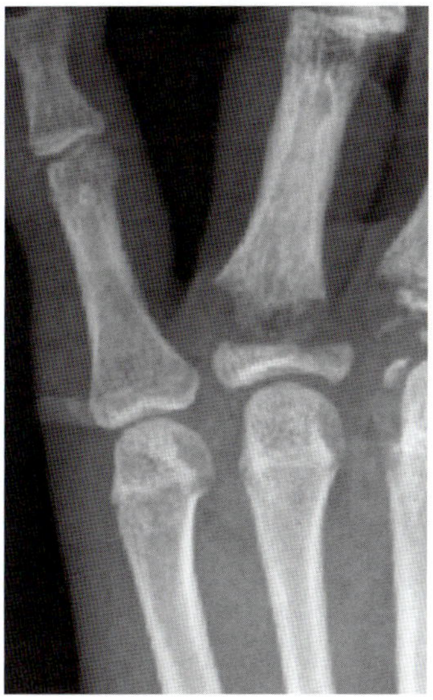

Extra-articular, comminuted

78-A Phalanx proximal and distal extra-articular and diaphysis noncomminuted

78-A2
Diaphysis noncomminuted
5,817 fractures
M: 4,567 (78.51%)
F: 1,250 (21.49%)
1.55% of total adult fractures
9.88% of adult hand fractures
17.19% of adult phalanx fractures
27.71% of type 78-A fractures

78-A2.1

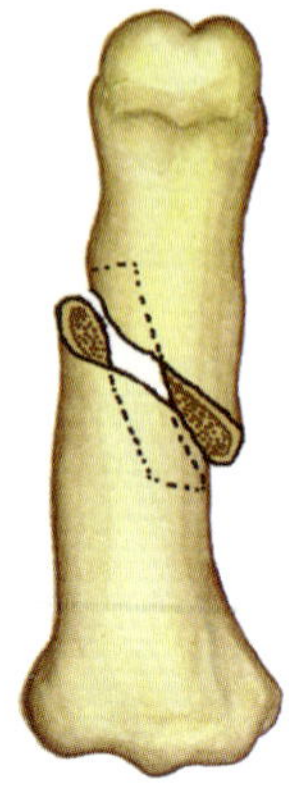

Spiral

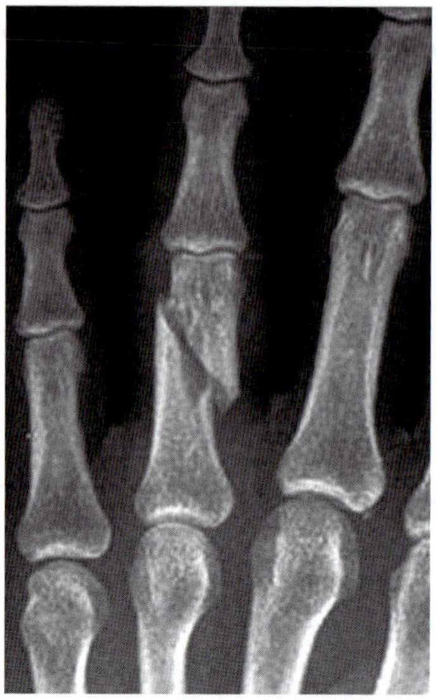

78-A2.2

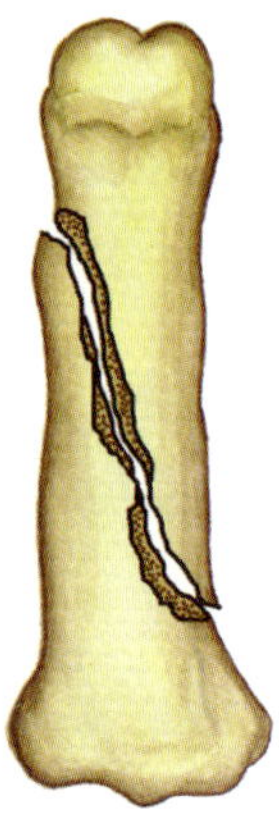

Oblique

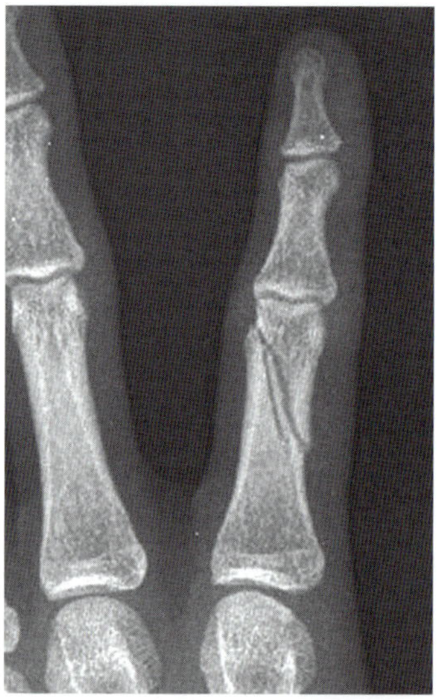

78-A2.3

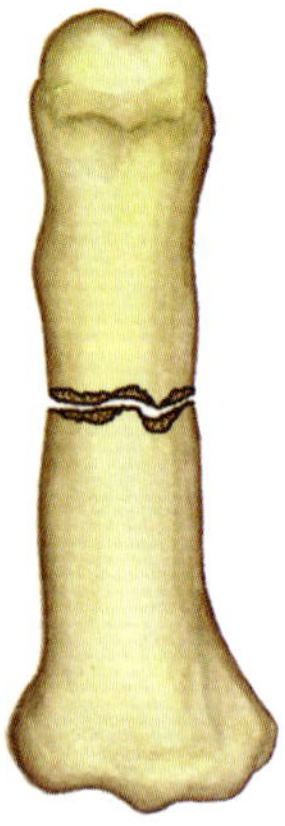

Transverse

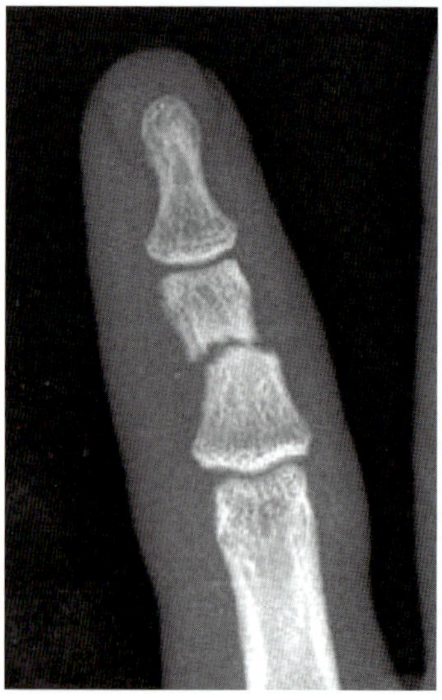

78-A Phalanx proximal and distal extra-articular and diaphysis noncomminuted	
78-A3 **Distal extra-articular** 11,620 fractures M: 9,034 (77.75%) F: 2,586 (22.25%) 3.10% of total adult fractures 19.75% of adult hand fractures 34.34% of adult phalanx fractures 55.34% of type 78-A fractures	**78-A3.1** 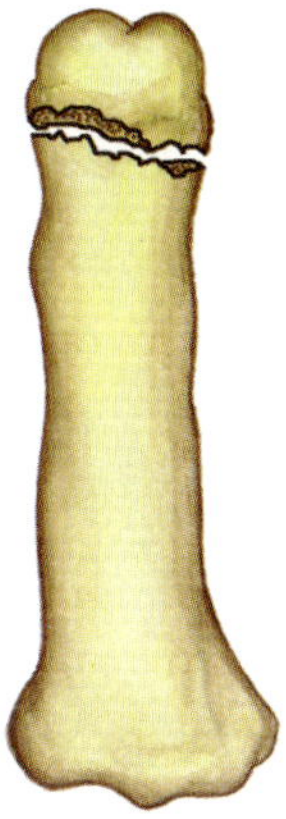 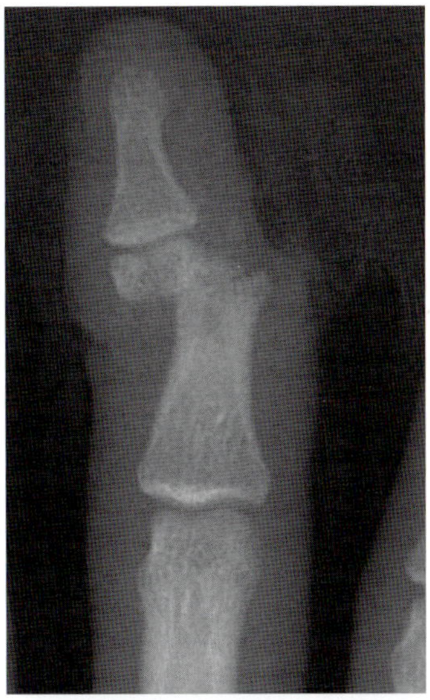 Spiral, simple **78-A3.2** 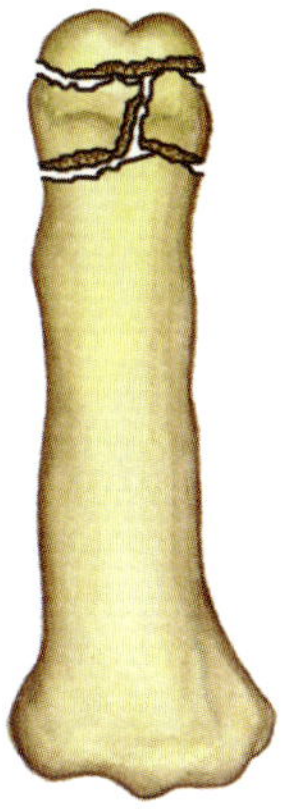 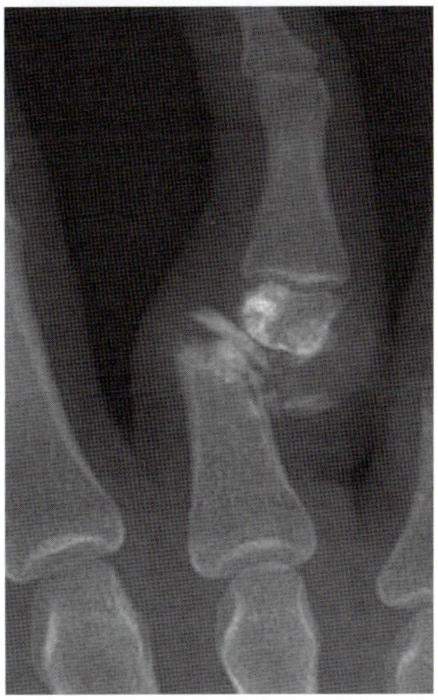 Comminuted

78-B Phalanx proximal and distal partial articular and diaphysis wedge comminution

78-B1
Proximal partial articular
3,900 fractures
M: 2,797 (71.72%)
F: 1,103 (28.28%)
1.04% of total adult fractures
6.63% of adult hand fractures
11.52% of adult phalanx fractures
49.39% of type 78-B fractures

78-B1.1

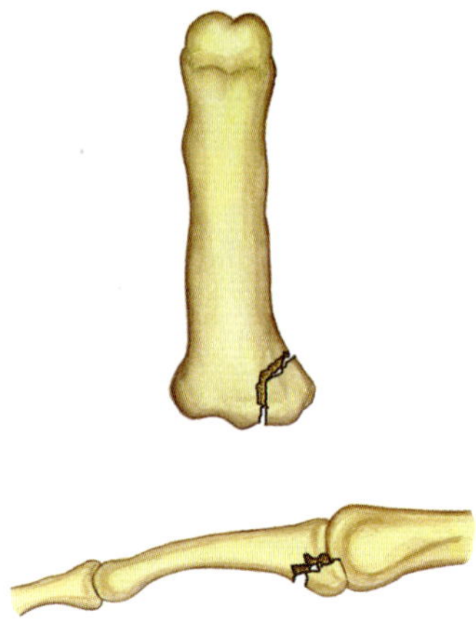

Avulsion or split

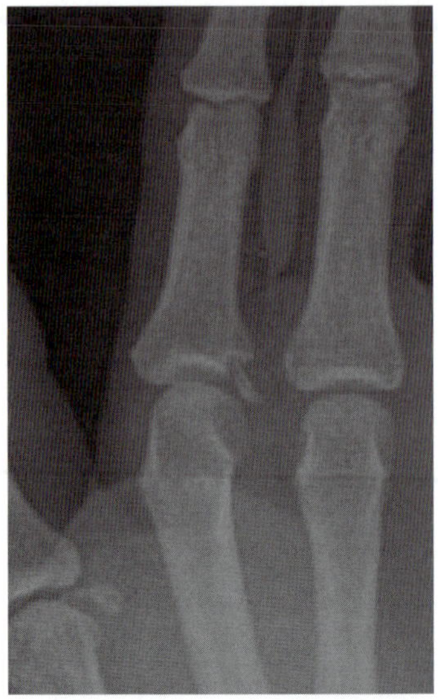

78-B1.2

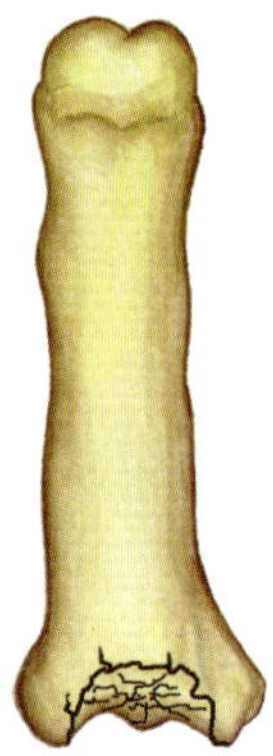

Depression

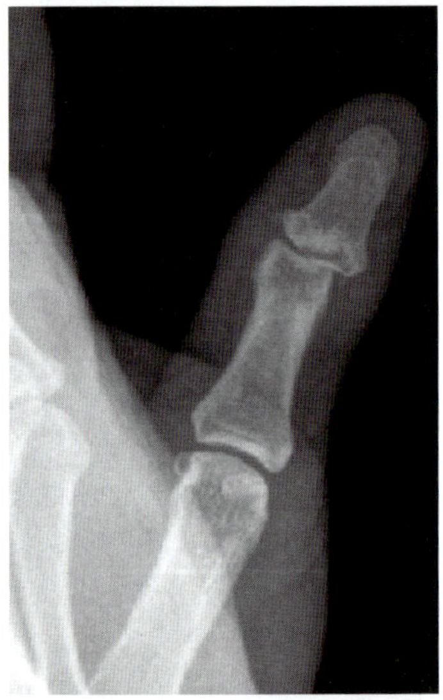

78-B1.3

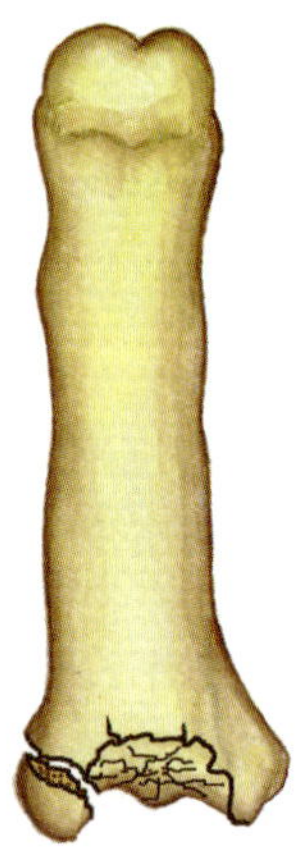

Split/depression

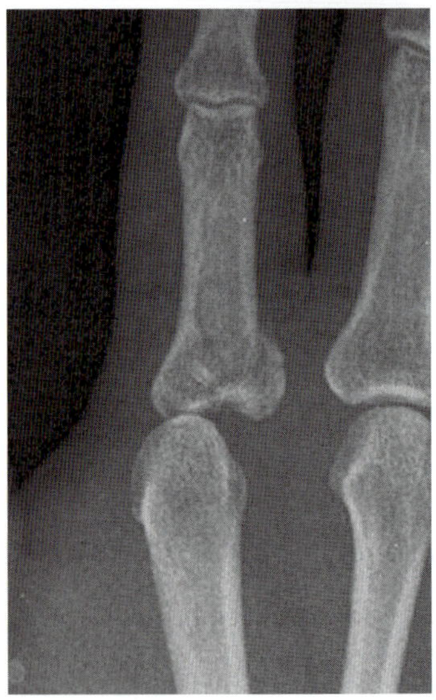

78-B Phalanx proximal and distal partial articular and diaphysis wedge comminution

78-B2
Diaphysis wedge
1,561 fractures
M: 1,278 (81.87%)
F: 283 (18.13%)
0.42% of total adult fractures
2.65% of adult hand fractures
4.61% of adult phalanx fractures
19.77% of type 78-B fractures

78-B2.1

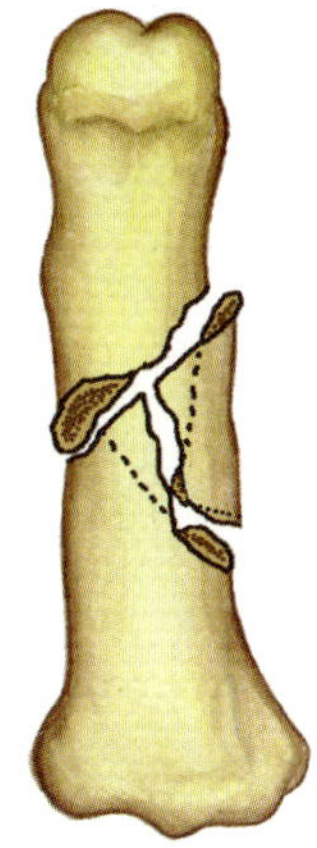

Spiral

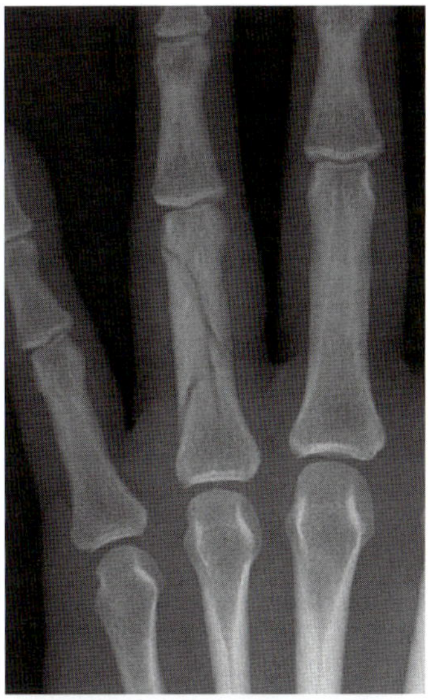

78-B2.2

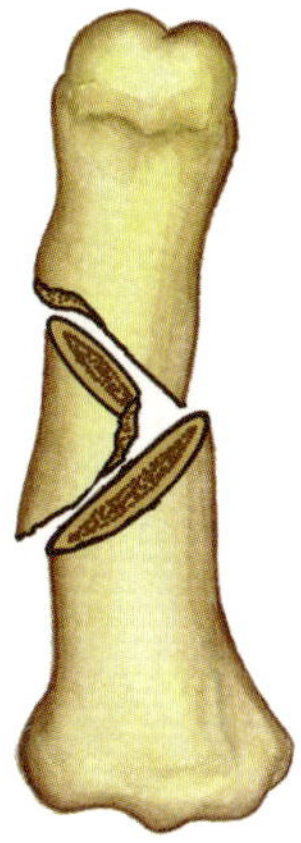

Bending

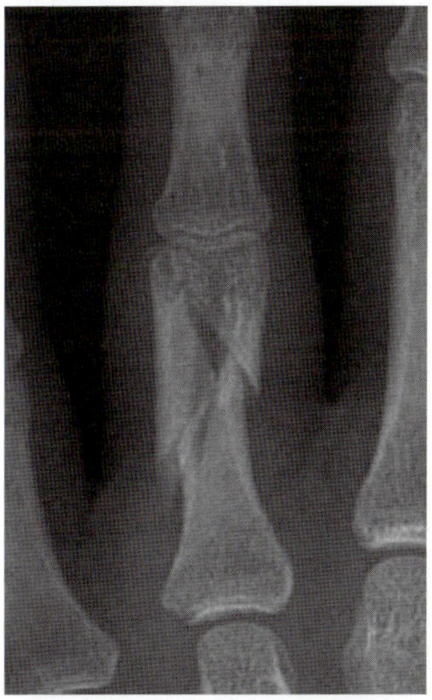

78-B2.3

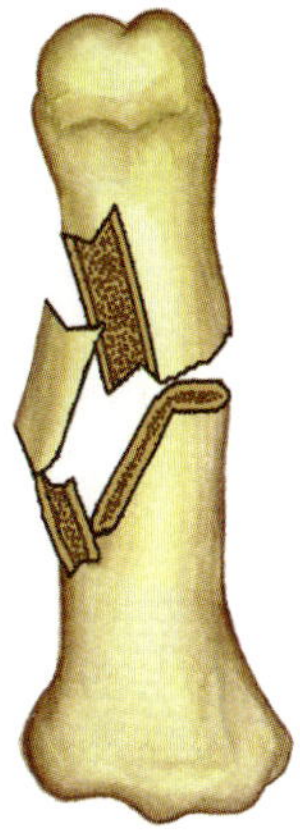

Fragmented

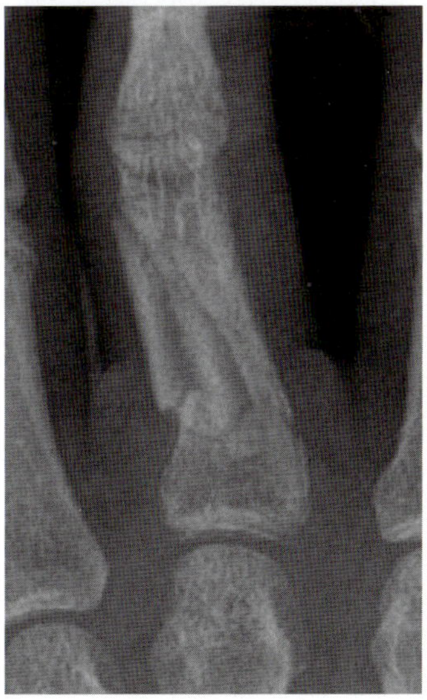

78-B Phalanx proximal and distal partial articular and diaphysis wedge comminution

78-B3
Distal partial articular
2,436 fractures
M: 1,889 (77.55%)
F: 547 (22.45%)
0.65% of total adult fractures
4.14% of adult hand fractures
7.20% of adult phalanx fractures
30.85% of type 78-B fractures

78-B3.1

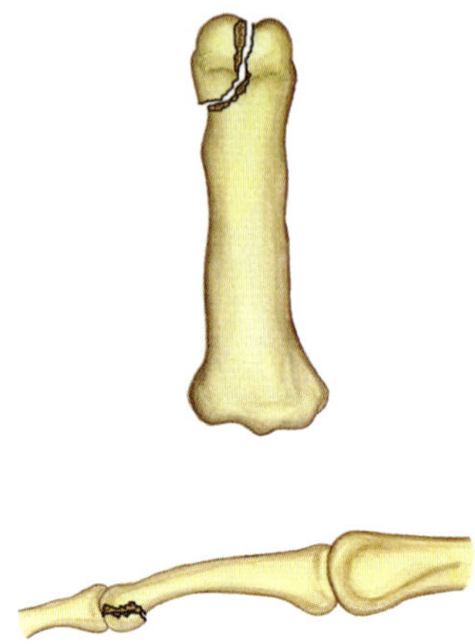

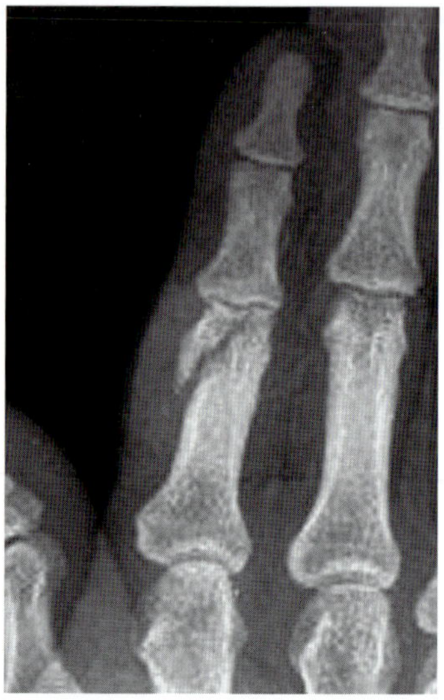

Avulsion or split

78-B3.2

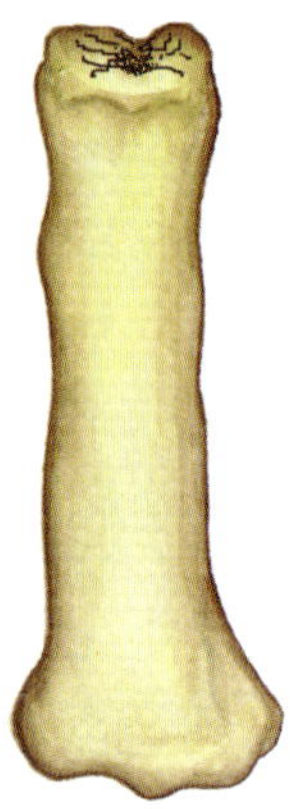

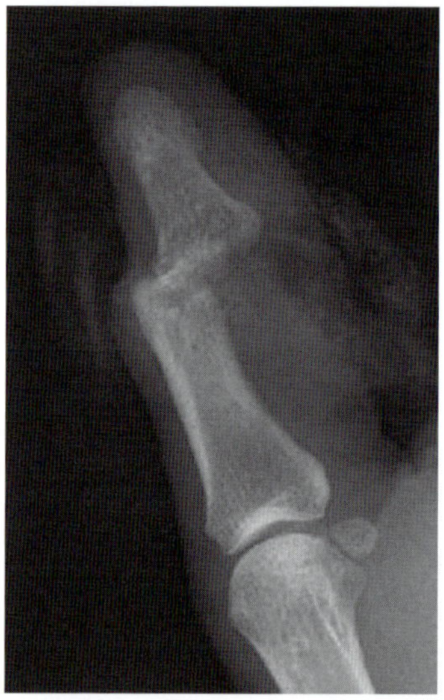

Depression

78-B3.3

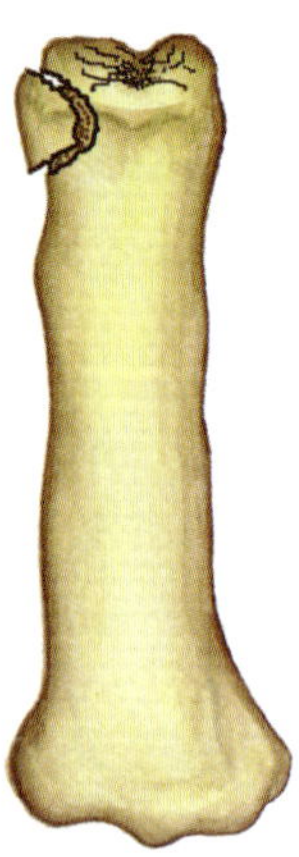

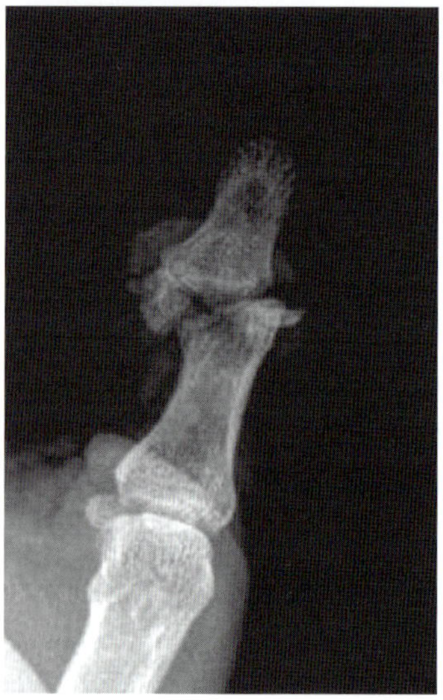

Split/depression

78-C Phalanx proximal and distal complete articular and diaphysis comminuted

78-C1
Proximal complete articular

1,420 fractures
M: 1,114 (78.45%)
F: 306 (21.55%)
0.38% of total adult fractures
2.41%of adult hand fractures
4.20% of adult phalanx fractures
28.69% of type 78-C fractures

78-C1.1

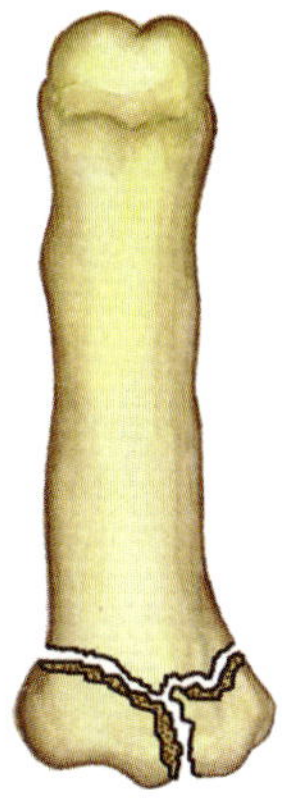

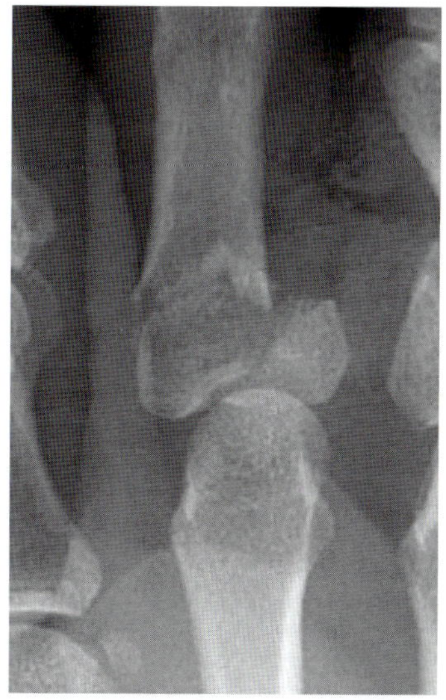

Noncomminuted articular metaphysis

78-C1.2

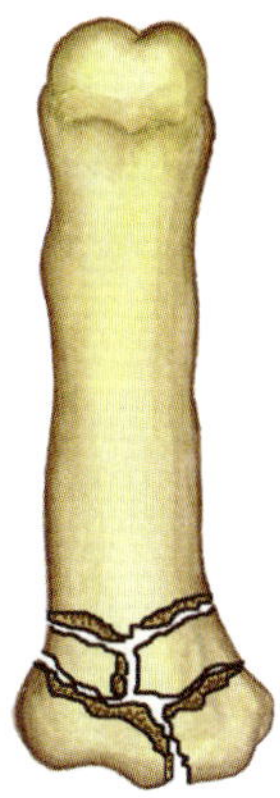

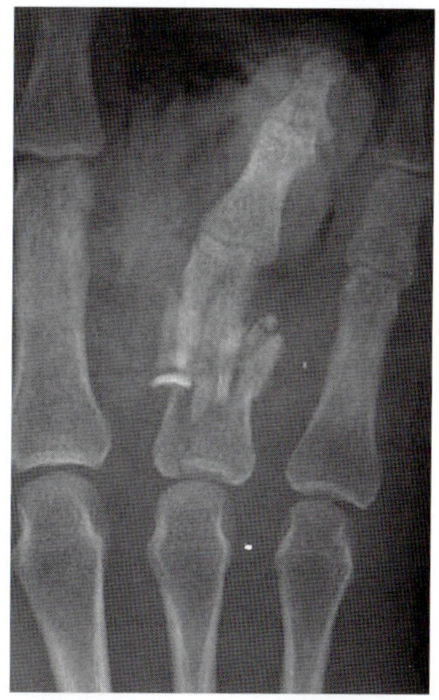

Noncomminuted articular/
comminuted metaphysis

78-C1.3

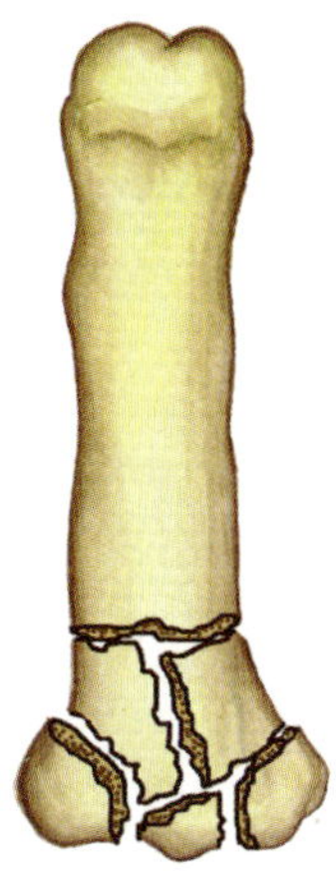

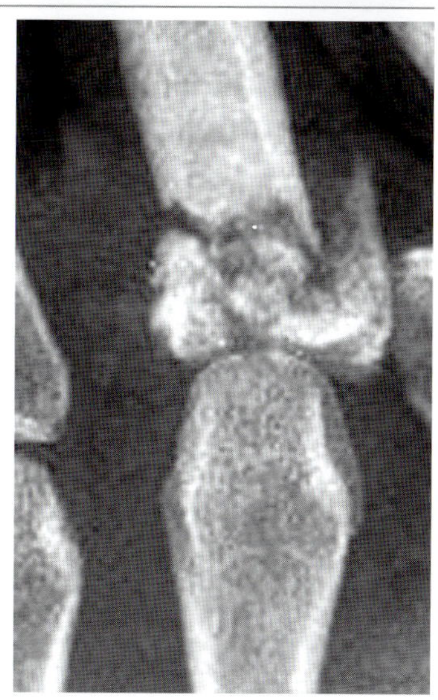

Comminuted articular and metaphysis

78-C Phalanx proximal and distal complete articular and diaphysis comminuted

78-C2
Diaphysis comminuted
2,422 fractures
M: 1,899 (78.41%)
F: 523 (21.59%)
0.65% of total adult fractures
4.12% of adult hand fractures
7.16% of adult phalanx fractures
48.93% of type 78-C fractures

78-C2.1

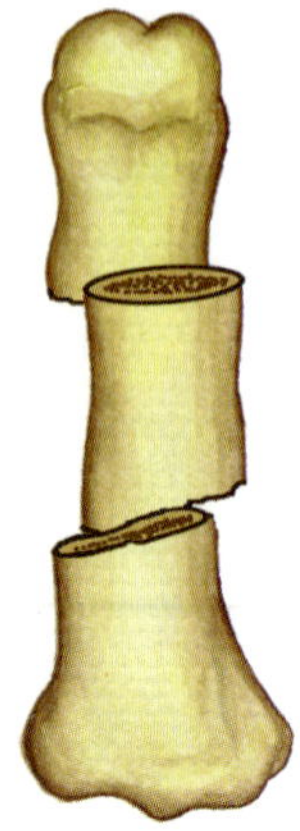

Segmental

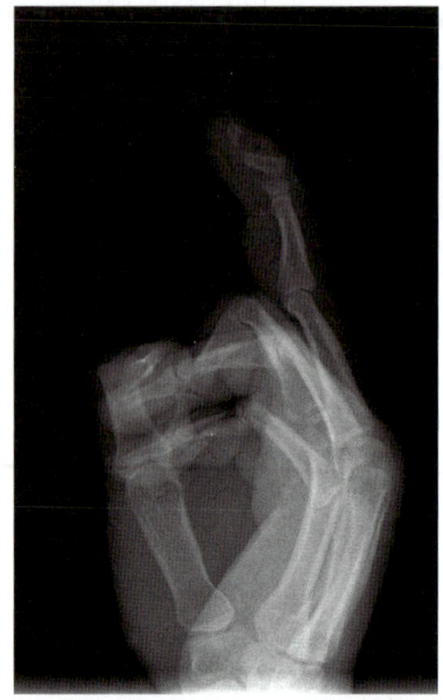

78-C2.2

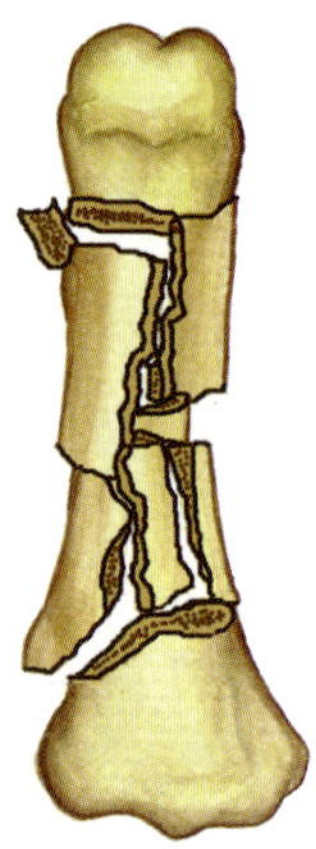

Complex comminuted

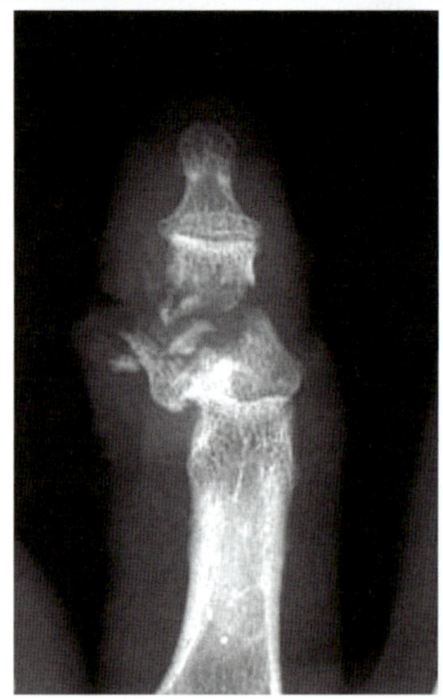

78-C Phalanx proximal and distal complete articular and diaphysis comminuted

78-C3
Distal articular
1,108 fractures
M: 885 (79.87%)
F: 223 (20.13%)
0.30% of total adult fractures
1.88% of adult hand fractures
3.27% of adult phalanx fractures
22.38% of type 78-C fractures

78-C3.1

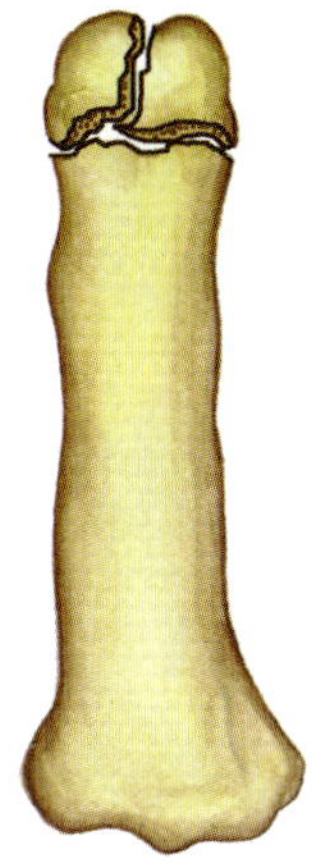

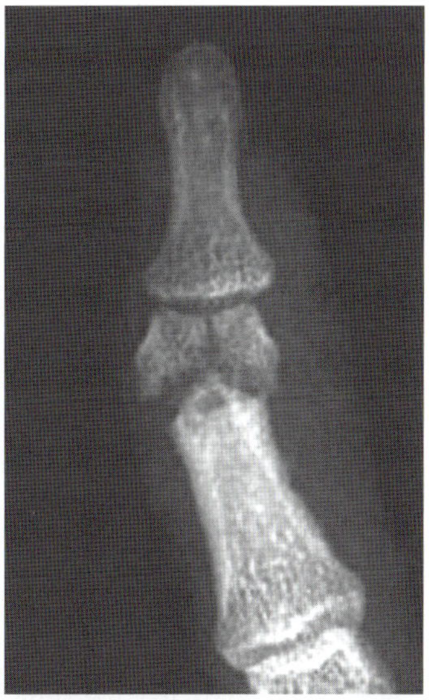

Noncomminuted articular/metaphysis

78-C3.2

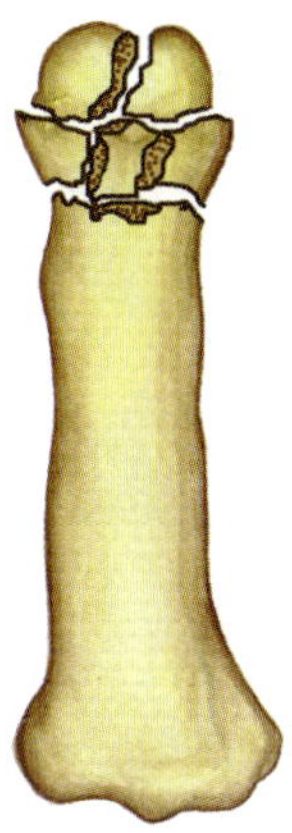

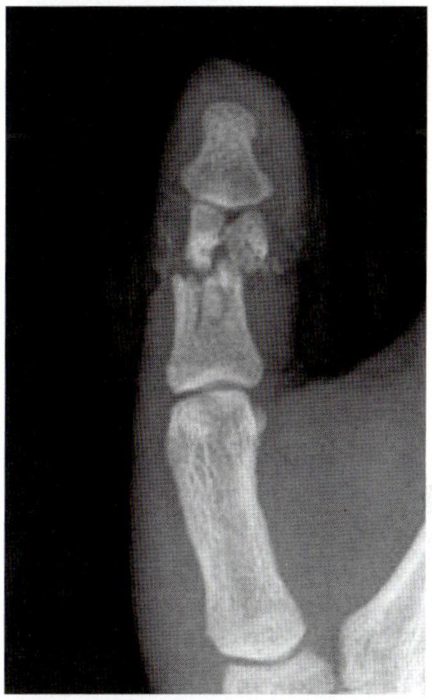

Noncomminuted articular/comminuted metaphysis

78-C3.3

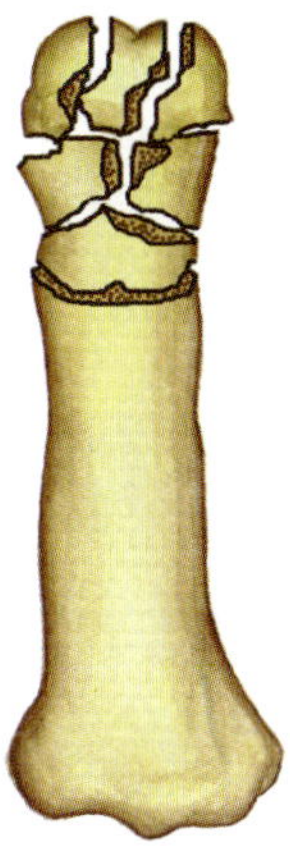

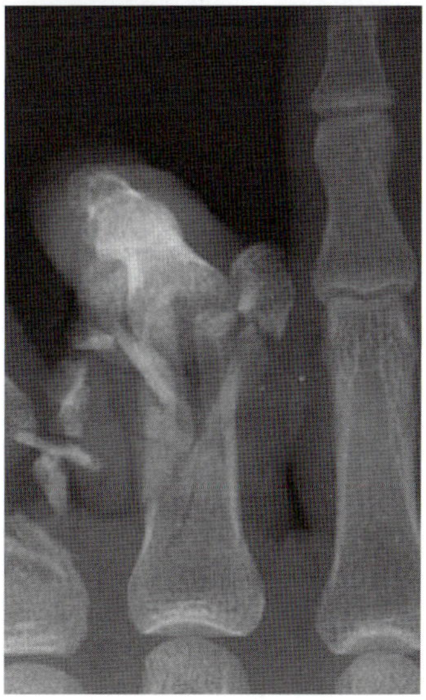

Comminuted articular

Injury Mechanism

This type of injury typically results in dorsal angulation (apex volar) because of the palmar force of the intrinsic muscles on the proximal fragment and the dorsal force of the extensor mechanism on the distal fragment. Middle phalanx base fractures result in dorsal or volar angulation in relation to the insertion of the flexor digitorum superficialis. Fractures that are proximal to the phalanx tendon result in dorsal angulation, while distal fractures result in volar angulation from deforming muscle forces. Most distal phalangeal fractures are results of perpendicular force, as in injuries from a car door, a hammer, or in contact sports. Fractures are often transverse or comminuted.

Diagnosis

Diagnosis is usually not difficult, with a clear history of trauma and a thorough clinical examination. Common indications of fracture include pain, swelling, and abnormality of motion, as well as apparent deformities. AP and lateral view radiographs of the hand help confirm the diagnosis.

Treatment

Among the three types of phalanges, fractures of the proximal phalanx have the greatest impact on the function and configuration of the finger, while fractures of the distal phalanx have the least impact.

Nondisplaced proximal phalangeal fractures are treated with small splinting for 4–6 weeks, followed by motion exercise. For irreducible and unstable fractures (oblique or spiral), open reduction and internal fixation with microplating or K-wire should be considered.

Distal phalangeal fractures are often unicondylar or bicondylar fractures. Isolated nondisplaced unicondylar or bicondylar fractures can be immobilized with the adjacent finger, which acts as a splint. Open reduction using K-wire fixation or microplating should be implemented for displaced condylar fractures after failed attempts at closed reduction.

Proximal phalangeal fractures are difficult to reduce, and open reduction using K-wire or microplating is required.

Multiple Fractures (Segment 79)

OTA Classification of Multiple Fractures of the Hand

The OTA classified multiple fractures of the hand into three types: 79-A, multiple fractures of the carpals; 79-B, multiple fractures of the metacarpals; and 79-C, multiple fractures of the phalanges.

Clinical Epidemiologic Features of Multiple Fractures (Segment 79)

A total of 11,504 adult patients with 11,797 multiple fractures of the hand were treated in 83 hospitals in China over a 2-year period from 2010 to 2011. All cases were reviewed and statistically studied, and accounted for 19.93% of all adult patients with hand fractures and 20.05% of all hand fractures in adults. Their epidemiologic features are as follows:

- More males than females
- There are two high-risk age groups. One is 21–25 years, the same age group for males. The other is 41–45 years, the same age group for females.
- The most common multiple fracture is Type 79-C—the same fracture type for both males and females.

Multiple Fractured Patients by Sex

Table 8.27 Sex distribution of 11,504 patients with multiple fractures (segment 79)

Sex	Number of patients	Percentage (%)
Male	9,014	78.36
Female	2,490	21.64
Total	11,504	100.00

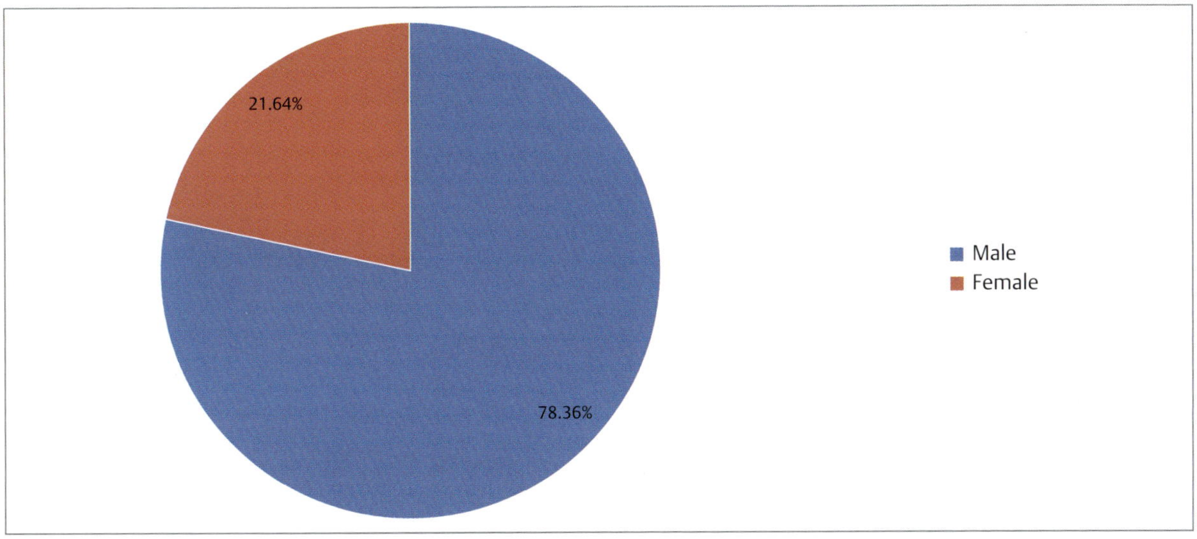

Fig. 8.27 Sex distribution of 11,504 patients with multiple fractures (segment 79).

Multiple Fractured Patients by Age Group

Table 8.28 Age and sex distribution of 11,504 patients with multiple fractures (segment 79)

Age group (years)	Male	Female	Total	Percentage (%)
16–20	999	182	1,181	10.27
21–25	1,376	208	1,584	13.77
26–30	1,134	226	1,360	11.82
31–35	968	275	1,243	10.80
36–40	1,133	405	1,538	13.37
41–45	1,117	439	1,556	13.53
46–50	862	300	1,162	10.10
51–55	569	176	745	6.48
56–60	486	111	597	5.19
61–65	188	67	255	2.22
66–70	83	40	123	1.07
71–75	65	29	94	0.82
76–80	22	22	44	0.38
81–85	10	6	16	0.14
≥86	2	4	6	0.05
Total	9,014	2,490	11,504	100.00

8

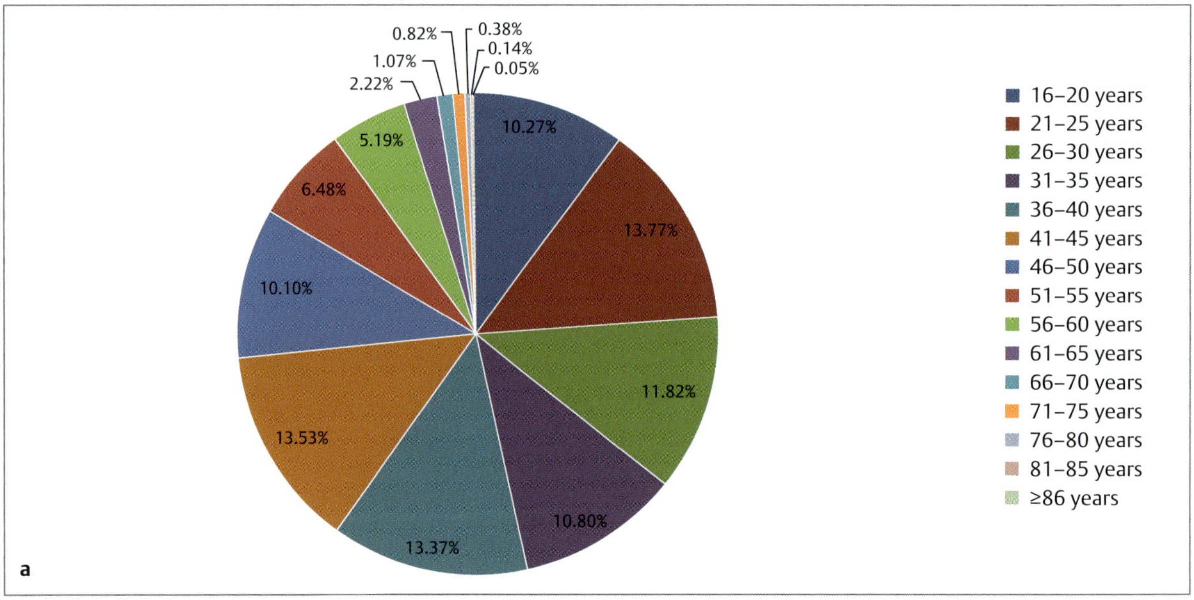

Fig. 8.28 **(a)** Age distribution of 11,504 patients with multiple fractures (segment 79).

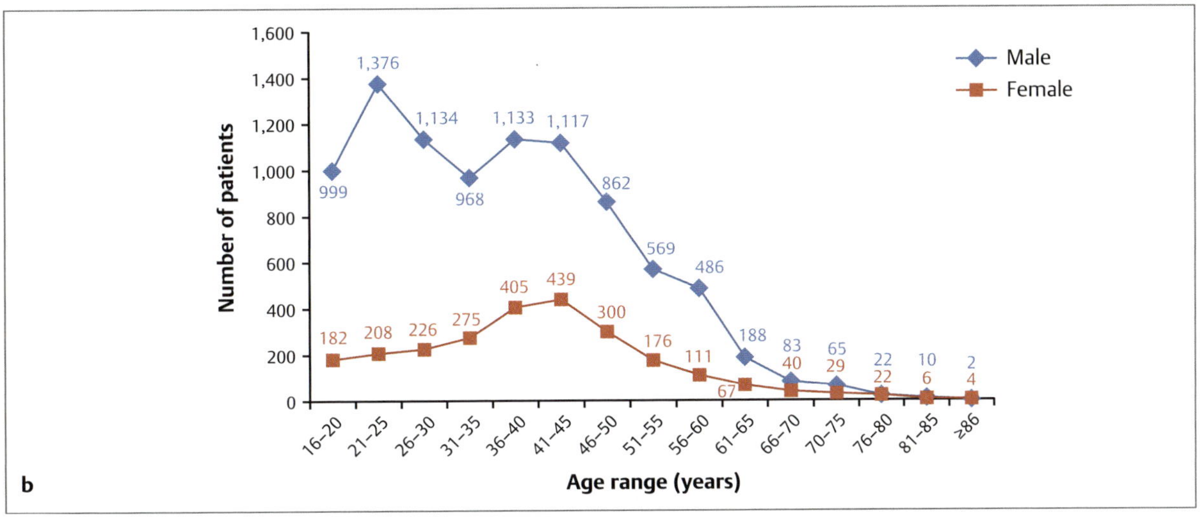

Fig. 8.28 (*continued*) **(b)** Age and sex distribution of 11,504 patients with multiple fractures (segment 79).

Multiple Fractures by Fracture Type

Table 8.29 Sex and fracture type distribution of 11,797 multiple hand fractures (segment 79)

Fracture type	Male	Female	Number of patients	Percentage (%)
79-A	278	75	353	2.99
79-B	1,939	472	2,411	20.44
79-C	7,023	2,010	9,033	76.57
Total	9,240	2,557	11,797	100.00

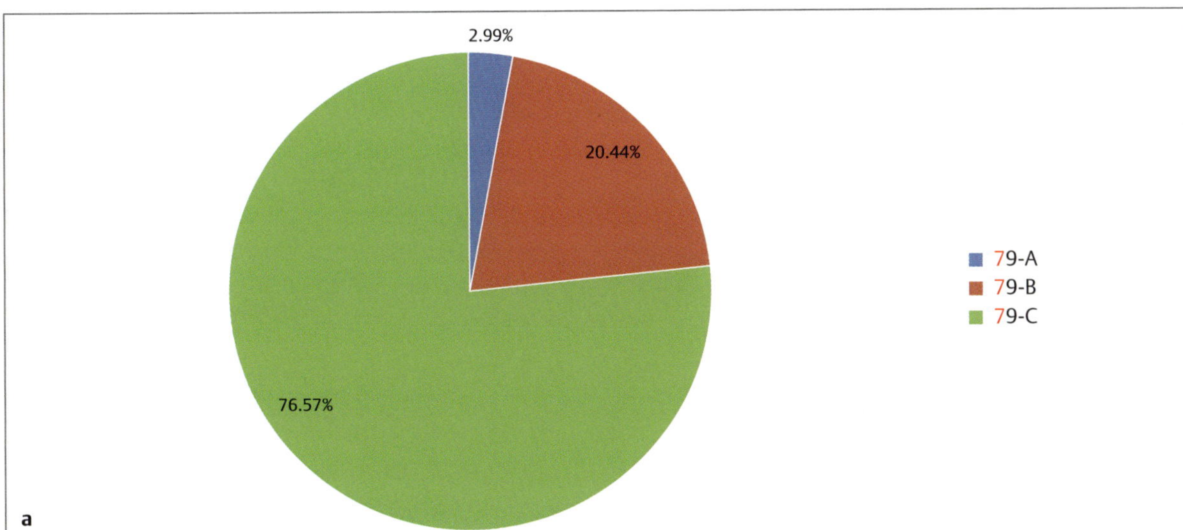

Fig. 8.29 **(a)** Fracture type distribution of 11,797 multiple hand fractures (segment 79). (*Continued*)

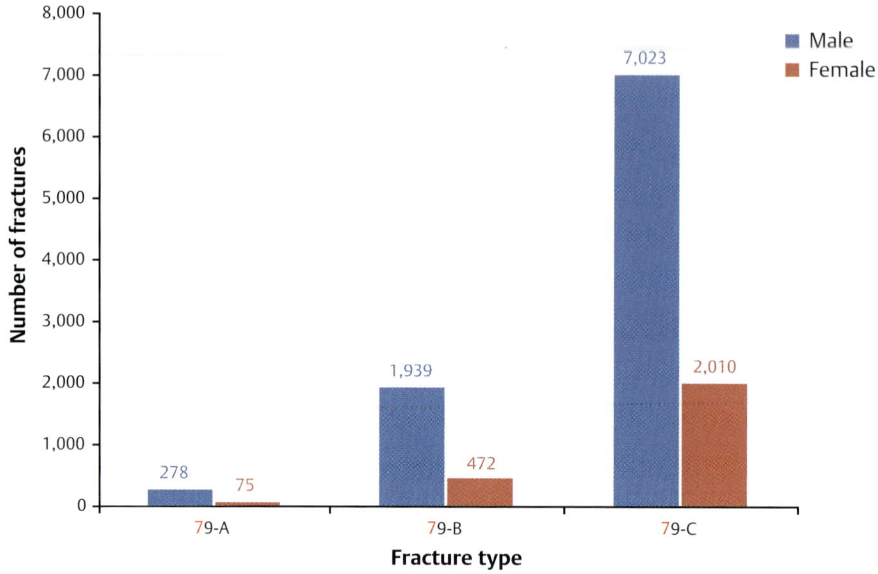

b

Fig. 8.29 (*continued*) **(b)** Sex and fracture type distribution of 11,797 multiple hand fractures (segment 79).

8

79 Multiple fractures of the hand

79-A
Multiple fractures of carpals
353 fractures
M: 278 (78.75%)
F: 75 (21.25%)
0.09% of total adult fractures
0.60% of adult hand fractures
2.99% of segment 79 fractures

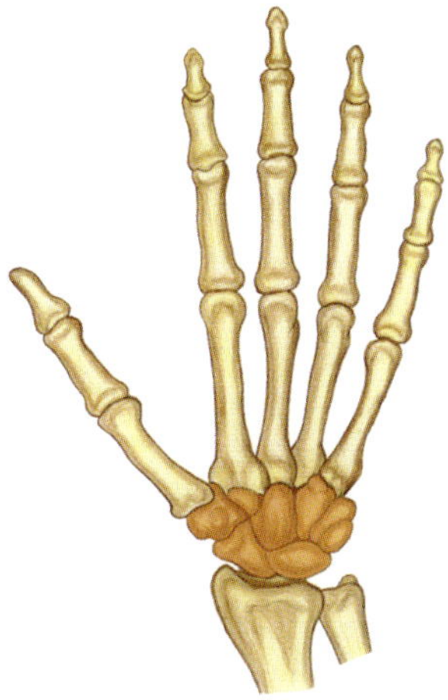

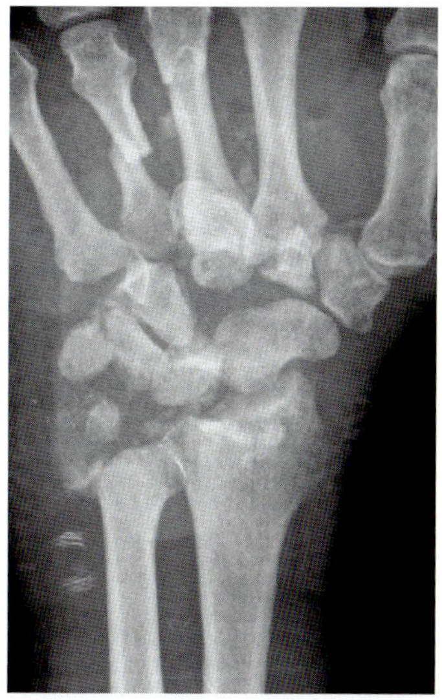

79-B
Multiple fractures of metacarpals
2,411 fractures
M: 1,939 (80.42%)
F: 472 (19.58%)
0.64% of total adult fractures
4.10% of adult hand fractures
20.44% of segment 79 fractures

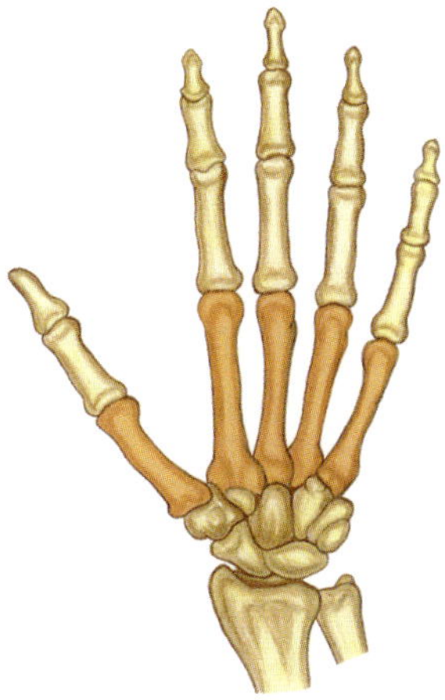

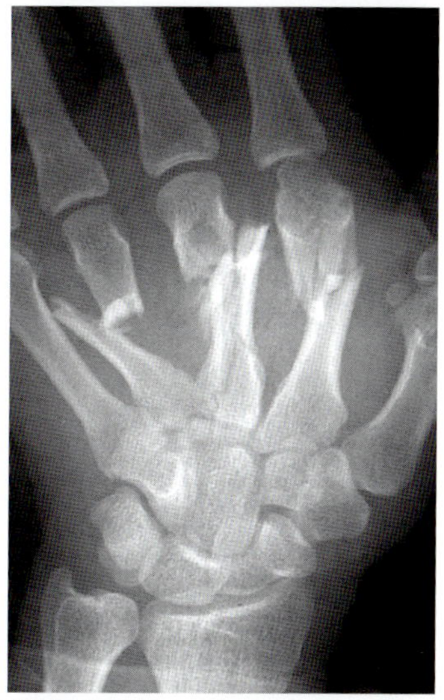

79-C
Multiple fractures of the phalanx
9,033 fractures
M: 7,023 (77.75%)
F: 2,010 (22.25%)
2.41% of total adult fractures
15.35% of adult hand fractures
76.57% of segment 79 fractures

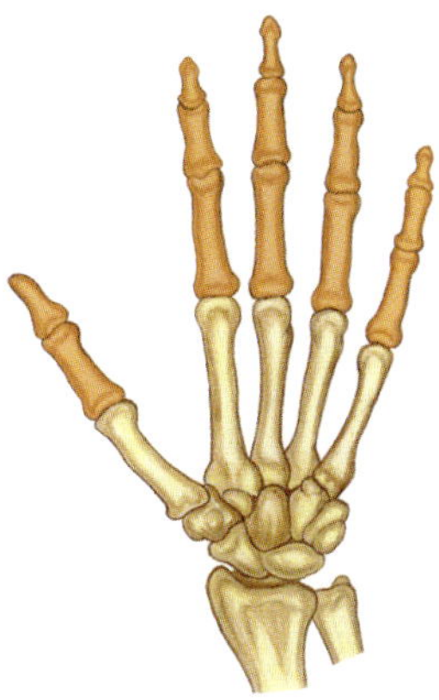

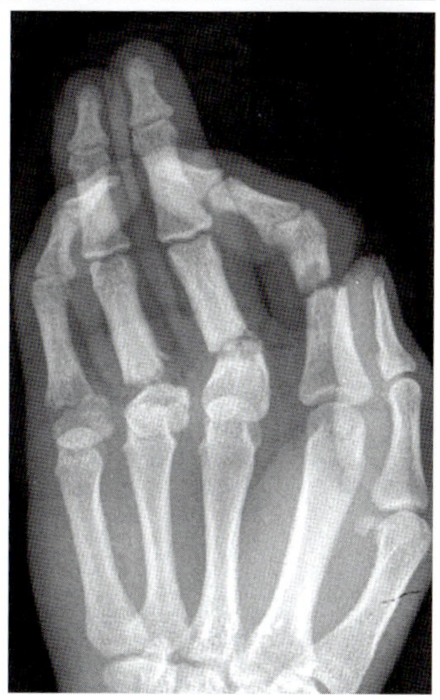

9 Fractures of the Foot

Overview

Anatomical Features

The foot is made up of a total of 26 bones of different shapes, which are supported by a network of approximately 32 muscles and tendons, 109 ligaments, and 45 articulations.

The foot is divided into three sections: the forefoot, midfoot, and hindfoot. The forefoot is composed of 5 metatarsal bones and 14 phalanges that make up the toes. The midfoot consists of five out of a total number of seven tarsal bones, including three cuneiforms, one tarsal navicular, and one cuboid bone. The hindfoot includes the calcaneus and talus bone. There are five metatarsal bones (labeled 1–5 starting at the big toe), each consisting of a shaft or body, and a base and head. The base is wedge shaped, expanding posteriorly. The head presents a convex articular surface, articulating distally with the phalangeal bones. There are 14 phalangeal bones of the foot, 3 in each toe except the big toe which has 2, and each bone consists of a base, a body, and a head (**Plate 9.1**).

OTA Classification and Coding System for Foot Fractures

According to the Orthopaedic Trauma Association (OTA) classification, a foot fracture is coded as the number 8 for its anatomical location; the talus, calcaneus, tarsal navicular, cuboid, cuneiforms, metatarsals, and phalanges are coded as the numbers 81, 82, 83, 84, 85, 87, and 88, respectively. In addition, multiple fractures of the foot are coded as the number 89. The classification varies with individual bones of the foot, due to complex anatomical features of each bone (**Plate 9.2**).

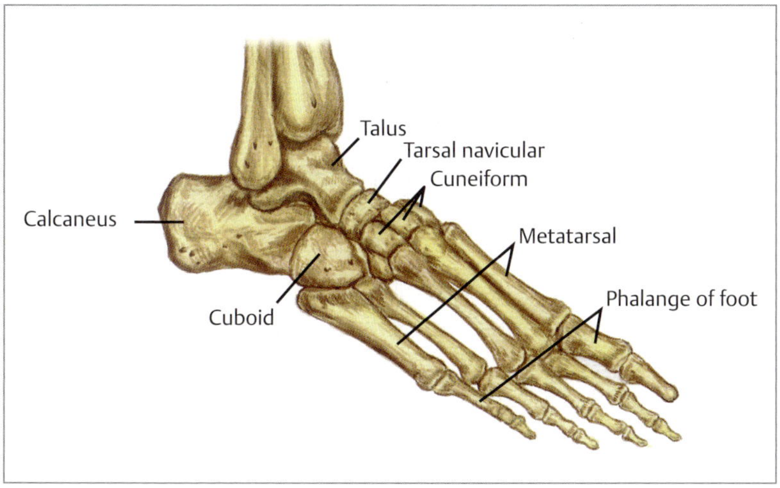

Plate 9.1

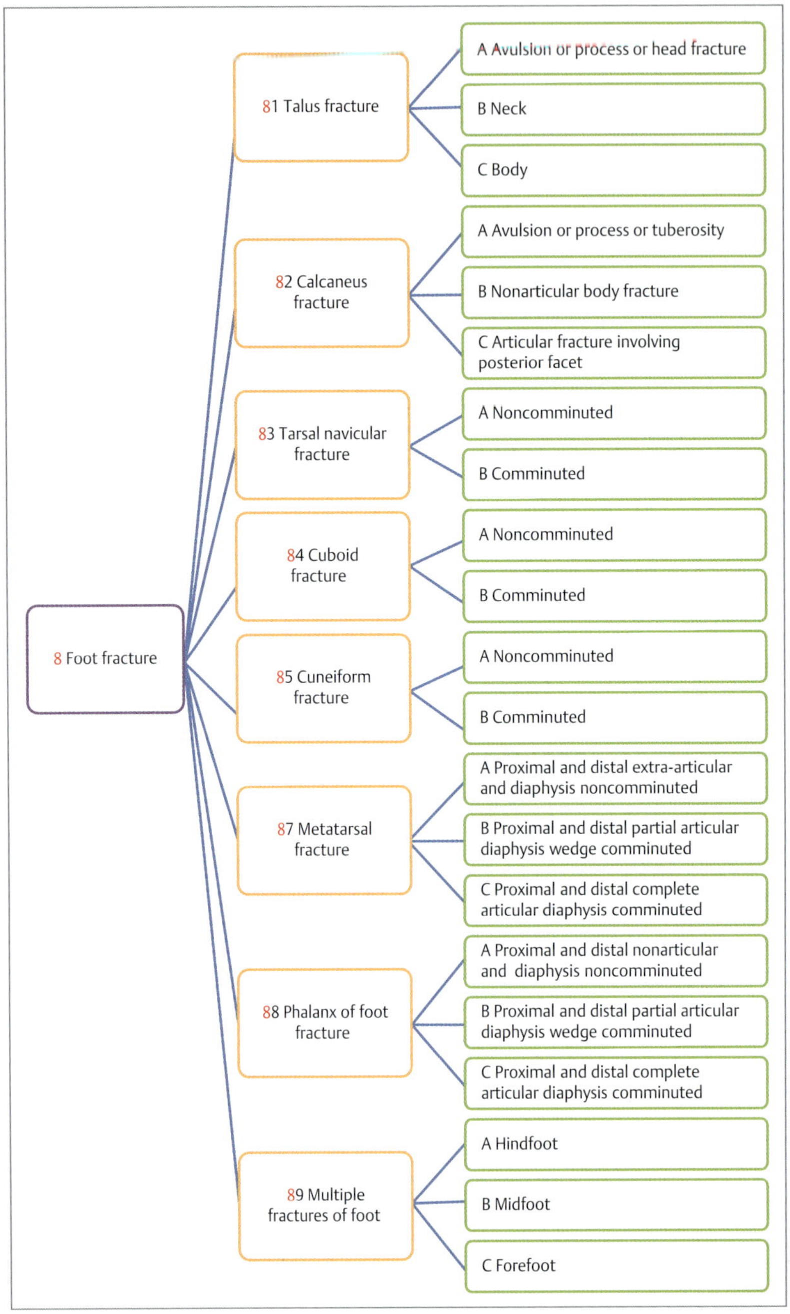

Plate 9.2

Clinical Epidemiologic Features of Foot Fractures

A total of 39,867 patients with 41,136 foot fractures were treated in 83 hospitals in China over a 2-year period from 2010 to 2011. All cases were reviewed and statistically studied; the fractures accounted for 9.61% of all patients with fractures and 9.53% of all types of fractures. Among these 39,867 patients, there were 2,466 pediatric patients (2,502 foot fractures) and 37,401 adult patients (38,634 foot fractures).

Epidemiologic features of foot fractures are as follows:

- More males than females
- Slightly more left-side than right-side fractures
- The high-risk age group is 36–40 years—the same age group for males, whereas the high-risk age group for females is 46–50 years.
- The most common foot fractures among adults are calcaneus fractures, in contrast to children, where the most common fractures are metatarsal.

Fractures of Foot by Sex

Table 9.1 Sex distribution of 39,867 patients with foot fractures

Sex	Number of patients	Percentage (%)
Male	28,385	71.20
Female	11,482	28.80
Total	39,867	100.00

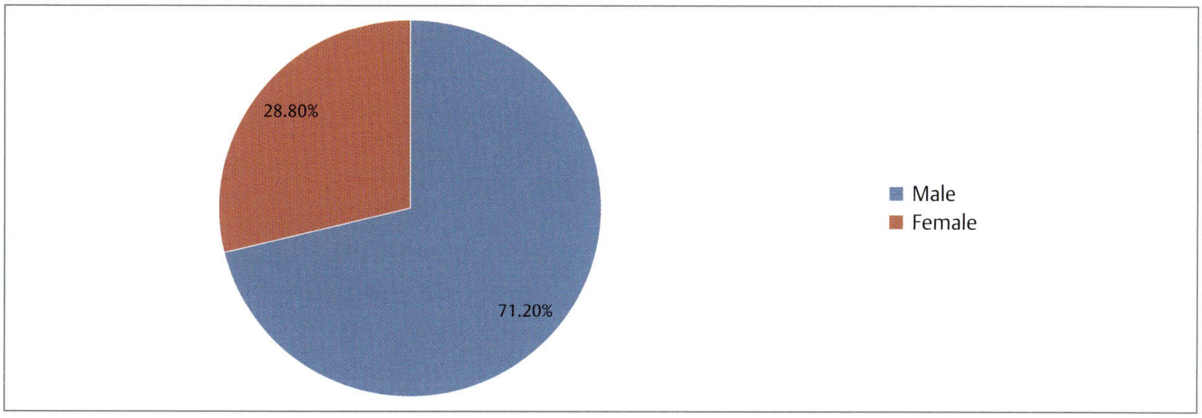

Fig. 9.1 Sex distribution of 39,867 patients with foot fractures.

Fractures of the Foot by Fracture Side

Table 9.2 Fracture side distribution of 39,867 patients with foot fractures

Fracture side	Number of patients	Percentage (%)
Left	19,331	48.49
Right	19,628	49.23
Bilateral	908	2.28
Total	39,867	100.00

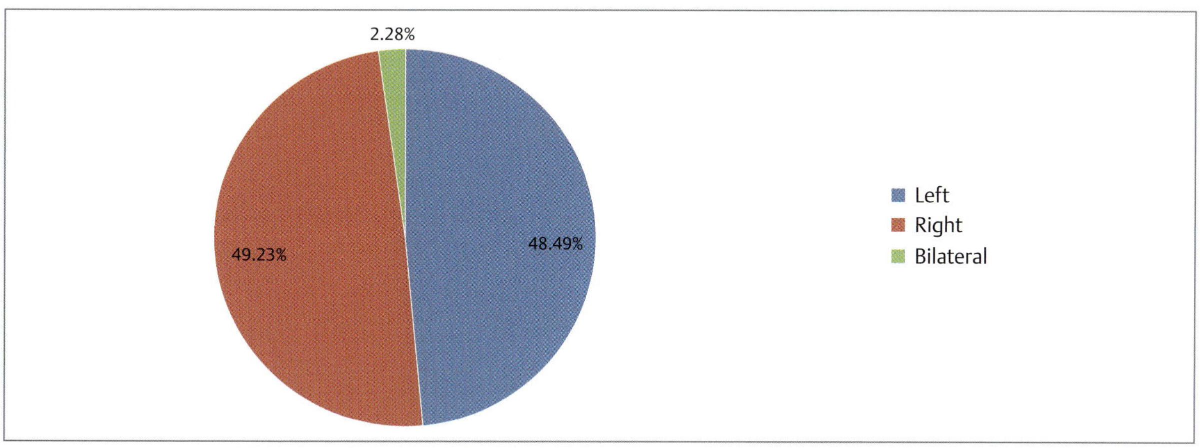

Fig. 9.2 Fracture side distribution of 39,867 patients with foot fractures.

Fractures of the Foot by Age Group

Table 9.3 Age and sex distribution of 39,867 patients with foot fractures

Age group (years)	Male	Female	Number of patients	Percentage (%)
0–5	369	193	562	1.41
6–10	460	335	795	1.99
11–15	793	316	1,109	2.78
16–20	2,006	514	2,520	6.32
21–25	2,979	878	3,857	9.67
26–30	2,997	924	3,921	9.84
31–35	2,930	835	3,765	9.44
36–40	3,904	1,104	5,008	12.56
41–45	3,647	1,176	4,823	12.10
46–50	2,998	1,268	4,266	10.70
51–55	2,079	1,116	3,195	8.01
56–60	1,548	1,131	2,679	6.72
61–65	761	648	1,409	3.53
66–70	365	434	799	2.00
71–75	244	293	537	1.35
76–80	184	193	377	0.95
81–85	83	91	174	0.44
≥86	38	33	71	0.18
Total	28,385	11,482	39,867	100.00

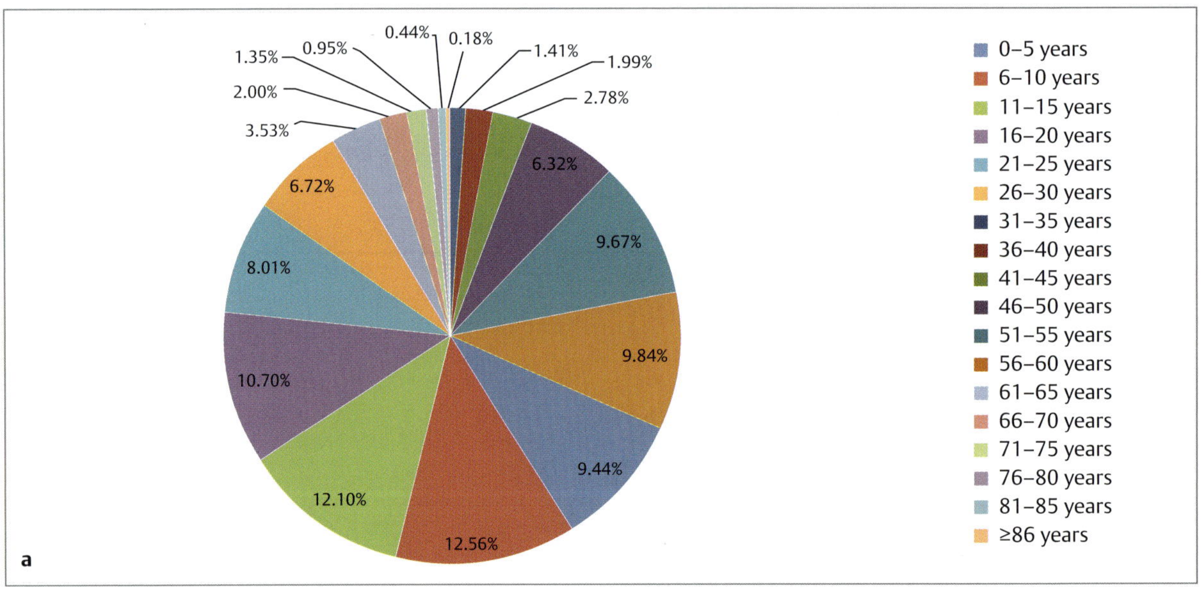

Fig. 9.3 **(a)** Age distribution of 39,867 patients with foot fractures.

9

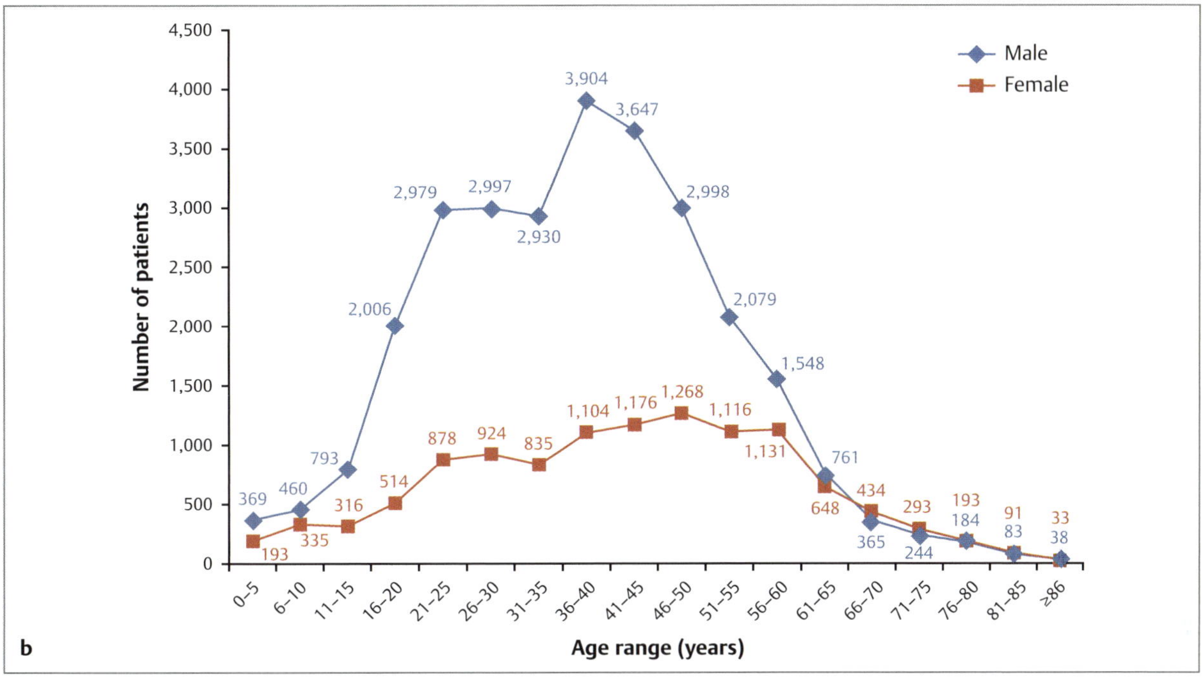

Fig. 9.3 (*continued*) **(b)** Age and sex distribution of 39,867 patients with foot fractures.

Foot Fractures in Children and Adults by Individual Foot Bone

Table 9.4 Distribution of 41,136 patients with fractures by individual foot bone in children and adults

Foot bone	Children	Adults	Number of patients	Percentage (%)
Talus	85	1,143	1,228	2.99
Calcaneus	522	11,720	12,242	29.76
Tarsal navicular	63	1,022	1,085	2.64
Cuneiform	28	532	560	1.36
Cuboid	30	552	582	1.41
Metatarsal	832	8,996	9,828	23.89
Phalanges	591	7,397	7,988	19.42
Multiple fratures	351	7,272	7,623	18.53
Total	2,502	38,634	41,136	100.00

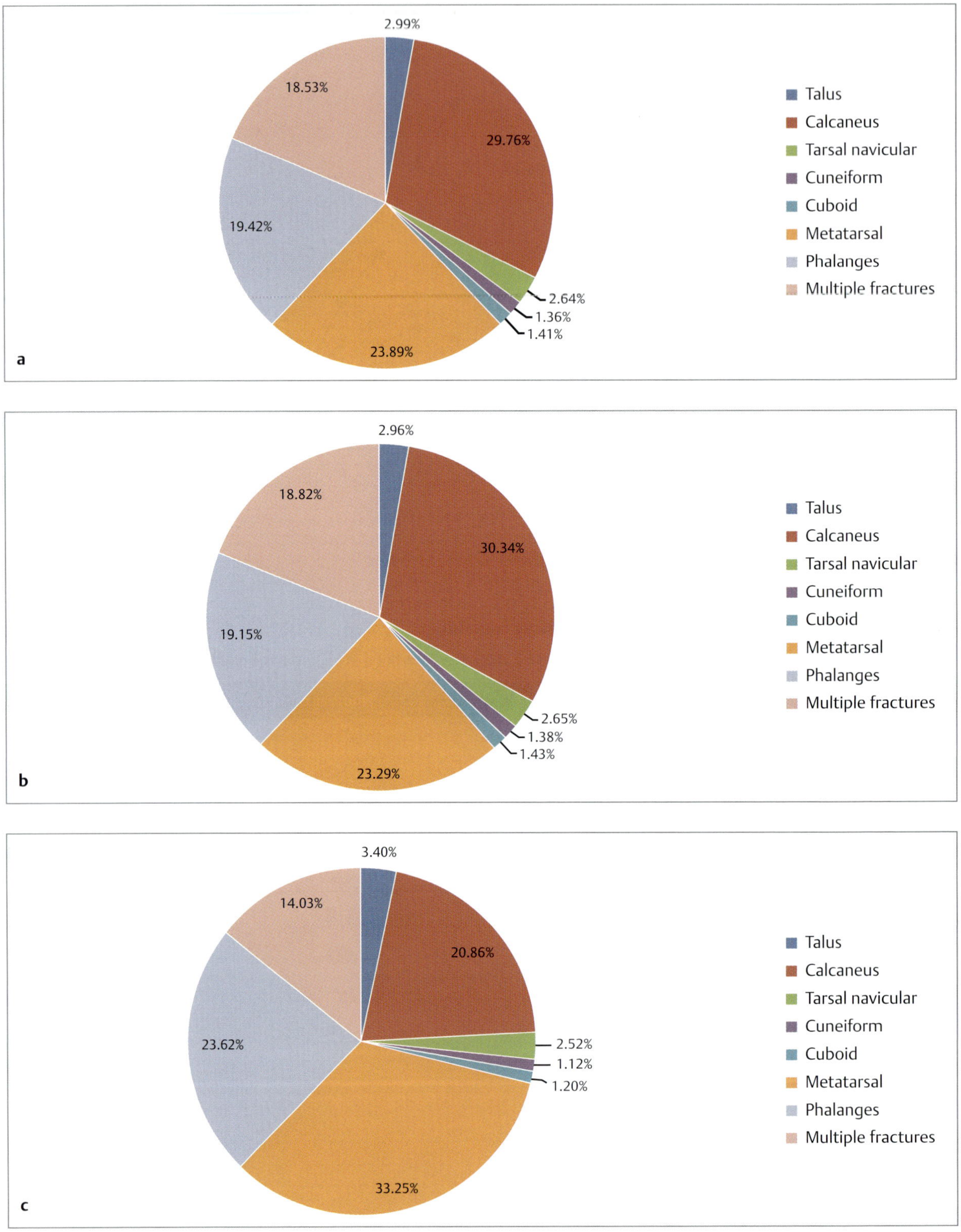

Fig. 9.4 **(a)** Distribution of 41,136 patients with foot fractures by individual foot bone.
(b) Distribution of 38,634 adult patients with foot fractures by individual foot bone.
(c) Distribution of 2,502 pediatric patients with foot fractures by individual foot bone.

Talus Fractures (Segment 81)

Anatomical Features

Examining its anatomical region, the talus bone can be subdivided into three parts: head, neck, and body. Between 60 and 70% of the talus surface is articular, forming seven articulations with adjacent bones.

The head is semicircular in form, carrying the articulate surface of the navicular bone. The neck, the constricted area between the body and head, is roughened for the attachment of the joint capsule. The irregular body is cuboid in shape, wide in the front and narrow in the back, which gives stability when the ankle is dorsiflexed. While its superior, medial, and lateral articulate surfaces join together to make up the trochlea of the talus, the posterior surface (facies articularis calcanea posterior) is separated by a furrow, the sulcus tali, which, together with the sulcus calcanei, forms a cavity, the sinus tarsi. Behind the trochlea is a posterior process with a medial and lateral tubercle separated by a groove for the flexor hallucis longus tendon. The medial and lateral tubercles give attachment to the medial talocalcaneal ligament and the posterior talofibular ligament, respectively. The medial articulate surface of the body, which is semilunar in shape, is only half the area of the lateral triangle surface of the body. The lateral surface projects laterally as a broad-based, wedge-shaped prominence, referred to as the lateral talar process, from which the lateral talocalcaneal ligament originates and passes immediately beneath its fibular facet to the lateral surface of the calcaneus.

The subtalar joint consists of three articulating surfaces: the anterior, middle, and posterior facets, with the posterior facet representing the major weight-bearing surface. The anterior and the middle facets usually conjoin as one anterior articulation facet (**Plate 9.3**).

OTA Classification of Talus Fractures

Based on the OTA classification, the talus is coded as the number 81 for its anatomical location. According to fracture location, talus fractures can be divided into three types: 81-A, avulsion, process, or head fractures; 81-B, neck fractures; and 81-C, body fractures (**Plate 9.4**).

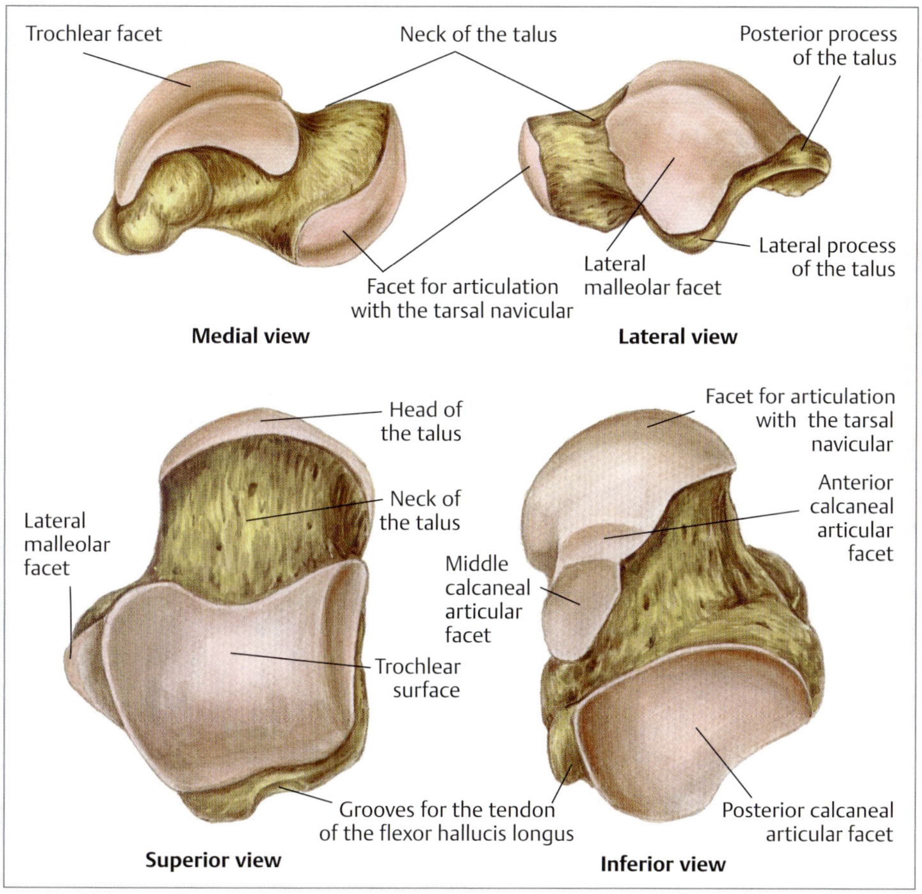

Plate 9.3

9

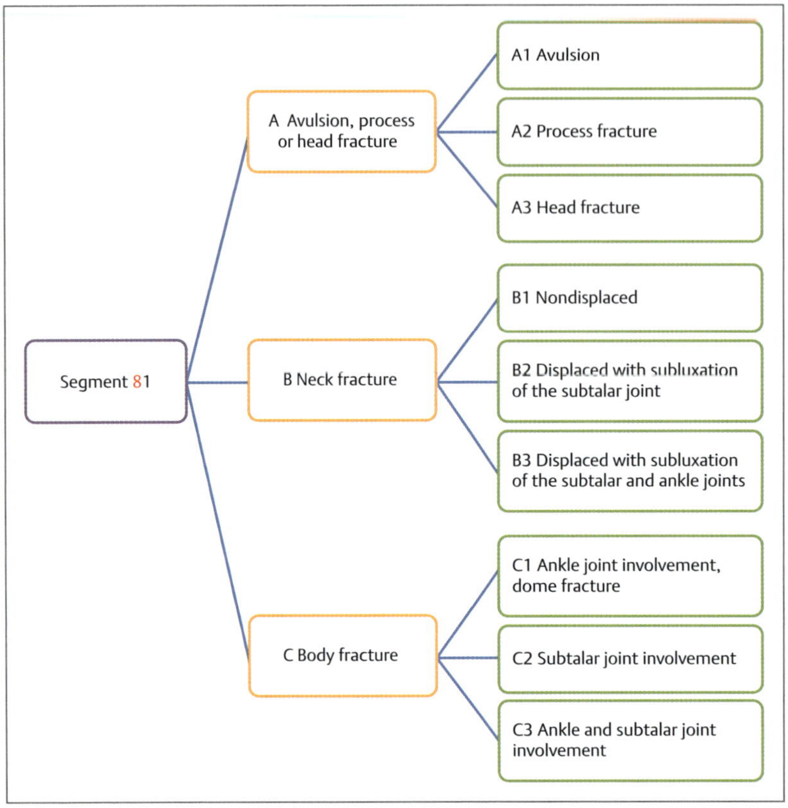

Plate 9.4

Clinical Epidemiologic Features of Talus Fractures

A total of 1,140 adult patients with 1,143 talus fractures were treated in 83 hospitals in China over a 2-year period from 2010 to 2011. All cases were reviewed and statistically studied, including 561 patients with left-side fractures, 576 with right-side fractures, and 3 with bilateral fractures. There were 803 males and 337 females, with a male-to-female ratio of 2.38:1.

Epidemiologic features of talus fractures are as follows:

- More males than females
- The high-risk age group is 26–30 years, the same age group for males, whereas the high-risk age group for females is 36–40 years.
- The most common fracture type is type 81-A—the same type for both males and females.
- The most common fracture group is group 81-A2, the same group for males, while the most common fracture group for females is group 81-A1.

Talus Fractures (Segment 81) by Sex

Table 9.5 Sex distribution of 1,140 patients with talus fractures

Sex	Number of patients	Percentage (%)
Male	803	70.44
Female	337	29.56
Total	1,140	100.00

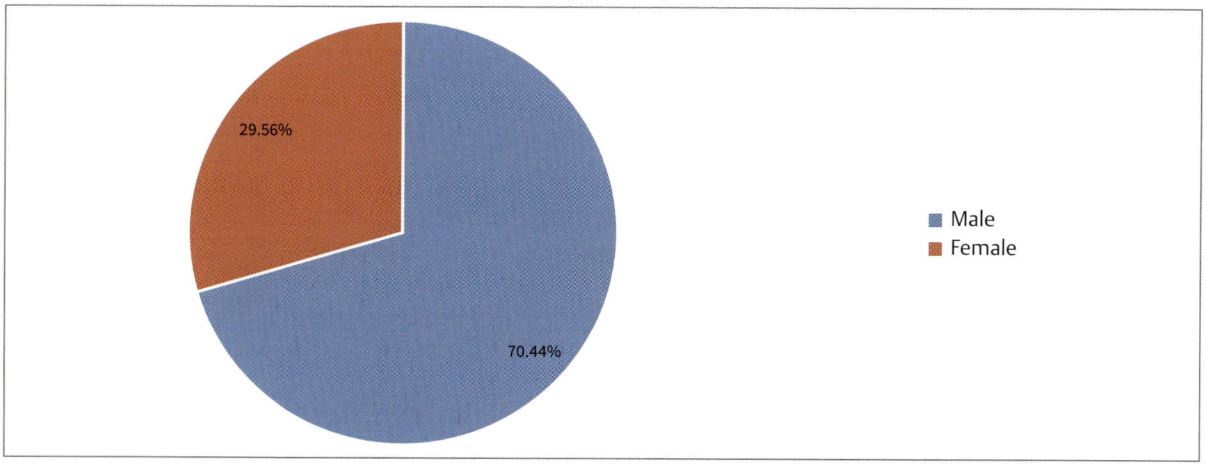

Fig. 9.5 Sex distribution of 1,140 patients with talus fractures.

Talus Fractures (Segment 81) by Age Group

Table 9.6 Age and sex distribution of 1,140 patients with talus fractures

Age group (years)	Male	Female	Number of patients	Percentage (%)
16–20	94	30	124	10.88
21–25	113	35	148	12.98
26–30	123	26	149	13.07
31–35	84	23	107	9.39
36–40	87	40	127	11.14
41–45	94	29	123	10.79
46–50	86	29	115	10.09
51–55	53	32	85	7.46
56–60	26	32	58	5.09
61–65	20	28	48	4.21
66–70	12	12	24	2.11
71–75	7	7	14	1.23
76–80	2	8	10	0.88
81–85	0	5	5	0.44
≥86	2	1	3	0.26
Total	803	337	1,140	100.00

9

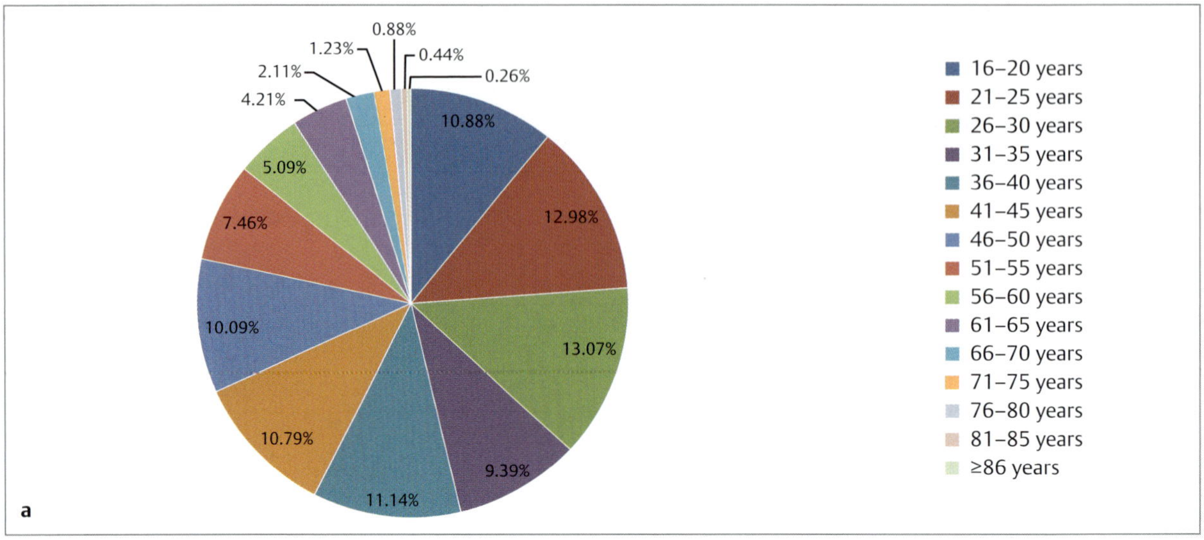

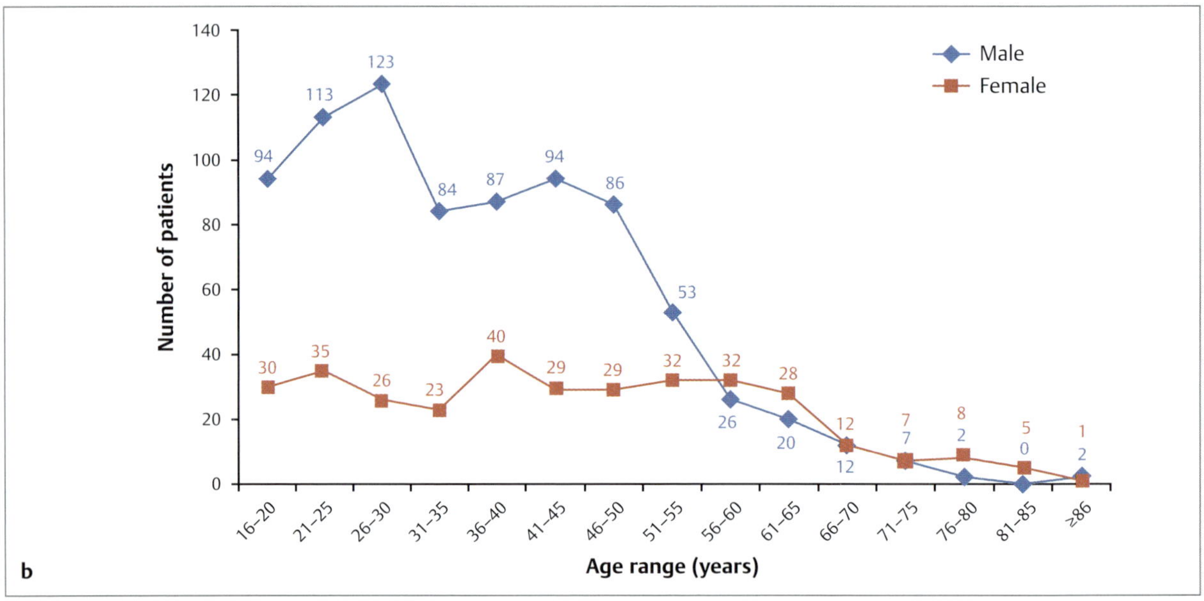

Fig. 9.6 **(a)** Age distribution of 1,140 patients with talus fractures.
(b) Age and sex distribution of 1,140 patients with talus fractures.

9

Talus Fractures (Segment 81) by Fracture Type

Table 9.7 Fracture type distribution of 1,143 talus fractures

Fracture type	Male	Female	Number of fractures	Percentage of talus fractures (%)
81-A	336	195	531	46.46
81-B	276	87	363	31.76
81-C	194	55	249	21.78
Total	806	337	1,143	100.00

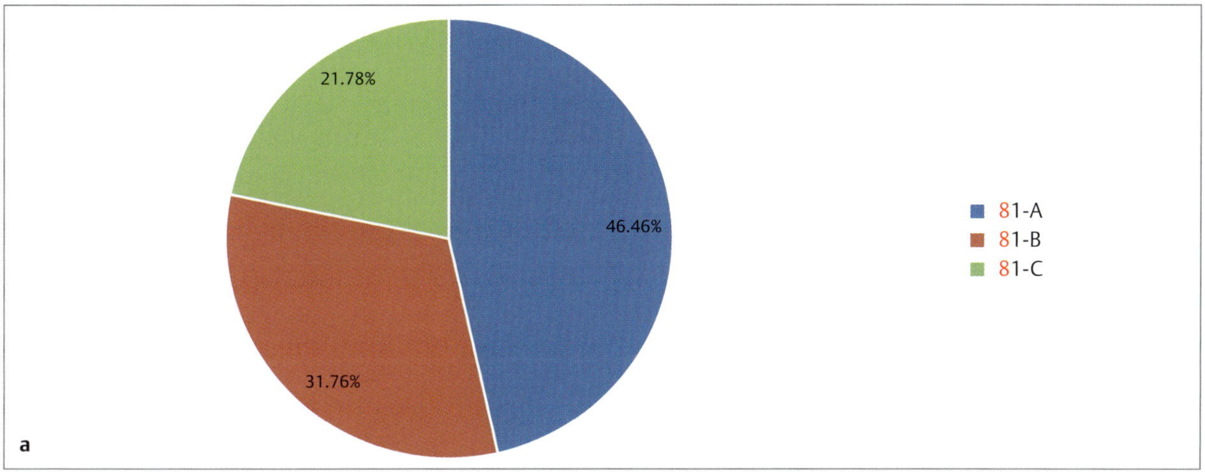

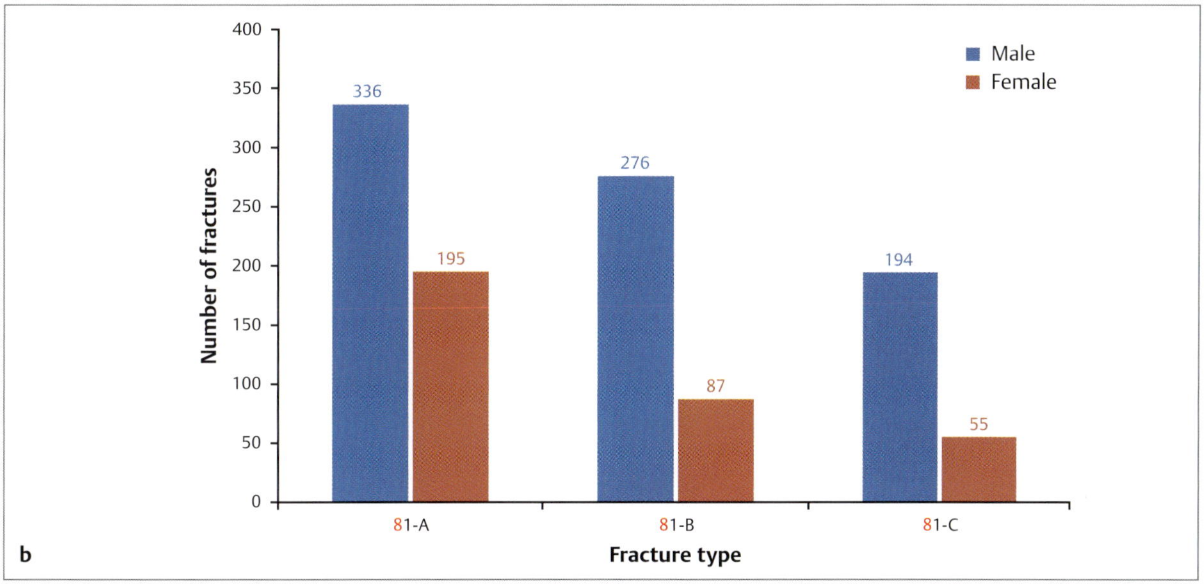

Fig. 9.7 **(a)** Fracture type distribution of 1,143 talus fractures.
(b) Sex and fracture type distribution of 1,143 talus fractures.

9

Table 9.8 Sex and fracture group distribution of 1,143 talus fractures

Fracture group	Male	Female	Number of fractures	Percentage of talus fractures (%)	Percentage of foot fractures (%)
81-A1	117	92	209	18.29	0.54
81-A2	190	88	278	24.32	0.72
81-A3	29	15	44	3.85	0.11
81-B1	69	38	107	9.36	0.28
81-B2	122	24	146	12.77	0.38
81-B3	85	25	110	9.62	0.28
81-C1	44	18	62	5.42	0.16
81-C2	56	19	75	6.56	0.19
81-C3	94	18	112	9.80	0.29
Total	806	337	1,143	100.00	2.96

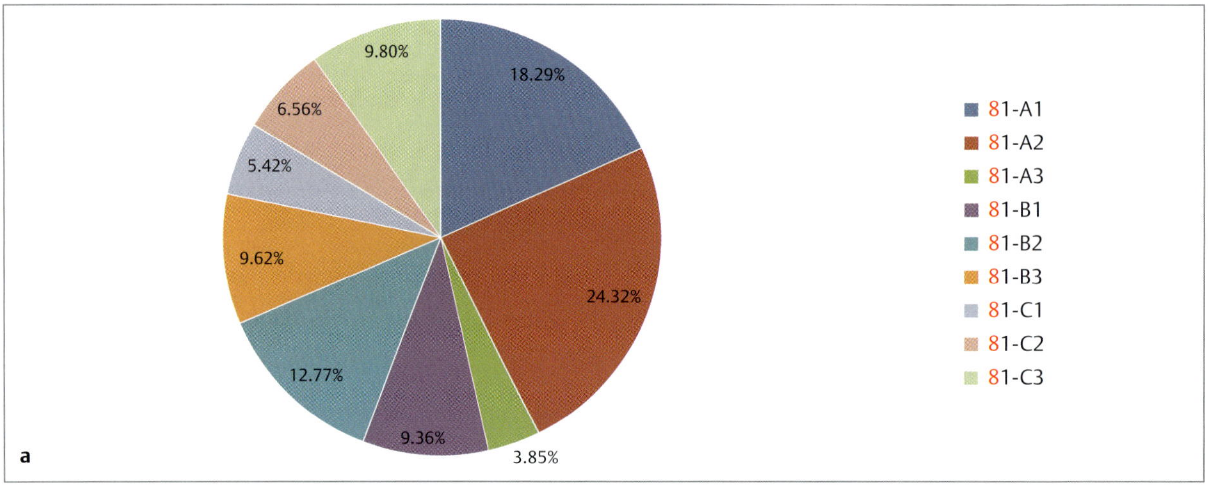

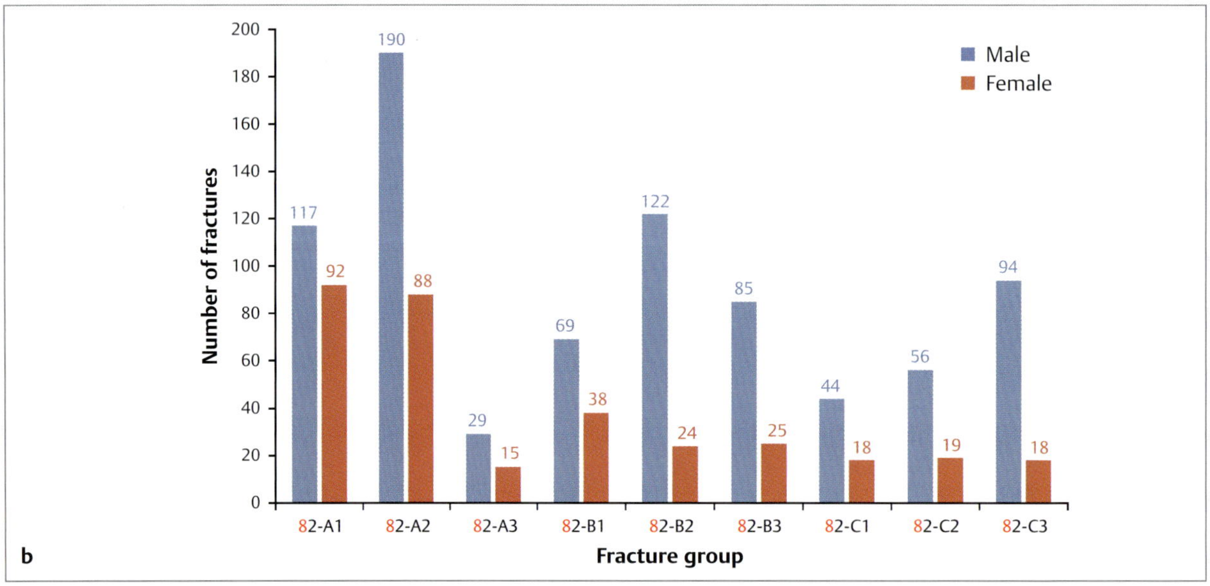

Fig. 9.8 **(a)** Fracture group distribution of 1,143 talus fractures.
(b) Sex and fracture group distribution of 1,143 talus fractures.

81-A Talus, avulsion, process, or head fractures		
81-A1 **Avulsion** 209 fractures M: 117 (55.98%) F: 92 (44.02%) 0.06% of total adult fractures 0.54% of adult foot fractures 18.29% of talus 39.36% of type 81-A	**81-A1.1** 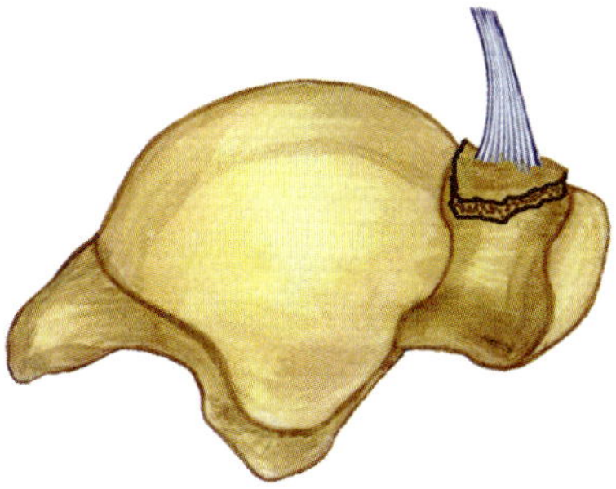 Anterior	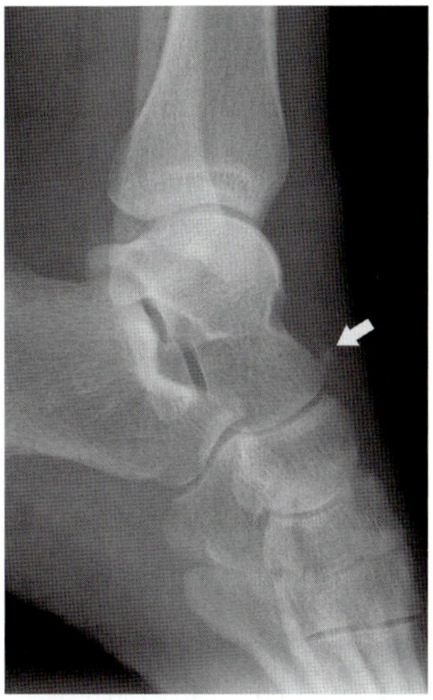
	81-A1.2 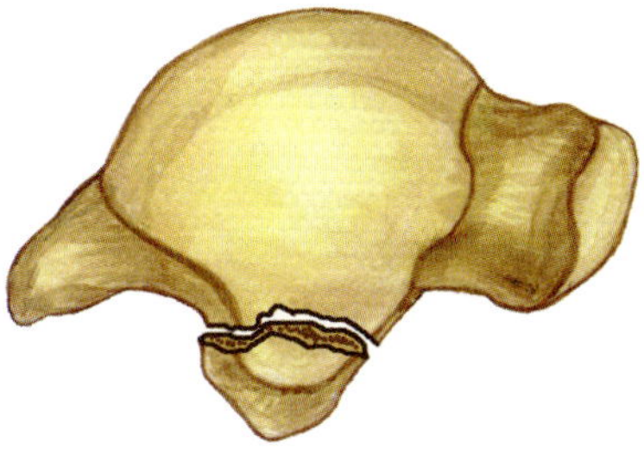 Other	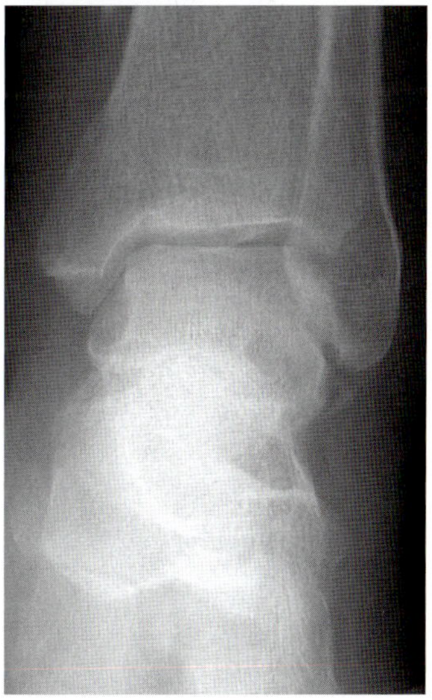

81-A Talus, avulsion, process, or head fractures

81-A2
Process
278 fractures
M: 190 (68.35%)
F: 88 (31.65%)
0.07% of total adult fractures
0.72% of adult foot fractures
24.32% of talus
52.35% of type 81-A

81-A2.1

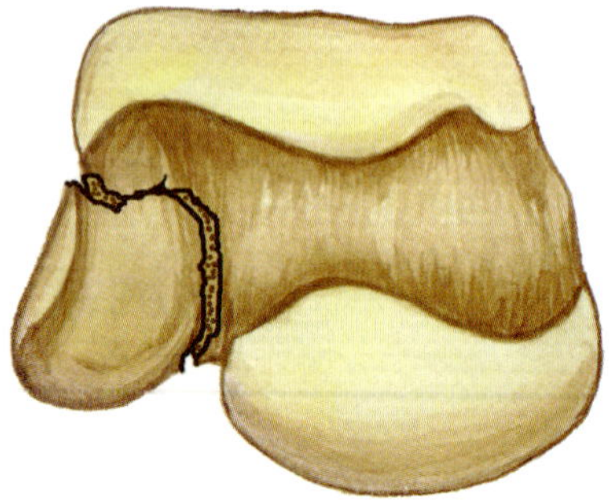

Lateral

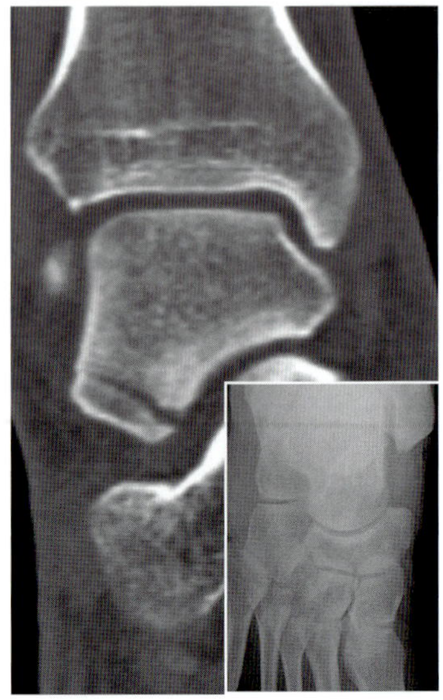

81-A2.2

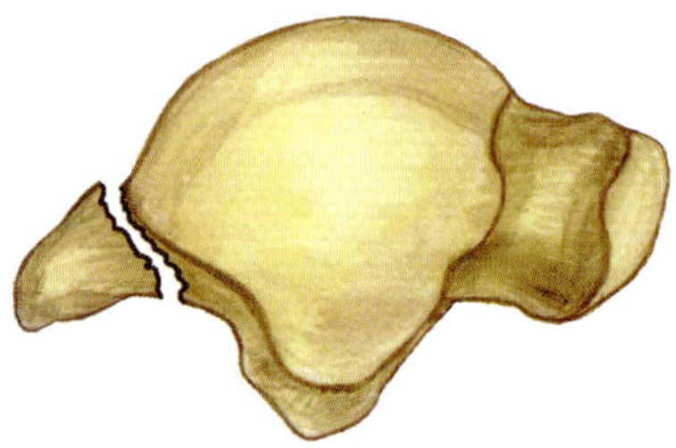

Posterior

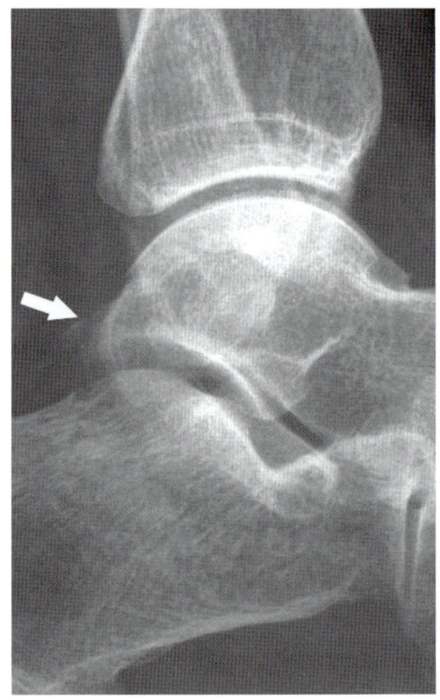

81-A Talus, avulsion, process, or head fractures

81-A3
Head fracture (without neck fracture)
44 fractures
M: 29 (65.91%)
F: 15 (34.09%)
0.01% of total adult fractures
0.11% of adult foot fractures
3.85% of talus
8.29% of type 81-A

81-A3.1

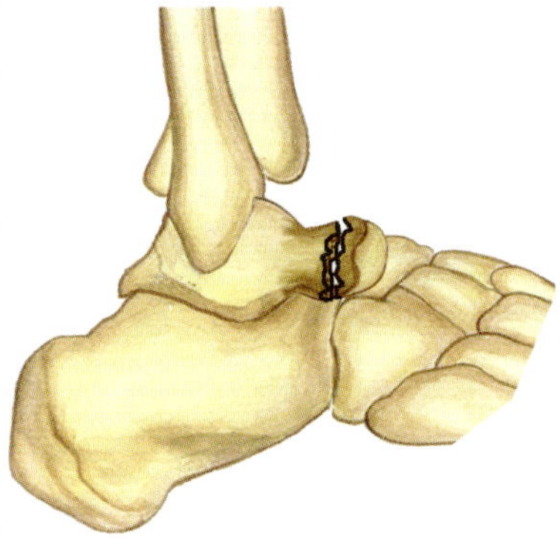

Noncomminuted

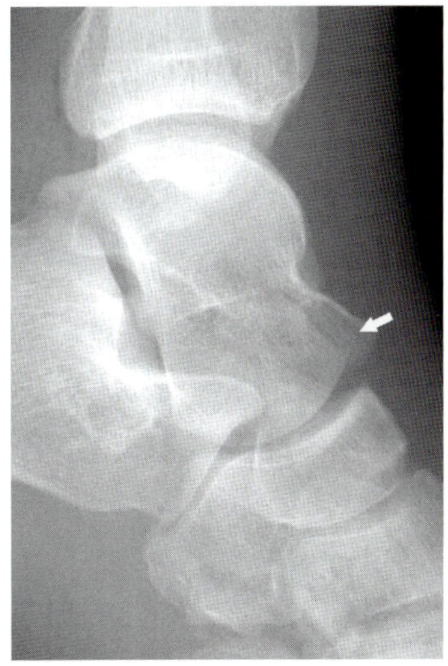

81-A3.2

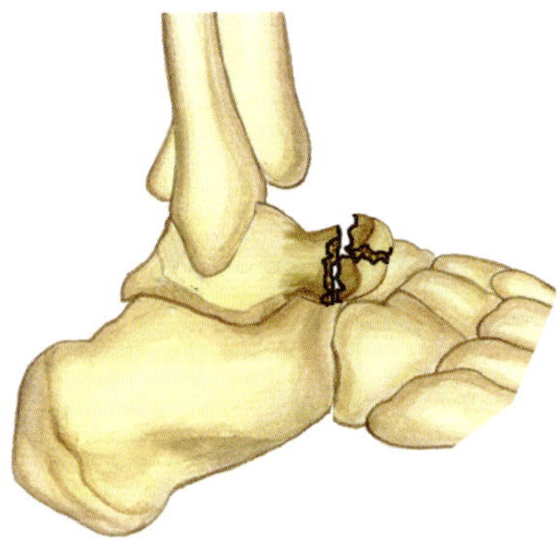

Comminuted

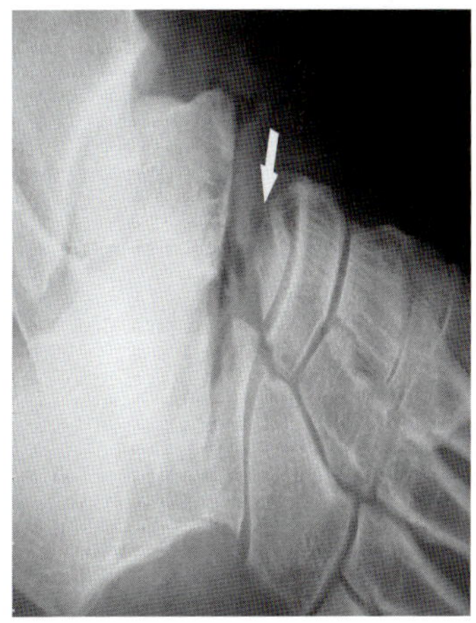

81-B Talus, neck fractures

81-B1
Nondisplaced
107 fractures
M: 69 (64.49%)
F: 38 (35.51%)
0.03% of total adult fractures
0.28% of adult foot fractures
9.36% of talus
29.48% of type 81-B

81-B1

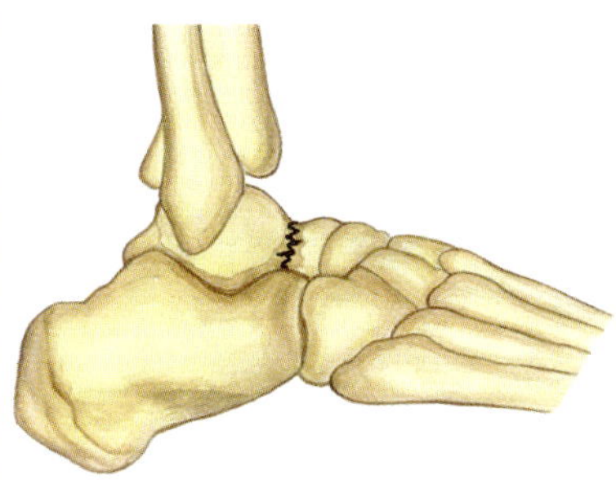

Nondisplaced

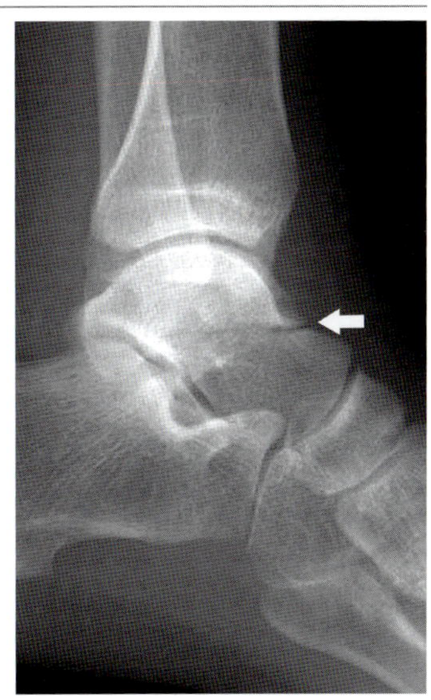

81-B Talus, neck fractures

81-B2
Displaced with subluxation of subtalar joint

146 fractures
M: 122 (83.56%)
F: 24 (16.44%)
0.04% of total adult fractures
0.38% of adult foot fractures
12.77% of talus
40.22% of type 81-B

81-B2.1

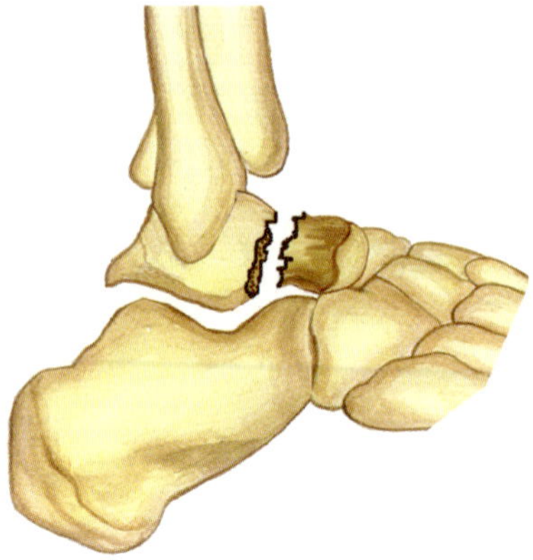

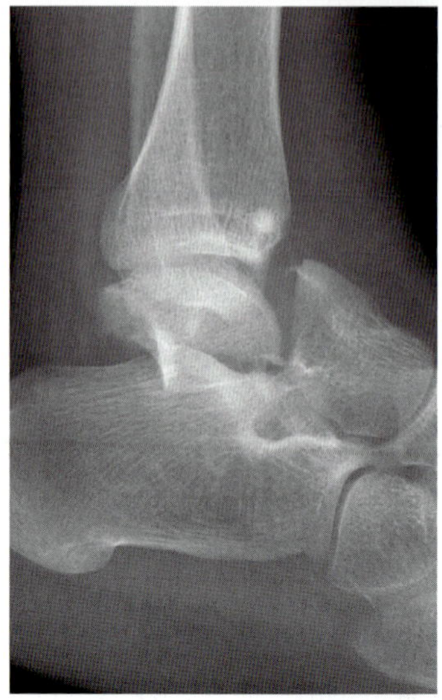

Noncomminuted

81-B2.2

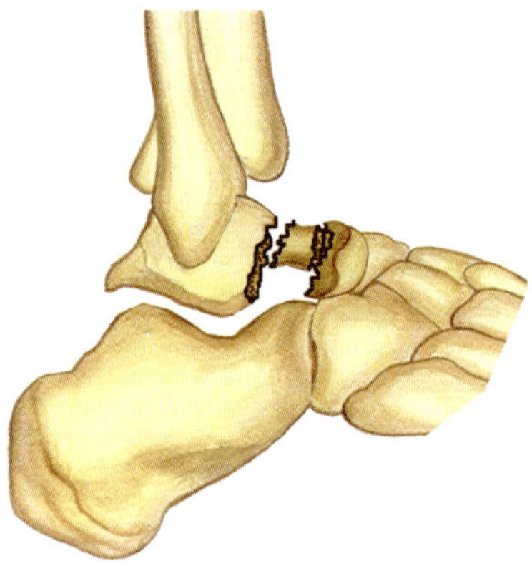

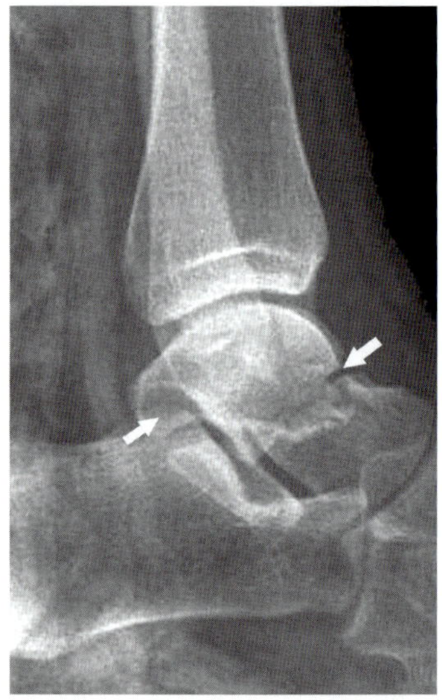

Comminuted

81-B2.3

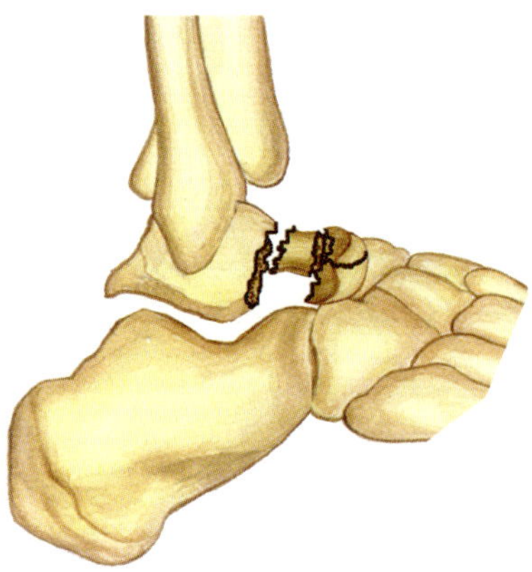

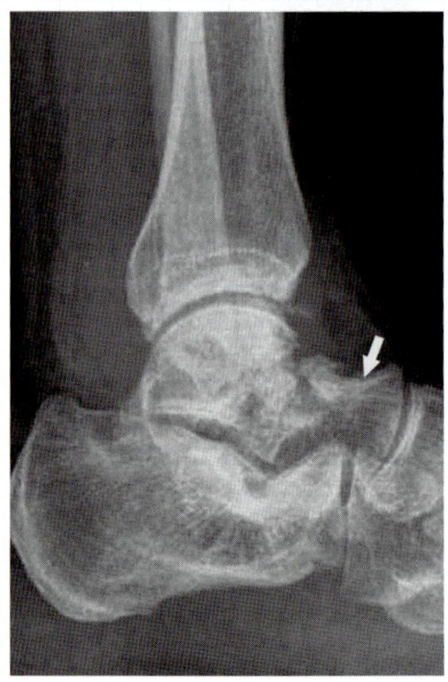

Involves talar head

81-B Talus, neck fractures

81-B3
Displaced with subluxation of subtalar and ankle joints
110 fractures
M: 85 (77.27%)
F: 25 (22.73%)
0.03% of total adult fractures
0.28% of adult foot fractures
9.62% of talus
30.3% of type 81-B

81-B3.1

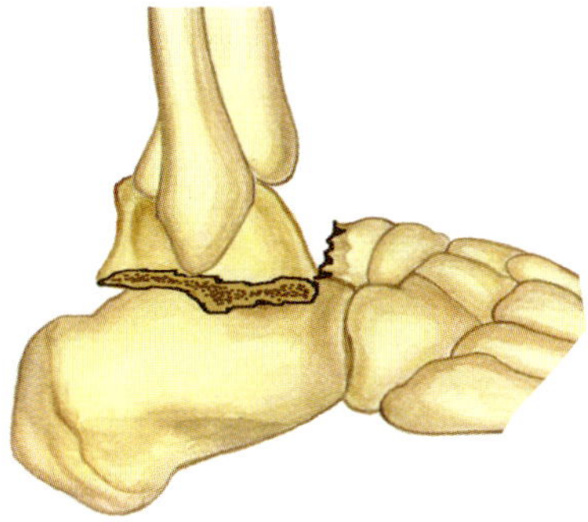

Noncomminuted

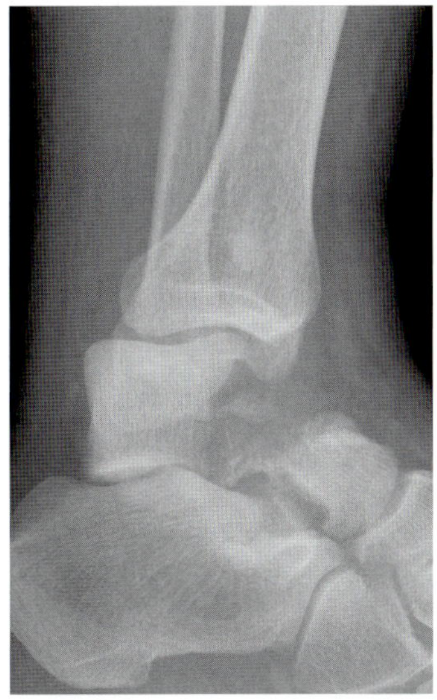

81-B3.2

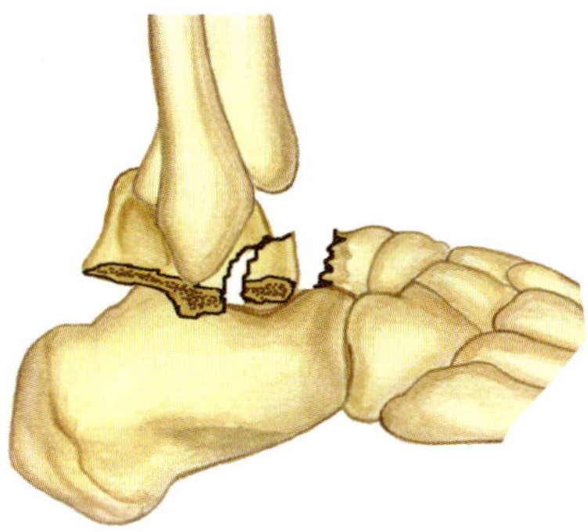

Comminuted

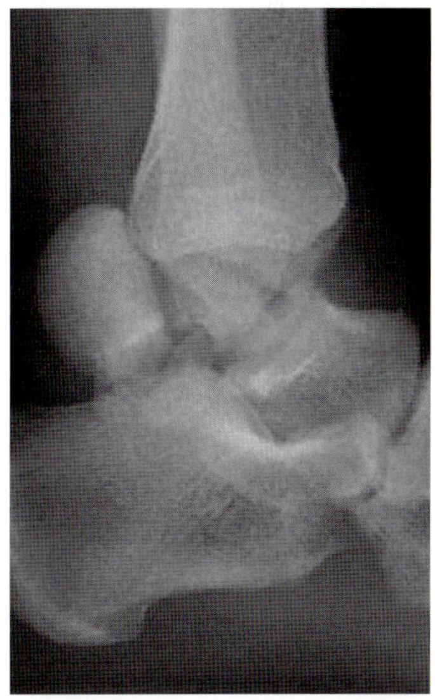

81-B3.3

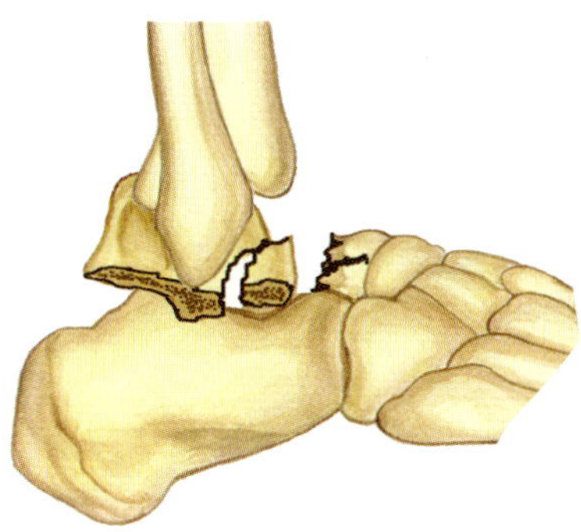

Involves talar head

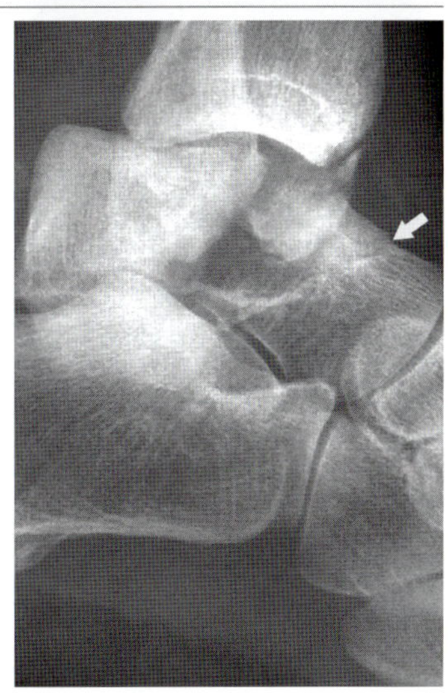

81-C Talus, body fractures

81-C1
Ankle joint involvement, dome fractures
62 fractures
M: 44 (70.97%)
F: 18 (29.03%)
0.02% of total adult fractures
0.16% of adult foot fractures
5.42% of talus
24.9% of type 81-C

81-C1.1

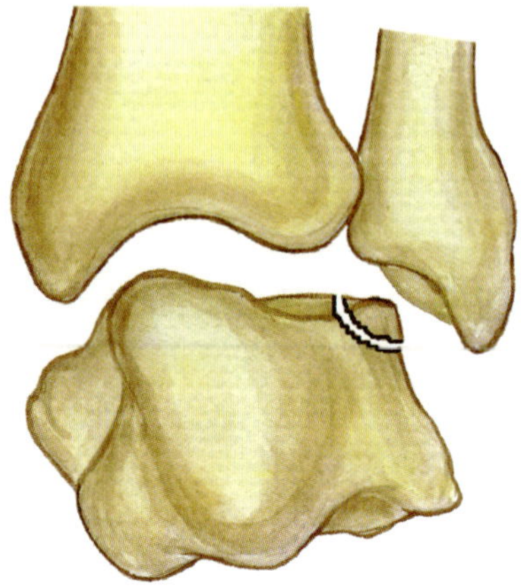

Noncomminuted

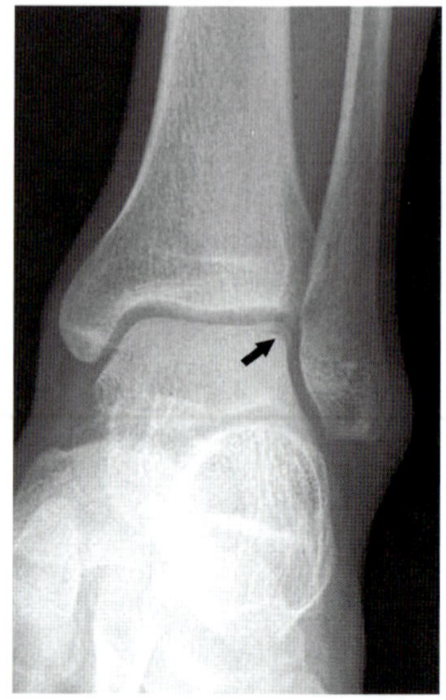

81-C1.2

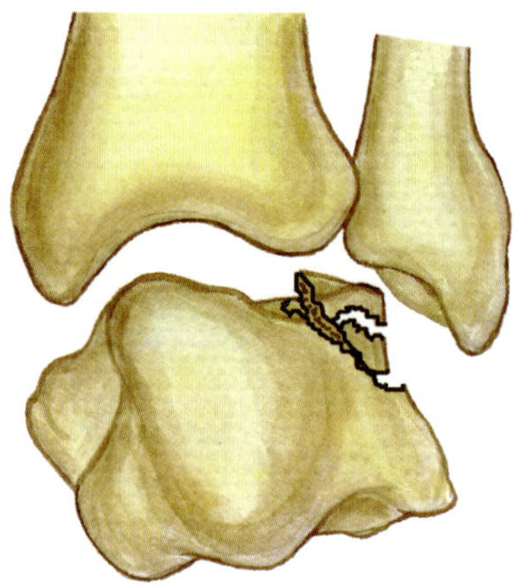

Comminuted

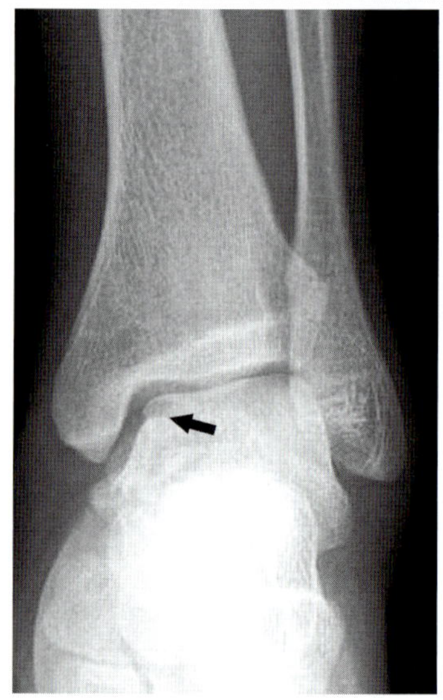

81-C Talus, body fractures

81-C2
Subtalar joint involvement
75 fractures
M: 56 (74.67%)
F: 19 (25.33%)
0.02% of total adult fractures
0.19% of adult foot fractures
6.56% of talus
30.12% of type 81-C

81-C2.1

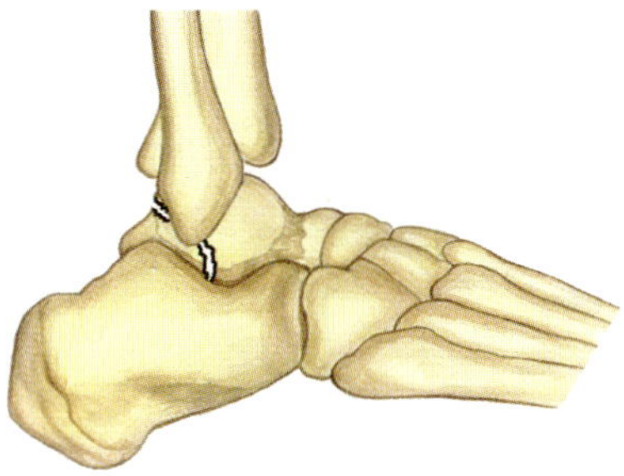

Noncomminuted

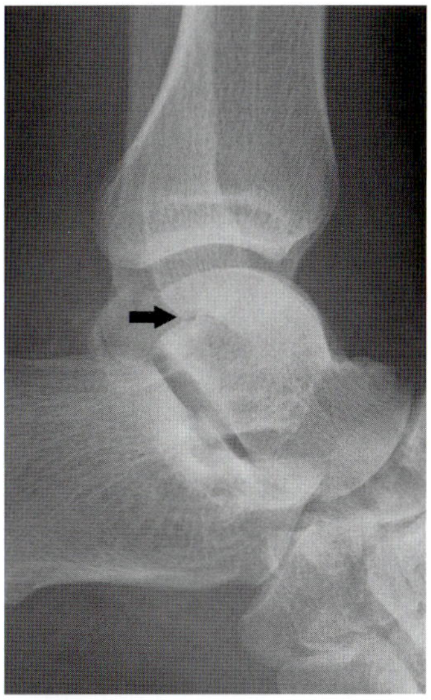

81-C2.2

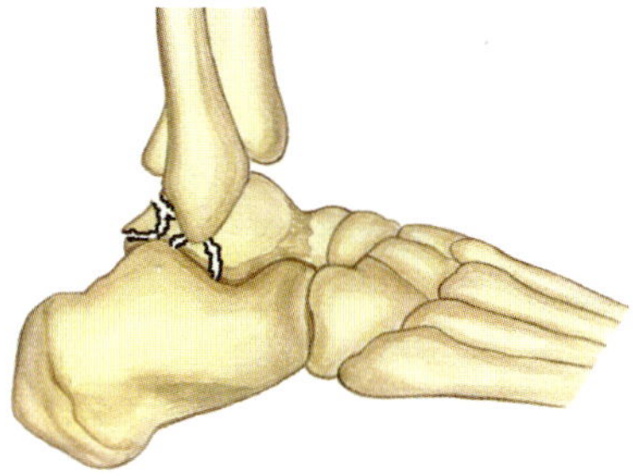

Comminuted

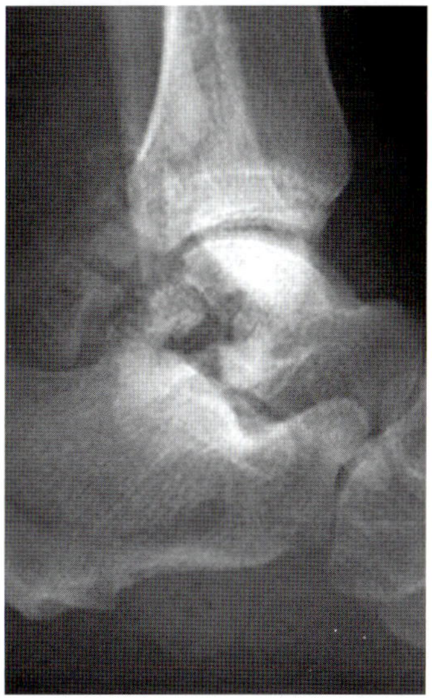

81-C Talus, body fractures

81-C3
Ankle and subtalar joint involvement
112 fractures
M: 94 (83.93%)
F: 18 (16.07%)
0.03% of total adult fractures
0.29% of adult foot fractures
9.8% of talus
44.98% of type 81-C

81-C3.1

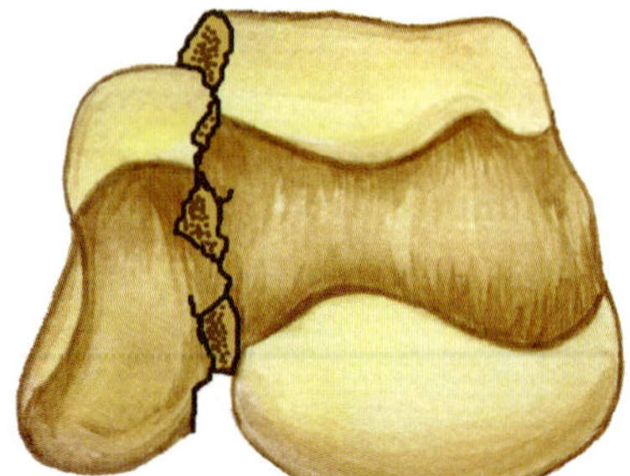

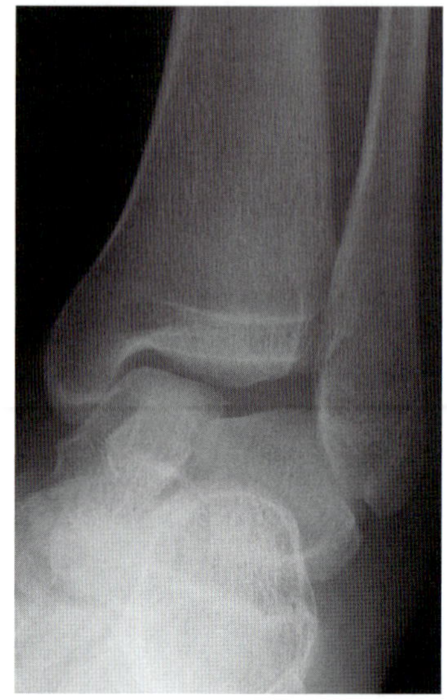

Noncomminuted

81-C3.2

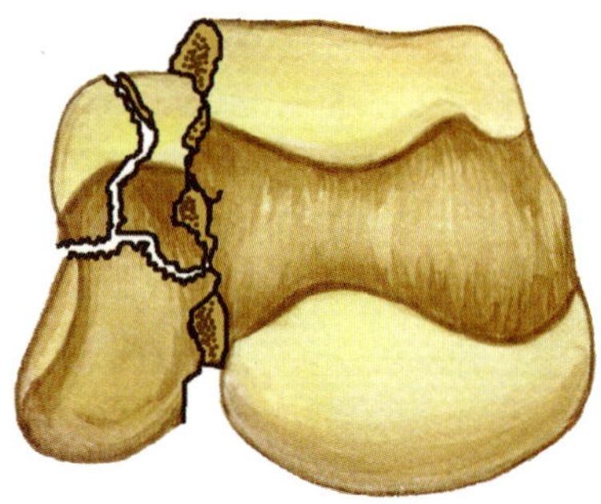

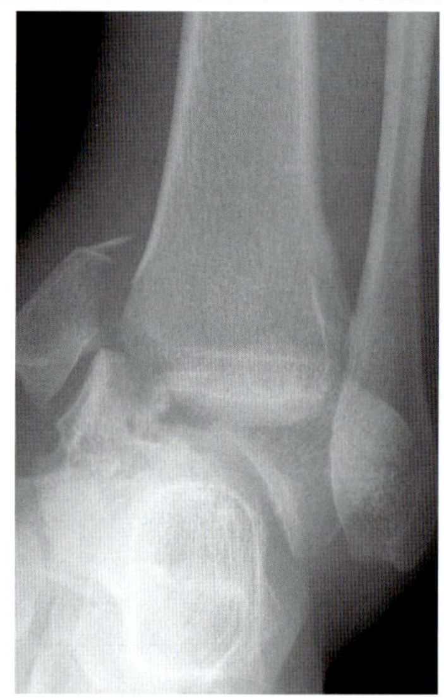

Comminuted

Injury Mechanism

Neck fractures are the most common talar fractures. The usual mechanism is associated with hyperdorsiflexion of the ankle as the talar neck impacts the anterior margin of the tibia, as may occur in an automobile accident or a fall from a height. The body of the talus locks in the ankle mortise following a talar neck fracture, and the remaining portion of the foot, including the head and calcaneus, is displaced medially. The continuous axial load may rupture the interosseous talocalcaneal ligament, the posterior talofibular ligament, and the posterior talocalcaneal ligament, causing the body of the talus to move out of the ankle mortise posteromedially. The resultant fracture line will run obliquely upward and laterally.

Body fractures of the talus occur most commonly as the result of axial compression load, as seen in a fall from a significant height. Ankle joint fractures may also accompany this injury. Fractures of the posterior and lateral processes are often results of violent contraction of nearby attached muscles as the injury occurs.

Talar head fractures are relatively uncommon, usually resulting from force transmitted along the metatarsal rays to the talar head.

Diagnosis

Most talar fractures are marked by acute pain, considerable swelling and tenderness, and limited or partially limited motion. If fractures are displaced markedly or the injury results in dislocation, deformity may present. The anteroposterior (AP) view of the ankle joint can reveal most talar fractures, while the oblique view provides better visualization of the head and neck of the talus, even with small fragments. It is important to note the extension and direction of fracture displacement and the presence of fractures of adjacent articulations. Particular attention should be given to the ankle mortise, the distal tibia, and the remaining tarsal to rule out possible fractures. Computed tomography (CT) scans and magnetic resonance imaging (MRI) can better reveal the nature of the fractures and provide accurate assessment of the articular involvement, as well as the degree of fracture displacement.

Treatment

Stable nondisplaced talar body fractures and avulsion fractures can be treated with immobilization with casting. Nondisplaced, unstable fractures and displaced talar body fractures can be managed by fixation of compression screws with minimally invasive techniques. Comminuted fractures can be treated with secondary arthrodesis if there is persistent pain or swelling. Stable nondisplaced talar neck fractures can be treated nonsurgically, in contrast to displaced talar neck fractures, which require surgical intervention. A displaced talar neck fracture with associated dislocation may be treated first with closed reduction. Emergency open reduction and internal fixation may be indicated if closed reduction fails.

Other Common Classifications of Talus Fractures

Types of Talus Fractures Classified According to Fracture Location

Hawkins Classification of Talar Neck Fractures

- *Type I:* Nondisplaced
- *Type II:* Associated subtalar subluxation or dislocation
- *Type III:* Associated subtalar and ankle dislocation
- *Type IV:* Canale and Kelley
- *Type IV:* with associated talonavicular subluxation of dislocation (see **Plate 9.5**)

Clinical Epidemiologic Features of Talus Fractures

According to Fracture Location

A total of 1,143 adult talus fractures were treated in 83 hospitals in China over a 2-year period from 2010 to 2011. All cases were reviewed and statistically studied. Their epidemiologic features are as follows:

- Talar process fractures are the most common talus fractures.
- Type II fractures are the most common type of talar neck fracture.
- Talar head fractures are rare, only accounting for 3.85% of talus fractures.

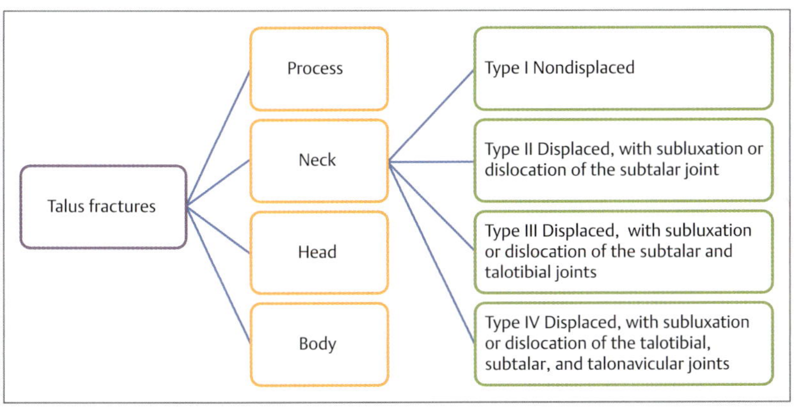

Plate 9.5

9

Talus Fractures by Fracture Location

Table 9.9 Sex and fracture location distribution of 1,143 talus fractures

Fracture location of talus	Male	Female	Number of fractures	Percentage of talus fractures (%)
Process	307	180	487	42.61
Neck	276	87	363	31.76
Head	29	15	44	3.85
Body	194	55	249	21.78
Total	806	337	1,143	100.00

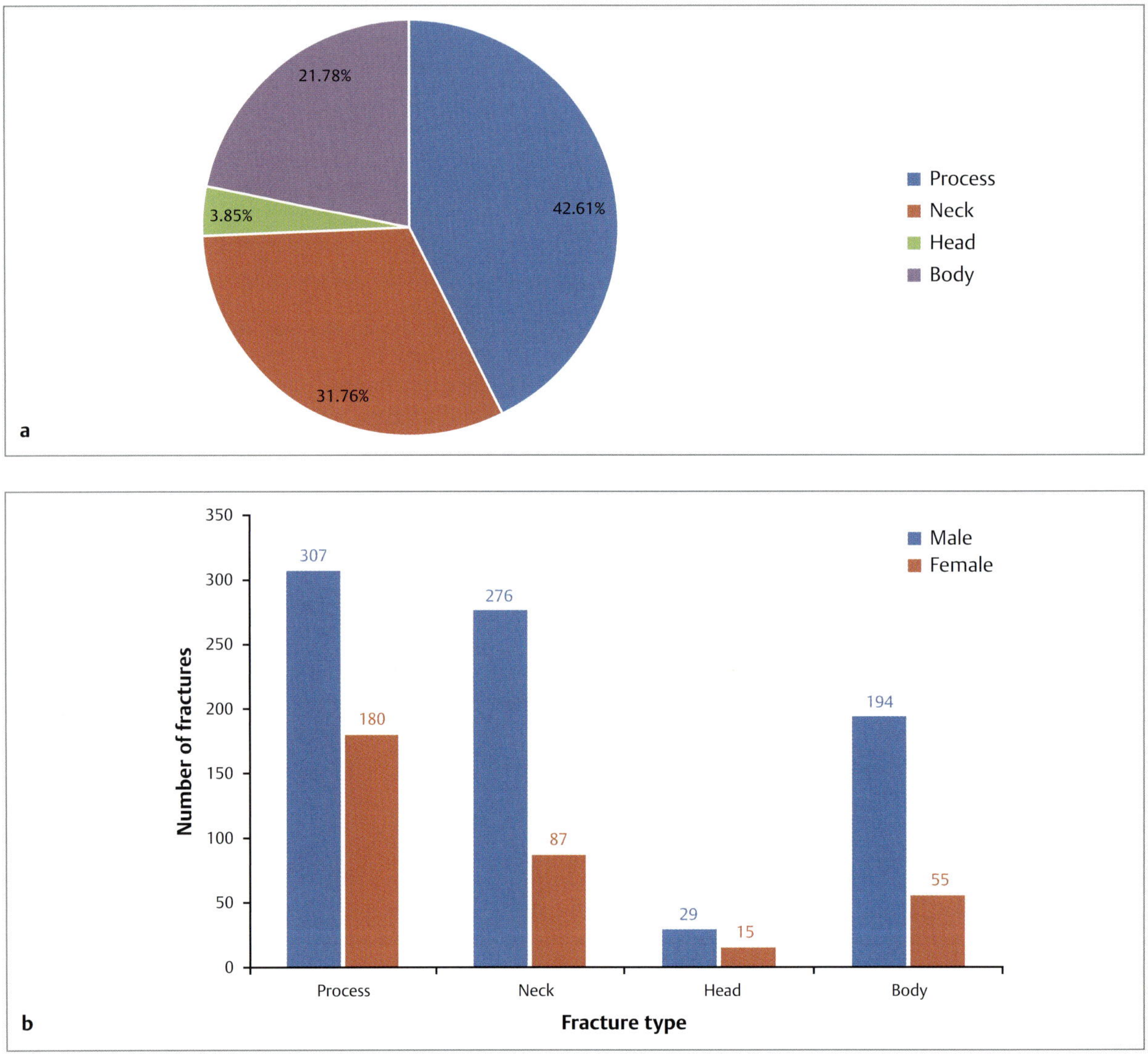

Fig. 9.9 **(a)** Fracture location distribution of 1,143 talus fractures.
(b) Sex and fracture location distribution of 1,143 talus fractures.

Talus fractures

Fractures of the talar process
487 fractures
M: 307 (63.04%)
F: 180 (36.96%)
0.13% of total adult fracture
1.26% of adult foot fracture
42.61% of talus

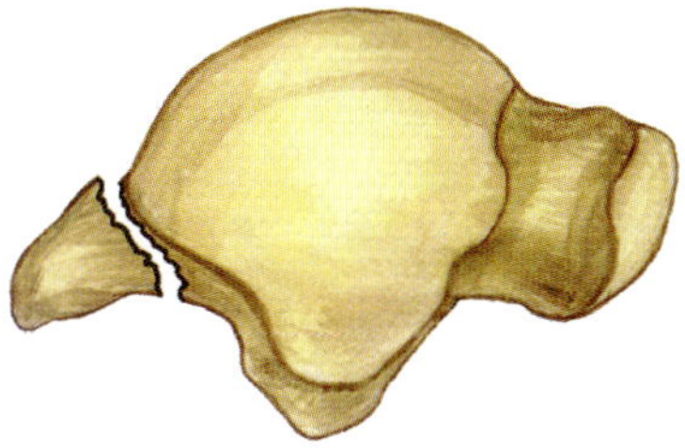

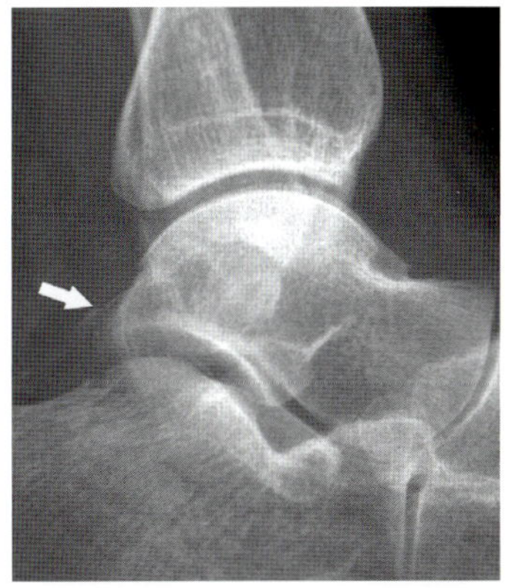

Fractures of the talar neck
363 fractures
M: 276 (76.03%)
F: 87 (23.97%)
0.1% of total adult fracture
0.94% of adult foot fracture
31.76% of talus

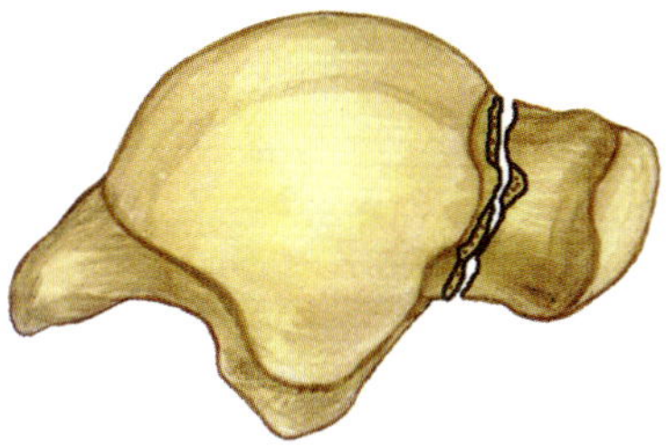

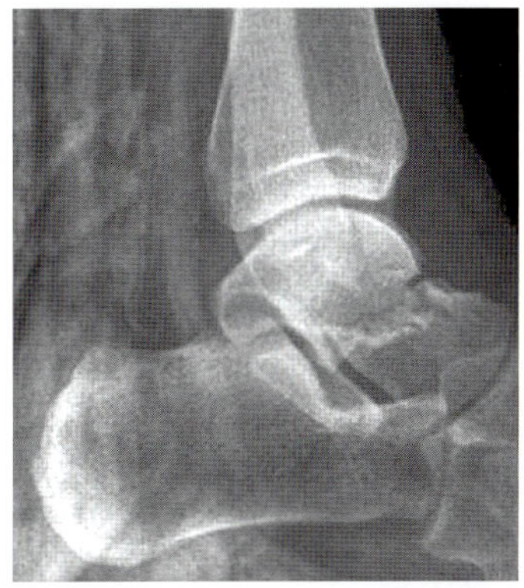

Fractures of the talar head
44 fractures
M: 29 (65.91%)
F: 15 (34.09%)
0.01% of total adult fracture
0.11% of adult foot fracture
3.85% of talus

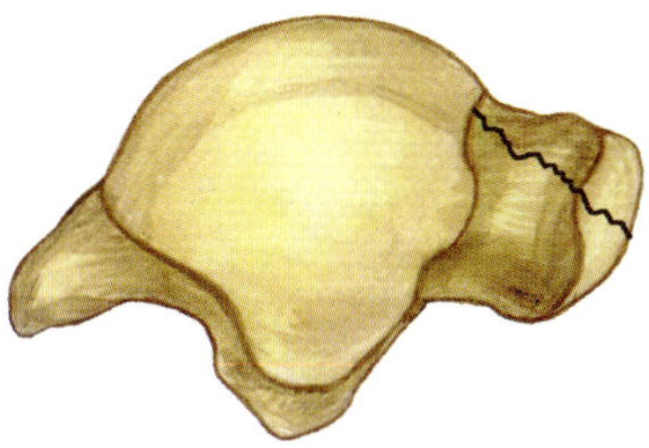

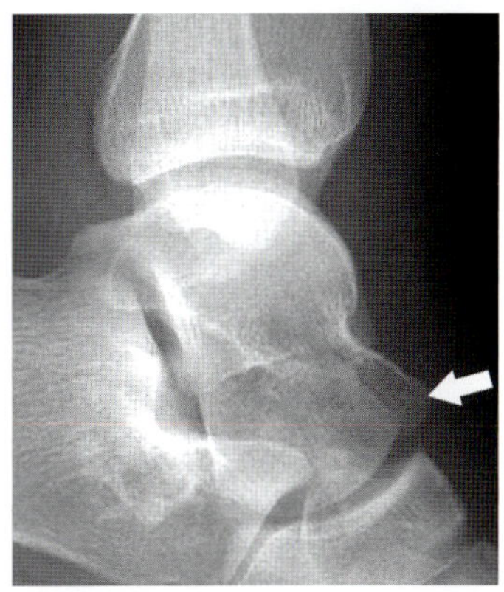

Fractures of the talar body
249 fractures
M: 194 (77.91%)
F: 55 (22.09%)
0.07% of total adult fracture
0.64% of adult foot fracture
21.78% of talus

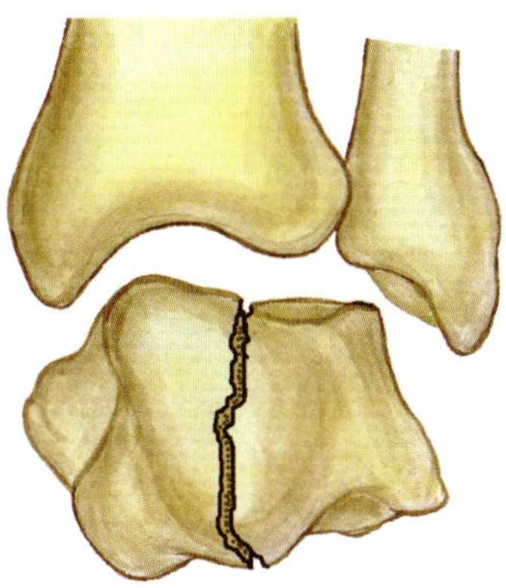

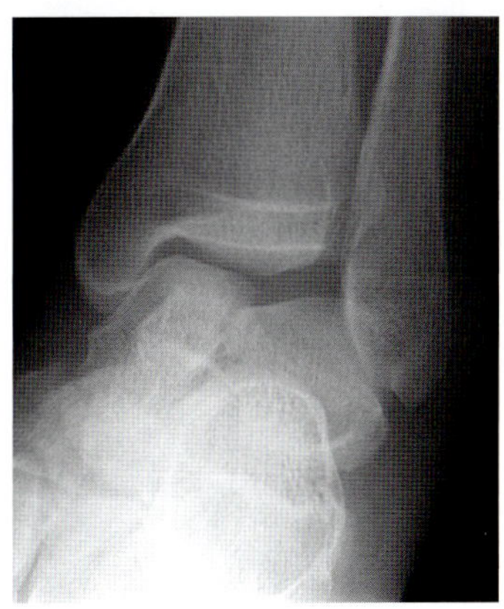

Talar neck fractures (Hawkins classification)		
Type I **Nondisplaced** 107 fractures 0.03% of total 0.28% of foot 9.36% of talus 29.48% of talar neck	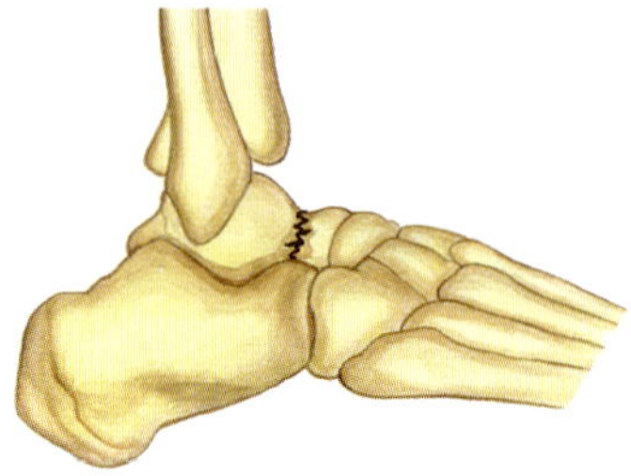	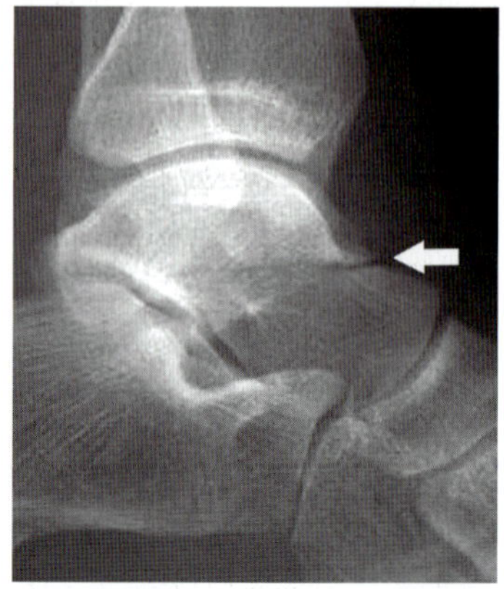
Type II **Displaced, with subluxation and dislocation of the subtalar joint** 146 fractures 0.04% of total 0.38% of foot 12.77% of talus 40.22% of talar neck	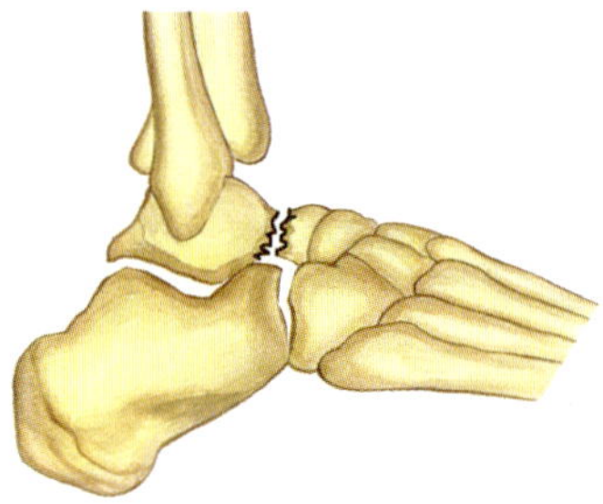	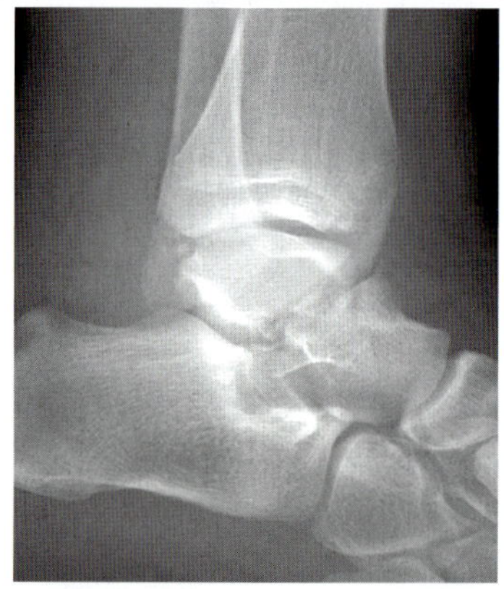
Type III **Displaced, with subluxation and dislocation of the subtalar and talotibial joints** 87 fractures 0.02% of total 0.23% of foot 7.61% of talus 23.97% of talar neck	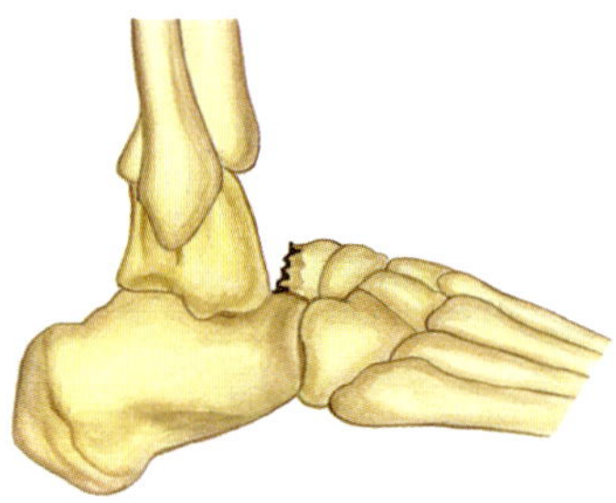	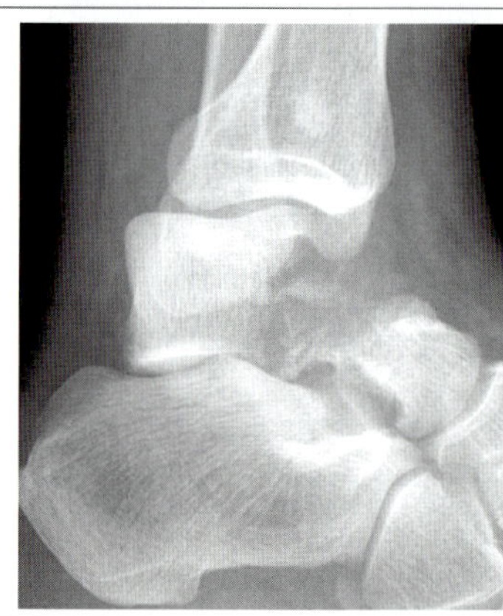
Type IV **Displaced, with subluxation and dislocation of the talotibial, subtalar, and talonavicular joints** 23 fractures 0.01% of total 0.06% of foot 2.01% of talus 6.34% of talar neck	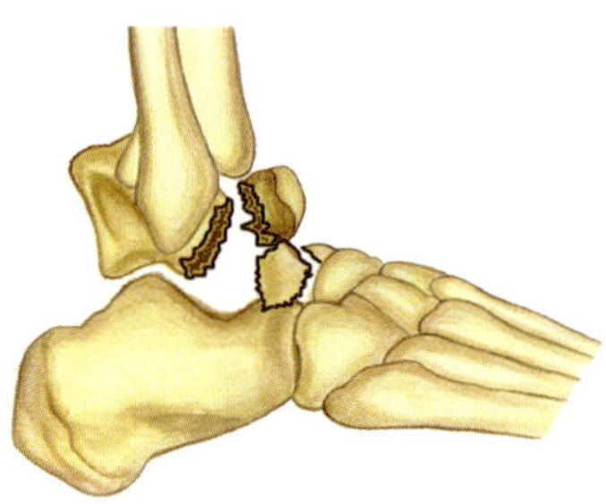	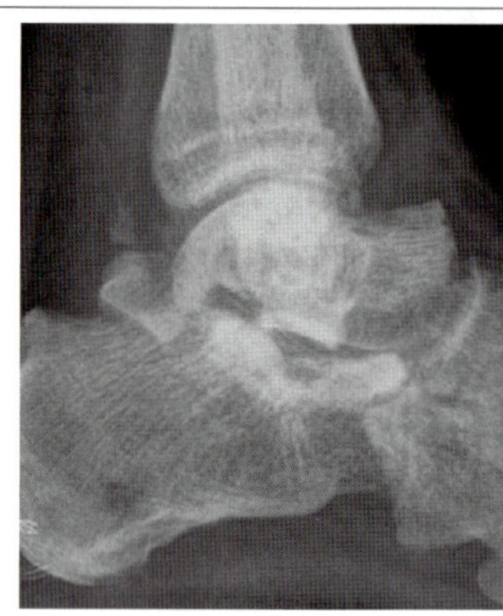

Calcaneus Fractures (Segment 82)

Anatomical Features

The calcaneus is the largest of the tarsal bones, rectangular in shape, and lies inferior to the talus. The calcaneus has six surfaces: superior, inferior, anterior, posterior, medial, and lateral—it has three talocalcaneal facets on its upper surface, and one calcaneocuboid facet on its front.

Superior: On its upper surface are three smooth facets—posterior, middle, and anterior—that articulate with the lower surface of the talus to form the subtalar joint. The middle one-third of the surface is the posterior facet, which is large and oval or oblong. It is anteriorly tilted, at an angle of 45 degrees from the midsagittal plane. The middle and anterior facets are located on the medial side of the upper calcaneal surface and are usually continuous with each other. On the medial side of the bone, below the middle talocalcaneal facet, is a shelflike projection, the sustentaculum tali, which supports the talar neck and also serves for the attachment of several ligaments. The posterior one-third of the upper calcaneal surface is roughened and is in between the posterior aspect of the ankle joint and the Achilles tendon.

Inferior: The inferior roughened area of the calcaneus gives attachment for the long plantar ligament and the quadratus plantae. The plantar surface forepart of the calcaneus is a small rounded projection known as the small

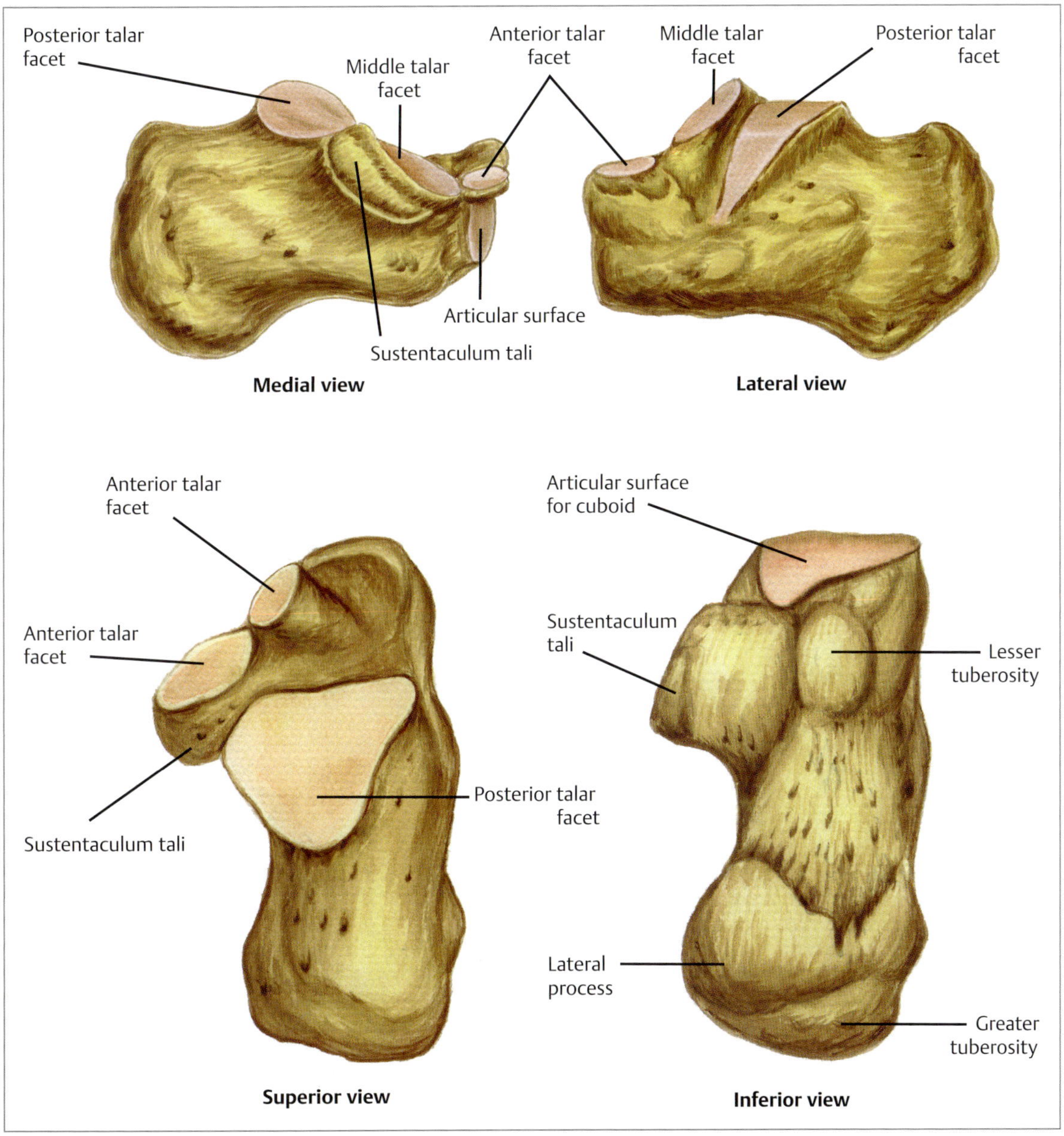

Plate 9.6

9

calcaneal tubercle, which gives attachment to the plantar calcaneocuboid ligament. The back part of the plantar surface is an eminence called the calcaneal tubercle.

Medial: The medial wall of the calcaneus is depressed. Under the surface of the sustentaculum tali of the calcaneus, there is a groove running obliquely downward from posterior to anterior, which contains the flexor hallucis longus tendon.

Lateral: The lateral wall of the calcaneus is flat and smooth, except for a small ridge called the peroneal tubercle. Passing below the peroneal tubercle of the calcaneus is the groove for the peroneus longus tendon.

Anterior: The anterior surface of the calcaneus, which is square in shape, has the smallest surface of all and has a saddle-shaped articulation, forming the calcaneocuboid joint with the cuboid bone.

Posterior: The posterior half of the calcaneus is an oval-shaped projection, which can be subdivided into three parts: upper, middle, and lower. The upper part of the posterior surface of the calcaneus is separated from the Achilles tendon by the subtendinous bursa and fat tissue; the middle part of the posterior surface, broad and rough, is the insertion point of the Achilles tendon; while the lower part is at a forward decline and continues with the calcaneal tuberosity. On the lower edge of the calcaneal tuberosity, on either side, are its lateral and medial processes serving as the origins of the abductor hallucis and abductor digit minimi (**Plate 9.6**).

OTA Classification of Calcaneal Fractures

Based on OTA classification, the calcaneus is coded as the number 82 for its anatomical location. According to fracture location, calcaneal fractures are classified into three types: 82-A, avulsion, process, or tuberosity; 82-B, extra-articular body fractures; and 82-C, articular fractures involving the posterior facet (**Plate 9.7**).

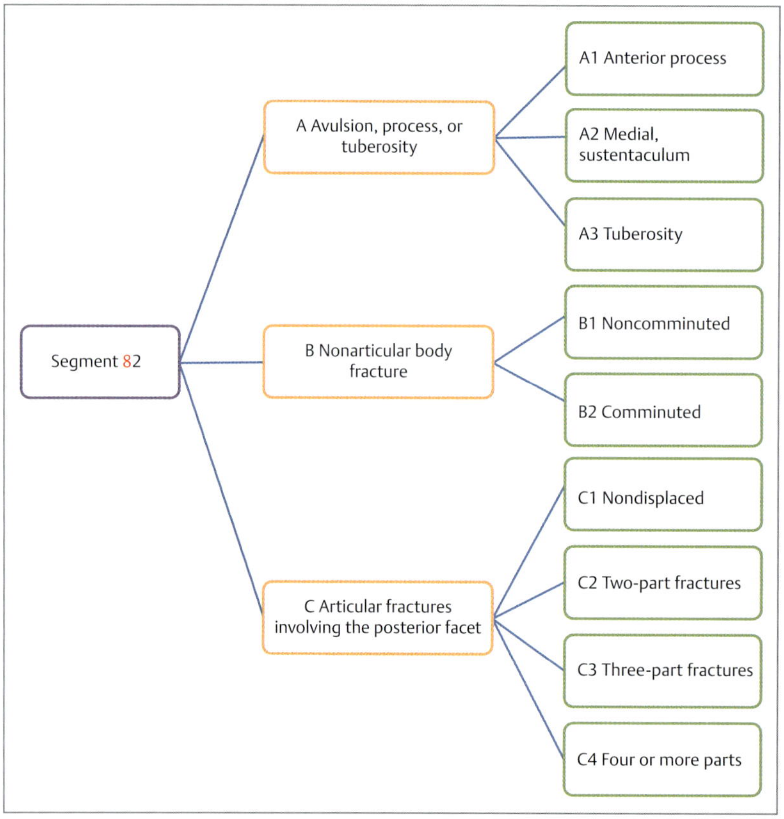

Plate 9.7

Clinical Epidemiologic Features of Calcaneal Fractures (Segment 82)

A total of 11,008 adult patients with 11,720 calcaneal fractures were treated in 83 hospitals in China over a 2-year period from 2010 to 2011. All cases were reviewed and statistically studied, including 5,092 patients with fractures on the left side, 5,204 on the right side, and 712 bilateral. There were 9,228 males and 1,780 females, with a male-to-female ratio of 5.18:1.

Epidemiologic features of calcaneal fractures are as follows:

- More males than females
- The high-risk age group is 36–40 years—the same age group for males, whereas the high-risk age groups for female are 36–40 years and 46–50 years.
- The most common fracture type is type 82-C.

Calcaneal Fractures by Sex

Table 9.10 Sex distribution of 11,008 patients with calcaneus fractures

Sex	Number of patients	Percentage (%)
Male	9,228	83.83
Female	1,780	16.17
Total	11,008	100.00

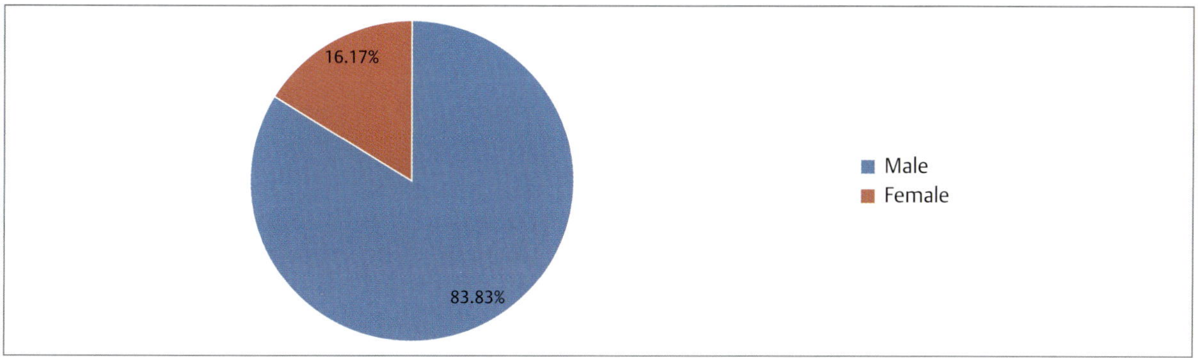

Fig. 9.10 Sex distribution of 11,008 patients with calcaneal fractures.

Calcaneal Fractures by Age Group

Table 9.11 Age and sex distribution of 11,008 patients with calcaneus fractures

Age group (years)	Male	Female	Number of patients	Percentage (%)
16–20	530	103	633	5.75
21–25	774	141	915	8.31
26–30	951	130	1,081	9.82
31–35	1,104	134	1,238	11.25
36–40	1,687	216	1,903	17.29
41–45	1,438	216	1,654	15.03
46–50	1,142	220	1,362	12.37
51–55	674	175	849	7.71
56–60	514	150	664	6.03
61–65	223	95	318	2.89
66–70	97	77	174	1.58
71–75	43	58	101	0.92
76–80	32	40	72	0.65
81–85	14	15	29	0.26
≥86	5	10	15	0.14
Total	9,228	1,780	11,008	100.00

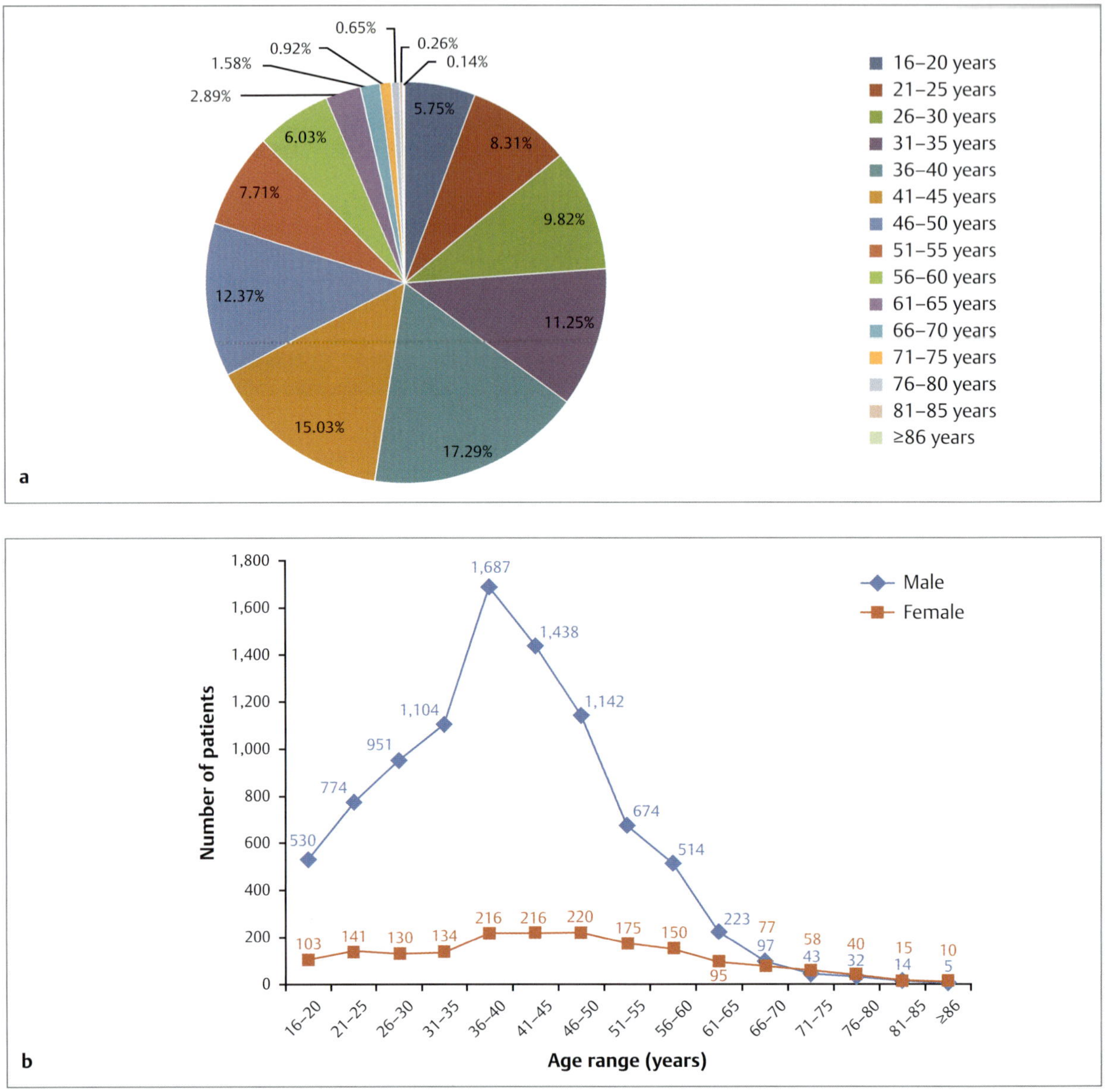

Fig. 9.11 **(a)** Age distribution of 11,008 patients with calcaneal fractures.
(b) Age and sex distribution of 11,008 patients with calcaneal fractures.

9

Calcaneal Fractures by Fracture Type

Table 9.12 Sex and fracture type distribution of 11,720 calcaneus fractures

Fracture type	Male	Female	Number of fractures	Percentage of calcaneus fracture (%)
82-A	1,632	536	2,168	18.50
82-B	2,262	498	2,760	23.55
82-C	5,978	814	6,792	57.95
Total	9,872	1,848	11,720	100.00

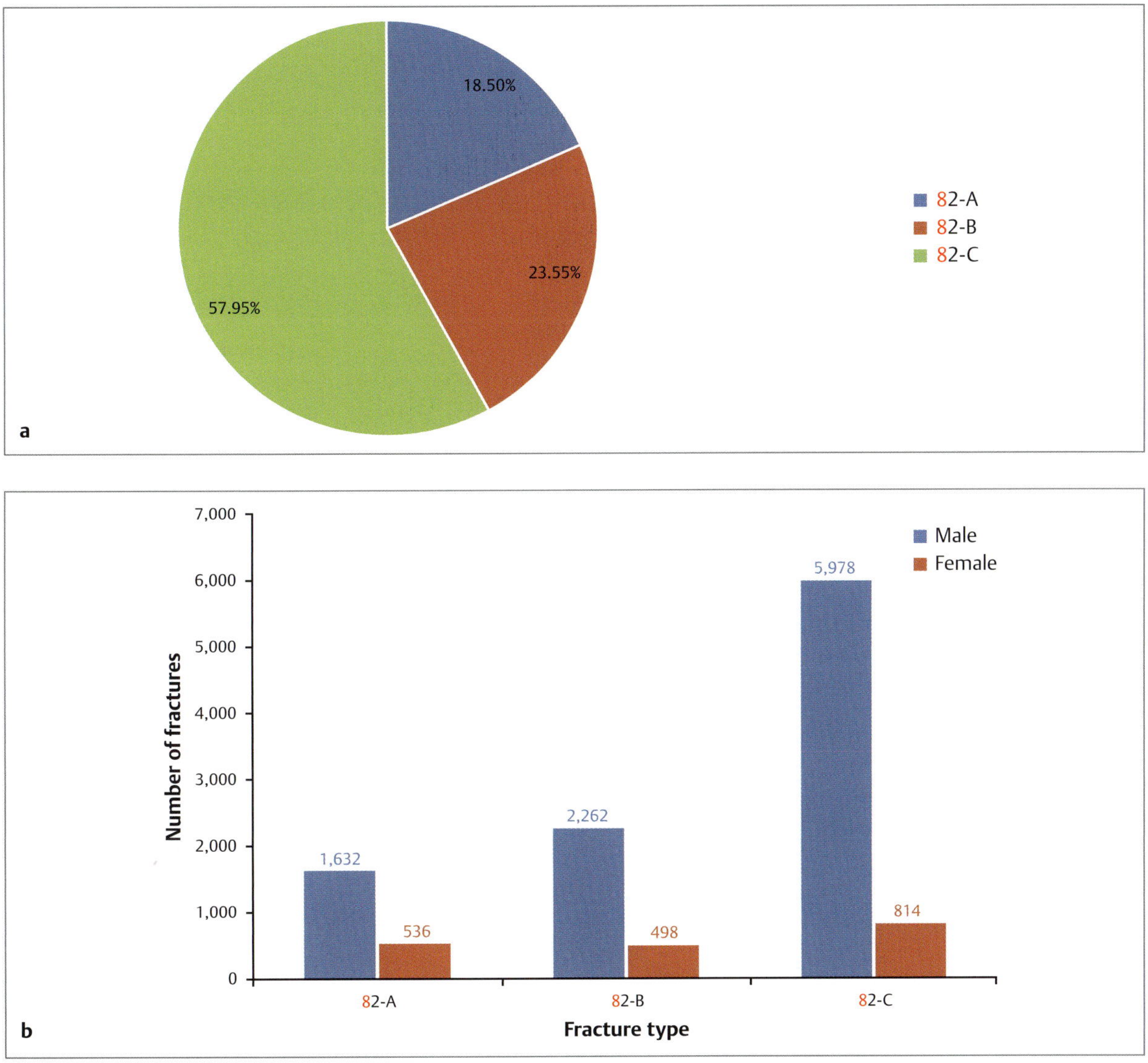

Fig. 9.12 **(a)** Fracture type distribution of 11,720 calcaneal fractures.
(b) Sex and fracture type distribution of 11,720 calcaneal fractures.

Table 9.13 Sex and fracture group distribution of 11,720 calcaneus fractures

Fracture group	Male	Female	Number of fractures	Percentage of calcaneus fractures (%)	Percentage of foot fractures (%)
82-A1	451	216	667	5.69	1.73
82-A2	254	85	339	2.89	0.88
82-A3	927	235	1,162	9.91	3.01
82-B1	1,161	275	1,436	12.25	3.72
82-B2	1,101	223	1,324	11.30	3.43
82-C	5,978	814	6,792	57.95	17.58
Total	9,872	1,848	11,720	100.00	30.34

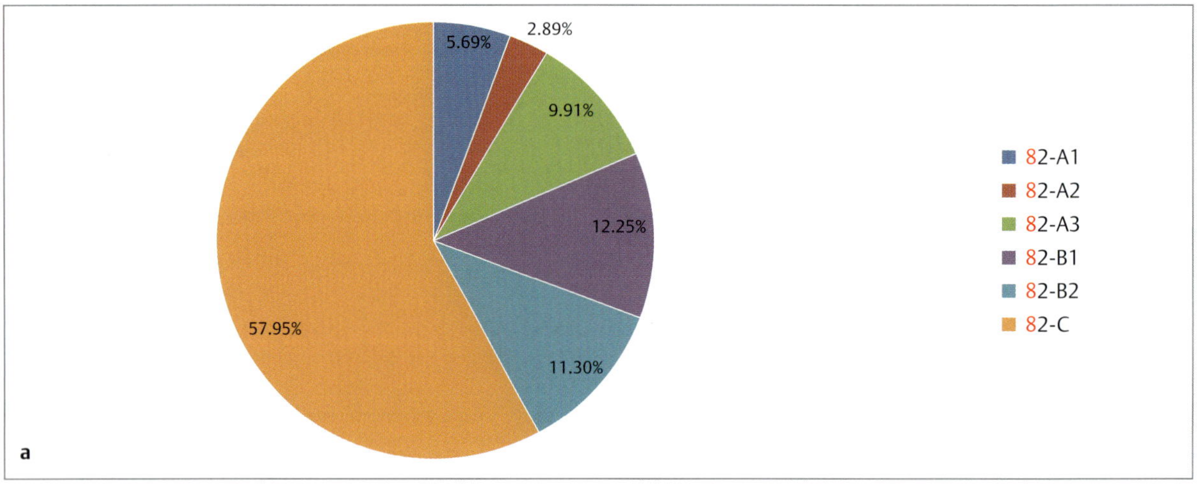

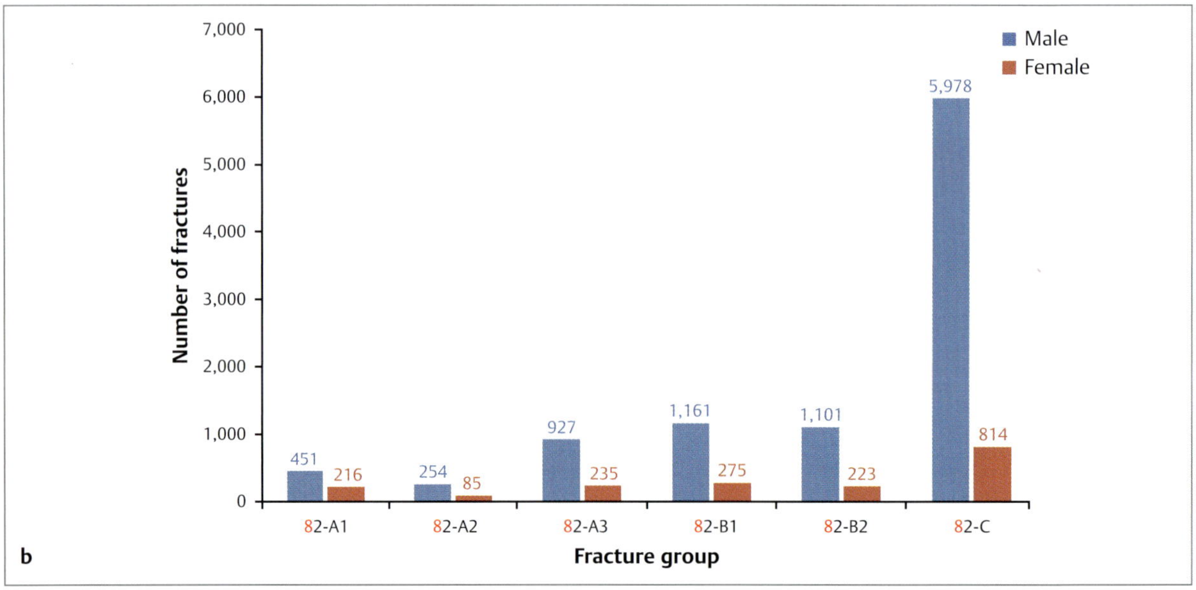

Fig. 9.13 **(a)** Fracture group distribution of 11,720 calcaneus fractures.
(b) Sex and fracture group distribution of 11,720 calcaneus fractures.

82-A Calcaneus, avulsion, process, or tuberosity

82-A1
Anterior process
667 fractures
M: 451 (67.62%)
F: 216 (32.38%)
0.18% of total adult fractures
1.73% of adult foot fractures
5.69% of calcaneus
30.77% of type 82-A

82-A1.1

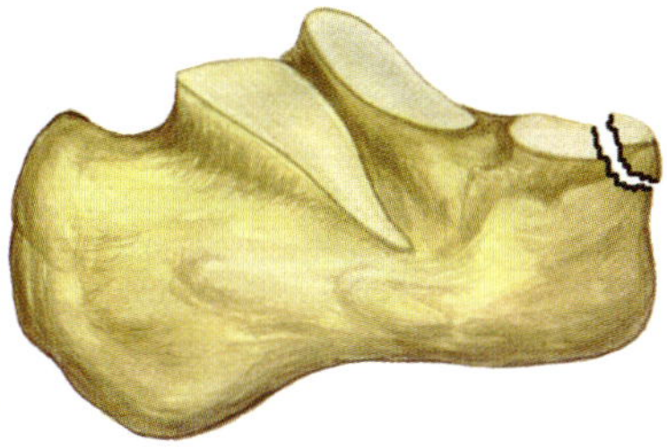

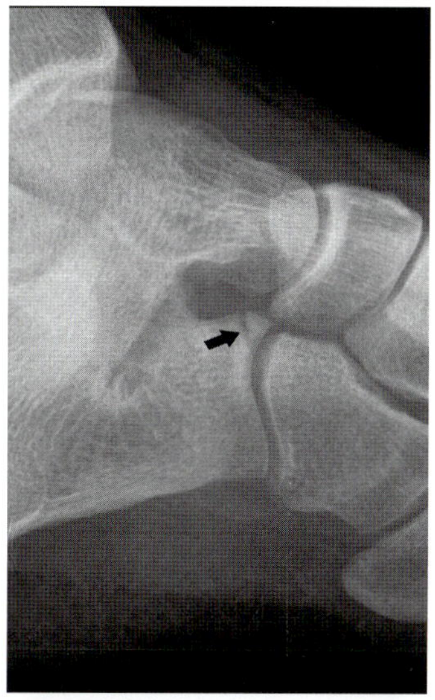

Noncomminuted

82-A1.2

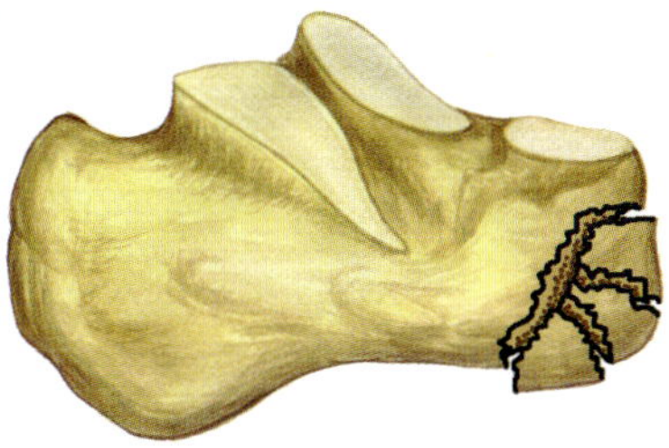

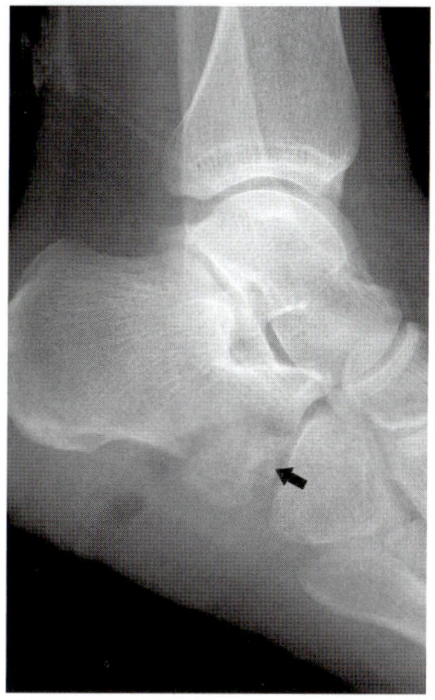

Comminuted

82-A Calcaneus, avulsion, process, or tuberosity

82-A2
Medial, sustentaculum
339 fractures
M: 254 (74.93%)
F: 85 (25.07%)
0.09% of total adult fracture
0.88% of adult foot fracture
2.89% of calcaneus
15.64% of type 82-A

82-A2.1

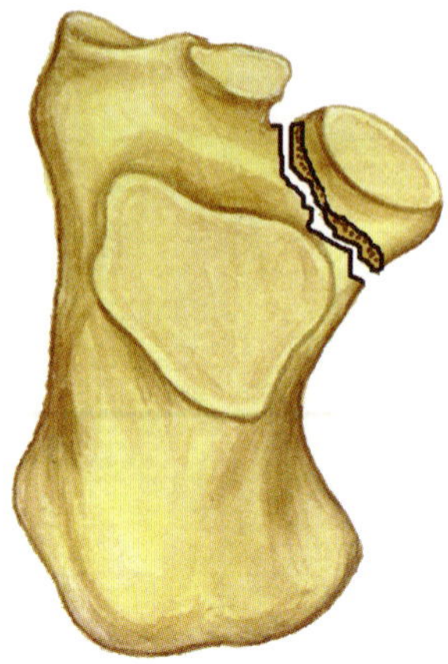

Noncomminuted

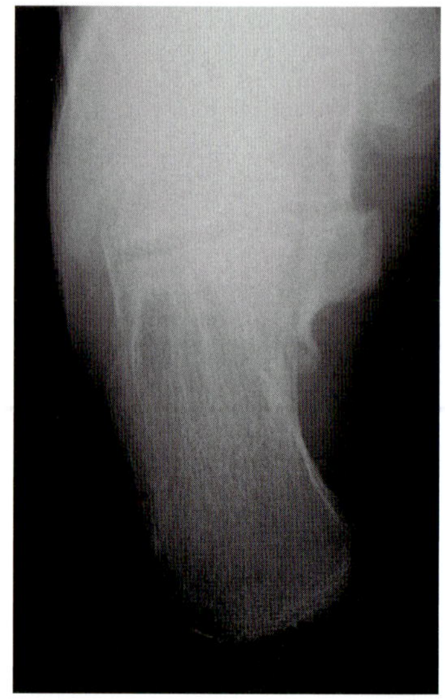

82-A2.2

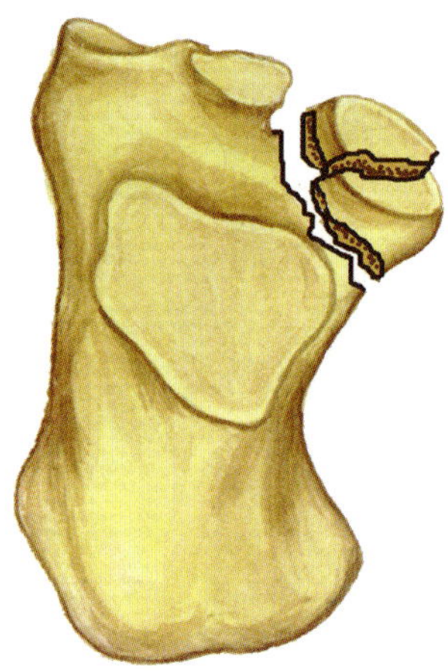

Comminuted

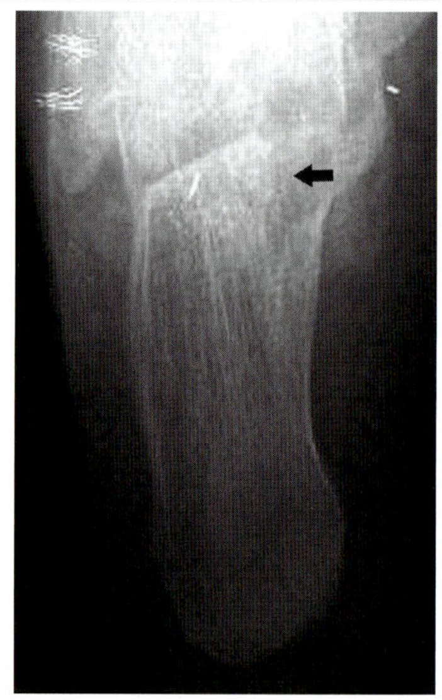

82-A Calcaneus, avulsion, process, or tuberosity

82-A3
Tuberosity
1,162 fractures
M: 927 (79.78%)
F: 235 (20.22%)
0.31% of total adult fracture
3.01% of adult foot fracture
9.91% of calcaneus
53.6% of type 82-A

82-A3.1

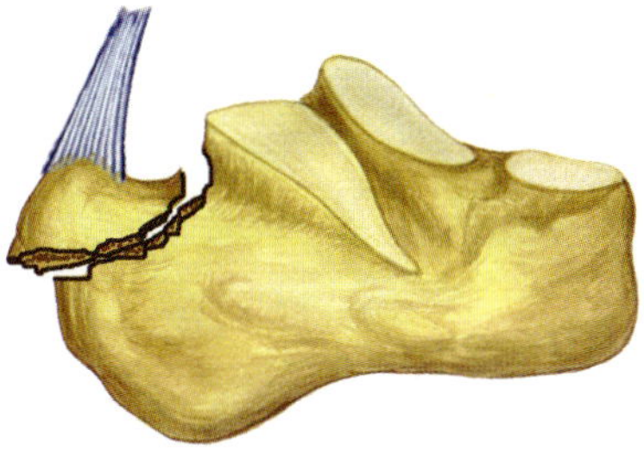

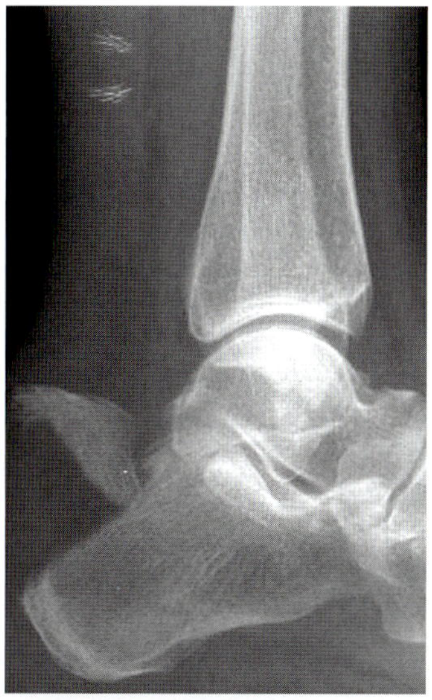

Noncomminuted

82-A3.2

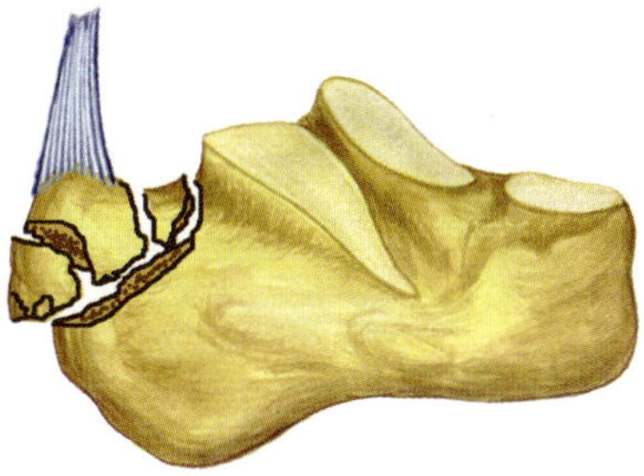

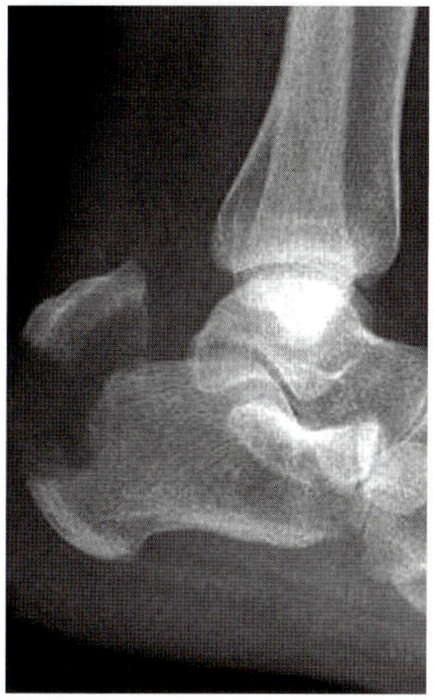

Comminuted

82-B Calcaneus, extra-articular body fractures

82-B1 **Noncomminuted** 1,436 fractures M: 1,161 (80.85%) F: 275 (19.15%) 0.38% of total adult fractures 3.72% of adult foot fractures 12.25% of calcaneus 52.03% of type 82-B	**82-B1** 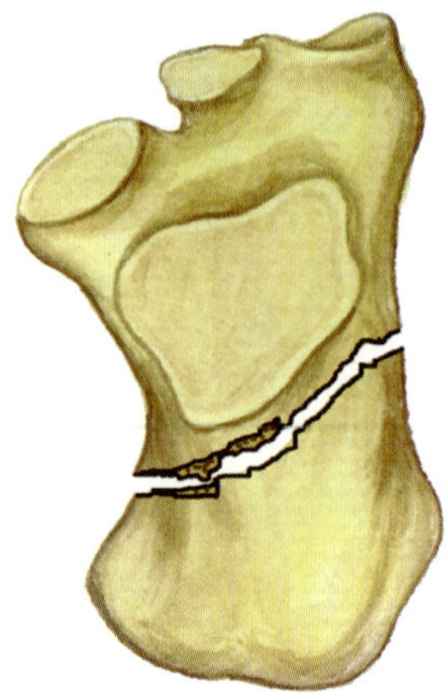 Noncomminuted 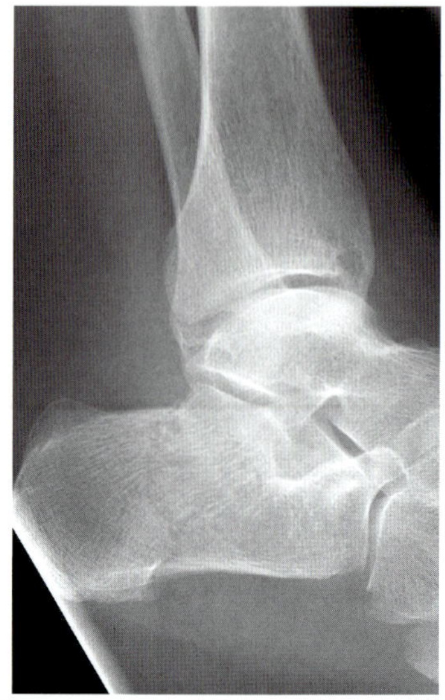
82-B2 **Comminuted** 1,324 fractures M: 1,101 (83.16%) F: 223 (16.84%) 0.35% of total adult fractures 3.43% of adult foot fractures 11.3% of calcaneus 47.97% of type 82-B	**82-B2** 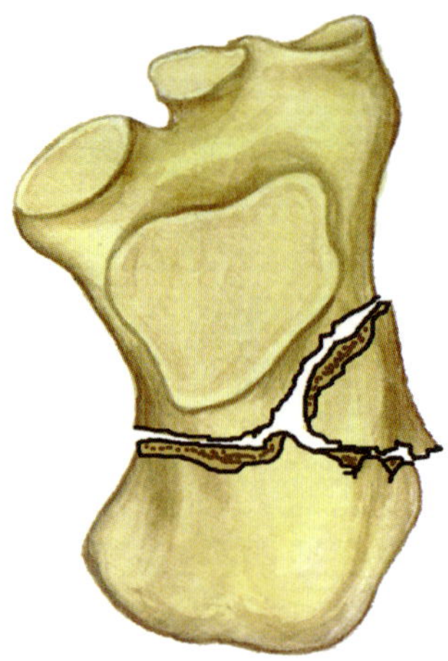 Comminuted 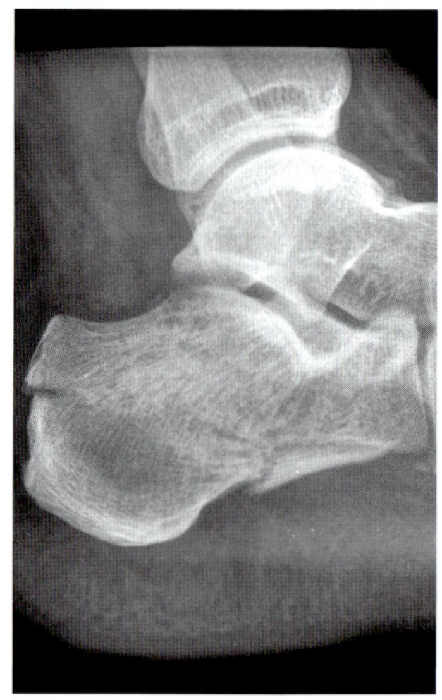

82-C Calcaneus, articular fractures involving posterior facet

82-C
Articular fractures involving posterior facet
6,792 fractures
M: 5,978 (88.02%)
F: 814 (11.98%)
1.81% of total adult fractures
17.58% of adult foot fractures
57.95% of calcaneus

82-C1

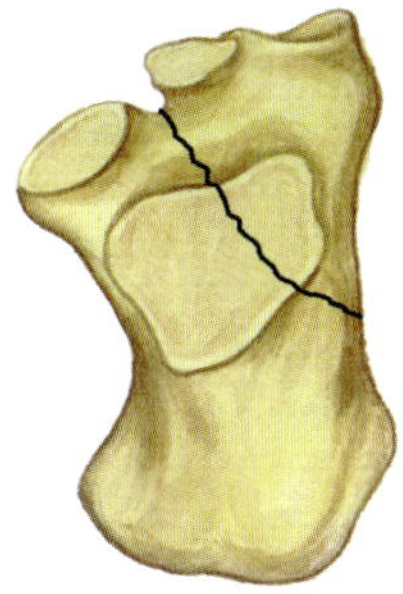
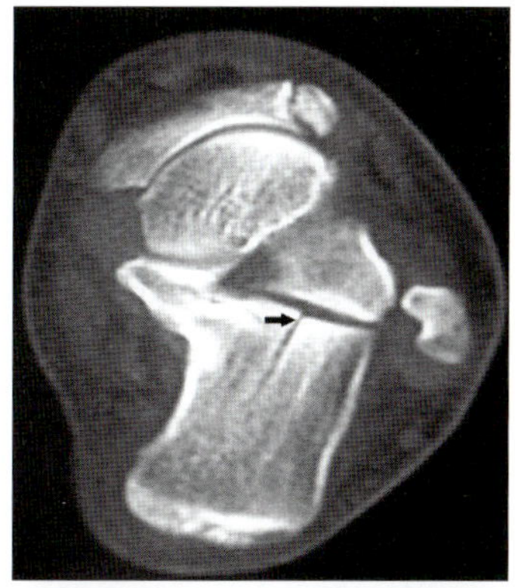

Nondisplaced

82-C2

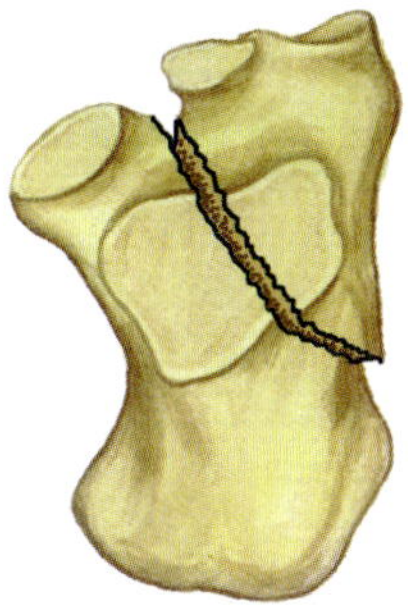
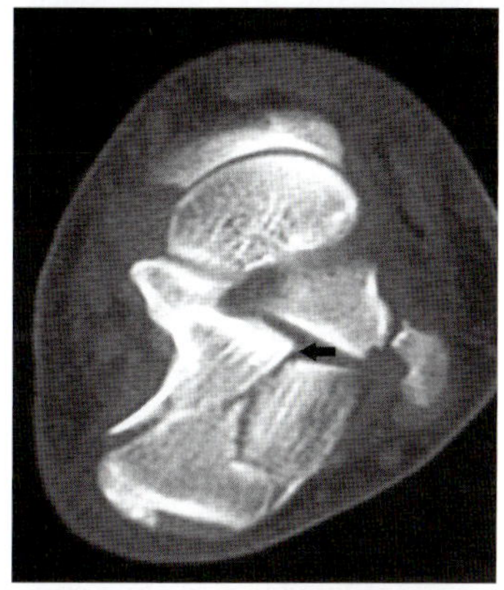

Two-part fractures

82-C3

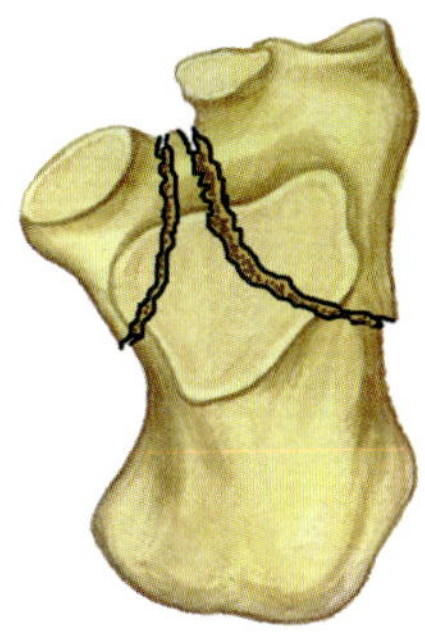
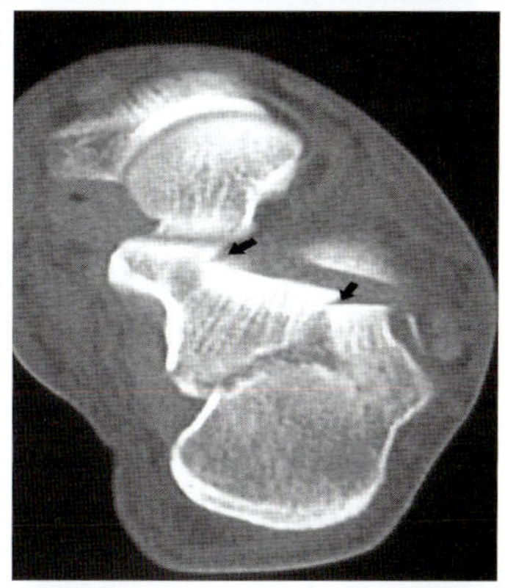

Three-part fractures

82-C4

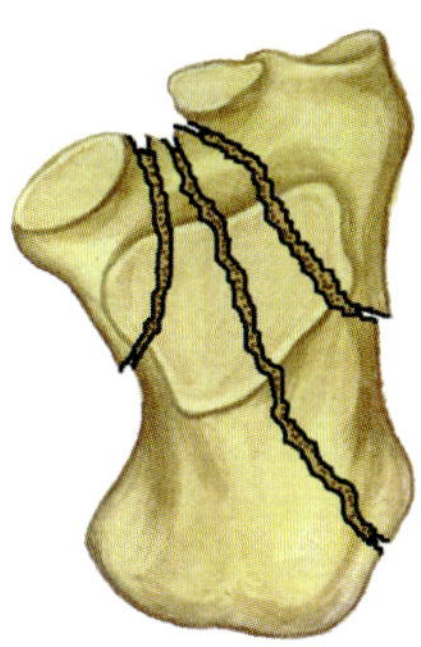
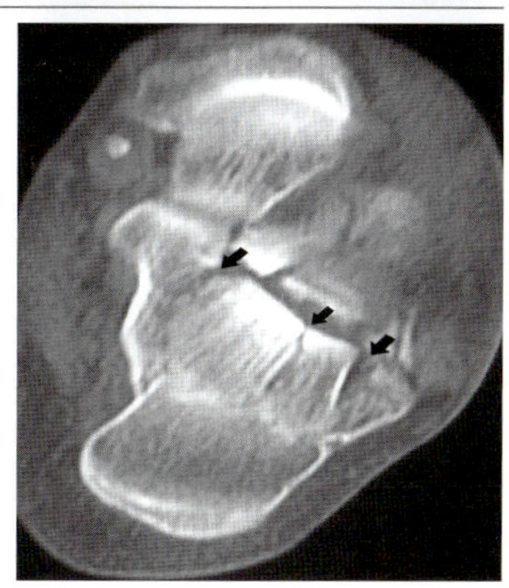

Four or more parts

Injury Mechanism

The patterns of foot fractures vary, depending on the direction of the force that acted on the foot and the position of the foot at the time of injury.

Fractures of the anterior part of the calcaneus usually involve avulsion and depression of the anterior process, with avulsion being the most common fracture of the anterior process. Avulsion fractures of the anterior process usually result from a strong tensile force from the bifurcate ligament, when axial load is applied at the calcaneus while the foot is dorsiflexed and inverted. Depression fractures of the anterior process usually occur as the result of a strong abduction force on the calcaneocuboid articulation surface.

Avulsion fractures of the calcaneal tuberosity tend to occur from avulsion of the Achilles tendon with its bony insertion, due to an abrupt contraction. Less commonly, it can also be the result of a direct force applied on the calcaneus.

Fracture of the sustentaculum tali is usually caused by an axial loading mechanism, which is directed through the laterally situated plantar tuberosity of the calcaneus with the foot inverted. Calcaneal body fractures are the result of axial loading when the heel hits the ground, as occurs in a fall from height; the fracture line usually is vertical or oblique, passing through the back of the subtalar articulation, and producing simple or comminuted fractures.

Most intra-articular fractures of the calcaneus involve the posterior facet of the subtalar joint, and are caused by an axial loading mechanism, as occurs in a fall from height or motor vehicle collision. Besides the axial loading force, rotation forces such as abduction or external rotation forces will also contribute to this type of injury. The axial loading force will produce a fracture line passing along the long axis of the calcaneus, obliquely upward from medial to lateral. If the axial loading force continues, the cortex of the lateral process of the calcaneus may start to rupture, followed by further fragmentation-, depression-, and displacement-type fractures.

9

Diagnosis

Patients with a fracture of the calcaneus may present with pain, edema, ecchymosis, deformity of the heel or plantar arch, and an inability to bear weight on the injured foot. Standard radiographic evaluations, including lateral and axial views of the calcaneus, are helpful in revealing general information about the fracture. Lateral radiographs of the foot are needed to evaluate the Böhler and Gissane angle, as well as dislocation of the subtalar joint. Axial views depict the primary and secondary fracture line, posterior facet step-off, and lateral wall displacement, providing good visualization of the sustentaculum tali. In addition, Broden views of the foot are needed to evaluate the posterior facet of the subtalar joint and can be used as a postoperative evaluation of fracture reduction. CT scans or three-dimensional CT of the calcaneus enable better visualization of the sustentaculum tali and the posterior facet, and are helpful in determining the fracture line and the displacement of the posterior facet. CT can provide valuable information, which is essential in selecting a surgical approach and determining whether the fracture can be reduced and stabilized through internal fixation. For fall injuries, where a foot hits the ground, attention should be given to the presence of a possible hip or spinal injury, because force can transmit along the lower extremities to the pelvis and spine. X-rays can help to rule out other possible injuries and confirm the diagnosis.

- ***Böhler angle:*** formed by the intersection of a line drawn from the tuberosity's most cephalic point to the posterior facet's peak point with a line from the latter to the most cephalic part of the anterior process of the calcaneus; a normal range for this angle is 25 to 40 degrees.

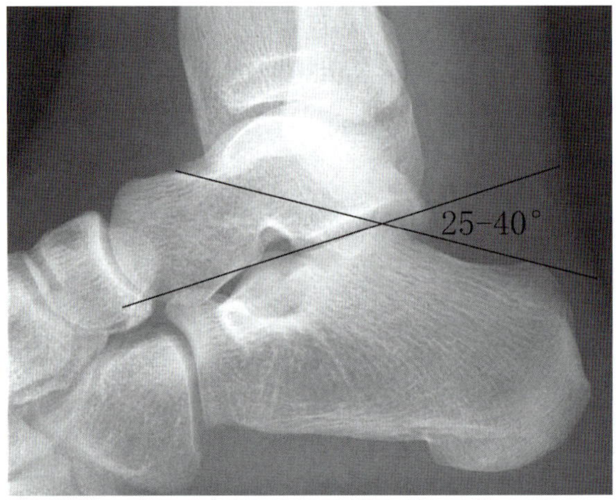

- ***Gissane angle:*** formed by the intersection of a line drawn along the dorsal aspect of the anterior process of the calcaneus, and a line drawn along the dorsal slope of the posterior facet; a normal value of the Gissane angle is 120 to 145 degrees.

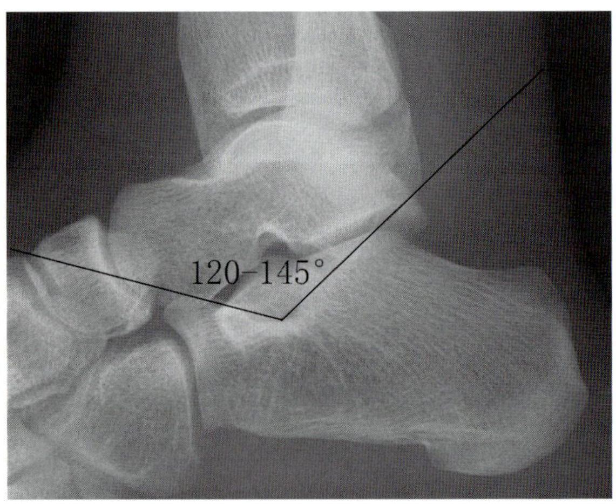

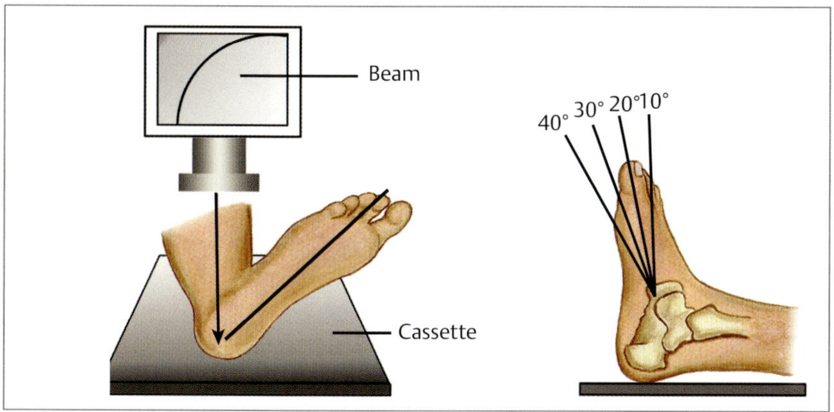

- ***Broden views of the foot*** (see above)**:** internally rotating the leg 45 degrees with the ankle in a neutral position. The beam may then be directed toward the lateral malleolus and advanced cephalad at intervals of 10, 20, 30, and 40 degrees to fully evaluate the posterior facet.

Treatment

The goal of treatment for calcaneal fractures is to restore the congruity of the subtalar joint and Böhler angle, to restore the height and width of the calcaneus as far as possible, and to maintain normal arch height and weight-bearing functionality. Nondisplaced calcaneal fractures only require nonsurgical treatment, while avulsion fractures of the tuberosity and displaced intra-articular fractures should be treated surgically. Commonly used surgical options include open reduction with internal fixation, and minimally invasive reduction and internal fixation. According to fracture location and pattern, multiple internal fixation devices can be selected, such as the H- plate, Y-plate, 3.5-mm constructive plate, anatomical plate, etc. Noncomminuted calcaneal fractures with a transverse fracture line can be treated with percutaneous reduction by leverage. However, internal fixation is still needed in some cases, even if reduction was obtained by percutaneous leverage. A group of talented orthopaedic surgeons led by Dr. Zhang Yingze has developed a minimally invasive internal fixation technique with plates, screws, and a compression system to treat calcaneal fractures and obtain a favorable clinical outcome.

Other Classifications for Calcaneal Fractures

Traditional Classification: Essex-Lopresti Classification

- Type I: extra-articular calcaneal fractures, accounting for 42.05% of calcaneal fractures (so-called tongue-type injury)
- Type II: intra-articular fractures involving the subtalar joint, accounting for 57.95% of calcaneal fractures (so-called joint depression–type injury, equivalent to type 82-C of the OTA classification)

Sanders Classification

Sanders classification of calcaneal fractures is based on fracture pattern—essentially, the number and location of calcaneal posterior facet articular fracture fragments through the widest portion of the posterior facet as seen on coronal CT. Sander classified calcaneal fractures into four types.

- *Type I*: fractures are nondisplaced.
- *Type II*: fractures are two-part fractures of the posterior facet, and are further classified into three subtypes—IIa, IIb, and IIc—based on location of the fracture line.
- *Type III*: fractures are three-part fractures of the posterior facet, and are further classified into three subtypes—IIIab, IIIac, and IIIbc—based on location and extension of the depression.
- *Type IV*: fractures are highly comminuted with four or more fractures of the posterior facet.

9

Sanders classification (intra-articular calcaneal fractures)		
Type I 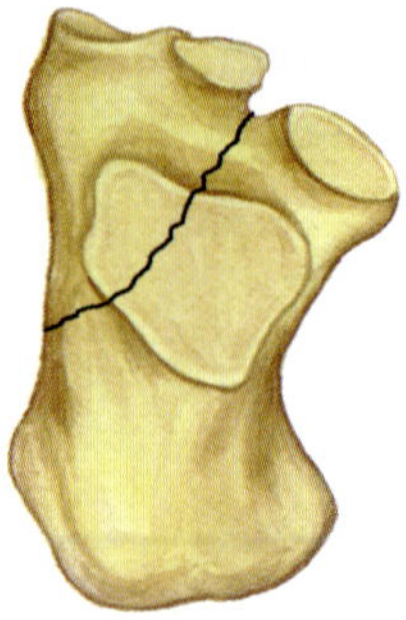 Nondisplaced	**Ia** 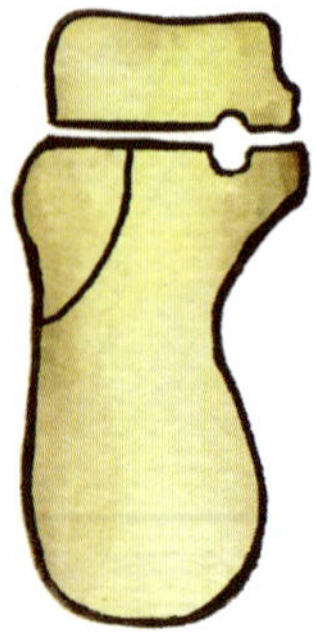	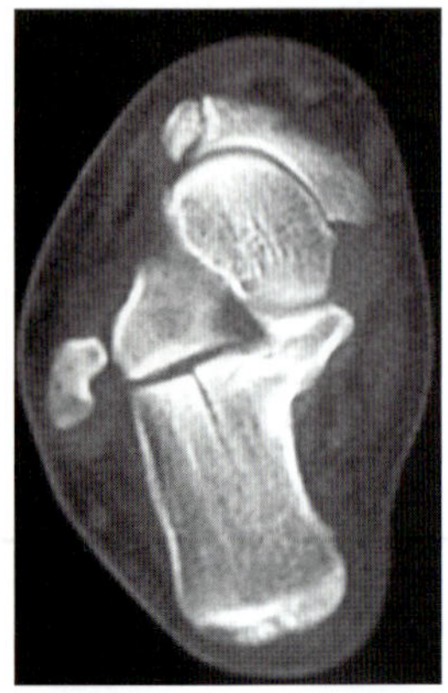
Type II 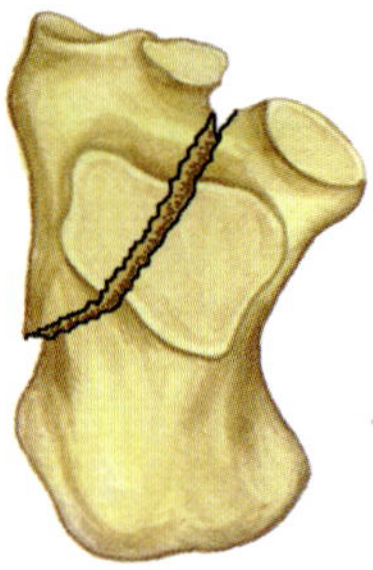 Two-part fractures of the posterior facet	**IIa** 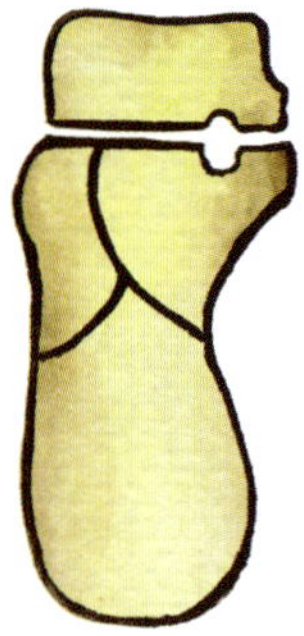	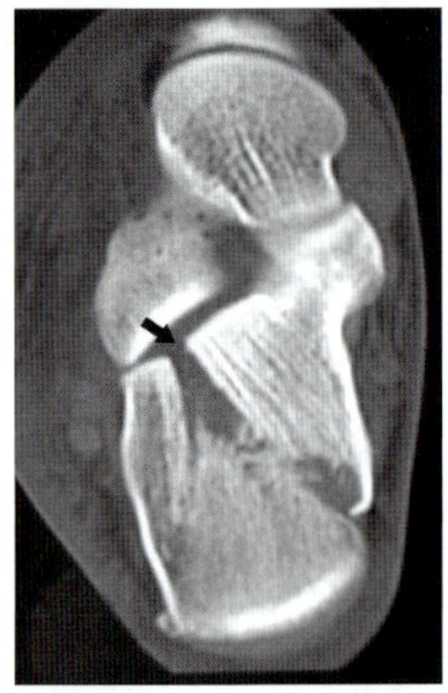
	IIb 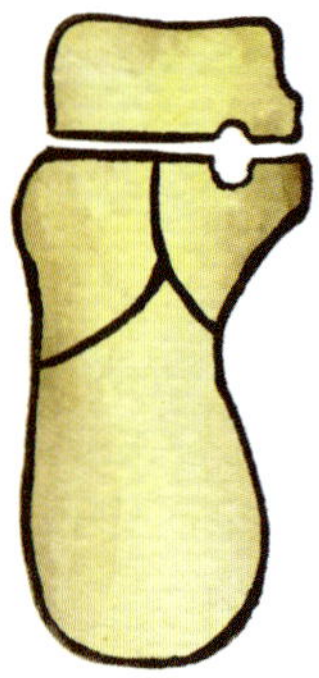	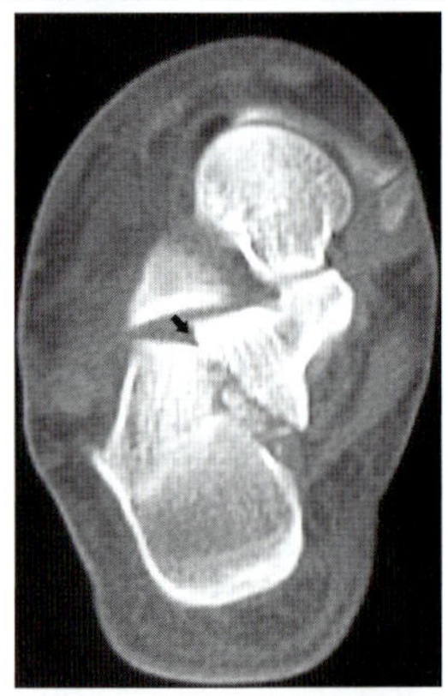
	IIc 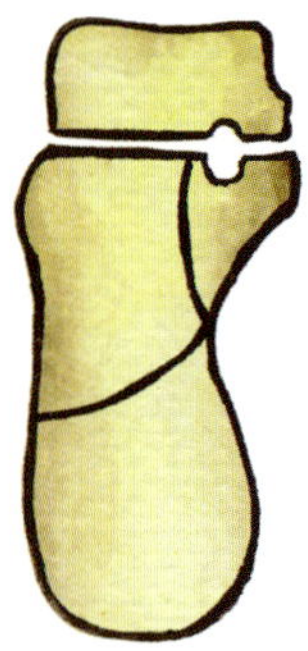	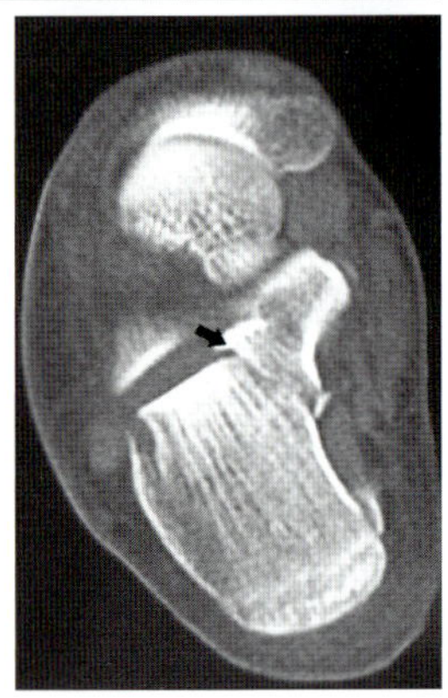

Sanders classification (intra-articular calcaneal fractures)

Type	Subtype	Diagram	CT
Type III 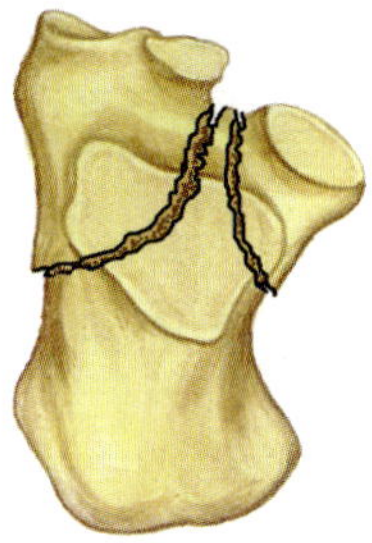 Three-part fractures of the posterior facet	**IIIab**	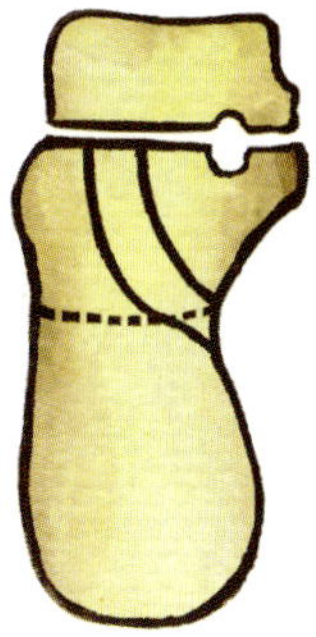	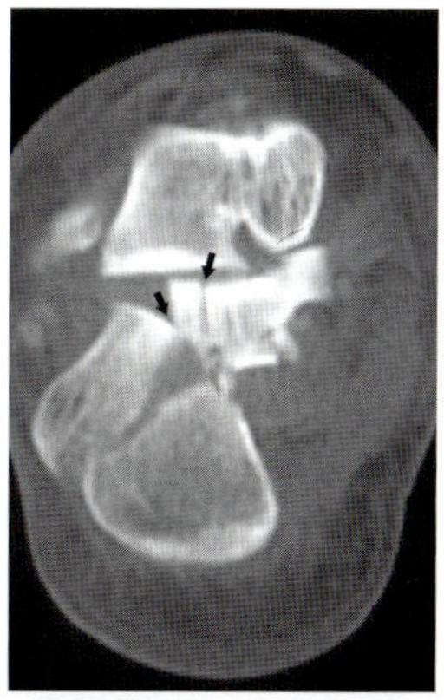
	IIIac	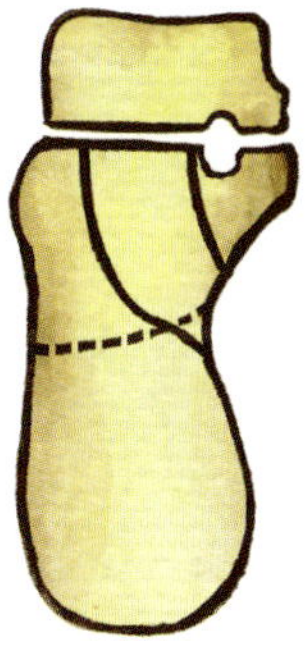	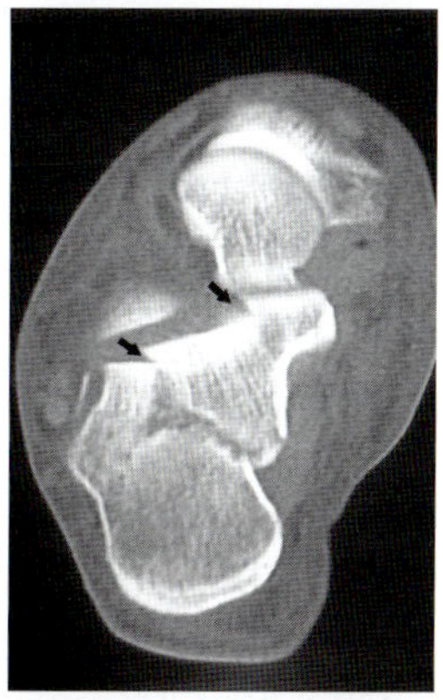
	IIIbc	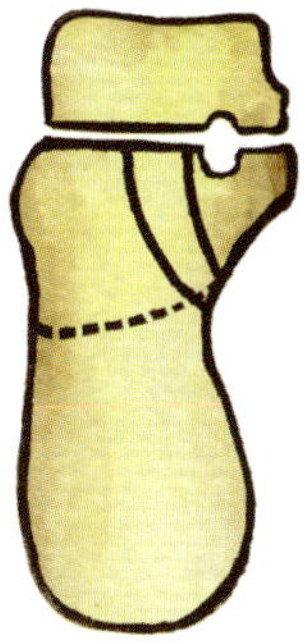	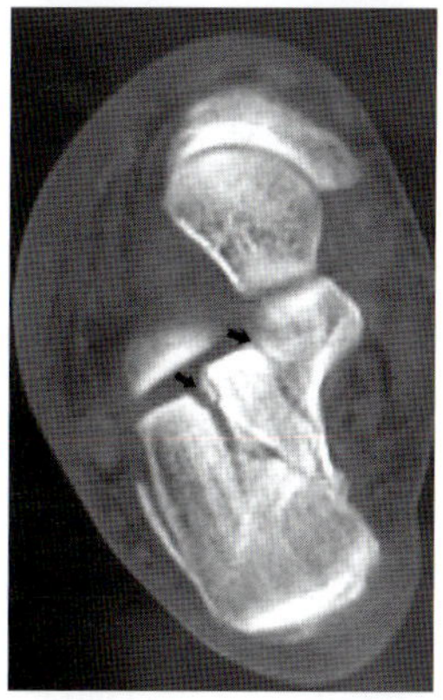
Type IV 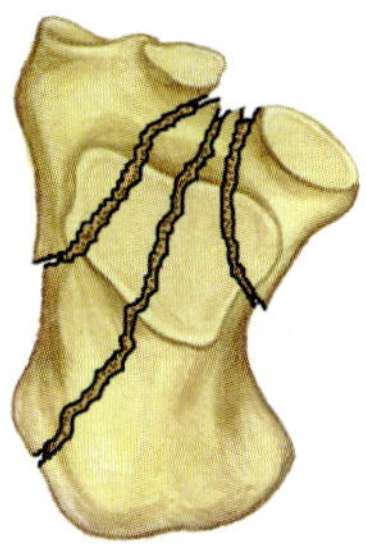 Highly comminuted fractures with four or more fragments of the posterior facet		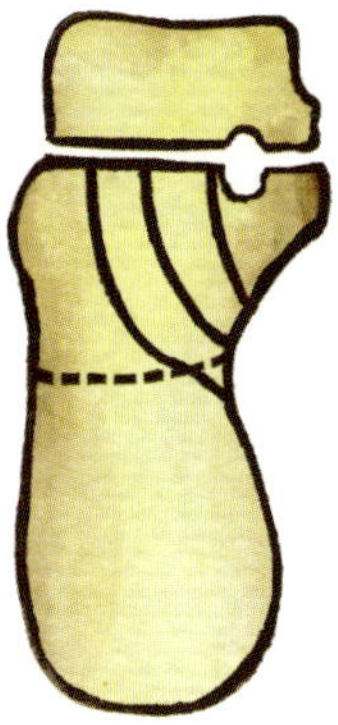	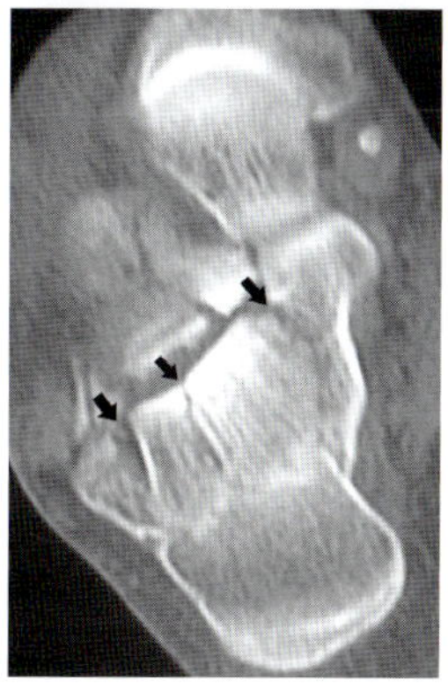

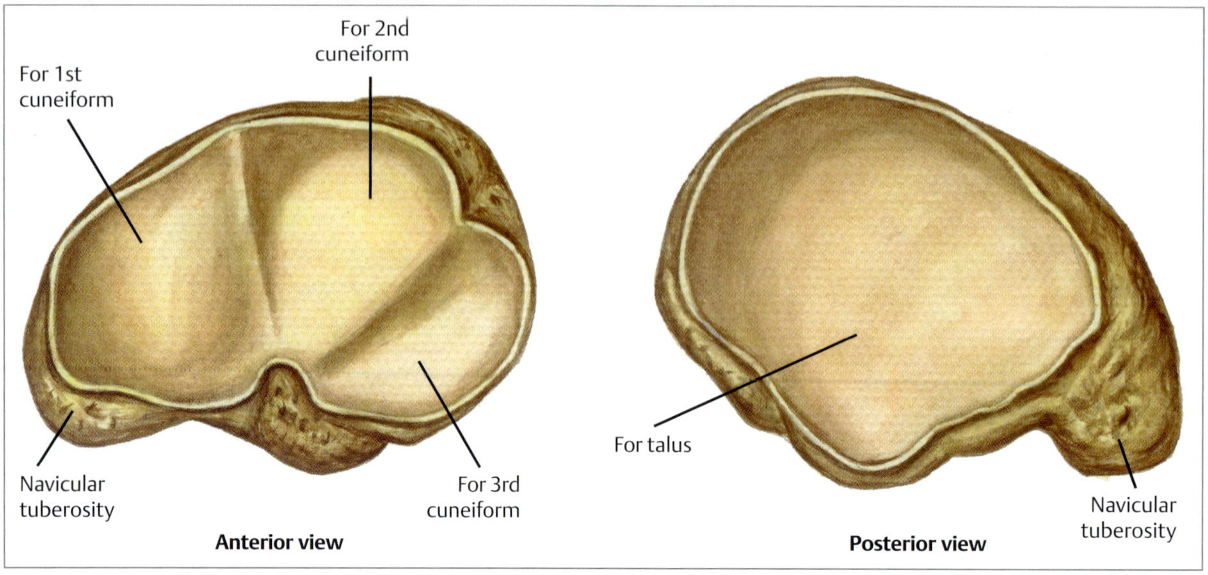

Plate 9.8

Fractures of the Tarsal Navicular Bone (Segment 83)

Anatomical Features

The tarsal navicular is a flattened, oval, boat-shaped bone between the talus posteriorly and the three cuneiform bones anteriorly. It is wide on the medial side and narrow on the lateral side. The posterior surface of the tarsal navicular is oval and concave, and articulates with the rounded head of the talus. The anterior surface is convex from side to side and has three facets for articulation with the three cuneiform bones. The dorsal surface is convex and rough for the attachment of a number of ligaments, such as the talonavicular ligament, dorsal cuneonavicular ligaments, and the dorsal cuboideonavicular ligament. The plantar surface is concave and irregular. The medial surface presents a rounded tuberosity, the lower part of which gives attachment to part of the tendon of the tibialis posterior. The rough lateral surface is the attachment site of the calcaneonavicular band of the bifurcated ligament, and occasionally presents a small facet for articulation with the cuboid bone. The navicular bone, situated at the middle of the tarsus, is on the top of the medial longitudinal arch, and transmits the entire body weight from the ankle joint to the first three metatarsal bones (**Plate 9.8**).

OTA Classification of Tarsal Navicular Fractures

Based on OTA classification, the tarsal navicular is coded as the number 83 for its anatomical location. Tarsal navicular fractures are classified into two types: 83-A, noncomminuted; and 83-B, comminuted (**Plate 9.9**).

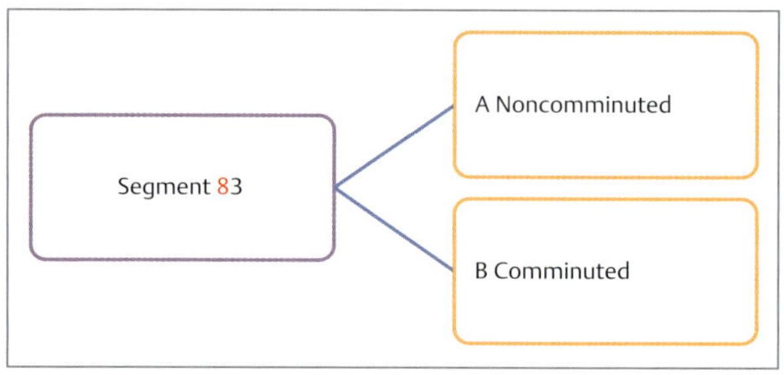

Plate 9.9

Clinical Epidemiologic Features of Tarsal Navicular (Segment 83)

A total of 1,017 adult patients with 1,022 tarsal navicular fractures were treated in 83 hospitals in China over a 2-year period from 2010 to 2011. All cases were reviewed and statistically studied, including 509 patients with fractures on the left side, 503 on the right, and 5 bilateral. There were 590 males and 427 females, with a male-to-female ratio of 1.38:1.

Epidemiologic features of tarsal navicular fractures are as follows:

- More males than females
- The high risk age group is 31–35 years; the age group 31–35 years is highest for males while 26–30 years and 31–35 years are highest for females.
- The most common fracture type is type 83-A.

Tarsal Navicular Fractures (Segment 83) by Sex

Table 9.14 Sex distribution of 1,017 patients with tarsal navicular fractures

Sex	Number of patients	Percentage (%)
Male	590	58.01
Female	427	41.99
Total	1,017	100.00

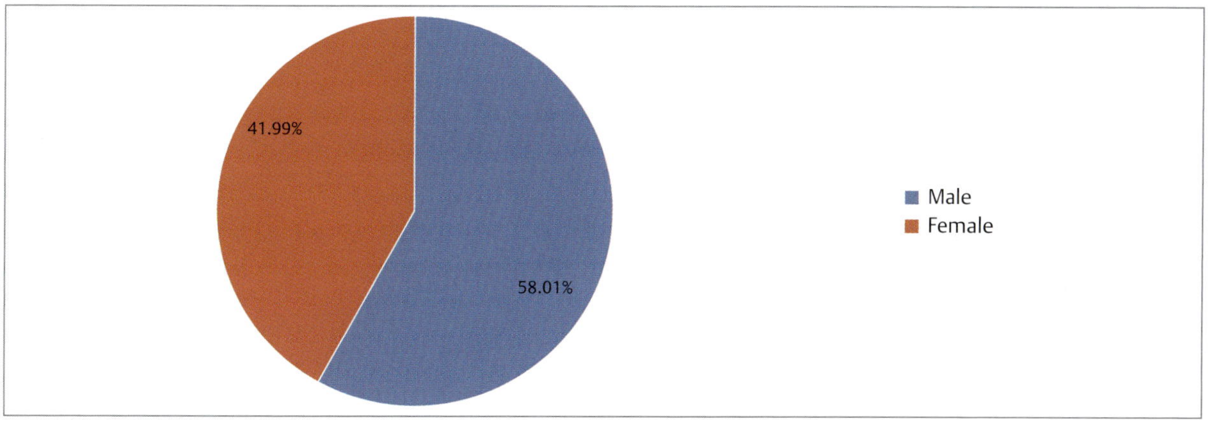

Fig 9.14 Sex distribution of 1,017 patients with tarsal navicular fractures.

9

Tarsal Navicular Fractures (Segment 83) by Age Group

Table 9.15 Age and sex distribution of 1,017 patients with tarsal navicular fractures

Age group (years)	Male	Female	Number of patients	Percentage (%)
16–20	60	32	92	9.05
21–25	72	41	113	11.11
26–30	67	48	115	11.31
31–35	79	48	127	12.49
36–40	72	45	117	11.50
41–45	67	44	111	10.91
46–50	58	40	98	9.64
51–55	49	37	86	8.46
56–60	28	28	56	5.51
61–65	8	26	34	3.34
66–70	9	16	25	2.46
71–75	7	10	17	1.67
76–80	8	10	18	1.77
81–85	4	2	6	0.59
≥86	2	0	2	0.20
Total	590	427	1,017	100.00

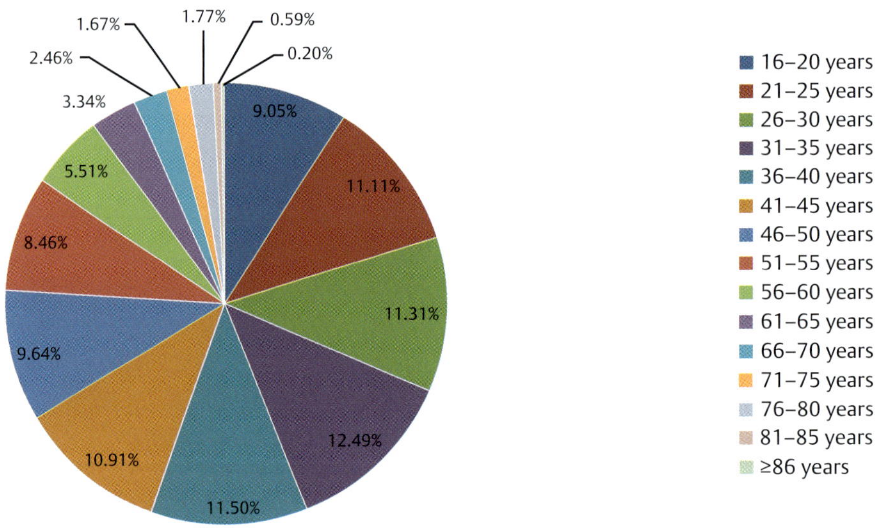

a

Fig. 9.15 **(a)** Age distribution of 1,017 patients with tarsal navicular fractures.

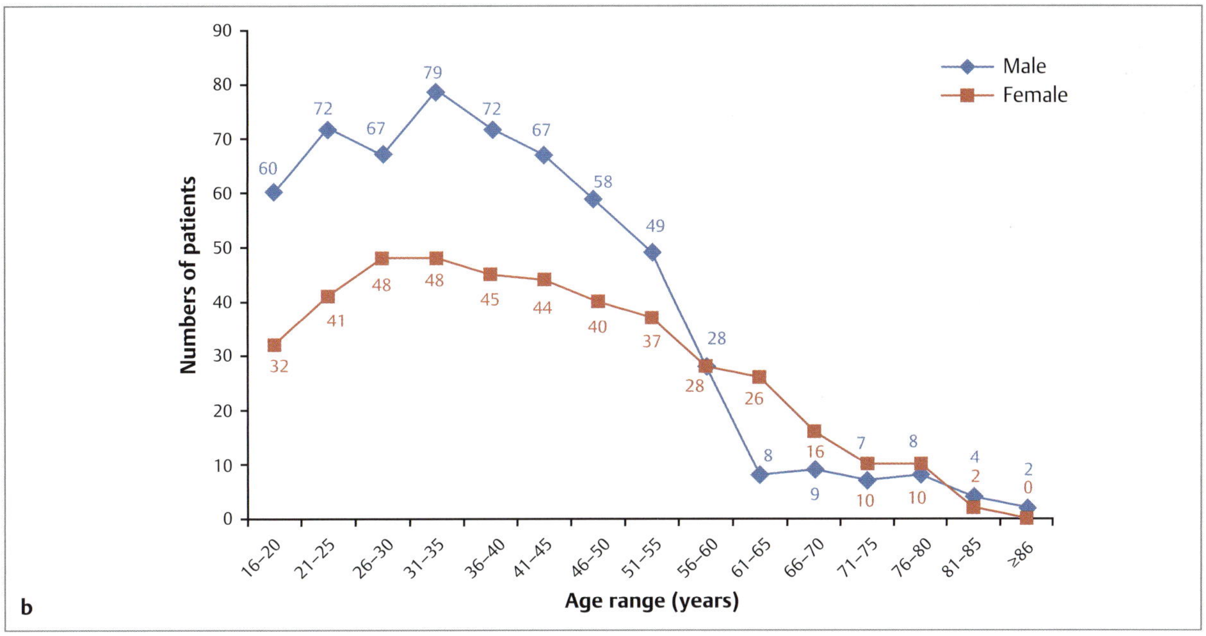

Fig. 9.15 (*continued*) **(b)** Age and sex distribution of 1,017 patients with tarsal navicular fractures.

Tarsal Navicular Fractures (Segment 83) by Fracture Type

Table 9.16 Sex and fracture type distribution of 1,022 tarsal navicular fractures

Fracture type	Male	Female	Number of fractures	Percentage of tarsal navicular fractures (%)
83-A	449	368	817	79.94
83-B	145	60	205	20.06
Total	594	428	1,022	100.00

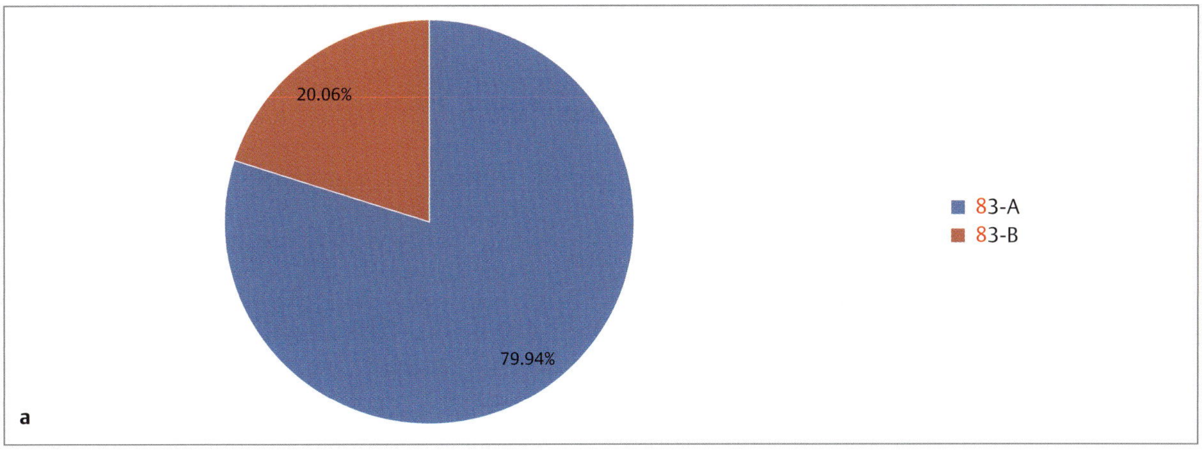

Fig. 9.16 **(a)** Fracture type distribution of 1,022 tarsal navicular fractures. (*Continued*)

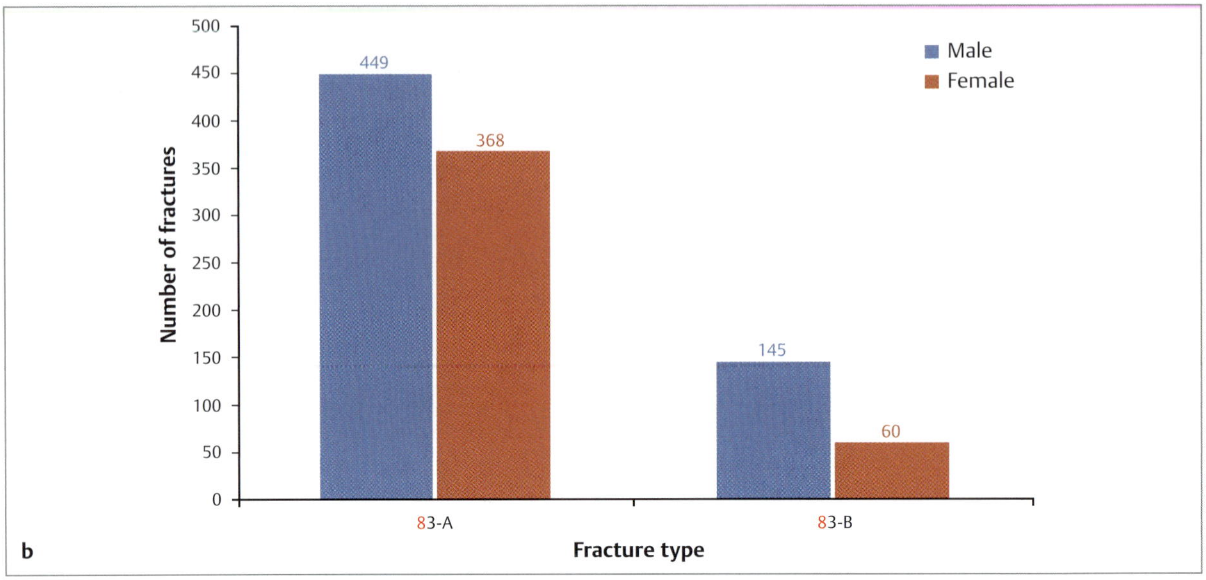

Fig. 9.16 (*continued*) **(b)** Sex and fracture type distribution of 1,022 tarsal navicular fractures.

83 Tarsal navicular fractures

83-A
Noncomminuted
817 fractures
M: 449 (54.96%)
F: 368 (45.04%)
0.22% of total adult fractures
2.11% of adult foot fractures
79.94% of tarsal navicular

83-A

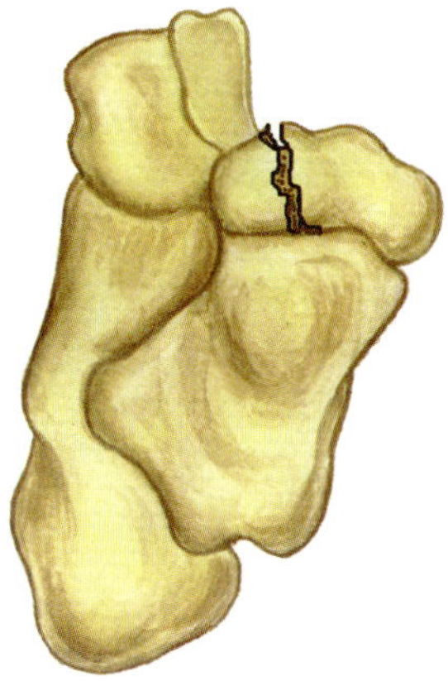

Noncomminuted

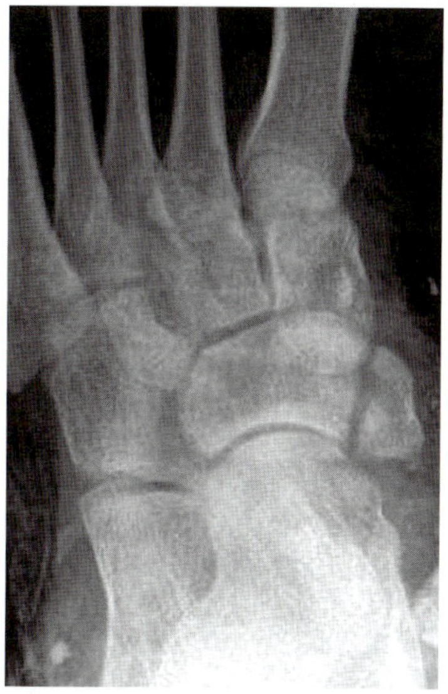

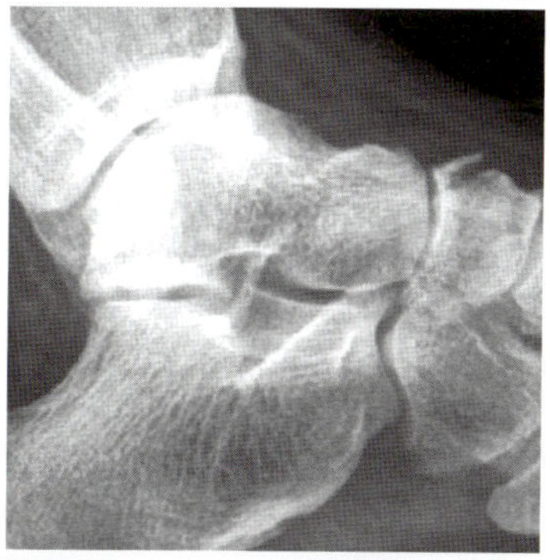

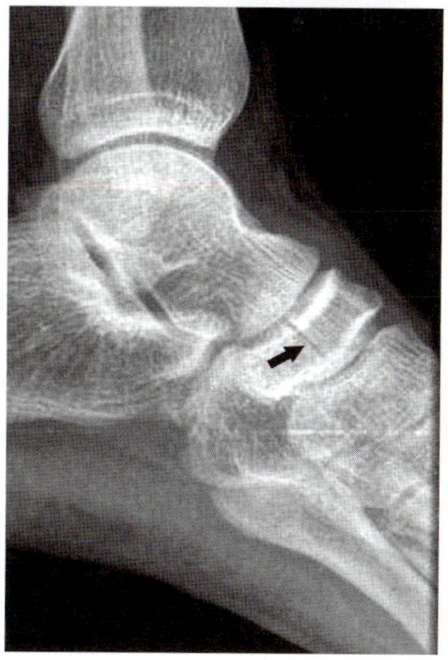

83 Tarsal navicular fracture

83-B
Comminuted
205 fractures
M: 145 (70.73%)
F: 60 (29.27%)
0.05% of total adult fractures
0.53% of adult foot fractures
20.06% of tarsal navicular

83-B

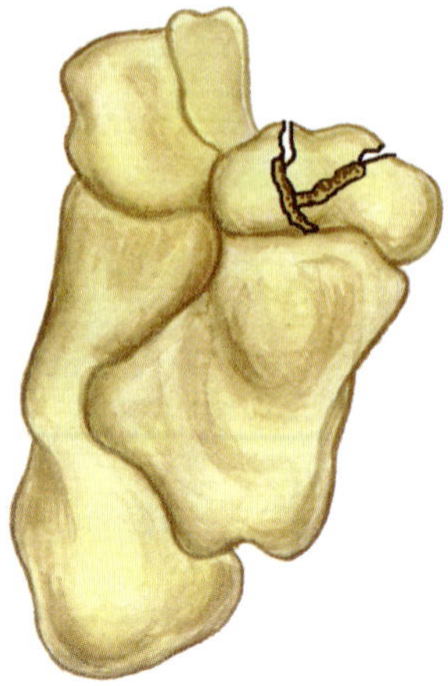

Comminuted

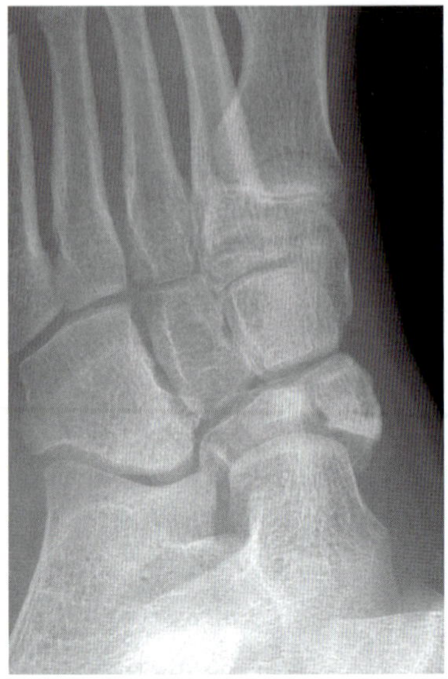

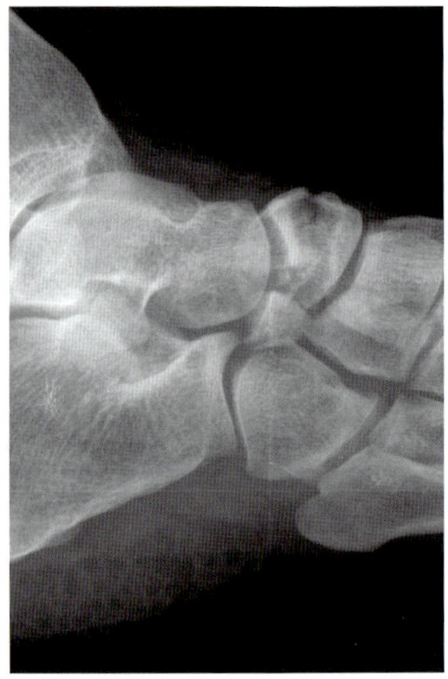

Injury Mechanism

Avulsion fracture is the most common fracture of the navicular bone. Dorsal lip fracture typically occurs as the result of tension of the dorsal talonavicular ligament, secondary to plantar flexion with inversion or eversion injuries. Navicular tuberosity avulsion fractures typically result from sudden eversion and/or valgus injuries, which lead to a sudden increased stress on the posterior tibial tendon. Usually, cuboid compression fractures occur concomitantly due to the resulting compression of the lateral column and tensile stretching of the medial column. Depending on the direction of the impacting force, navicular body fractures can occur in the horizontal, coronal, or sagittal plane. Subluxation of the talonavicular joint may present if fractures are displaced.

Diagnosis

Patients usually present with pain, swelling over the navicular bone, partial-to-complete limitation of motion, and deformity if there is marked fracture displacement or dislocation. Standard X-rays including AP, oblique, and lateral views of the foot generally demonstrate fracture. Attention should be given to the position of the navicular bone in relation to its adjacent tarsal bones. CT scans or MRI should be considered if indicated.

Treatment

Nondisplaced navicular fractures can be treated with short-leg casting for 6 weeks. If fractures involve 20–30% of the articulation surface, or the proximal tuberosity has been displaced more than 5 mm, open reduction and internal fixation with K-wire or screws should be considered. Displaced body fractures of the navicular bone require open reduction and internal fixation with screws. Arthrodesis of navicular articulations are indicated in severely comminuted intra-articular fractures.

Cuboid Fractures (84)

Anatomical Features

The cuboid bone is irregularly cubical in shape, and is situated at the lateral side of the foot. The posterior surface has a saddle-shaped articular surface, for articulation with the anterior surface of the calcaneus; its inferomedial angle projects backward as a process that underlies and supports the anterior end of the calcaneus. On the middle and upper part of the medial surface, there is a smooth oval facet, for articulation with the third cuneiform. The remainder of its surface is rough, and is the attachment site of the strong interosseous cuneocuboid ligament and cuboideonavicular ligament. The lateral surface presents a deep groove formed by the beginning of the peroneal sulcus. The rough dorsal surface is the attachment site of multiple ligaments: the dorsal calcaneocuboid ligament, dorsal cuboideonavicular ligament, and dorsal cuneocuboid ligament. The plantar surface has a prominent ridge to which the long plantar ligament is attached; the ridge ends laterally in an eminence, the cuboid tuberosity (**Plate 9.10**).

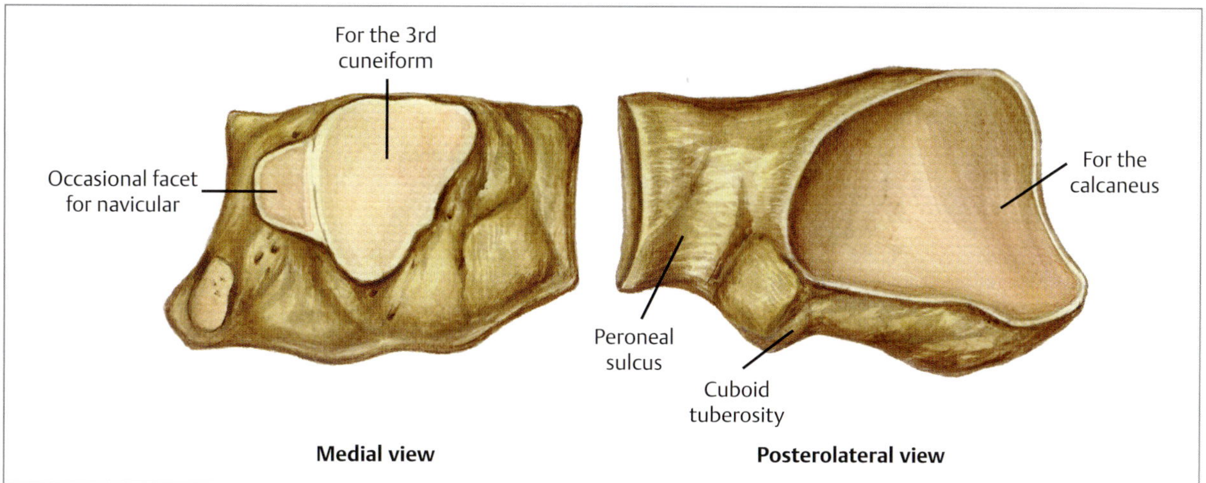

Plate 9.10

9

OTA Classification of Cuboid Fractures

Based on OTA classification, the cuboid bone is coded as the number 84 for its anatomical location. Cuboid fractures are classified into two types: 84-A, noncomminuted; and 84-B, comminuted (**Plate 9.11**).

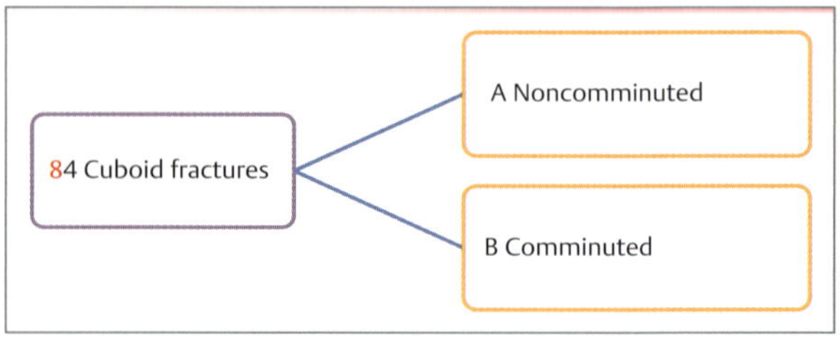

Plate 9.11

Clinical Epidemiologic Features of Cuboid Fractures

A total of 532 adult patients with 532 cuboid fractures were treated in 83 hospitals in China over a 2-year period from 2010 to 2011. All cases were reviewed and statistically studied, including 260 patients with fractures on the left side, 272 on the right, and no bilateral fractures. There were 310 males and 222 females, with a male-to-female ratio of 1.40:1.

Epidemiologic features of cuboid fractures are as follows:

- More males than females
- The high-risk age group is between ages 36 and 40, with ages 36–40 being the highest for males and 26–30 the highest for females
- The most common fracture type is type 84-A.

Cuboid Fractures (Segment 84) by Sex

Table 9.17 Sex distribution of 532 patients with cuboid fractures

Sex	Number of patients	Percentage (%)
Male	310	58.27
Female	222	41.73
Total	532	100.00

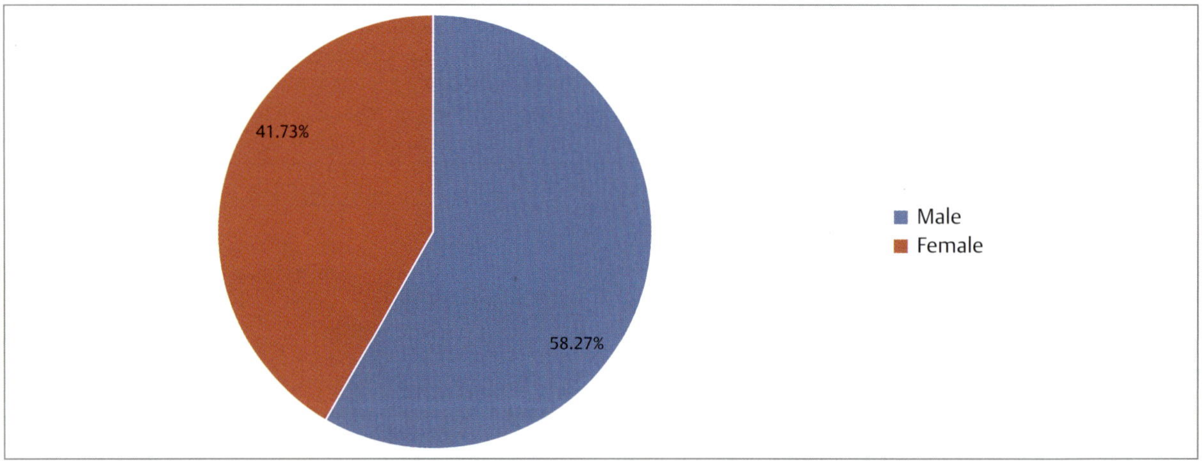

Fig. 9.17 Sex distribution of 532 patients with cuboid fractures.

Cuboid Fractures (Segment 84) by Age Group

Table 9.18 Age and sex distribution of 532 patients with cuboid fractures

Age group (years)	Male	Female	Number of patients	Percentage (%)
16–20	22	9	31	5.83
21–25	26	13	39	7.33
26–30	41	27	68	12.78
31–35	36	20	56	10.53
36–40	44	25	69	12.97
41–45	30	25	55	10.34
46–50	33	21	54	10.15
51–55	18	21	39	7.33
56–60	19	26	45	8.46
61–65	17	16	33	6.20
66–70	8	6	14	2.63
71–75	3	7	10	1.88
76–80	10	3	13	2.44
81–85	2	3	5	0.94
≥86	1	0	1	0.19
Total	310	222	532	100.00

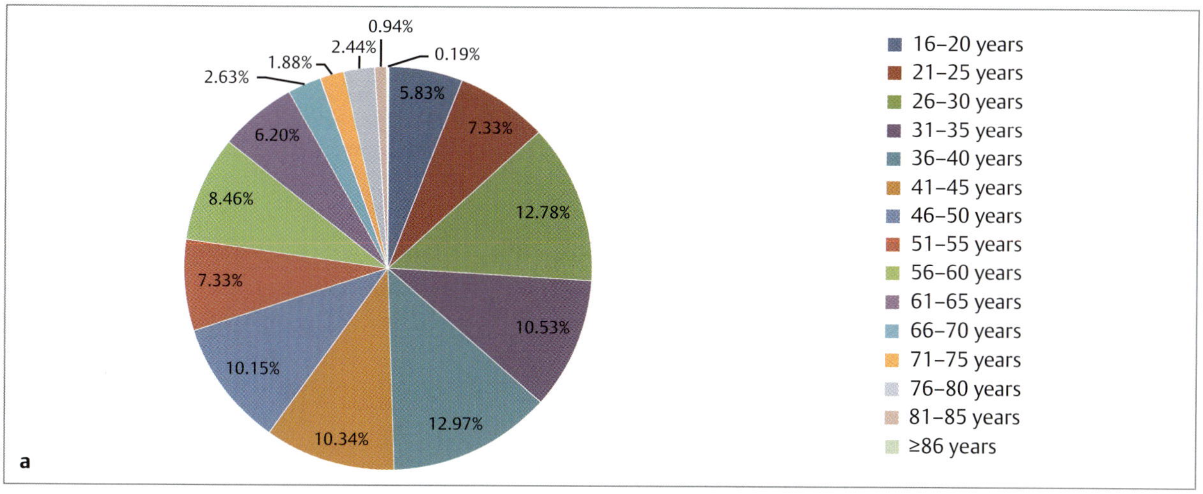

Fig. 9.18 **(a)** Age distribution of 532 patients with cuboid fractures. (*Continued*)

9

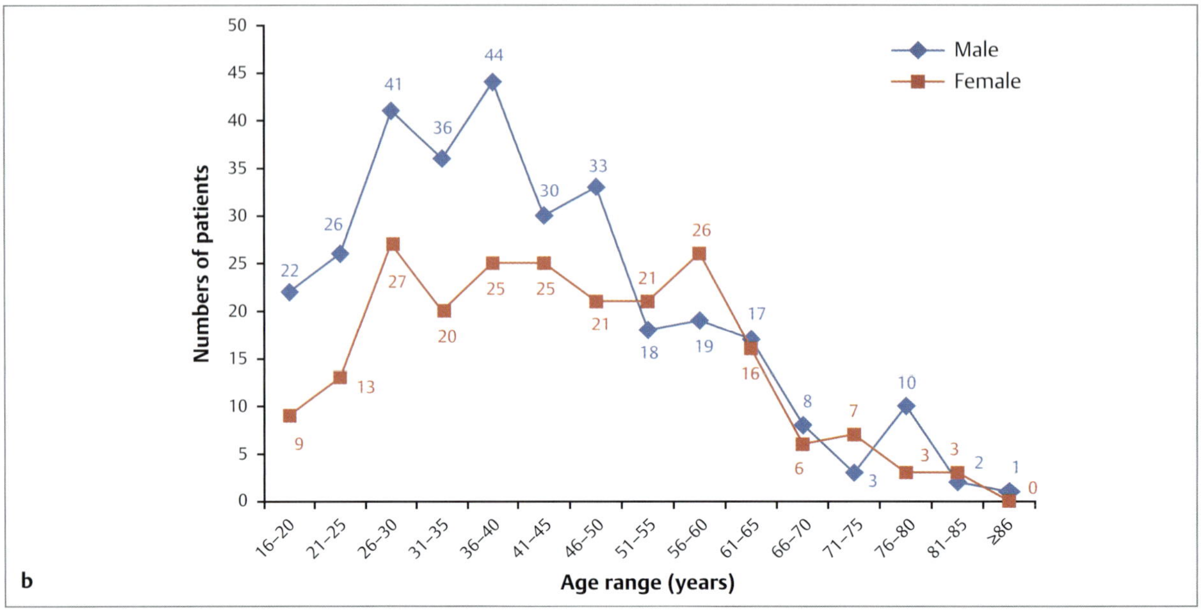

Fig. 9.18 (*continued*) **(b)** Age and sex distribution of 532 patients with cuboid fractures.

Cuboid Fractures (Segment 84) by Fracture Type

Table 9.19 Sex and fracture type distribution of 532 cuboid fractures

Fracture type	Male	Female	Number of fractures	Percentage (%)	Percentage of foot fractures (%)
84-A	264	179	443	83.27	1.15
84-B	46	43	89	16.73	0.23
Total	310	222	532	100.00	1.38

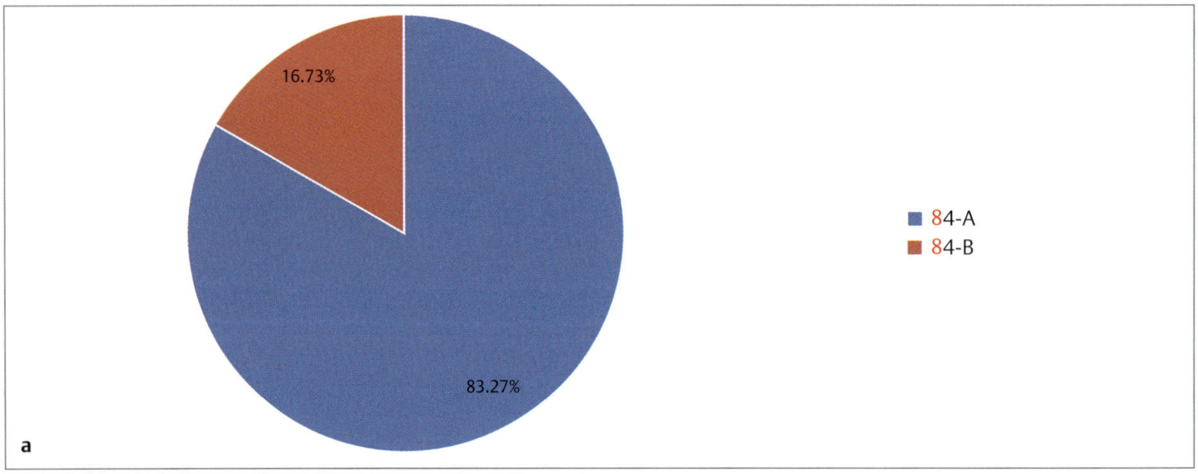

Fig. 9.19 **(a)** Fracture type distribution of 532 cuboid fractures.

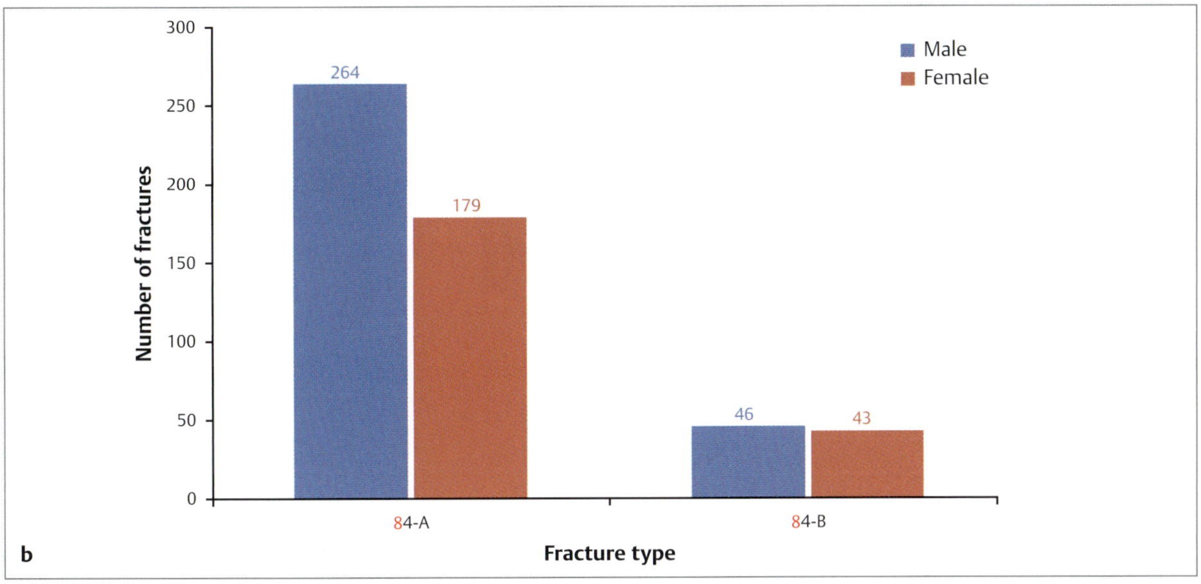

Fig. 9.19 (*continued*) **(b)** Sex and fracture type distribution of 532 cuboid fractures.

84 Cuboid fractures

84-A
Noncomminuted
443 fractures
M: 264 (59.59%)
F: 179 (40.41%)
0.12% of total adult fractures
1.15% of adult foot fractures
83.27% of cuboid

84-A

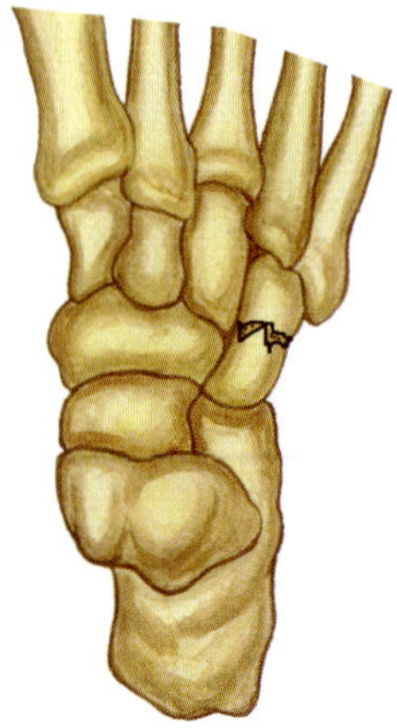

Noncomminuted

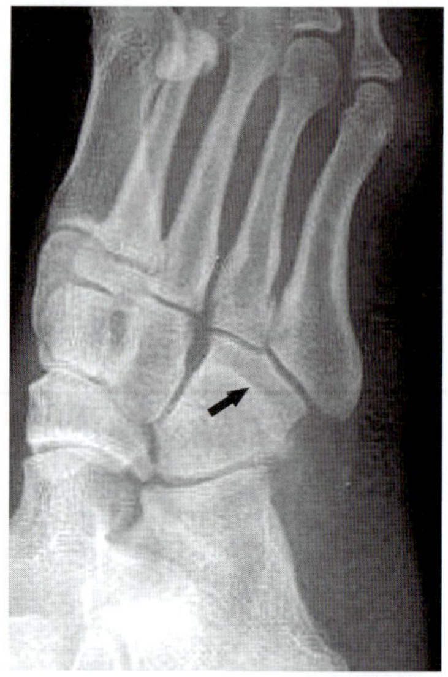

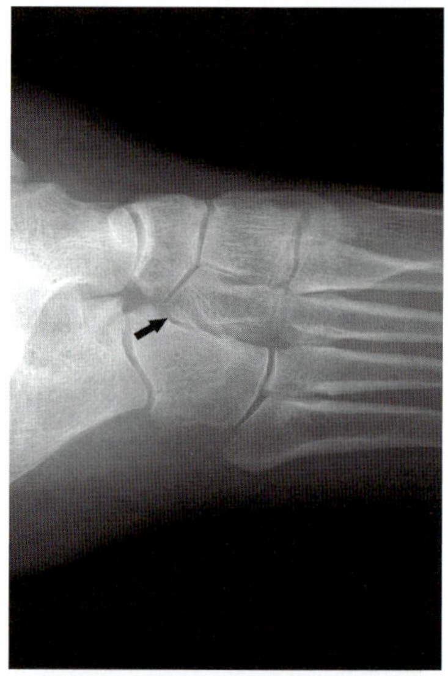

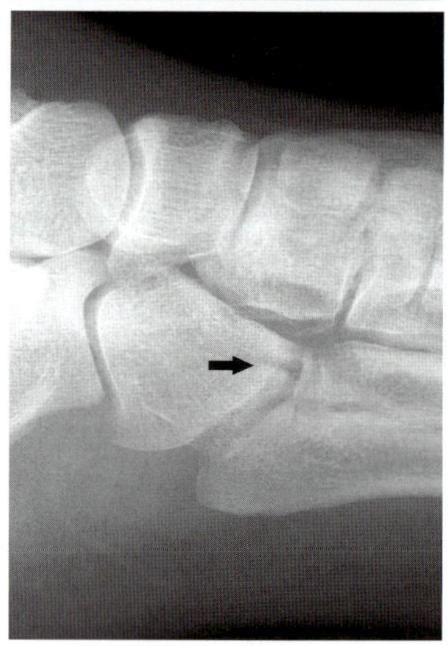

84 Cuboid fractures		
84-B **Comminuted** 89 fractures M: 46 (51.69%) F: 43 (48.31%) 0.02% of total adult fractures 0.23% of adult foot fractures 16.73% of cuboid	**84-B** 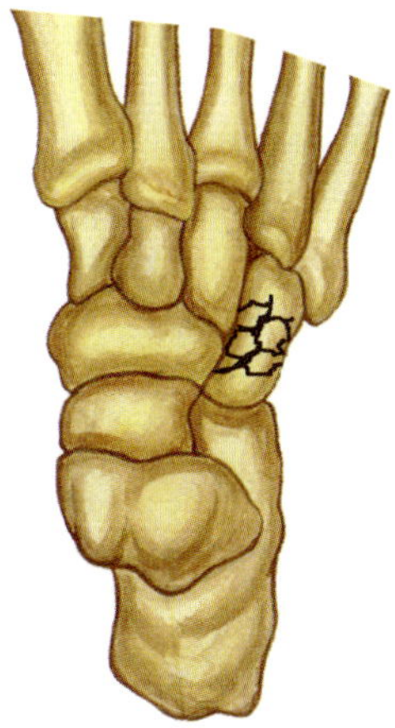 Comminuted	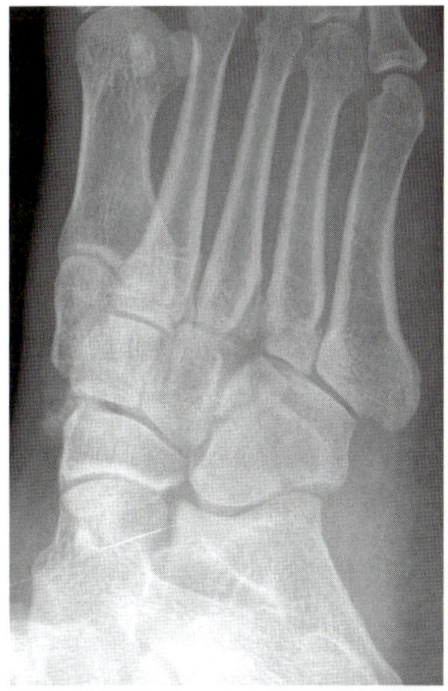 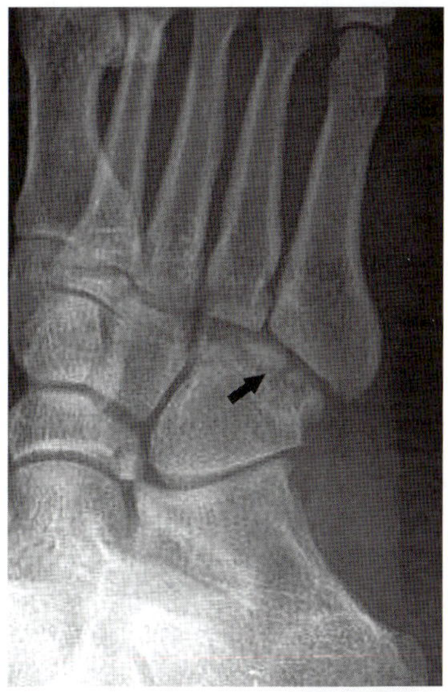 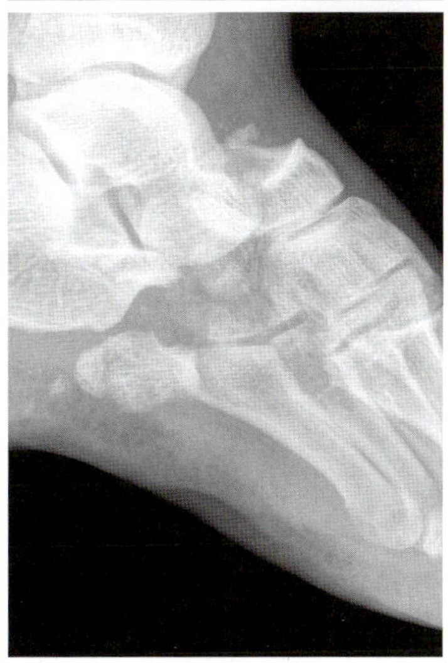

Injury Mechanism

Isolated fractures to the cuboid are not common, and are usually concomitant with fractures of the cuneiform, calcaneus, or the base of the lateral metatarsal. Fractures of the cuboid can occur through direct or indirect mechanisms. Indirect injury usually occurs when the cuboid is crushed between the calcaneus and metatarsals by forced plantar flexion and abduction. Direct injuries occur by direct blow or high-energy crush injuries to the area. Subluxation or luxation of tarsometatarsal or intertarsal may be seen in this injury. Because the cuboid is protected by surrounding ligamentous tissue and a capsule, total dislocation of the cuboid is rare. Avulsion fractures often occur as a result of ligamentous tension secondary to forced adduction of the cuboid. Compression fractures, so-called nutcracker effect injuries, occur when the cuboid is compressed between the base of the fourth and fifth metatarsals and the calcaneus as a result of severe abduction of the forefoot, or when body weight is transferred to the fixed and plantar-flexed foot. In severe cases, an associated middle tarsal dislocation may occur.

Diagnosis

Physical examination and radiographic evaluation are the tools used to determine the presence of a fracture. Patients may present with swelling, pain over the midfoot area, partial-to-complete limitation of motion, and deformity if there is marked displacement or dislocation. Standard radiographic views including AP and lateral views of the foot usually confirm the diagnosis. However, an isolated cuboid fracture is rare and is often associated with other fractures and dislocations of the midfoot. Particular attention should be given to associated fractures to avoid misdiagnosis. CT scan and MRI may be considered if indicated.

Treatment

Nondisplaced cuboid or avulsion fractures can be treated with immobilization by a short-leg cast for 4–6 weeks. Fractures with marked displacement, comminuted articular fractures, or subluxation of the cuboid require surgical intervention. Articular arthrodesis should be considered for severe articular comminution. The biological morphology of the foot arch and length of the lateral column should be preserved during the arthrodesis.

Cuneiform Fractures (Segment 85)

Anatomical Features

There are three cuneiform bones in the human foot. They are located between the navicular bone posteriorly and the metatarsals anteriorly. Irregularly cubic in shape, they are designated the medial, intermediate, and lateral cuneiform from medial to lateral. The medial cuneiform bone is the largest of the three. Its dorsal surface is the narrow end of the wedge, directly upward and lateralward and its rough surface is the site of ligament attachment. The rough plantar surface is the site of attachment for the peroneus longus, part of the anterior tibialis tendon and the posterior tibialis. The middle cuneiform, the smallest of the three cuneiforms, has a regular, wedgelike form with its narrow end directed downward. It is situated between the other two cuneiforms, and articulates with the navicular bone posteriorly and the second metatarsal anteriorly. The lateral cuneiform is quadrilateral in shape, its base at the uppermost end. Its rough dorsal surface is the site of attachment for its ligaments; its plantar surface has a rounded margin and serves for the attachment of the plantar muscles (**Plate 9.12**).

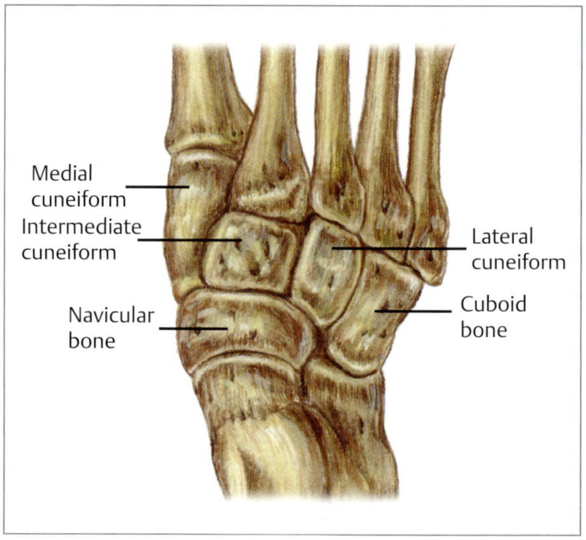

Plate 9.12

OTA Classification of Cuneiform Fractures

Based on OTA classification, the cuneiform is coded as the number 85 for its anatomical location. Cuneiform fractures are classified into two types: 85-A, noncomminuted fractures; and 85-B, comminuted fractures (**Plate 9.13**).

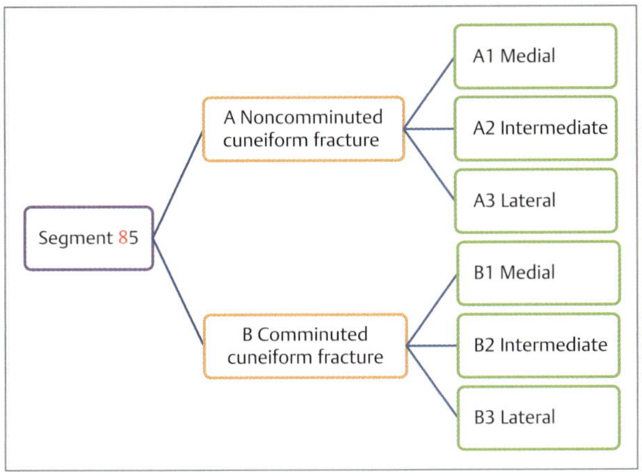

Plate 9.13

Clinical Epidemiologic Features of Cuneiform Fractures (Segment 85)

A total of 552 adult patients with 552 cuneiform fractures were treated in 83 hospitals in China over a 2-year period from 2010 to 2011. All cases were reviewed and statistically studied; the fractures accounted for 0.15% of all adult fractures, including 281 patients with fractures on the left side, 271 on the right side. There were 343 males and 209 females, with a male-to-female ratio of 1.64:1.

Epidemiologic features of cuneiform fractures are as follows:

- More males than females
- The highest-risk age group is 36–40 years, with ages 26–30 years being highest for males and 46–50 being highest for females.
- The most common fracture type is type 85-A.
- The most common fracture group is group 85-A1.
- The medial cuneiform is the most commonly fractured cuneiform.

Cuneiform Fractures (Segment 85) by Sex

Table 9.20 Sex distribution of 552 patients with cuneiform fractures

Sex	Number of patients	Percentage (%)
Male	343	62.14
Female	209	37.86
Total	552	100.00

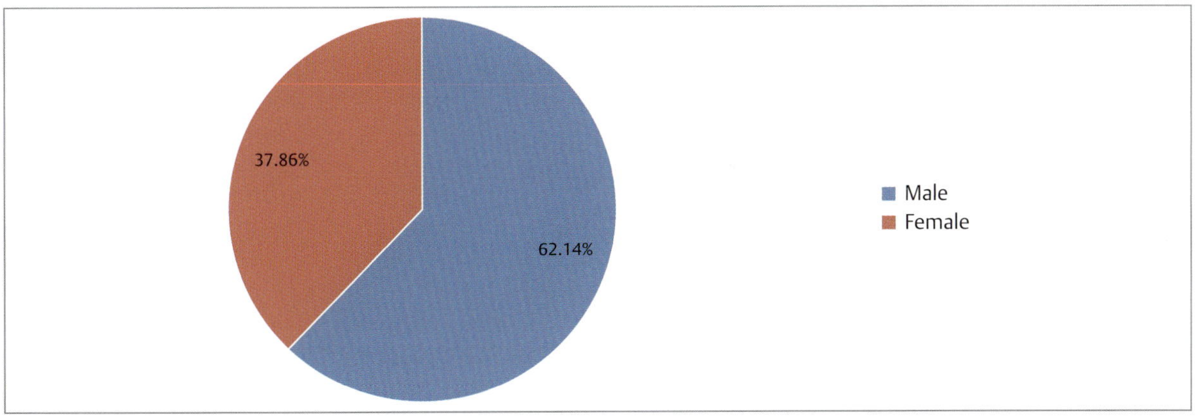

Fig. 9.20 Sex distribution of 552 patients with cuneiform fractures.

Cuneiform Fractures (Segment 85) by Age

Table 9.21 Age and sex distribution of 552 patients with cuneiform fractures

Age group (years)	Male	Female	Number of patients	Percentage (%)
16–20	38	9	47	8.51
21–25	48	15	63	11.41
26–30	55	15	70	12.68
31–35	32	30	62	11.23
36–40	50	22	72	13.04
41–45	33	26	59	10.69
46–50	27	31	58	10.51
51–55	24	17	41	7.43
56–60	16	11	27	4.89
61–65	11	17	28	5.07
66–70	4	5	9	1.63
71–75	2	4	6	1.09
76–80	0	5	5	0.91
81–85	3	2	5	0.91
≥86	0	0	0	0.00
Total	343	209	552	100.00

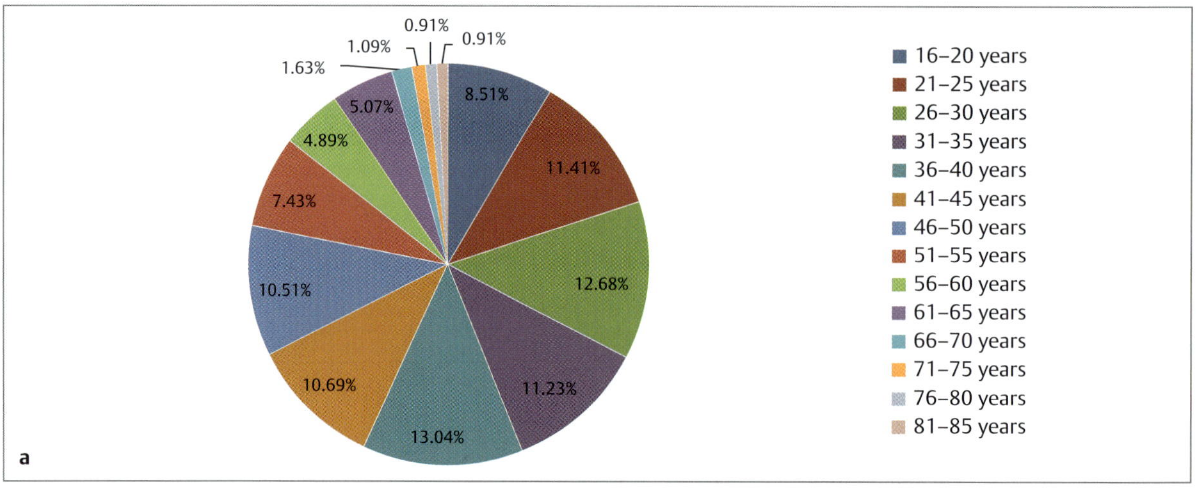

Fig. 9.21 **(a)** Age distribution of 552 patients with cuneiform fractures.

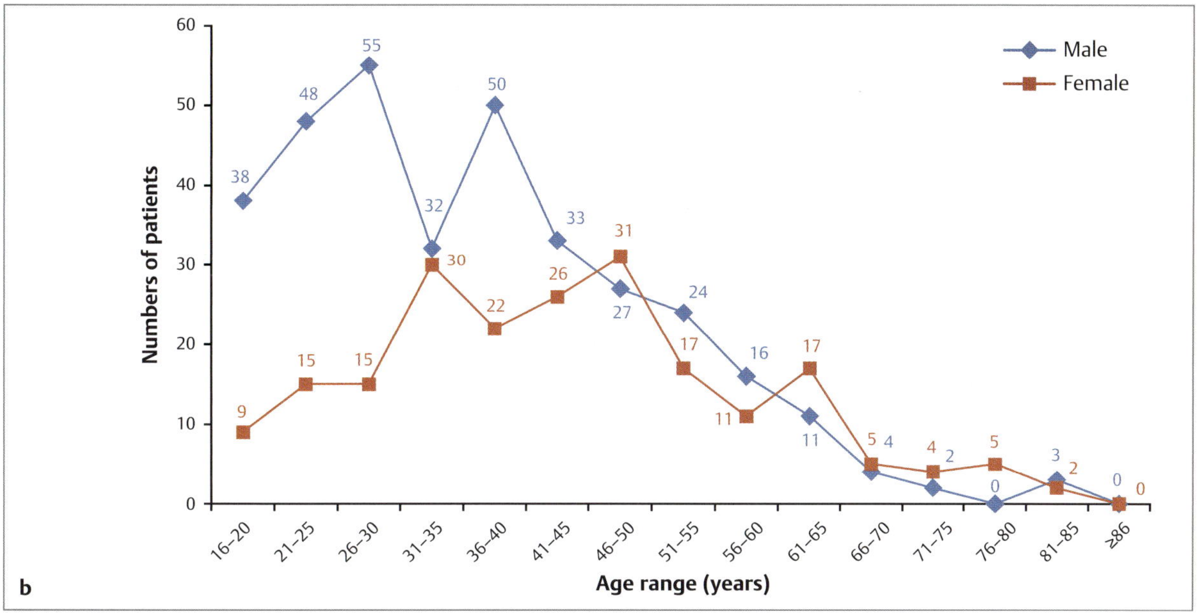

Fig. 9.21 (*continued*) **(b)** Age and sex distribution of 552 patients with cuneiform fractures.

Cuneiform Fracture (Segment 85) by Fracture Type

Table 9.22 Sex and fracture type distribution of 552 cuneiform fractures

Fracture type	Male	Female	Number of fractures	Percentage (%)
85-A	282	165	447	80.98
85-B	61	44	105	19.02
Total	343	209	552	100.00

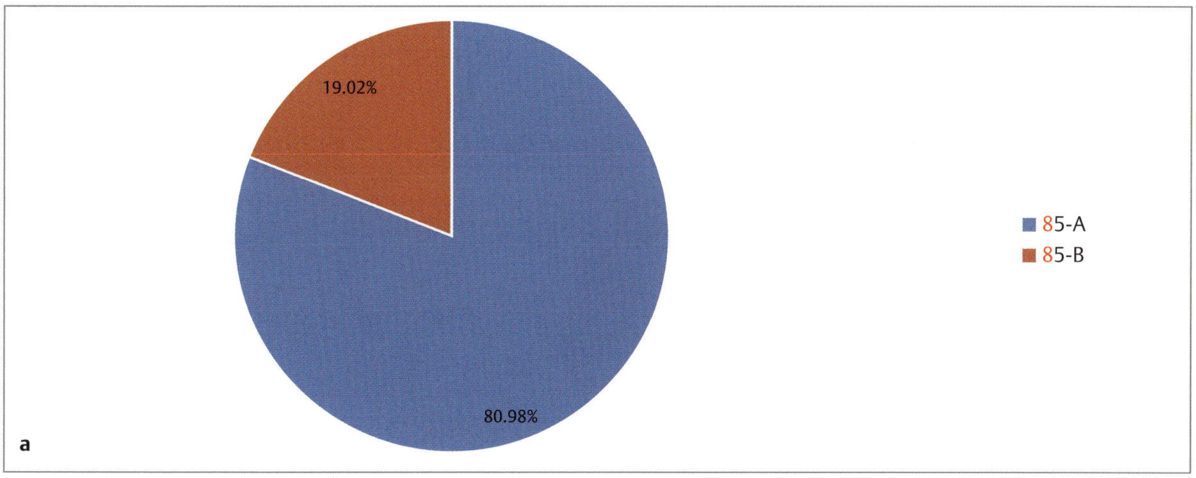

Fig. 9.22 **(a)** Fracture type distribution of 552 cuneiform fractures. (*Continued*)

9

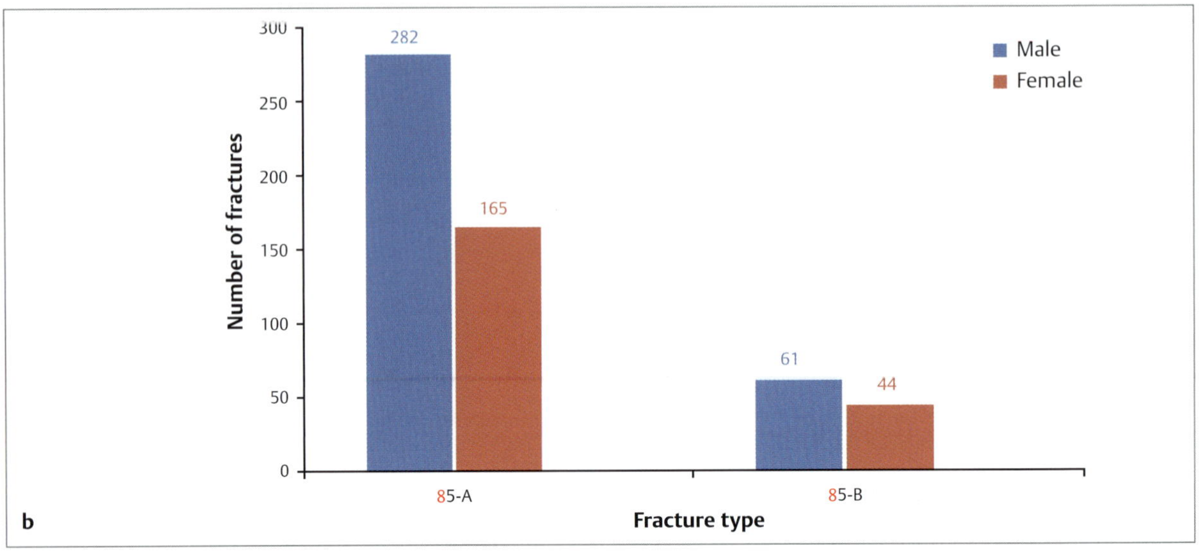

Fig. 9.22 (*continued*) **(b)** Sex and fracture type distribution of 552 cuneiform fractures.

Table 9.23 Sex and fracture group distribution of 552 cuneiform fractures

Fracture group	Male	Female	Number of fractures	Percentage of cuneiforms (%)	Percentage of foot fractures (%)
85-A1	216	118	334	60.51	0.86
85-A2	46	25	71	12.86	0.18
85-A3	20	22	42	7.61	0.11
85-B1	42	36	78	14.13	0.20
85-B2	15	4	19	3.44	0.05
85-B3	4	4	8	1.45	0.02
Total	343	209	552	100.00	1.43

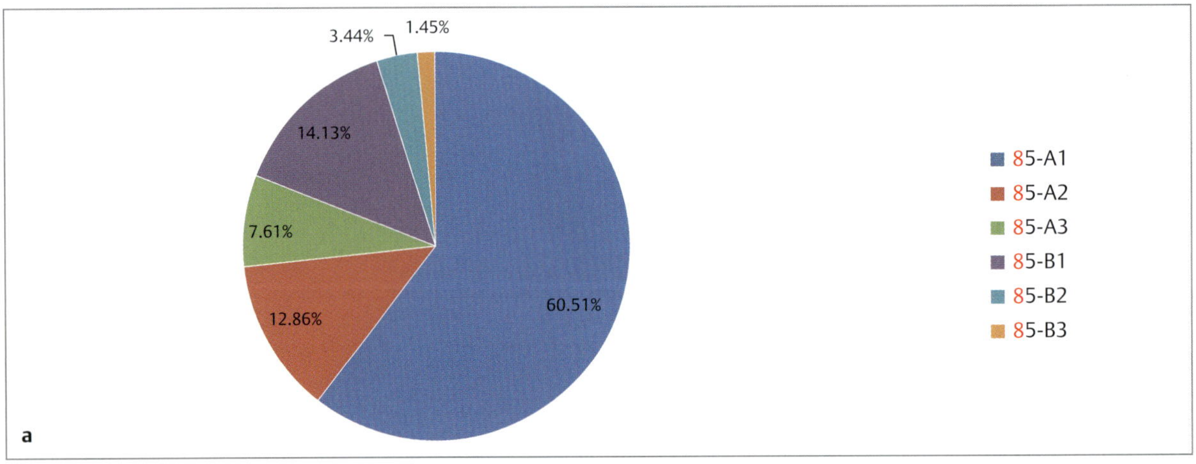

Fig. 9.23 **(a)** Fracture group distribution of 552 cuneiform fractures.

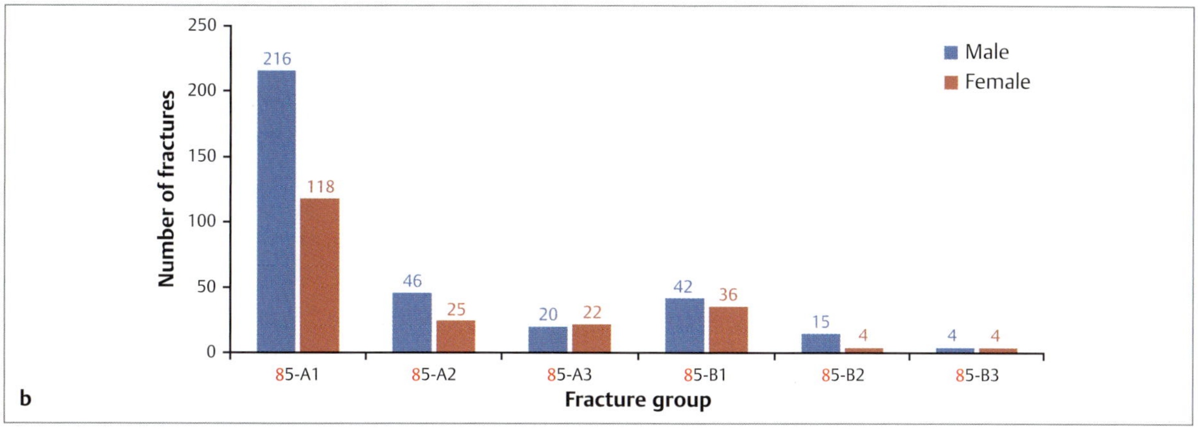

Fig. 9.23 (*continued*) **(b)** Sex and fracture group distribution of 552 cuneiform fractures.

Cuneiform Fracture (Segment 85) by Individual Cuneiform

Table 9.24 Distribution of 552 cuneiform fractures by individual cuneiform

Cuneiform	Number of fractures	Percentage (%)
Medial	412	74.64
Middle	90	16.30
Lateral	50	9.06
Total	552	100.00

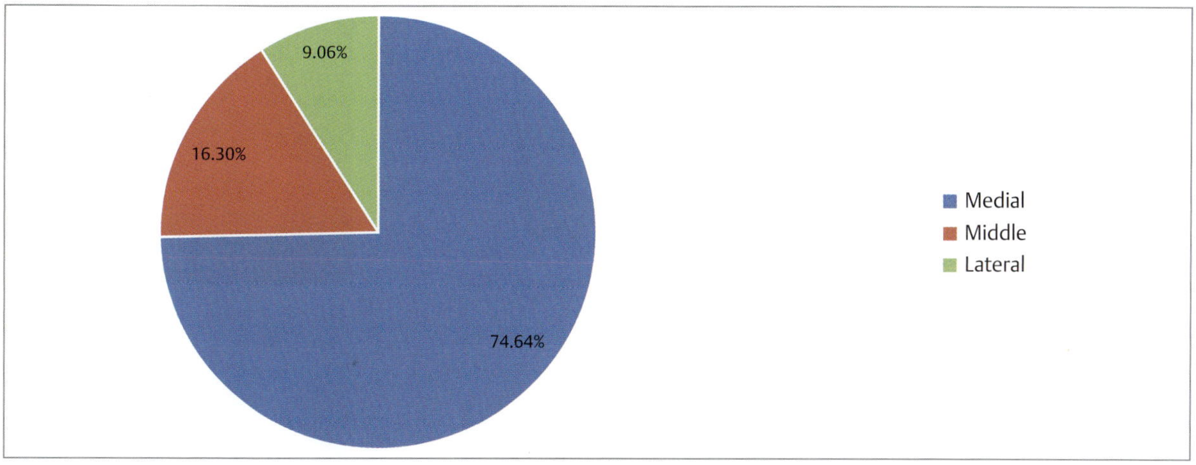

Fig. 9.24 Distribution of 552 cuneiform fractures by individual cuneiform.

85-A Cuneiform, noncomminuted fractures

85-A
Noncomminuted
447 fractures
M: 282 (63.09%)
F: 165 (36.91%)
0.12% of total adult fractures
1.16% of adult foot fractures
80.98% of cuneiform

85-A1

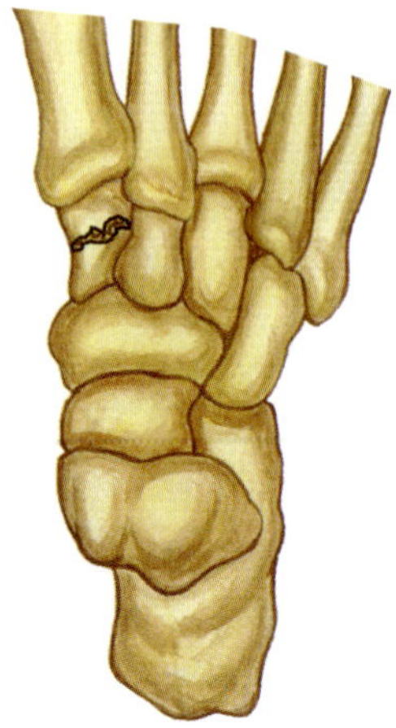

Medial

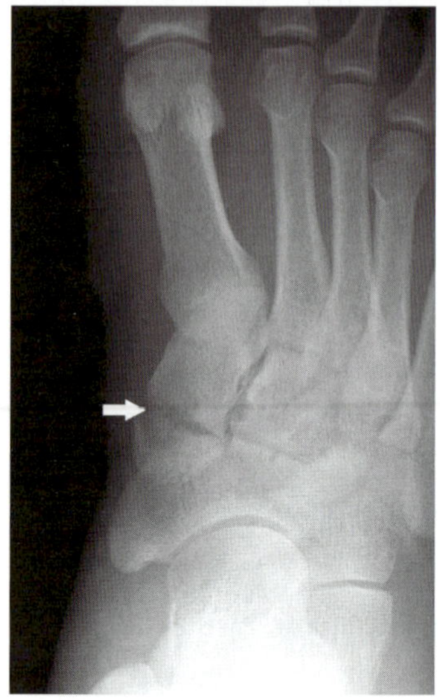

85-A2

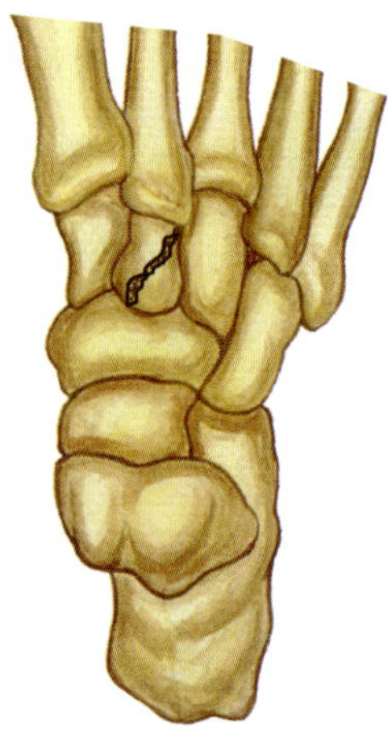

Intermediate

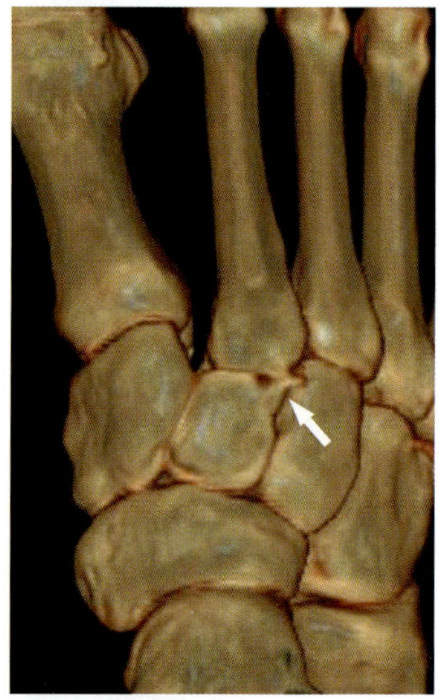

85-A3

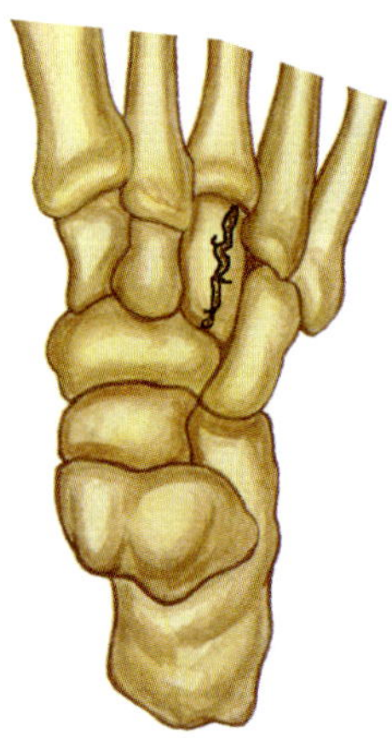

Lateral

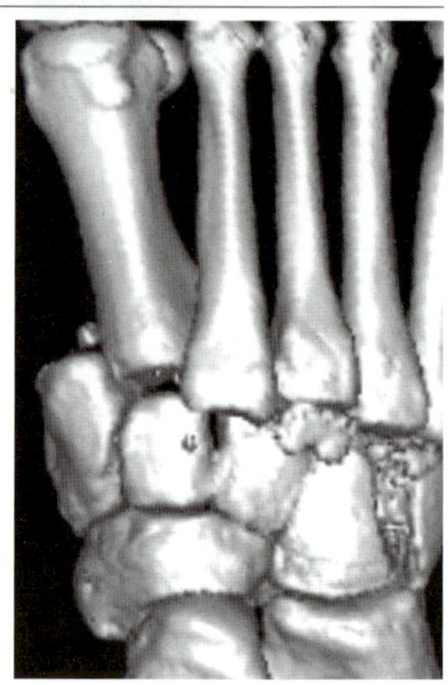

85-B Cuneiform, comminuted fractures

85-B
Comminuted
105 fractures
M: 61 (58.1%)
F: 44 (41.9%)
0.03% of total adult fractures
0.27% of adult foot fractures
19.02% of cuneiform

85-B1

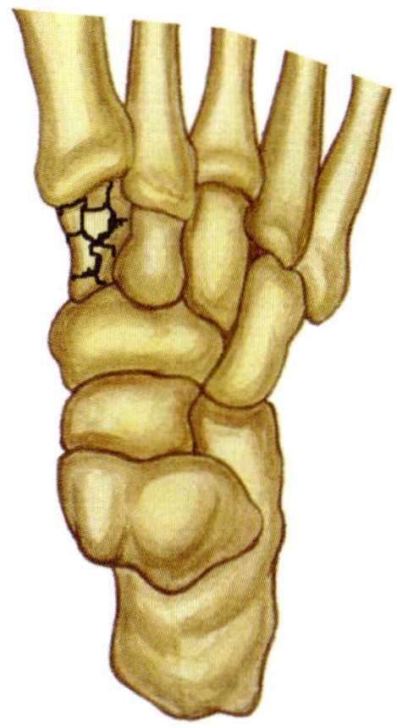

Medial

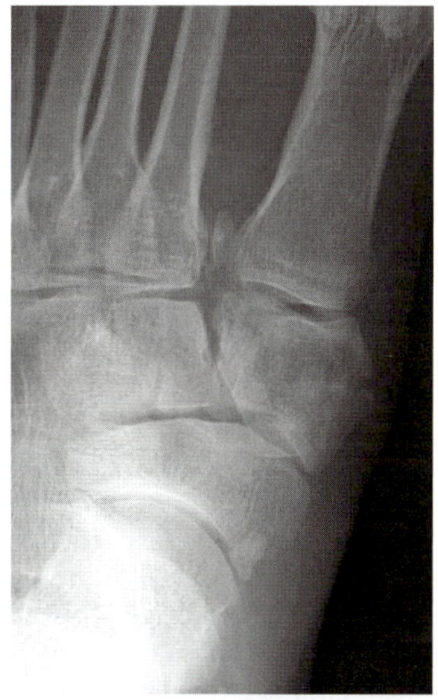

85-B2

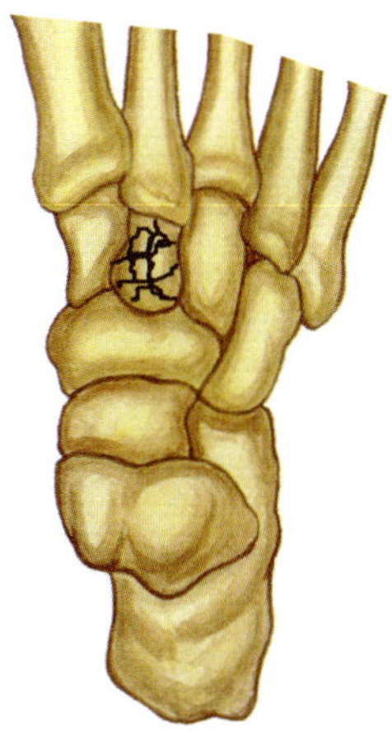

Intermediate

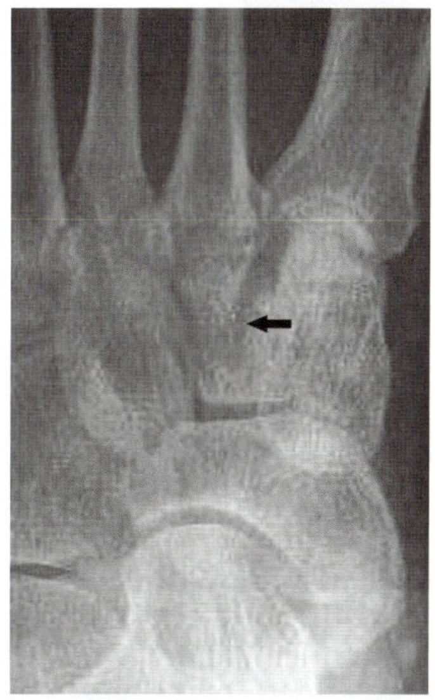

85-B3

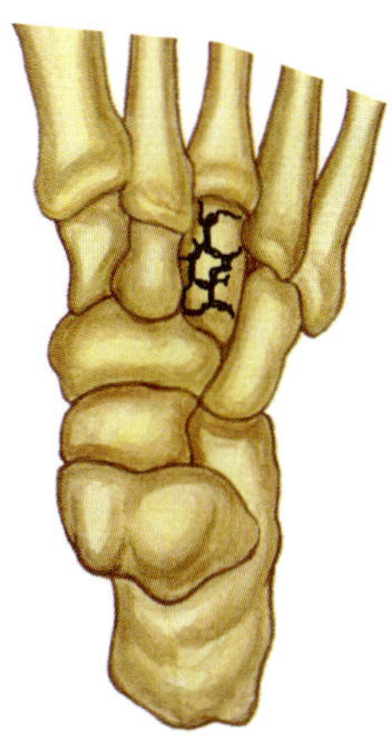

Lateral

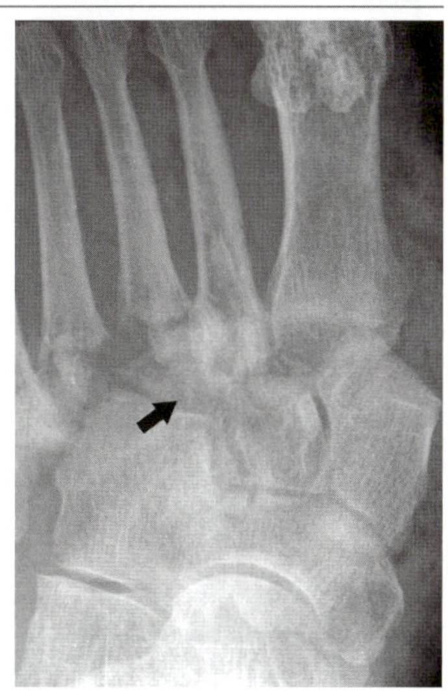

Injury Mechanism

Avulsion cuneiform fracture is the most common type of cuneiform fracture, and usually occurs as the result of abrupt tensile force of the intertarsal ligament secondary to the combination of plantar flexion, inversion, and abduction of the foot. Some patients may present with subluxation or dislocation of the cuneiform.

Diagnosis

History and physical examination plus radiographs make the diagnosis. Patients present with swelling, pain over the midfoot area, partial-to-complete limitation of motion, and deformity if there is marked displacement or dislocation. Radiographs of the foot, including AP, lateral, and oblique views, can usually confirm the diagnosis. If plain radiographs are inconclusive, CT and MRI are indicated.

Treatment

Nondisplaced cuneiform fractures or those with associated subluxation or dislocation of the intertarsal joints can be treated with a short-leg walking cast for 4–6 weeks, if the reduction can be achieved successfully by manipulative methods. Open reduction and internal fixation or arthrodesis is indicated for comminuted fractures or fractures with dislocated tarsometatarsal or intertarsal joints that cannot be reduced manually.

Metatarsal Fractures (Segment 87)

Anatomical Features

The metatarsus consists of five short tubular bones, each having three parts: a base, a body, and a head. Although individually different, all five metatarsal bones share common characteristics. The base, or posterior extremity, is wedge shaped, and broader behind than in front, articulating proximally with the tarsal bones, and with the continuous metatarsal bones on its sides. Its rough dorsal and plantar surfaces are for the sites of attachment of its ligaments. The distal part of the metatarsal bone is the head or anterior extremity, which presents a convex articular surface that articulates with the phalanx. On each side of the head, there is a depression, surmounted by a tubercle, for the attachment of the ligaments and capsule. Between the head and the base is the prismoid-shaped body, which tapers gradually from the tarsal to the phalangeal extremity. The body presents three surfaces: medial, lateral, and dorsal. The dorsal surface has a flattened area in the middle, while the medial and lateral surfaces are broad and concave; all three surfaces are attached by muscles (**Plate 9.14**).

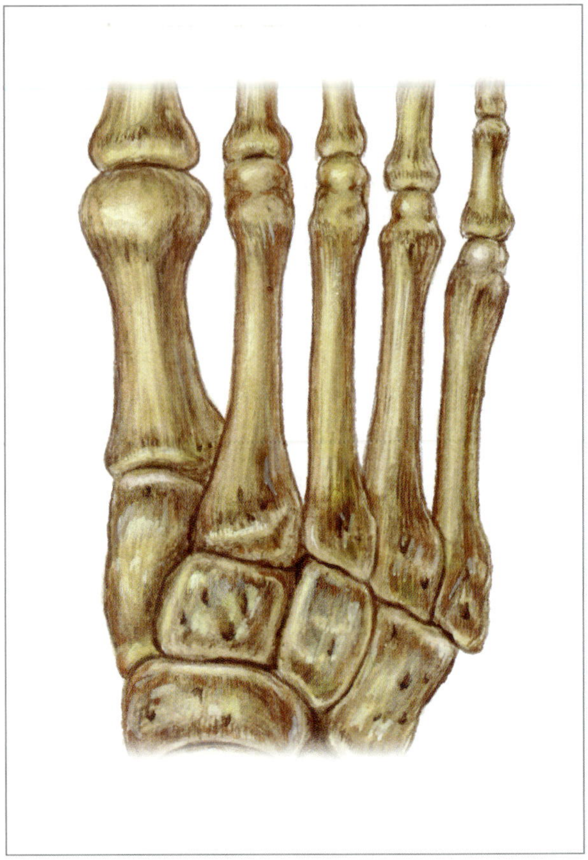

Plate 9.14

9

OTA Classification of Metatarsal Fractures

Based on OTA classification, the metatarsus is coded as the number 87 for its anatomical location. Metatarsal fractures are classified into three types: 87-A, metatarsal proximal, distal extra-articular, and diaphysis noncomminuted; 87-B, metatarsal proximal, distal partial articular, and diaphysis wedge comminuted; and 87-C, metatarsal proximal, distal complete, and articular diaphysis comminuted (**Plate 9.15**).

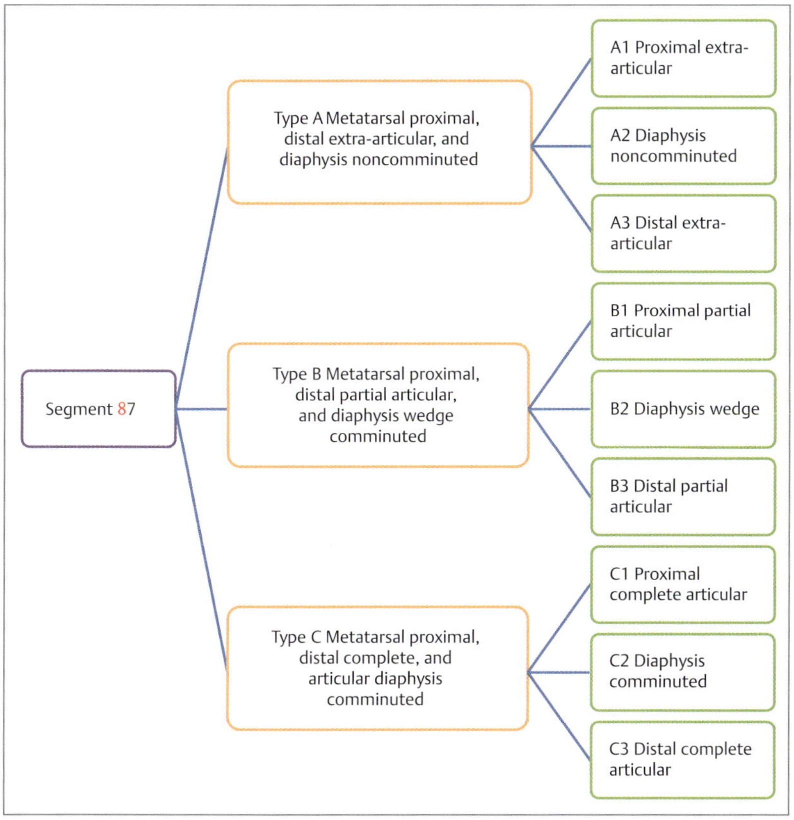

Plate 9.15

9

Clinical Epidemiologic Features of Metatarsal Fractures (Segment 87)

A total of 8,996 adult patients with 8,996 metatarsal fractures were treated in 83 hospitals in China over a 2-year period from 2010 to 2011. All cases were reviewed and statistically studied; the fractures accounted for 2.5% of all adult patients with fractures, including 4,599 patients with fractures on the left side, 4,397 on the right side. There were 4,960 males and 4,036 females, with a male-to-female ratio of 1.23:1.

Epidemiological features of metatarsal fractures are as follows:

- More males than females
- The highest risk age group is 41–45 years, with males aged 41–45 and females 56–60 at the highest risk.
- The most common fracture type is type 87-B.
- The most common fracture group is group 87-B1.
- The fifth metatarsal is the most frequently fractured metatarsal.
- The proximal metatarsal metaphysis is the most often fractured metatarsal component.

Metatarsal Fractures (Segment 87) by Sex

Table 9.25 Sex distribution of 8,996 patients with metatarsal fractures

Sex	Number of patients	Percentage (%)
Male	4,960	55.14
Female	4,036	44.86
Total	8,996	100.00

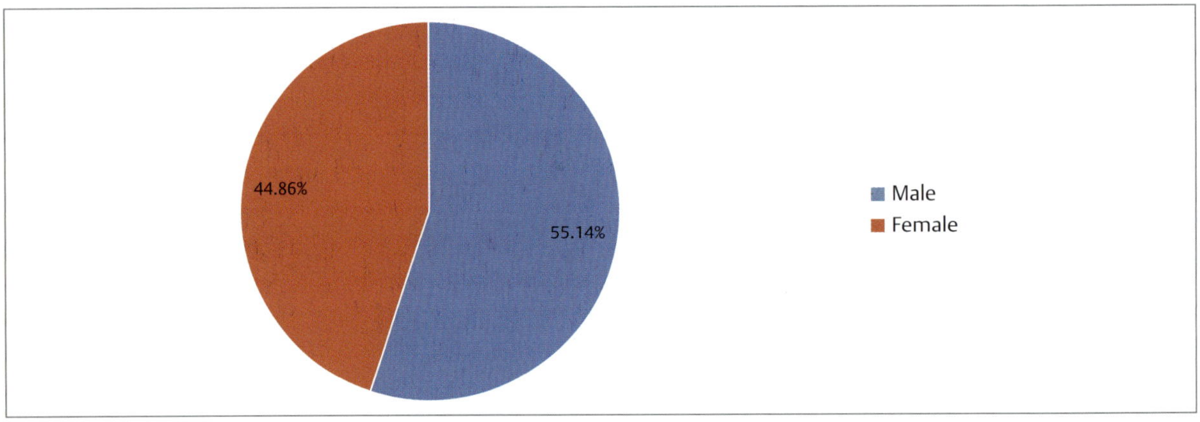

Fig. 9.25 Sex distribution of 8,996 patients with metatarsal fractures.

Metatarsal Fractures (Segment 87) by Age

Table 9.26 Age and sex distribution of 8,996 patients with metatarsal fractures

Age group (years)	Male	Female	Number of patients	Percentage (%)
16–20	393	153	546	6.07
21–25	561	292	853	9.48
26–30	523	350	873	9.70
31–35	508	260	768	8.54
36–40	598	345	943	10.48
41–45	619	427	1,046	11.63
46–50	491	497	988	10.98
51–55	431	502	933	10.37
56–60	346	514	860	9.56
61–65	181	284	465	5.17
66–70	108	173	281	3.12
71–75	90	120	210	2.33
76–80	71	74	145	1.61
81–85	28	34	62	0.69
≥86	12	11	23	0.26
Total	4,960	4,036	8,996	100.00

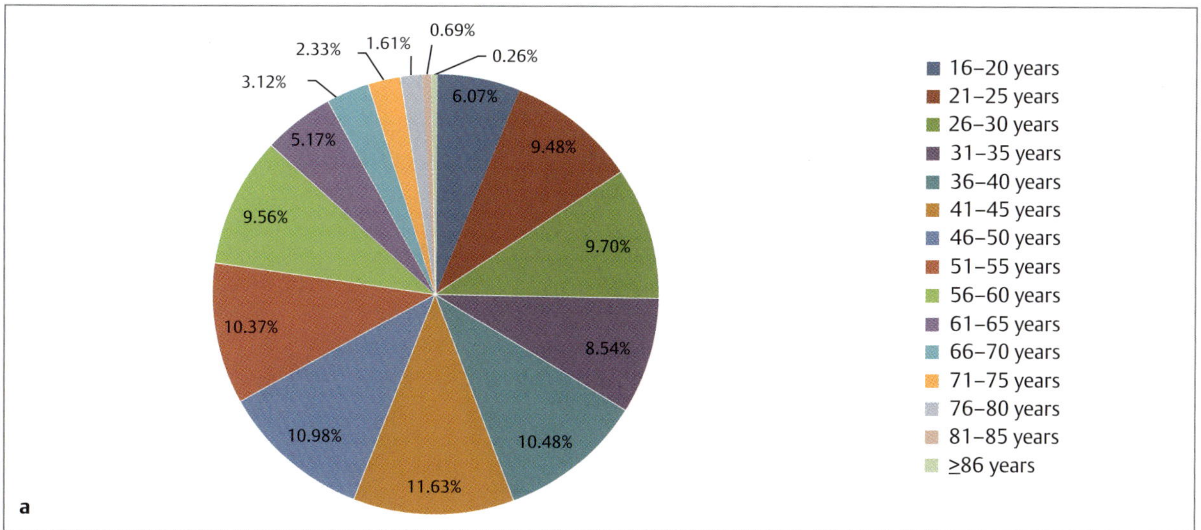

Fig. 9.26 **(a)** Age distribution of 8,996 patients with metatarsal fractures. (*Continued*)

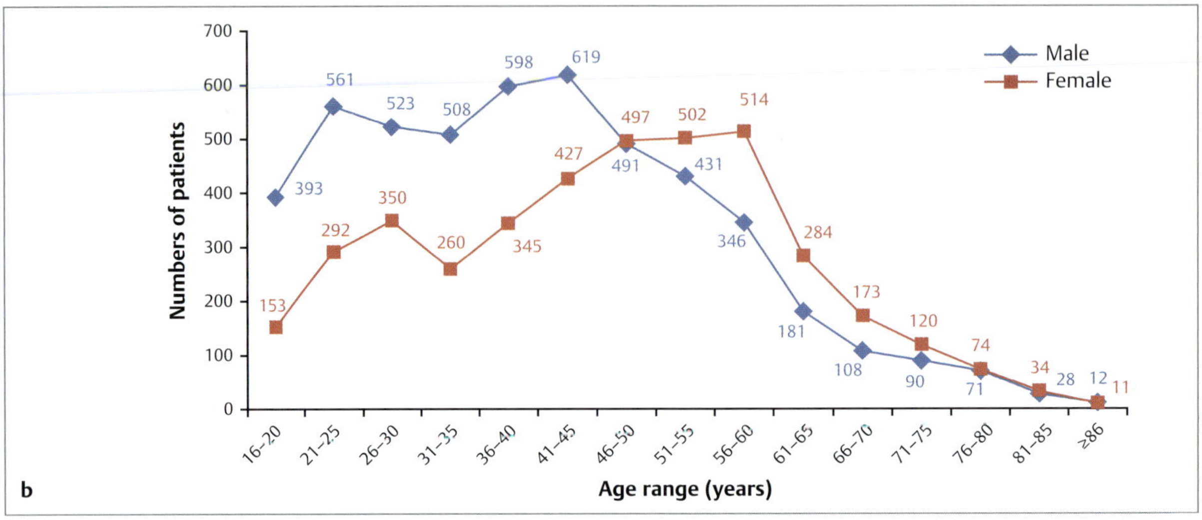

Fig. 9.26 (*continued*) **(b)** Age and sex distribution of 8,996 patients with metatarsal fractures.

Metatarsal Fractures (Segment 87) by Fracture Type

Table 9.27 Sex and fracture type distribution of 8,996 metatarsal fractures

Fracture type	Male	Female	Number of fractures	Percentage (%)
87-A	2,160	1,441	3,601	40.03
87-B	2,462	2,402	4,864	54.07
87-C	338	193	531	5.90
Total	4,960	4,036	8,996	100.00

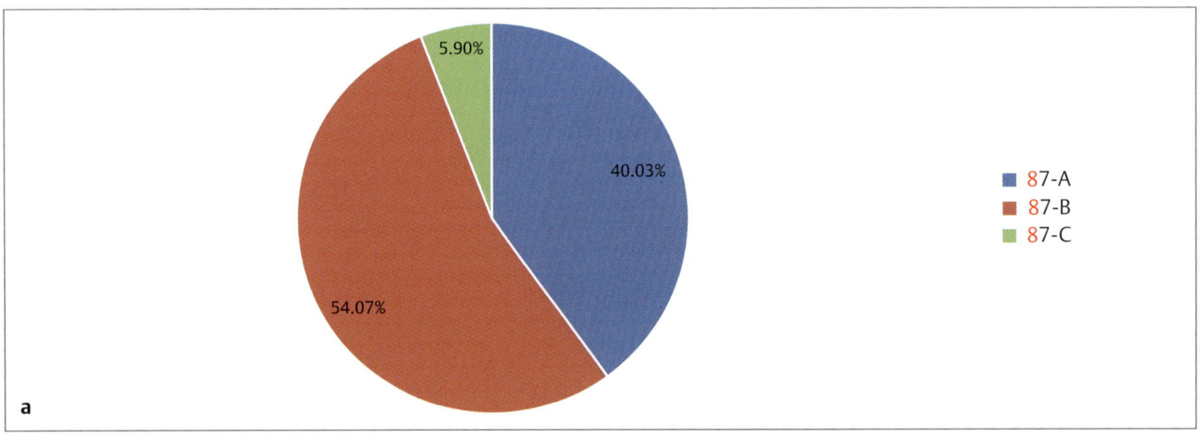

Fig. 9.27 **(a)** Fracture type distribution of 8,996 metatarsal fractures.

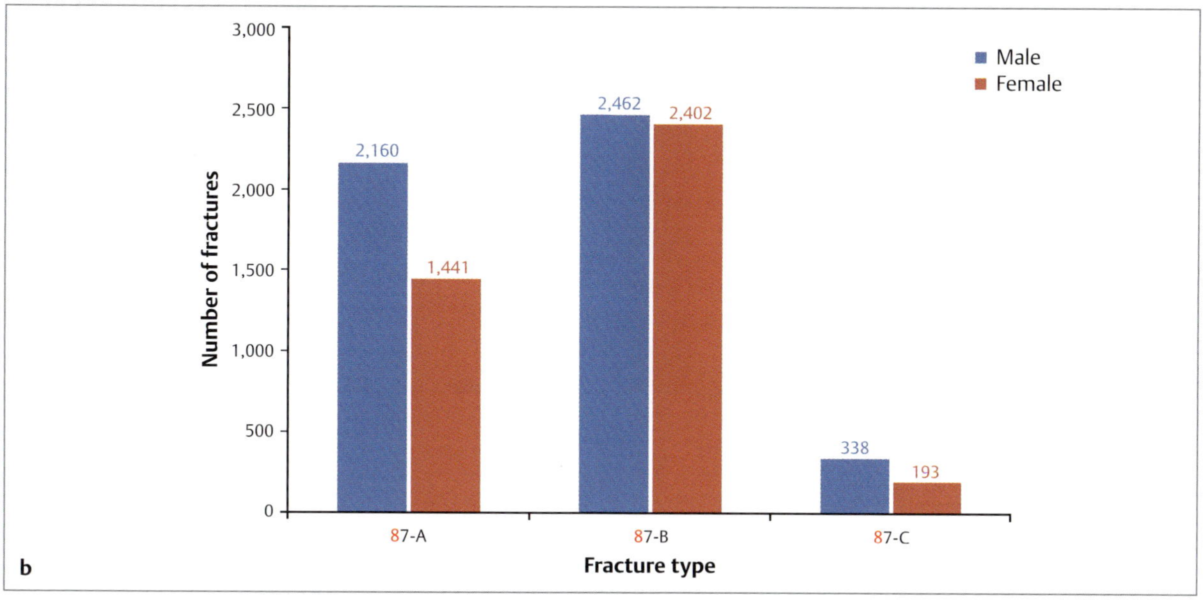

Fig. 9.27 (*continued*) **(b)** Sex and fracture type distribution of 8,996 metatarsal fractures.

Table 9.28 Sex and fracture group distribution of 8,996 metatarsal fractures

Fracture group	Male	Female	Number of fractures	Percentage of metatarsal fractures (%)	Percentage of foot fractures (%)
87-A1	1,011	798	1,809	20.11	4.68
87-A2	603	291	894	9.94	2.31
87-A3	546	352	898	9.98	2.32
87-B1	2,235	2,266	4,501	50.03	11.65
87-B2	156	95	251	2.79	0.65
87-B3	71	41	112	1.24	0.29
87-C1	173	116	289	3.21	0.75
87-C2	127	55	182	2.02	0.47
87-C3	38	22	60	0.67	0.16
Total	4,960	4,036	8,996	100.00	23.29

9

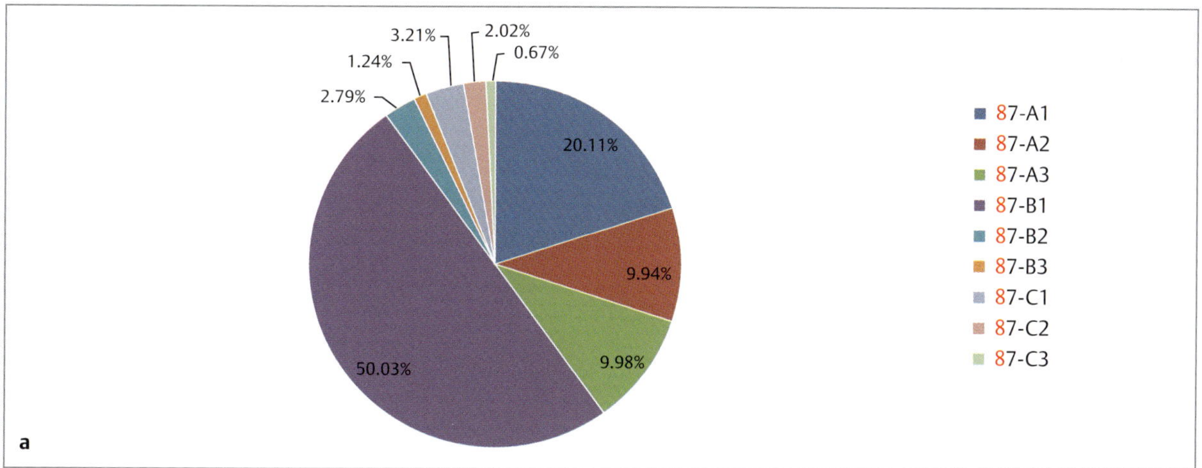

Fig. 9.28 **(a)** Fracture group distribution of 8,996 metatarsal fractures. (*Continued*)

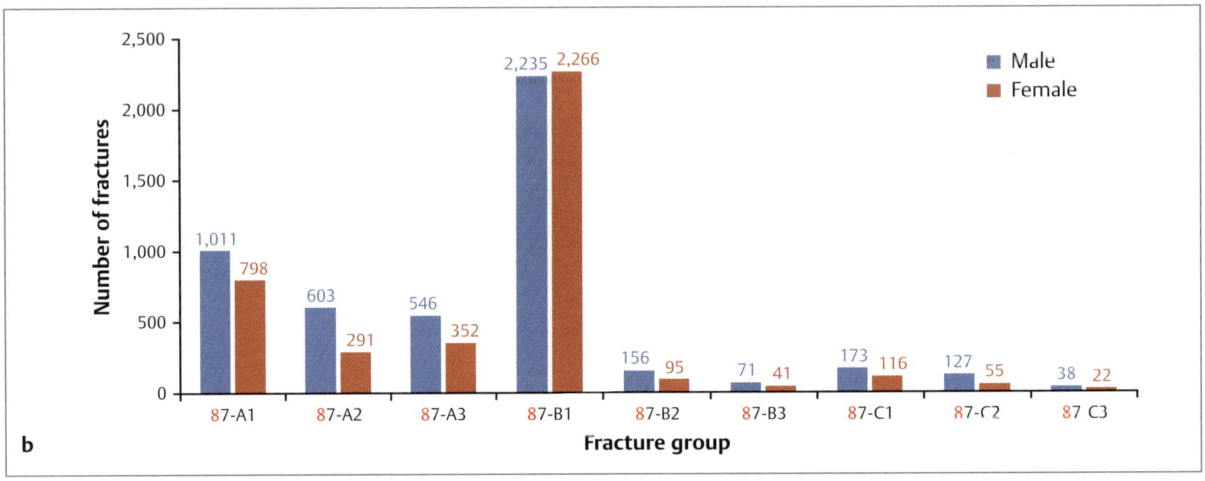

Fig. 9.28 (*continued*) **(b)** Sex and fracture group distribution of 8,996 metatarsal fractures.

Metatarsal Fractures (Segment 87) by Individual Metatarsal Bones

Table 9.29 Distribution of 8,996 metatarsal fractures by the number of the metatarsal bones

Metatarsal number	Number of fractures	Percentage of metatarsal fractures (%)
1st	813	9.04
2nd	744	8.27
3rd	652	7.25
4th	418	4.65
5th	6,369	70.80
Total	8,996	100.00

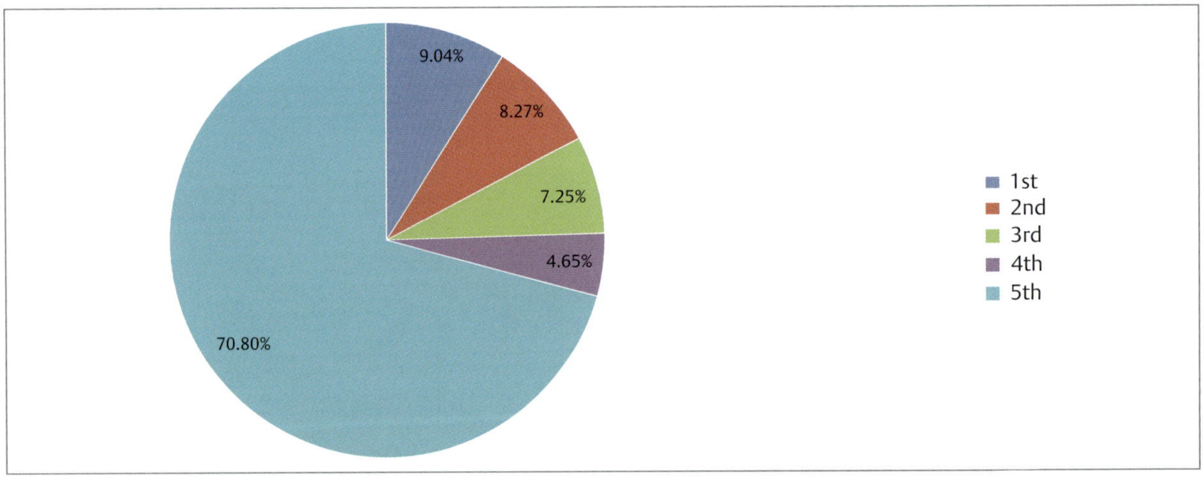

Fig. 9.29 Distribution of 8,996 metatarsal fractures by the number of the metatarsal bones.

Metatarsal Fractures by Segment (Segment 87)

Table 9.30 Sex and fracture segment distribution of 8,996 metatarsal fractures

Fracture segment	Male	Female	Number of fractures	Percentage (%)
Proximal	3,419	3,180	6,599	73.35
Diaphysis	886	441	1,327	14.75
Distal	655	415	1,070	11.89
Total	4,960	4,036	8,996	100.00

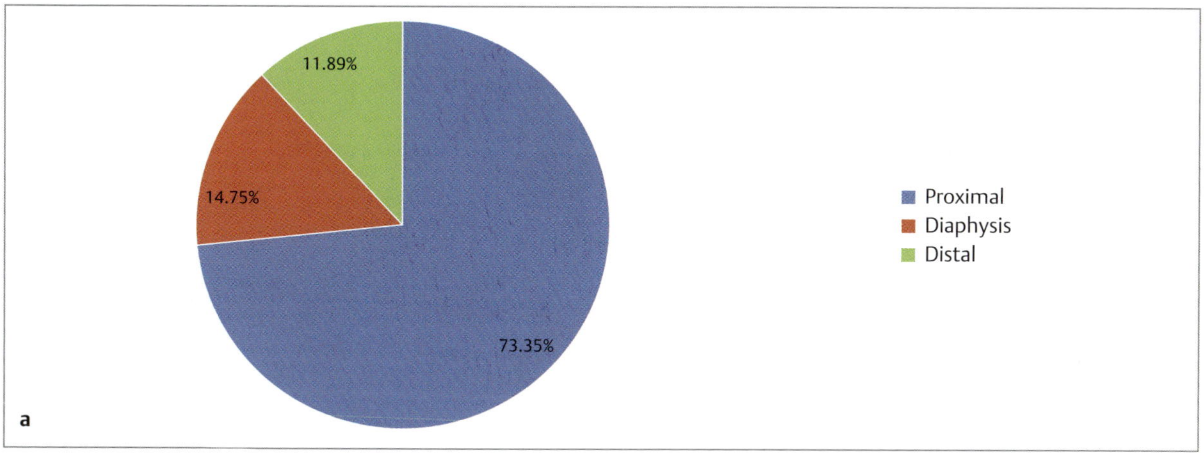

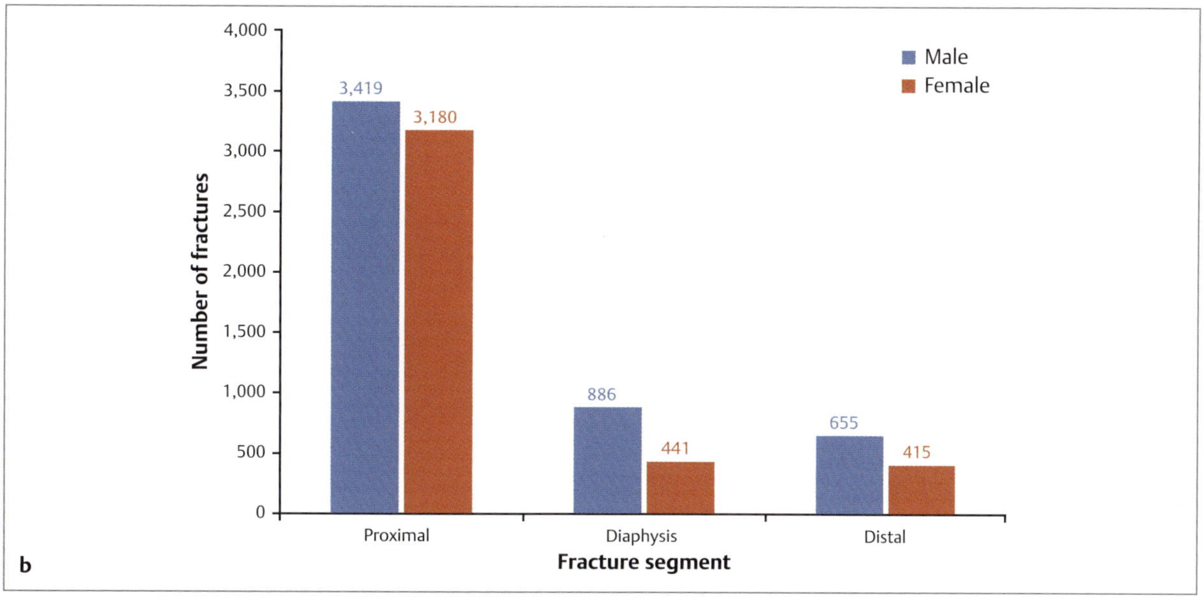

Fig. 9.30 **(a)** Fracture segment distribution of 8,996 metatarsal fractures.
(b) Sex and fracture segment distribution of 8,996 metatarsal fractures.

87-A Metatarsal proximal distal extra-articular, and diaphysis noncomminuted

87-A1
Proximal extra-articular
1,809 fractures
M: 1,011 (55.89%)
F: 798 (44.11%)
0.48% of total adult fractures
4.68% of adult foot fractures
20.11% of metatarsal
50.24% of type 87-A

87-A1.1

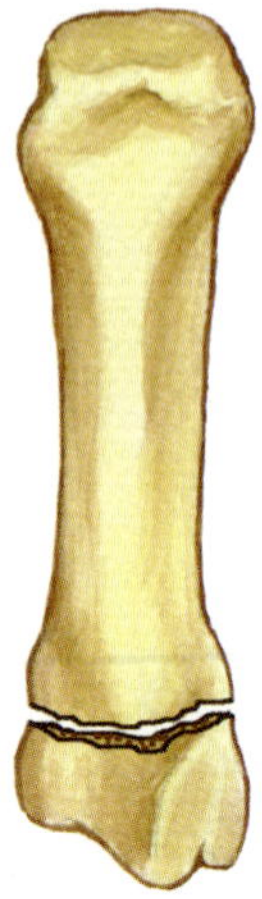

Noncomminuted

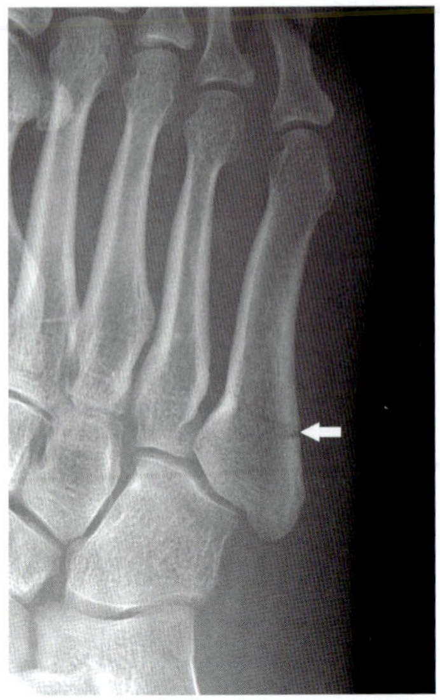

87-A1.2

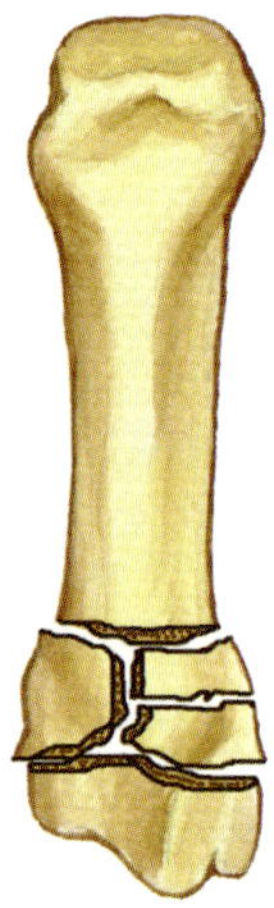

Comminuted

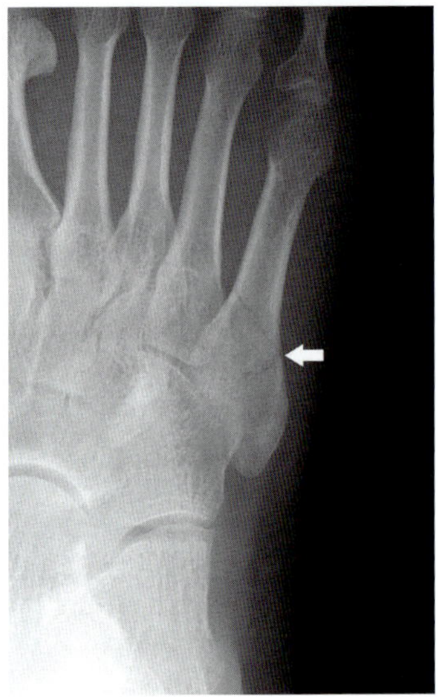

87-A Metatarsal proximal distal extra-articular, and diaphysis noncomminuted

87-A2
Diaphysis noncomminuted
894 fractures
M: 603 (67.45%)
F: 291 (32.55%)
0.24% of total adult fractures
2.31% of adult foot fractures
9.94% of metatarsal
24.83% of type 87-A

87-A2.1

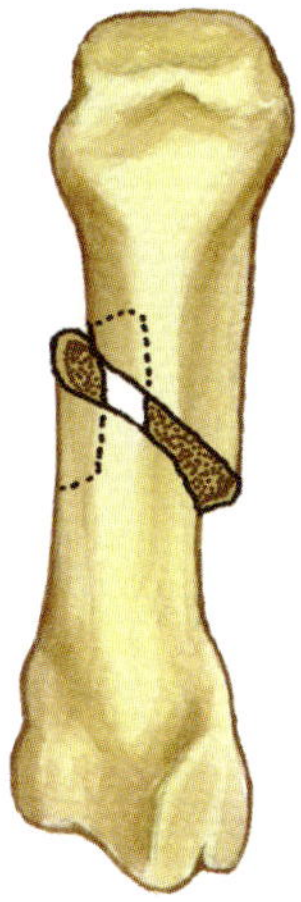

Spiral

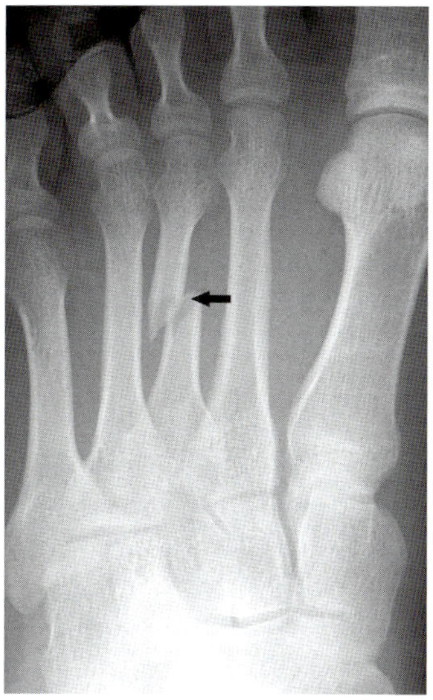

87-A2.2

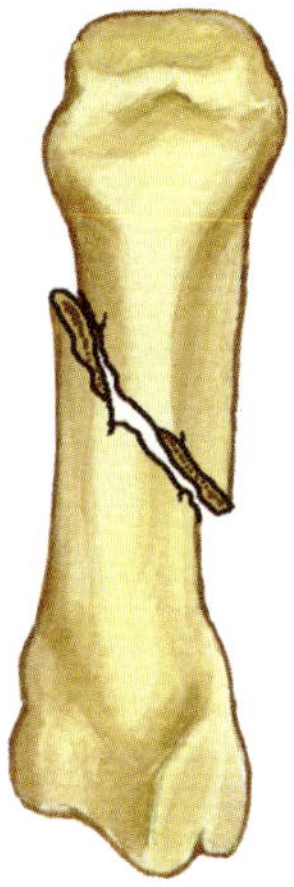

Oblique

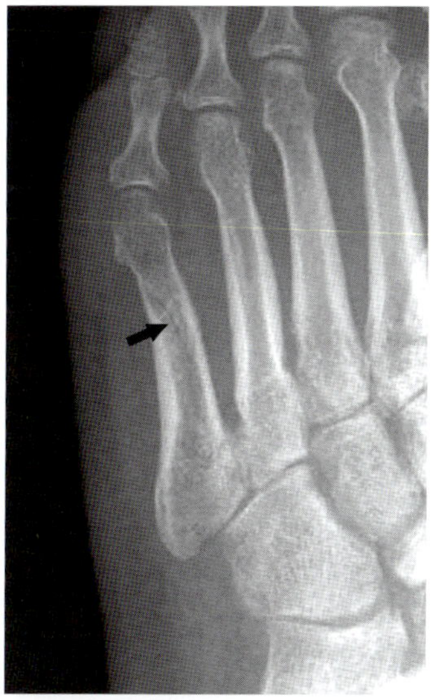

87-A2.3

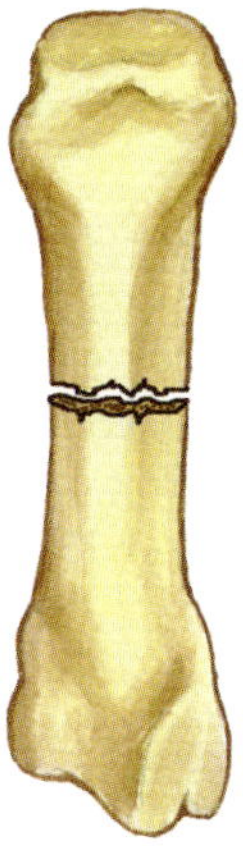

Transverse

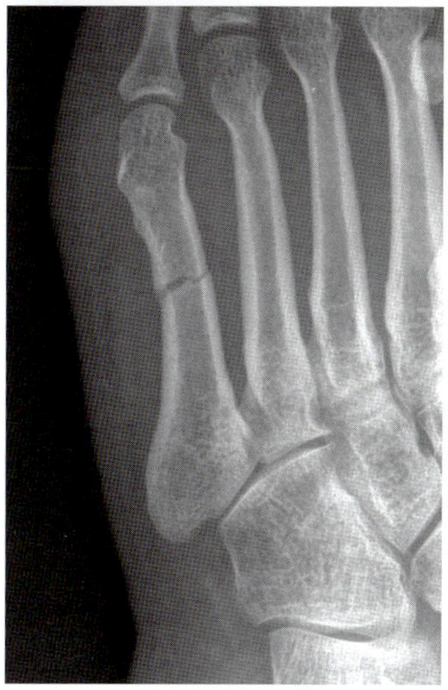

87-A Metatarsal proximal distal extra-articular, and diaphysis noncomminuted

87-A3
Distal extra-articular
898 fractures
M: 546 (60.8%)
F: 352 (39.2%)
0.24% of total adult fractures
2.32% of adult foot fractures
9.98% of metatarsal
24.94% of type 87-A

87-A3.1

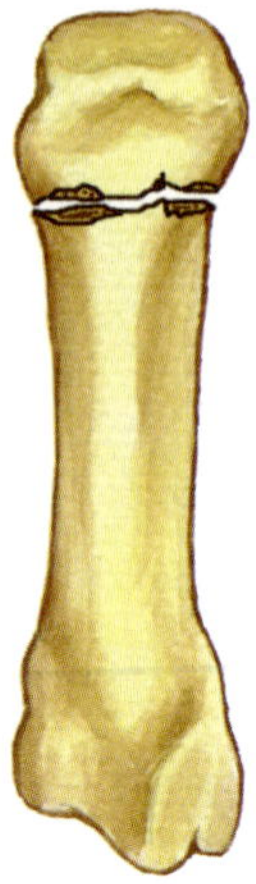

Noncomminuted

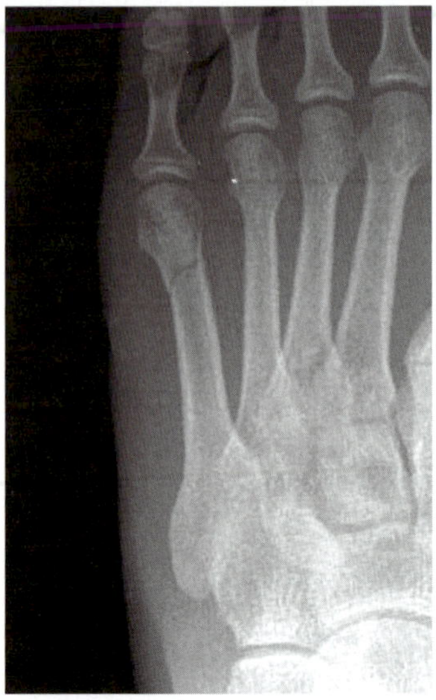

87-A3.2

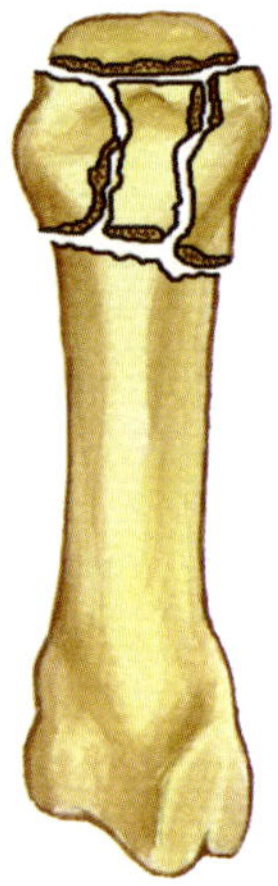

Comminuted

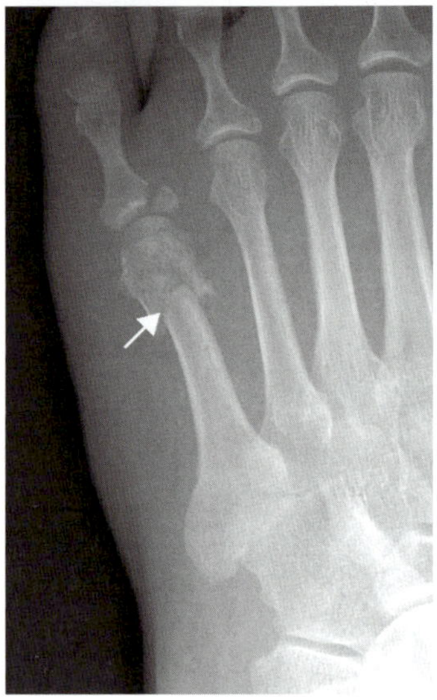

87-B Metatarsal proximal distal partial articular, and diaphysis wedge comminuted

87-B1
Proximal partial articular
4,501 fractures
M: 2,235 (49.66%)
F: 2,266 (50.34%)
1.2% of total adult fractures
11.65% of adult foot fractures
50.03% of metatarsal
92.54% of type 87-B

87-B1.1

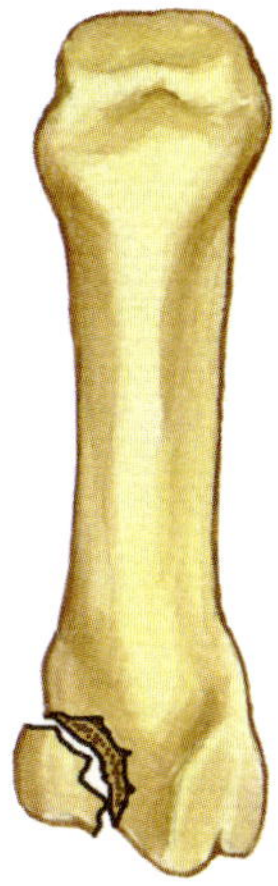

Avulsion or split

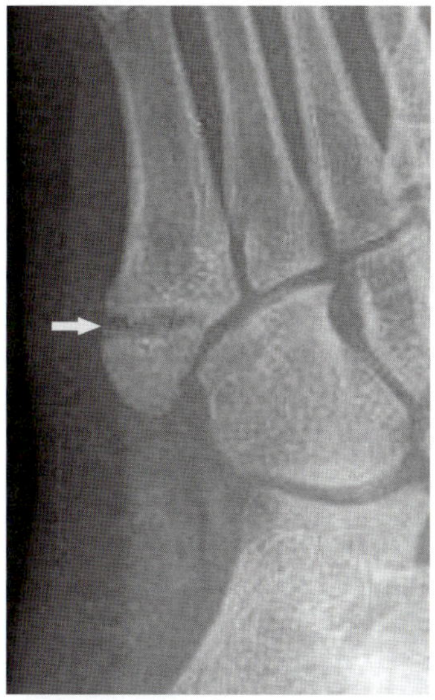

87-B1.2

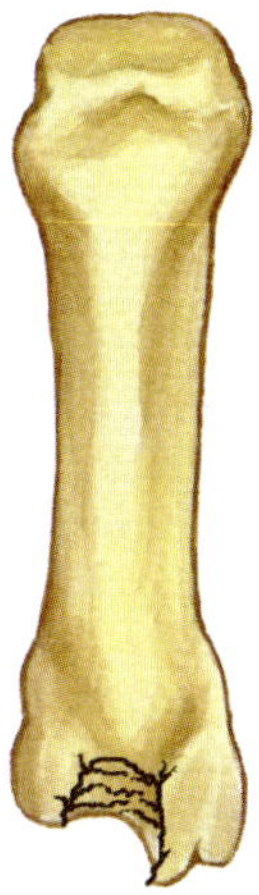

Depression

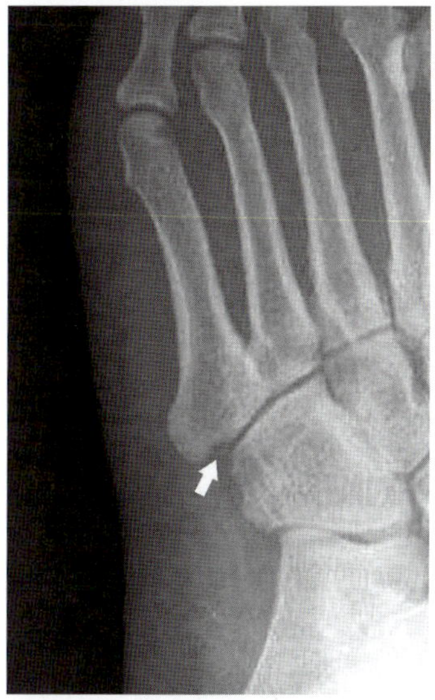

87-B1.3

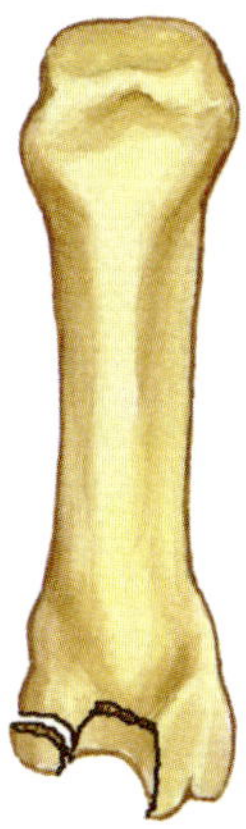

Split/depression

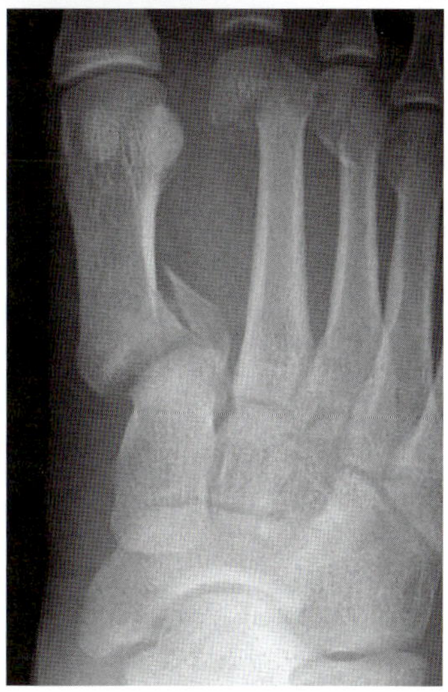

87-B Metatarsal proximal distal partial articular, and diaphysis wedge comminuted

87-B2
Diaphysis wedge
251 fractures
M: 156 (62.15%)
F: 95 (37.85%)
0.07% of total adult fractures
0.65% of adult foot fractures
2.79% of metatarsal
5.16% of type 87-B

87-B2.1

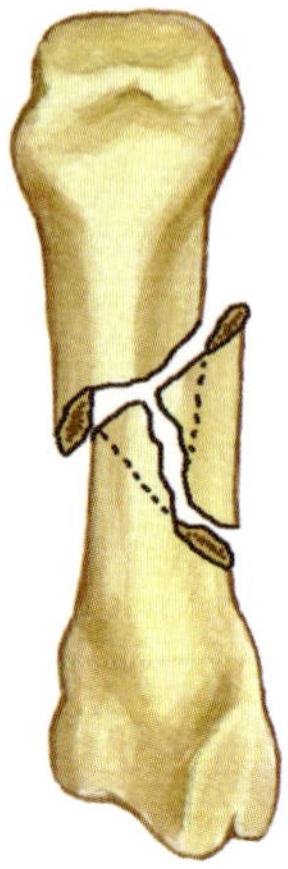

Spiral

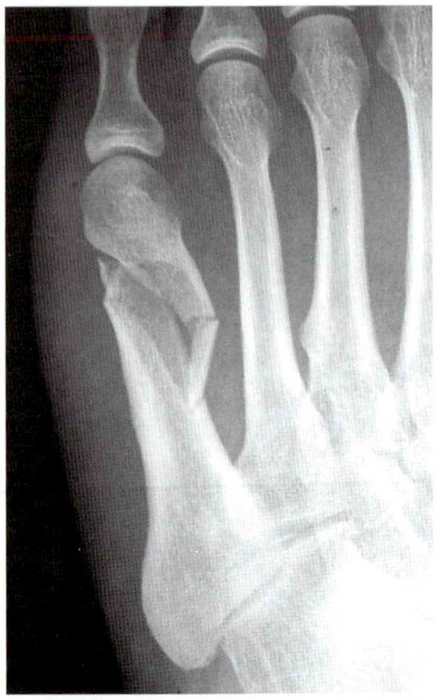

87-B2.2

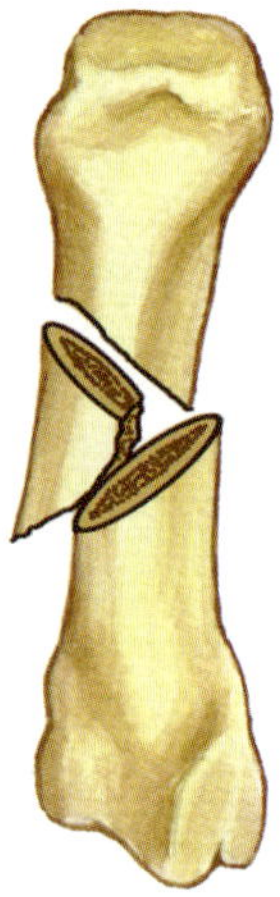

Bending

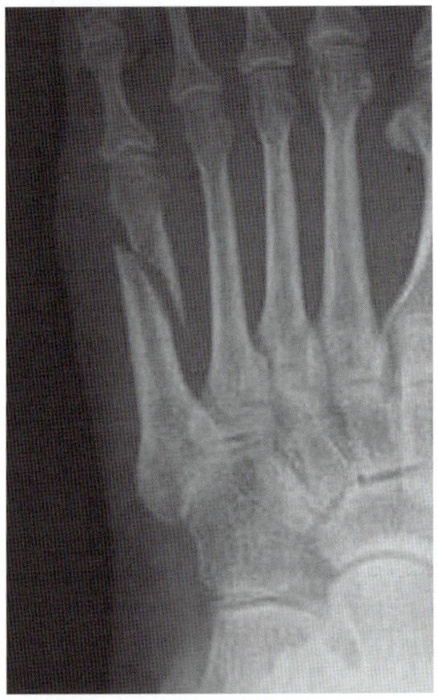

87-B2.3

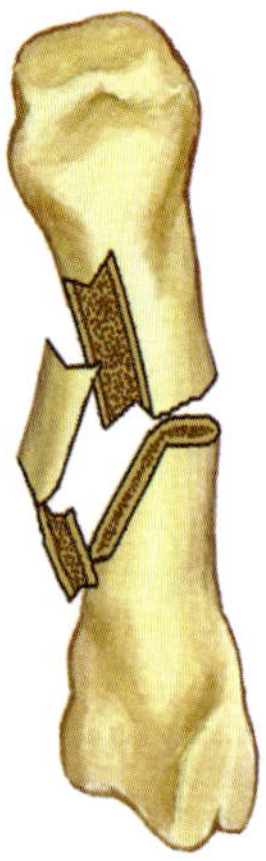

Comminuted wedge

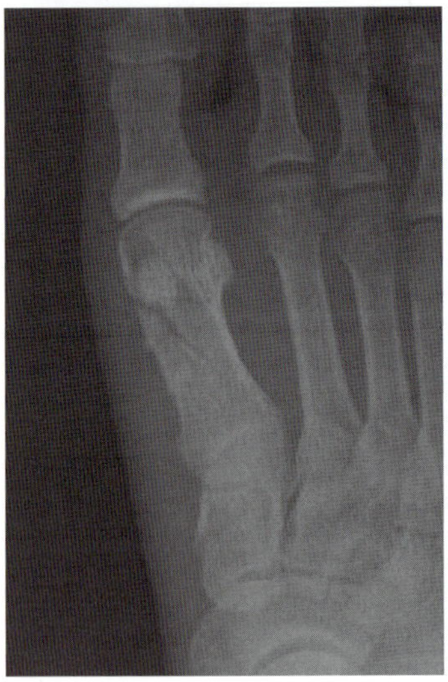

87-B Metatarsal proximal distal partial articular, and diaphysis wedge comminuted

87-B3
Distal partial articular
112 fractures
M: 71 (63.39%)
F: 41 (36.61%)
0.03% of total adult fractures
0.29% of adult foot fractures
1.24% of metatarsal
2.30% of type 87-B

87-B3.1

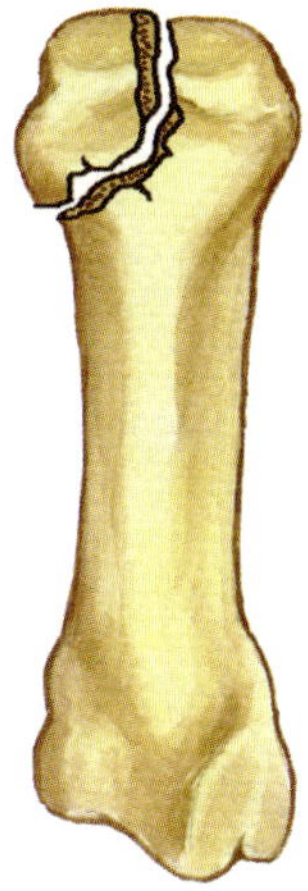

Avulsion or split

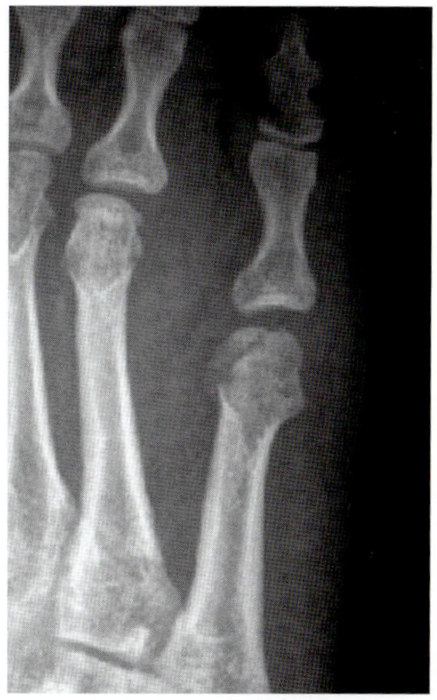

87-B3.2

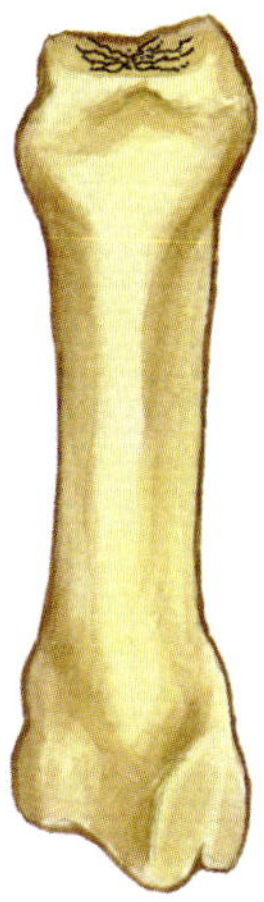

Depression

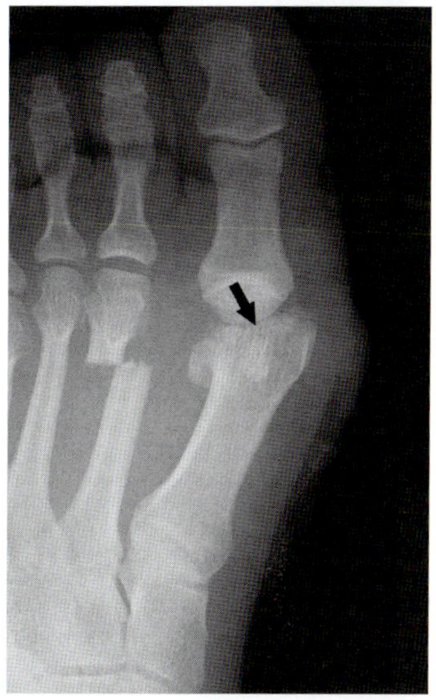

87-B3.3

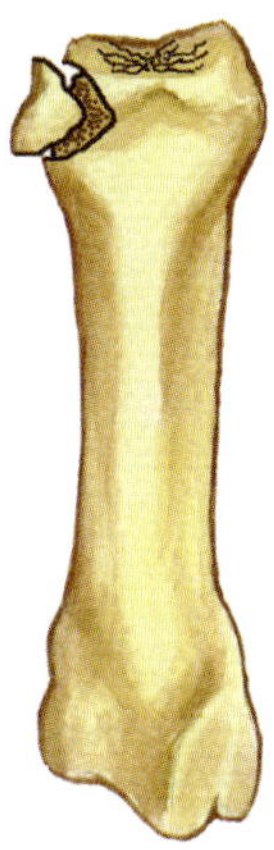

Split/depression

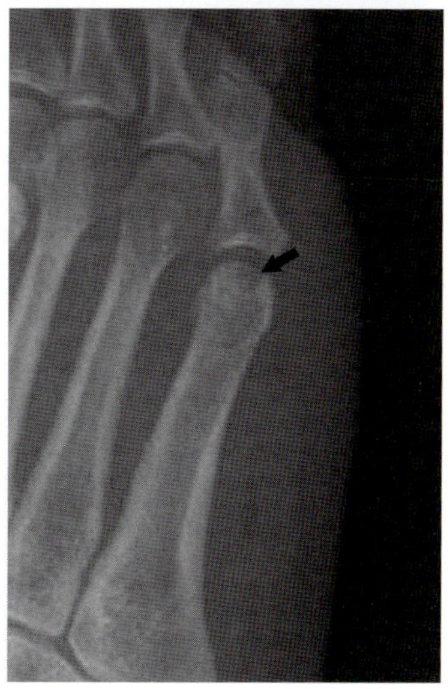

87-C Metatarsal proximal distal complete articular, and diaphysis comminuted

87-C1
Proximal complete articular
289 fractures
M: 173 (59.86%)
F: 116 (40.14%)
0.08% of total adult fractures
0.75% of adult foot fractures
3.21% of metatarsal
54.43% of type 87-C

87-C1.1

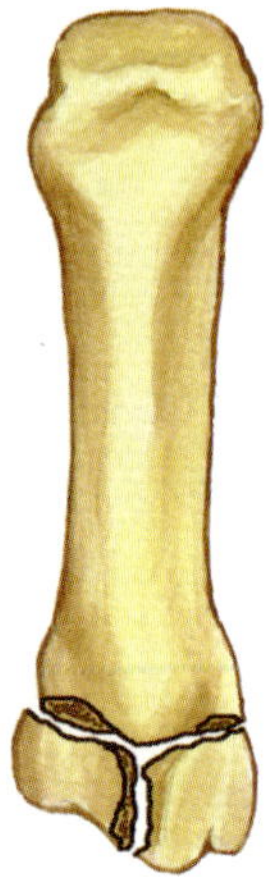

Noncomminuted articular and metaphysis

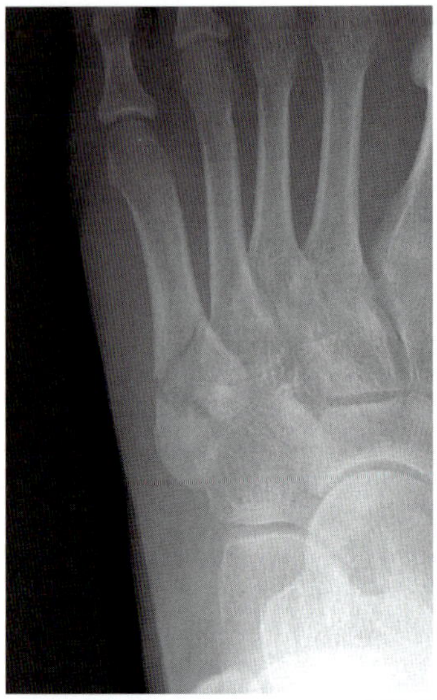

87-C1.2

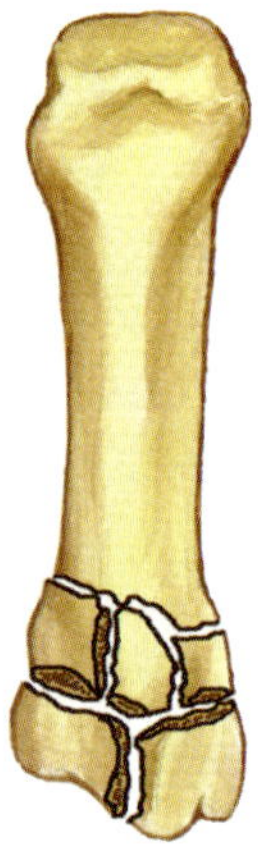

Noncomminuted articular, comminuted metaphysis

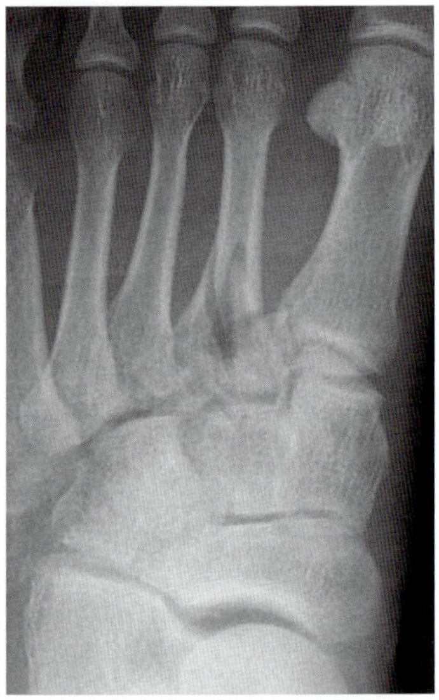

87-C1.3

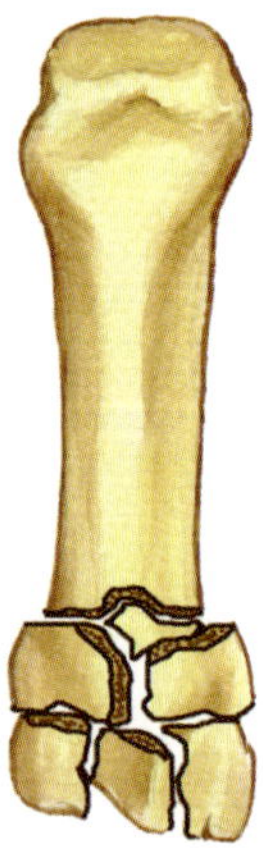

Comminuted articular

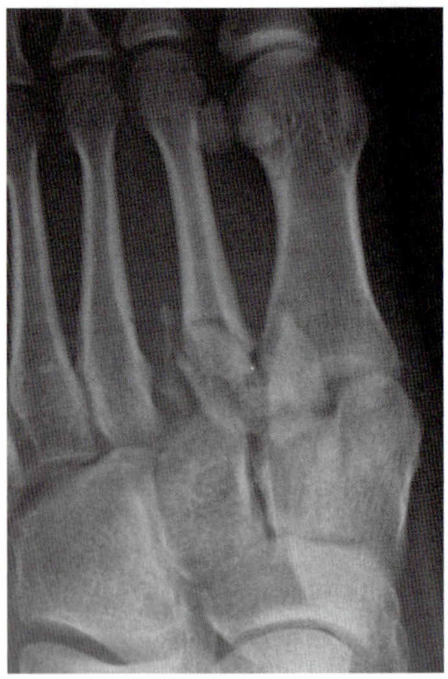

87-C Metatarsal proximal distal complete articular, and diaphysis comminuted

87-C2
Diaphysis comminuted
182 fractures
M: 127 (69.78%)
F: 55 (30.22%)
0.05% of total adult fractures
0.47% of adult foot fractures
2.02% of metatarsal
34.27% of type 87-C

87-C2.1

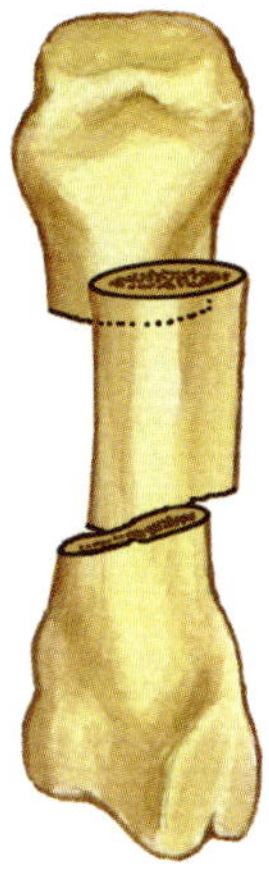

Segmental

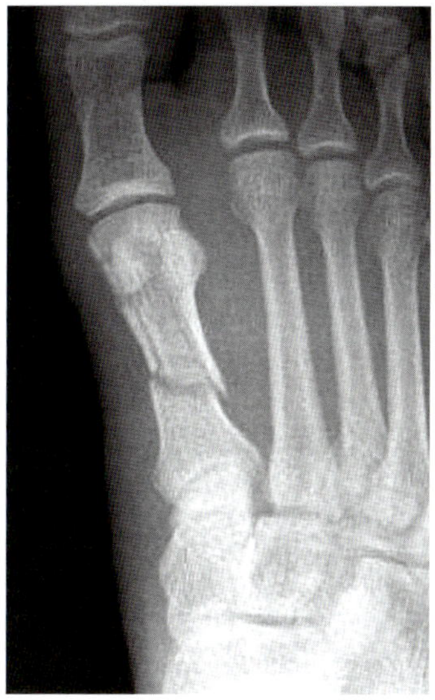

87-C2.2

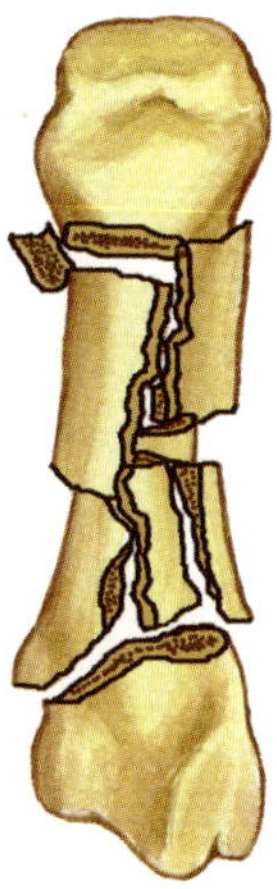

Complex comminuted

87-C Metatarsal proximal distal complete articular, and diaphysis comminuted

87-C3
Distal articular
60 fractures
M: 38 (63.33%)
F: 22 (36.67%)
0.02% of total adult fractures
0.16% of adult foot fractures
0.67% of metatarsal
11.3% of type 87-C

87-C3.1

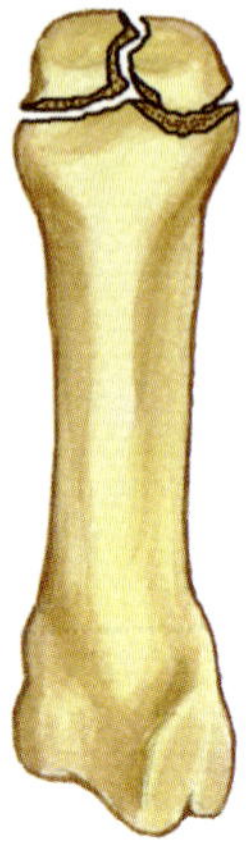

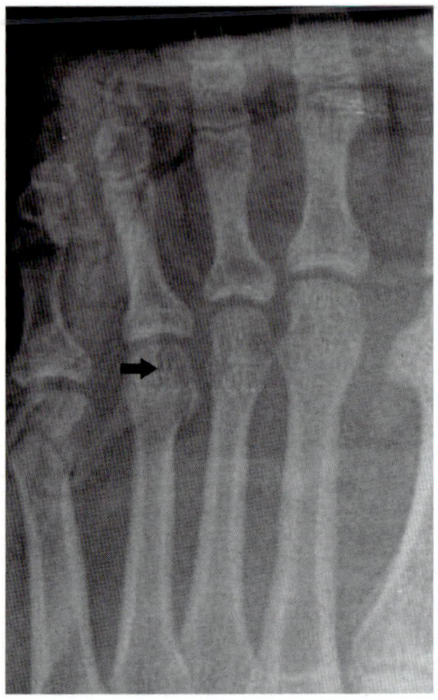

Simple articular/metaphysis

87-C3.2

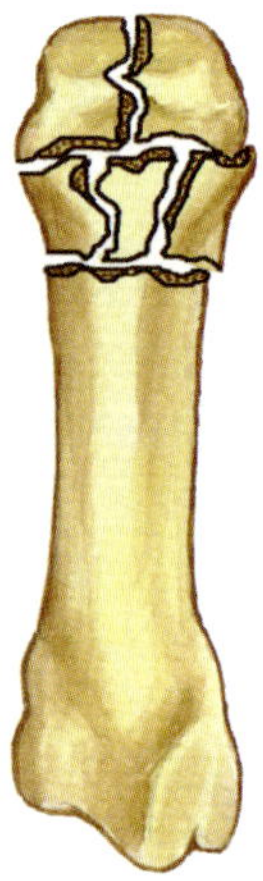

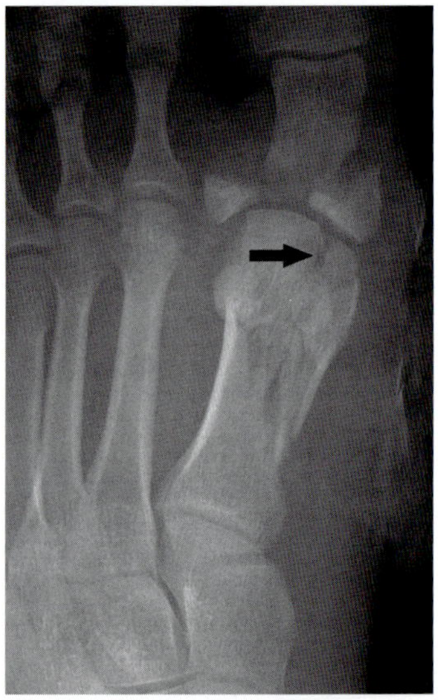

Simple articular/comminuted metaphysis

87-C3.3

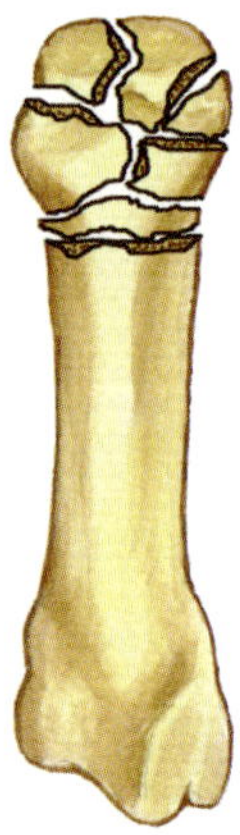

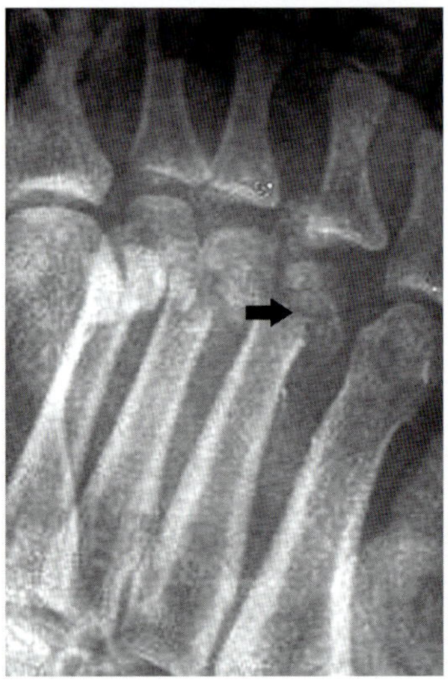

Comminuted articular

Injury Mechanism

Fractures of the metatarsal usually occur as a result of direct trauma from dropping a heavy object on an extremity, or having an extremity crushed by a car. Although the second, third, and fourth metatarsal bones are often injured from direct mechanisms, multiple fractures may present as well. Indirect trauma after torsional stress may result in spiral fractures. Fractures of the base of the fifth metatarsal bone are often caused by forced inversion of the foot, which produces substantial tension on the peroneus brevis tendon. The inferoposterior displacement of the distal fragment following the base fracture will likely compress or injure the plantar arterial arch. Transverse, oblique, or comminuted fractures of the metatarsal shaft may occur, depending on the magnitude and direction of the impacting force. A single-shaft fracture of the second to fourth metatarsals is weakly associated with marked displacement, while metatarsal neck fractures are often associated with inferoposterior displacement of the distal fragment, resulting in the lowering of the metatarsal head and a decreased weight-bearing capacity of the foot.

Diagnosis

Trauma history, physical examination findings, and radiographic evaluation usually lead to a diagnosis. Patients commonly present with pain, swelling, and ecchymosis over the forefoot area. Deformity may occur if there is marked displacement or dislocation. Various levels of motion limitation may be present, depending on the severity of the injury. Physical examination findings include local tenderness on palpation, abnormality of motion, and presence of bony crepitus. Standard radiographs include the AP, lateral, and oblique views of the foot, which are the most often used investigations required for the diagnosis of fractures. Particular attention should be focused on the direction of the fracture line, involvement of the articulation, presence of displacement, and the number of fractures.

Treatment

Fractures of the bases of the second to fourth metatarsal bones are often associated with dislocations and are often unstable. The inferoposterior displacement of the distal fragment may disturb the blood supply of the forefoot. Emergent closed reduction should be performed followed by casting as soon as possible to avoid any interruption of blood supply. If closed reduction fails, an intramedullary (IM) pin can be inserted from the head of the metatarsal bone across the fracture line into the tarsal bone for internal fixation. Isolated fractures of the base of the fifth metatarsal can be immobilized with the foot in abduction, followed by application of a bandage or cast for 4–6 weeks. Range-of-motion exercises can be initiated after the external fixation device is removed.

Single nondisplaced metatarsal shaft fractures can be treated by casting for 4–6 weeks. Multiple metatarsal shaft fractures with displacement should be treated with closed reduction first; if closed reduction fails, open reduction and internal fixation is indicated with insertion of an intramedullary pin from the inferior part of the head for 4–6 weeks.

Displaced metatarsal neck fractures can be treated by closed reduction initially, followed by casting if the reduction is successful; if not, open reduction and internal fixation is indicated. Particular attention should be given to the avoidance of dorsal angulation of the distal fragment. Weight-bearing exercises should start as soon as radiographs show adequate fracture healing.

Phalangeal Fractures (Segment 88)

Anatomical Features

The phalanges of the foot can be divided into three segments according to their distance from the body: proximal, middle, intermediate (the big toe does not have a middle phalanx), and distal phalanges. Each phalanx has a base, a shaft, and a head. The interphalangeal articulations of the foot are ginglymoid joints, and each has a plantar and two collateral ligaments. They are second to the ankle joint as the most mobile joints in the body, and are easy targets for injuries due to their anatomical location (**Plate 9.16**).

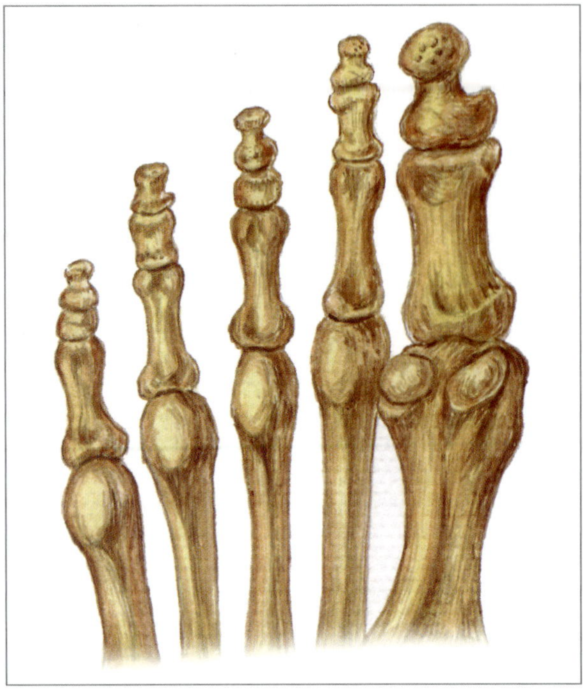

Plate 9.16

OTA Classification of Phalangeal Fractures

Based on OTA classification, the phalanx is coded as the number 88 for its anatomical location. Phalangeal fractures are classified into three types: 88-A, phalanx proximal and distal extra-articular, and diaphysis noncomminuted; 88-B, phalanx proximal and distal partial articular, and diaphysis wedge comminuted; and 88-C, phalanx proximal and distal complete articular, and diaphysis comminuted (**Plate 9.17**).

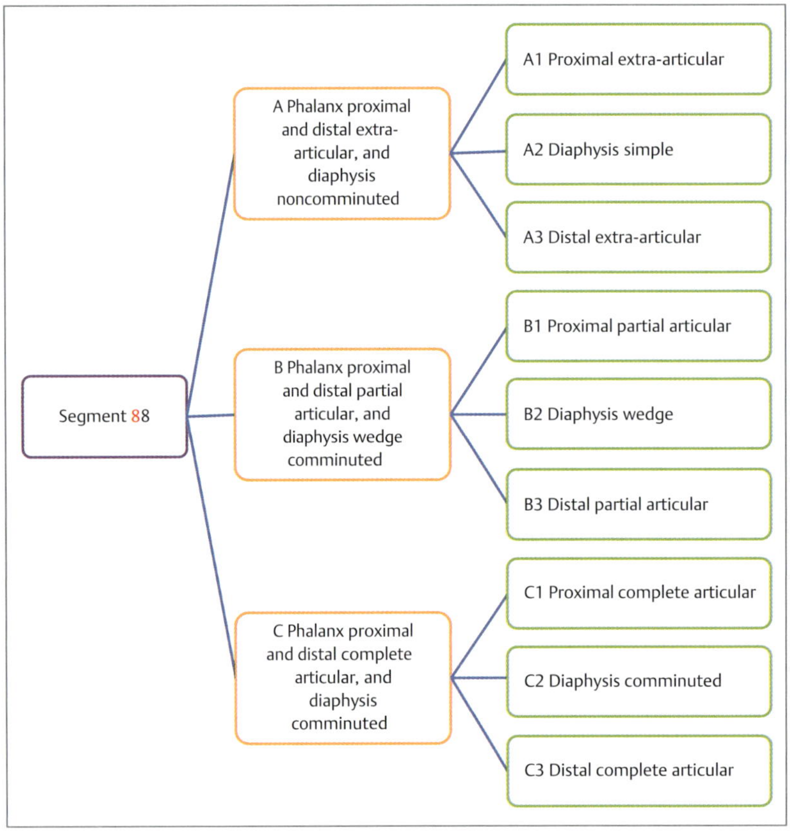

Plate 9.17

Clinical Epidemiologic Features of Phalangeal Fractures (Segment 88)

A total of 7,397 adult patients with 7,397 phalanx fractures were treated in 83 hospitals in China over a 2-year period from 2010 to 2011. All cases were reviewed and statistically studied; the fractures accounted for 2.05% of all patients with fractures, including 3,591 patients with fractures on the left side and 3,806 on the right side. There were 5,243 males and 2,154 females, with a male-to-female ratio of 2.43:1.

Epidemiologic features of phalanx fractures are as follows:

- More males than females
- The high-risk age group is 21–25 years, with ages 21–25 years the highest for males and 36–40 years the highest for females.
- The most common fracture type is type 88-A.
- The most common fracture group is group 88-A3.
- The first digit is the most commonly fractured foot digit.
- The distal phalanx is the most commonly fractured phalanx.

Phalanx Fractures (Segment 88) by Sex

Table 9.31 Sex distribution of 7,397 patients with fractures of the phalanx of the foot

Sex	Number of patients	Percentage (%)
Male	5,243	70.88
Female	2,154	29.12
Total	7,397	100.00

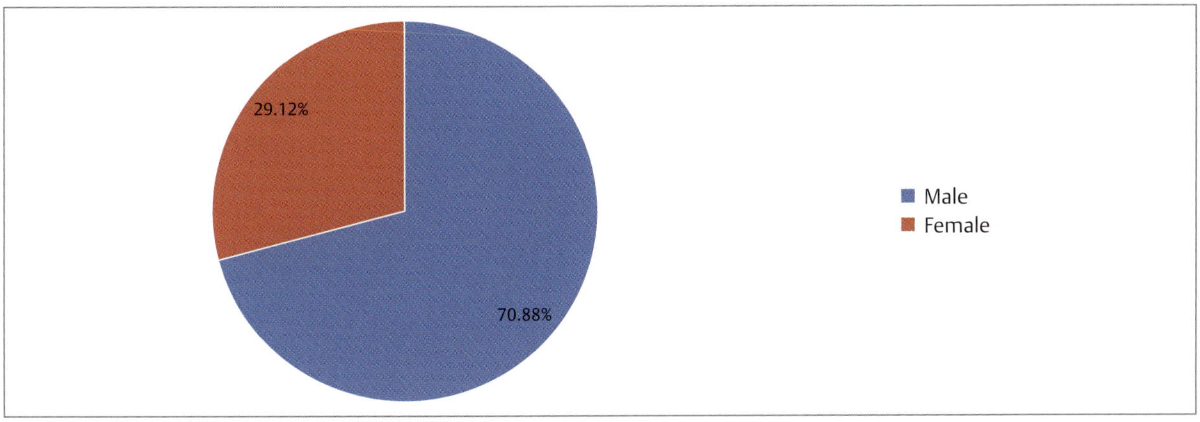

Fig. 9.31 Sex distribution of 7,397 patients with fractures of the phalanx of the foot.

Phalanx Fractures (Segment 88) by Age Group

Table 9.32 Age and sex distribution of 7,397 patients with fractures of the phalanx of the foot

Age group (years)	Male	Female	Number of patients	Percentage (%)
16–20	489	89	578	7.81
21–25	714	236	950	12.84
26–30	648	225	873	11.80
31–35	551	190	741	10.02
36–40	674	264	938	12.68
41–45	674	232	906	12.25
46–50	544	249	793	10.72
51–55	388	200	588	7.95
56–60	296	214	510	6.89
61–65	141	101	242	3.27
66–70	40	64	104	1.41
71–75	41	45	86	1.16
76–80	22	24	46	0.62
81–85	14	16	30	0.41
≥86	7	5	12	0.16
Total	5,243	2,154	7,397	100.00

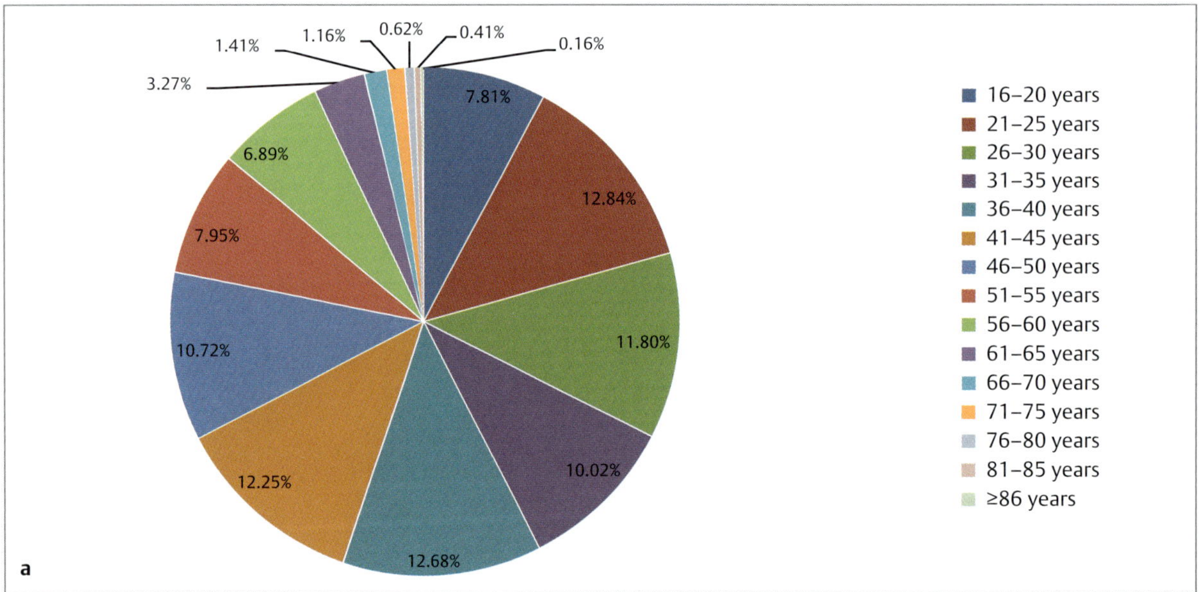

Fig. 9.32 **(a)** Age distribution of 7,397 patients with fractures of the phalanx of the foot.

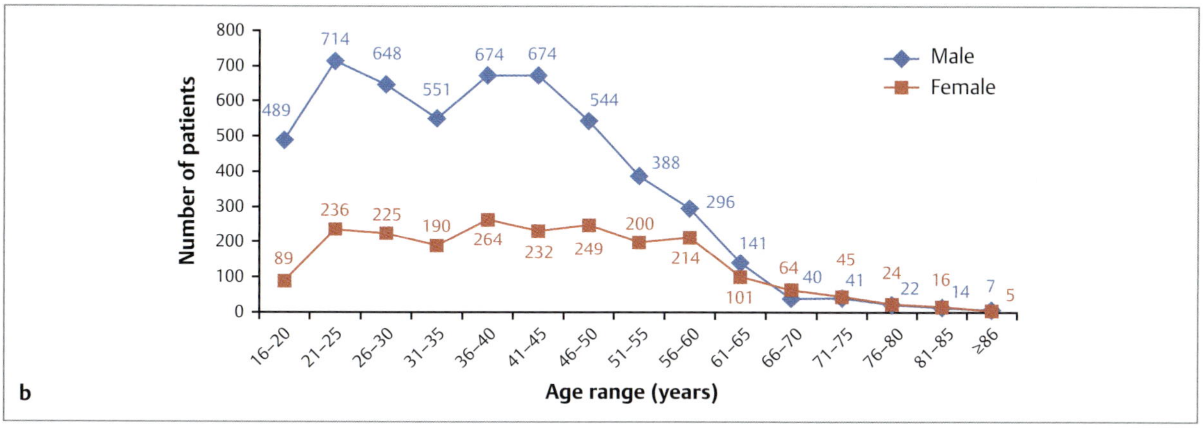

Fig. 9.32 (*continued*) **(b)** Age and sex distribution of 7,397 patients with fractures of the phalanx of the foot.

Phalanx Fractures (Segment 88) by Fracture Type

Table 9.33 Sex and fracture type distribution of 7,397 fractures of the phalanx of the foot

Fracture type	Male	Female	Number of fractures	Percentage (%)
88-A	2,637	1,122	3,759	50.82
88-B	1,536	755	2,291	30.97
88-C	1,070	277	1,347	18.21
Total	5,243	2,154	7,397	100.00

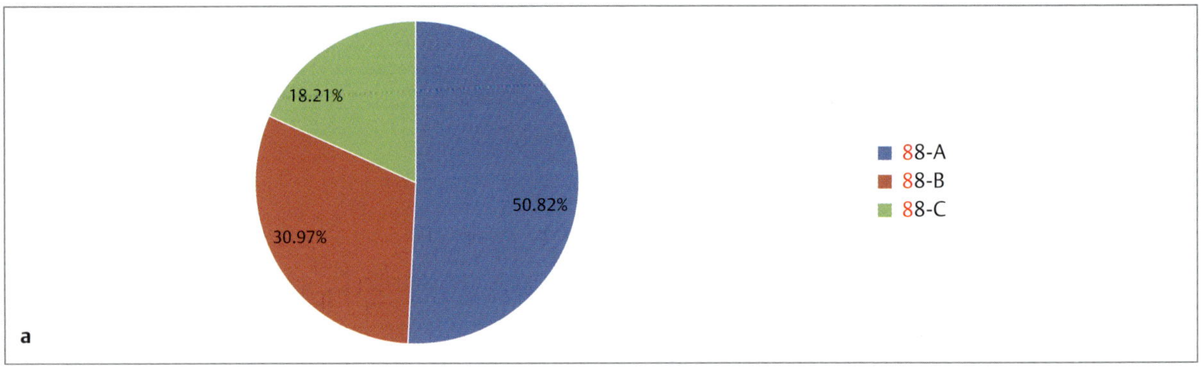

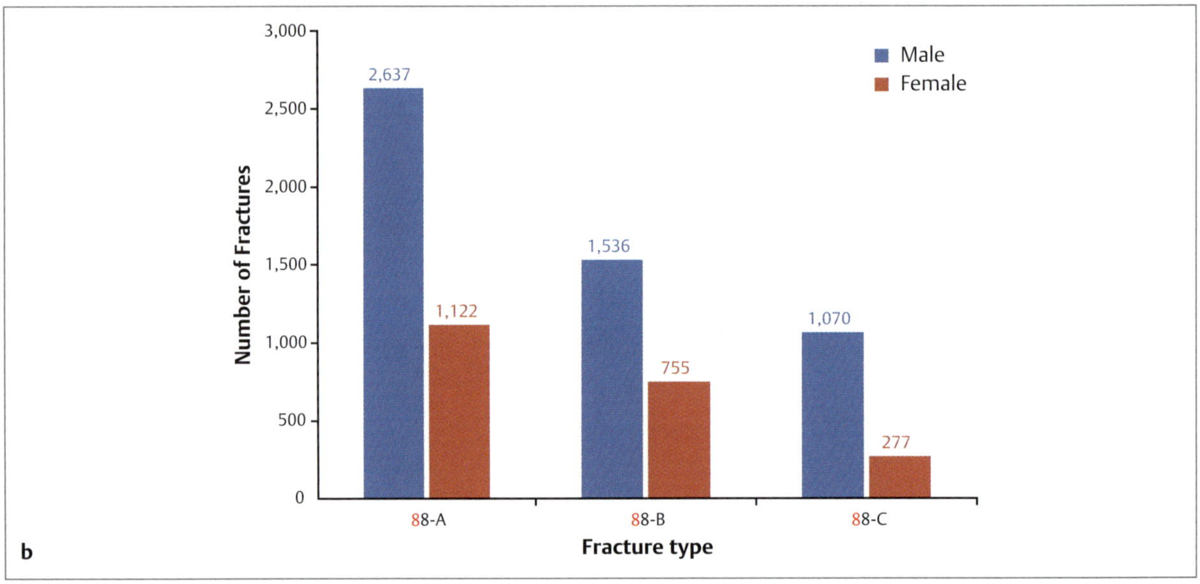

Fig. 9.33 **(a)** Fracture type distribution of 7,397 fractures of the phalanx of the foot.
(b) Sex and fracture type distribution of 7,397 fractures of the phalanx of the foot.

Table 9.34 Sex and fracture group distribution of 7,397 fractures of the phalanx of the foot

Fracture group	Male	Female	Number of fractures	Percentage of phalanx fractures (%)	Percentage of foot fractures (%)
88-A1	299	194	493	6.66	1.28
88-A2	903	439	1,342	18.14	3.47
88-A3	1,435	489	1,924	26.01	4.98
88-B1	827	441	1,268	17.14	3.28
88-B2	242	80	322	4.35	0.83
88-B3	467	234	701	9.48	1.81
88-C1	205	65	270	3.65	0.70
88-C2	448	103	551	7.45	1.43
88-C3	417	109	526	7.11	1.36
Total	5,243	2,154	7,397	100.00	19.15

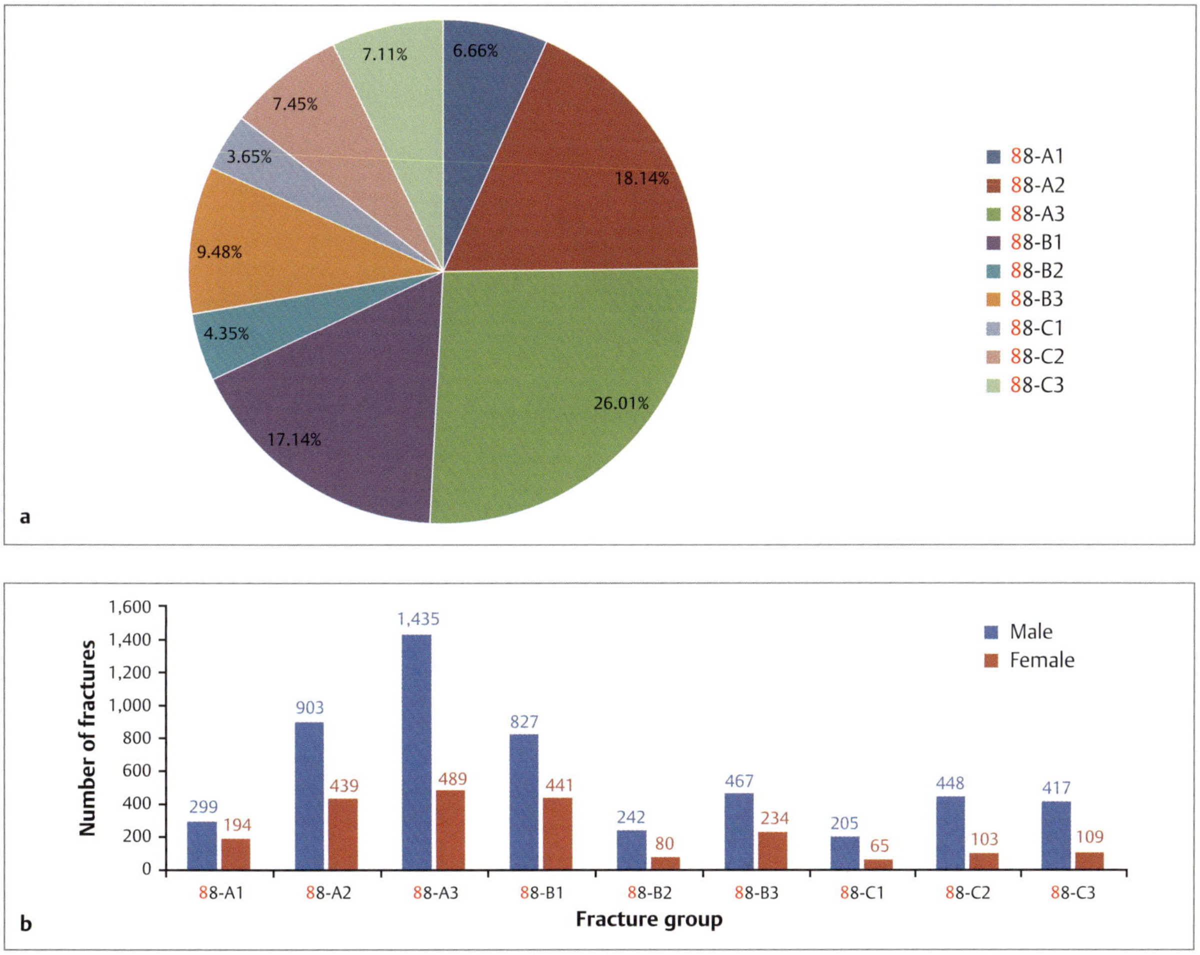

Fig. 9.34 **(a)** Fracture group distribution of 7,397 fractures of the phalanx of the foot. **(b)** Sex and fracture group distribution of 7,397 fractures of the phalanx of the foot.

Phalanx Fractures (Segment 88) by Individual Foot Digit

Table 9.35 Distribution of 7,397 fractures of the phalanx of the foot by individual foot digit

The number of the phalanx of the foot	Number of digits with fractures	Percentage of phalangeal fractures (%)
1st	4,637	62.69
2nd	700	9.46
3rd	414	5.60
4th	401	5.42
5th	1,245	16.83
Total	7,397	100.00

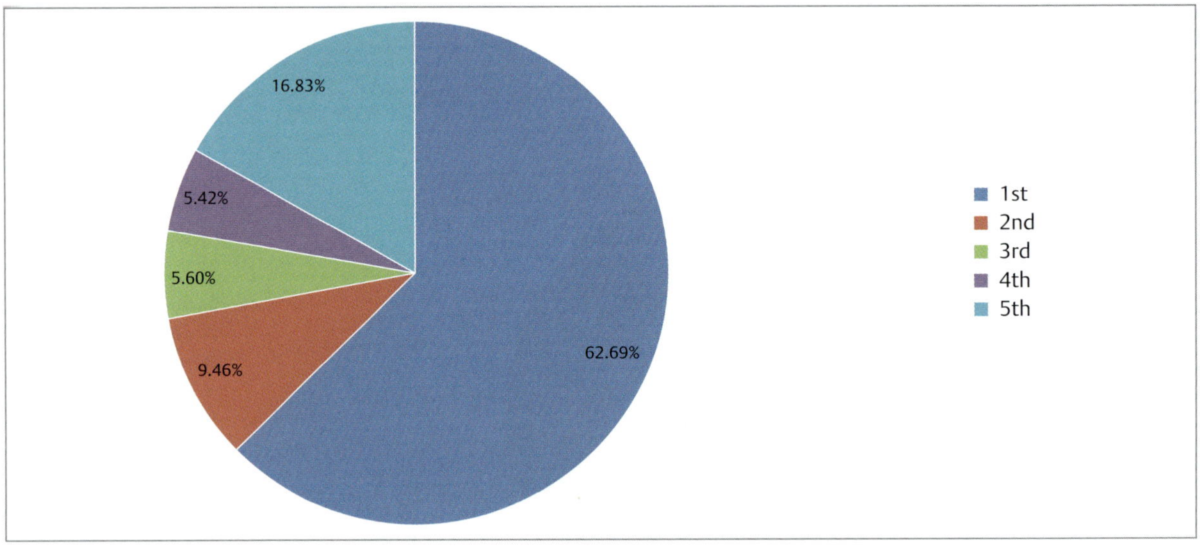

Fig. 9.35 Distribution of 7,397 fractures of the phalanx of the foot by individual foot digit.

Phalanx Fractures by Segment (Segment 88)

Table 9.36 Sex and fracture segment distribution of 7,397 fractures of the phalanx of the foot

Fracture segment	Male	Female	Number of fractures	Percentage (%)
Proximal	1,331	700	2,031	27.46
Diaphysis	1,593	622	2,215	29.94
Distal	2,319	832	3,151	42.60
Total	5,243	2,154	7,397	100.00

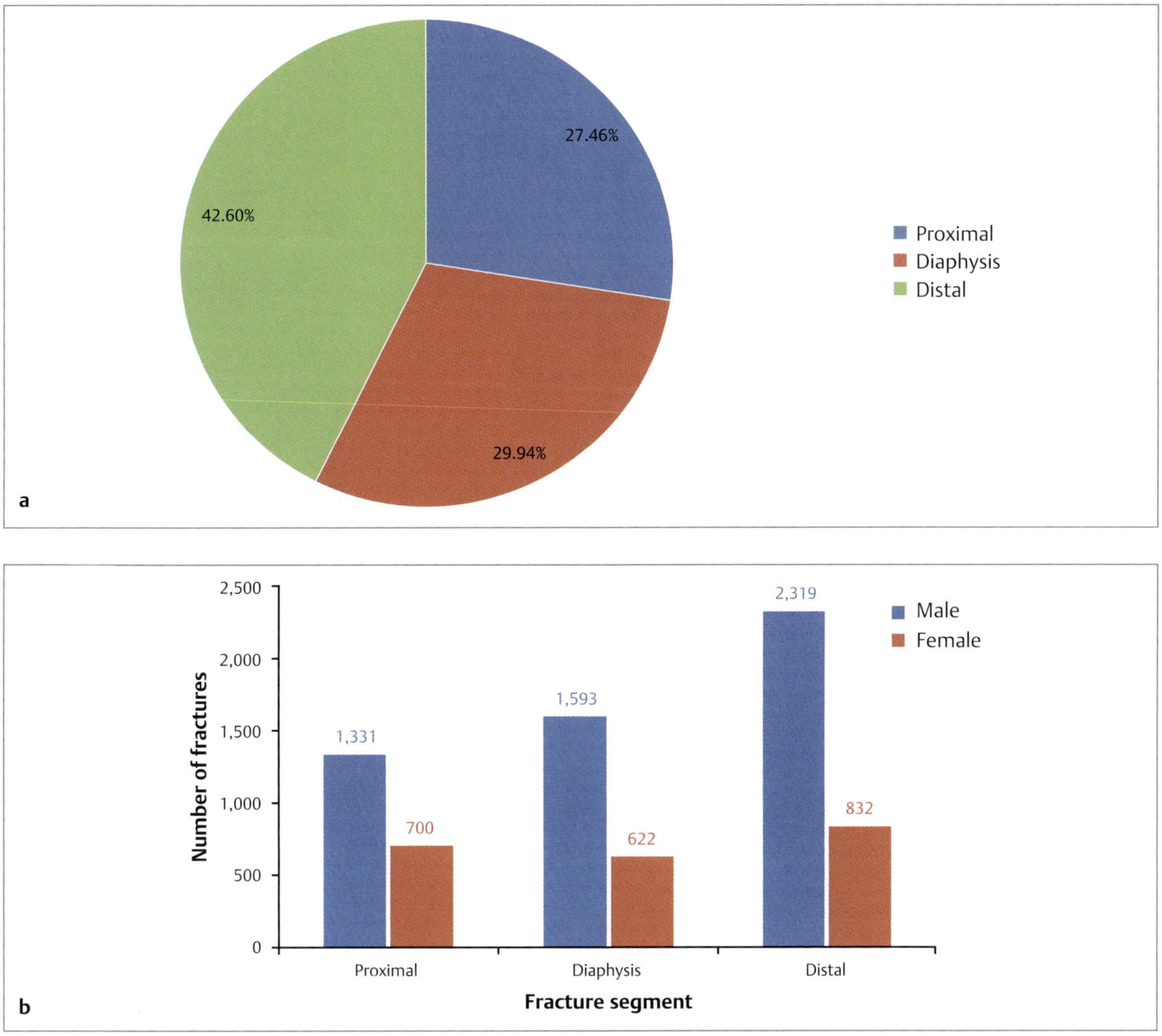

Fig. 9.36 **(a)** Fracture segmental distribution of 7,397 fractures of the phalanx of the foot. **(b)** Sex and fracture segment distribution of 7,397 fractures of the phalanx of the foot.

88-A Phalanx proximal and distal extra-articular, and diaphysis noncomminuted

88-A1
Proximal extra-articular
493 fractures
M: 299 (60.65%)
F: 194 (39.35%)
0.13% of total adult fractures
1.28% of adult foot fractures
6.66% of phalanx
13.12% of type 88-A

88-A1.1

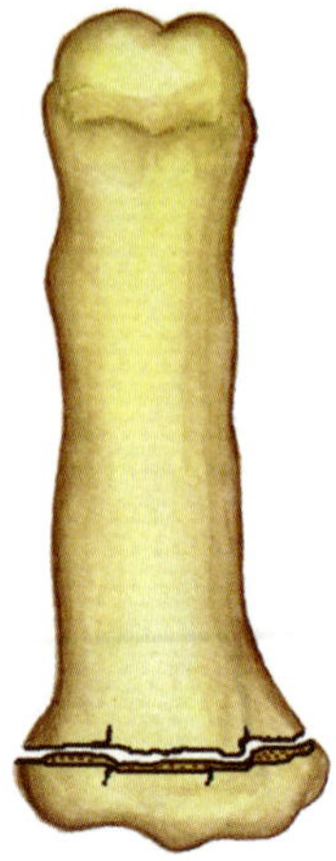

Noncomminuted

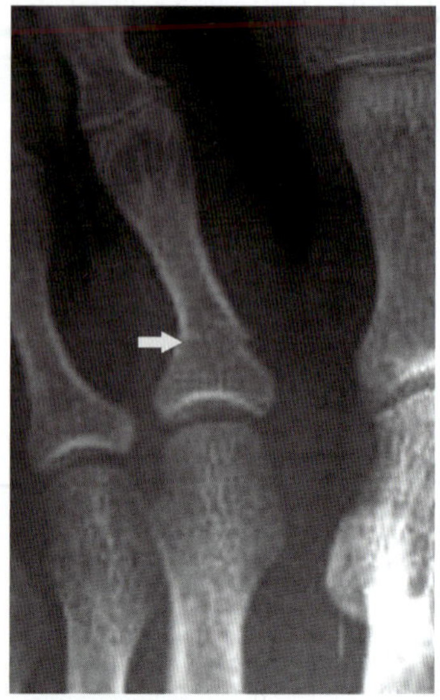

88-A1.2

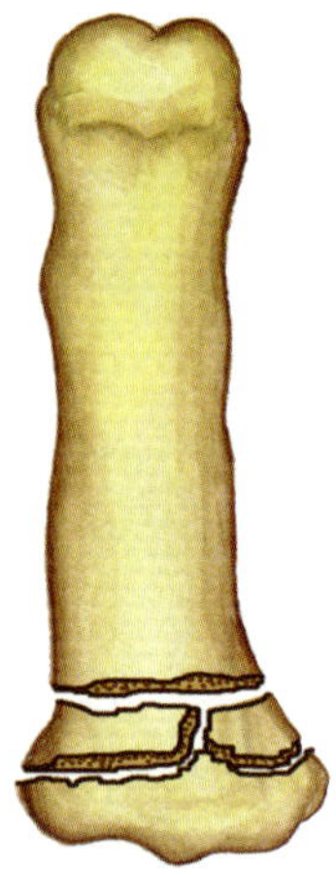

Comminuted

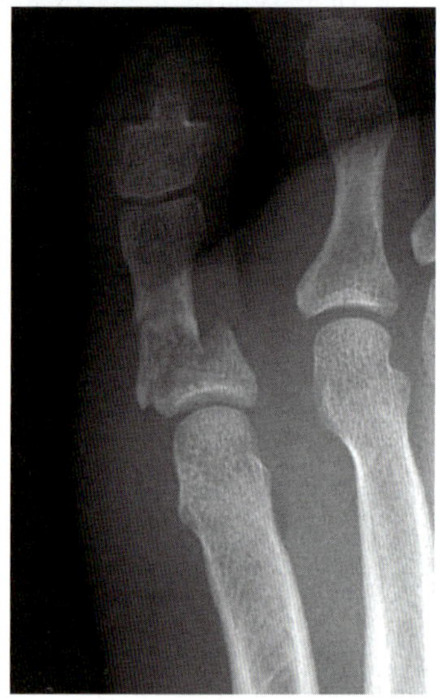

88-A Phalanx proximal and distal extra-articular, and diaphysis noncomminuted

88-A2
Diaphysis simple
1,342 fractures
M: 903 (67.29%)
F: 439 (32.71%)
0.36% of total adult fractures
3.47% of adult foot fractures
18.14% of phalanx
35.7% of type 88-A

88-A2.1

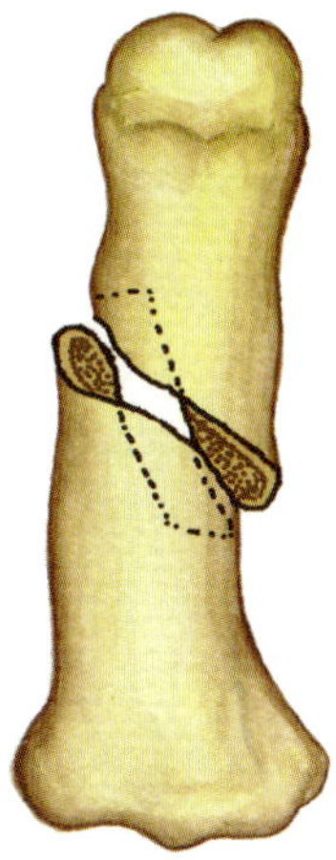

Spiral

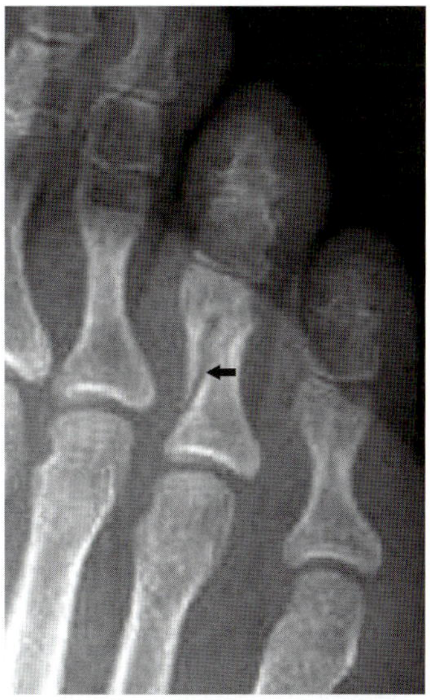

88-A2.2

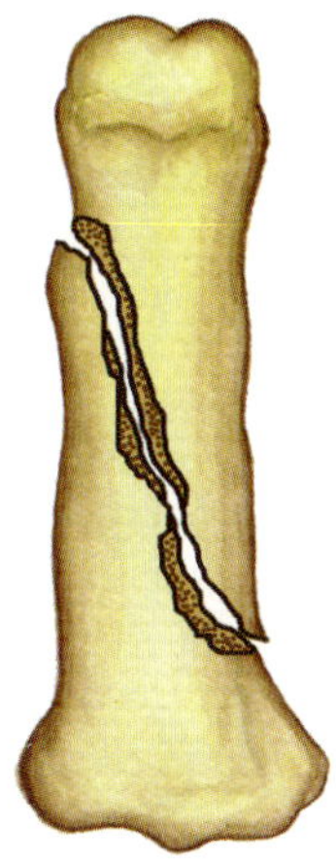

Oblique

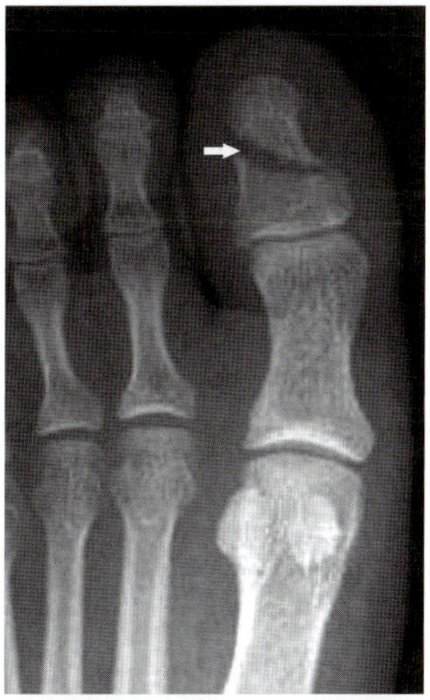

88-A2.3

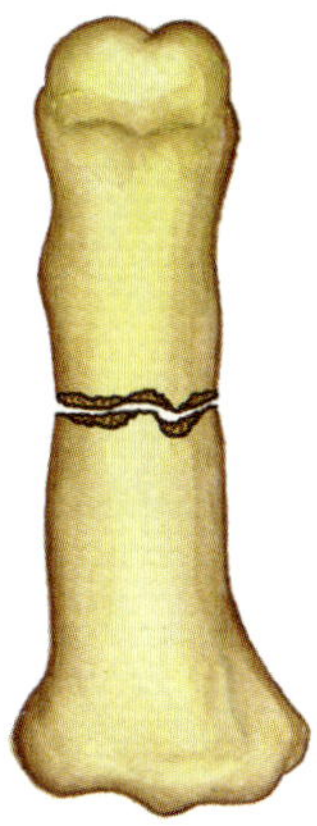

Transverse

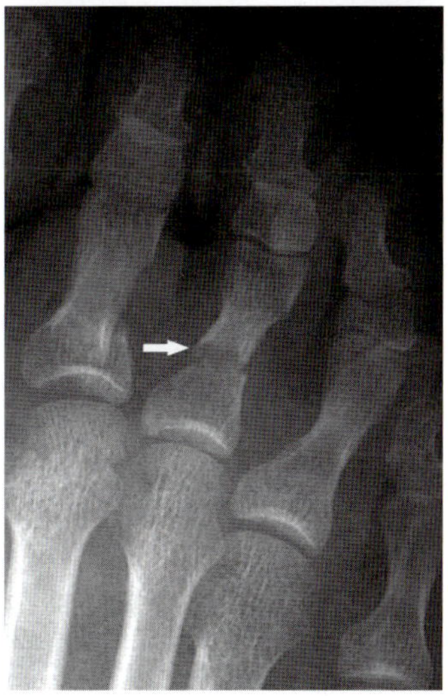

88-A Phalanx proximal and distal extra-articular, and diaphysis noncomminuted

88-A3
Distal extra-articular
1,924 fractures
M: 1,435 (74.58%)
F: 489 (25.42%)
0.51% of total adult fractures
4.98% of adult foot fractures
26.01% of phalanx
51.18% of type 88-A

88-A3.1

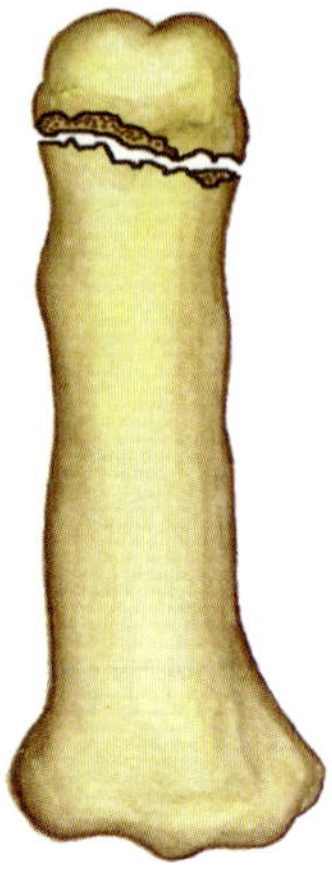

Noncomminuted

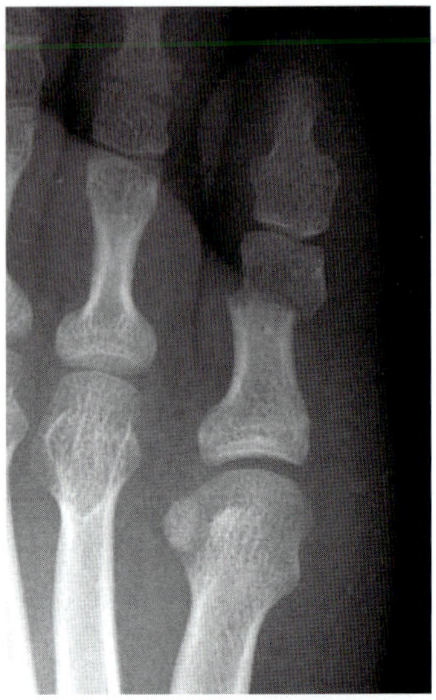

88-A3.2

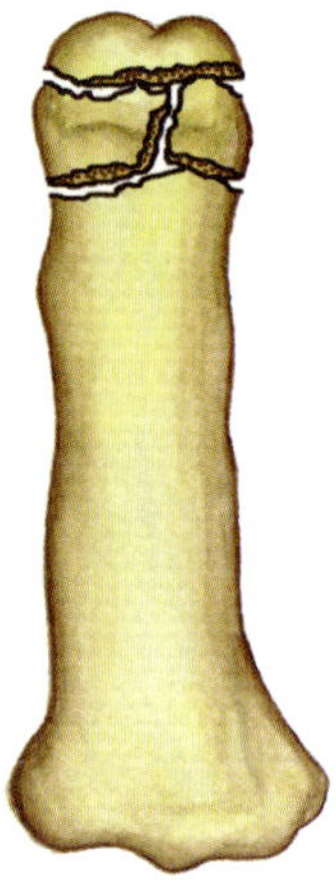

Comminuted

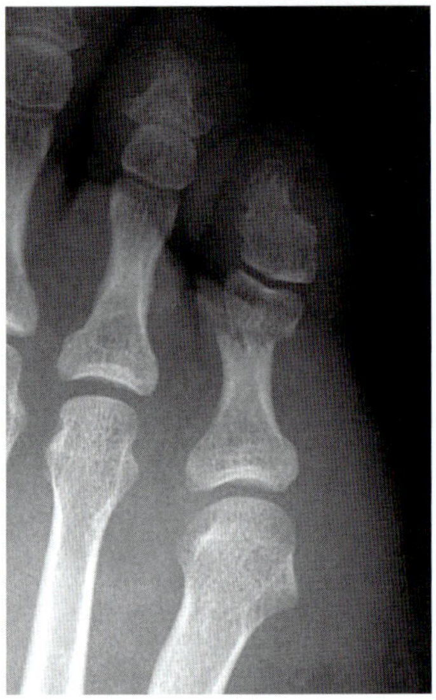

88-B Phalanx proximal and distal partial articular, and diaphysis wedge comminuted

88-B1
Proximal partial articular

1,268 fractures
M: 827 (65.22%)
F: 441 (34.78%)
0.34% of total adult fractures
3.28% of adult foot fractures
17.14% of phalanx
55.35% of type 88-B

88-B1.1

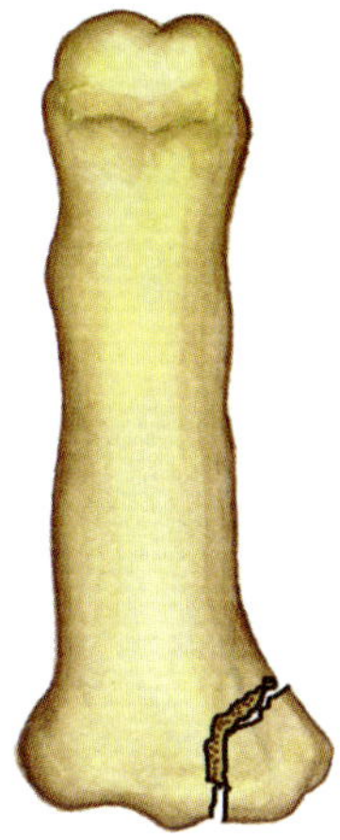

Avulsion or split

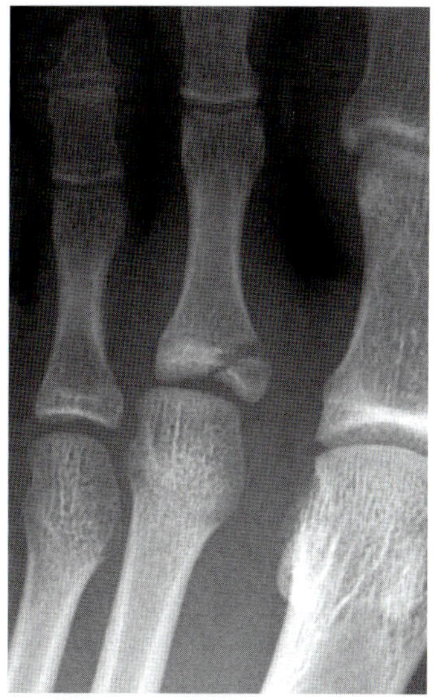

88-B1.2

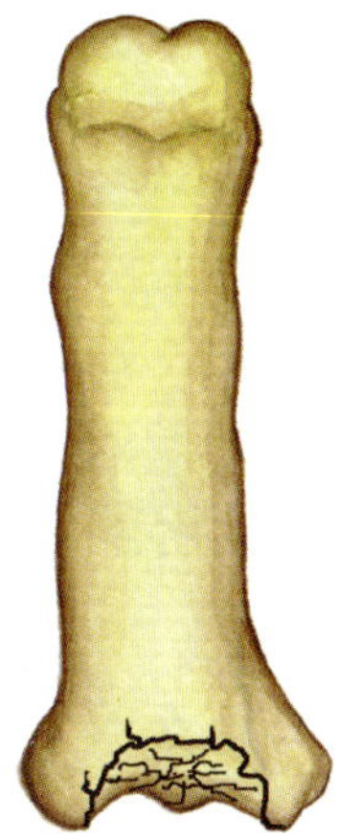

Depression

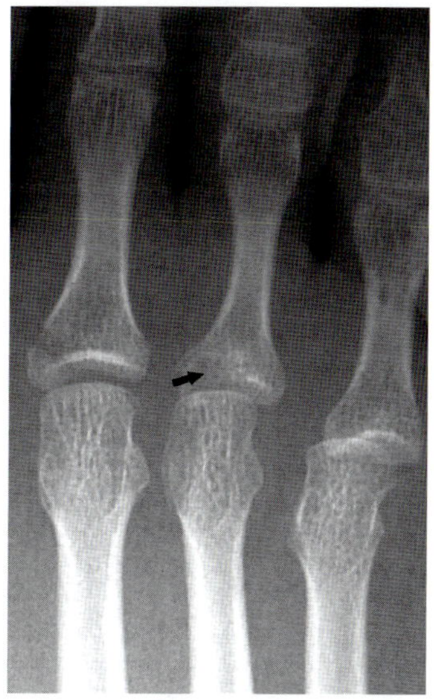

88-B1.3

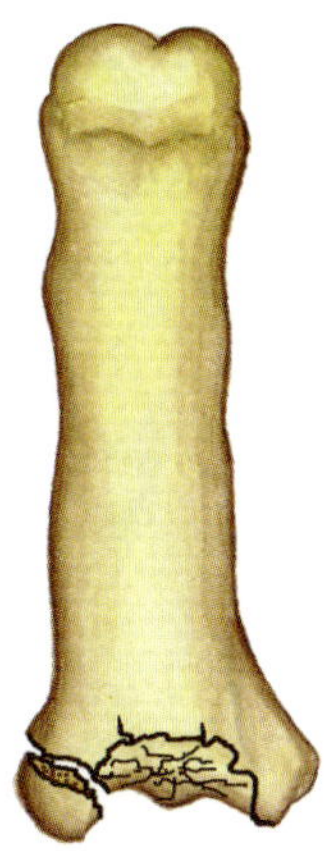

Split/depression

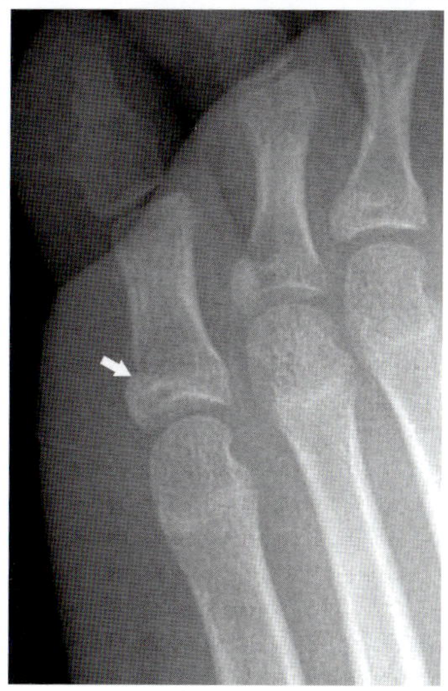

88-B Phalanx proximal and distal partial articular, and diaphysis wedge comminuted

88-B2
Diaphysis wedge
322 fractures
M: 242 (75.16%)
F: 80 (24.84%)
0.09% of total adult fractures
0.83% of adult foot fractures
4.35% of phalanx
14.05% of type 88-B

88-B2.1

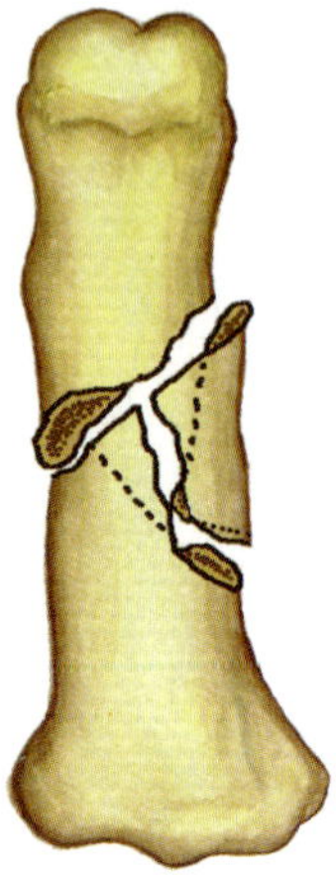

Spiral

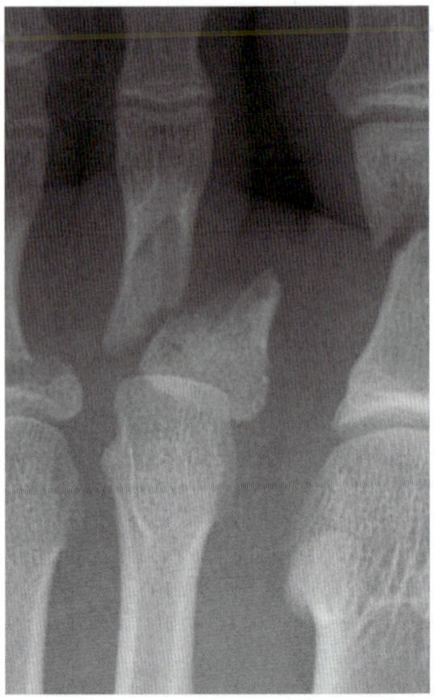

88-B2.2

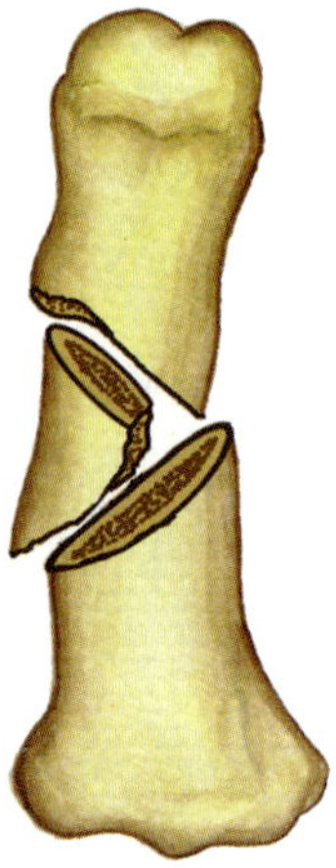

Bending

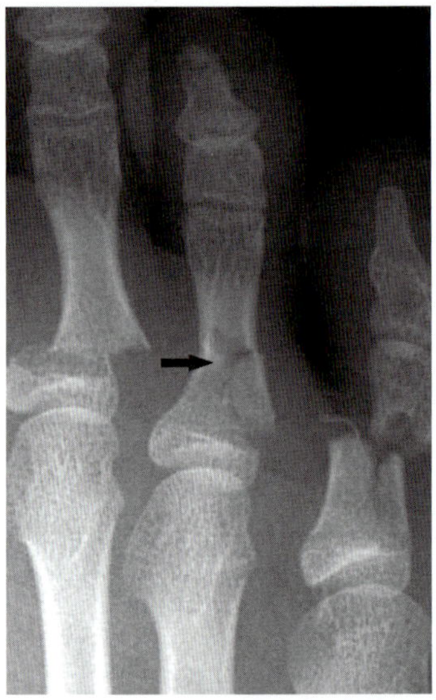

88-B2.3

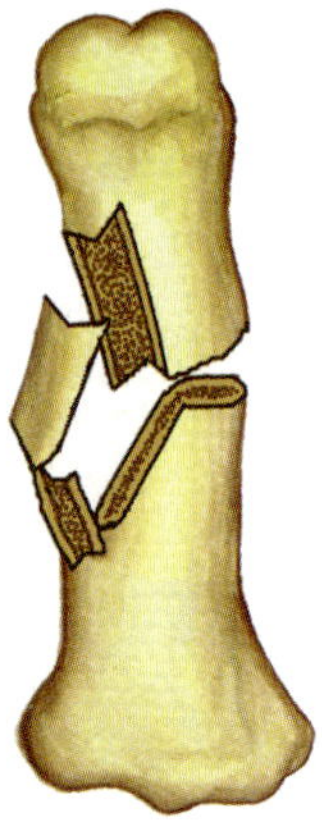

Fragmented

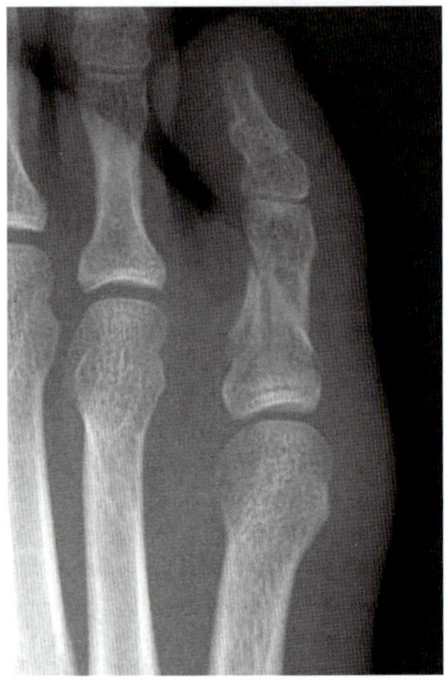

88-B Phalanx proximal and distal partial articular, and diaphysis wedge comminuted

88-B3
Distal partial articular
701 fractures
M: 467 (66.62%)
F: 234 (33.38%)
0.19% of total adult fractures
1.81% of adult foot fractures
9.48% of phalanx
30.6% of type 88-B

88-B3.1

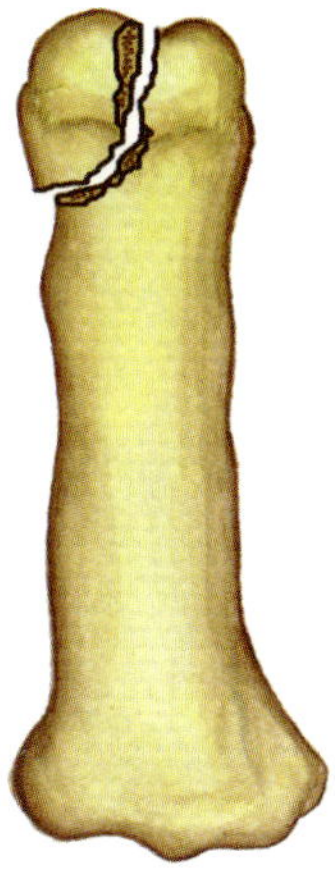

Avulsion or split

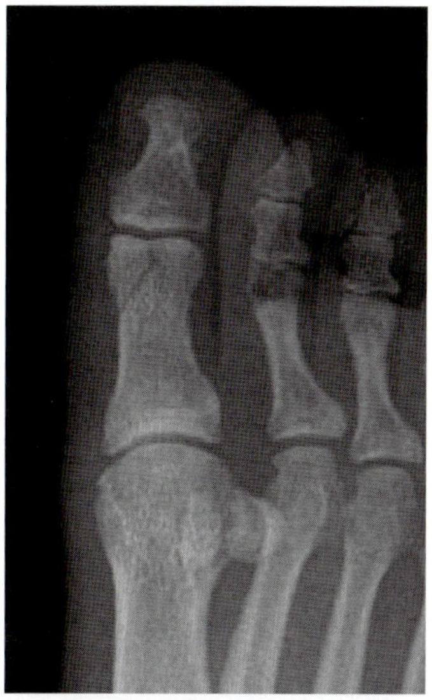

88-B3.2

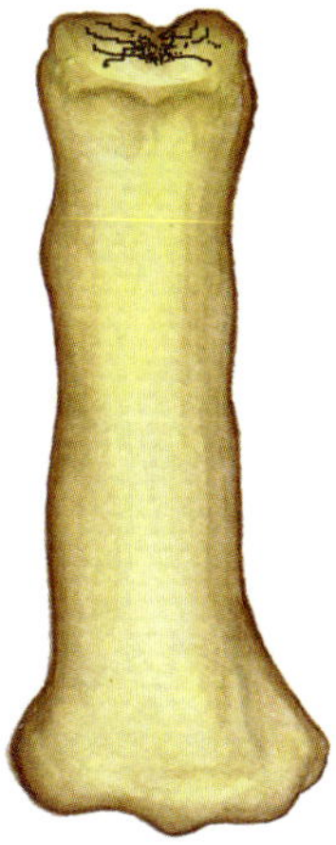

Depression

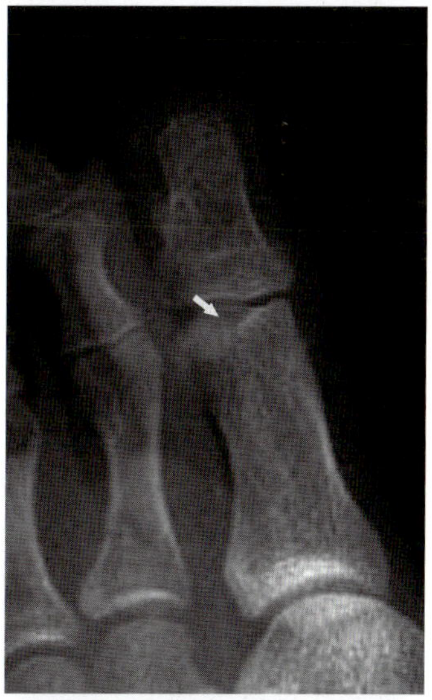

88-B3.3

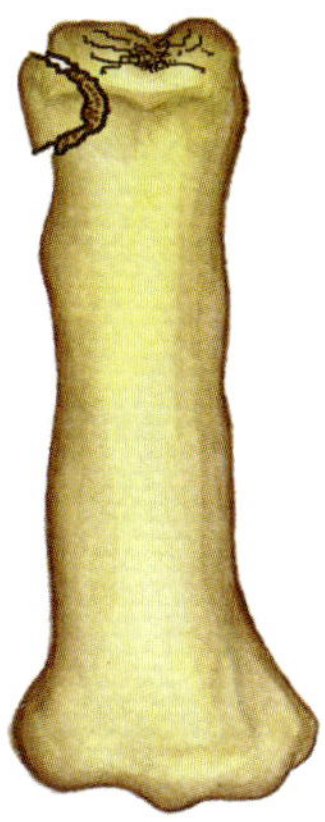

Split/depression

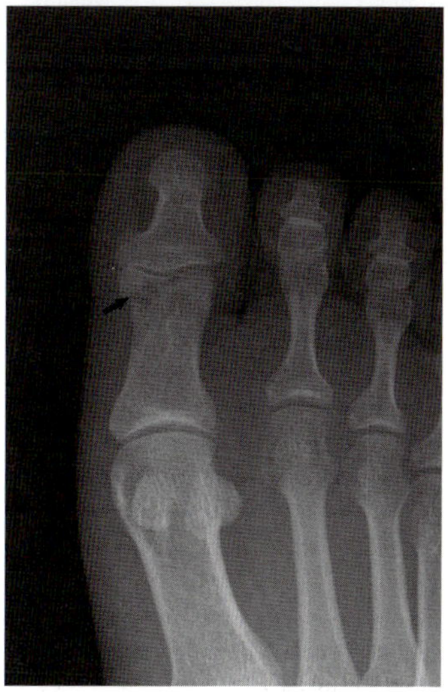

88-C Phalanx proximal and distal complete articular, and diaphysis comminuted

88-C1
Proximal complete articular
270 fractures
M: 205 (75.93%)
F: 65 (24.07%)
0.07% of total adult fractures
0.7% of adult foot fractures
3.65% of phalanx
20.04% of type 88-C

88-C1.1

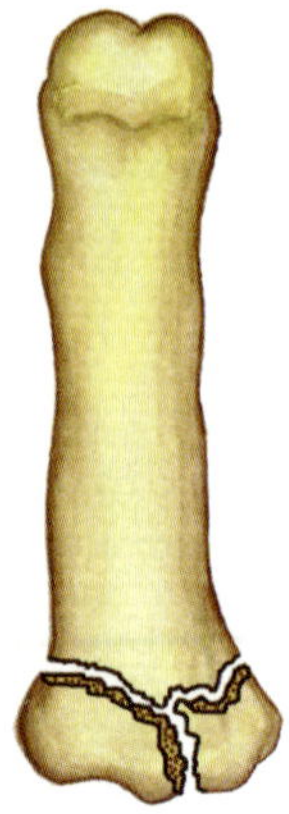

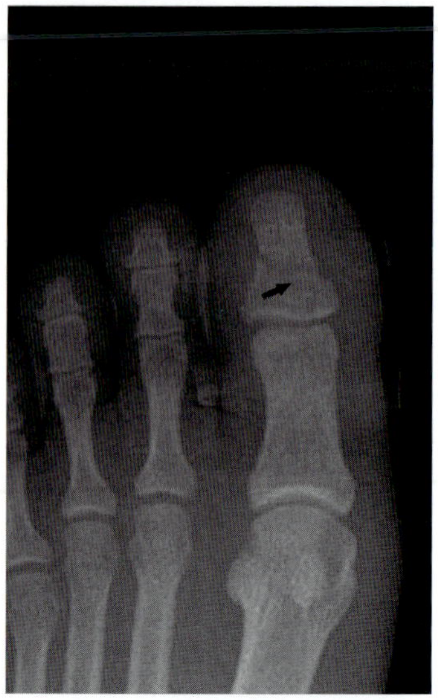

Noncomminuted articular/metaphysis

88-C1.2

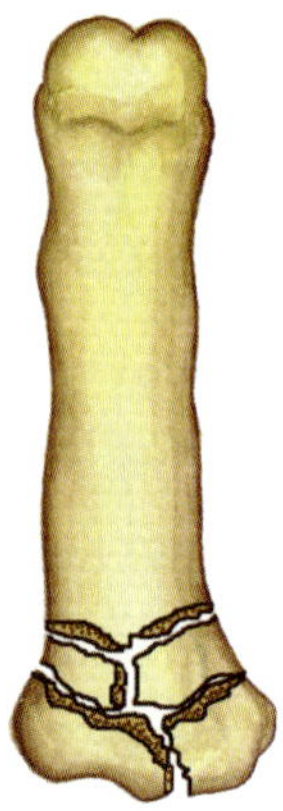

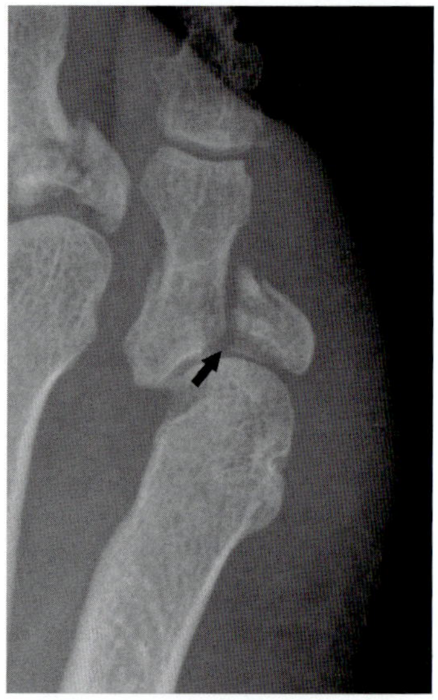

Noncomminuted articular/comminuted metaphysis

88-C1.3

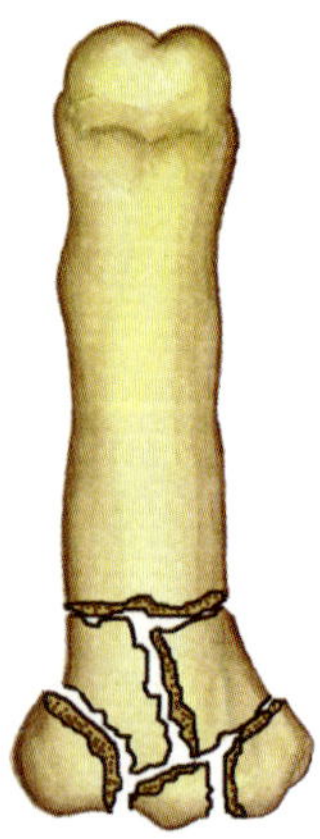

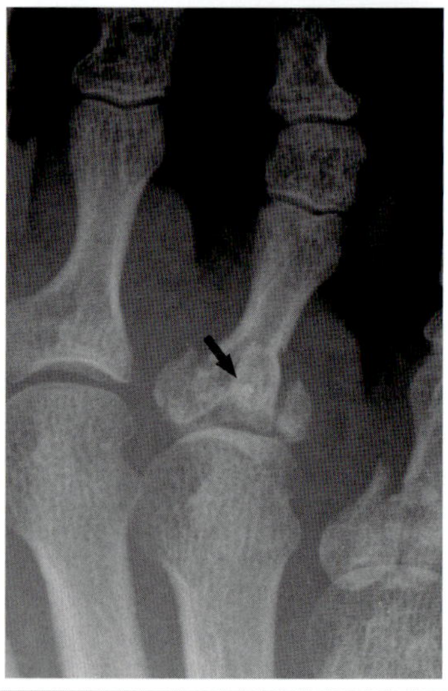

Comminuted articular and metaphysis

88-C Phalanx proximal and distal complete articular, and diaphysis comminuted

88-C2
Diaphysis comminuted
551 fractures
M: 448 (81.31%)
F: 103 (18.69%)
0.15% of total adult fractures
1.43% of adult fractures foot
7.45% of phalanx
40.91% of type 88-C

88-C2.1

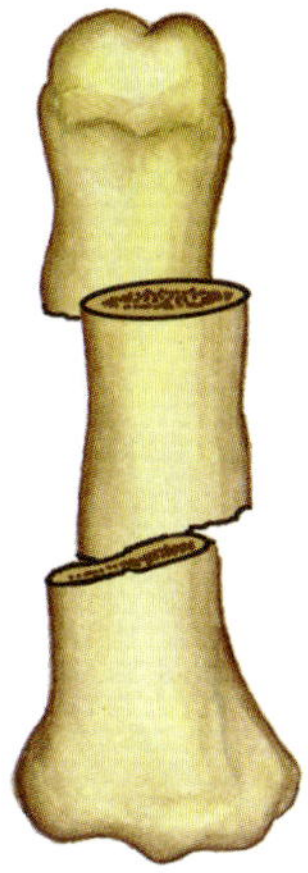

Segmental

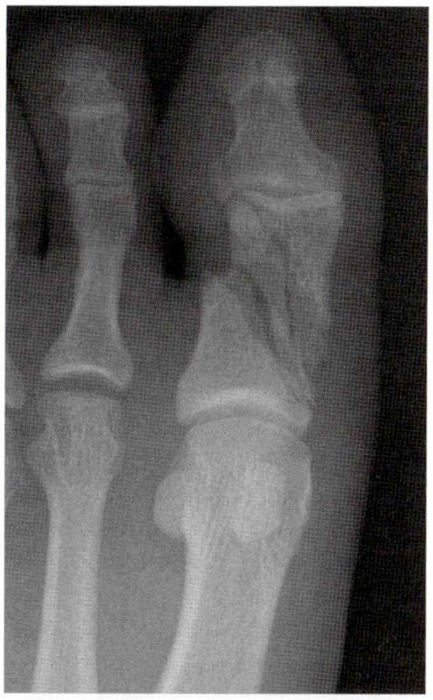

88-C2.2

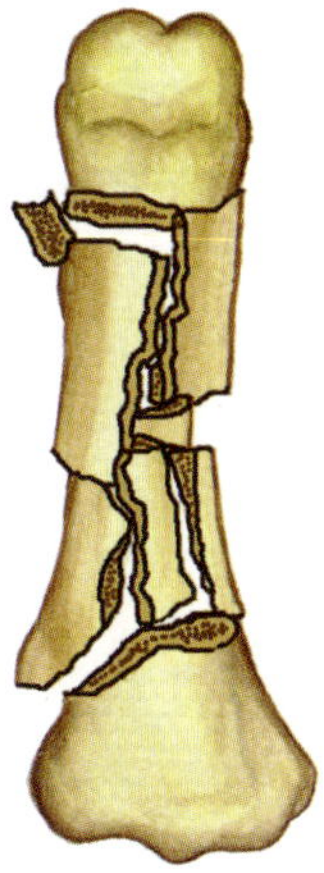

Complex comminuted

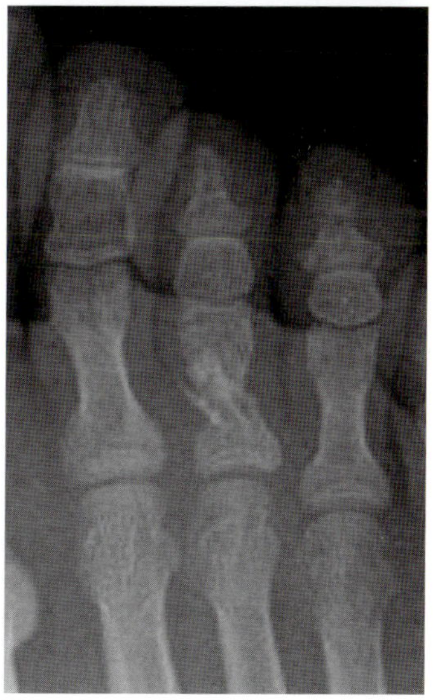

88-C Phalanx proximal and distal complete articular, and diaphysis comminuted

88-C3
Distal complete articular
526 fractures
M: 417 (79.28%)
F: 109 (20.72%)
0.14% of total adult fractures
1.36% of adult foot fractures
7.11% of phalanx
39.05% of type 88-C

88-C3.1

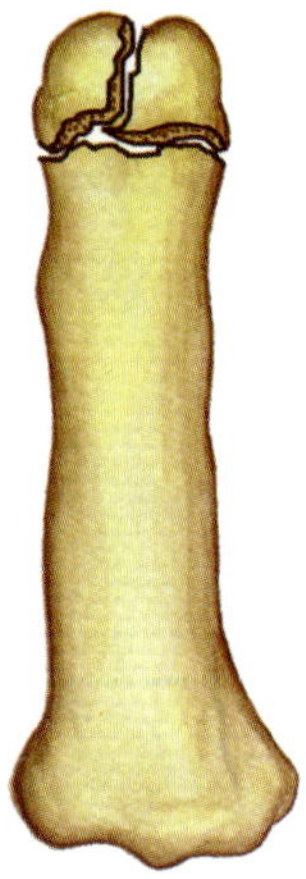

Noncomminuted articular/metaphysis

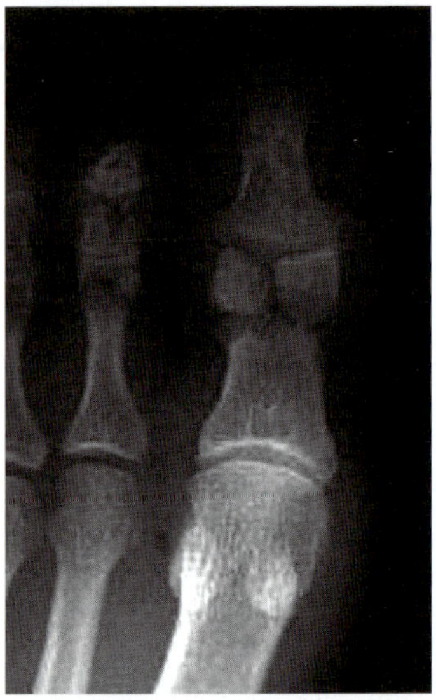

88-C3.2

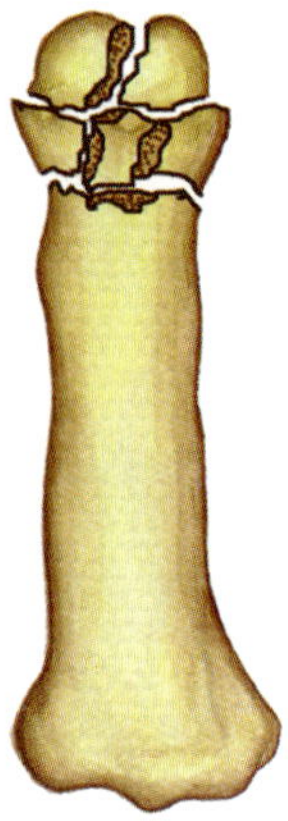

Noncomminuted articular comminuted metaphysis

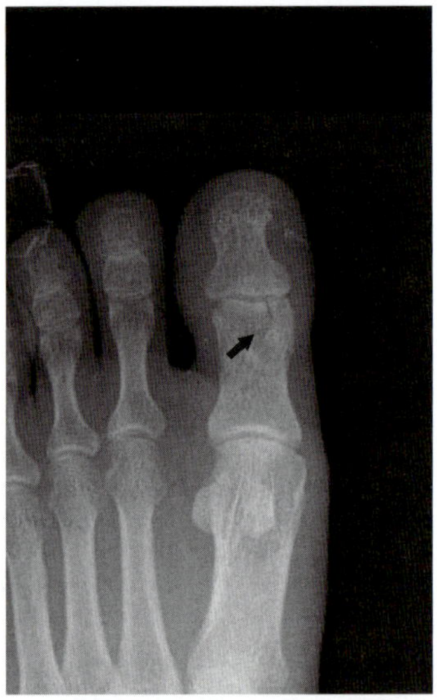

88-C3.3

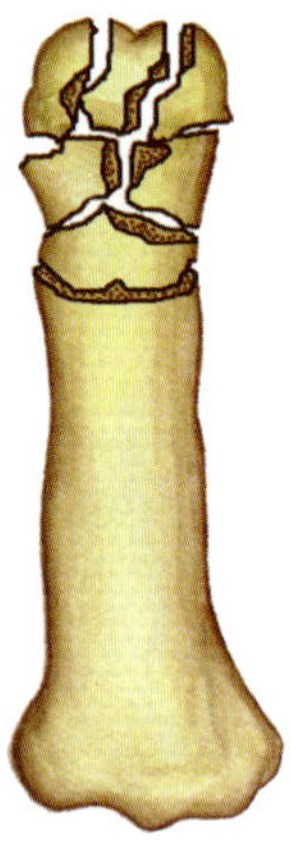

Comminuted articular

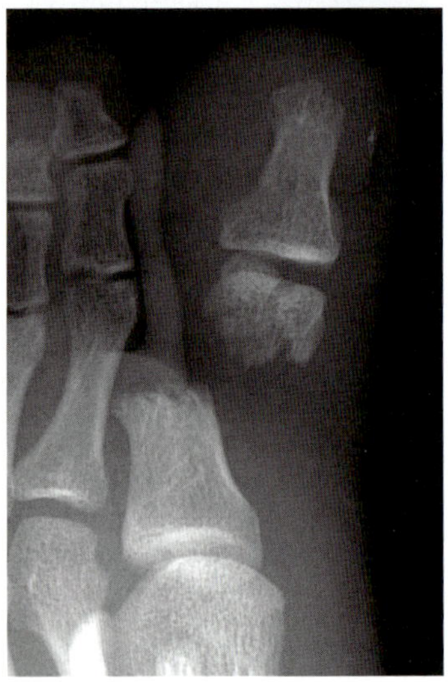

Injury Mechanism

Fractures and dislocation of the phalanx usually occur as the result of direct trauma, such as from a heavy object falling on an extremity, kicking a hard surface, or crush injuries. A direct blow to the area will lead to comminuted fractures or longitudinal fractures, and is associated with open fractures and toenail damage. Kicking a hard surface usually results in transverse or oblique fractures. Depression fractures or avulsion of the capsular ligament are more associated with indirect trauma, as seen in soccer or ballet when the metatarsophalangeal joints are forcibly plantar flexed.

Diagnosis

Due to the anatomical location of the phalanx, diagnosis usually can be made without much difficulty. Swelling, pain, ecchymosis, or deformity may be present. Radiographs usually confirm the presence of a fracture.

Treatment

Nondisplaced phalangeal fractures do not require specific treatment, instead, 2–3 weeks of bed rest is usually required before beginning to walk again. A displaced single phalangeal fracture should be treated with closed reduction, and the fractured digit should be taped to an adjacent digit for immobilization, which permits early active motion. After reduction, most phalangeal fractures can be treated by cast plating, using a plate made by extending the casting material beyond the distal toes; this process prohibits plantar flexion and limits dorsiflexion. Weight-bearing exercise, started at 2–3 weeks after the immobilization, is recommended. Caution is necessary to correct rotational deformity and to avoid dorsal or palmar angulation, thereby minimizing functional limitation due to misalignment of the digit.

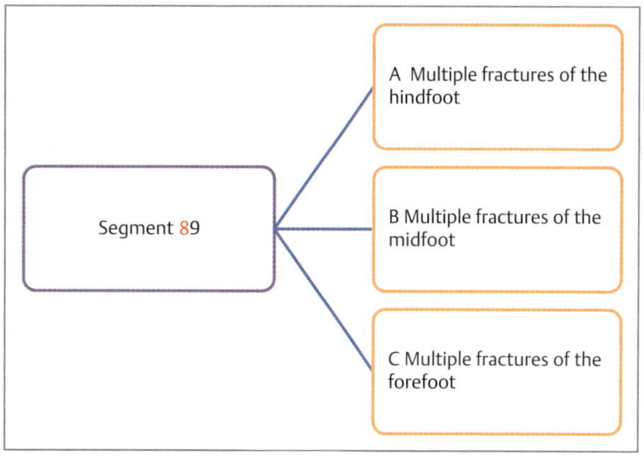

Plate 9.18

Multiple Fractures of the Foot (Segment 89)

Based on OTA classification, multiple fractures of the foot are coded as the number 89, which is then divided into three types: 89-A, multiple fracture of the hindfoot; 89-B, multiple fracture of the midfoot; and 89-C, multiple fracture of the forefoot (**Plate 9.18**).

Clinical Epidemiologic Features of Multiple Fractures of the Foot (Segment 89)

OTA Classification of Multiple Fractures of the Foot

A total of 7,272 adult patients with multiple fractures of the foot (OTA) were treated in 83 hospitals in China over a 2-year period from 2010 to 2011.

Epidemiologic features of multiple foot fractures are as follows:

- More males than females
- The most common fracture type is 89-C; thus, multiple fractures of the forefoot occur most often.

Table 9.37 Sex and fracture type distribution of 7,272 multiple foot fractures

Fracture type	Male	Female	Number of patients	Percentage (%)
89-A	236	59	295	4.06
89-B	644	193	837	11.51
89-C	4,801	1,339	6,140	84.43
Total	5,681	1,591	7,272	100.00

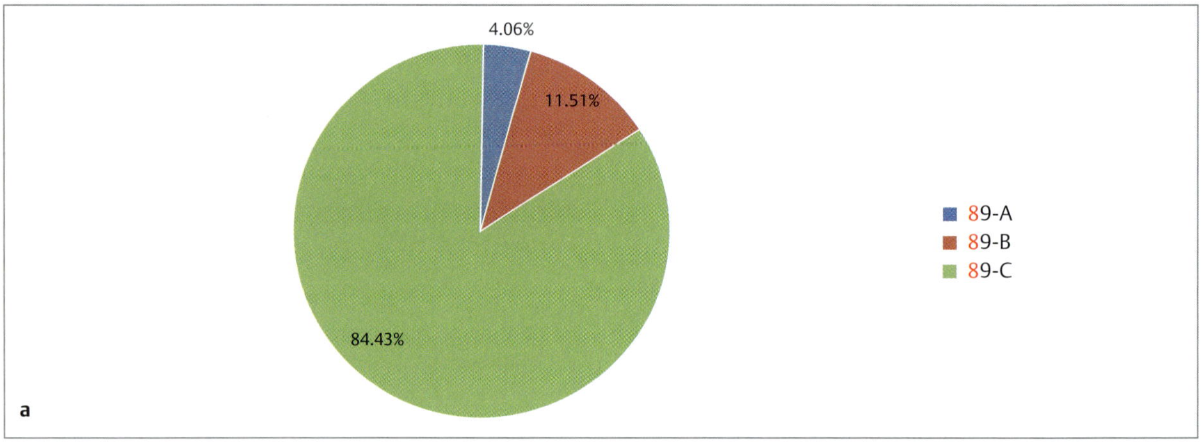

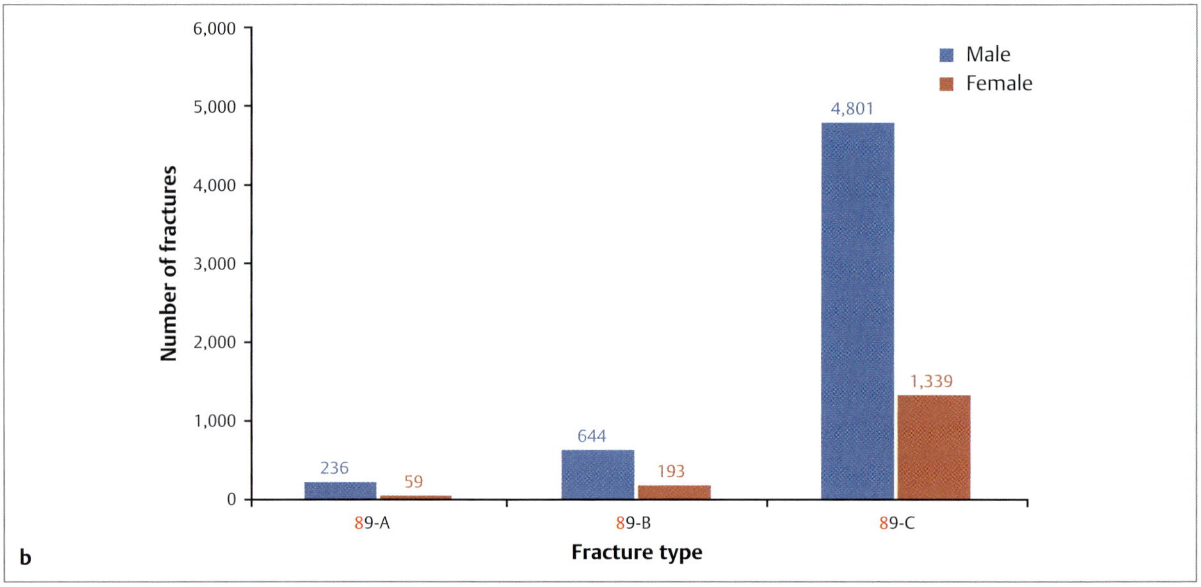

Fig. 9.37 **(a)** Fracture type distribution of 7,272 multiple foot fractures.
(b) Sex and fracture type distribution of 7,272 multiple foot fractures.

89 Multiple fractures of the foot

89
Multiple fractures of the foot
7,272 fractures
M: 5,681 (78.12%)
F: 1,591 (21.88%)

89-A

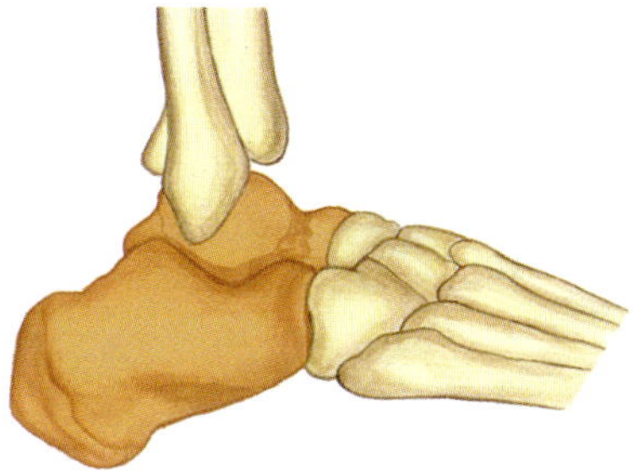

Hindfoot

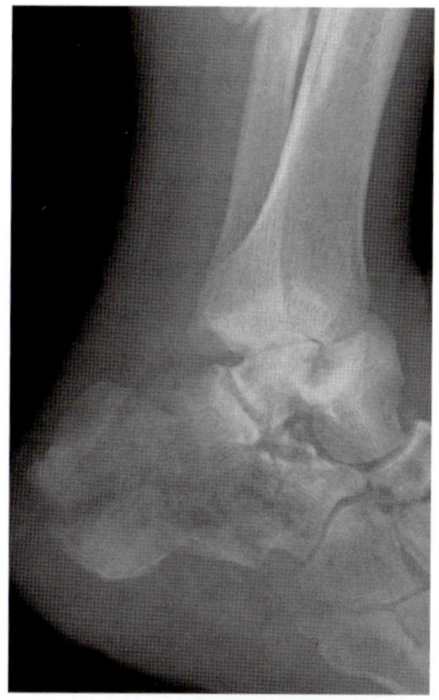

89-B

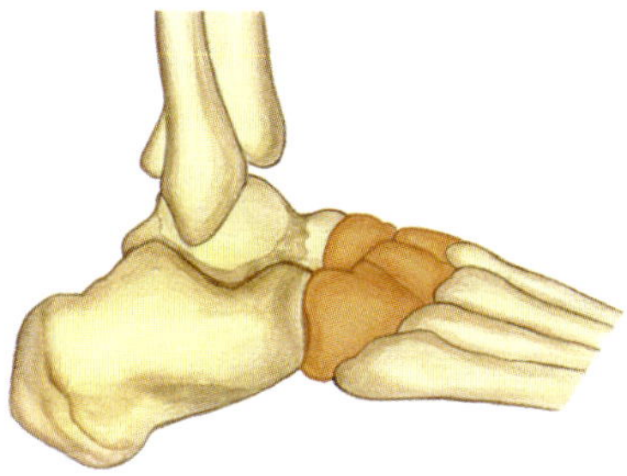

Midfoot

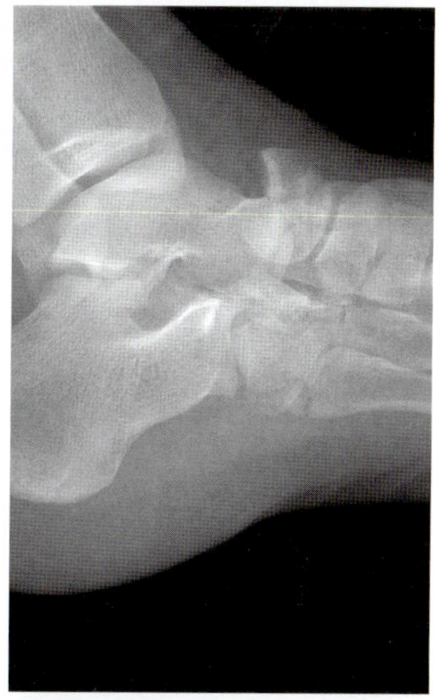

89-C

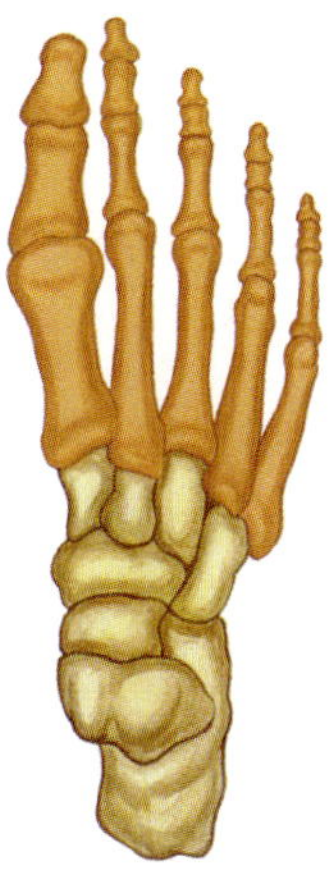

Forefoot

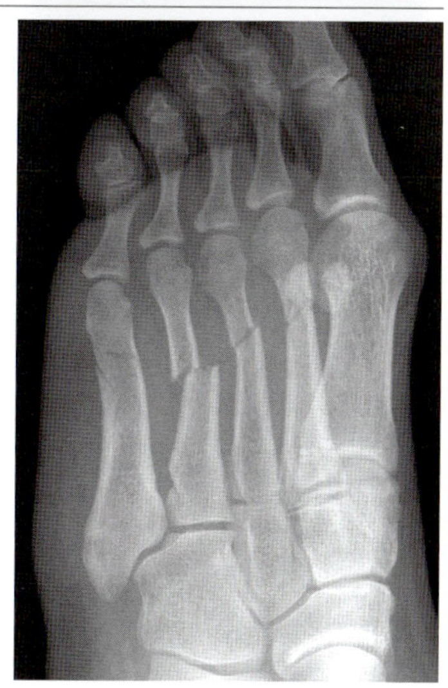

10 Fractures of Other Locations

Fractures of the Patella (Segment 34)

Anatomical Features

The patella is the largest sesamoid bone in the human body, and is an important component of the knee joint. It serves to increase the leverage of the quadriceps femoris as a fulcrum, protects the front of the joint, and maintains joint stability. It is a flat, triangular bone; its superior border is thick, while the medial and lateral borders are thinner, and it gives attachment to the tendon of the quadriceps femoris and the medial and lateral patellar retinacula. The lateral borders converge below to the apex, which gives attachment to the ligamentum patellae; the anterior surface is convex and rough, and covered by the expansion from the tendon of the quadriceps femoris; the posterior surface is a smooth, oval, articular area, and for the most part is covered with smooth, slippery cartilage; and it is divided into two facets, medial and lateral, by a vertical ridge. Each facet is further subdivided into three facets: superior, middle and inferior. Lateral to the inner facet is another longitudinal facet. These seven facets in total make contacts with the femur at various angles during extension-flexion of the knee joint (**Plate 10.1**).

OTA Classification and Coding System for Patellar Fractures

Based on Orthopaedic Trauma Association (OTA classification, the patella is coded as the number 34 for its anatomical location. Patellar fractures are classified into three types

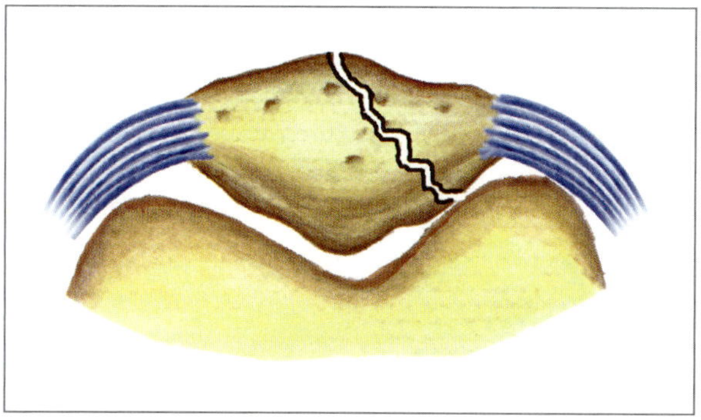

Plate 10.2

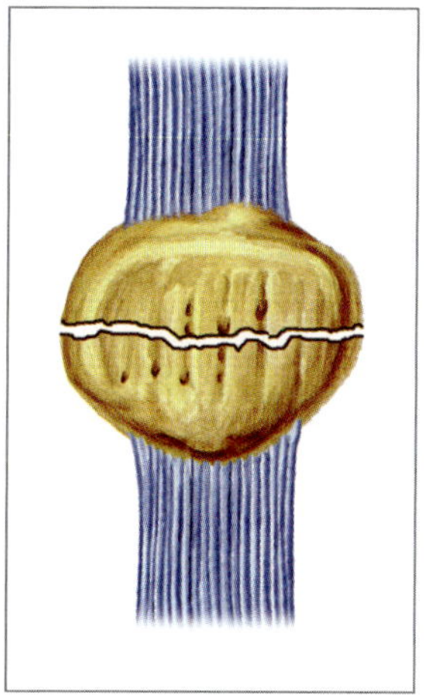

Plate 10.3

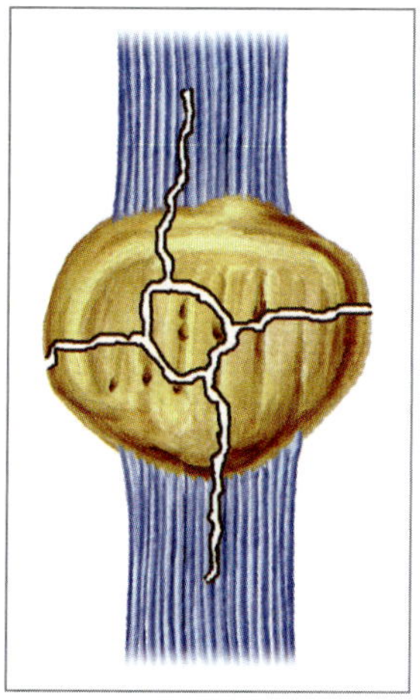

Plate 10.4

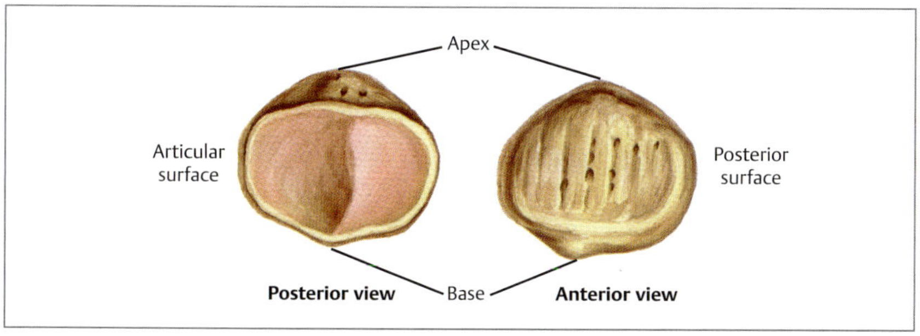

Plate 10.1

according to the fracture pattern: 34-A, extra-articular; 34-B, partial articular, vertical; and 34-C, complete articular, nonvertical (**Plate 10.5**).

Clinical Epidemiologic Features of Patellar Fractures (Segment 34)

A total of 11,332 patients with 11,378 patellar fractures were treated in 83 hospitals in China over a 2-year period from 2010 to 2011. All cases were reviewed and statistically studied, accounting for 2.73% of all patients with fractures, and 2.63% of all kinds of fractures, respectively; of a total 11,332 patients, there were 279 pediatric patients (290 patellar fractures) and 11,053 adult patients with 11,088 fractures.

Epidemiologic features of patellar fractures are the following:

- More males than females
- More left side than right side fractures
- The high-risk age group is between ages 41 and 50 years, the same age group for males while for females, the high risk age group is between ages 51 and 60 years.
- The most common fracture type is type 34-C, the same fracture type for both males and females.
- The most common fracture group is group 34-C1, the same fracture group for both males and females.

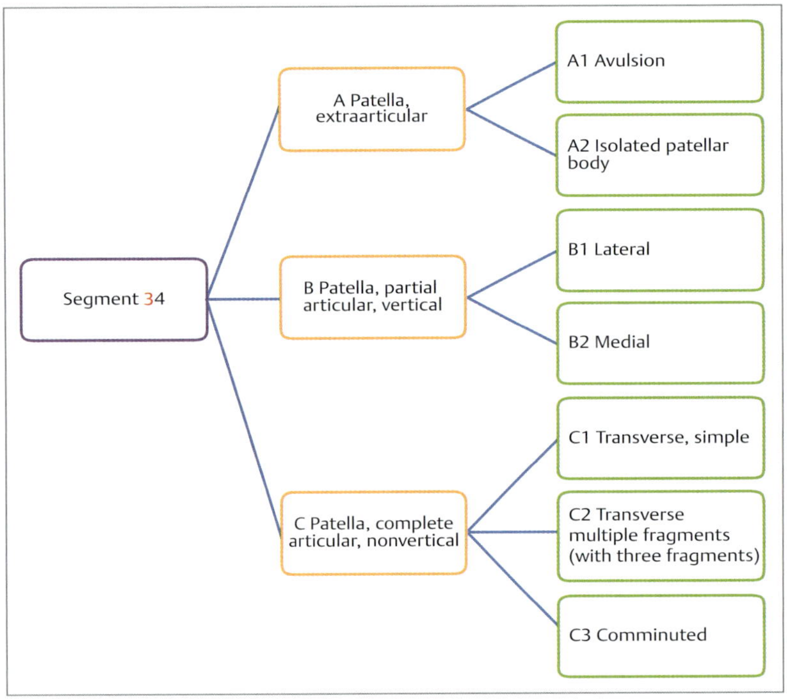

Plate 10.5

Patellar Fractures by Sex

Table 10.1 Sex distribution of 11,332 patients with patellar fractures

Sex	Number of patients	Percentage (%)
Male	6,791	59.93
Female	4,541	40.07
Total	11,332	100.00

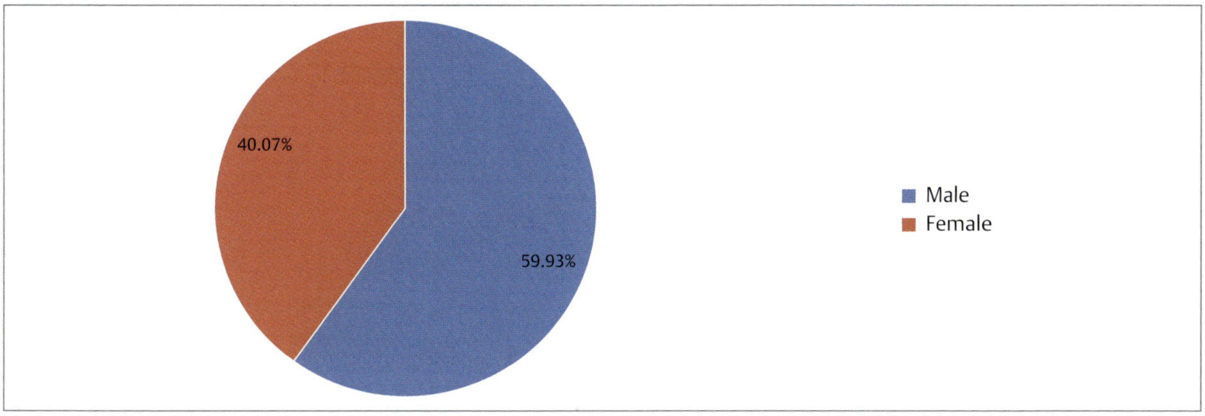

Fig. 10.1 Sex distribution of 11,332 patients with patellar fractures.

Patellar Fractures by Fracture Side

Table 10.2 Fracture side distribution of 11,332 patients with patellar fractures

Fracture side	Number of patients	Percentage (%)
Left	5,972	52.70
Right	5,314	46.89
Bilateral	46	0.41
Total	11,332	100.00

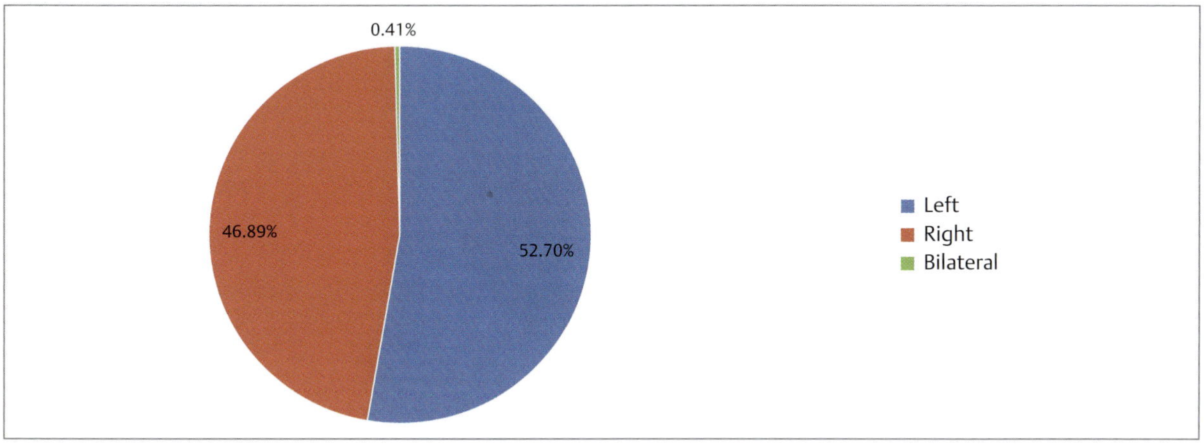

Fig. 10.2 Fracture side distribution of 11,332 patients with patellar fractures.

10

Patellar Fractures by Age Group

Table 10.3 Age and sex distribution of 11,332 patients with patellar fractures

Age group (years)	Male	Female	Number of patients	Percentage (%)
0–5	41	17	58	0.51
6–10	51	16	67	0.59
11–15	121	33	154	1.36
16–20	278	65	343	3.03
21–25	456	146	602	5.31
26–30	482	164	646	5.70
31–35	567	249	816	7.20
36–40	772	337	1,109	9.79
41–45	861	398	1,259	11.11
46–50	886	539	1,425	12.58
51–55	634	592	1,226	10.82
56–60	579	704	1,283	11.32
61–65	388	471	859	7.58
66–70	230	338	568	5.01
71–75	182	241	423	3.73
76–80	144	151	295	2.60
81–85	91	48	139	1.23
≥86	28	32	60	0.53
Total	6,791	4,541	11,332	100.00

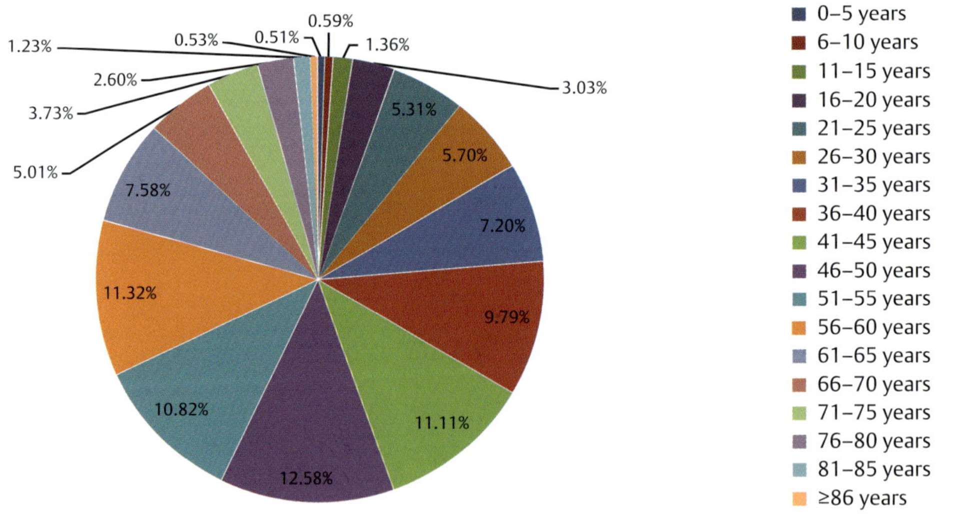

a

Fig. 10.3 **(a)** Age distribution of 11,332 patients with patellar fractures.

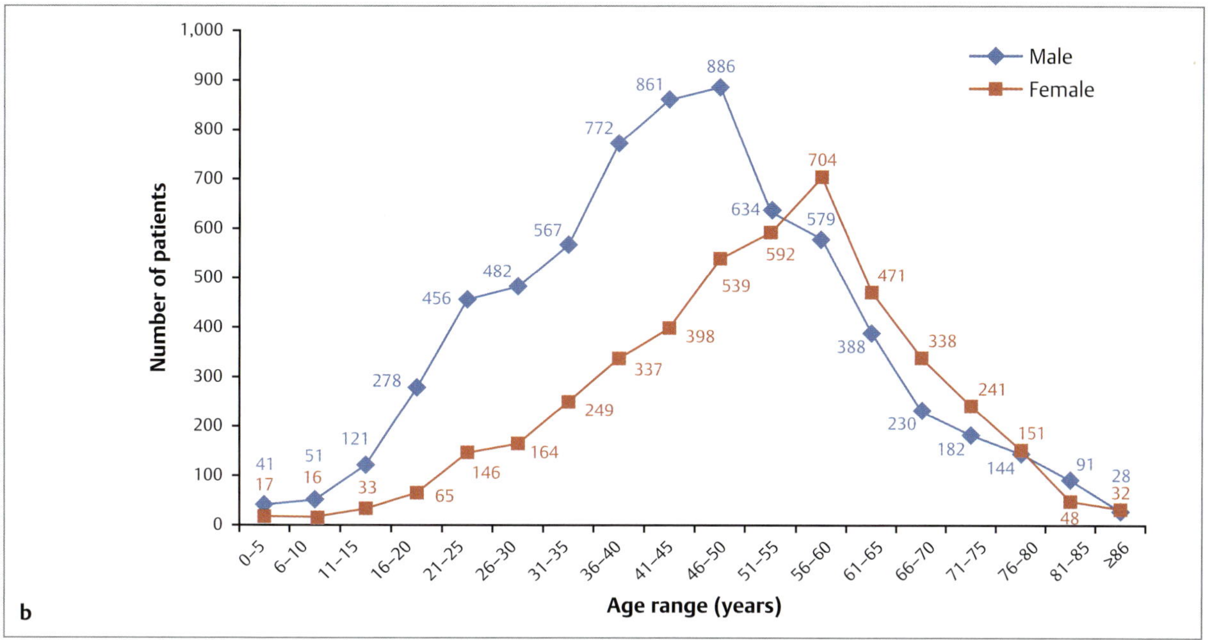

Fig. 10.3 (*continued*) **(b)** Age and sex distribution of 11,332 patients with patellar fractures.

Adult Patellar Fractures by Fracture Type

Table 10.4 Fracture type distribution of 11,088 adult patellar fractures

Fracture type	Male	Female	Number of fractures	Percentage/talus (%)
34-A	1,034	767	1,801	16.24
34-B	701	481	1,182	10.66
34-C	4,872	3,233	8,105	73.10
Total	6,607	4,481	11,088	100.00

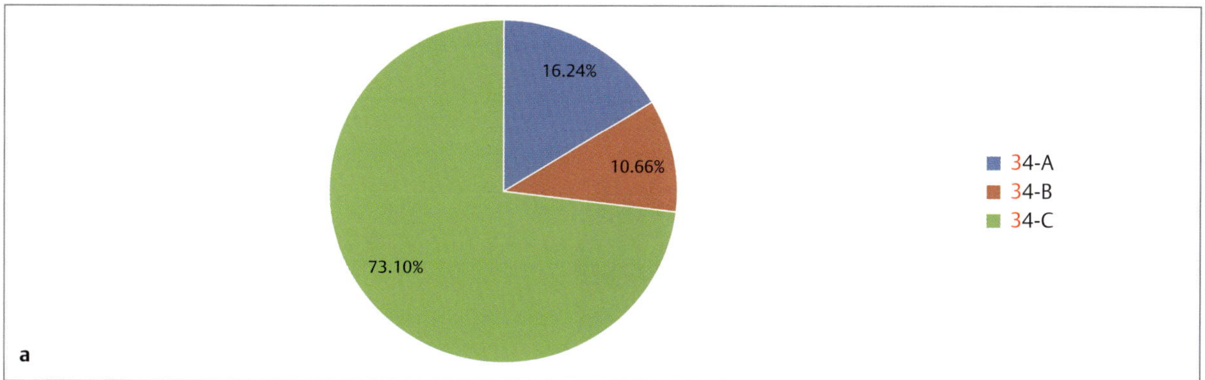

Fig. 10.4 **(a)** Fracture type distribution of 11,088 adult patellar fractures by OTA classification. (*Continued*)

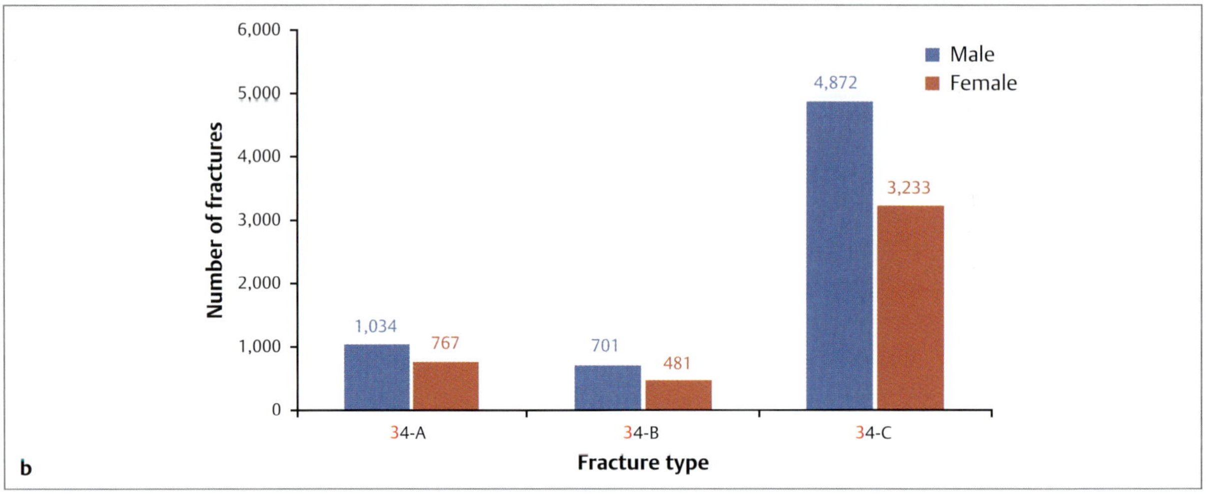

Fig. 10.4 (*continued*) **(b)** Sex and fracture type distribution of 11,088 adult patellar fractures by OTA classification.

Adult Patellar Fractures by Fracture Group

Table 10.5 Fracture group and sex distribution of 11,088 adult patellar fractures

Fracture group	Male	Female	Number of fractures	Percentage (%)
34-A1	852	610	1,462	13.19
34-A2	182	157	339	3.06
34-B1	461	293	754	6.80
34-B2	240	188	428	3.86
34-C1	2,443	2,073	4,516	40.73
34-C2	930	490	1,420	12.81
34-C3	1,499	670	2,169	19.56
Total	6,607	4,481	11,088	100.00

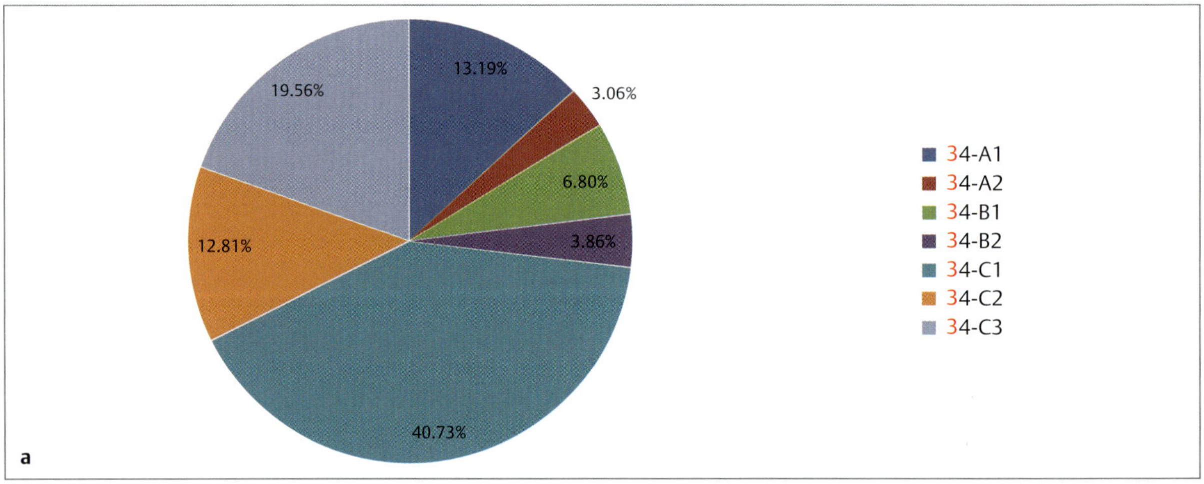

Fig. 10.5 **(a)** Fracture group distribution of 11,088 adult patellar fractures by OTA classification.

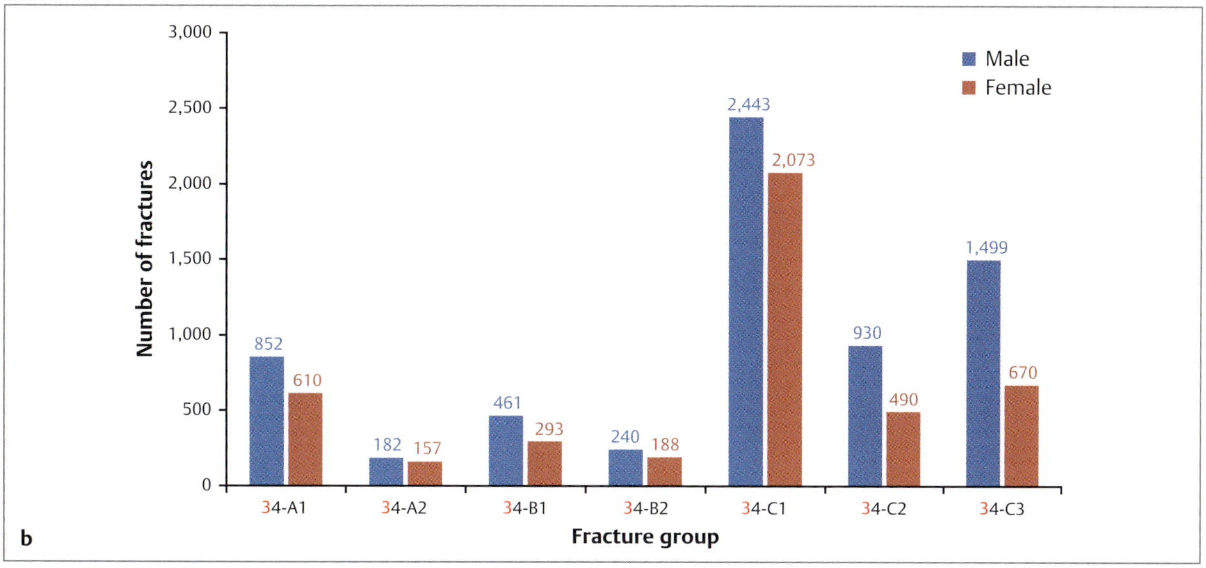

Fig. 10.5 (*continued*) **(b)** Sex and fracture group distribution of 11,088 adult patellar fractures by OTA classification.

34-A Patella extra-articular fractures

34-A1
Avulsion
1,462 fractures
M: 852 (58.28%)
F: 610 (41.72%)
0. 39% of total adult fractures
13.19% of adult patellar fractures
81.18% of type 34-A adult fractures

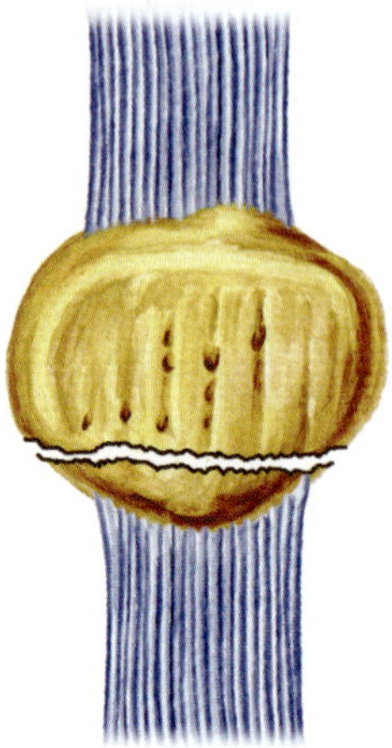

Avulsion

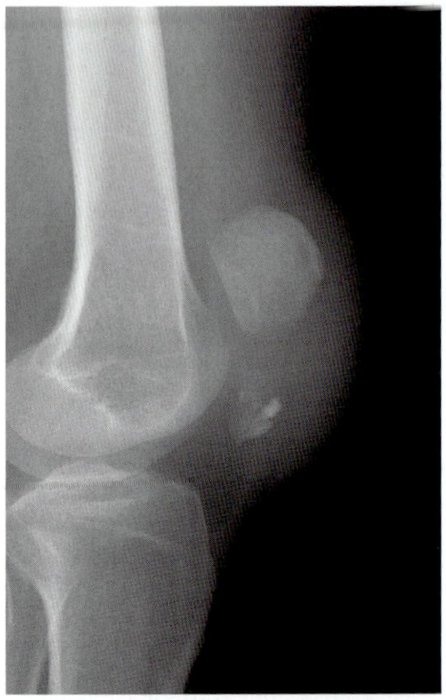

34-A2
Isolated patellar body
339 fractures
M: 182 (53.69%)
F: 157 (46.31%)
0.09% of total adult fractures
3.06% of adult patellar fractures
18.82% of type 34-A adult fractures

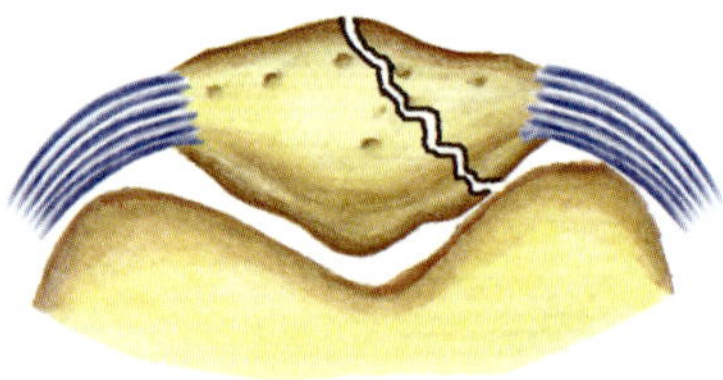

Body fractures simple

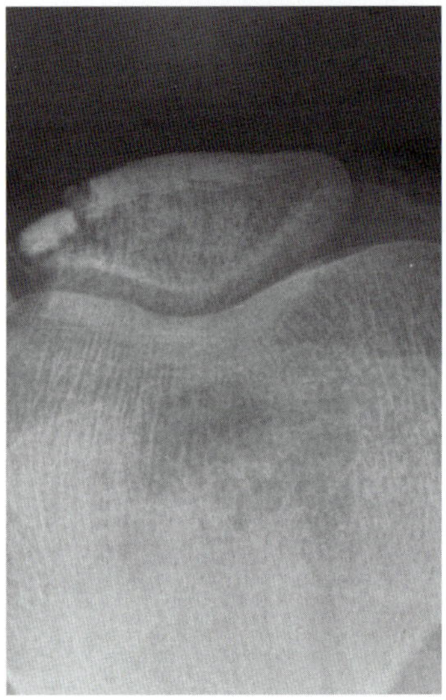

Axial view of patella

34-B Patella partial articular fractures, vertical

34-B1
Lateral
754 fractures
M: 461 (61.14%)
F: 293 (38.86%)
0.2% of total adult fractures
6.8% of adult patellar fractures
63.79% of type 34-B adult fractures

34-B1.1

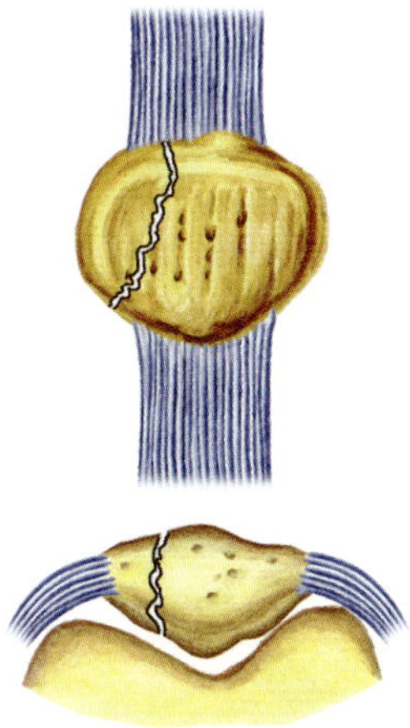

Simple

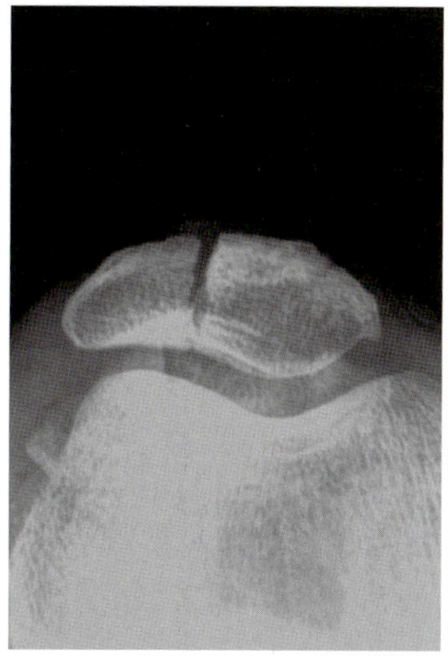

Axial view of patella

34-B1.2

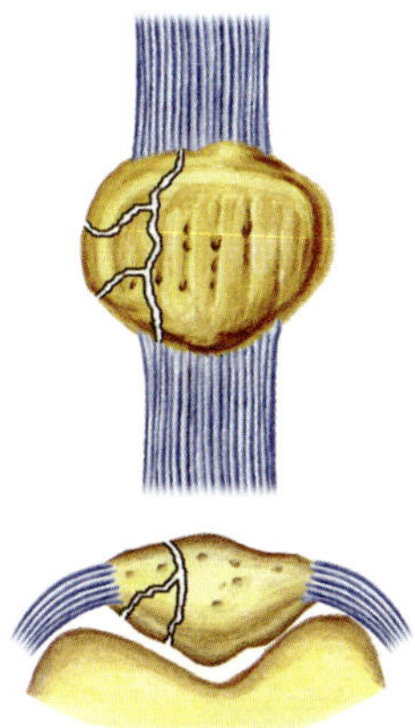

Comminuted

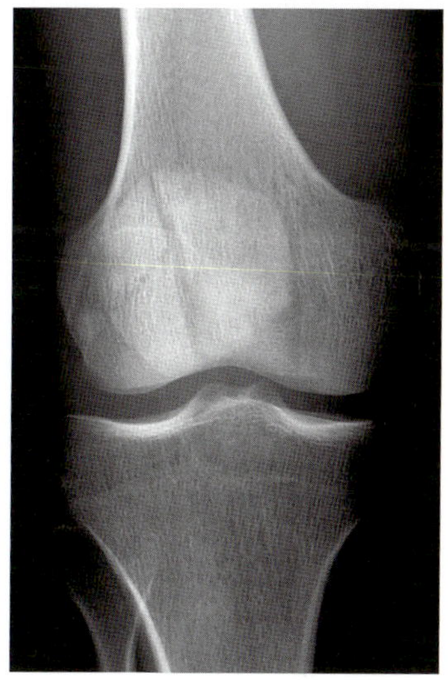

34-B Patella partial articular fractures, vertical

34-B2
Medial
428 fractures
M: 240 (56.07%)
F: 188 (43.93%)
0.11% of total adult fractures
3.86% of adult patellar fractures
36.21% of type 34-B adult fractures

34-B2.1

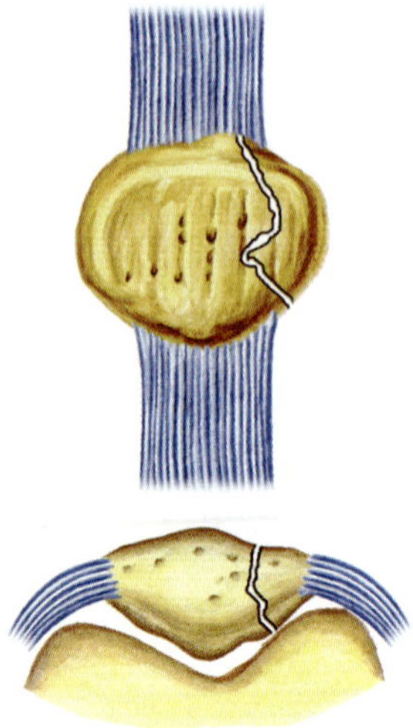

Simple

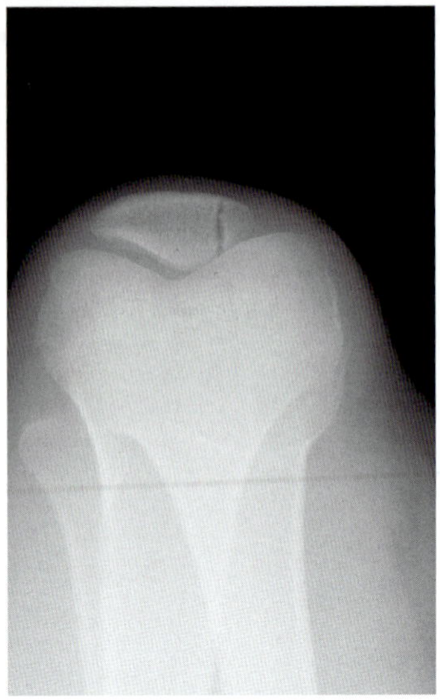

Axial view of patella

34-B2.2

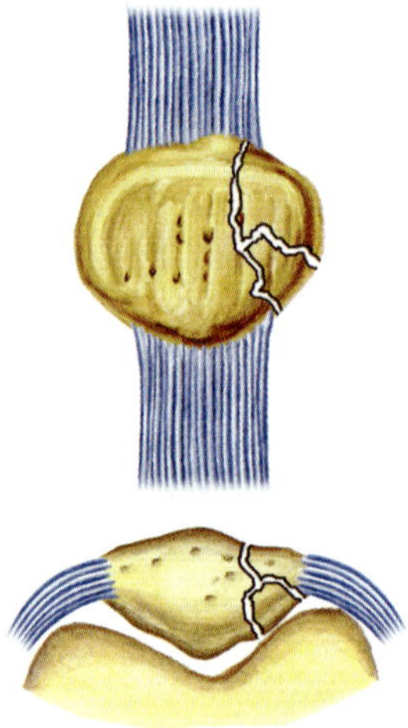

Comminuted

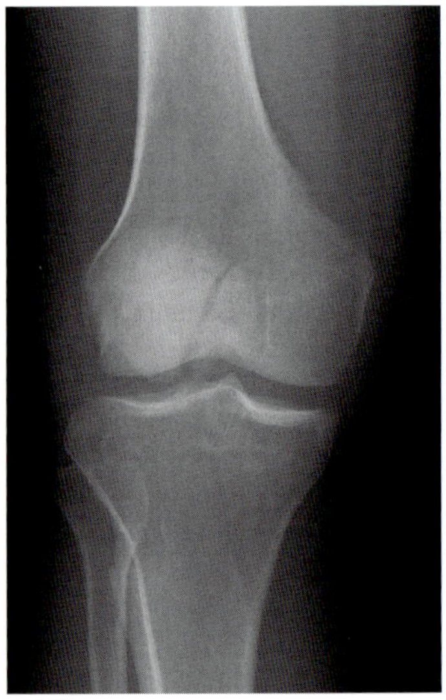

34-C Patella complete articular fractures, nonvertical

34-C1
Transverse, simple
4,516 fractures
M: 2,443 (54.1%)
F: 2,073 (45.9%)
1.21% of total adult fractures
40.73% of adult patella fractures
55.72% of type 34-C adult fractures

34-C1.1

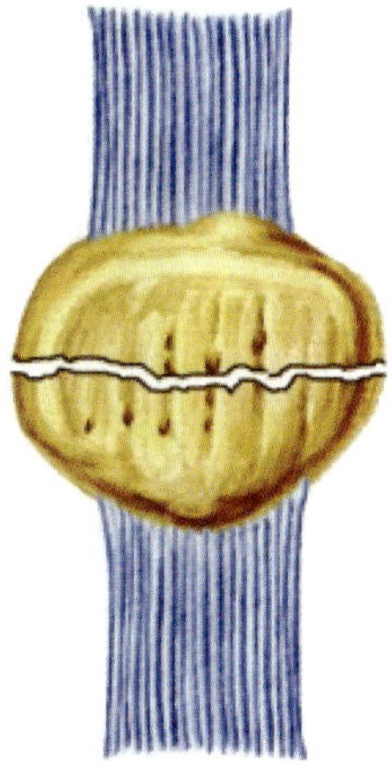

Middle

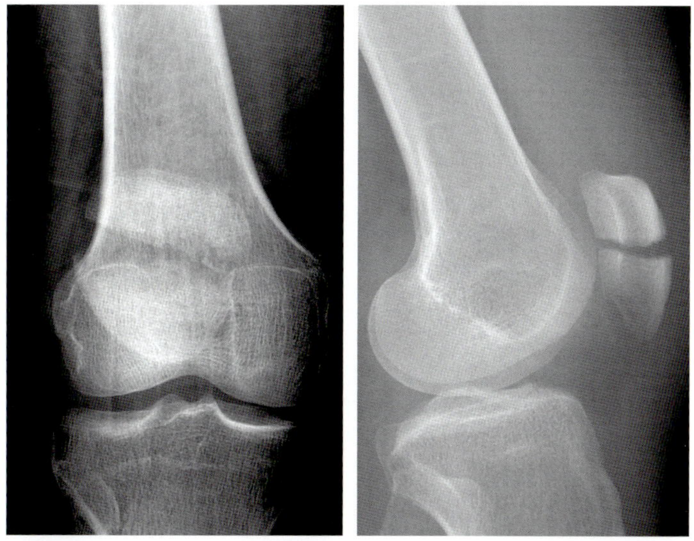

34-C1.2

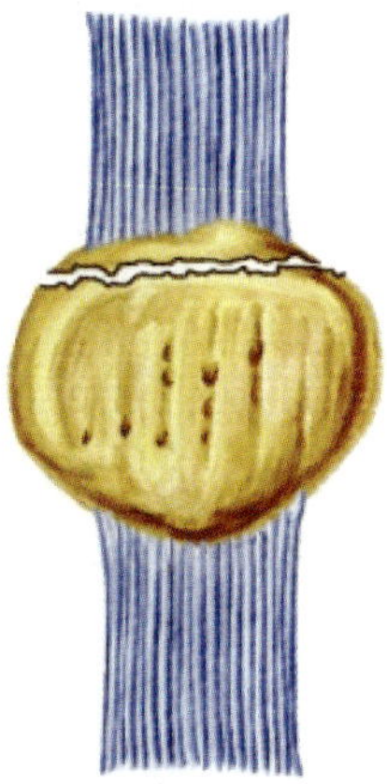

Proximal

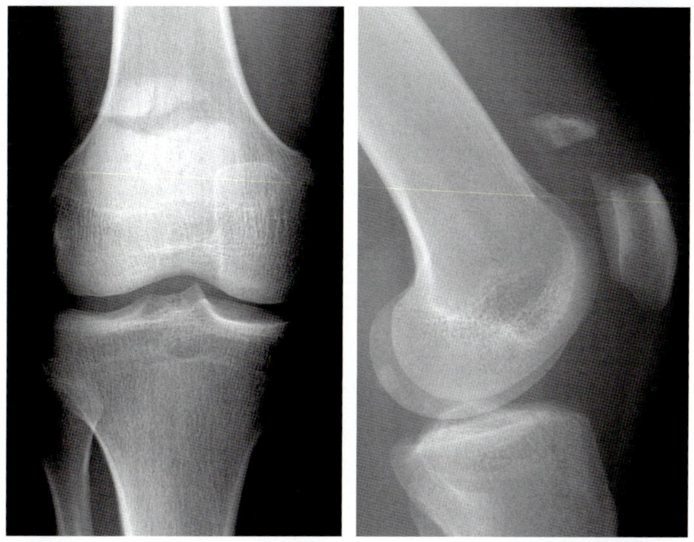

34-C1.3

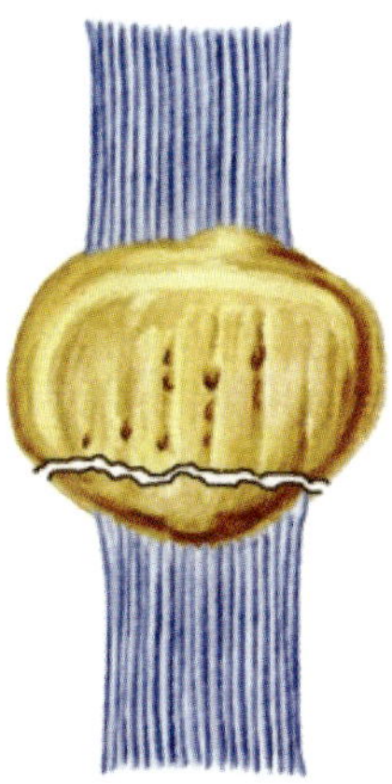

Distal

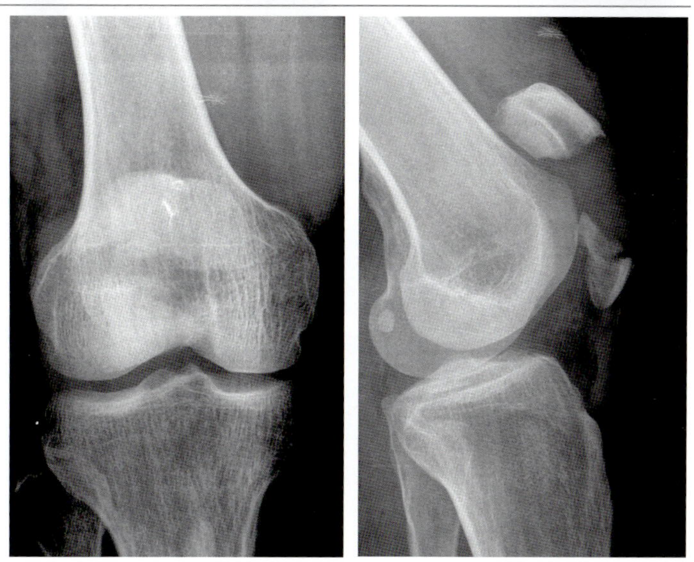

34-C Patella complete articular fractures, nonvertical

34-C2
Transverse, fragmented (with three fragments)
1,420 fractures
M: 930 (65.49%)
F: 490 (34.51%)
0.38% of total adult fractures
12.81% of adult patella fractures
17.52% of type 34-C adult fractures

34-C2.1

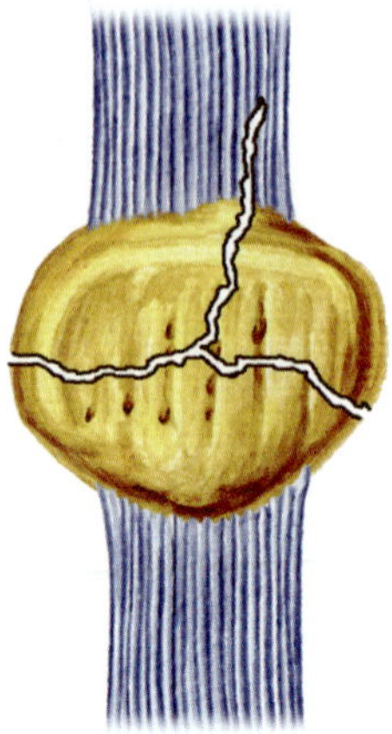

Middle

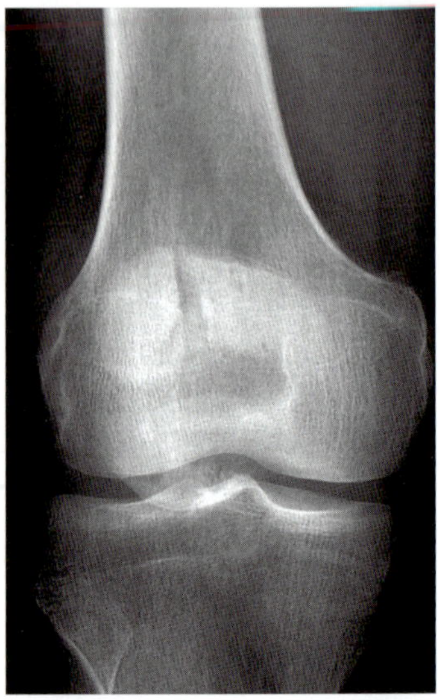

34-C2.2

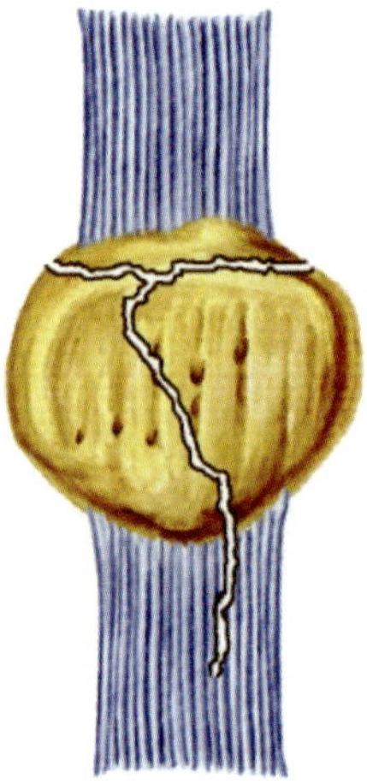

Proximal

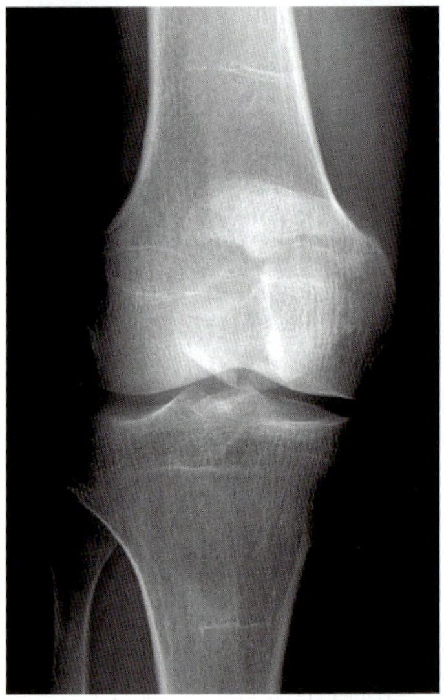

34-C2.3

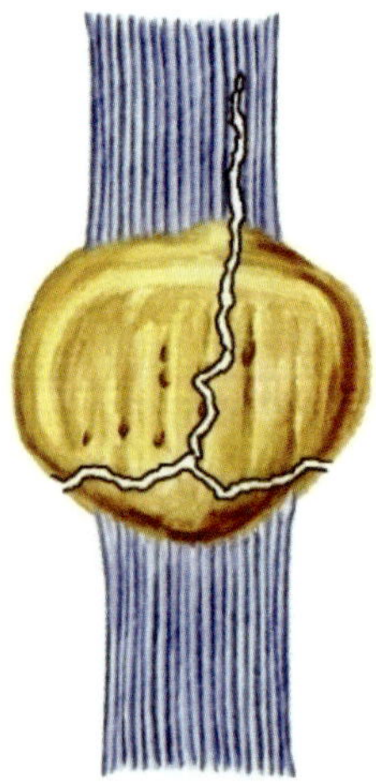

Distal

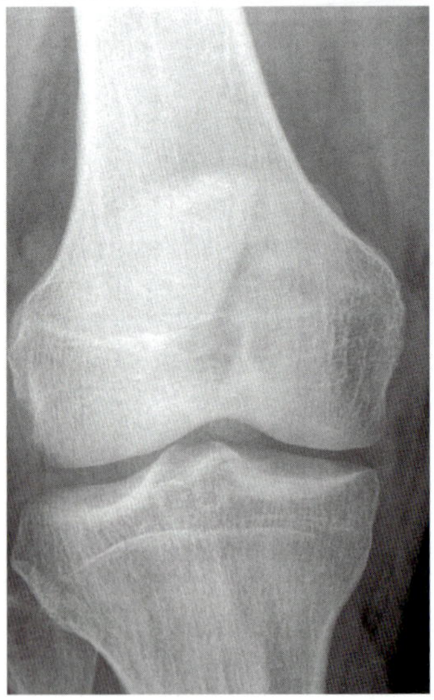

34-C Patella complete articular fractures, nonvertical

34-C3
Comminuted (with > three fragments)
2,169 fractures
M: 1,499 (69.11%)
F: 670 (30.89%)
0.58% of total adult fractures
19.56% of adult patella fractures
26.76% of type 34-C adult fractures

34-C3.1

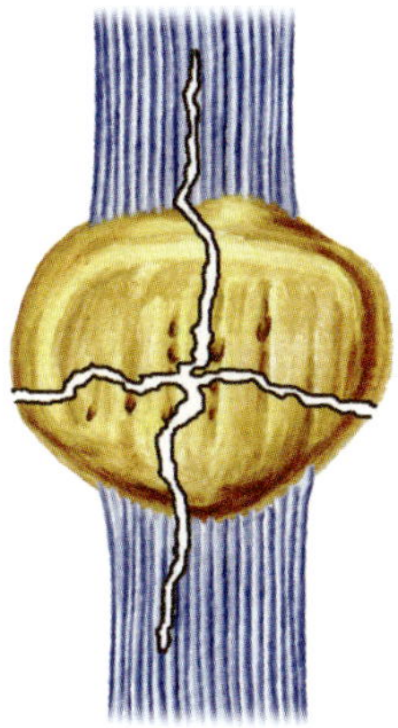

With four fragments

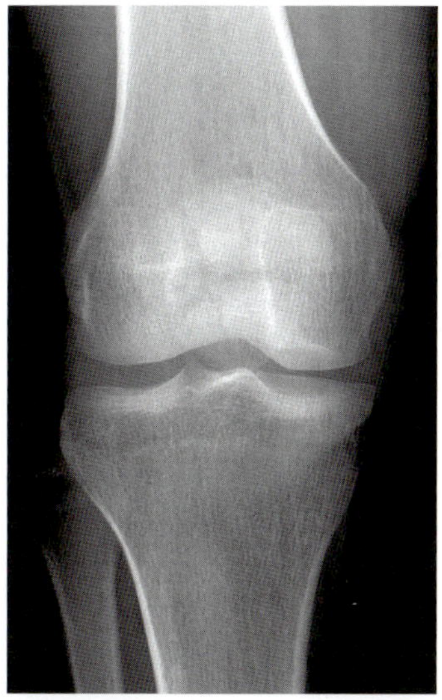

34-C3.2

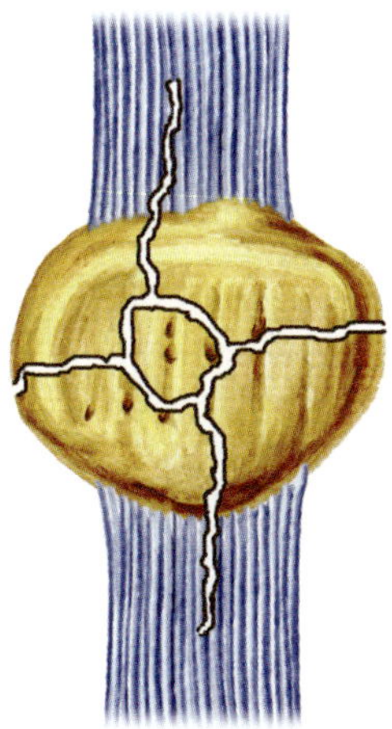

With > four fragments

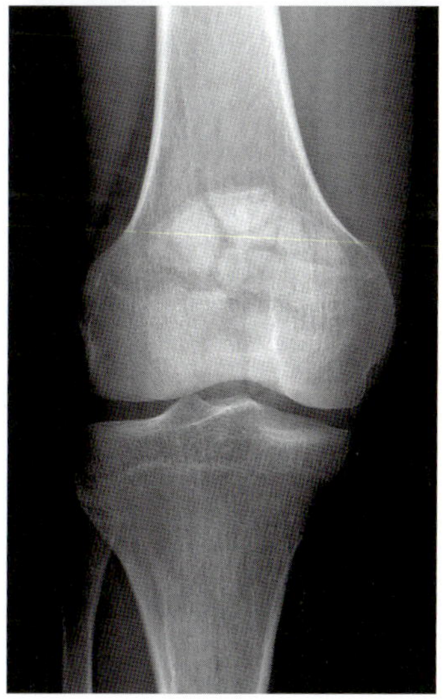

Injury Mechanism

Transverse fractures of the patella and avulsion fractures of the superior and inferior poles are often caused by indirect mechanisms, seen with hyperflexion of the knee due to sudden tensile force of the quadriceps. Comminuted, vertical, and oblique fractures are more clearly associated with direct mechanisms, such as from direct blows and crush injuries. The energy of the impacting force, which results in comminuted fractures of the patella, may also cause damage to the articular cartilage of both the patella and the femoral condyles.

Diagnosis

Patellar fractures usually present with a history of trauma. Physical exam reveals ecchymosis over the anterior aspect of the knee, hemarthrosis, swelling, tenderness, and partial-to-complete limitation of knee joint mobility. If fracture displacement is present, a gap between fragments and retropatellar crepitus can be noted. Radiographs of anteroposterior (AP) and lateral views of the knee joint usually confirm the diagnosis. If vertical or border fractures are clinically suspected, an axial view or CT scan of the knee joint may be indicated. Magnetic resonance imaging (MRI) is necessary for comminuted patellar fractures due to damage of the articular cartilage of both the patella and the femoral condyles. The diagnosis of a vertical fracture of the patella should be differentiated from that of a patellar variation. Vertical fractures present with a clear trauma history, positive physical exam findings, fracture lines, and a jagged surface of the broken ends; this is in contrast to variations of the patella (binary or trinary patella), which are known to have wide gaps, smooth broken ends, or mild to absent physical signs/syndrome. In addition, the thin layer of cortex can be exposed.

Treatment

If the fracture is displaced less than 3 mm, or the intra-articular step-off is less than 2 mm, the fracture may be treated with a nonoperative modality. However, for elderly patients, operative management with rigid internal fixation should be considered to allow early postoperative mobilization and to minimize knee fibro-adhesive scar formation. In young healthy patients, patellar fractures can be treated with immobilization followed by casting, external fixation devices, and tuck loop fixation, etc. Surgical treatment is advised for displaced fractures, which are defined as fractures that have an intra-articular step-off of more than 2 mm or a separation of more than 3 mm. Additional caution should be taken for pediatric patients with patella fractures when considering an operative approach because operative procedures have the potential to damage growth cartilage, and subsequently impact the growth and development of the patella. Because children have a greater potential for tissue bone repair and molding, fractures with marked displacement, or even with a comminuted pattern, should initially be treated with nonoperative management. Partial surgical removal of the patella should be considered for severe comminuted fractures that are not able to be anatomically reduced. Severe comminuted patellar fractures in elderly patients should be treated with primary total surgical removal of the patella.

Further Classifications of Patellar Fractures

Regazzoni Classification

Based on the fracture location, pattern, and the presence of displacement, Regazzoni classified patellar fractures into three types with three subgroups for each fracture type:

- *Type A:* Vertical fracture: A1 with no displacement; A2 with displacement; A3 comminuted.
- *Type B:* Transverse fracture: B1 avulsion fracture of the superior and inferior poles of the patella (< 5 mm in diameter of the superior pole, < 15 mm in diameter of the inferior pole); B2 simple; B3 comminuted.
- *Type C:* Comminuted fractures: C1 with no displacement; C2 with displacement of < 2 mm; C3 Burst fractures with displacement of more than 2 mm.

Clinical Epidemiologic Features of Patellar Fractures by the Regazzoni Classification

A total of 11,088 adult patellar fractures were treated in 83 hospitals in China over a 2-year period from 2010 to 2011, all cases were reviewed and statistically studied. Their epidemiologic features are as follows:

- More males than females
- The most common fracture type was type B (transverse).

Table 10.6 Sex and fracture type distribution of 11,088 adult patellar fractures by Regazzoni classification

Fracture type	Male	Female	Number of fractures	Percentage (%)
A	701	481	1,182	10.66
B	4,407	3,330	7,737	69.78
C	1,499	670	2,169	19.56
Total	6,607	4,481	11,088	100.00

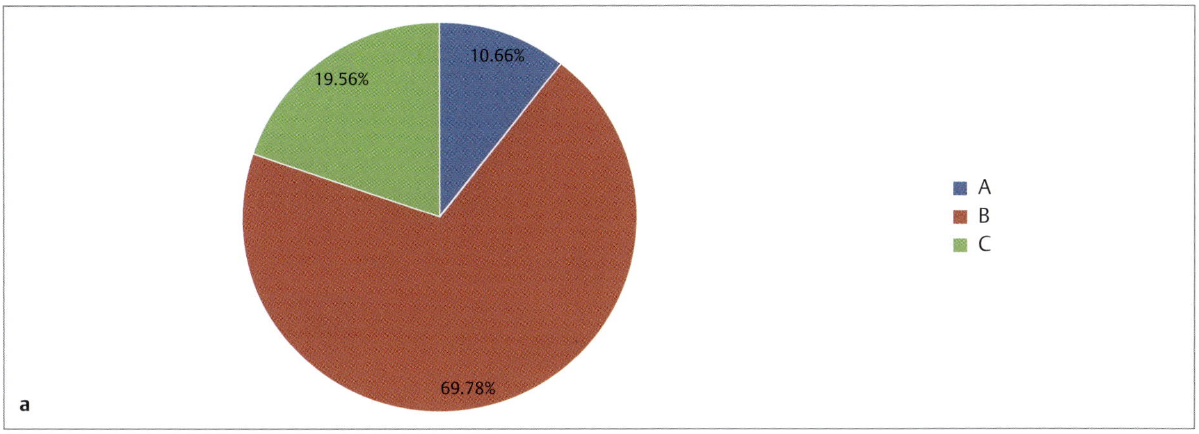

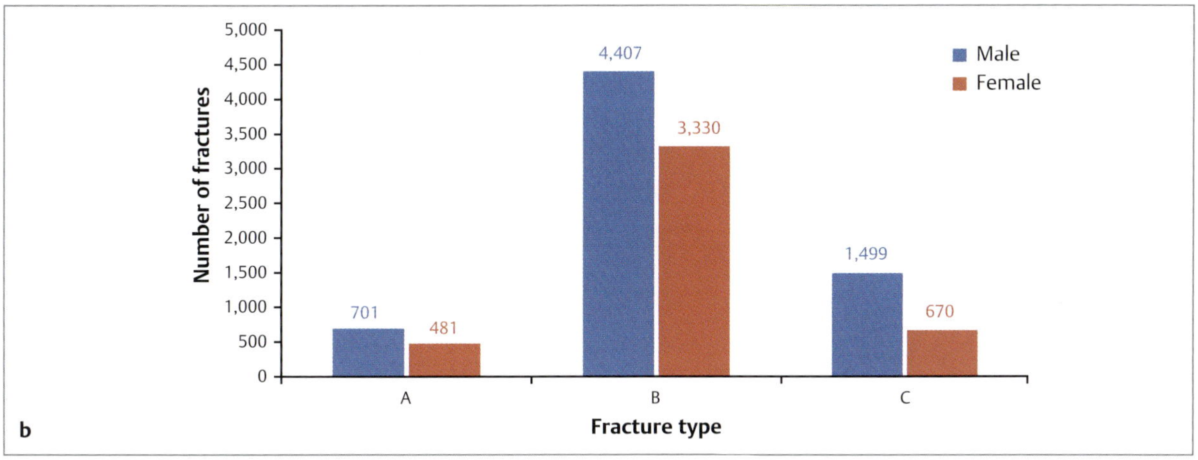

Fig. 10.6 **(a)** Fracture type distribution of 11,088 adult patellar fractures by Regazzoni classification. **(b)** Sex and fracture type distribution of 11,088 adult patellar fractures by Regazzoni classification.

Regazzoni classification of patellar fractures		
Type A **Vertical** 1,182 fractures M: 701 (59.31%) F: 481 (40.69%) 0.32% of total adult fractures 10.66% of adult patellar fractures	**A1** 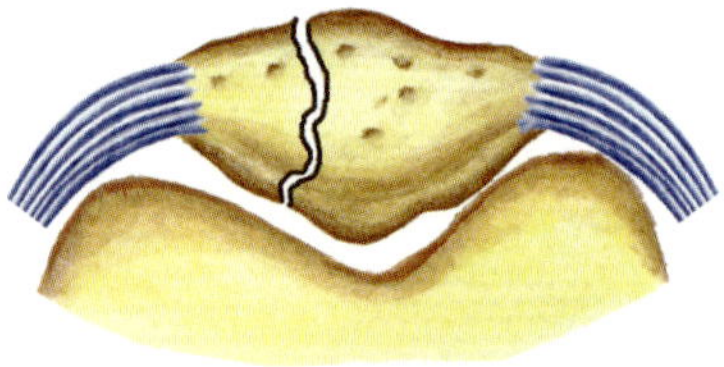 Without displacement	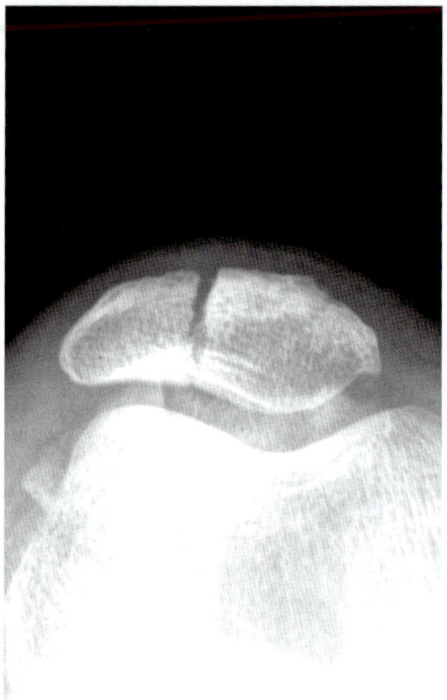
	A2 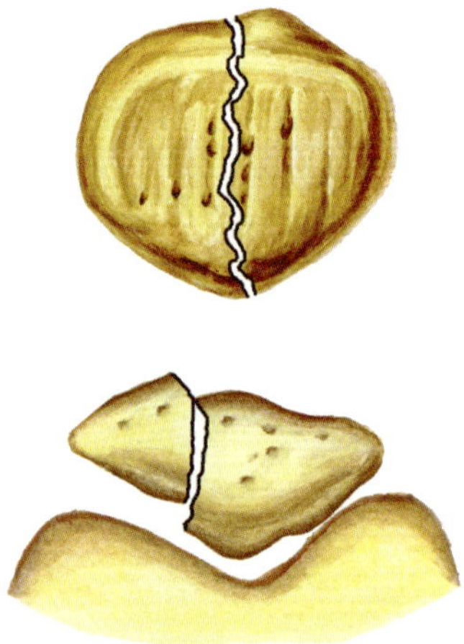 With displacement	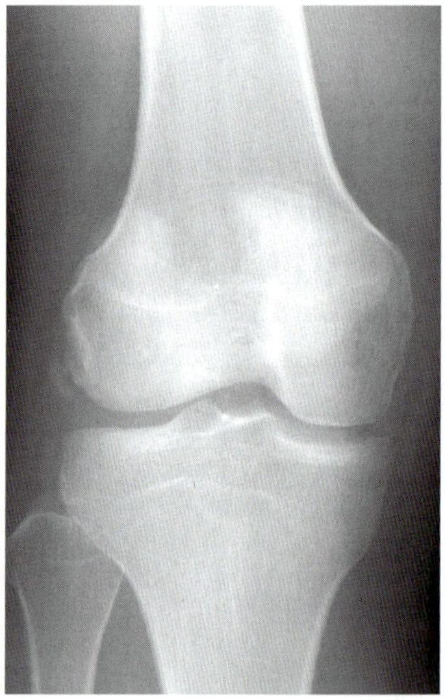
	A3 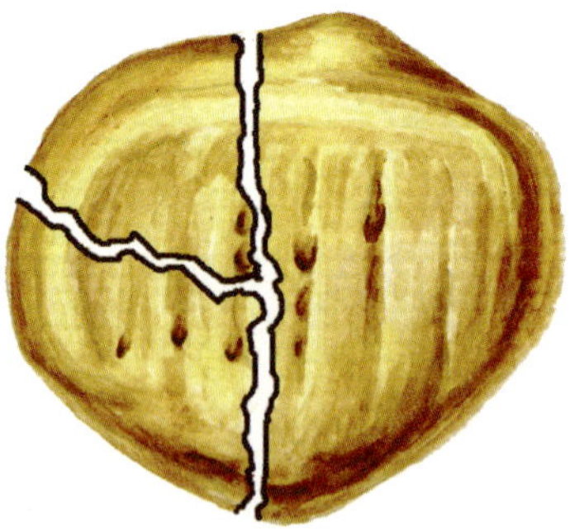 Comminuted	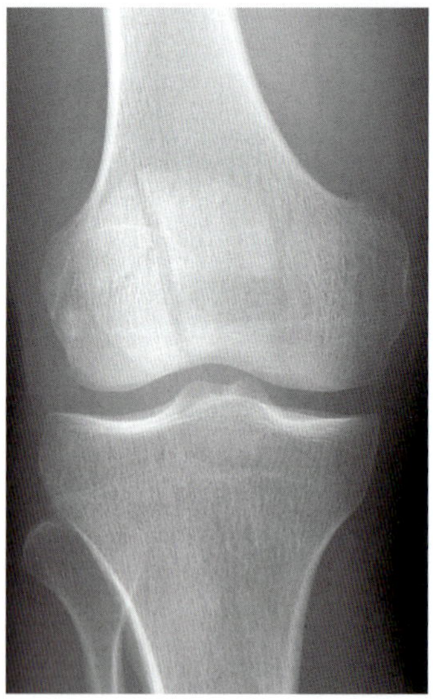

Regazzoni classification of patellar fractures			
Type B **Transverse** 7,737 fractures M: 4,407 (56.96%) F: 3,330 (43.04%) 2.07% of total adult fractures 69.78% of adult patellar fractures	**B1**	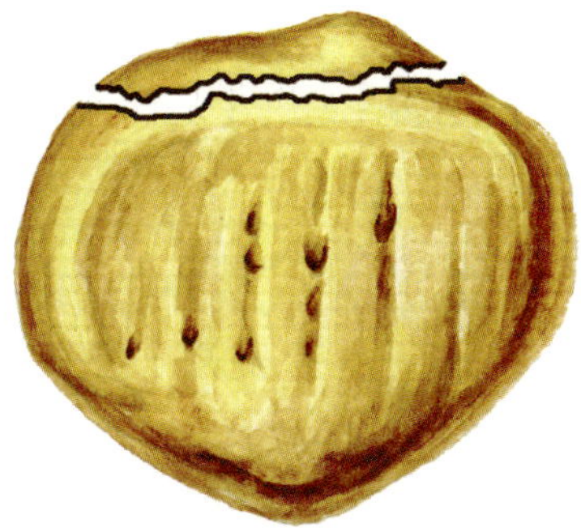 Avulsion fracture of superior and inferior poles (< 5 mm in diameter of superior pole; < 15 mm in diameter of inferior pole)	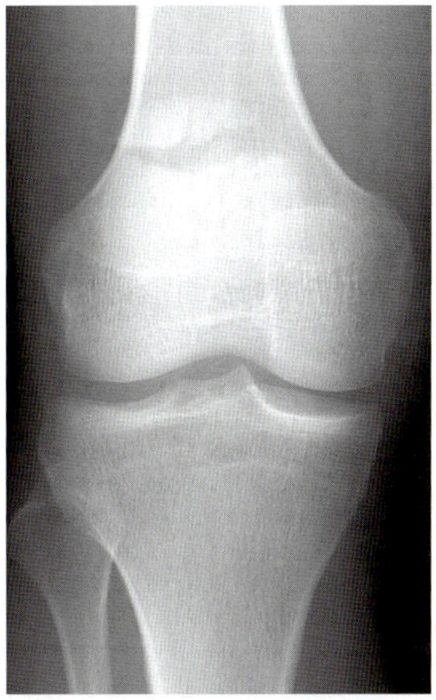
	B2	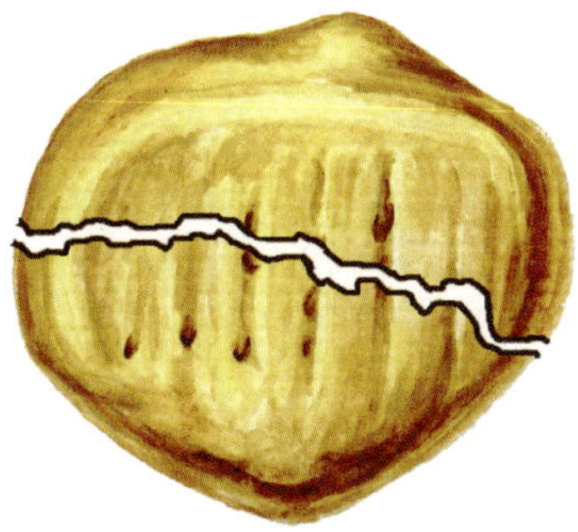 Simple	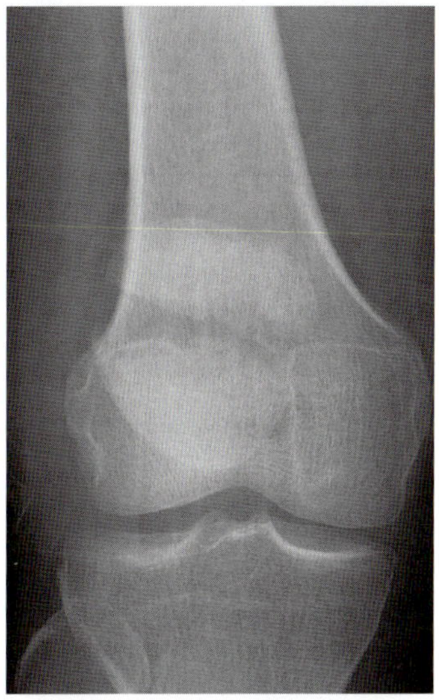
	B3	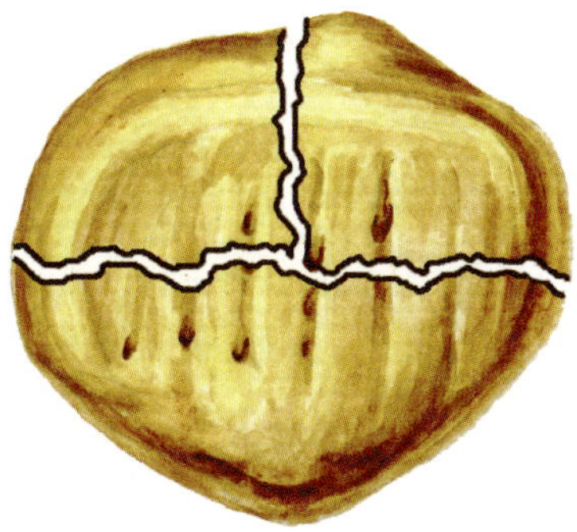 Comminuted	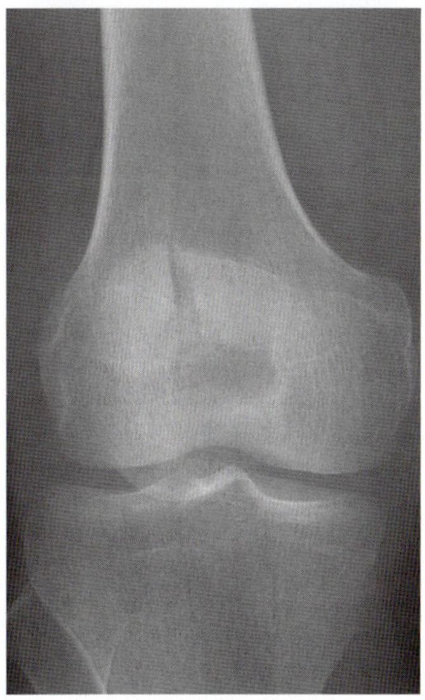

Regazzoni classification of patellar fractures

Type C
Comminuted fractures
2,169 fractures
M: 1,499 (69.11%)
F: 670 (30.89%)
0.58% of total adult fractures
19.56% of adult patellar fractures

C1

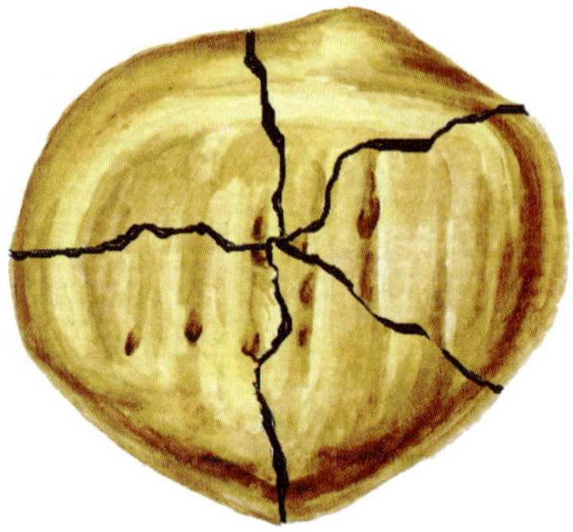

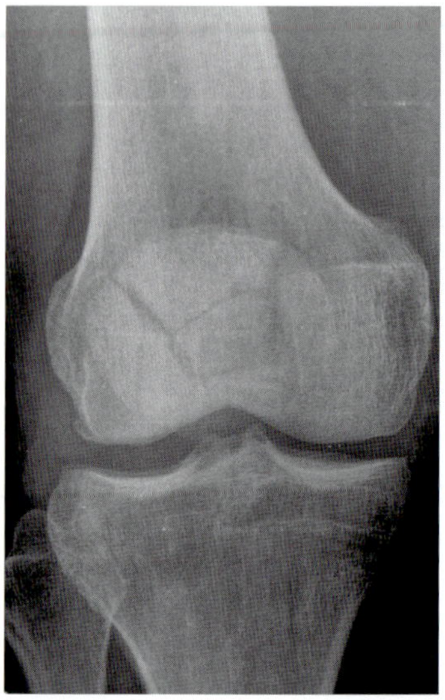

Without marked displacement

C2

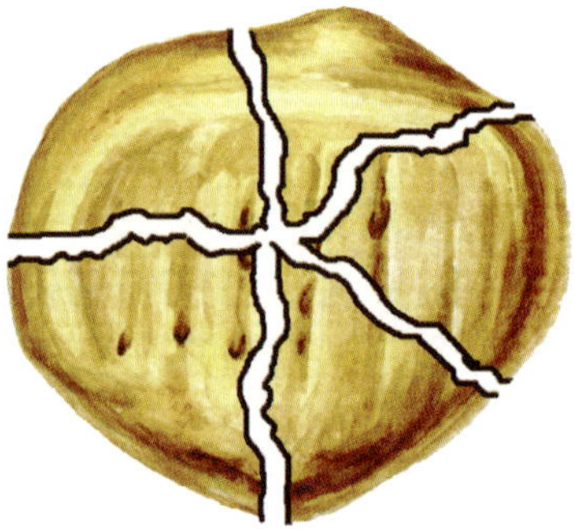

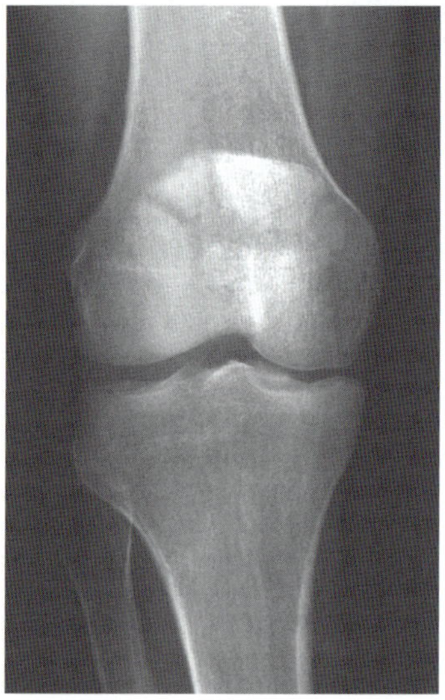

With displacement of < 2 mm

C3

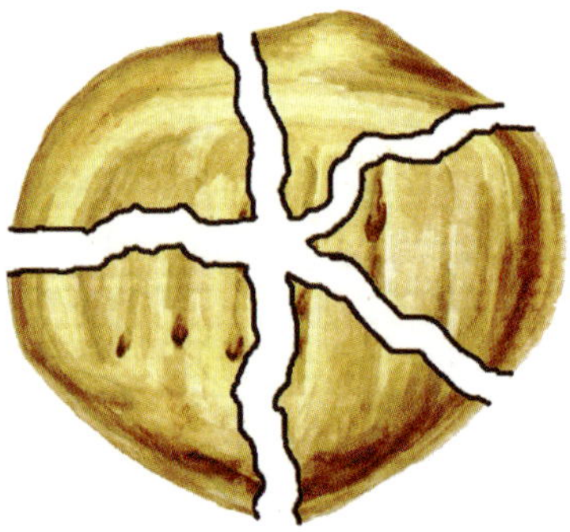

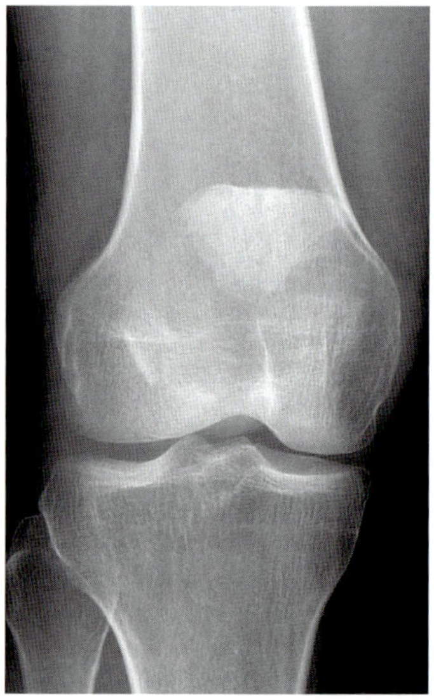

Combined with burst fractures with displacement of > 2 mm

Clavicle Fractures (Segment 15)

Anatomical Features

The clavicle forms the anterior portion of the shoulder girdle, and is placed nearly horizontally at the upper and anterior part of the thorax. It serves as the only direct bony attachment of the arm to the trunk. The clavicle is connected strongly to a number of muscles and accordingly to facets, most of which are essential for the stability of the shoulder girdle. It is a long bone, curved somewhat like the letter "s" in the superior view, but appears straight in the anterior view. The lateral third of the clavicle is flattened from above and downward, to accommodate the attachment and traction of muscles; furthermore, its middle third is tubular, and its medial third has a prismatic form to withstand the axial compression load and traction (**Plate 10.6**).

The lateral third of the clavicle gives attachment to the trapezius and deltoid muscles. On the posterosuperior border of the medial third is a rough area for attachment of the sternocleidomastoid muscle. The clavicular portion of the pectoralis major originates off of the anterior surface of medial border of the medial third. The subclavius muscle originates from the inferior border of the middle third of the clavicle and inserts on the first rib, just dorsal to the subclavian surface (**Plate 10.7**).

Anatomical Features and Muscular Attachment of the Clavicle

From an anatomical point of view, a few factors that result in the displacement of clavicle fractures can be summarized as follows: (1) the proximal fragment is typically displaced upward because of the pull of the sternocleidomastoid muscle; (2) although there may be some upward movement of the clavicle due to the pull of the trapezius muscle, the major displacement is caused by the downward pull of the upper extremity, since most patients would not be able to withstand the weight of the upper arm due to the pain; (3) however, if the upward pull of the trapezius muscle surpasses the weight of the upper arm, or patients are using a sling to support the arm, then the distal fragment may also be displaced upward; and (4) the pull of the pectoralis major, pectoralis minor, and the latissimus dorsi draw the distal fragment medially (**Plate 10.8**).

The clavicle articulates medially with the clavicular notch of the manubrium sterni, forming the sternoclavicular joint, which is supported by the anterior and posterior sternoclavicular and interclavicular ligaments. The lateral end of the clavicle articulates with the acromion of the scapula, forming the acromioclavicular joint, which is stabilized by the acromioclavicular, coracoacromial, and coracoclavicular ligaments; these three ligaments form the coracoacromial arch. The coracoclavicular ligament consists of two fasciculi, the trapezoid and conoid ligaments, which are attached between the coracoid process of the scapula and the underside of the clavicle; they primarily provide stabilization of the acromioclavicular joint and prevent superior dislocation of the shoulder joint (**Plate 10.9**).

OTA Classification and Coding System for Clavicle Fractures

Based on OTA classification, the clavicle is coded as the number 15 for its anatomical location, and is divided into three segments: proximal, shaft, and distal according to the Heim square method. The OTA classification of clavicle fractures is as shown in **Plate 10.10**.

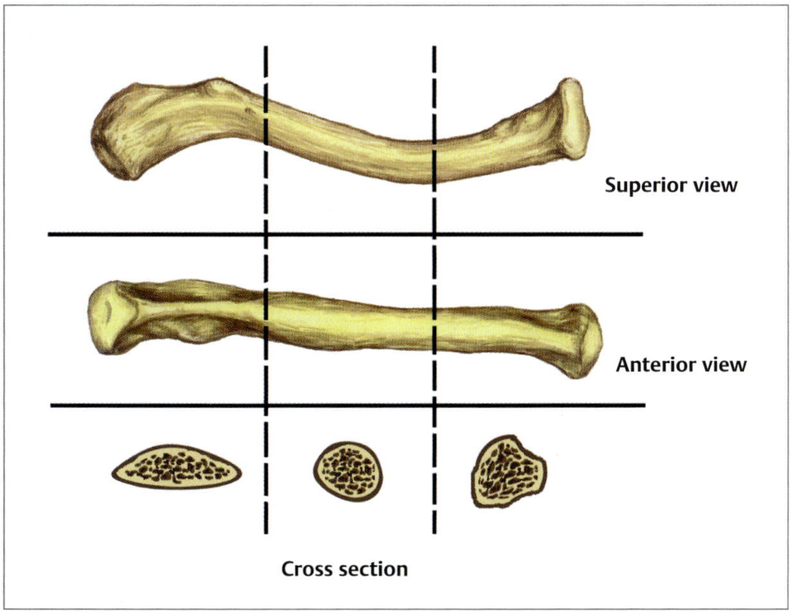

Plate 10.6

Plate 10.7

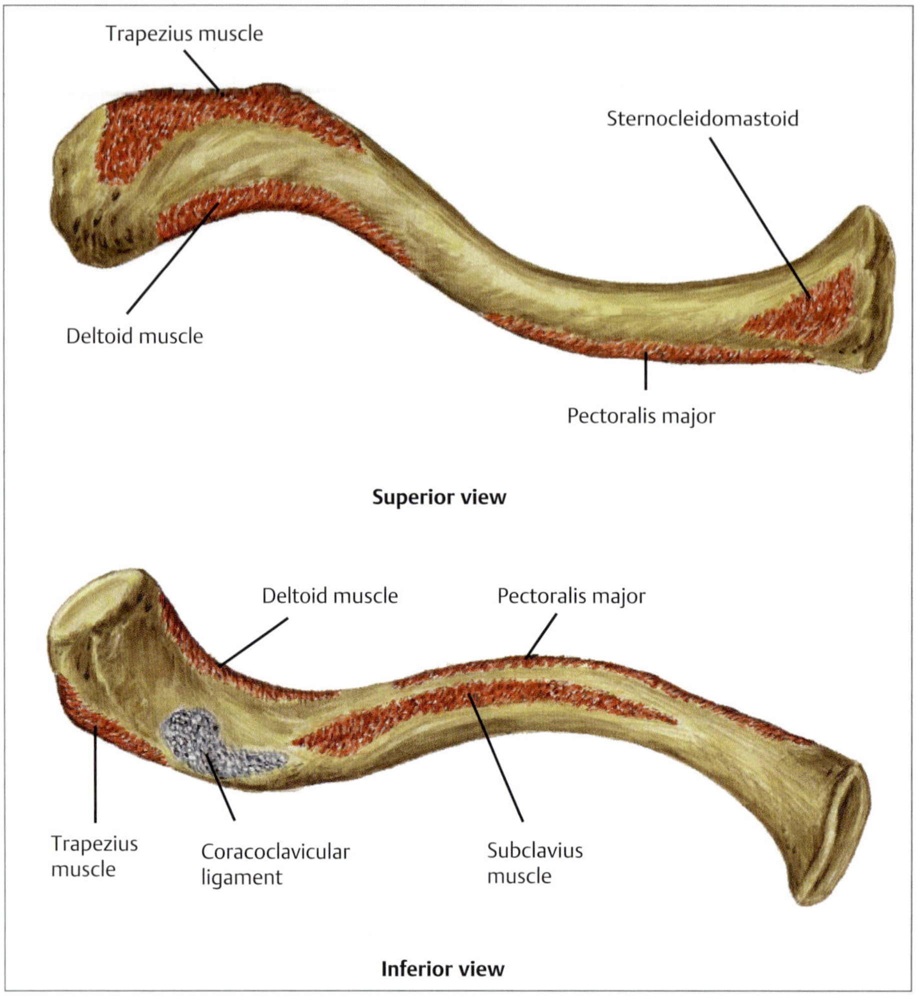
Trapezius muscle
Sternocleidomastoid
Deltoid muscle
Pectoralis major
Superior view
Deltoid muscle
Pectoralis major
Trapezius muscle
Coracoclavicular ligament
Subclavius muscle
Inferior view

Plate 10.8

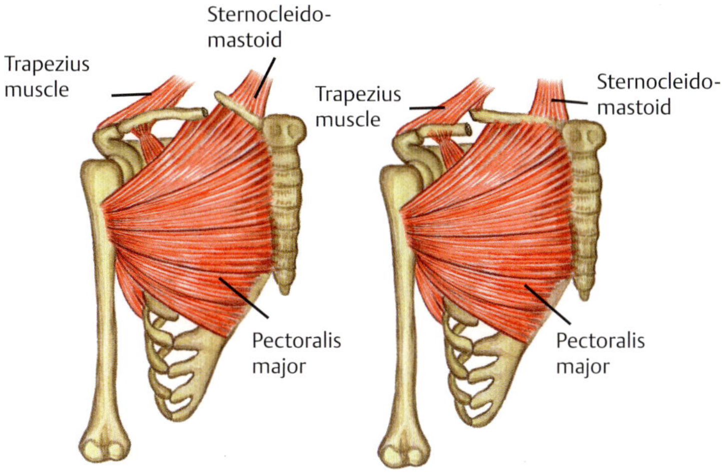

Fracture displacement of clavicle

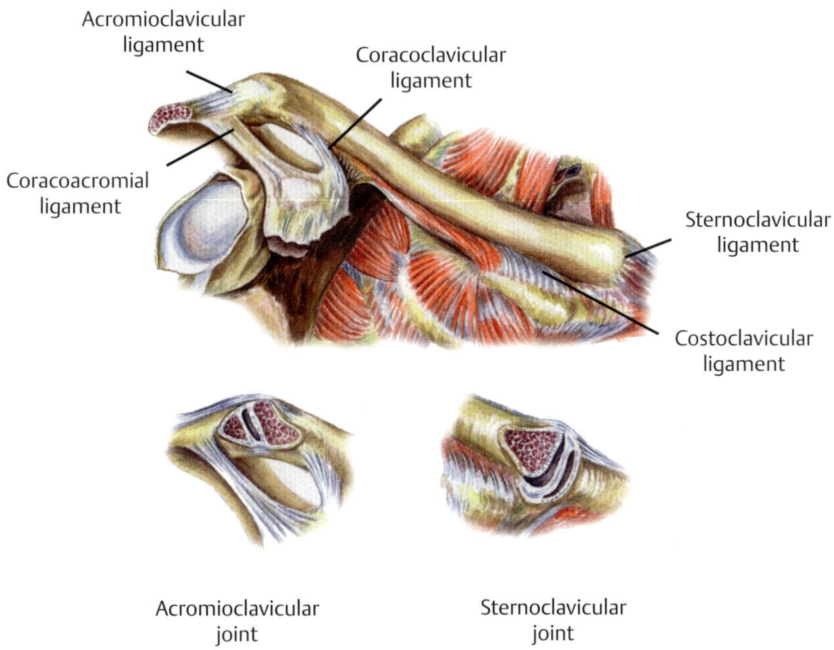

Joint and ligament of clavicle

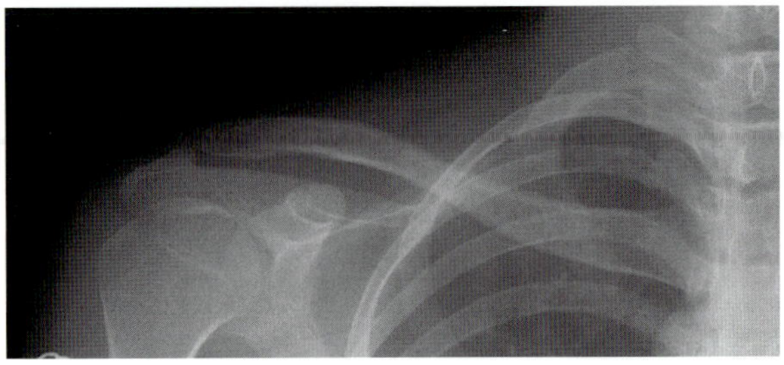

Plate 10.9

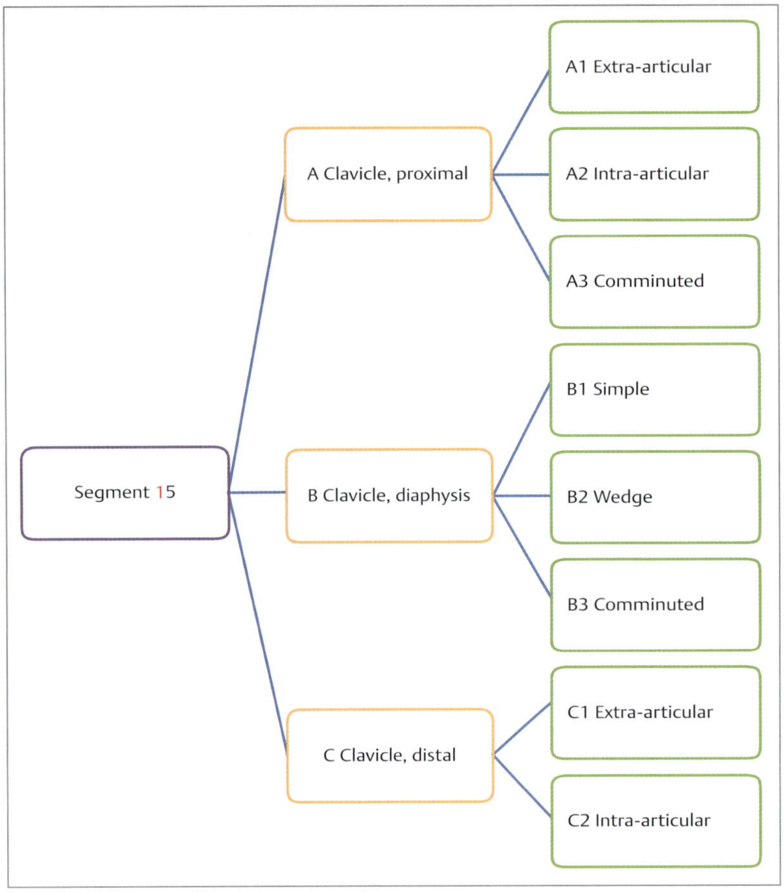

Plate 10.10

Clinical Epidemiologic Features of Clavicle Fractures (Segment 15)

A total of 18,502 patients with 18,587 clavicle fractures were treated in 83 hospitals in China over a 2-year period from 2010 to 2011. All cases were reviewed and statistically studied, accounting for 4.46% of all patients with fractures and 4.3% of all kinds of fractures, respectively. Among 18,502 patients, there were 4,424 pediatric patients (4,430 clavicle fractures) and 14,078 adult patients with 14,157 clavicle fractures.

Epidemiologic features of clavicle fractures are as follows:

- More males than females
- More left side than right side fractures
- The high risk age group is between ages 0 and 5 years, the same age group for females, while for males the high risk age group is between ages 41 and 50 years.
- The most common fracture type is type B.

Clavicle Fractures by Sex

Table 10.7 Sex distribution of 18,502 patients with clavicle fractures

Sex	Number of patients	Percentage (%)
Male	12,827	69.33
Female	5,675	30.67
Total	18,502	100.00

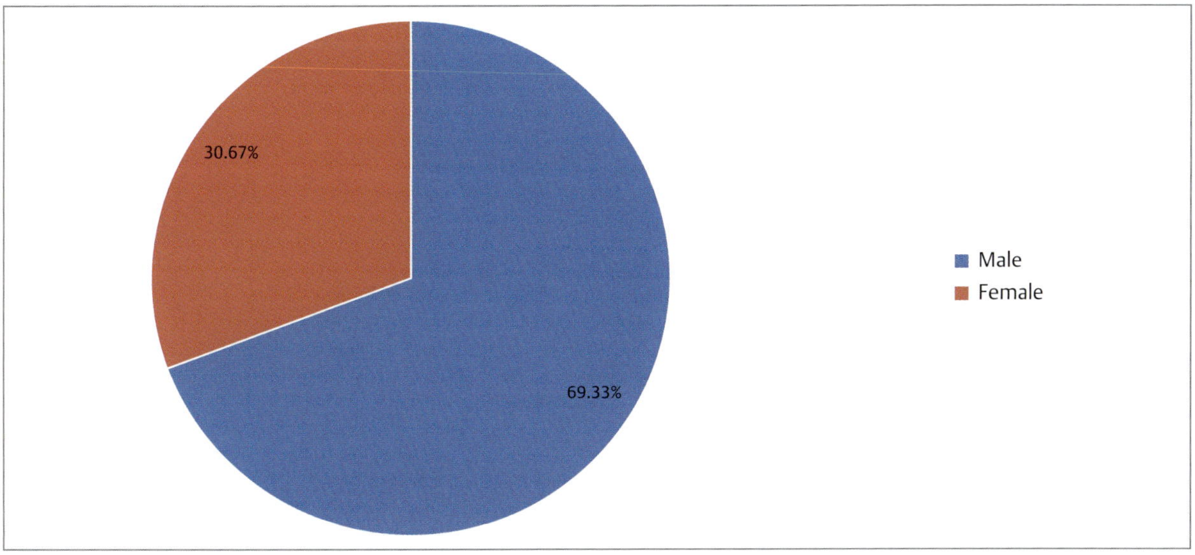

Fig. 10.7 Sex distribution of 18,502 patients with clavicle fractures.

Clavicle Fractures by Fracture Side

Table 10.8 Fracture side distribution of 18,502 patients with clavicle frac tures

Fracture side	Number of patients	Percentage (%)
Left	10,100	54.59
Right	8,317	44.95
Bilateral	85	0.46
Total	18,502	100.00

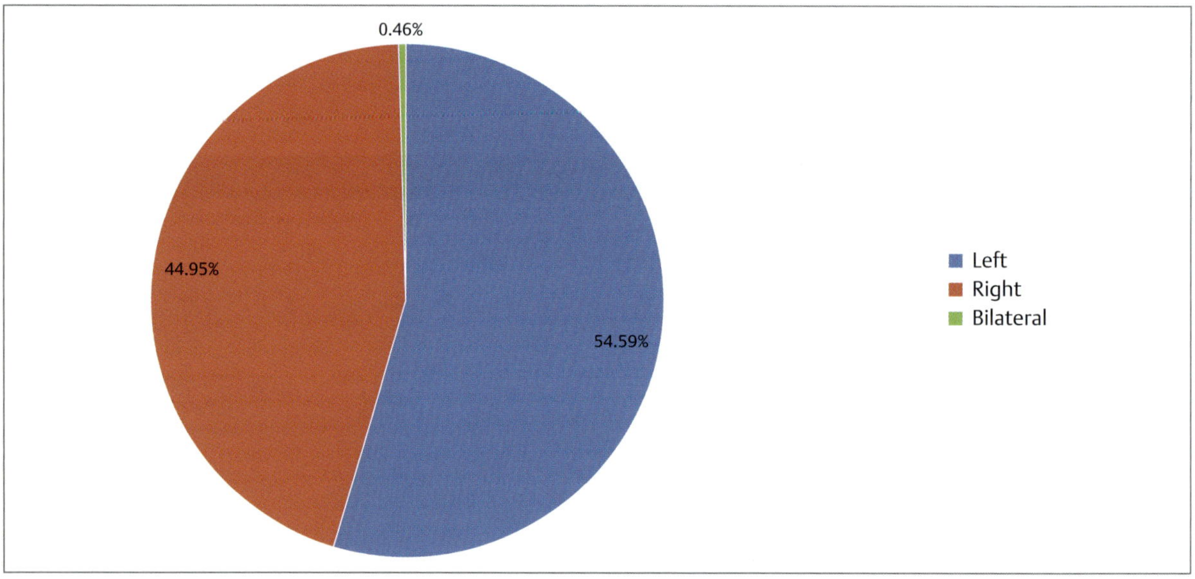

Fig. 10.8 Fracture side distribution of 18,502 patients with clavicle fractures.

Clavicle Fractures by Age Group

Table 10.9 Age and sex distribution of 18,502 patients with clavicle fractures

Age group (years)	Male	Female	Number of patients	Percentage (%)
0–5	1,183	883	2,066	11.17
6–10	869	407	1,276	6.90
11–15	804	278	1,082	5.85
16–20	760	250	1,010	5.46
21–25	892	352	1,244	6.72
26–30	913	320	1,233	6.66
31–35	978	351	1,329	7.18
36–40	1,093	376	1,469	7.94
41–45	1,396	381	1,777	9.60
46–50	1,224	362	1,586	8.57
51–55	908	379	1,287	6.96
56–60	776	392	1,168	6.31
61–65	381	333	714	3.86
66–70	235	216	451	2.44
71–75	164	169	333	1.80
76–80	122	114	236	1.28
81–85	78	68	146	0.79
≥86	51	44	95	0.51
Total	12,827	5,675	18,502	100.00

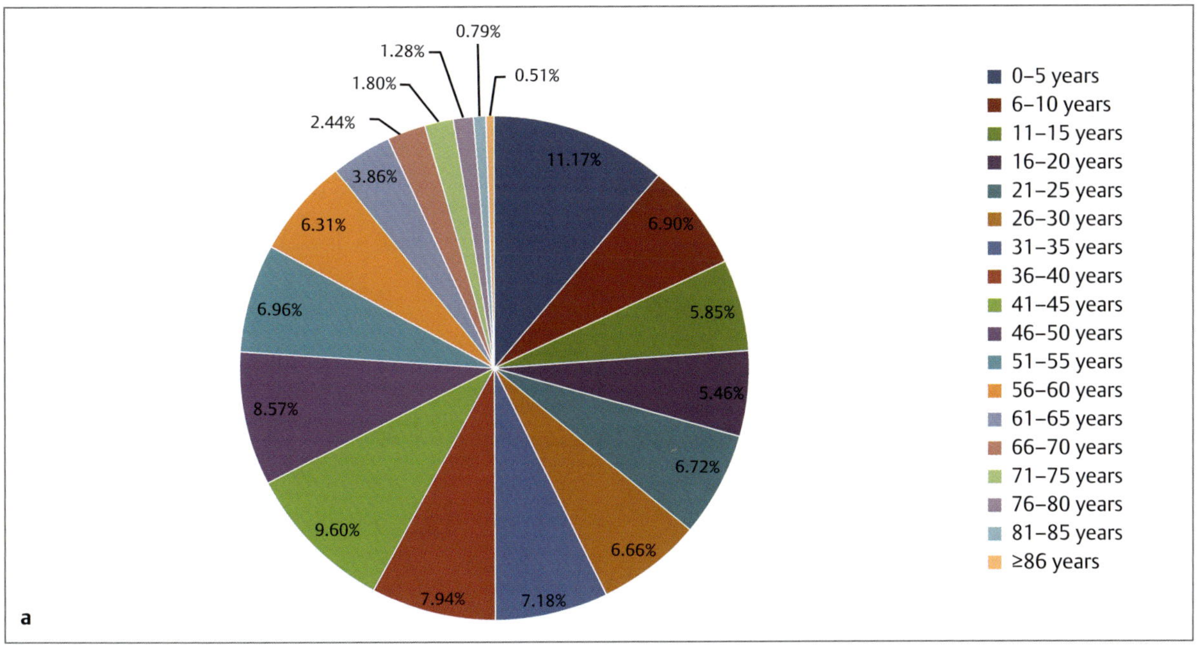

Fig. 10.9 **(a)** Age distribution of 18,502 patients with clavicle fractures. (*Continued*)

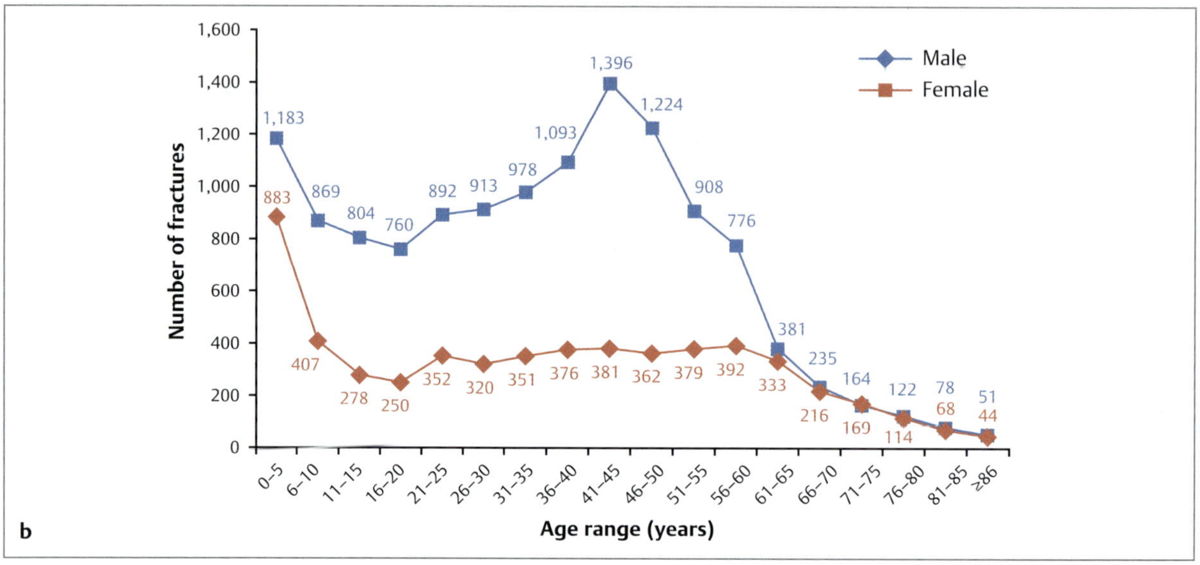

Fig. 10.9 (*continued*) **(b)** Age and sex distribution of 18,502 patients with clavicle fractures.

Clavicle fractures by fracture type based on OTA classification

Table 10.10 Sex and fracture type distribution of 14,157 adult clavicle fractures by OTA classification

Fracture type	Male	Female	Number of fractures	Percentage (%)
15-A	183	60	243	1.72
15-B	7,472	2,835	10,307	72.80
15-C	2,370	1,237	3,607	25.48
Total	10,025	4,132	14,157	100.00

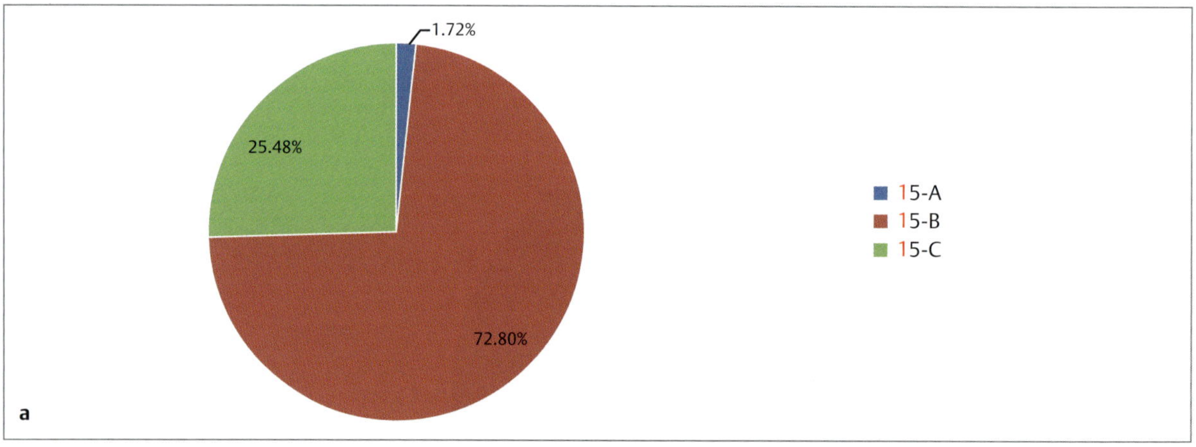

Fig 10.10 **(a)** Fracture type distribution of 14,157 adult clavicle fractures by OTA classification.

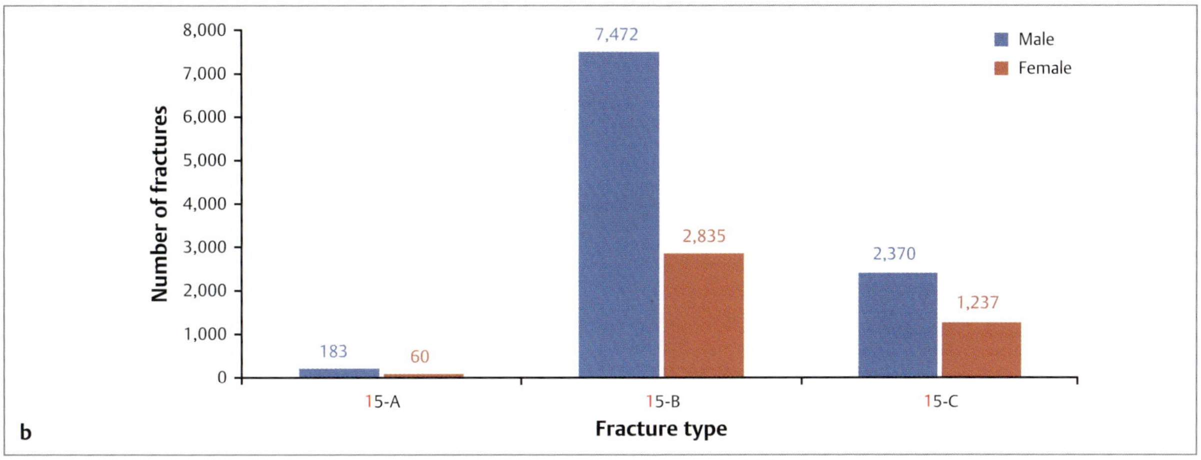

Fig 10.10 (*continued*) **(b)** Sex and fracture type distribution of 14,157 adult clavicle fractures by OTA classification.

OTA Classification of Clavicle Fractures	
15-A **Proximal** 243 fractures M: 183 (75.31%) F: 60 (24.69%) 1.72% of adult clavicle fractures 0.06% of total adult fractures	**15-A** 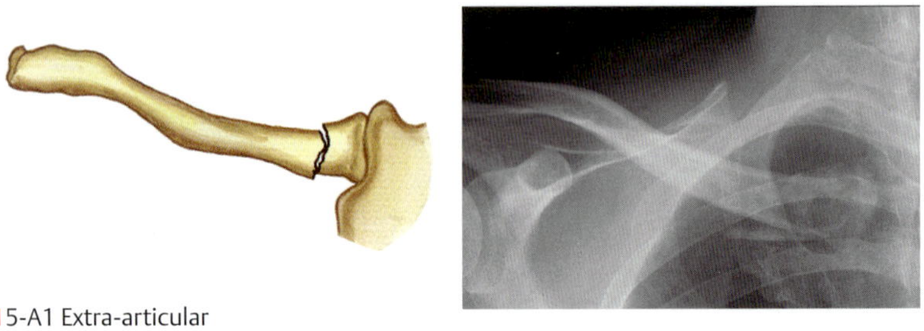 15-A1 Extra-articular 15-A2 Intra-articular 15-A3 Comminuted
15-B **Diaphysis** 10,307 fractures M: 7,472 (72.49%) F: 2,835 (27.51%) 72.8% of adult clavicle fractures 2.75% of total adult fractures	**15-B1** 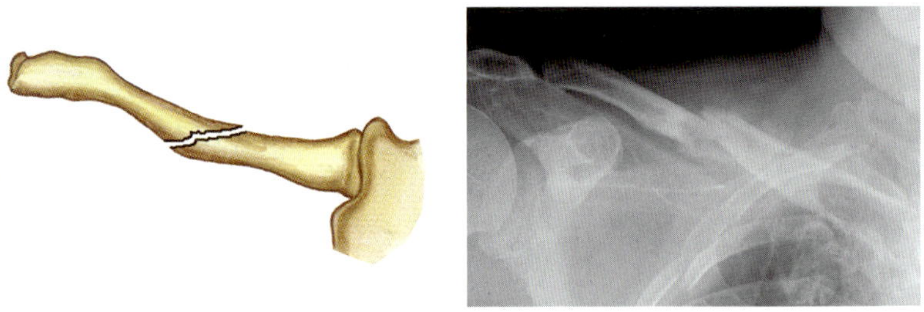 Simple
	15-B2 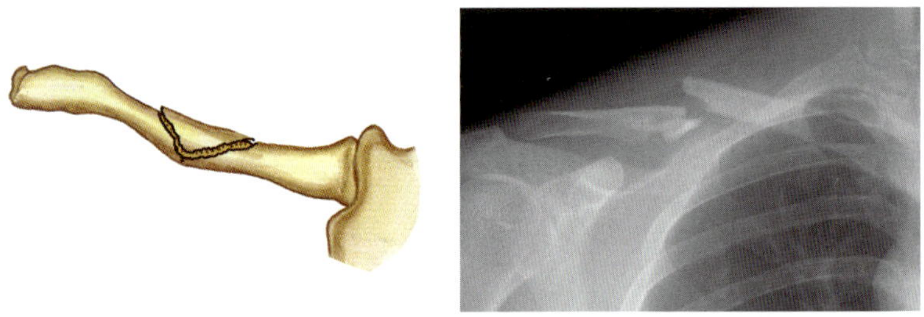 Wedge
	15-B3 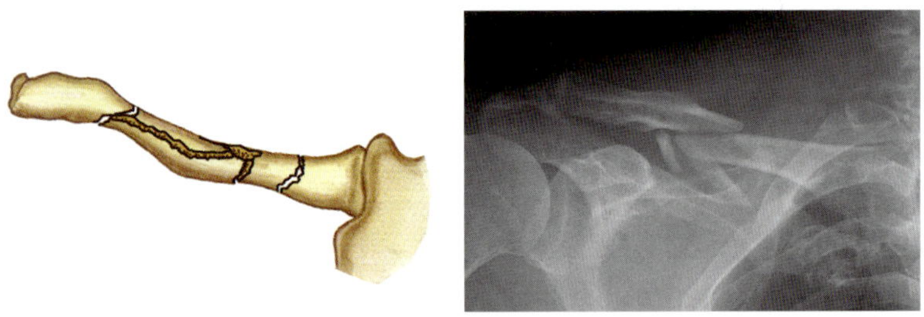 Comminuted

OTA Classification of Clavicle Fractures

15-C **Distal** 3,607 fractures M: 2,370 (65.71%) F: 1,237 (34.29%) 25.48% of adult clavicle fractures 0.96% of total adult fractures	**15-C1** 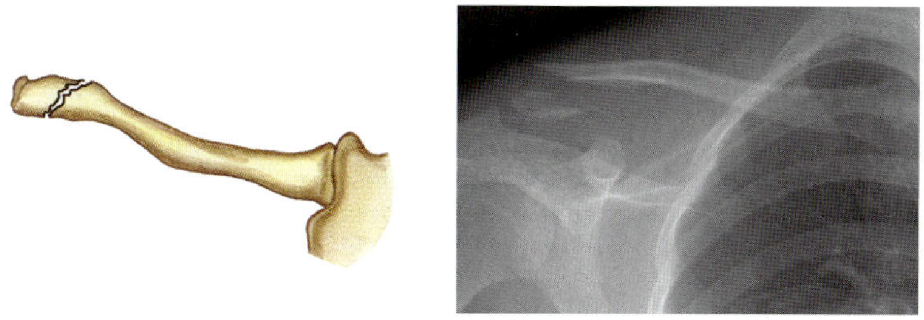 Extra-articular
	15-C2 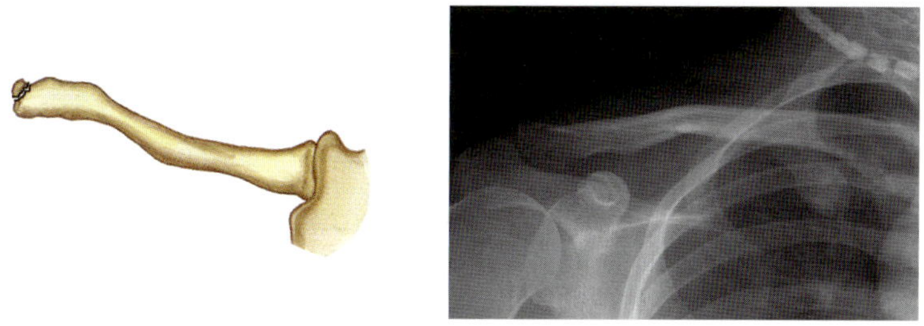 Intra-articular

Injury Mechanism

Clavicle fractures in adults and youths usually occur as the result of a direct force from high-energy trauma. In children and elderly patients, indirect trauma with a low force of energy is the usual cause. The most common mechanism of injury is a fall onto the shoulder or onto an outstretched hand, whereby the force of the fall is transmitted up the arm through the shoulder to the clavicle.

Diagnosis

Adult patients with clavicle fractures will present with obvious swelling and deformity along the clavicle. Fractures without displacement, commonly seen in pediatric patients, usually do not present obvious deformity. Physicians should perform visual examination and palpation along the clavicle to determine the fracture line. Patients typically present with the following signs: worsening loss of shoulder mobility, actively supporting the elbow and forearm with the opposite hand, and tilting of one's head to the affected side.

A standard AP view of the clavicle usually confirms the diagnosis of a fracture. X-rays should include the acromioclavicular and sternoclavicular joints to rule out any associated injury of adjacent structures. Surrounding structures such as the scapula and ribs should be inspected for injury as well. In addition, an oblique view of the clavicle is helpful in defining the direction and degree of the displacement. The apical lordotic view (an AP view with the tube tilted 45 degrees cephalad) can minimize overlap of the thoracic structures and allow for better assessment of the clavicle fracture.

Treatment

If the fracture is displaced, then an operative approach may be the best choice. There are several indications for operative management of clavicle fractures: (1) fracture of the lateral clavicle with associated torn coracoclavicular ligaments; (2) gross displacement and angulation of the fracture with tenting of skin; (3) comminuted fracture of the middle third or if there is marked displacement; (4) injury to the brachial plexus or subclavian artery by a fragment of bone following fracture of the clavicle; (5) patients unable to withstand long periods of immobilization; (6) open clavicle fractures; (7) occurring concurrently with multiple associated injuries; (8) nonunion of clavicle fractures; (9) for cosmetic purposes; (10) incarceration of soft tissue between widely spaced fragments; and (11) posterior displacement of the proximal fragment to the sternum, and difficultly reducing and maintaining the reduction. The operative approach is best chosen from minimally invasive methods, especially when treating female patients. The forms of available internal fixation for clavicle fractures are plate, screw, intramedullary (IM) nail, memory alloy internal fixation, tension band, and Kirschner wire (K-wire).

Nondisplaced clavicle fractures can be treated nonsurgically. A figure-of-eight bandage and cast, clavicle strap, or simple sling can provide comfort and immobilization.

Further Classifications of Clavicle Fractures

Allman Classification of Clavicle Fractures

Based on the Allman classification, the clavicle is divided into thirds: middle third injuries (Allman I), lateral third injuries (Allman II), and medial third injuries (Allman III). Each group is further divided into two subgroups (**Plate 10.11**): (a) those with no displacement and (b) those with displacement. The middle third group has an additional subgroup: (c) comminuted fractures. The Allman classification is the most common classification system for clavicle fractures (**Plate 10.12**).

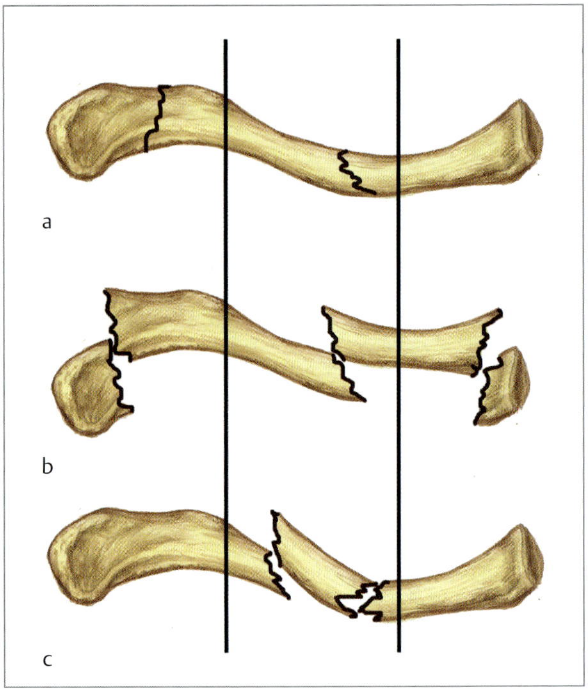

Plate 10.11

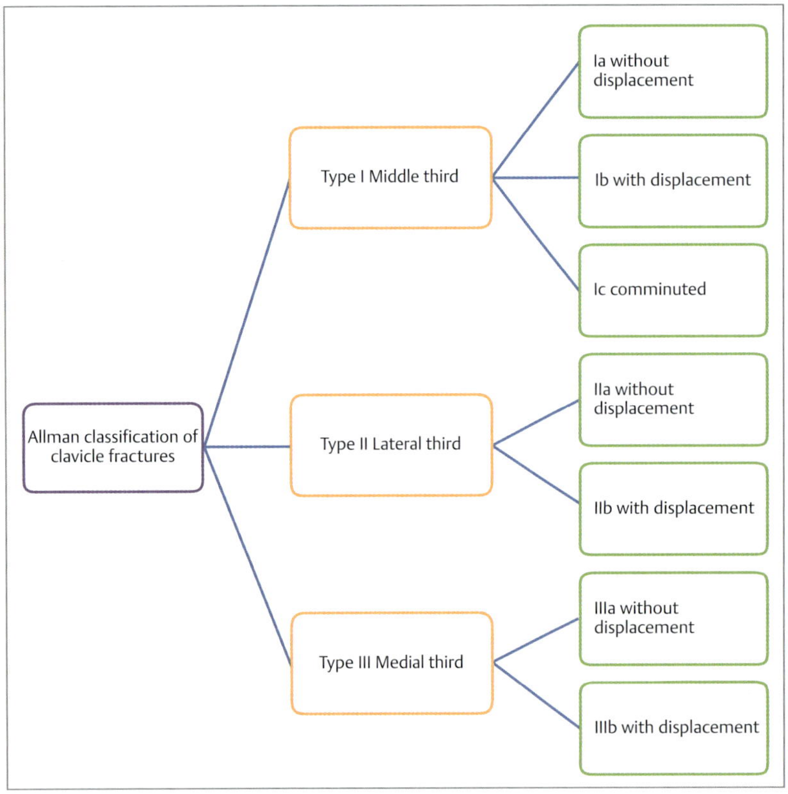

Plate 10.12

Clinical Epidemiologic Features of Clavicle Fractures by the Allman Classification

A total of 14,157 clavicle fractures were treated in 83 hospitals in China over a 2-year period from 2010 to2011; all cases were reviewed and statistically studied. Their epidemiologic features are as follows:

- More males than females
- The most common fracture type is type I, while type Ib is the most common subgroup.

Table 10.11 Sex and fracture type distribution of 14,157 clavicle fractures by Allman classification

Fracture type	Male	Female	Number of fractures	Percentage (%)
I	7,403	2,801	10,204	72.08
II	2,308	1,178	3,486	24.62
III	314	153	467	3.30
Total	10,025	4,132	14,157	100.00

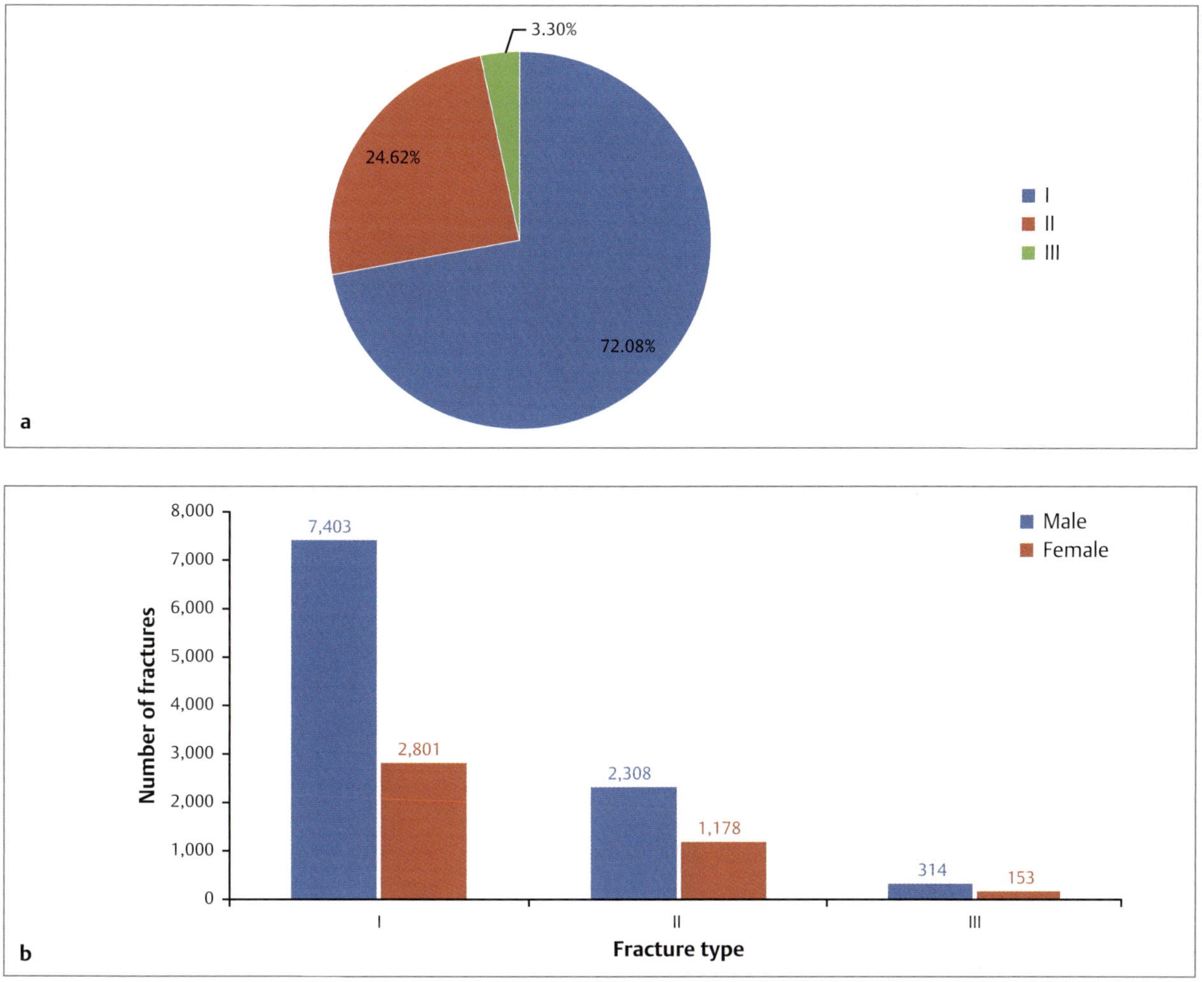

Fig. 10.11 **(a)** Fracture type distribution of 14,157 clavicle fractures by Allman classification.
(b) Sex and fracture type distribution of 14,157 clavicle fractures by Allman classification.

Table 10.12 Sex and fracture subtype distribution of 14,157 clavicle fractures by Allman classification

Fracture type	Male	Female	Number of fractures	Percentage (%)
Ia	1,885	758	2,643	18.67
Ib	3,302	1,259	4,561	32.22
Ic	2,216	784	3,000	21.19
IIa	1,103	572	1,675	11.83
IIb	1,205	606	1,811	12.79
IIIa	186	102	288	2.03
IIIb	128	51	179	1.26
Total	10,025	4,132	14,157	100.00

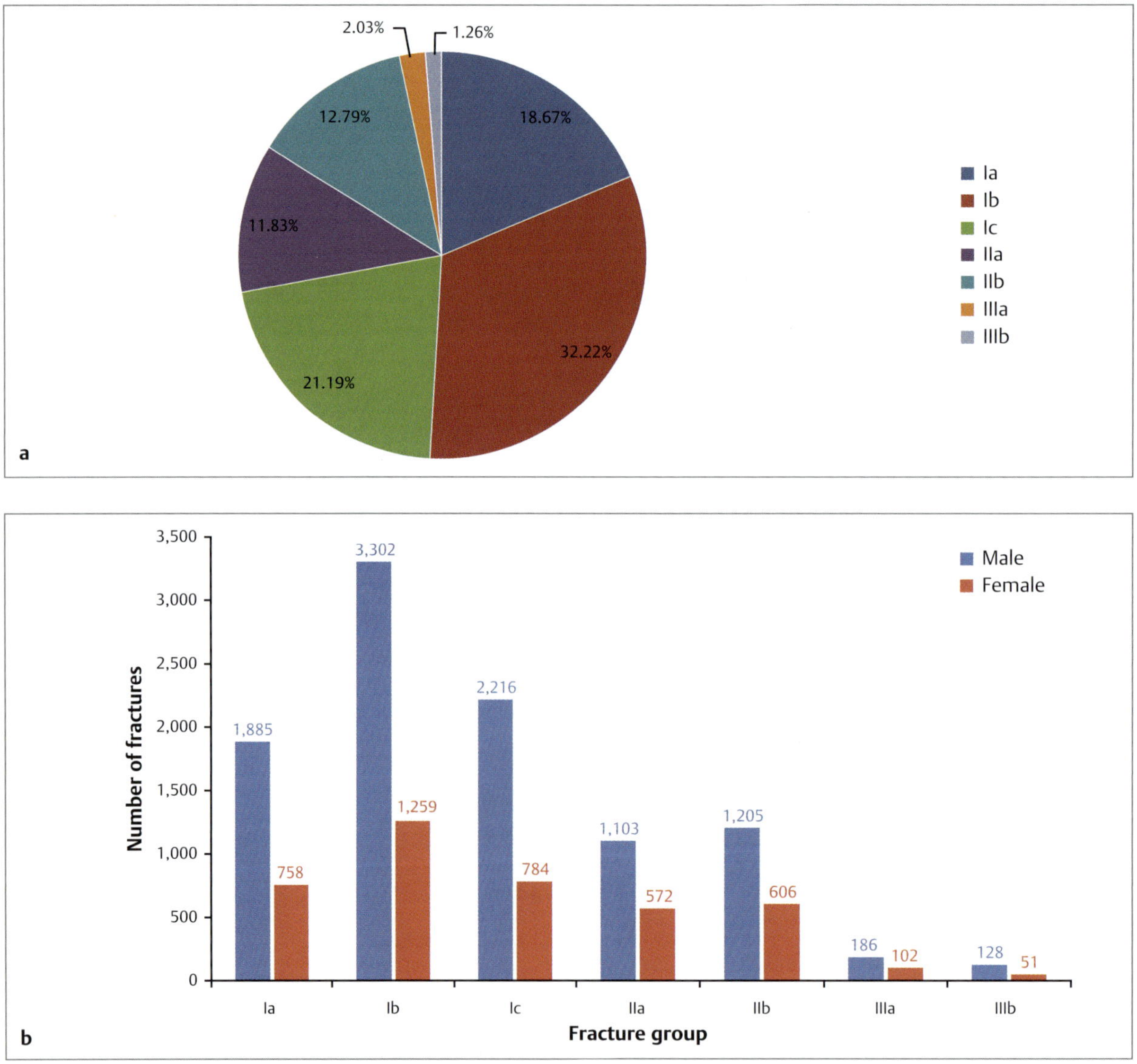

Fig. 10.12 **(a)** Fracture subtype distribution of 14,157 clavicle fractures by Allman classification. **(b)** Sex and fracture subtype distribution of 14,157 clavicle fractures by Allman classification.

Allman Classification of Clavicle Fractures	
Type I **Middle third** 10,204 fractures M: 7,403 (72.55%) F: 2,801 (27.45%) 72.08% of adult clavicle fractures 2.73% of total adult fractures	**Ia** 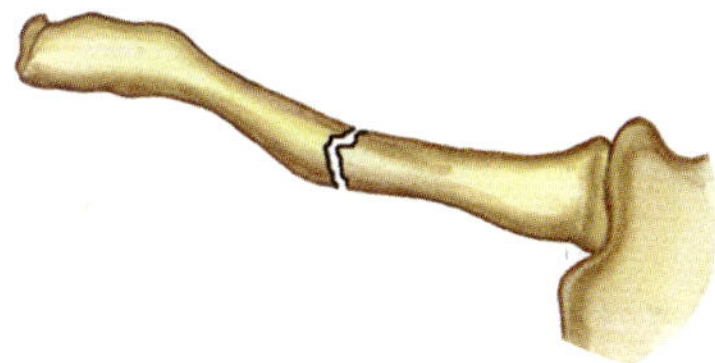 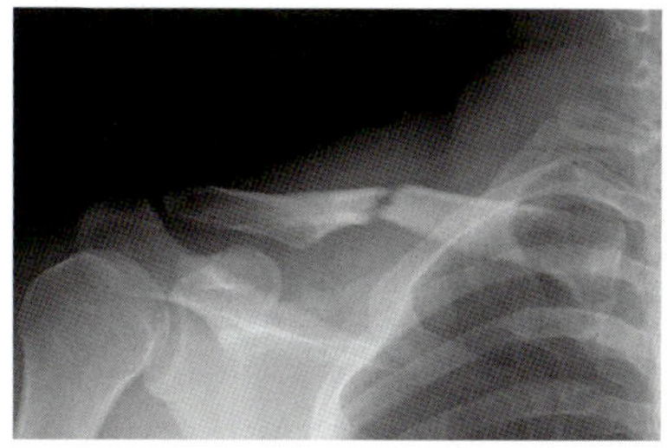 With no displacement
	Ib 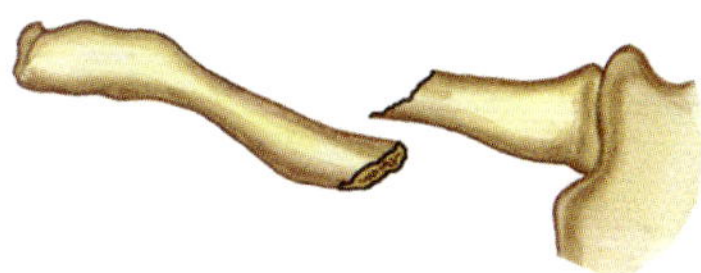 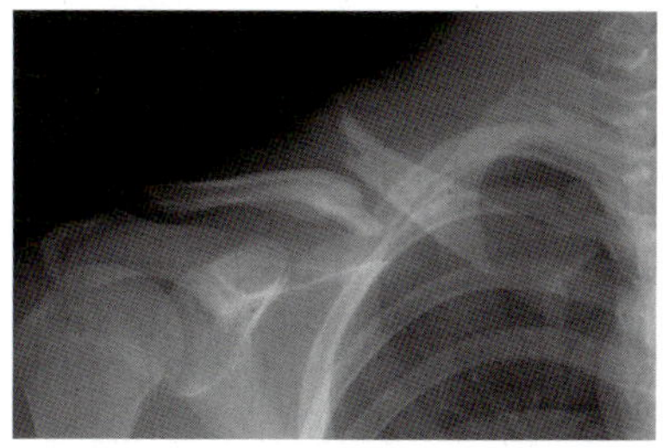 With displacement
	Ic 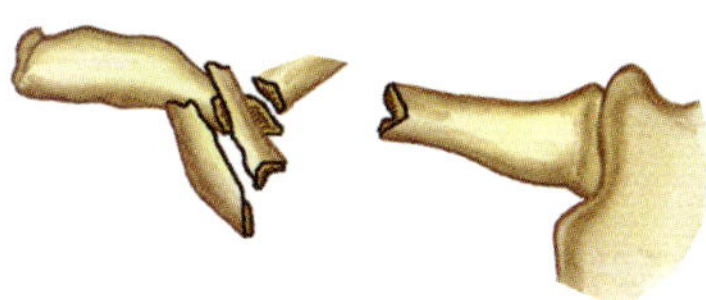 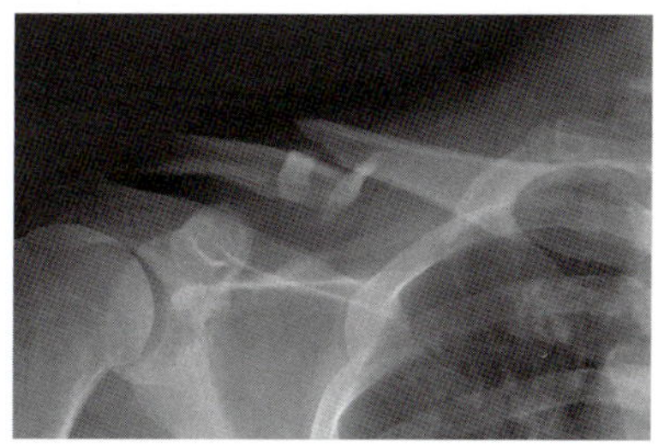 Comminuted

Allman Classification of Clavicle Fractures	
Type II **Lateral third** 3,486 fractures M: 2,308 (66.21%) F: 1,178 (33.79%) 24.62% of adult clavicle fractures 0.93% of total adult fractures	**IIa** 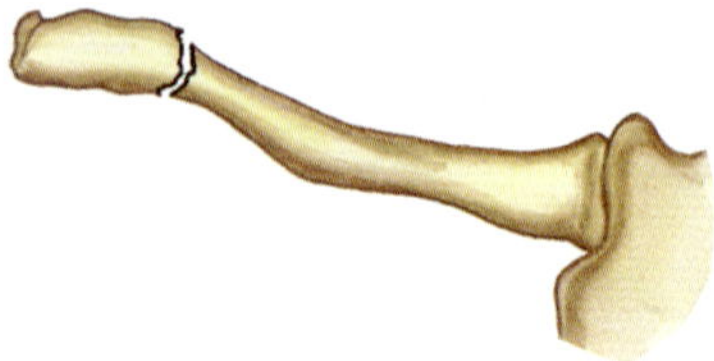 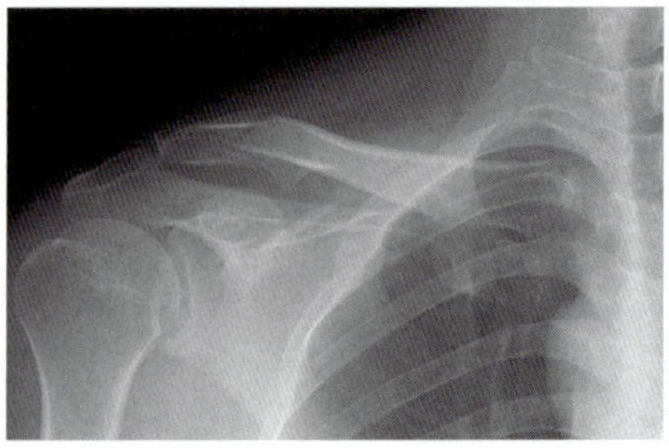 With no displacement
	IIb 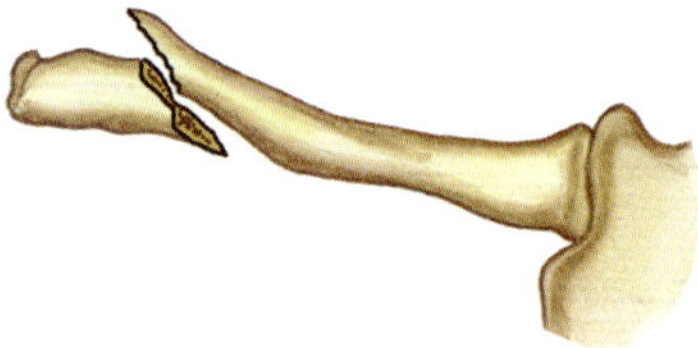 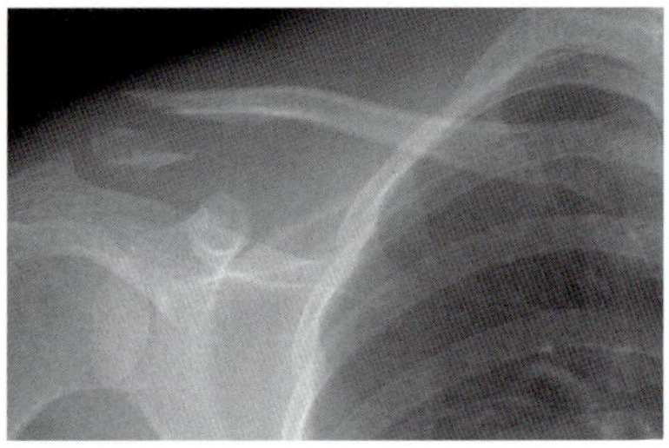 With displacement
Type III **Medial third** 467 fractures M: 314 (67.24%) F: 153 (32.76%) 3.30% of adult clavicle fractures 0.12% of total adult fractures	**IIIa** 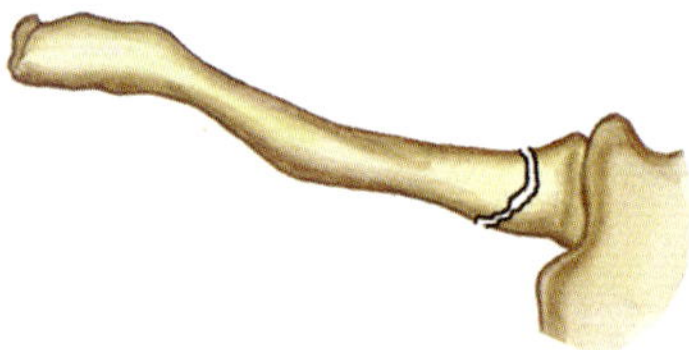 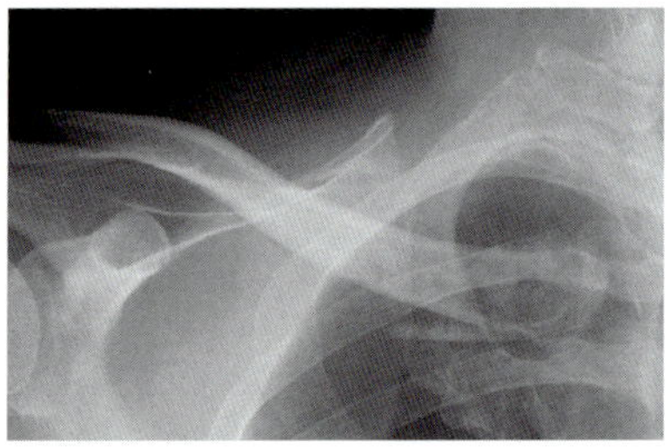 With no displacement
	IIIb 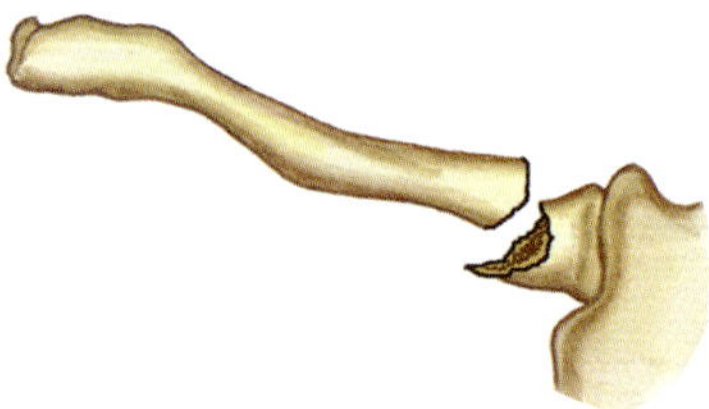 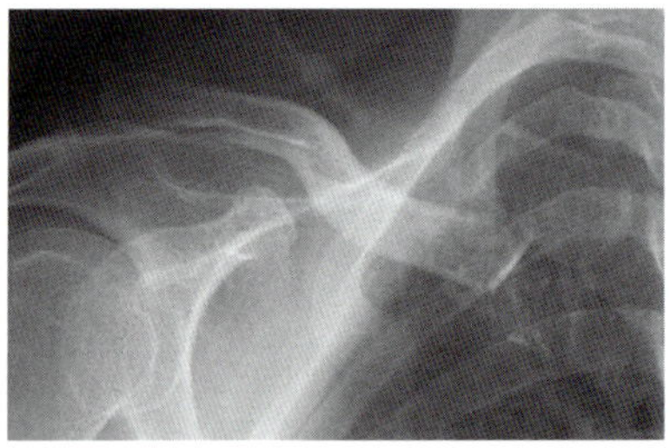 With displacement

Robinson Classification of Clavicle Fractures

In 1988, Robinson proposed the following classification scheme for clavicle fractures:

- *Type 1*: fractures of the medial fifth
- *Type 2*: diaphyseal fractures
- *Type 3*: fractures of the outer fifth (the fifth of the bone lateral to a vertical line drawn upward from the center of the base of the coracoid process, a point normally marked by the conoid tuberosity)

Each type of fracture was broken down further into two subtypes, A and B, depending on displacement (greater or less than 100% translation) of the major fragments. Type 1A and type 1B fractures were further subdivided into (1) extra-articular or (2) intra-articular. Type 2A fractures were subdivided according to the presence of angulation but in all these injuries there was residual bony contact. Two subgroups of type 2B were simple or wedge comminuted fractures (type 2B1), and isolated segmental or segmentally comminuted fractures (type 2B2). Type 3A and type 3B fractures were also subdivided according to their articular involvement (**Plate 10.13**).

Clinical Epidemiologic Features of Clavicle Fractures by the Robertson Classification

A total of 14,157 clavicle fractures were treated in 83 hospitals in China from 2010 to 2011. The epidemiologic features of clavicle fractures by the Robinson classification are:

- More males than females
- The most common fracture type is type 2.

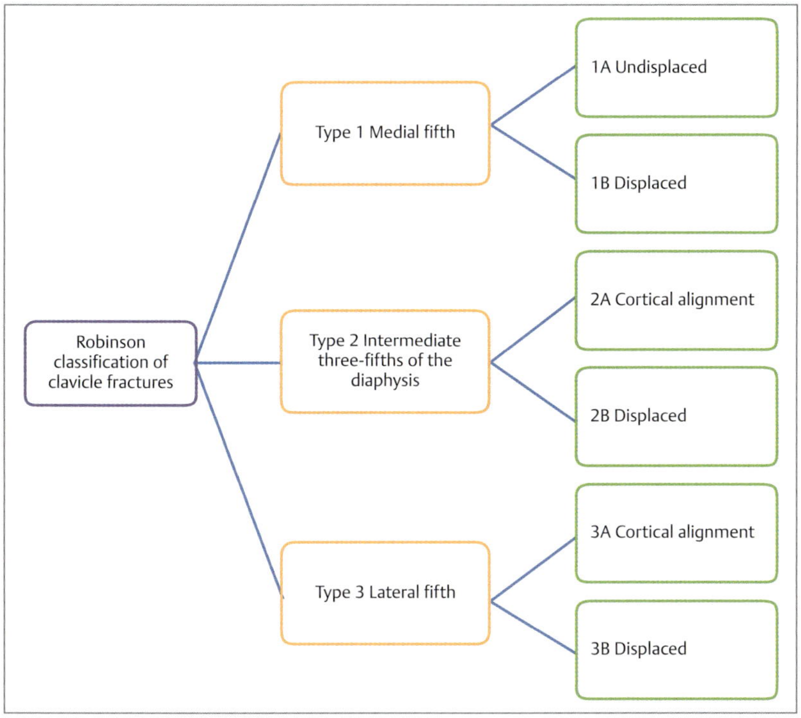

Plate 10.13

Table 10.13 Sex and fracture type distribution of 14,157 clavicle fractures by Robinson classification

Fracture type	Male	Female	Number of fractures	Percentage (%)
1	164	55	219	1.55
2	7,523	2,839	10,362	73.19
3	2,338	1,238	3,576	25.26
Total	10,025	4,132	14,157	100.00

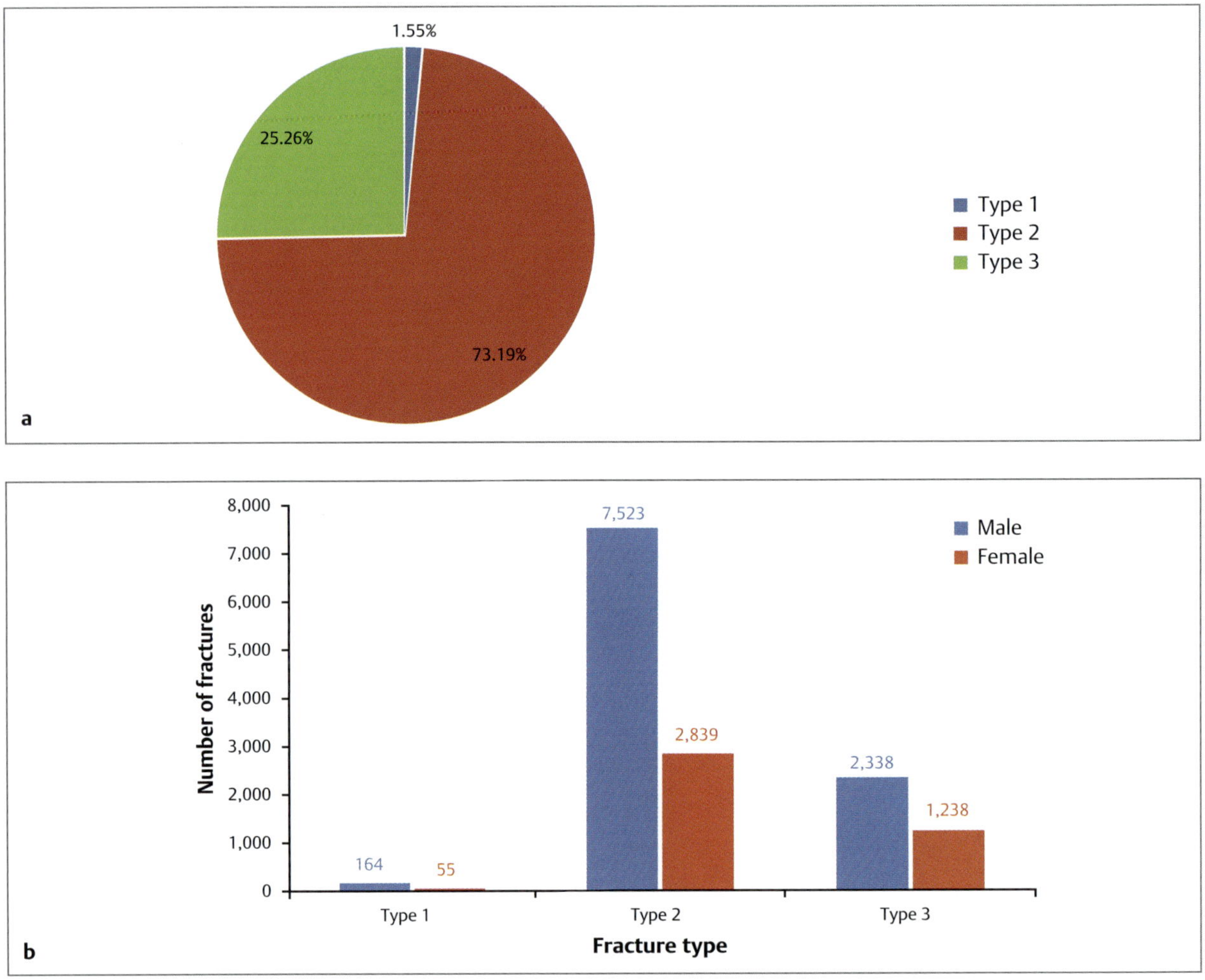

Fig. 10.13 **(a)** Fracture type distribution of 14,157 clavicle fractures by Robinson classification.
(b) Sex and fracture type distribution of 14,157 clavicle fractures by Robinson classification.

Robinson classification of clavicle fractures	
Type 1 **Medial fifth** 219 fractures M: 164 (74.89%) F: 55 (25.11%) 1.55% of adult clavicle fractures 0.06% of total adult fractures	**1A** 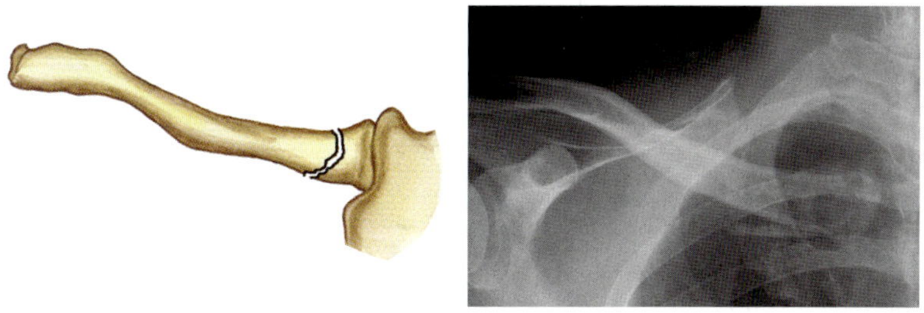 Nondisplaced fractures
	1B 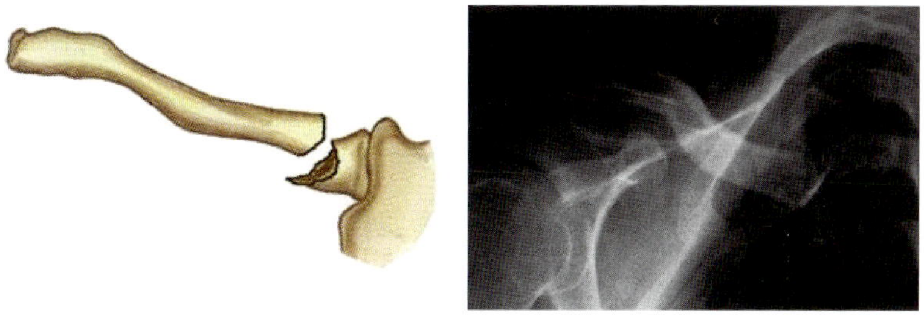 Displaced fractures
Type 2 **Intermediate three-fifths of diaphysis** 10,362 Fractures M: 7,523 (72.6%) F: 2,839 (27.4%) 73.19% of adult clavicle fractures 2.77% of total adult fractures	**2A** 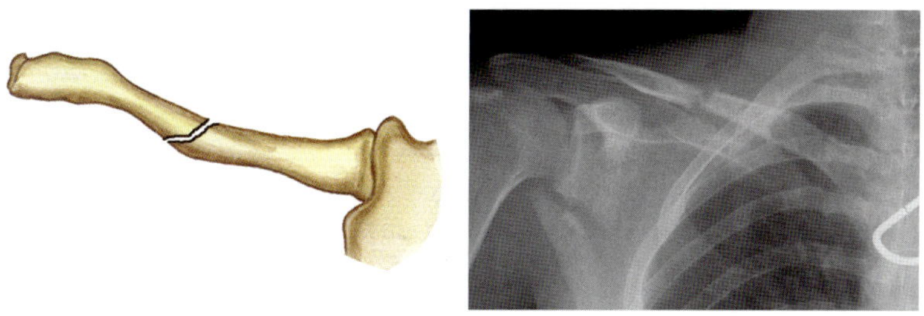 Cortical alignment fractures
	2B 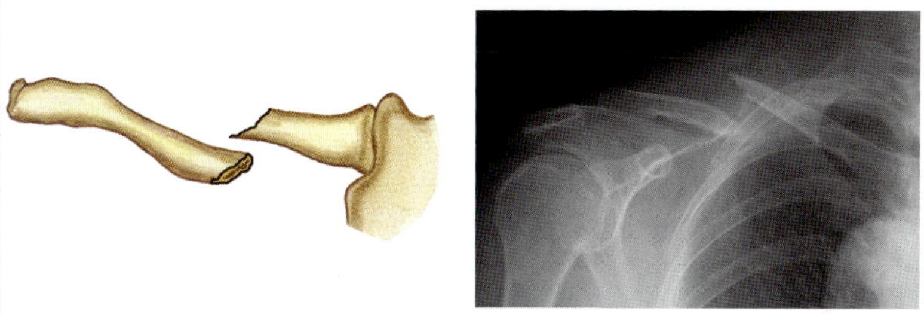 Displaced fractures

10

Robinson classification of clavicle fractures	
Type 3 **Lateral fifth** 3,576 Fractures M: 2,338 (65.38%) F: 1,238 (34.62%) 25.26% of adult clavicle fractures 0.96% of total adult fractures	**3A** 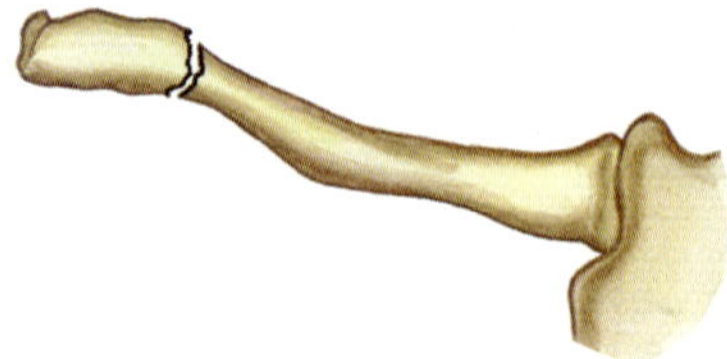 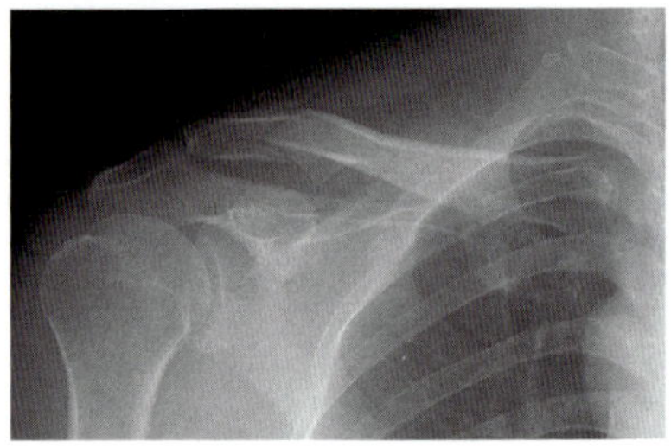 Cortical alignment fractures
	3B 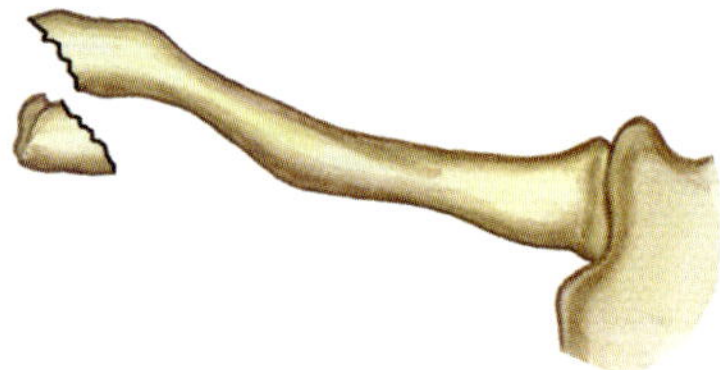 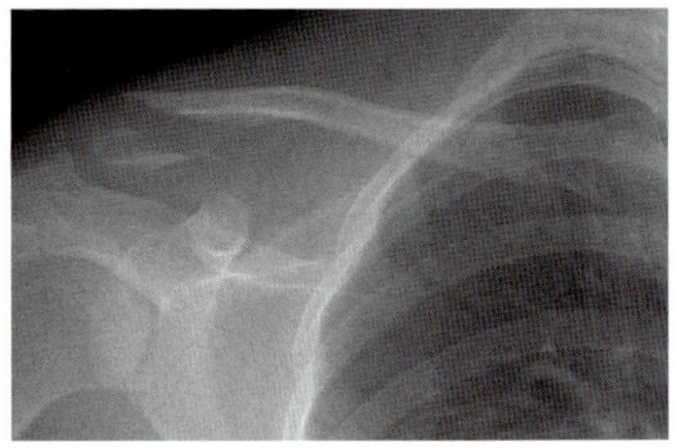 Displaced fractures

Scapular Fractures (Segment 14)

Scapular fractures are uncommon and usually result from major blunt trauma. These fractures not only affect shoulder motion but are also associated with other injuries.

Anatomical Features

The scapula forms the posterior part of the shoulder girdle, the anterior part of which is formed by the clavicle. Prominent areas of the scapula serve as attachment points for many muscles and ligaments, which each provide support and protection for the scapula. The supraspinatus muscle lies in the supraspinatus fossa. The infraspinatus fossa below the spine is mostly covered by the infraspinatus muscle. The anterior surface of the scapula facing the ribs has a broad concavity, the subscapular fossa; the medial two-thirds of this fossa is marked by an oblique ridge that serves as the attachment site of the subscapularis. There are a few projections from the border of the scapula-coracoid process, acromion, and the glenoid cavity; the coracobrachialis and short head of the biceps muscles originate from the coracoid, and the pectoralis minor inserts on the coracoid. Scapular fractures are more closely associated with fragment displacement and fracture deformity due to the pull of the three muscles attached to the coracoid.

The acromion first projects lateralward and then curves forward and upward, so as to overhang the glenoid cavity. The medial border of the acromion presents a small, oval surface for articulation with the acromial end of the clavicle. The supraspinatus and infraspinatus muscles both pass beneath the acromion and insert on the greater tubercle of the humerus. On the lateral angle of the scapula is a shallow articular surface, the glenoid fossa, which articulates with the head of the humerus. The margins of the cavity surface, which give attachment to a fibrocartilaginous structure and the glenoid labrum, are slightly raised, thereby deepening the cavity. The tendon of the long head of the biceps brachii attaches to the scapula at the supraglenoid tubercle, while the long head of the triceps brachii muscle arises from the infraglenoid tubercle of the scapula. While passing through the spinoglenoid notch to supply the infraspinatus, the suprascapular nerve and vessels are susceptible to traction injuries, which occur from fracture displacement of the glenoid cavity or shoulder joint manipulation from the posterior approach (**Plate 10.14**).

OTA Classification and Coding System for Scapular Fractures

Based on OTA classification, the scapula is coded as the number 14 for its anatomical location. Scapular fractures are classified into three types: 14-A, extra-articular; 14-B, partial articular; and 14-C, complete articular (**Plate 10.15**).

Epidemiologic Features of Scapular Fractures (Segment 14)

A total of 3,107 patients with 3,123 scapular fractures were treated in 83 hospitals in China over a 2-year period from 2010 to 2011. All cases were reviewed and statistically studied, the fractures accounted for 0.75% of all patients with fractures, and 0.72% of all kinds of fractures, respectively; among 3,107 patients, there were 150 pediatric patients (151 scapular fractures) and 2,957 adult patients with 2,972 scapular fractures.

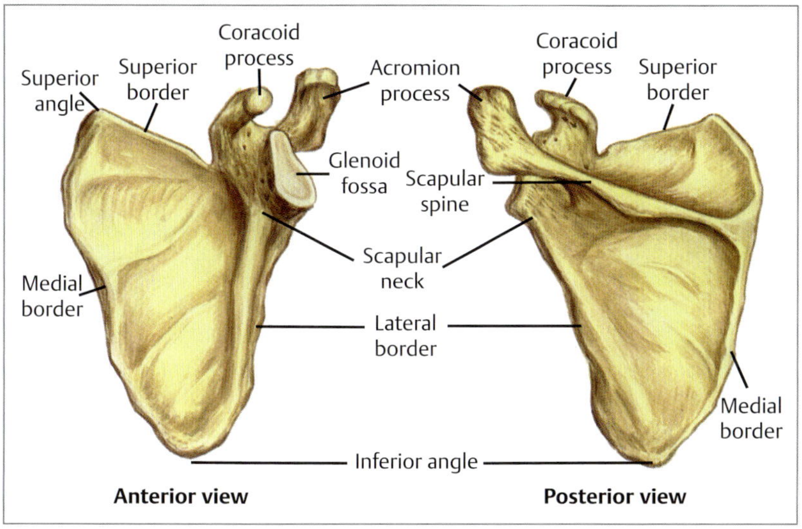

Plate 10.14

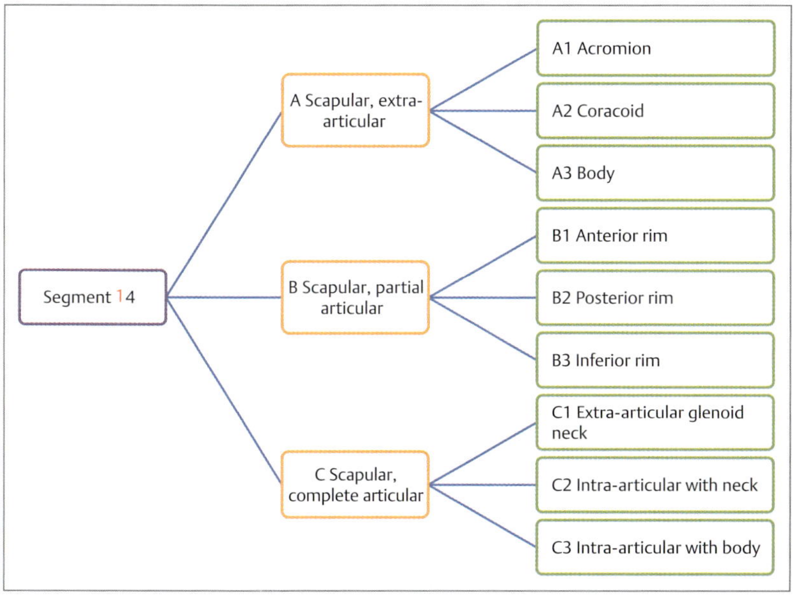

Plate 10.15

Epidemiologic features of scapular fractures are follows:

- More males than females
- More left side than right side injuries
- The high-risk age group is 41–45 years, the same age group for males while for females, the high-risk age group is 46–50 years.
- The most common fracture type is type 14-A, the same fracture type for both males and females.
- The most common fracture group is group 14-A3, the same fracture group for both males and females.

Scapular Fractures by Sex

Table 10.14 Sex distribution of 3,107 patients with scapular fractures

Sex	Number of patients	Percentage (%)
Male	2,349	75.60
Female	758	24.40
Total	3,107	100.00

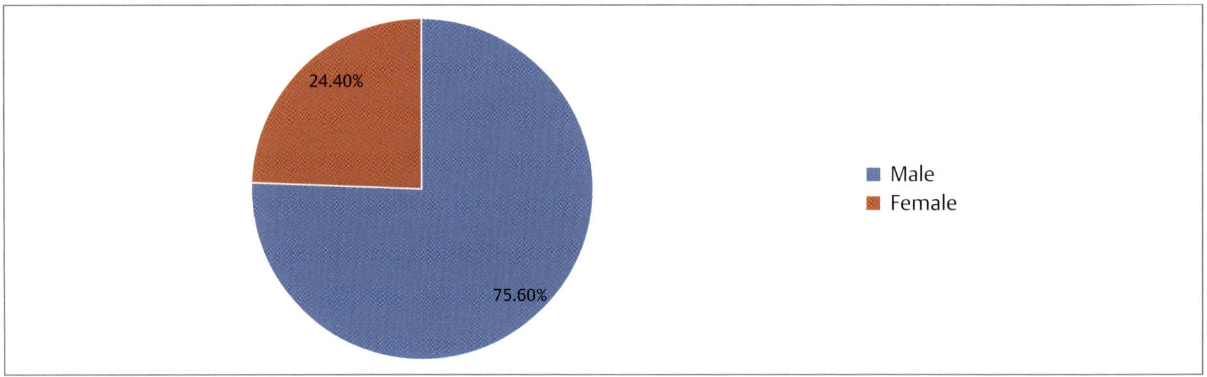

Fig. 10.14 Sex distribution of 3,107 patients with scapular fractures.

Scapular Fractures by Fracture Side

Table 10.15 Fracture side distribution of 3,107 patients with scapular fractures

Fracture side	Number of patients	Percentage (%)
Left	1,601	51.53
Right	1,490	47.96
Bilateral	16	0.51
Total	3,107	100.00

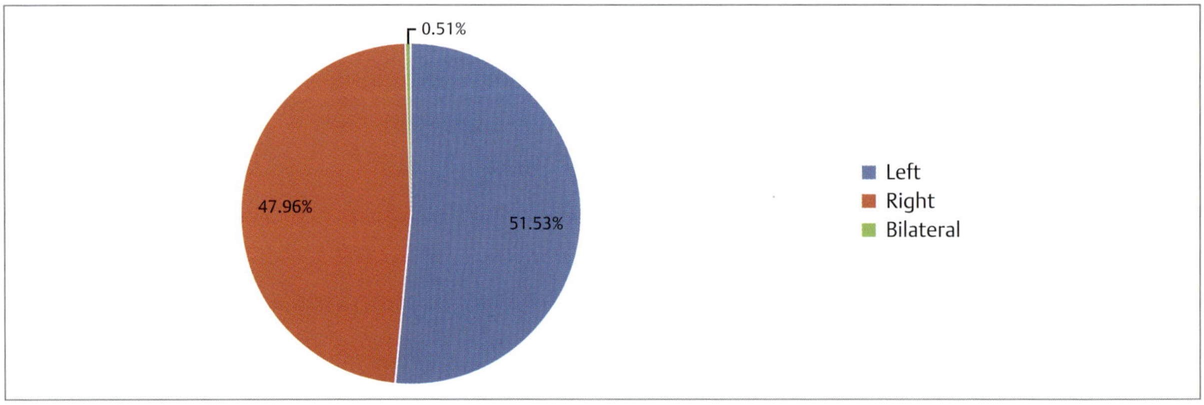

Fig. 10.15 Fracture side distribution of 3,107 patients with scapular fractures.

Scapular Fractures by Age Group

Table 10.16 Age and sex distribution of 3,107 patients with scapular fractures

Age group (years)	Male	Female	Number of patients	Percentage (%)
0–5	13	9	22	0.71
6–10	20	9	29	0.93
11–15	72	27	99	3.19
16–20	137	21	158	5.09
21–25	165	30	195	6.28
26–30	208	29	237	7.63
31–35	221	51	272	8.75
36–40	246	85	331	10.65
41–45	358	83	441	14.19
46–50	264	86	350	11.26
51–55	192	67	259	8.34
56–60	202	80	282	9.08
61–65	98	51	149	4.80
66–70	75	50	125	4.02
71–75	33	38	71	2.29
76–80	26	24	50	1.61
81–85	9	11	20	0.64
≥86	10	7	17	0.55
Total	2,349	758	3,107	100.00

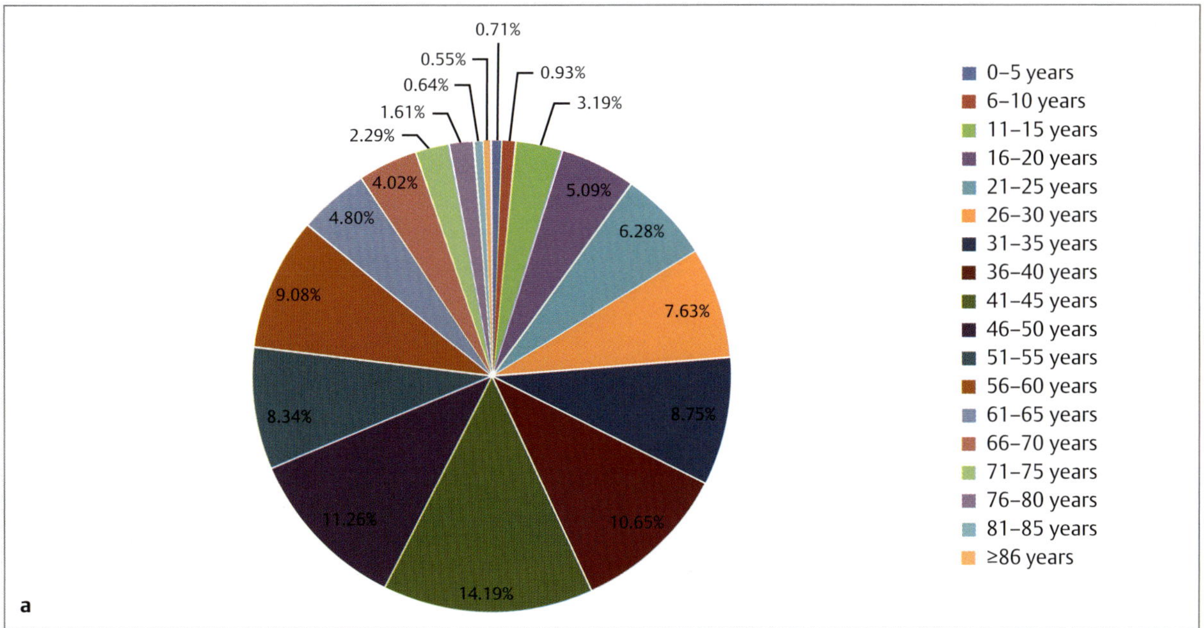

Fig. 10.16 **(a)** Age distribution of 3,107 patients with scapular fractures. (*Continued*)

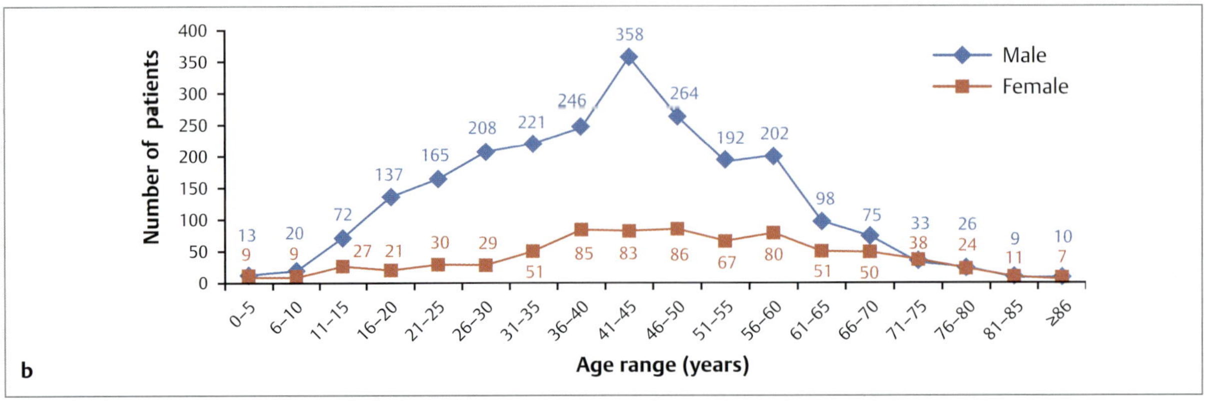

Fig. 10.16 (*continued*) **(b)** Age and sex distribution of 3,107 patients with scapular fractures.

Adult Scapular Fractures by Fracture Type

Table 10.17 Fracture type distribution of 2,972 adult scapular fractures

Fracture type	Male	Female	Number of fractures	Percentage (%)
14-A	1,425	409	1,834	61.71
14-B	257	117	374	12.58
14-C	575	189	764	25.71
Total	2,257	715	2,972	100.00

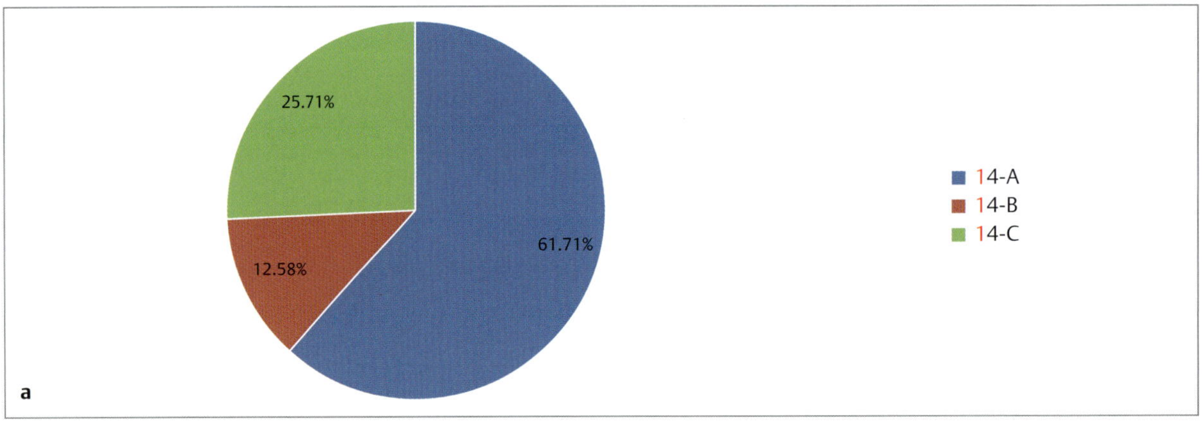

Fig. 10.17 **(a)** Fracture type distribution of 2,972 scapular fractures.

10

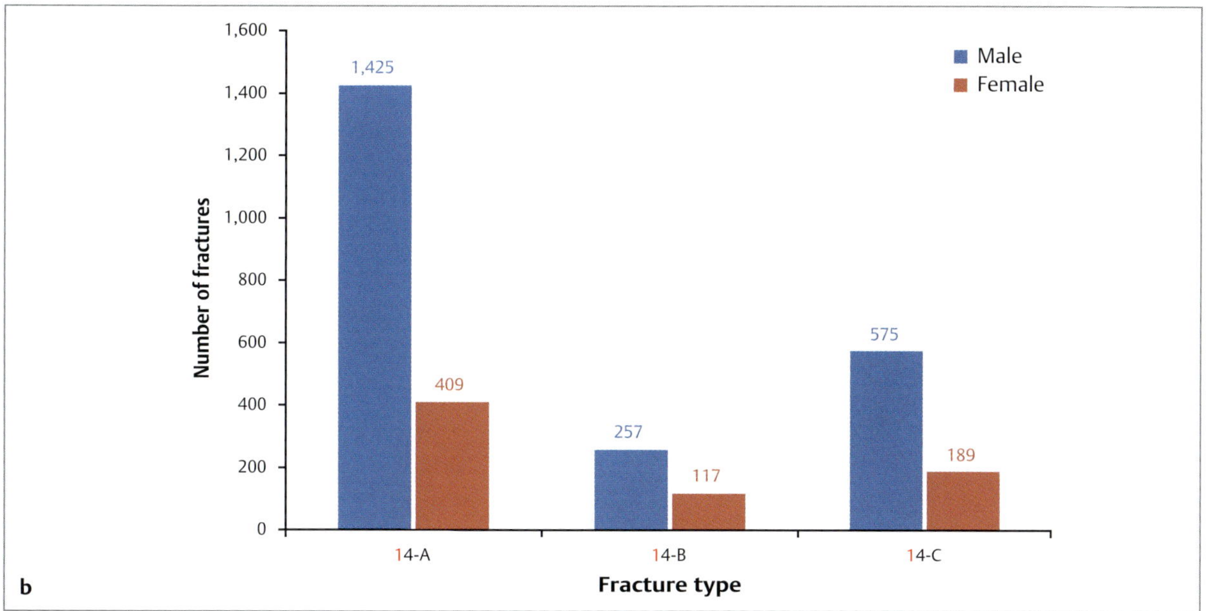

Fig. 10.17 (*continued*) **(b)** Sex and fracture type distribution of 2,972 scapular fractures.

Table 10.18 Sex and fracture group distribution of 2,972 scapular fractures

Fracture group	Male	Female	Number of patients	Percentage (%)
14-A1	412	127	539	18.14
14-A2	128	49	177	5.96
14-A3	885	233	1,118	37.62
14-B1	36	24	60	2.02
14-B2	40	27	67	2.25
14-B3	181	66	247	8.31
14-C1	362	125	487	16.39
14-C2	68	18	86	2.89
14-C3	145	46	191	6.43
Total	2,257	715	2,972	100.00

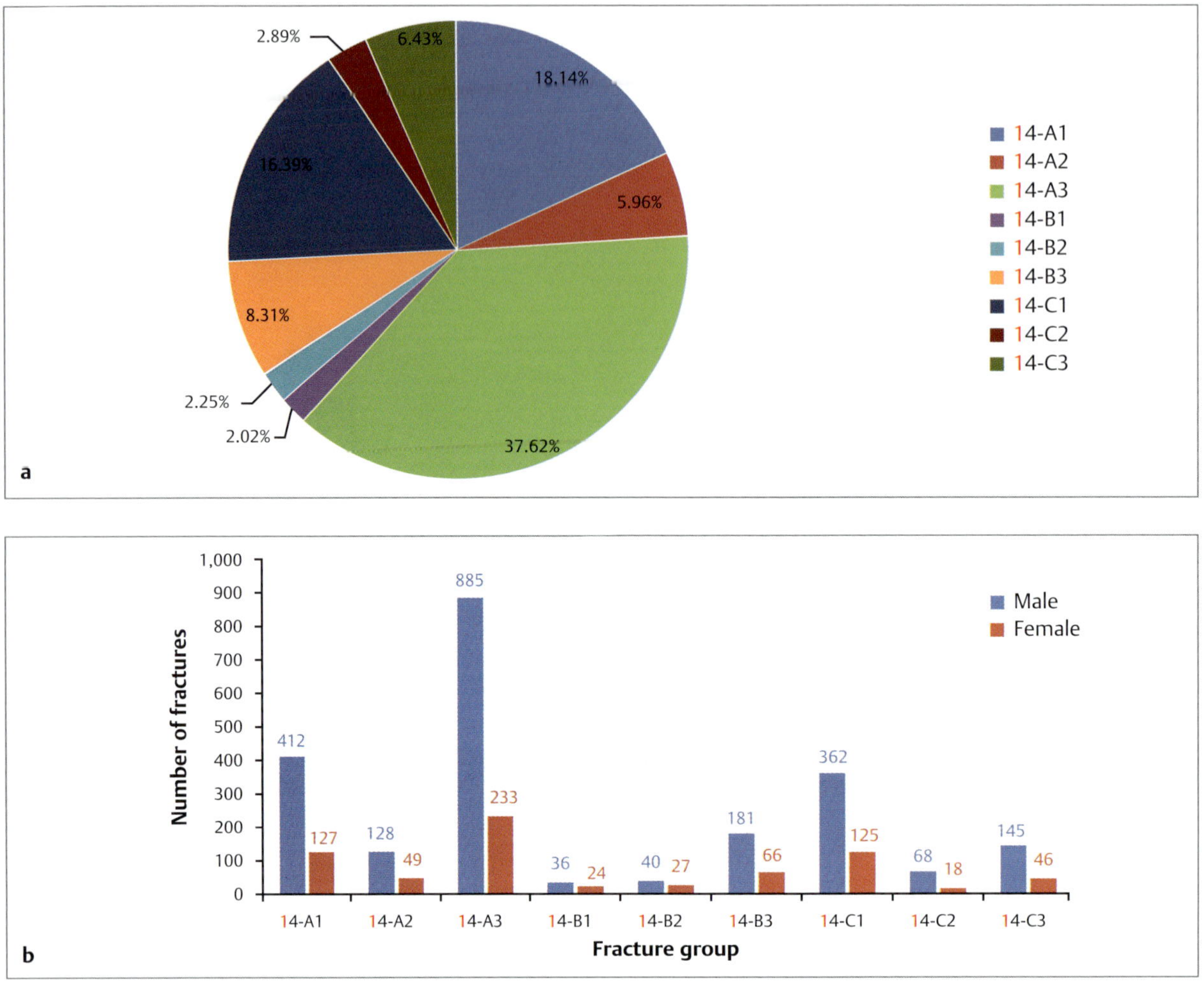

Fig. 10.18 **(a)** Fracture group distribution of 2,972 scapular fractures.
(b) Sex and fracture group distribution of 2,972 scapular fractures.

14-A Scapula, extra-articular fractures		
14-A1 Acromion 539 fractures M: 412 (76.44%) F: 127 (23.56%) 0.14% of total adult fractures 18.14% of adult scapula fractures 29.39% of type 14-A	**14-A1.1** 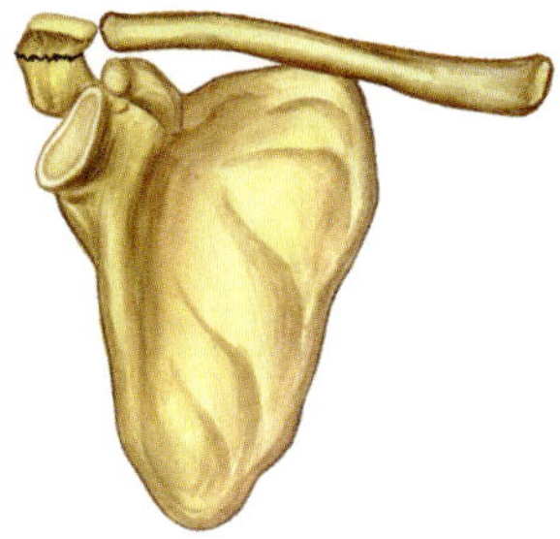 Simple	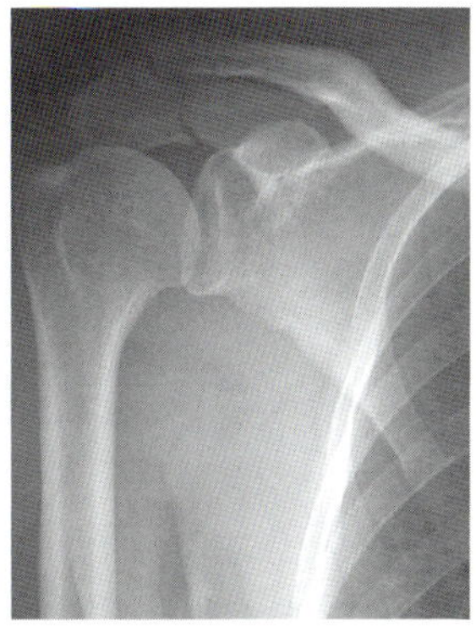
	14-A1.2 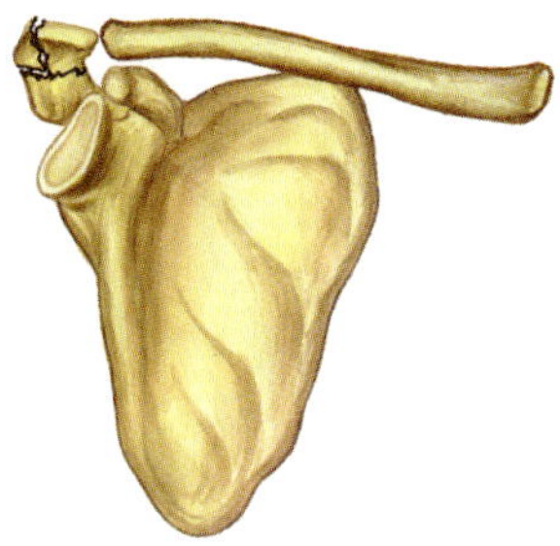 Comminuted	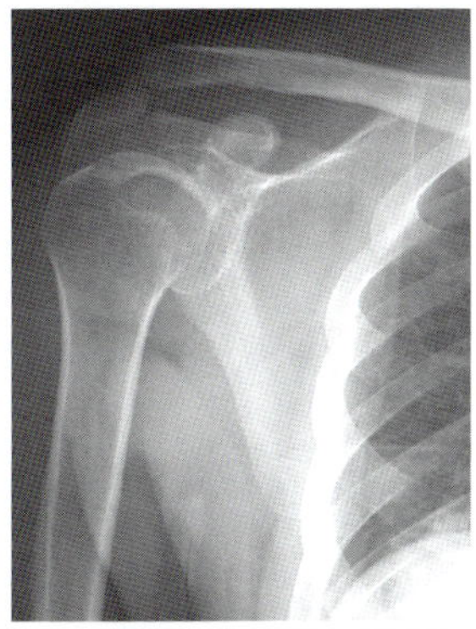
14-A2 **Coracoid** 177 fractures M: 128 (72.32%) F: 49 (27.68%) 0.05% of total adult fractures 5.96% of adult scapula fractures 9.65% of type 14-A	**14-A2.1** 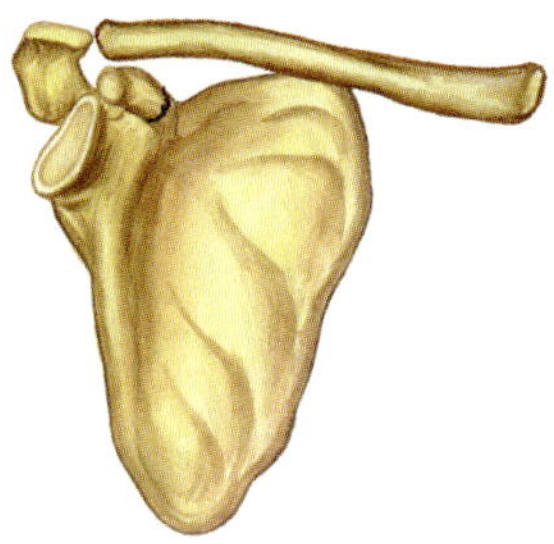 Simple	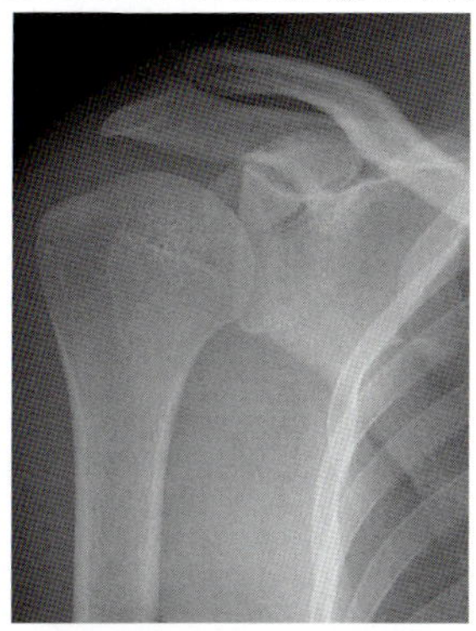
	14-A2.2 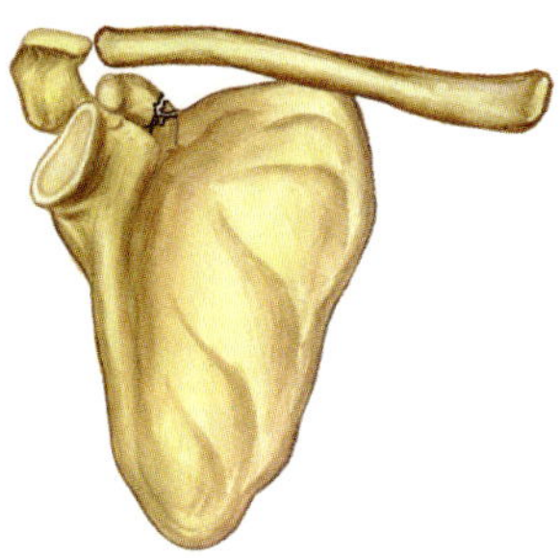 Comminuted	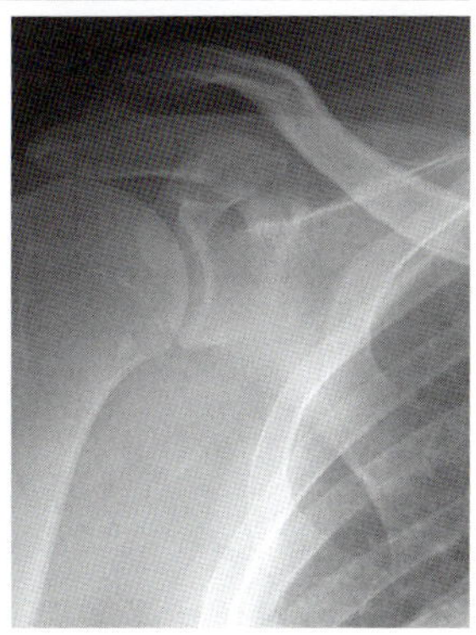

14-A Scapula, extra-articular fractures

14-A3 **Body** 1,118 fractures M: 885 (79.16%) F: 233 (20.84%) 0.3% of total adult fractures 37.62% of adult scapula fractures 60.96% of type 14-A	**14-A3.1**	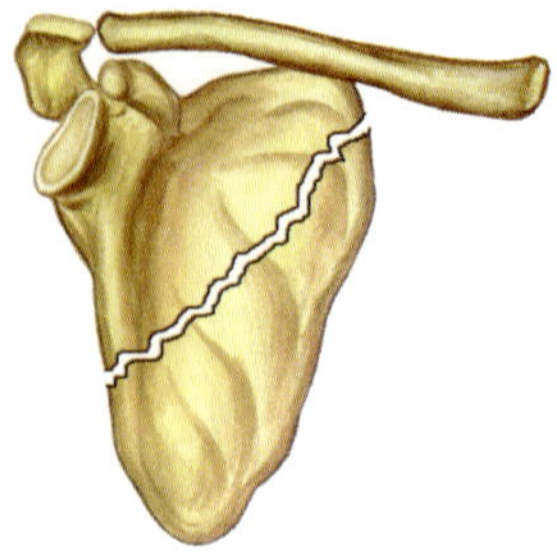 Simple	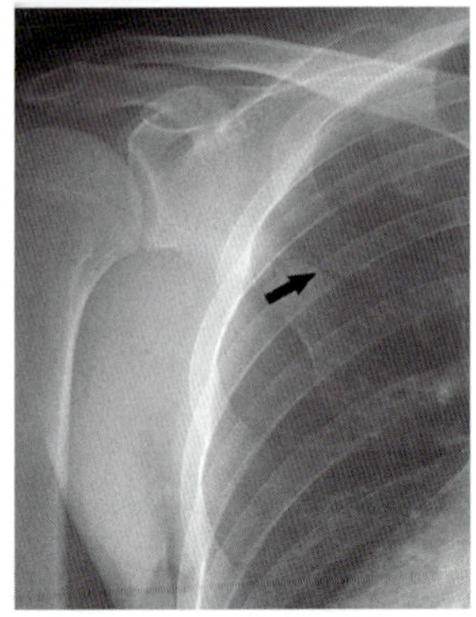
	14-A3.2	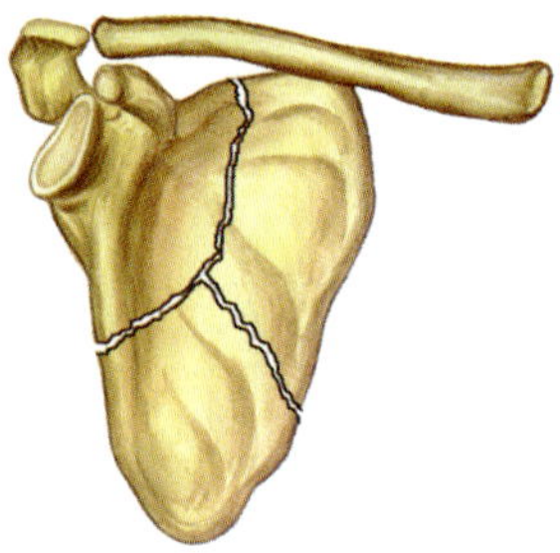 Comminuted	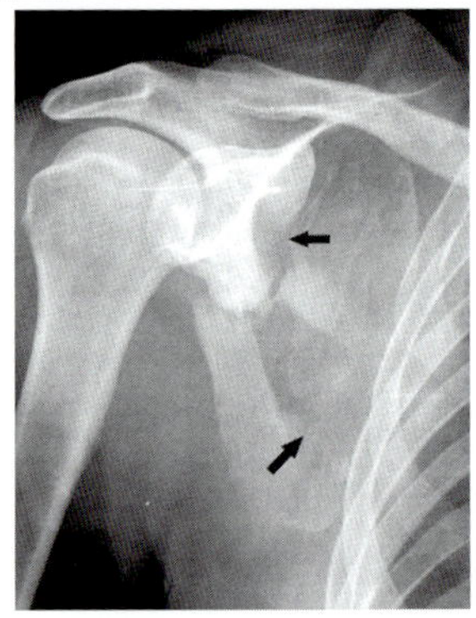
14-B1 **Anterior rim** 60 fractures M: 36 (60%) F: 24 (40%) 0.02% of total adult fractures 2.02% of adult scapula fractures 16.04% of type 14-B	**14-B1.1**	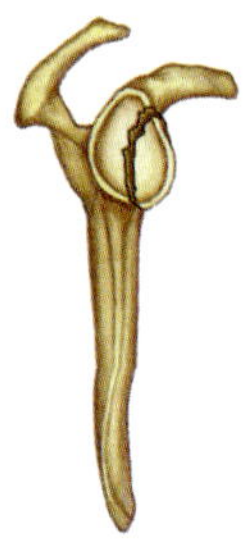 Simple	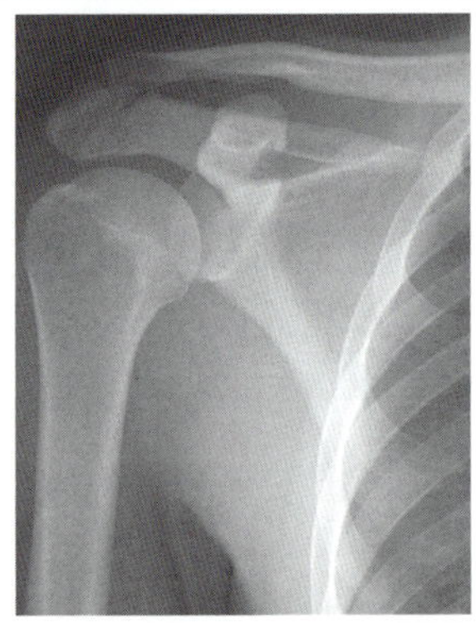
	14-B1.2	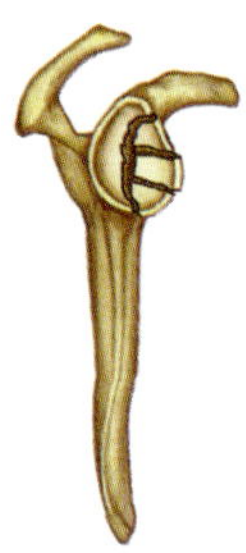 Comminuted	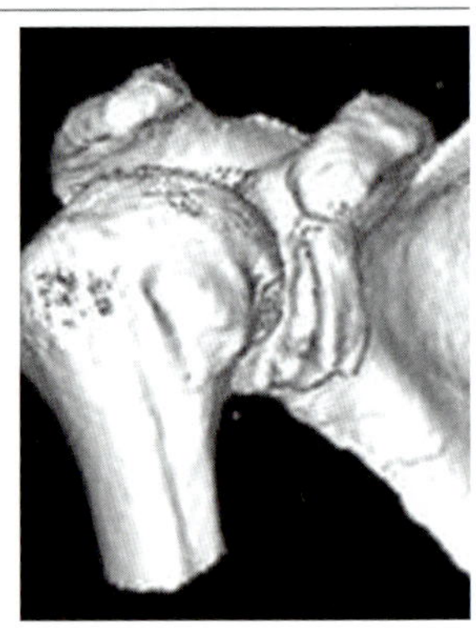

14-B Scapula, partial articular fractures

14-B2 **Posterior rim** 67 fractures M: 40 (59.7%) F: 27 (40.3%) 0.02% of total adult fractures 2.25% of adult scapula fractures 17.91% of type 14-B	**14-B2.1** 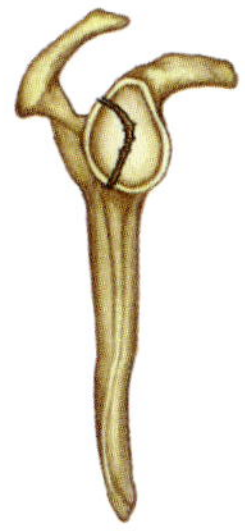 Simple	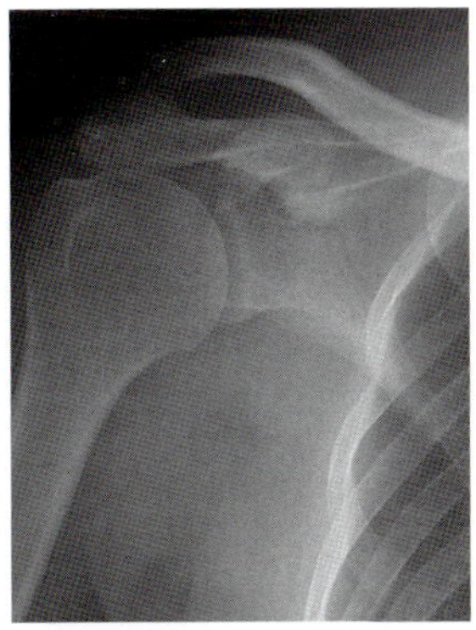
	14-B2.2 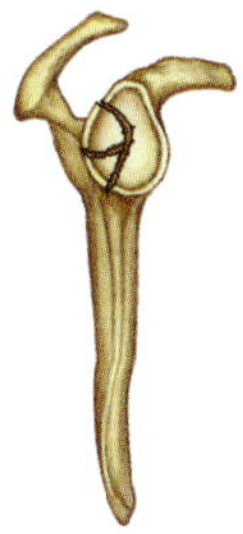 Comminuted	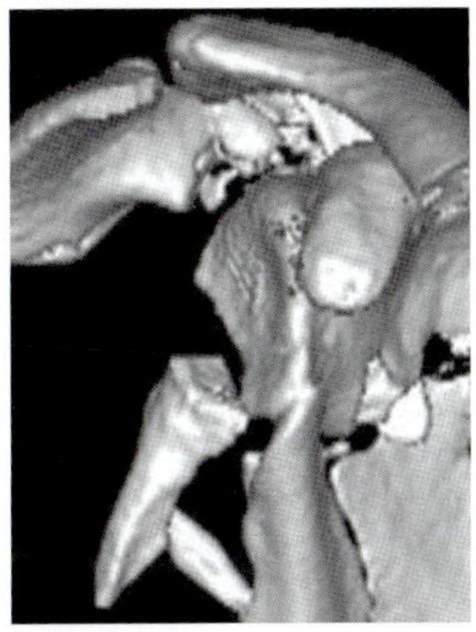
14-B3 **Inferior rim** 247 fractures M: 181 (73.28%) F: 66 (26.72%) 0.07% of total adult fractures 8.31% of adult scapula fractures 66.04% of type 14-B	**14-B3.1** 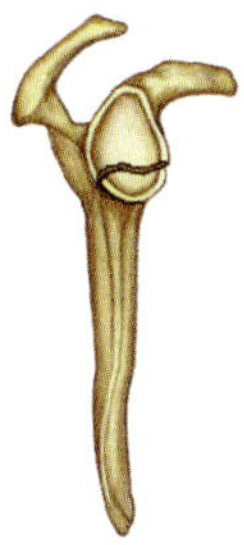 Simple	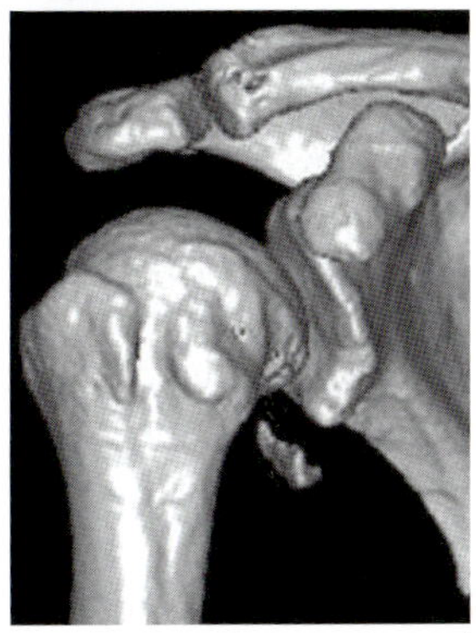
	14-B3.2 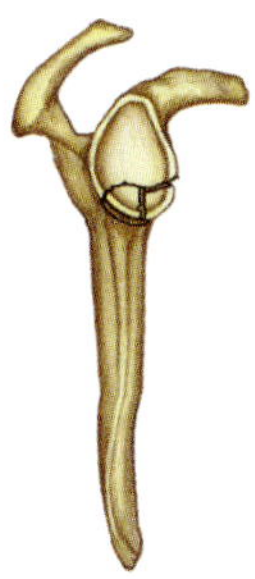 Comminuted	

14-C Scapula, complete articular fractures

14-C1
Extra-articular glenoid neck

487 fractures
M: 362 (74.33%)
F: 125 (25.67%)
0.13% of total adult fractures
16.39% of adult scapula fractures
63.74% of type 14-C

14-C1.1

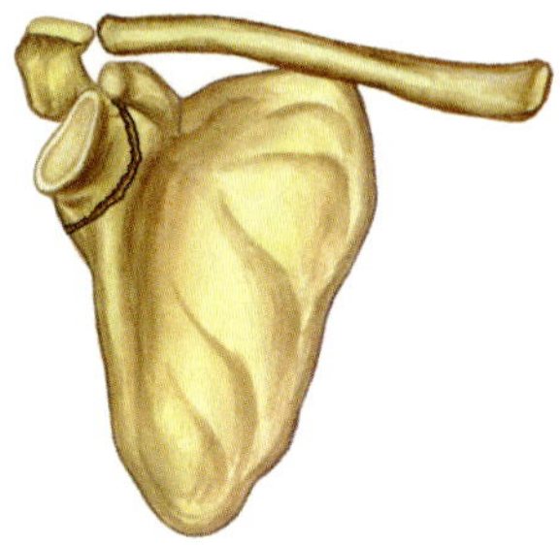

Simple

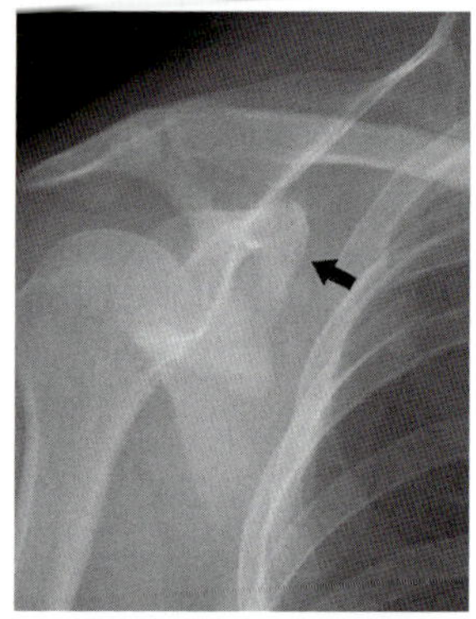

14-C1.2

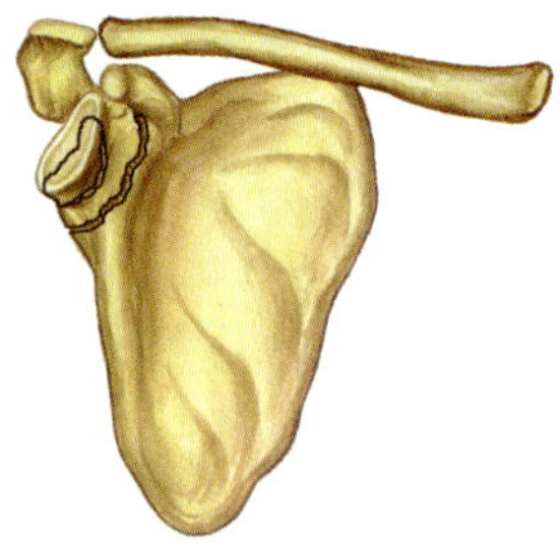

Comminuted

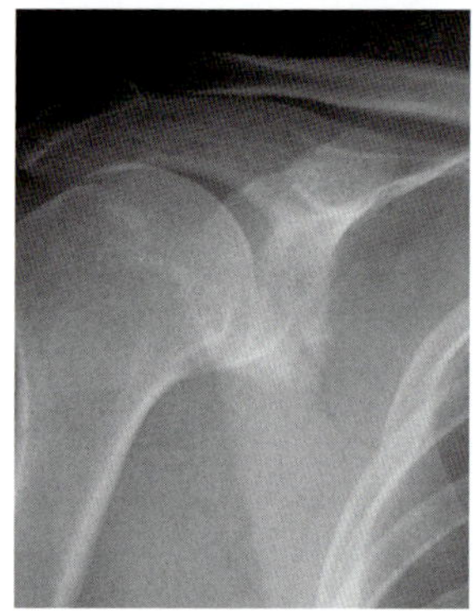

14-C Scapula, complete articular fractures

14-C2
Intra-articular with neck
86 fractures
M: 68 (79.07%)
F: 18 (20.93%)
0.02% of total adult fractures
2.89% of adult scapula fractures
11.26% of type 14-C

14-C2.1

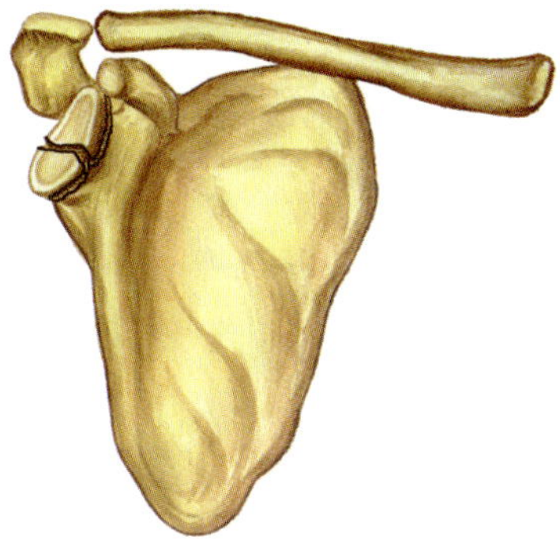

Intra-articular simple, neck simple

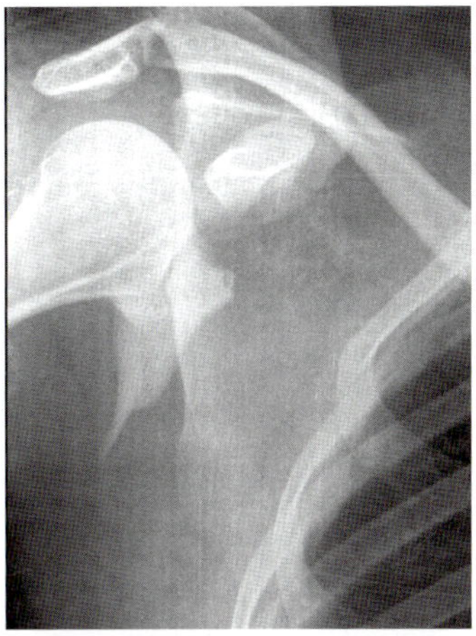

14-C2.2

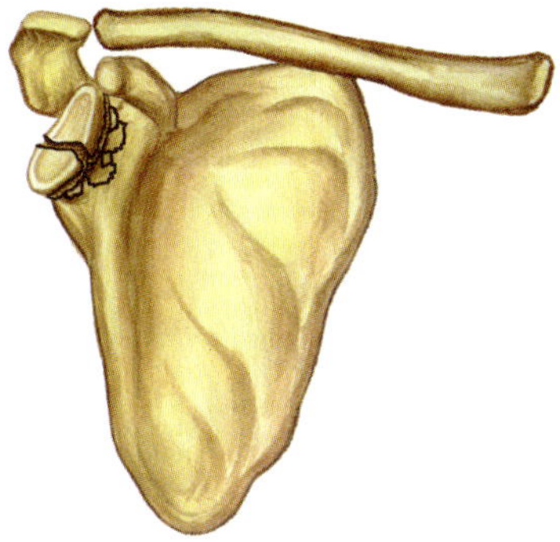

Intra-articular simple, neck comminuted

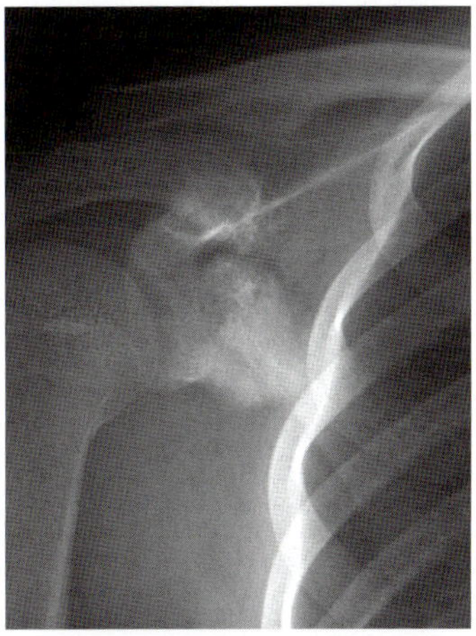

14-C2.3

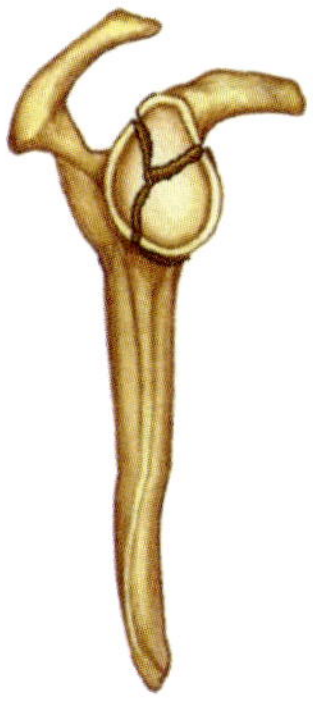

Articular comminuted

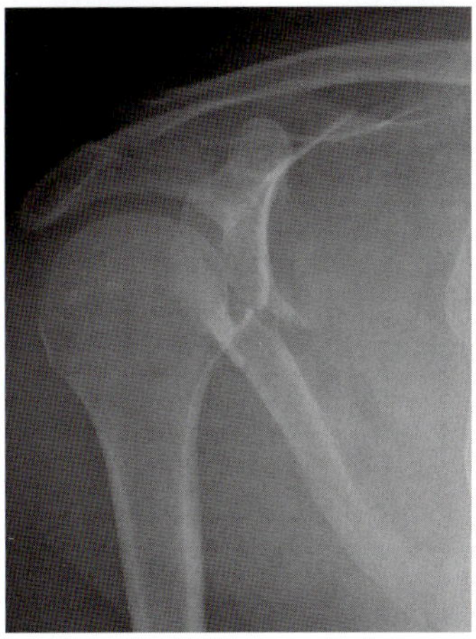

14-C Scapula, complete articular fractures

14-C3
Intra-articular with body
191 fractures
M: 145 (75.92%)
F: 46 (24.08%)
0.05% of total adult fractures
6.43% of adult scapula fractures
25% of type 14-B

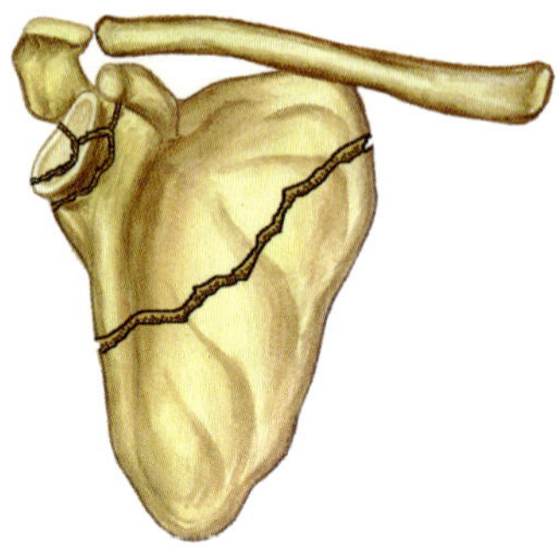

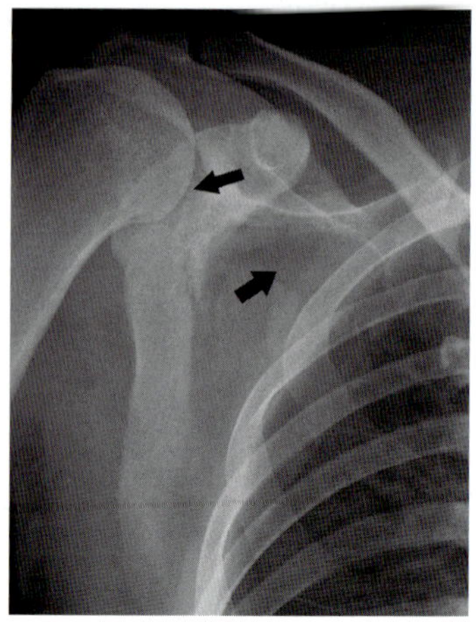

Injury Mechanism

Typically, scapula fractures result from high-energy trauma. Extensive muscle coverage serves as a cushion against any impact force and protects the scapula from low-energy trauma. Avulsion fractures of the coracoid and the superior angle of the scapula may be caused by tensile traction from the attached muscles.

Diagnosis

Patients with scapular fractures usually present with a clear trauma history. Physical examination reveals swelling, pain, tenderness, crepitus, and ecchymosis over the scapular region. The affected arm is usually adducted, and pain is aggravated by shoulder movement, especially lifting the arm up to the side.

Scapular fractures are easily misdiagnosed due to the presence of other obvious injuries. Studies report that the misdiagnosis rate of scapular fractures is as high as 43% when based on primary plain radiographic films alone. In practice, when patients complain of pain over the shoulder area after a traumatic event, particularly when there are concomitant fractures of multiple ribs or a pneumohemothorax, the scapula should be inspected for possible injury. An AP view of the shoulder or a chest radiograph is usually adequate to detect scapular fractures. For further classification, one should obtain lateral and axillary views of the shoulder/scapula. If an intra-articular injury is suspected, a CT scan or 3D CT will allow for better detection of fractures. If soft tissue injuries of the shoulder are clinically suspected, MRI is indicated.

Treatment

Scapular fractures are usually accompanied by multiple injuries from high-energy trauma. Medical treatment should aim to care for life-threatening injuries and stabilize the cardiopulmonary system prior to operative fixation of scapular fractures. Scapular fractures with minimal or no displacement should be treated nonsurgically. Treatment is for symptomatic purposes. Short-term immobilization in a sling and swathe bandage is provided for comfort. Early shoulder motion exercise in moderation should be initiated as pain subsides. Open reduction and internal fixation should be performed for fractures with marked displacement or with compromised shoulder motion to restore shoulder function and prevent the development of traumatic arthritis.

For displaced glenoid neck fractures, closed reduction is utilized followed by immobilization with an abduction splint or traction when the patient is in bed. The affected arm should be externally rotated to maintain the anatomical reduction. If closed reduction or traction fails, operative treatment should be considered.

For glenoid rim fractures, if the intra-articular step-off is greater than 5–8 mm, or if the triceps is torn and needs repair, operative reduction and internal fixation is required. Restoration of the articulation congruence is essential to prevent development of posttraumatic arthritis by cleaning up bone debris left on the articular surface.

Further Classifications of Scapular Fractures

Coracoid Process Fractures

In 1995, Eyres and colleagues proposed a classification scheme for coracoid process fractures that divided into five types according to the degree of extension of the fracture into the base of the coracoid. Types I, II, and III, which are often caused by avulsion injuries, do not involve the body of the scapula. Type IV fractures involve the body of the scapula while type V involves the glenoid fossa; both types of fractures are typically caused by shearing injuries.
In addition, Ogawa et al (1997) classified coracoid fractures into two types (**Plate 10.16**):

- *Type I:* basal fractures of the coracoid and fractures behind the attachment of the coracoclavicular ligament with disturbance of the scapuloclavicular connection.
- *Type II:* avulsion fractures of the coracoid and fractures anterior to the attachment of the coracoclavicular ligament with no disturbance of the scapuloclavicular connection.

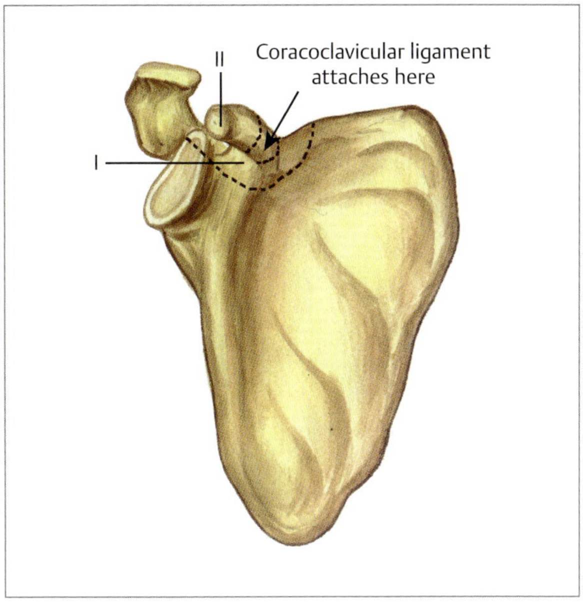

Plate 10.16

Clinical Epidemiologic Features of Coracoid Process Fractures

A total of 183 coracoid fractures were treated in 83 hospitals in China over a 2-year period from 2010 to 2011, the fractures accounted for 5.86% of scapular fractures. Their epidemiologic features are as follows:

- More males than females
- The high-risk age group is 46–50 years.

Coracoid Fractures by Sex

Table 10.19 Sex distribution of 183 coracoid fractures

Sex	Number of fractures	Percentage (%)
Male	128	69.95
Female	55	30.05
Total	183	100.00

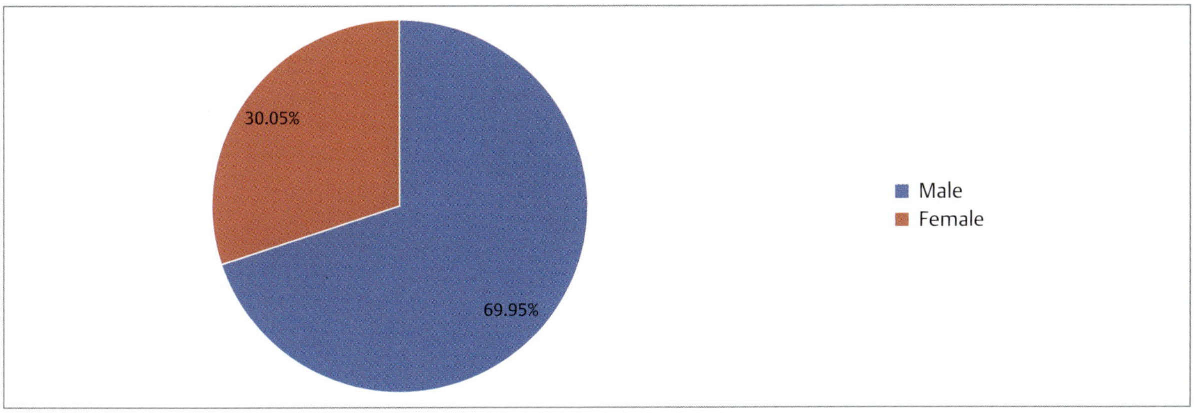

Fig. 10.19 Sex distribution of 183 coracoid fractures.

Coracoid Fractures by Age Group

Table 10.20 Age and sex distribution of 183 coracoid fractures

Age group (years)	Male	Female	Number of fractures	Percentage (%)
0–5	0	1	1	0.55
6–10	3	2	5	2.73
11–15	4	3	7	3.83
16–20	7	6	13	7.10
21–25	15	3	18	9.84
26–30	12	0	12	6.56
31–35	14	4	18	9.84
36–40	9	6	15	8.20
41–45	14	4	18	9.84
46–50	14	7	21	11.48
51–55	13	2	15	8.20
56–60	11	8	19	10.38
61–65	0	2	2	1.09
66–70	4	2	6	3.28
71–75	2	2	4	2.19
76–80	4	1	5	2.73
81–85	1	2	3	1.64
≥86	1	0	1	0.55
Total	128	55	183	100.00

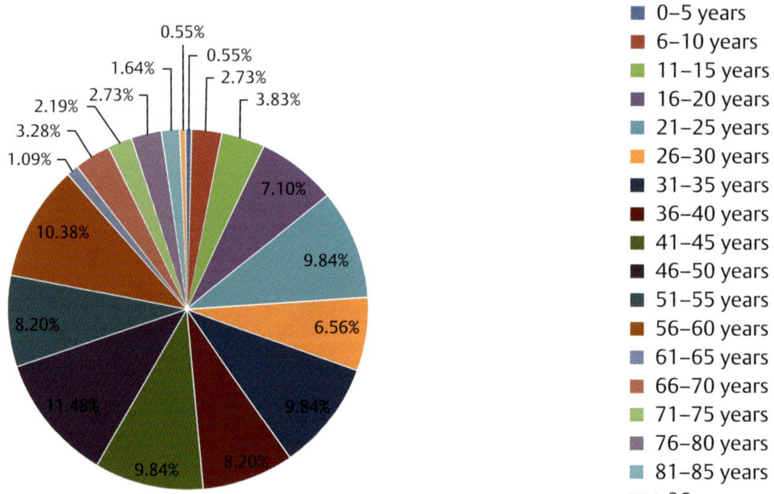

Fig. 10.20 **(a)** Age distribution of 183 coracoid fractures.

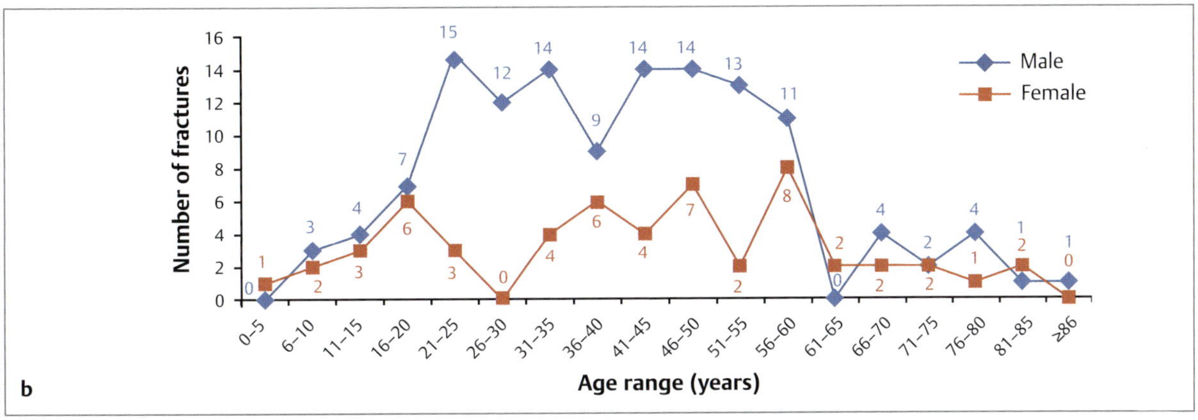

Fig. 10.20 (*continued*) **(b)** Age and sex distribution of 183 coracoid fractures.

Coracoid Fractures by Fracture Type

Table 10.21 Sex and fracture type distribution of 183 coracoid fractures

Fracture type	Male	Female	Number of fractures	Percentage (%)
I	68	23	91	49.73
II	60	32	92	50.27
Total	128	55	183	100.00

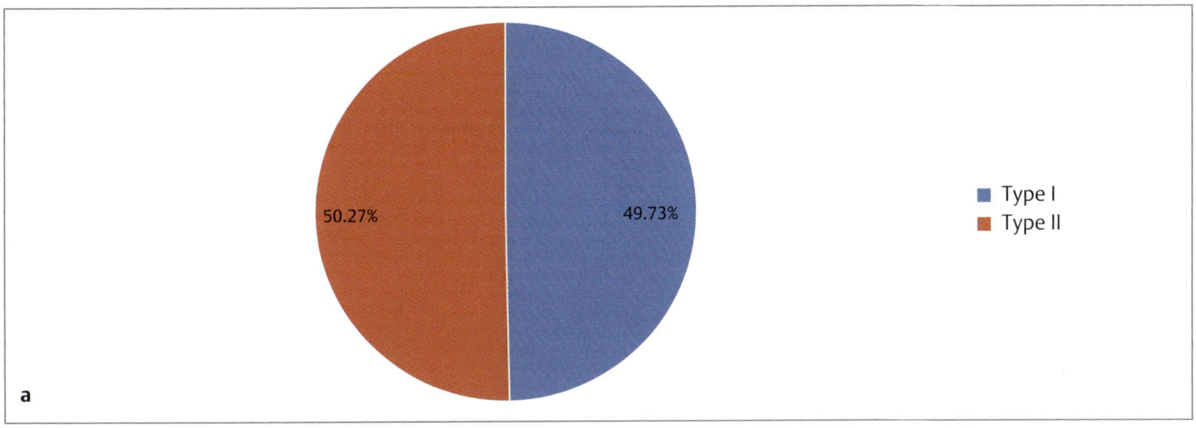

Fig. 10.21 **(a)** Fracture type distribution of 183 coracoid fractures. (*Continued*)

10

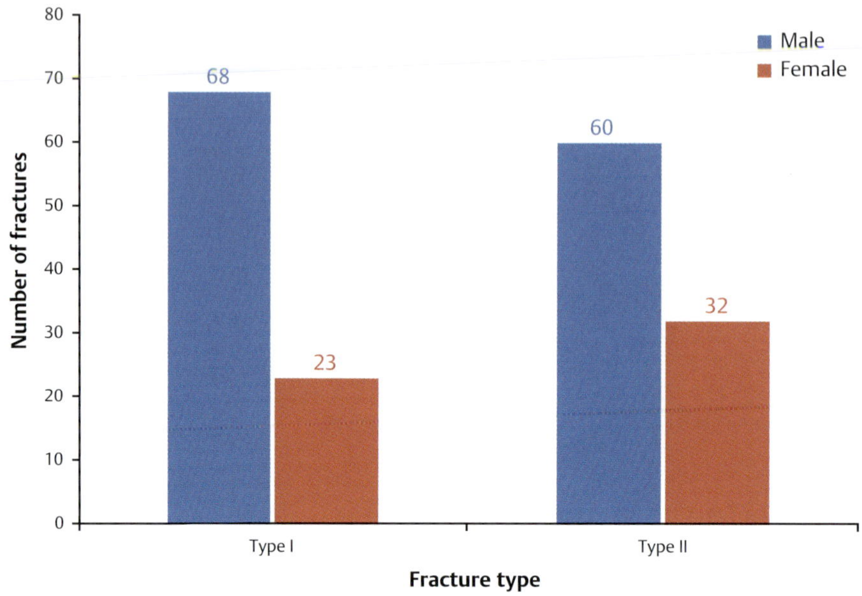

b

Fig. 10.21 (*continued*) **(b)** Sex and fracture type distribution of 183 coracoid fractures.

Coracoid process fractures types I–V		
Type I: Coracoid tip or epiphyseal fracture	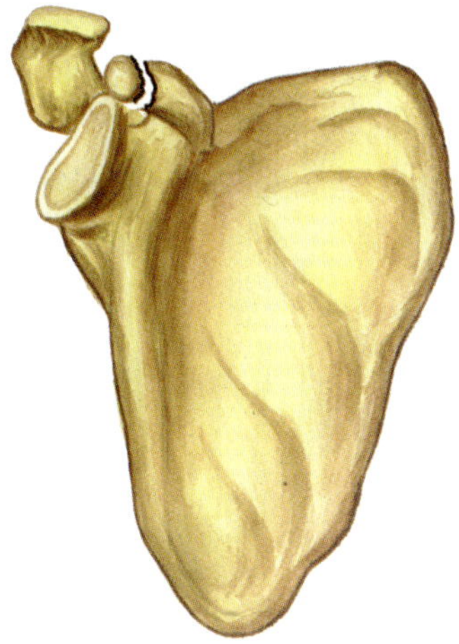	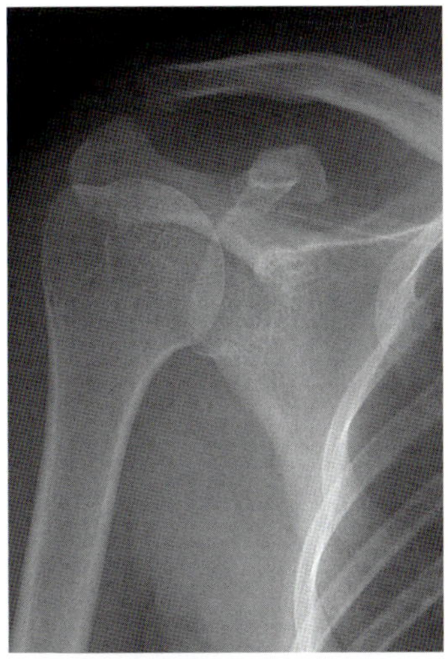
Type II: Mid process	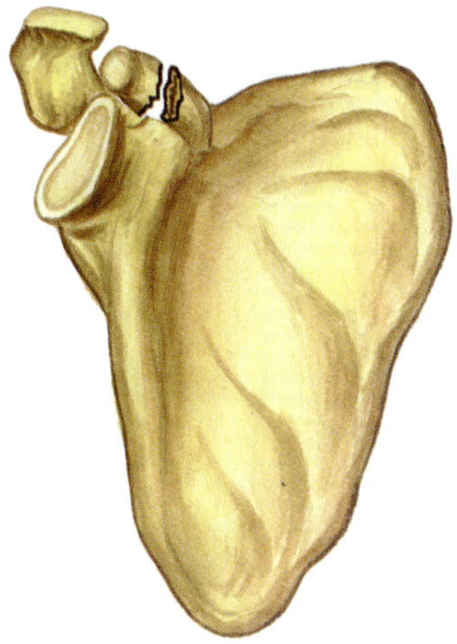	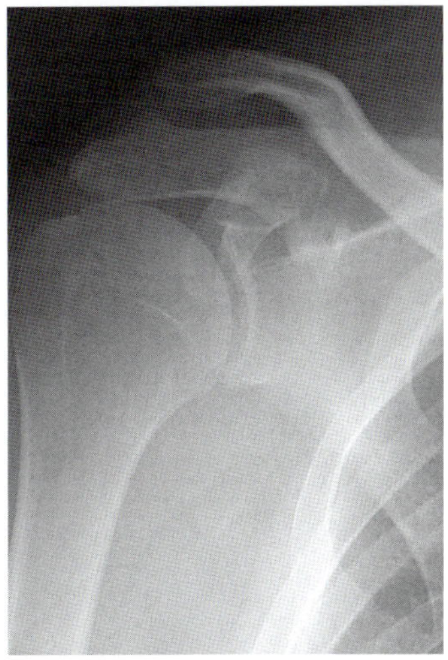
Type III: Basal fracture	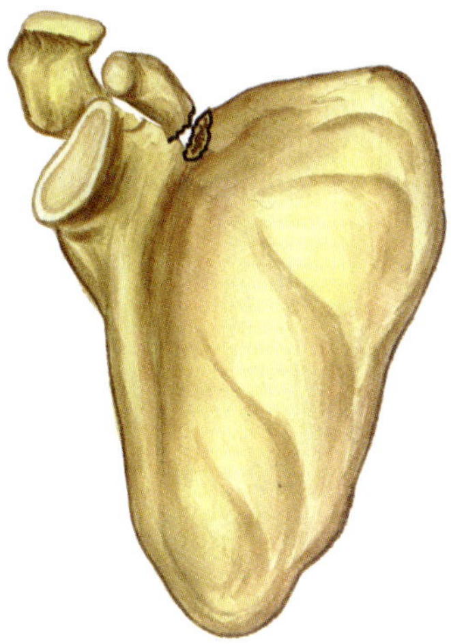	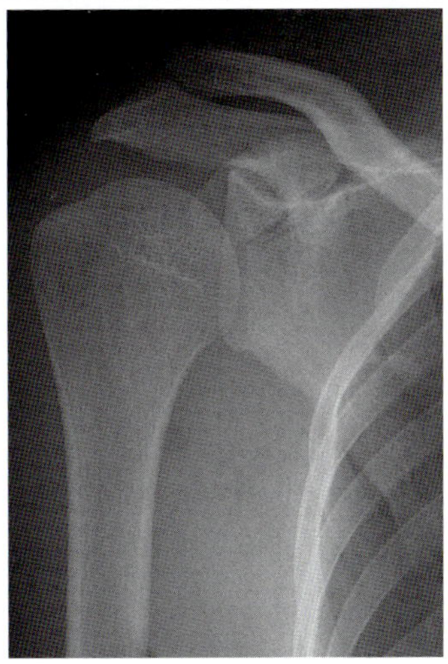

Coracoid process fractures types I–V	
Type IV: Involvement of the superior body of the scapula	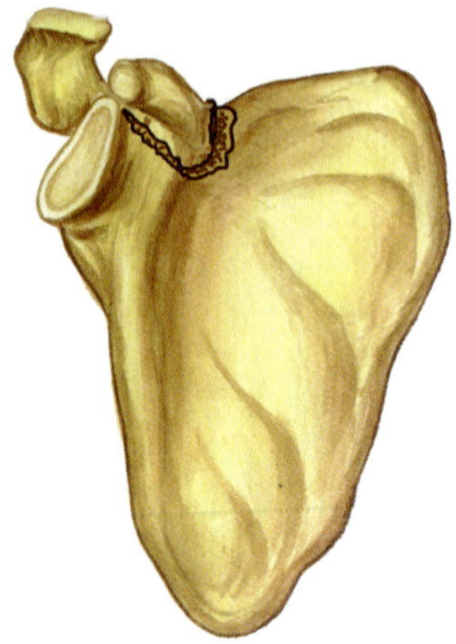 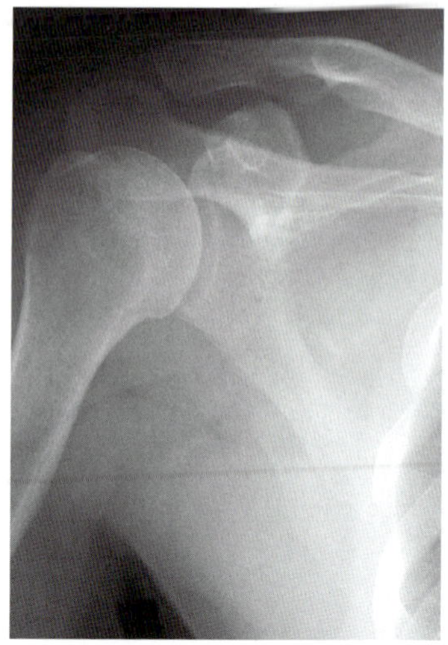
Type V: Extension into the glenoid fossa	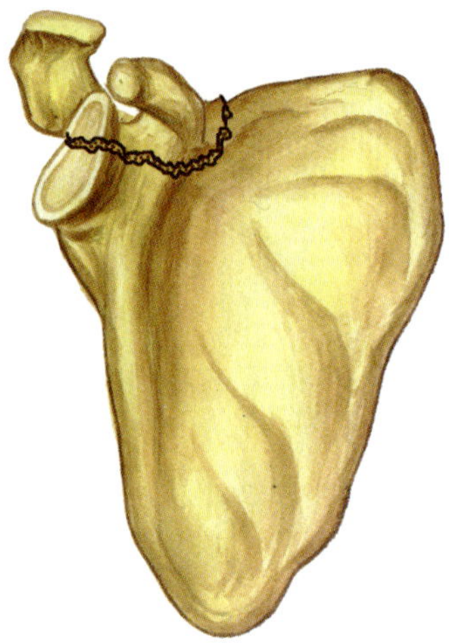 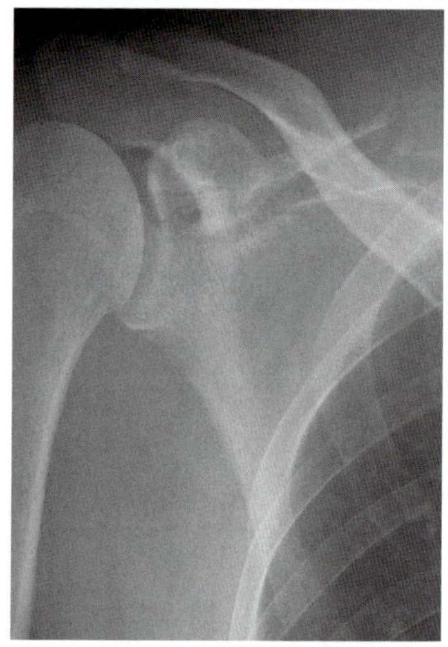 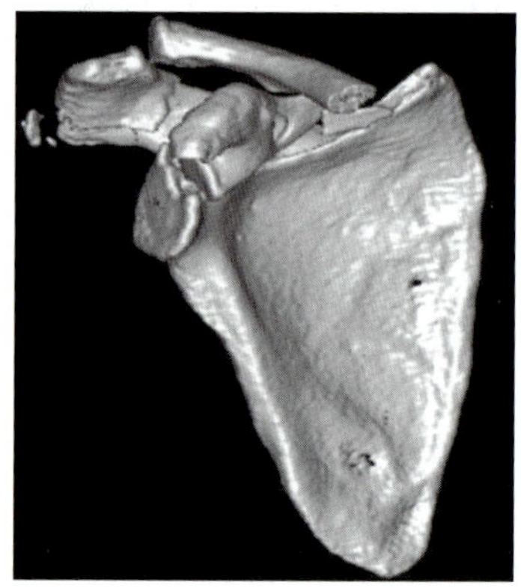

Ogawa classification of coracoid fractures	
Type I **Basal fracture** 91 fractures M: 68 (74.73%) F: 23 (25.27%) 49.73% of coracoid	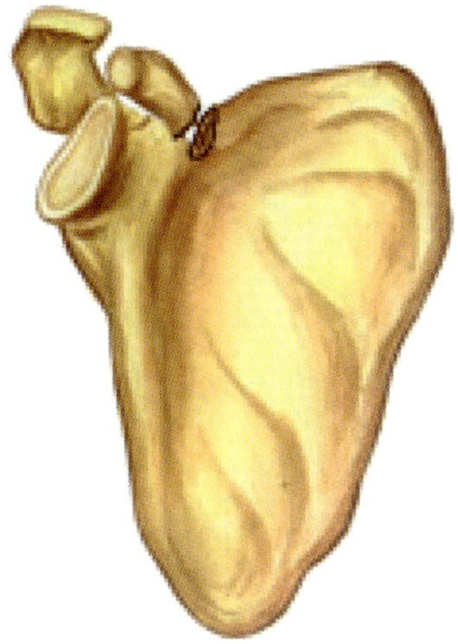 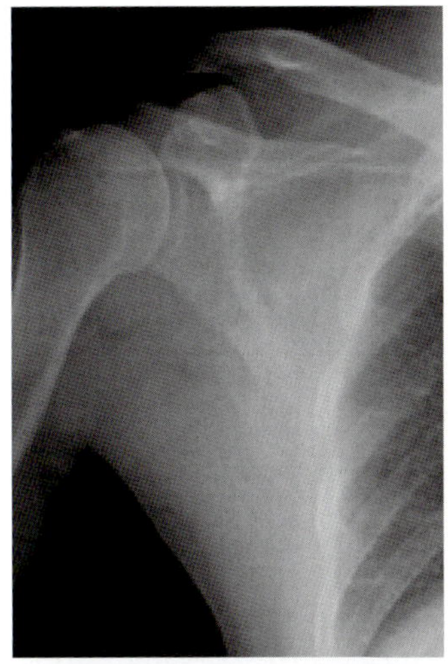
Type II **Avulsion fracture** 92 fractures M: 60 (65.22%) F: 32 (34.78%) 50.27% of coracoid	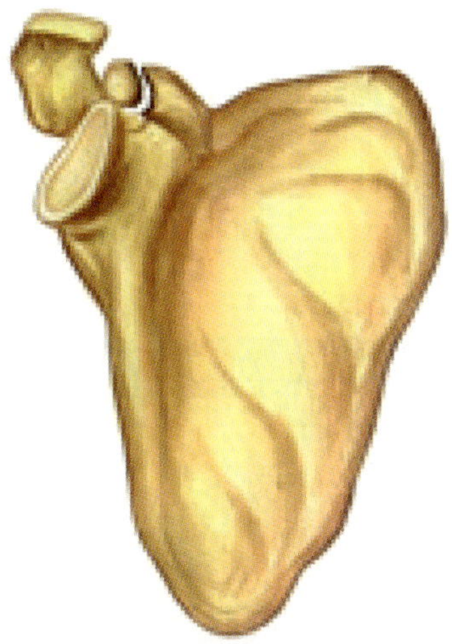 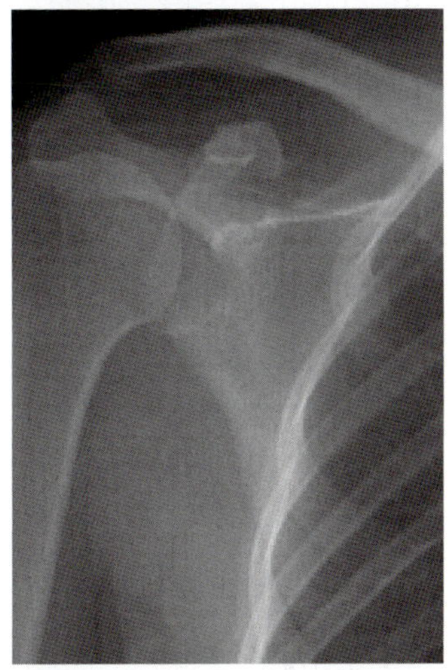 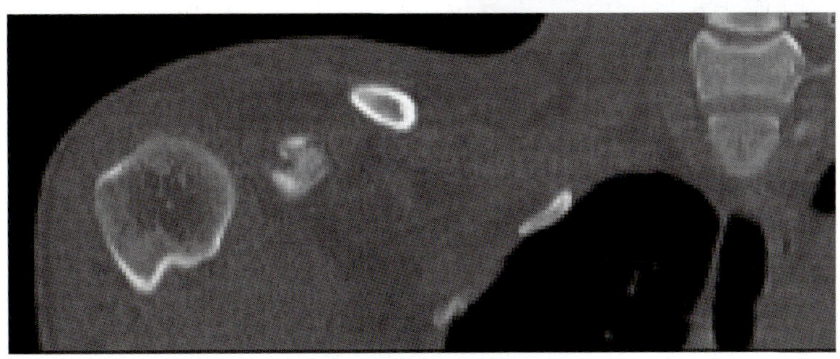

Acromion Fractures

Acromion fractures usually occur in two anatomical zones (**Plate 10.17**).

Fractures of zone I are classified into three types:

- *Type IA*: avulsion fractures
- *Type IB*: nondisplaced fractures
- *Type II*: displaced fractures with no reduction of the subacromial space
- *Type III*: displaced fractures, with reduction of the subacromial space

Fractures of zone II are basal fractures of the acromion.

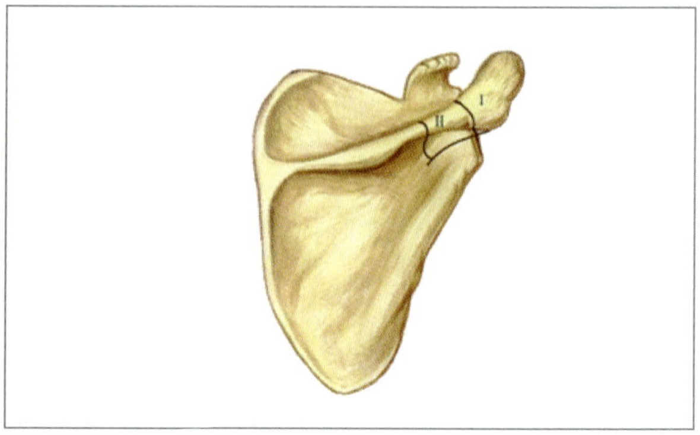

Plate 10.17

Clinical Epidemiologic Features of Acromion Fractures

A total of 592 acromion fractures were treated in 83 hospitals in China over a 2-year period from 2010 to 2011; the fractures accounted for 18.96% of scapular fractures. Their epidemiologic features are as follows:

- More males than females
- The high-risk age group is 16–20 years.
- Fractures occur mostly in zone I, with type IB as the most common fracture type.

Acromion Fractures by Sex

Table 10.22 Sex distribution of 592 acromion fractures

Sex	Number of fractures	Percentage (%)
Male	450	76.01
Female	142	23.99
Total	592	100.00

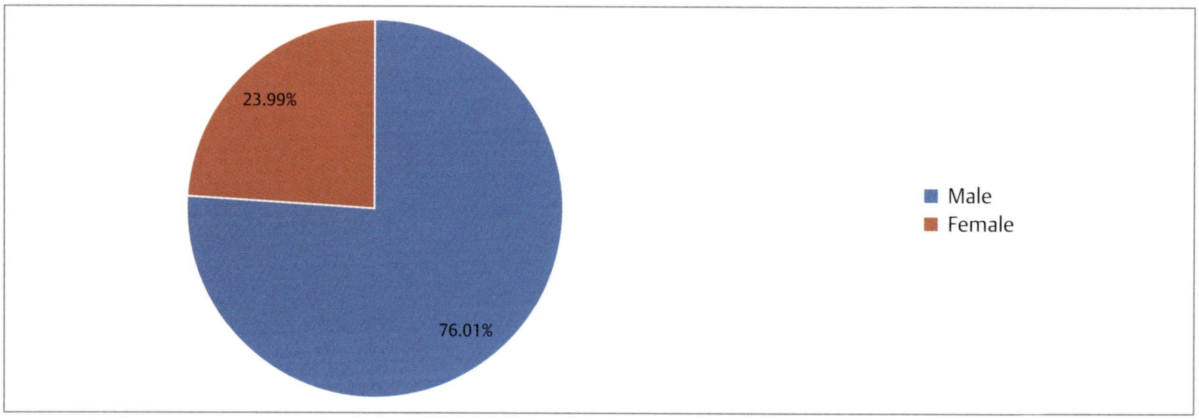

Fig. 10.22 Sex distribution of 592 acromion fractures.

Acromion Fractures by Age Group

Table 10.23 Age and sex distribution of 592 acromion fractures

Age group (years)	Male	Female	Number of fractures	Percentage (%)
0–5	0	2	2	0.34
6–10	5	1	6	1.01
11–15	28	10	38	6.42
16–20	70	4	74	12.50
21–25	42	10	52	8.78
26–30	31	3	34	5.74
31–35	49	6	55	9.29
36–40	43	12	55	9.29
41–45	51	21	72	12.16
46–50	37	18	55	9.29
51–55	30	8	38	6.42
56–60	28	13	41	6.93
61–65	15	7	22	3.72
66–70	9	6	15	2.53
71–75	5	10	15	2.53
76–80	4	6	10	1.69
81–85	2	2	4	0.68
≥86	1	3	4	0.68
Total	450	142	592	100.00

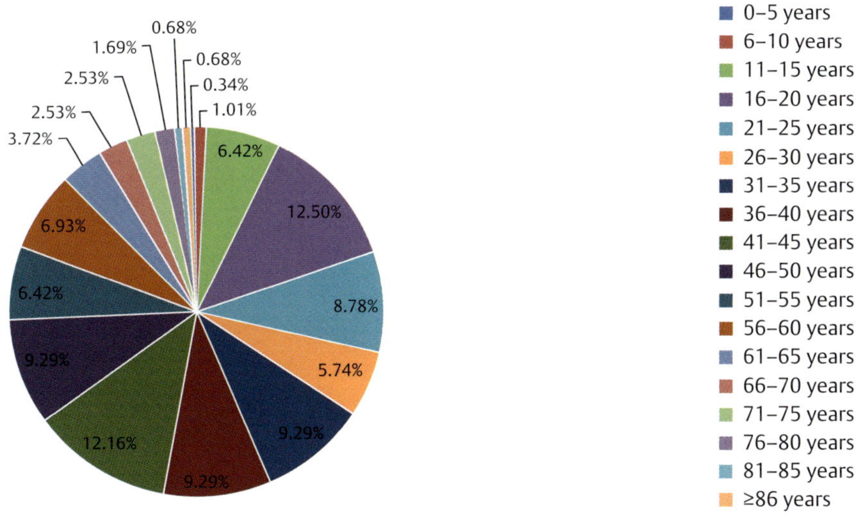

a

Fig. 10.23 **(a)** Age distribution of 592 acromion fractures. (*Continued*)

10

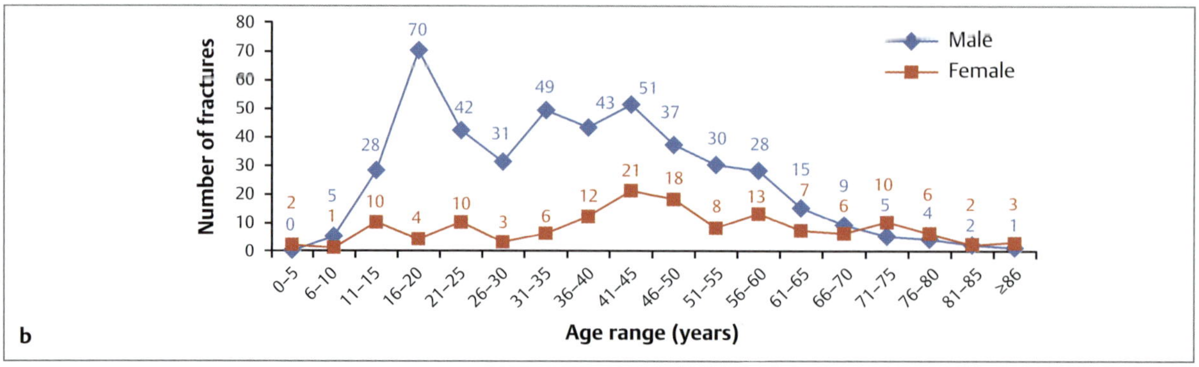

Fig. 10.23 (*continued*) **(b)** Age and sex distribution of 592 acromion fractures.

Acromion Fractures by Fracture Type

Table 10.24 Fracture type distribution of 592 acromion fractures

Fracture type		Male	Female	Number of fractures	Percentage (%)
Zone I	**IA**	140	43	183	30.91
	IB	151	48	199	33.61
	II	65	22	87	14.70
	III	32	9	41	6.93
Zone II		62	20	82	13.85
Total		450	142	592	100.00

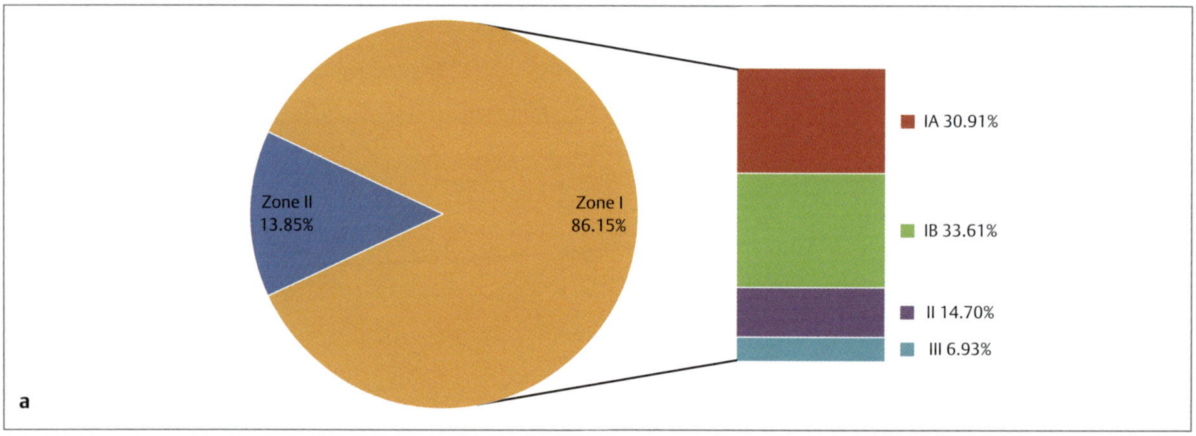

Fig. 10.24 **(a)** Fracture type distribution of 592 acromion fractures.

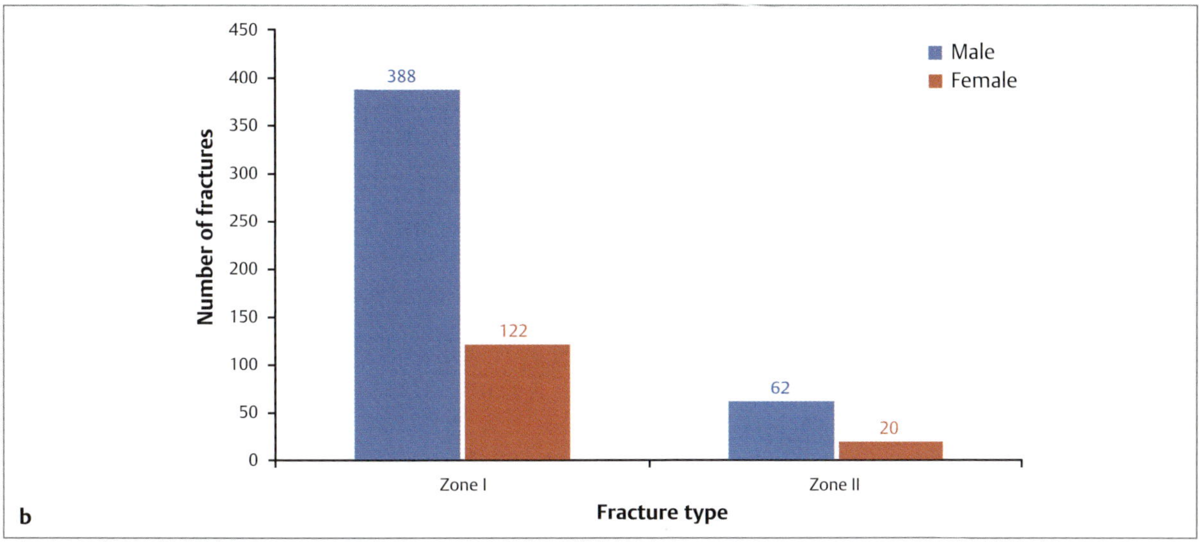

Fig. 10.24 (*continued*) **(b)** Sex and fracture type distribution of 592 acromion fractures.

Classification of acromion fractures

Zone I
510 fractures
M: 388 (76.08%)
F: 122 (23.92%)
86.15% of acromion

Type IA
Avulsion fractures
183 fractures
M: 140 (76.50%)
F: 43 (23.50%)
35.88% of zone I
30.91% of acromion

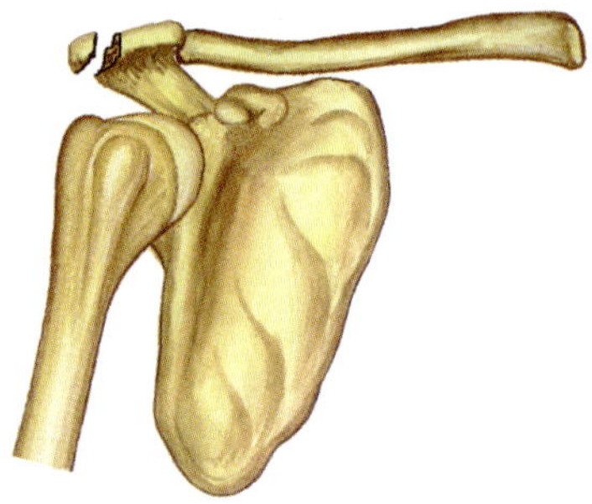

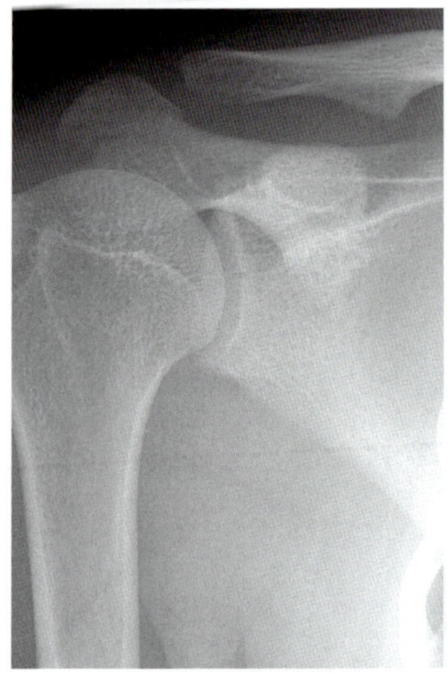

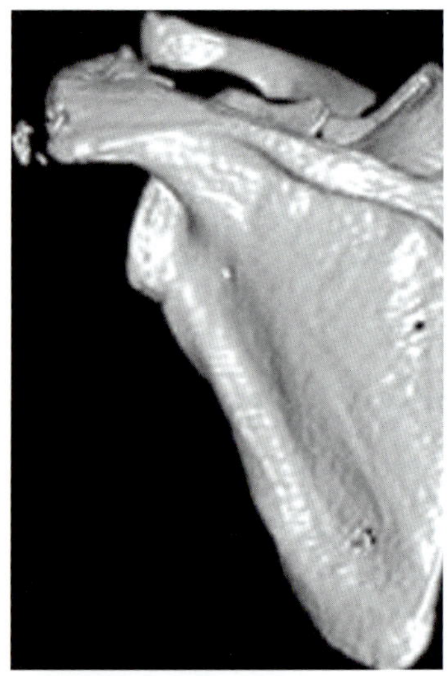

Type IB
Nondisplaced fractures
199 fractures
M: 151 (75.88%)
F: 48 (24.12%)
39.02% of zone I
33.61% of acromion

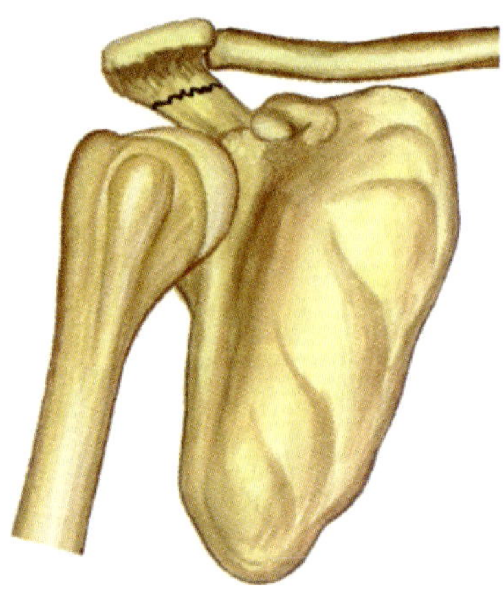

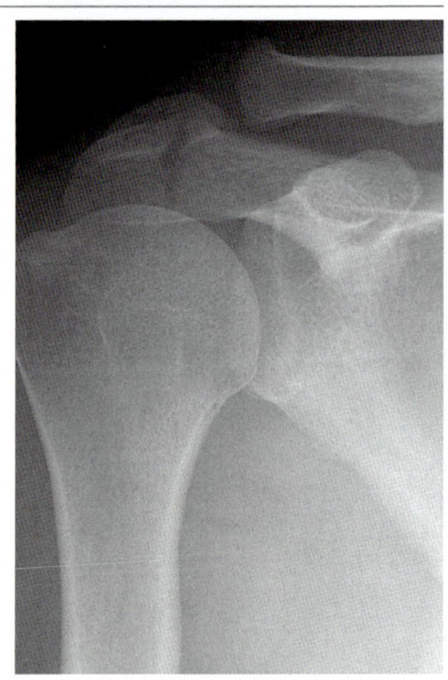

Type II
Displaced fractures with no reduction of the subacromial space
87 fractures
M: 65 (74.71%)
F: 22 (25.29%)
17.06% of zone I
14.70% of acromion

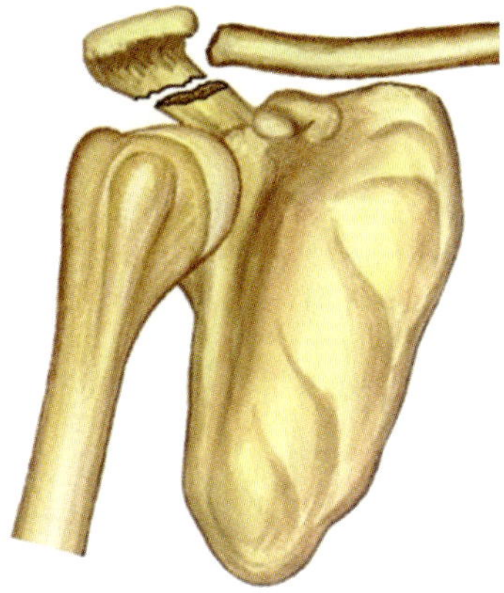

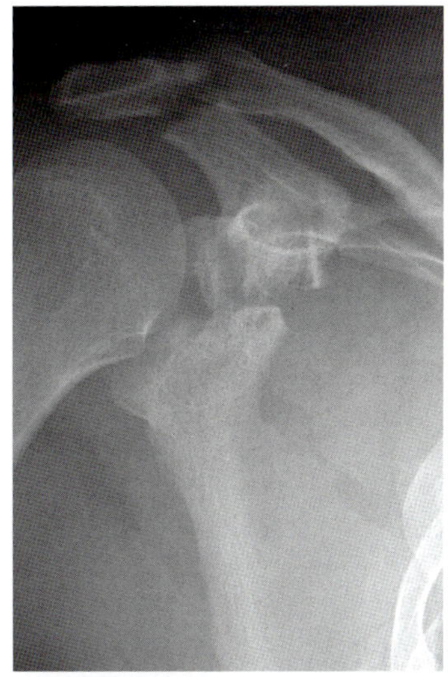

Type III
Displaced fractures with reduction of the subacromial space
41 fractures
M: 32 (78.05%)
F: 9 (21.95%)
8.04% of zone I
6.93% of acromion

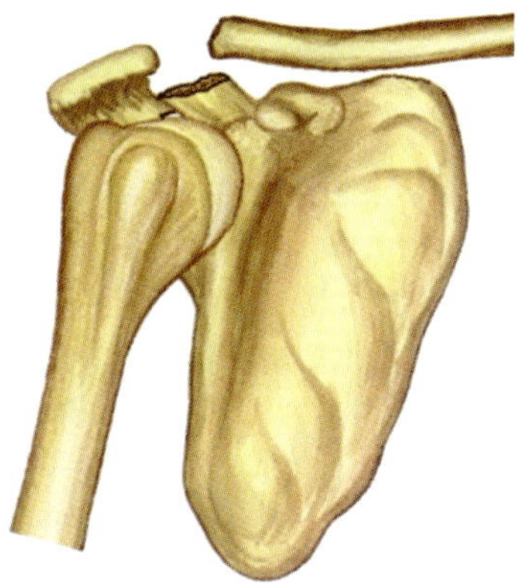

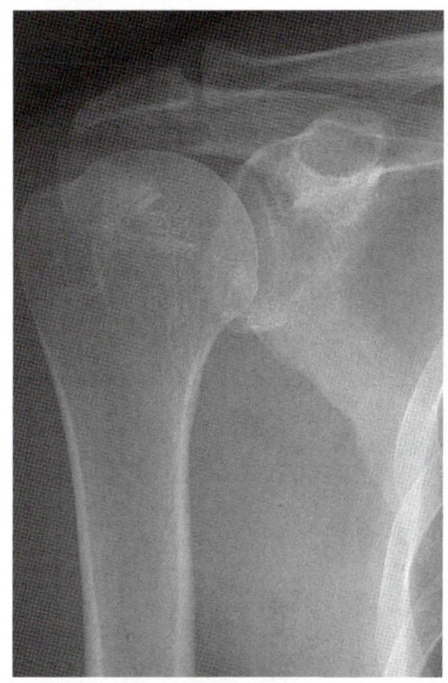

Zone II
Basal fractures of the acromion
82 fractures
M: 62 (75.61%)
F: 20 (24.39%)
13.85% of acromion

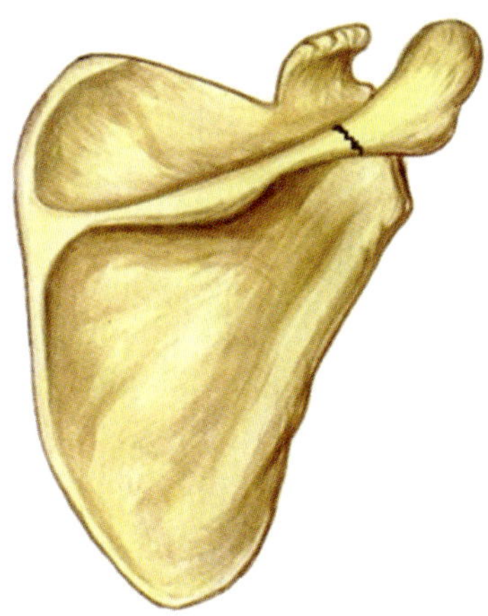

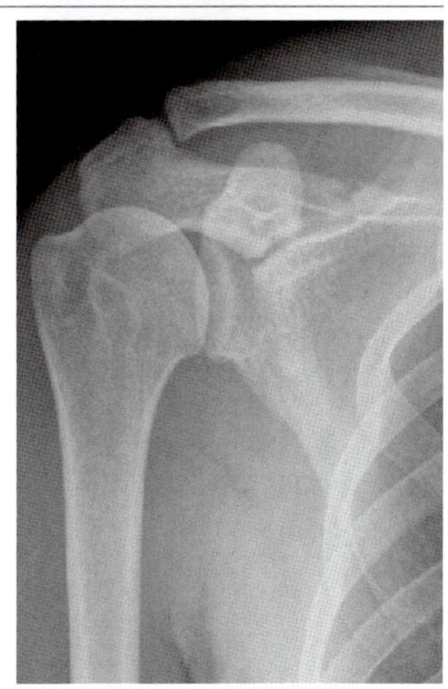

Scapular Neck Fractures

Miler and coworkers classified scapular neck fractures into three types according to degree and directionality (translational or angulatory) of displacement (**Plate 10.18**).

- *Type I:* Anatomical neck fractures. The fracture line lies between the acromion-basal portion of the scapular spine (spinoglenoid notch) and the lateral coracoid. After the fracture occurs, the distal fragment and upper arm lose bony support from the clavicle and are usually displaced lateralward and downward, due to the persistent pull of the long head of the triceps, which originates on the infraglenoid tubercle. Closed reduction alone cannot restore the anatomical alignment of the bony fragments.
- *Type II:* Surgical neck fractures involving the base of the acromion or the scapular spine. The fracture line runs downward and lateralward from the suprascapular notch medial to the coracoid process, and crosses the neck to the inferior glenoid. The lateral angle of the scapula can be displaced significantly; the degree of displacement is based upon the presence of an associated ipsilateral clavicle fracture and/or a coracoclavicular ligament tear. The latter results in the "functional imbalance" of the superior suspensory shoulder complex (SSSC) and instability of the entire shoulder and arm. When the coracoclavicular ligament tears, the distal fragment along with the shoulder separate from the clavicle due to muscle traction and the weight of the upper limb, which is displaced forward, downward, and rotated medially. Clinically, ipsilateral fractures of the clavicle and scapular neck, or dislocation of the acromioclavicular joint are called floating shoulder injuries.
- *Type III:* Transverse fractures of the inferior scapular neck. The fracture line extends from the inferior portion of the scapular spine to the medial border of the scapula.

Additionally, this type of fracture is classified into two types:

- Stable fracture: Fracture displacement of less than 1 cm with angulations of less than 40 degrees.
- Unstable fracture: Fracture displacement of greater than 1 cm with angulations of more than 40 degrees.

Clinical Epidemiologic Features of Scapular Neck Fractures

A total number of 841 scapular neck fractures were treated in 83 hospitals in China over a 2-year period from 2010 to 2011, the fractures accounted for 26.93% of scapular fractures. Their epidemiologic features are as follows:

- More males than females
- The high-risk age group is 41–45 years.
- Surgical neck fractures are the most common type of scapular neck fractures, the majority of which are stable fractures.

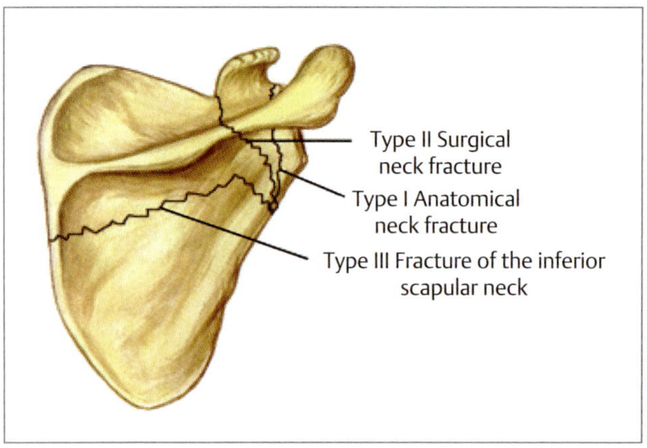

Plate 10.18

10

Scapular Neck Fractures by Sex

Table 10.25 Sex distribution of 841 scapular neck fractures

Sex	Number of fractures	Percentage (%)
Male	643	76.46
Female	198	23.54
Total	841	100.00

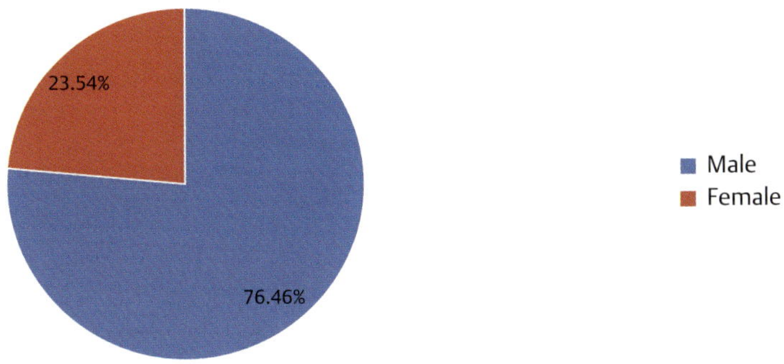

Fig. 10.25 Sex distribution of 841 scapular neck fractures.

Scapular Neck Fractures by Age Group

Table 10.26 Age and sex distribution of 841 scapular neck fractures

Age group (years)	Male	Female	Number of fractures	Percentage (%)
0–5	4	1	5	0.59
6–10	3	0	3	0.36
11–15	6	1	7	0.83
16–20	17	4	21	2.50
21–25	32	6	38	4.52
26–30	79	9	88	10.46
31–35	60	16	76	9.04
36–40	80	35	115	13.67
41–45	116	19	135	16.05
46–50	80	16	96	11.41
51–55	51	22	73	8.68
56–60	45	27	72	8.56
61–65	30	14	44	5.23
66–70	20	17	37	4.40
71–75	9	7	16	1.90
76–80	7	2	9	1.07
81–85	2	2	4	0.48
≥86	2	0	2	0.24
Total	643	198	841	100.00

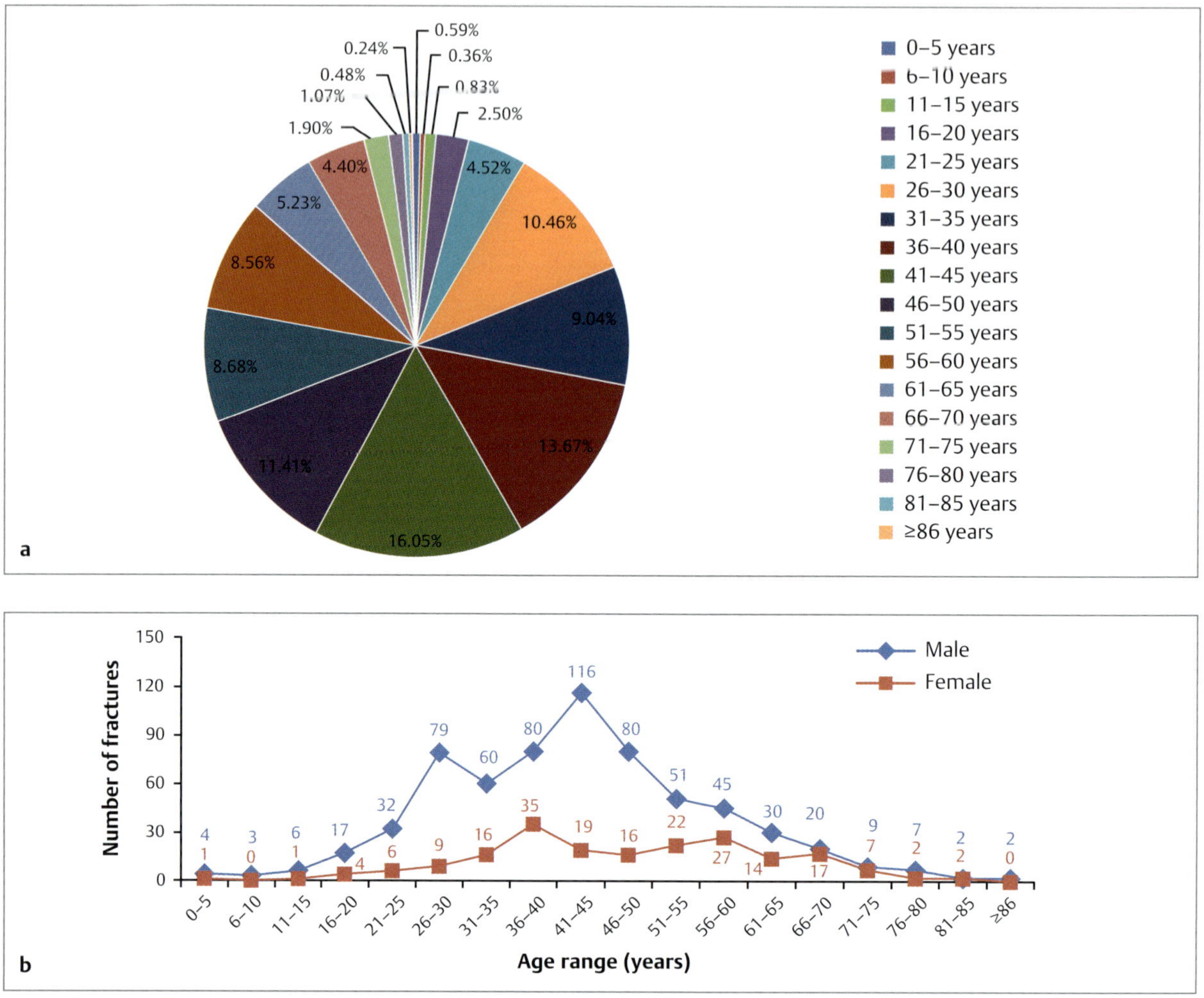

Fig. 10.26 **(a)** Age distribution of 841 scapular neck fractures.
(b) Sex and age distribution of 841 scapular neck fractures.

Scapular Neck Fractures by Fracture Type

Table 10.27 Sex and fracture type distribution of 841 scapular neck fractures by fracture line direction

Fracture type	Male	Female	Number of fractures	Percentage (%)
I	87	30	117	13.91
II	269	97	366	43.52
III	287	71	358	42.57
Total	643	198	841	100.00

10

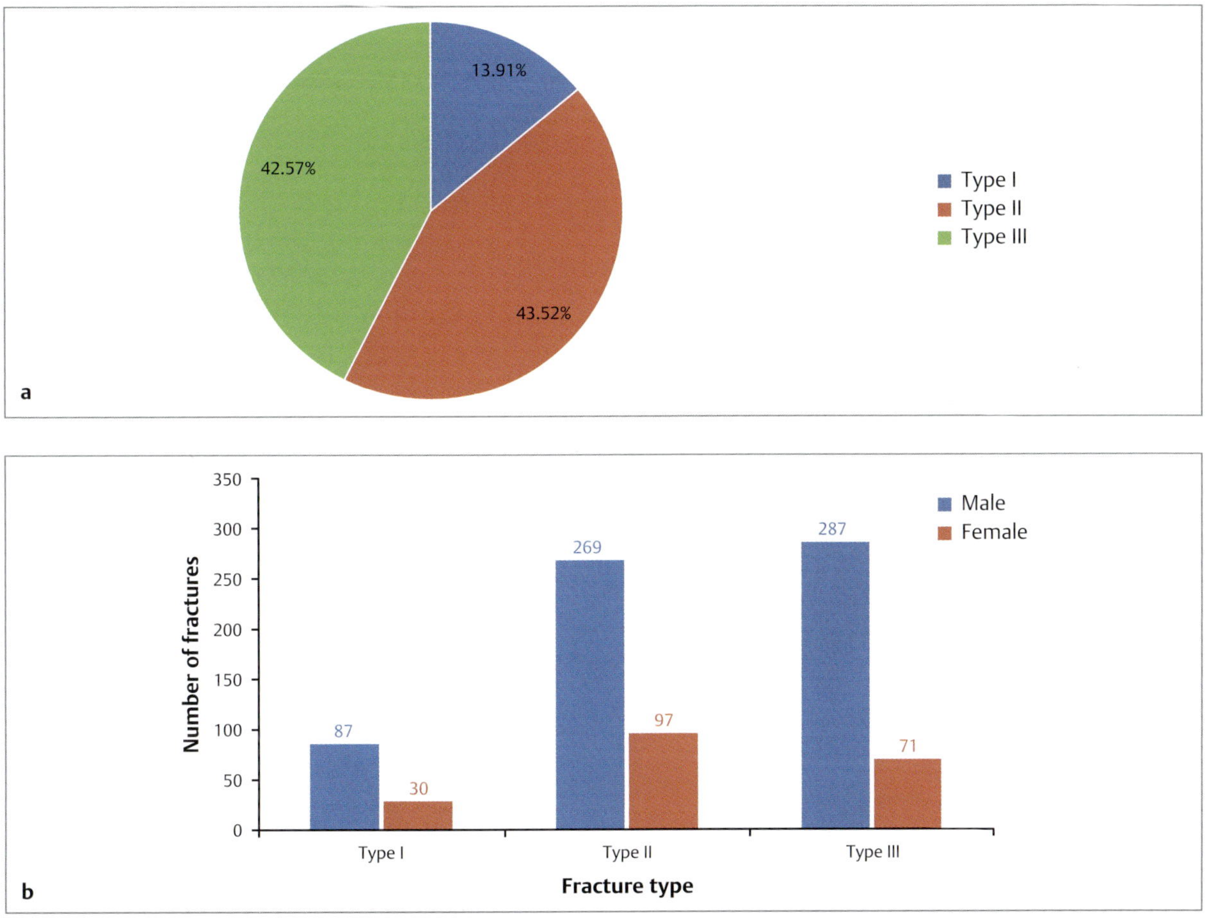

Fig. 10.27 **(a)** Fracture type distribution of 841 scapular neck fractures.
(b) Sex and fracture type distribution of 841 scapular neck fractures.

Table 10.28 Sex and fracture type distribution of scapular neck fractures by degree of fracture displacement

Fracture type	Male	Female	Number of fractures	Percentage (%)
Stable	311	119	430	51.13
Unstable	332	79	411	48.87
Total	643	198	841	100.00

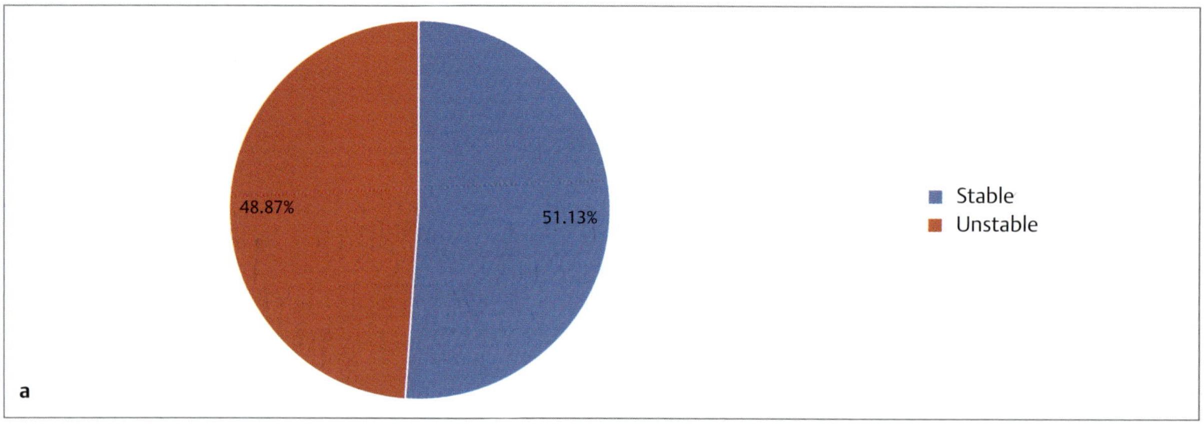

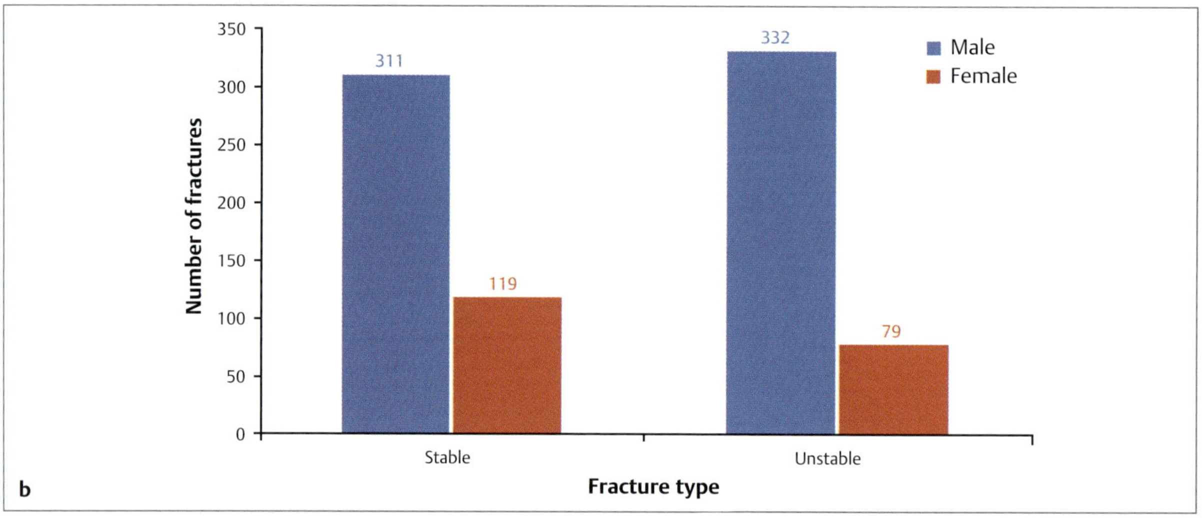

Fig. 10.28 **(a)** Fracture type distribution of 841 scapular neck fractures.
(b) Sex and fracture type distribution of 841 scapular neck fractures.

Classification of scapular neck fractures	
Anatomical neck fractures 117 fractures M: 87 (74.36%) F: 30 (25.64%) 13.91% of scapular neck	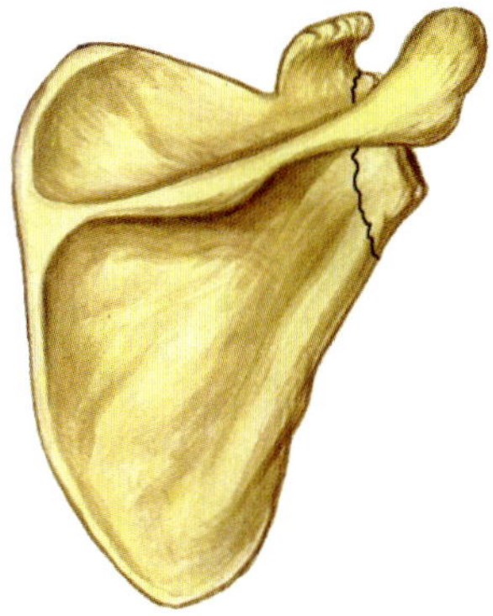 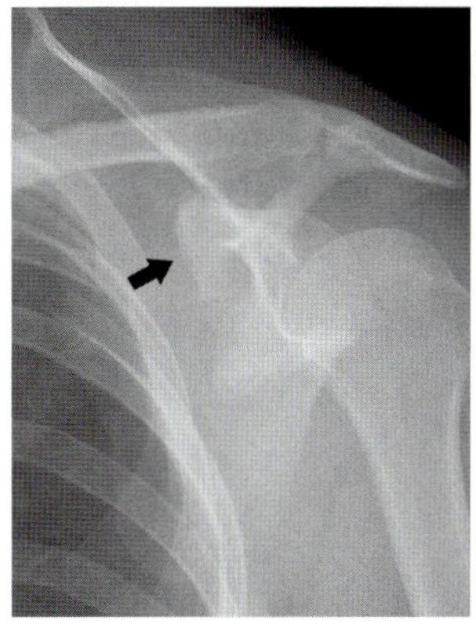
Surgical neck fractures 366 fractures M: 269 (73.5%) F: 97 (26.5%) 43.52% of scapular neck	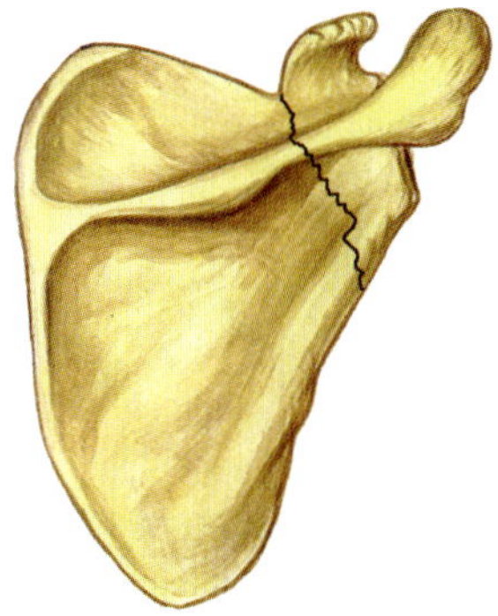 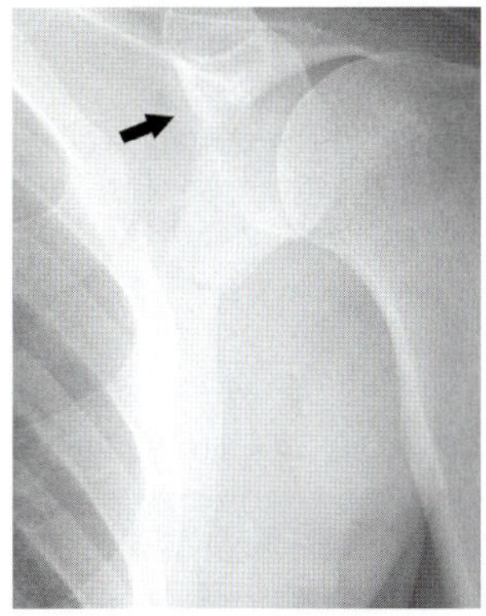
Inferior scapular neck fractures 358 fractures M: 287 (80.17%) F: 71 (19.83%) 42.57% of scapular neck	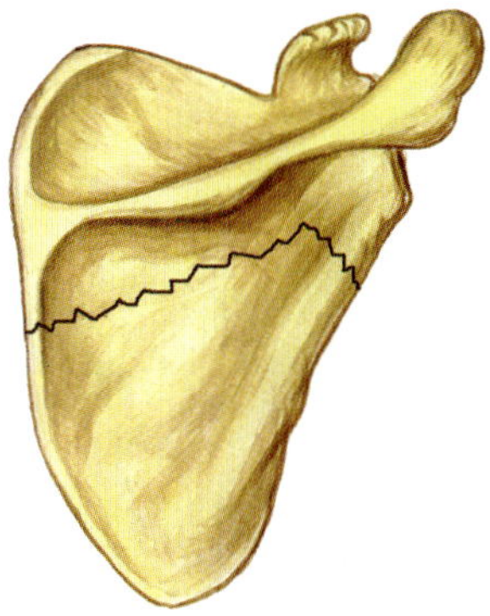 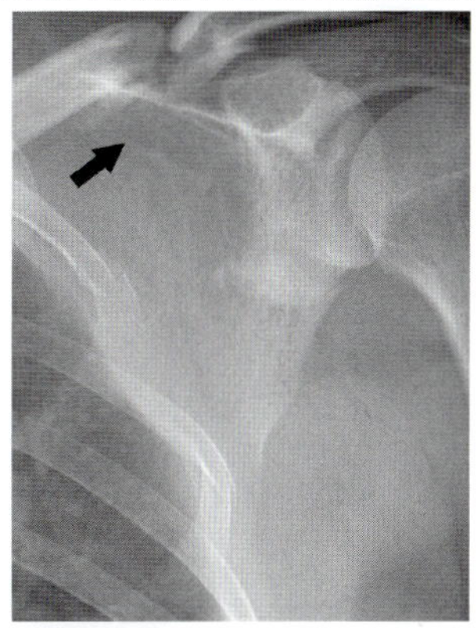 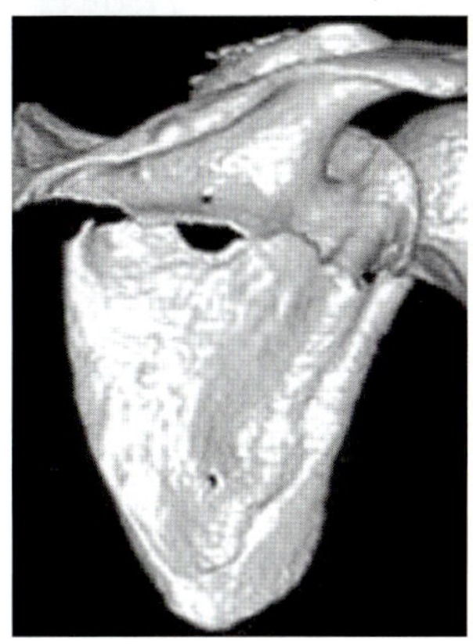

Glenoid Fractures

Ideberg classified glenoid fractures into six types based on fracture location and injury mechanism.

- *Type I*: fractures of the glenoid rim
  - *Type Ia*: anterior
  - *Type Ib*: posterior
- *Type II*: with an external force applied the humeral head impacts the glenoid fossa obliquely downward, resulting in fractures through the glenoid fossa.
  - *Type IIa*: transverse fracture through the glenoid fossa exiting inferiorly.
  - *Type IIb*: oblique fracture through the glenoid fossa exiting inferiorly.
- *Type III*: an external force presses the humeral head against the glenoid fossa obliquely upward, resulting in oblique fractures through the glenoid that exit at the superior border of the scapula. This type is often associated with acromioclavicular fractures or dislocations.
- *Type IV*: a transverse fracture line exits through the medial border of the scapula. This type results from impaction of the humeral head into the center of the glenoid fossa; of two resulting fragments, the smaller one is at the top, the larger one on the bottom.
- *Type V*: combination of a type II, III, and IV pattern. The major fracture line extends from the glenoid fossa to the medial border of the scapula, and is commonly caused by a strong external force.
  - *Type Va*: combination of type II and type IV pattern.
  - *Type Vb*: combination of type III and type IV pattern.
  - *Type Vc*: combination of type II, III, and IV pattern.
  - *Type VI*: severe comminution of the glenoid surface.

Clinical Epidemiologic Features of Glenoid Fractures

A total of 519 glenoid fractures were treated in 83 hospitals in China over a 2-year period from 2010 to 2011, the fractures accounted for 16.62% of scapular fractures. Their epidemiologic features are as follows:

- More males and females
- The high-risk age group is 41–45 years.
- The most common fracture type is type II.

Glenoid Fractures by Sex

Table 10.29 Sex distribution of 519 glenoid fractures

Sex	Number of fractures	Percentage (%)
Male	371	71.48
Female	148	28.52
Total	519	100.00

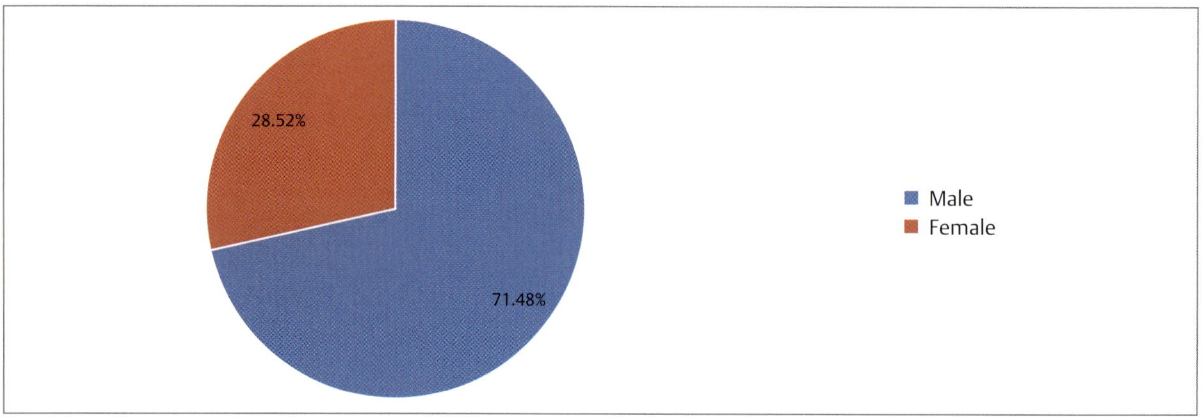

Fig. 10.29 Sex distribution of 519 glenoid fractures.

Glenoid Fractures by Age Group

Table 10.30 Age and sex distribution of 519 glenoid fractures

Age group (years)	Male	Female	Number of fractures	Percentage (%)
0–5	0	0	0	0.00
6–10	0	0	0	0.00
11–15	4	3	7	1.35
16–20	16	2	18	3.47
21–25	25	2	27	5.20
26–30	31	6	37	7.13
31–35	26	8	34	6.55
36–40	37	15	52	10.02
41–45	47	17	64	12.33
46–50	41	17	58	11.18
51–55	38	15	53	10.21
56–60	37	17	54	10.40
61–65	29	8	37	7.13
66–70	20	11	31	5.97
71–75	8	13	21	4.05
76–80	6	8	14	2.70
81–85	3	4	7	1.35
≥86	3	2	5	0.96
Total	371	148	519	100.00

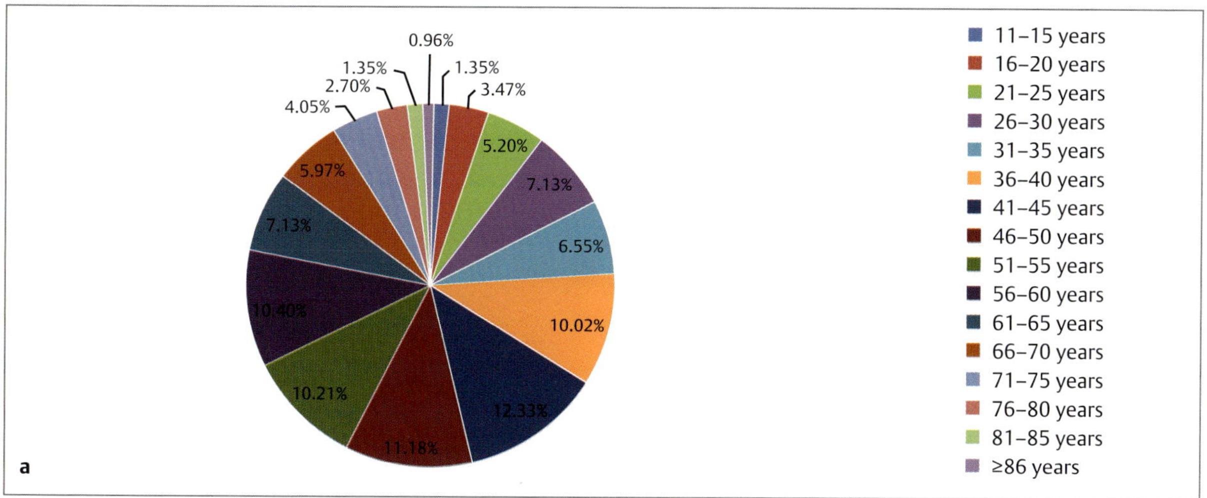

Fig. 10.30 **(a)** Age distribution of 519 glenoid fractures. (*Continued*)

10

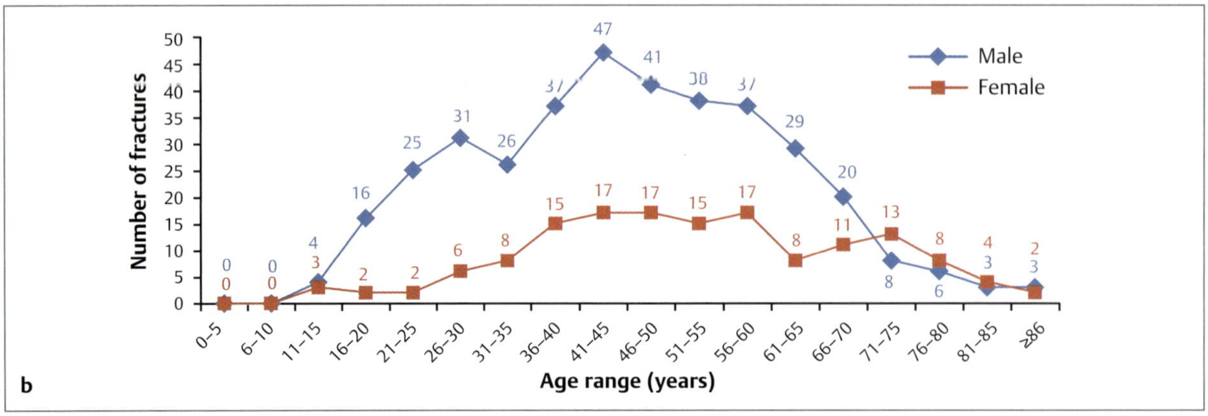

Fig. 10.30 (*continued*) **(b)** Age and sex distribution of 519 glenoid fractures.

Glenoid Fractures by Fracture Type

Table 10.31 Sex and fracture type distribution of 519 glenoid fractures

Fracture type	Male	Female	Number of fractures	Percentage (%)
I	61	42	103	19.85
II	163	54	217	41.81
III	27	10	37	7.13
IV	24	11	35	6.74
V	66	23	89	17.15
VI	30	8	38	7.32
Total	371	148	519	100.00

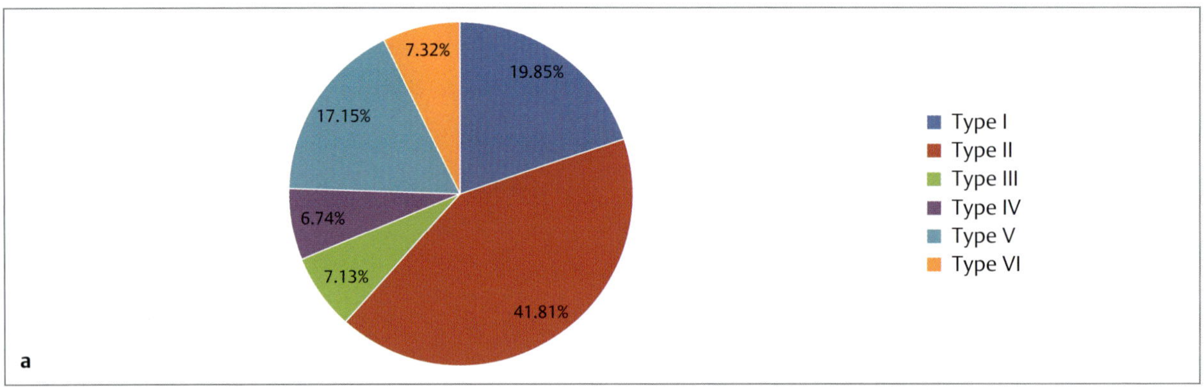

Fig. 10.31 **(a)** Fracture type distribution of 519 glenoid fractures.

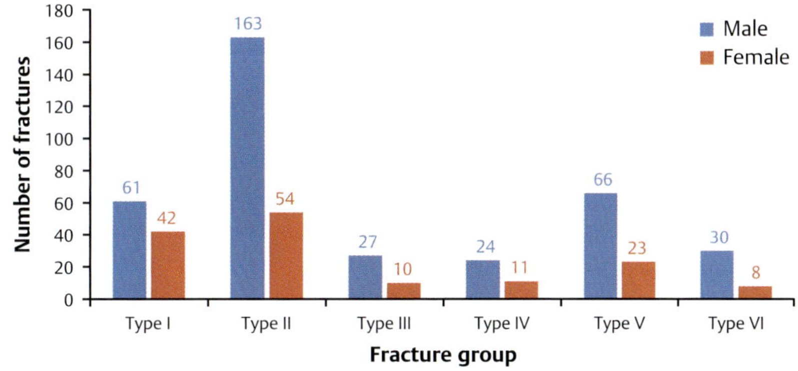

b

Fig. 10.31 (*continued*) **(b)** Sex and fracture type distribution of 519 glenoid fractures.

Ideberg classification of glenoid fractures	
Type I **Glenoid rim** 103 fractures M: 61 (59.22%) F: 42 (40.78%) 19.85% of glenoid	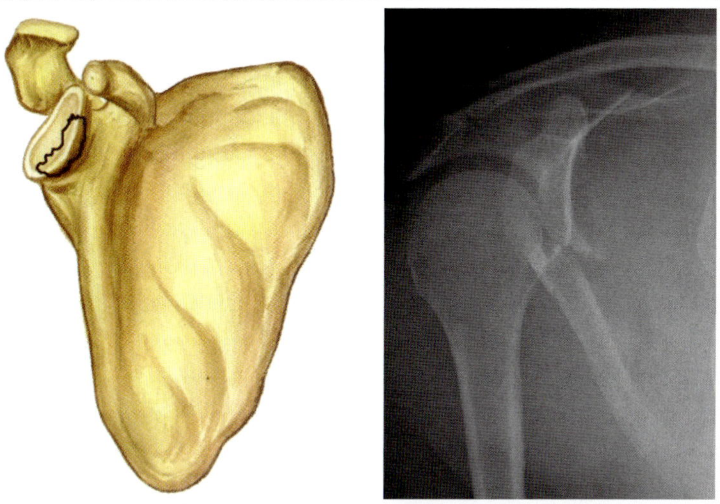
Type II **Fracture line exiting inferior part of glenoid fossa** 217 fractures M: 163 (75.12%) F: 54 (24.88%) 41.81% of glenoid	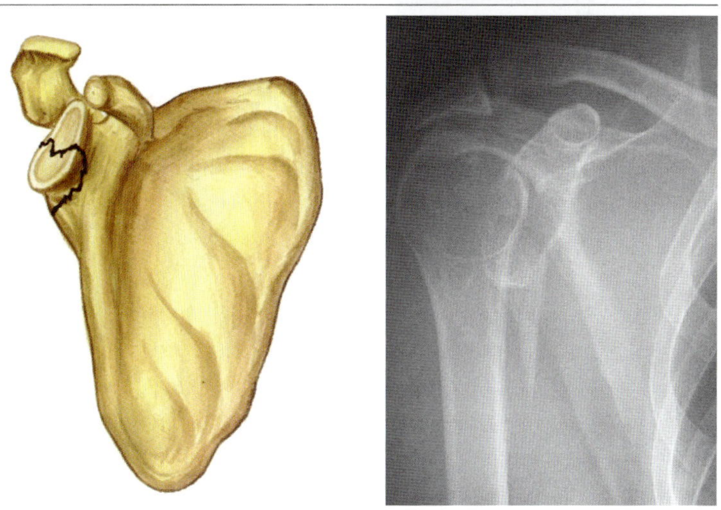

Ideberg classification of glenoid fractures		
Type III **Fracture line exiting** **superior part of glenoid fossa** 37 fractures M: 27 (72.97%) F: 10 (27.03%) 7.13% of glenoid	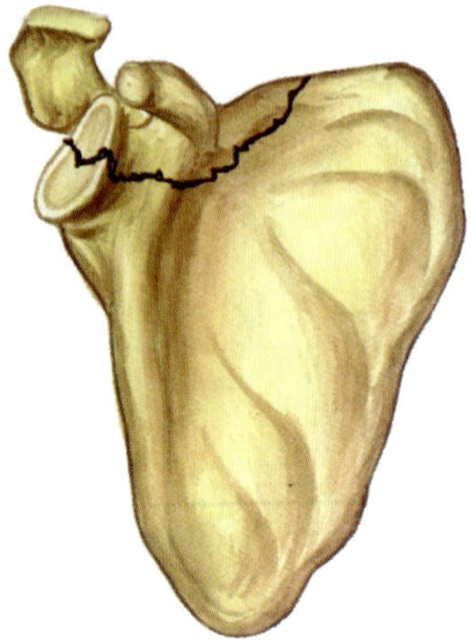	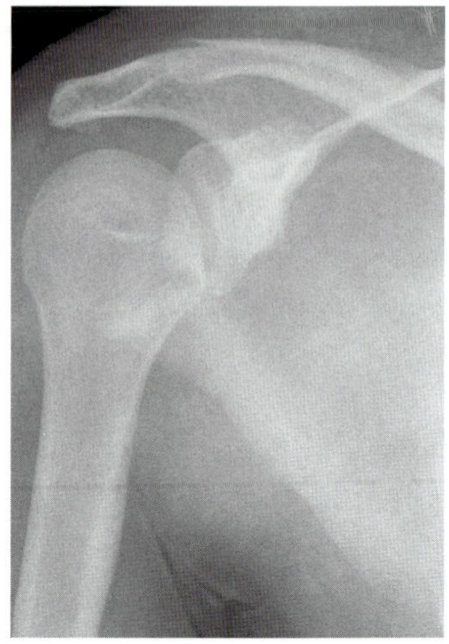 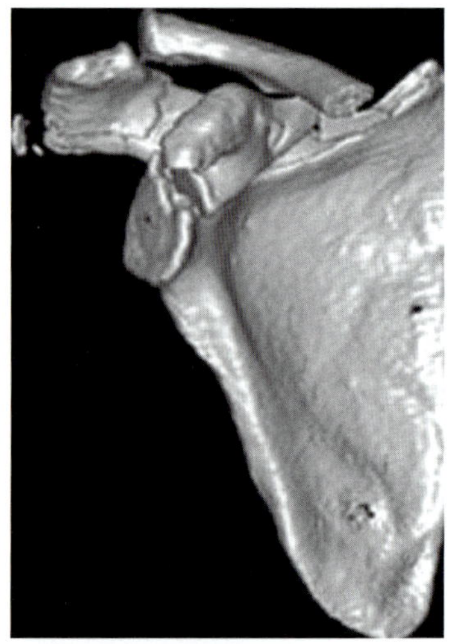
Type IV **Transverse fracture from the glenoid fossa** **to the medial border of the scapula** 35 fractures M: 24 (68.57%) F: 11 (31.43%) 6.74% of glenoid	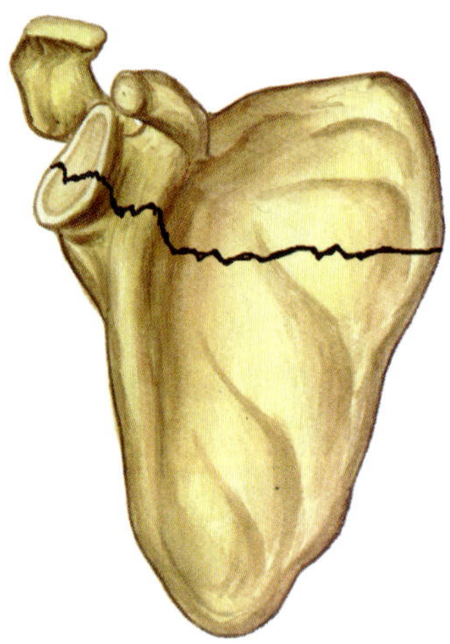	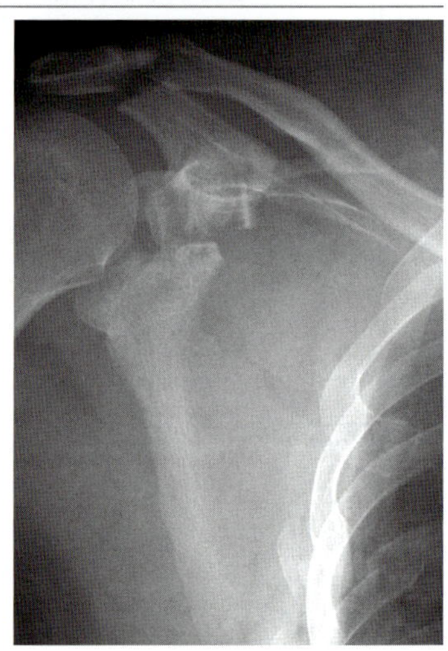

Ideberg classification of glenoid fractures		
Type V **Combination of fractures of the glenoid fossa and the body of the scapula** 89 fractures M: 66 (74.16%) F: 23 (25.84%) 17.15% of glenoid	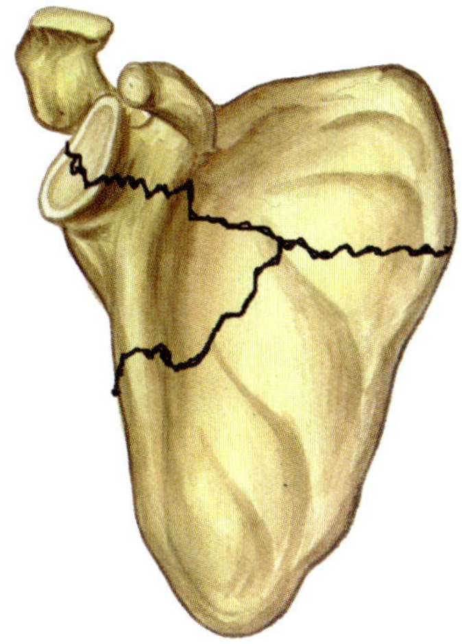	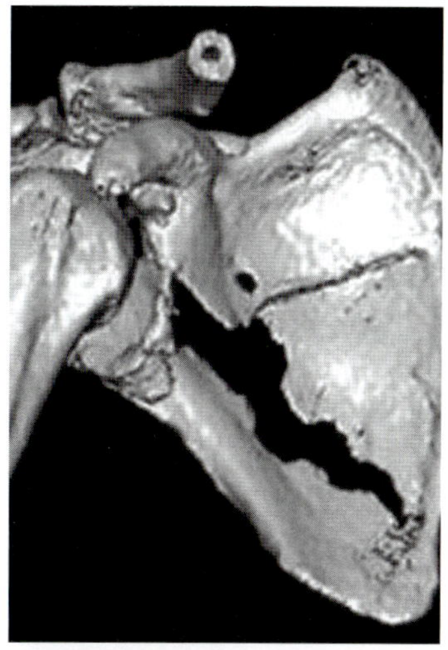
Type VI **Severe comminution of the glenoid fossa** 38 fractures M: 30 (78.95%) F: 8 (21.05%) 7.32% of glenoid	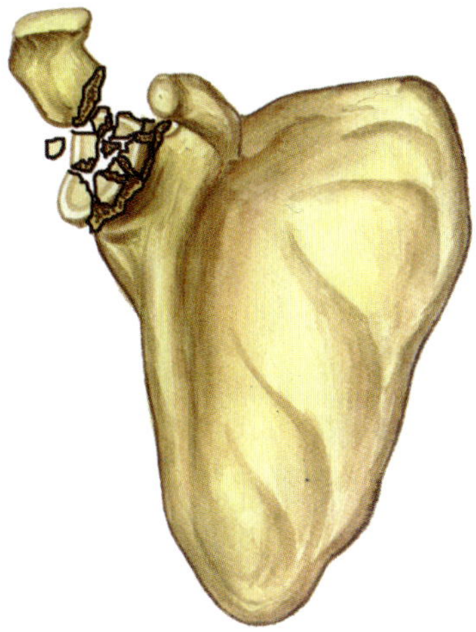	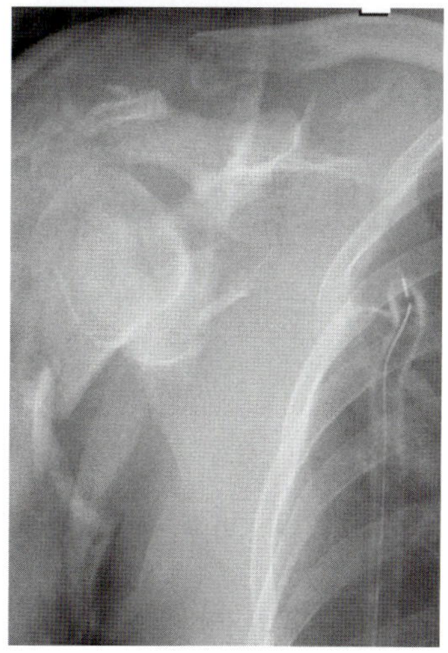

Index

Page numbers in *italics* refer to illustrations or tables.

D

E

F

Q

R

U

V

W

Y